Mucosal Vaccines

MUCOSAL VACCINES

Edited by

Hiroshi Kiyono
Immunobiology Vaccine Center
University of Alabama at Birmingham
Birmingham, Alabama
and Department of Mucosal Immunology
Research Institute for Microbial Diseases
Osaka University
Osaka, Japan

Pearay L. Ogra
Department of Pediatrics
Children's Hospital
University of Texas Medical Branch
Galveston, Texas

Jerry R. McGhee
Department of Microbiology
Immunobiology Vaccine Center
University of Alabama at Birmingham
Birmingham, Alabama

Academic Press
San Diego London Boston New York
Sydney Tokyo Toronto

This book is printed on acid-free paper. ∞

Academic Press, Inc.
525 B Street, Suite 1900, San Diego, California 92101-4495, USA
http://www.apnet.com

Academic Press Limited
24-28 Oval Road, London NW1 7DX, UK
http://www.hbuk.co.uk/ap/

Library of Congress Cataloging-in-Publication Data

Mucosal vaccines / edited by Hiroshi Kiyono, Jerry R. McGhee, Pearay L. Ogra.
p. cm.
Includes bibliographical references and index.
ISBN 0-12-410580-7 (alk. paper)
1. Mucous membrane--Immunology. 2. Vaccines. I. Kiyono, H. (Hiroshi) II. McGhee, Jerry R. III. Ogra, Pearay L.
[DNLM: 1. Vaccines--immunology. 2. Vaccines--administration & dosage. 3. Mucous Membrane--immunology. 4. Adjuvants, Immunologic--physiology. 5. Immunity, Mucosal. QW 805 M942 1996]
QR185.9.M83M86 1996
615'.372--dc20
DNLM/DLC
for Library of Congress 96-19774
CIP

PRINTED IN THE UNITED STATES OF AMERICA
96 97 98 99 00 01 EB 9 8 7 6 5 4 3 2 1

This book is dedicated to our families,

Momoyo and Erika Kiyono;

Kathy, Monica, Maria, and Sanjay Ogra;

Mary Lou, Jerry Jr., Kimberly, Patricia, and Mary Rachael McGhee;

for their support and understanding during the preparation of this book.

Contents

Contributors

Numbers in parentheses indicate the pages on which the authors' contributions begin.

William W. Agace (389), Department of Medical Microbiology, Division of Clinical Immunology, Lund University, S-223 62 Lund, Sweden

Marie J. Anderson (137), Department of Microbiology, The University of Alabama at Birmingham, Birmingham, Alabama 35294

Robert B. Belshe (311), Division of Infectious Diseases and Immunology, Saint Louis University Health Sciences Center, St. Louis, Missouri 63110

Peter K. Brown (105), Department of Biology, Washington University, St. Louis, Missouri 63130

Thomas R. Cate (303), Departments of Microbiology and Immunology and Medicine, Baylor College of Medicine, Houston, Texas 77030

H. Fred Clark (325), Department of Pediatrics, School of Medicine, University of Pennsylvania, Philadelphia, Pennsylvania 19104

John D. Clements (73), Department of Microbiology and Immunology, Tulane University Medical Center, New Orleans, Louisiana 70112

Margaret E. Conner (325), Division of Molecular Virology, Baylor College of Medicine, Houston, Texas 77030; and Houston Veterans Administration Medical Center, Houston, Texas 77030

Karen F. T. Copeland (147), Department of Pathology, McMaster University, Hamilton, Ontario L8N 3Z5, Canada

Robert B. Couch (303), Department of Microbiology and Immunology, Baylor College of Medicine, Houston, Texas 77030

Cecil Czerkinsky (89), Department of Medical Microbiology, University of Göteborg, S413-46 Göteborg, Sweden

Steven J. Czinn (255), Department of Pediatrics, Case Western Reserve University, Cleveland, Ohio 44106

Bonny L. Dickinson (73), Department of Microbiology and Immunology, Tulane University Medical Center, New Orleans, Louisiana 70112

Teresa A. Doggett (105), Department of Biology, Washington University, St. Louis, Missouri 63130

John J. Donnelly (119), Department of Virus and Cell Biology, Merck Research Laboratories, West Point, Pennsylvania 19486

Jacqueline D. Duncan (159), Pharmaceutical Formulations Department, Southern Research Institute, Birmingham, Alabama 35205

Charles O. Elson (59), Division of Gastroenterology and Hepatology, Department of Medicine, University of Alabama at Birmingham, Birmingham, Alabama 35294

Peter B. Ernst (255), Department of Pediatrics and Sealy Center for Molecular Sciences, University of Texas Medical Branch, Galveston, Texas 77555

Mary K. Estes (325), Division of Molecular Virology, Baylor College of Medicine, Houston, Texas 77030

Ninggou Feng (325), Division of Gastroenterology, Stanford School of Medicine, Stanford, California 94305; and Palo Alto Veterans Administration Medical Center, Palo Alto, California 94304

Manuel Franco (325), Division of Gastroenterology, Stanford School of Medicine, Stanford, California 94305; and Palo Alto Veterans Administration Medical Center, Palo Alto, California 94304

W. Scott Gallichan (147), Department of Biology, McMaster University, Hamilton, Ontario L8N 3Z5, Canada

Robert J. Genco (437), Department of Oral Biology, School of Dental Medicine, State University of New York, Buffalo, New York 14214

Marina Gheorghiu (269), Laboratoire du BCG, Institut Pasteur, 75724 Cedex, Paris, France

Richard M. Gilley (159), Pharmaceutical Formulations Department, Southern Research Institute, Birmingham, Alabama 35205

Harry B. Greenberg (325), Division of Gastroenterology, Stanford School of Medicine, Stanford, California 94305; and Palo Alto Veterans Administration Medical Center, Palo Alto, California 94304

Shigeyuki Hamada (187), Department of Oral Microbiology, Faculty of Dentistry, Osaka University, Suita, Osaka 565, Japan

Thomas L. Hearn (175), Division of Laboratory Systems Public Health Program Office, Centers for Disease Control and Prevention, Atlanta, Georgia 30333

Daniel F. Hoft (269), Division of Infectious Diseases Department of Internal Medicine, Saint Louis University Health Sciences Center, Saint Louis, Missouri 63110

Jan Holmgren (241), Department of Medical Microbiology and Immunology, University of Göteborg, 413 46 Göteborg, Sweden

Albert Z. Kapikian (345), Epidemiology Section, Laboratory of Infectious Diseases, National Institute of Allergy and Infectious Diseases, National Institutes of Health, Bethesda, Maryland 20892

Charu Kaushic (375), Department of Physiology, Dartmouth Medical School, Lebanon, New Hampshire 03756

Wendy A. Keitel (303), Departments of Microbiology and Immunology and Medicine, Baylor College of Medicine, Houston, Texas 77030

Hiroshi Kiyono (89), Immunobiology Vaccine Center, University of Alabama at Birmingham Medical Center, Birmingham, Alabama 35294; and Department of Mucosal Immunology, Research Institute for Microbial Diseases, Osaka University, Suita, Osaka 565, Japan

Yoshikatsu Kodama (187), Immunology Research Institute in Gifu, Sano, Gifu 501-11, Japan

Jean-Pierre Kraehenbuhl (41), Swiss Institute for Experimental Cancer Research and Institute of Biochemistry, University of Lausanne, CH-1066 Epalinges, Switzerland

Takeshi Kurata (425), Department of Pathology, National Institute of Health, Shinju-ku, Tokyo 162, Japan

Yuichi Kurono (451), Department of Otolaryngology, Oita Medical University, Hasama-machi, Oita 879-55, Japan

Solomon Langermann (129), Department of Mucosal Immunity and Vaccines, MedImmune, Inc., Gaithersburg, Maryland 20878

Thomas Lehner (357), Department of Immunology, United Medical and Dental Schools at Guy's and St. Thomases' Hospital, London SE1 9RT, United Kingdom

Myron M. Levine (201), Center for Vaccine Development, University of Maryland School of Medicine, Baltimore, Maryland 21201

Alf A. Lindberg (213), Pasteur Mérieux Connaught Group, Pasteur Mérieux Serums and Vaccines, 69280 Marcy, l'Étoile, France

Margaret A. Liu (119), Department of Virus and Cell Biology, Merck Research Laboratories, West Point, Pennsylvania 19486

Jerry R. McGhee (17), Department of Microbiology and Immunobiology Vaccine Center, University of Alabama at Birmingham, Birmingham, Alabama 35294

John J. Mekalanos (229), Department of Microbiology and Molecular Genetics and Shipley Institute of Medicine, Harvard Medical School, Boston, Massachusetts 02115

Jiri F. Mestecky (159), Department of Microbiology, University of Alabama at Birmingham, Birmingham, Alabama 35294

Christopher J. Miller (357), California Regional Primate Research Center, Virology and Immunology Unit, University of California, Davis, California 95616

Goro Mogi (451), Department of Otolaryngology, Oita Medical University, Hasama-machi, Oita 879-55, Japan

Zina Moldoveanu (137, 159), Department of Microbiology, University of Alabama at Birmingham, Birmingham, Alabama 35294

Paul C. Montgomery (403), Department of Immunology and Microbiology, School of Medicine, Wayne State University, Detroit, Michigan 48201

Casey D. Morrow (137), Department of Microbiology, University of Alabama at Birmingham, Birmingham, Alabama 35294

J. G. Nedrud (255), Institute of Pathology , Case Western Reserve University, Cleveland, Ohio 44106

Marian R. Neutra (41), Department of Pediatrics, Harvard Medical School and Children's Hospital, Boston, Massachusetts 02115

Frances K. Newman (311), Division of Infectious Diseases and Immunology, Saint Louis University Health Sciences Center, St. Louis, Missouri 63110

Paul A. Offit (325), Division of Infectious Diseases, The Children's Hospital of Philadelphia, Philadelphia, Pennsylvania 19104

Pearay L. Ogra (3, 283), Department of Pediatrics, Children's Hospital, University of Texas Medical Branch, Galveston, Texas 77555

Roy C. Page (437), Research Center in Oral Biology, University of Washington, Seattle, Washington 98195

Tibor Pál (213), Department of Microbiology, Faculty of Medicine, University of Kuwait, 13100 Safat, Kuwait

Donna C. Porter (137), Department of Microbiology, University of Alabama at Birmingham, Birmingham, Alabama 35294

Ranjit Ray (311), Division of Infectious Diseases and Immunology, Saint Louis University Health Sciences Center, St. Louis, Missouri 63110

Victor E. Reyes (255), Department of Pediatrics, University of Texas Medical Branch, Galveston, Texas 77555

Kenneth Rosenthal (147), Molecular Virology and Immunology Program, Department of Pathology, McMaster University, Hamilton, Ontario L8N 3Z5, Canada

Dennis P. Schafer (159), Zynaxis, Inc., Malvern, Pennsylvania 19355

John W. Shiver (119), Department of Virus and Cell Biology, Merck Research Laboratories, West Point, Pennsylvania 19486

Herman F. Staats (17), Department of Medicine, Center for AIDS Research, Duke University Medical Center, Durham, North Carolina 27710

Catharina Svanborg (389), Department of Medical Microbiology and Clinical Immunology, Lund University, S-223 62 Lund, Sweden

Ann-Mari Svennerholm (241), Department of Medical Microbiology and Immunology, University of Göteborg, South-413 46 Göteborg, Sweden

Marcello B. Sztein (201), Center for Vaccine Development, University of Maryland School of Medicine, Baltimore, Maryland 21201

Shini-chi Tamura (425), Department of Pathology, National Institute of Health, Shinju-ku, Tokyo 162, Japan

Maurizio Tomasi (175), Laboratorio di Biologia Cellulare, Istituto Superiore di Sanita, Rome, 00161, Italy

Jeffrey B. Ulmer (119), Department of Virus and Cell Biology, Merck Research Laboratories, West Point, Pennsylvania 19486

Matthew K. Waldor (229), Department of Microbiology and Molecular Genetics and Shipley Institute of Medicine, Harvard Medical School, Boston, Massachusetts 02115

Carolyn Weeks-Levy (283), Biostar Inc., Saskatoon, Saskatchewan S7N 3R2 Canada

Judith Whittum-Hudson (403), The Wilmen Institute, Johns Hopkins University, Baltimore, Maryland 21287

Charles Wira (375), Department of Physiology, Dartmouth Medical School, Lebanon, New Hampshire 03756

Peter F. Wright (295), Departments of Pediatrics and Microbiology and Immunology, Vanderbilt Medical Center, Nashville, Tennessee 37232

Preface

From a historical perspective, 1996 is an important year in the annals of vaccinology and immunology. Nearly 200 years to date, Edward Jenner discovered that cowpox/vaccinia virus successfully induced protection against smallpox, a fatal and common infectious disease until about 3 decades ago. The disease was essentially eradicated with the use of the vaccine and the technology proposed almost 2 centuries ago. Jenner named the procedure "vaccination." The development of smallpox vaccine is considered to be the cornerstone for the subsequent evolution of modern concepts of vaccine-induced approaches to protection against infectious diseases. The term vaccination is derived from the original observation of cowpox immunization (*vacca* L = cow) and has been used to describe the administration in healthy subjects of weakened and/or attenuated infectious microorganisms to provide protection or immunity against the development of disease. This discovery is also considered to be the beginning of the new field immunology.

Mucosal Vaccines summarizes the most current and updated views and concepts related to the development of new generations of vaccines. As described within, the concepts of mucosal immunization offer several benefits for mass immunization. For example, an appropriate mucosal vaccine could provide immunity at both mucosal and systemic components of the mammalian immune system. Thus, protection can be expected against reinfection at the mucosal level as well as against disease at systemic sites.

The year 2000 has been designated by WHO as the target date for global eradication of poliomyelitis. This mucosally acquired infectious disease has already been eradicated in Europe, the American hemisphere, and many other parts of the world. The successful control of poliomyelitis to date has been achieved to a large extent with the global use of orally administered live attenuated poliovaccine, the only mucosal vaccine available for routine use to date. As we begin to take into account the magnitude and existing load of infectious diseases in many parts of the world, the emergence of new infectious disease syndromes, and the difficulties encountered in prevention, control, or eradication of serious infectious agents by available chemotherapeutic agents or available vaccines, it is apparent that we must consider the development of other effective mucosal vaccines.

Considerable effort is devoted in this volume to the discussion of infectious agents that gain entry into the human host via the mucosal portals and that produce disease selectively at the mucosal surfaces of respiratory, gastrointestinal, or genital tracts. Several chapters in this volume explore the concepts of mucosal vaccination in other areas of disease prevention. These include induction of systemic hyporesponsiveness to mucosally introduced antigens (mucosally induced tolerance). Currently there is significant interest in this approach in the prevention and/or treatment of autoimmune diseases, the regulation of systemic inflammatory processes, and the control of homograft rejection. The concepts of mucosal immunization represent a new generation of immunologic approaches that may have a very broad scope of application in the control of human disease.

Individual chapters in this book are contributed by both basic scientists and clinical scholars who are actively contributing to the field of mucosal immunology and vaccine evaluation or development. This book will be of benefit to diverse groups of clinicians and investigators whose interests are based in the fields of immunology, basic biology of the mucosal immune system, or vaccines.

Proceeds from the sale of this book will support the Society for Mucosal Immunology. We thank our expert contributors, who have devoted their time to the preparation of this first comprehensive and modern view of mucosal vaccines. Our special appreciation goes to Ms. Wendy Jackson, at the University of Alabama at Birmingham, who spent numerous hours editing individual chapters. Without her willingness and hard work, this publication would not exist. We also thank Dr. Jasna Markovac, Mr. Craig Panner, and Ms. Charlotte Brabants at Academic Press, who assisted in the publication of this book.

Hiroshi Kiyono
Pearay L. Ogra
Jerry R. McGhee

I

Introduction

1

Mucosal Immunoprophylaxis: An Introductory Overview

PEARAY L. OGRA
Department of Pediatrics and Microbiology,
University of Texas Medical Branch,
Galveston, Texas 77555

I. Introduction

"The idea of local immunity as we conceive it, that is, an immunity without the obligatory participation of antibodies, has barely made its appearance. This conception already rests upon a large number of facts. Many of the phenomena, which cannot be explained by the accepted theories, are cleared up in the light of this new conception. As a result of these researches, applications to vaccination and vaccinotherapy have followed, and are now being employed in daily practice."

The statement above is not based on developments during the 1990s, but appeared in the Preface of a classic monograph over six decades ago entitled "Local Immunization" by Professor A. Besredka (Besredka, 1927). He thus proposed the framework for modern concepts of mucosal immunity, based on his own studies, and by other contemporary investigators, including Shiga, Dumas and Combiesco, Chvostek, and Metchnikoff (Metchnikoff and Besredka, 1911). Professor Besredka further states in this monograph (Besredka, 1927) that

"As far back as we may look into the early history of our science, we find evidence of the idea of vaccination and immunity. The primitive people, actuated by the instinct of self-preservation, developed ideas that would be worthy of our contemporaries. The savage Vatuas from oriental Africa showed evidence of this remarkable intuition, in treating serpent bites by making cutaneous incisions in the arms and legs and then applying a paste, which contained the specific poison. We must also consider the Achantis as our predecessors, the Siamese, and the Chinese, who from time immemorial put specific crusts into the nose and lesions of the skin for protection against smallpox. It is also interesting to note the active technic employed by the Maures of the Senegambia, who protected their animals against peripneumonia, by plunging a spear into the lungs of an infected animal and then applying the material obtained to the skin of healthy animals. Does not the method of Willelm consist in producing an incision under the surface of the tail of a healthy animal and applying the serous liquid obtained from an animal infected with peripneumonia? Our ancestors then possessed methods of vaccination in their prophylactic armamentarium, which were just as effective as those employed by us today. Hence they practiced cutaneous vaccination a long time before we did."

In a similar historical perspective, ingestion of Rhus leaves to modify the severity of reactions to exposure to poison ivy has been reported to be an age old practice in the United States (Duncan, 1916; French, 1916; Shelmire, 1941). These remarkable clinical observations preceded by decades the discovery of IgA, the identification of secretory IgA (S-IgA) as a unique immunoglobulin in human external secretions, and the discovery of the secretory component and the J chain allowed the characterization of the bronchus-associated lymphoid tissue (BALT) and the gut associated lymphoid tissue (GALT) in many mammalian species. During the past decade, the concept of local immunity has been expanded to include M cells, intraepithelial lymphocytes, cytokines and neuropeptides, and other effector cellular mechanisms of immunoregulation. The bulk of this information is extensively reviewed in recent texts on mucosal immunology (Ogra *et al.*, 1994). This chapter will briefly highlight general concepts of mucosal immunity and the experience with available approaches to mucosal immunoprophylaxis. Further details on specific aspects of different mucosal vaccines will be discussed in the following chapters.

MUCOSAL VACCINES

II. Elements of Mucosal Immune System Involved in Immune Response

Several recent publications have reviewed this subject in some detail (Ogra *et al.*, 1994; Holmgren, 1991; Brandtzaeg, 1989; McGhee *et al.*, 1992; Shalaby, 1995). Briefly, the mucosal sites which comprise the common mucosal immune system include BALT, GALT, genital tract, salivary glands, ocular tissues, and mammary glands. These sites are in intimate and constant contact with the external environment, contain mucocilliary epithelium, possess secretory component and/or S-IgA in the epithelium and lamina propria, and contain organized lymphoid follicles in subepithelial regions. These tissues participate in circulation of antigen reactive IgA B lymphocytes and specifically sensitized T cells to other distant sites, after *in vivo* stimulation in the BALT or GALT.

The intestinal mucosa represents a major source of IgA precursor immunocompetent tissue in the body. It comprises over 80% of all immunoglobulin producing cells in the human body. The lymphoid aggregates in the Peyer's patches and in other parts of the gastrointestinal tract are the central focus of T- and B-cell responses following mucosal exposure to an antigen. The most organized lymphoid follicles, including Peyer's patches, lie below a specialized layer of membranous epithelial cells called M cells. M cells are more permeable than other epithelial cells overlying the villus and crypt epithelium, thus providing sites in which the luminal antigens can be sampled and processed immunologically. M cells have been shown to produce class II MHC molecules, which suggests that they may also play a role in presenting antigens to local T cells (Owen, 1977; Keljo and Hamilton, 1983). Once antigen has traversed the M cells, other conventional antigen-presenting cells within the Peyer's patch take it up and present it to adjacent regulatory T cells. Subsequently, B cells within the follicles are stimulated. The local antigen-presenting cells and regulatory T cells have been shown to selectively enhance IgA responses. The predominance of B cells in the Peyer's patches or lamina propria express IgA and respond to certain cytokines to produce IgA (Tonkonogy *et al.*, 1989). Thus, it appears that several independent forces act in concert to ensure that IgA responses predominate in mucosal tissues.

The regulatory T cells in the Peyer's patches include helper T cells of both the Th1 and Th2 phenotypes. Other cell populations include suppressor T cells that limit the immune response against chronically administered antigens and other macromolecules (Taguchi *et al.*, 1990). Other T-cell subsets associated with mucosal lymphoid follicles may abrogate local anergy associated with oral tolerance (referred to as contrasuppressor cells) (Green *et al.*, 1982; Suzuki *et al.*, 1986). Although controversial, the presence of regulatory circuits of T cells has been widely reported. The case for the presence of regulatory circuits can also be appreciated in view of the fact that IgA responses have been shown to be selected by cytokines produced by Th2 cells (Ernst *et al.*, 1988a). However, these cytokines are extremely pleiotrophic, and yet the multiple effects of these cytokines are not generally observed during the induction of IgA responses. Although the Peyer's patches play a leading role in the induction of mucosal immune responses, antigens can cross absorptive cells and contact other local antigen-presenting cells, such as enterocytes. Several studies have suggested the expression of accessory molecules such as class II MHC on intestinal villous enterocytes, that are normally associated with antigen-presenting cells.

Recent studies have documented the expression of an invariant chain (Ouellette *et al.*, 1991), a protein associated with the production and expression of MHC class II molecules. Several investigators have shown that T cells can be stimulated by enterocytes expressing class II molecules. However, enterocytes are not directly exposed to $CD4^+$ T cells; as an alternative role, they may lead to inhibitory signals to curtail the magnitude of the host response to luminal antigens that gain entry, particularly when the epithelial barrier is compromised during inflammation. This finding is substantiated by reports that enterocytes selectively activate $CD8^+$ T cells (Bland and Warren, 1986). Under conditions such as inflammatory bowel disease, enterocytes may thus preferentially stimulate rather than inhibit immune responses (Mayer and Eisenhardt, 1990).

In addition to MHC class II molecules, the gut epithelium has been shown to express relatively conserved class I-like molecules including, CD1, TL and Qa (Heshberg *et al.*, 1990; Blumberg *et al.*, 1991). The class I molecules provide a useful ligand for the intraepithelial lymphocytes (IELs), which express a more limited immunologic repertoire. Several observations support the hypothesis that intraepithelial T lymphocytes can recognize such class I-like molecules (Balk *et al.*, 1991). However, specific repertoires expressed within the intestinal lymphocytes are also found in mice expressing certain class II MHC phenotypes (Lefrancois *et al.*, 1990), suggesting that both types of ligands may be important. Within the epithelium of the intestine, approximately 1 in 10 cells is lymphoid. Eighty-five percent of these cells express a T-cell receptor and virtually none of them represent B cells. This compartment has been shown to contain antiviral NK cells or cytolytic T lymphocytes (CTLs), as well as mast cell precursors which may be important in immunity to local infections (Ernst *et al.*, 1985; Lefrancois, 1991). Many T and B cells in the lamina propria and epithelium appear to be typical of lymphocytes in other sites, although they do exhibit some heterogeneity.

As discussed earlier, in addition to their entry into

the Peyer's patches or lamina propria, mucosally delivered antigens may also enter the lymphatics which lead to the draining mesenteric lymph node. For example, some isolates of *Salmonella* can reach the mesenteric lymph nodes after intestinal infection. Such nodes have their own array of antigen-presenting cells, regulatory T cells, and effector T and B lymphocytes. Other antigens, including replicating viruses, may travel widely in the blood to other tissues for which they have particular tropism and wherein they can induce appropriate immune responses. Thus, redistributing a sufficient antigen load to different sites can lead to a widespread induction of immune responses following oral administration.

The proximity of immune effector cells within all mucosal tissues to nonimmunological tissues such as the nerves and smooth muscle (Marshall *et al.*, 1989) has generated considerable interest in their potential interactions *in vivo*. This association appears to be quite significant, and neuroendocrine influences have been shown to modulate the immune response at several distinct levels. Thus, these physiological systems confer afferent input which modulates the induction, magnitude, and type of immune response. Neuroendocrine tissues may also be associated with the efferent end of the immune response, and modulate epithelial cell proliferation or secretion (McDonald and Spencer, 1988) as well as muscle contractility (Vermillion *et al.*, 1991). It appears that these physiological systems collaborate with more traditional antigen-specific systems to broaden the effector responses that are protective in mucosal sites.

The antigen-sensitized T and B cells generated in the intestine enter the lymphatics, reach the mesenteric nodes and subsequently travel via the lymphatics to the blood and become disseminated in different mucosal tissues. These cells are found in the lamina propria and epithelium where they constitute the effector limb of the mucosal immune response. The intestinal lamina propria is distinguished by the large number of plasma cells and some B cells, almost all of which produce IgA. There are also large numbers of T cells, most of which express CD4 suggesting that they consist largely of helper T subsets.

III. Immunoprophylaxis by the Mucosal Route

The information summarized above suggests that mucosal surfaces, especially in the intestine and the respiratory tract, represent the sites of large accumulation of immunocompetent cells involved in host defense. Of particular importance is the fact that most infectious agents and environmental antigens gain entry into the host via the mucosal surfaces and the surfaces of the respiratory and gastrointestinal tract are able to present and process a diversity of antigens and mount specific local immune responses. Available information concerning the development of mucosal immune responses employing conventional vaccines and other experimental approaches is discussed briefly below.

A. Conventional Vaccines

The nature of serum and secretory immune responses induced after immunization by conventional live attenuated or killed (nonreplicating) vaccines has been reviewed previously (Ogra *et al.*, 1980; Czerkinsky *et al.*, 1993; Kagnoff, 1993) and is summarized in Table I. Earlier studies conducted with live attenuated orally administered (Sabin) poliovaccine (OPV), live enteric-coated adenovirus vaccines, inactivated Salk poliovirus vaccine (IPV-Salk) administered intranasally or intramuscularly, live attenuated rubella virus vaccines (Cedenhill, HPV-77, RA27/3) administered intranasally or intramuscularly, and live attenuated mumps and measles viruses administered intramuscularly have provided

TABLE I
Nature of Immunologic Reactivity after Systemic or Mucosal Immunization with Conventional Live or Inactivated (Killed) Viral Vaccines

	Response to immunization by indicated route and type of vaccine			
	Systemic		Mucosal (enteric or respiratory)	
Features of response	Live	Killed	Live	Killed
Immunologic response similar to natural infection	±	−	+	−
Development of systemic immune response	+	+	+	±
Persistence of systemic immune response	+	±	+	−
Detection of viral antigen in mucosal surfaces	±	−	+	±
Development of secretory immune response	±	±	+	±
Persistence of secretory immune response	±	−	+	±
Development of secretory immunity in other mucosal sites and milk	+	−	+	±
Protection against mucosal natural reinfection	±	−	+	+
Protection against systemic disease after natural reinfection	+	+	+	±
Development of herd immunity via spread of vaccine virus to contacts	−	−	+	−
Development of more severe disease after natural reinfection	−	±	−	−

Note. +, Always; ±, occasional or inconsistent; −, absent.

a wealth of evidence to support the concept of relative compartmentalization of systemic vs mucosal antibody as well as cell-mediated immune responses in most mammalian species (Ogra and Karzon, 1971). Immunization by replicating viral vaccines available for use by the respiratory or enteric mucosal routes (adenovirus, polioviruses) has been shown to induce secretory immune responses which are consistently superior to that observed after immunization with replicating or nonreplicating viral vaccines administered parenterally. Development of neutralizing antibody response in mucosal sites has been observed consistently with most orally administered replicating agents. Respiratory or enteric mucosal immunization with nonreplicating or attenuated viral vaccines which are currently recommended only for parenteral use, such as IPV, rubella, or measles vaccines, has also been shown to induce secretory antibody response which is superior (albeit transient) to immunization via the parental route (Table 1). The functional role of pathogen-specific secretory antibody response has been reviewed extensively in several recent publications (Ogra and Karzon, 1971; Bergmann and Waldman, 1988; Mestecky, 1987). A number of studies have suggested that protection against mucosal reinfection with a variety of respiratory and enteric pathogens is better correlated with the presence and the levels of S-IgA antibody rather than the serum antibody (Ogra and Karzon, 1971; Bergmann and Waldman, 1988; Mestecky, 1987). The levels of preexisting antibody have been shown to influence the extent of replication and outcome of infection after a subsequent challenge with a live pathogen (Ogra and Karzon, 1971).

Investigations employing other conventional vaccines have suggested that in general, the human mucosal immune system functions at different and possibly lower levels of efficiency in the neonatal period. Very little IgA is detectable in the mucosal secretions during the first few days after birth. It has been previously demonstrated that colostrum and milk contain specific antibody and cell-mediated immune reactivity against a wide variety of antigens present in the enteric and respiratory membranes. In breast-fed infants, the acquisition of such immmunologic activity represents an ideal mechanism to compensate for the lack of mucosal immunity. Numerous clinical and epidemiologic studies have suggested that breast-fed infants are less prone than bottle-fed infants to develop acute respiratory and enteric mucosal infection (Ogra *et al.*, 1994). The presence and levels of pathogen specific neutralizing antibody activity in S-IgA and in other immunoglobulin isotypes thus provide important antimicrobial functions at external mucosal surfaces. The appearance of such activity should be considered a vital attribute of any viral vaccine designed to prevent infection acquired via the respiratory, intestinal, or genital tracts. As a result of the superior immune response observed with mucosal administration of replicating viral vaccines, recent investigations have favored the use of immunization with a variety of microbial antigens via the oral route in order to selectively stimulate the vast resource of precursor immunocompetent cells in the GALT (Ogra *et al.*, 1980; Czerkinsky *et al.*, 1993; Kagnoff, 1993; Ogra and Karzon, 1971; Bergmann and Waldman, 1988; Mestecky, 1987).

Based on available information in human and other mammalian systems using conventional vaccines, it appears that following exposure to an antigen in the intestinal mucosa, the IgA-committed precursor immunocompetent cells from the GALT migrate to the regional lymph nodes and enter into the bloodstream via the major lymphatic ducts. Such antigen-sensitized cells eventually home as antibody-producing IgA plasma cells, to the lamina propria of intestinal, bronchopulmonary, genital mucosa, and other mucosal associated tissues, such as mammary glands, conjunctiva, salivary glands, and the middle ear cleft (Ogra *et al.*, 1994).

Stimulation of the GALT by oral immunization has now been used to induce specific immune response in one or more mucosal sites against a variety of microorganisms. These include, among others, polioviruses, adenoviruses, influenza viruses, parainfluenzae viruses, respiratory syncytial virus, *Chlamydia trachomatis, Escherichia coli, Streptococcus mutans, Vibrio cholerae, Shigella, Salmonella,* diphtheria, tetanus, *pertussis,* giardia, and toxoplasma as reviewed recently (Ogra *et al.*, 1994). In view of the relative paucity of immunocompetent tissue in the BALT, it has been suggested that priming of intestine followed by booster antigen exposure in the respiratory tissue may be more effective in inducing mucosal immune responses in the respiratory tract than immunization of the respiratory tract alone (Freihorst *et al.*, 1989).

B. Current Approaches to Mucosal Immunoprophylaxis

Mucosal immunization with replicating organisms appears to be the most effective means of inducing mucosal immune responses. However, many microbial agents are not amenable to delivery and replication in the intestinal mucosa when administered orally. Furthermore, several currently available vaccines pose potential delivery problems and may result in altered immune responses when administered via the mucosal route. New techniques using the tools of molecular biology and genetics offer the ability to overcome some of the limitations associated with conventional vaccines when administered mucosally. These include subunit vaccines, synthetic peptides, and generation of vaccine antigens by mutagenesis, chemical conjugation, and genetic reassortment. Experience with these products for oral immunization is described briefly.

1. Subunit Vaccines

The polysaccharide capsule used in the prepara- ... vaccines against *H. influenzae* and *N. menin-* ... well as *S. pneumoniae* are purified polysac- ...roducts generated in culture *in vitro*. Similarly, ...d G proteins have been purified from tissue ...rown viruses and subsequently tested in man ...e candidates (Belshe *et al.*, 1993; Tristram *et* ...). These products have not been used for mu- ...unization to date. However, purified diphthe- ...incorporated in egg proteins has been used for ...unization in rabbits (Mirchamsy *et al.*, 1994). ...imals were partially protected against lethal ... with diphtheria toxin. Rabbits and monkeys ...munized with diphtheria and tetanus antigens ...ated significant immune response and total ...n against lethal challenge (Mirchamsy *et al.*, ...imiliarly, mucosal immunization with filamen- ...aagglutinin of *B. pertussis* by either respiratory ... routes was found to protect mice against *B.* ...infection of the trachea and lungs (Shahin *et* ...).

... Synthetic Peptides

...tide antigens are of great interest as potential ... because they do not require live organisms for synthesis, and can be customized to specific antigenic determinants mediating protection against illness or infection. Currently, there are several possible candidate vaccines of this nature (Table II). Synthetic peptides for adherence pilus proteins of *N. gonorrhoeae* have been tested in pilot studies in man (Tramont *et al.*, 1984).

TABLE II
New Approaches to Vaccine Development

Approach	Potential candidate vaccine
1. Purified subunits	*H. influenzae*, *N. meningitidis*, *S. pneumoniae*, RSV, hepatitis B, *B. pertusis* toxin
2. Synthetic peptides	*N. gonorrhoeae* (Adherence-Pili) *V. cholerae* toxin (B subunit) HIV V_3 loop, Group A *Streptococcus*
3. Nucleic acid vaccines	Influenza A, hepatitis B, RSV
4. Mutagenesis, chemical, irradiation, site-directed, transposon	*S. typhi*, (Ty21a), *V. cholerae*
5. Reassortants	Influenza, RSV, rotavirus
6. Chemical conjugation with cholera toxin B subunit (CT-B), *E. coli* heat-labile toxin (LT)	HIV, *S. mutans*, hepatitis B
7. Recombinant bacteria and viruses vectors: *Salmonella*, *Yersinia*, *BCG*, adenovirus, yeast	*S. mutans*, *Shigella*, hepatitis B, RSV, poliovirus

Unfortunately the vaccine did not seem to offer protection against challenge. On the other hand, a peptide vaccine utilizing the conserved region of M protein of type 6 *Group A* streptococci was found to be protective against homologous challenge (Bessen and Fischetti, 1990). Studies are ongoing with the peptides of the V3 loop of gp120 envelope protein of HIV (Arnon and Van Regenmortel, 1992). Little information is available regarding the presence of the nature of mucosal immune responses to such peptide vaccines. Studies with cholera toxin, especially with peptides CTP1 and CTP3 of B subunit, have shown induction of significant antibody responses. The antibody possesses significant functional activity and can inhibit the biologic activity of the native toxin (Arnon and Van Regenmortel, 1992; Lewis *et al.*, 1994).

3. Nucleic Acid Vaccines

It has been known for some time that naked DNA can transmit infection (Hepatitis B, polyoma viruses) (Israel *et al.*, 1979; Chan *et al.*, 1979; Will *et al.*, 1982). However, the potential for nucleoproteins to induce immune responses has been demonstrated only in recent studies. For example, immunization with DNA encoding for influenza A viral-nucleoprotein has been shown to result in the development of specific CTL responses (Ulmer *et al.*, 1993). Immunization with purified genetic material allows presentation of antigens to the immune system in a natural form and the antigens synthesized after inoculation of the DNA are directed to the MHC class I- and II-associated pathways in a manner remarkably similar to natural infection. Although studies regarding their use in oral immunization are in progress, no data are currently available.

4. Mutagenesis

One of the best studied examples of vaccines generated by chemically or irradiation-induced mutagenesis is the ty21a strain *Salmonella typhi* vaccine, which contains mutations in several poorly defined genes important in the mechanisms of pathogenesis and disease. The vaccine has been found to be quite effective when administered orally. It induces significant intestinal antibody responses, and after a three-dose vaccination regimen, it confers immunity in up to 70% of vaccinees (Cryz *et al.*, 1993).

Site-directed mutagenesis employs restriction enzymes to cleave DNA at defined sites in order to facilitate removal of a portion of native DNA and its replacement with mutant DNA. Mutations designed to eliminate toxin production in *V. cholerae* have generated several candidate vaccines. These include the CVD 110 strain in which virtually all segments coding for cholera toxin A subunit production have been replaced. The effectiveness of such mutants as mucosal vaccine candidates remains to be determined (Tacket *et al.*, 1993).

Specific mutations in pathogenic organisms have also been induced by the use of transposons. *S. typhi aro A strain,* in which a Tn10 transposon was inserted in the *aro A* gene (the gene required for utilization of aromatic amino acids in bacteria), represents one such vaccine candidate. *S. typhi aro A* with additional mutations in *pur A* and *his G* has been tested as an orally administered replicating vaccine. Its effectiveness as a mucosal vaccine remains to be determined, although in preliminary studies the vaccine was found to be able to induce good CTL responses (Edelman and Levine, 1986; Levine *et al.*, 1989).

5. *Reassortants*

The ability of some viruses to acquire new genetic material by reassortment with other viruses coexisting in the environment has been employed effectively to generate specifically targeted antigens in reassortant vaccines. This approach is currently being employed in developing several viral vaccines including influenza virus. Cold adapted strains which cannot replicate well at body temperature, are examples of such vaccines (Edwards *et al.*, 1994). Several such mutants have been tested in humans employing mucosal routes of administration (Edwards *et al.*, 19945; Kuno-Sakai *et al.*, 1994; Murphy, 1993). Strains of cold adapted H1N1 and H3N2 influenza viruses have been found to induce protection against illness in 60 to 90% of vaccinees following intranasal immunization (Edwards *et al.*, 1994). A number of other reassortant vaccines including those for RSV (Tristram *et al.*, 1993) and rotavirus (Bishop, 1993) are undergoing intense scrutiny in different laboratories and are discussed elsewhere in this book (Bishop, 1993).

6. *Chemical Conjugation*

Certain chemical agents, environmental macromolecules, and microbial antigens are taken up more efficiently by the mucosal epithelial cells and M cells. For example, cholera toxin B subunit (CT-B) and LT of *E. coli* preferentially bind to the G_{M1} ganglioside receptors on M cells, and their conjugation with other mucosally introduced antigens appears to significantly improve their immunogenecity (Czerkinsky *et al.*, 1989). The conjugation with CT-B or LT has been studied using a number of vaccines, including hepatitis B, HIV, influenza virus, *Streptococcus mutans,* and simian immune deficiency virus (SIV) (Shalaby, 1995; Lewis *et al.*, 1994; Lehner *et al.*, 1992, 1994).

7. *Recombinant Bacteria and Viruses*

A number of microbial vectors have been evaluated according to the development of recombinant vaccines with single or multiple antigenic determinants, representing single or multiple pathogens. These include such vectors as adendovirus types IV and VII, *Vaccinia, BCG, Salmonella,* and *Yersinia* (Johnson, 1991; Moss, 1991; Hackett, 1990; Jacobs *et al.*, 1990) and *Listeria monocytogenes* (Slifka *et al.*, 1996). A large number of bacterial and viral antigens and other proteins have been expressed in such hosts (Table II). Studies of oral immunization with *Salmonella* and adenovirus recombinant vector vaccines have demonstrated induction of immune response and protection against reinfection when administered orally as candidate vaccines for RSV, *S. mutans,* and *S. pyogenes* (Meitin *et al.*, 1994; Mahr and Payne, 1992; *Newton et al.*, 1991; Wathen *et al.*, 1989; Curtiss *et al.*, 1989).

IV. Mucosal Adjuvants and Vaccine Delivery Systems

Mucosal application of antigens in general induces relatively low immune responses, with the exception of naturally acquired or vaccine-induced active infections. This is due in part to the mechanical elimination of the antigens in the feces, the presence of anatomic and chemical barriers, the degradation and denaturation of antigens, and variables such as systemic absorption and the presence of preexisting specific antibody activity. A number of adjuvants have been employed to enhance the immunogenicity of mucosally administered antigens (Table III). The most potent adjuvant currently under investigation is cholera toxin. As pointed out earlier, CT specifically binds to the M cells and to G_{M1}-ganglioside receptors on the mucosal epithelium. It also enhances the proliferation of immunocompentent B and T cells, and augments the antigen-presenting capacity of macrophages (Lycke and Holmgren, 1986; Bromander *et al.*,

TABLE III
Mucosal Adjuvants and Vaccine Delivery Systems

Adjuvants
Cholera toxin, *E. coli*-labile toxin (LT)
Other bacterial proteins
Lectins, polyelectrolytes
Muramyl dipeptide
Immunostimulatory complexes (ISCOMs)
Delivery systems
Liposomes
Microencapusulation
Synthetic polymers (microspheres)
hydrophobic—polystyrene acid (PLA), polylactic acid (PGA)
Hydrophilic (hydrogels)—polyacrylamide, polycyanoacrylates
Other
Enteric coated capsules
Inert particles

1991). Other bacterial products such as heat-labile *E. coli* toxin (LT), lectins, polyelectrolytes such as diethylaminoelhyl (-4-dextran), Polyornithine, and detergents sodium dodecyl sulfate possess varying degrees of adjuvant activity and have been employed to enhance immune responses following mucosal immunization (Shalaby, 1995; Clements *et al.*, 1988; de Aizpurua and Russell-Jones, 1988).

Concurrent to the efforts to enhance immune response to mucosally introduced antigens, studies are currently underway to develop effective delivery systems to overcome the natural barriers related to antigen retention and biodegradation in the intestine (Eldridge *et al.*, 1989, 1990; O'Hagan *et al.*, 1989). A listing of the delivery systems under investigation at this time and detailed elsewhere in this book is presented in Table III.

V. Potential Limitations of Mucosal Immunization

A. Oral Tolerance

Nonreplicating antigens, when administered by the oral route, are less efficient in inducing a serologic response than live replicating agents. Oral tolerance is a specific systemic hyporesponsiveness to parenteral challenge induced after oral priming with the homologous antigen (Chase, 1946; Challacombe and Tomasi, 1980). In many cases, oral tolerance can occur concurrent with the development of specific S-IgA responses at mucosal sites. The majority of evidence suggests that oral tolerance develops after oral administration of soluble protein antigens (heterologous red cells, chemical, haptens and nonreplicating microbial agents. There is little or no evidence to support the development of oral tolerance to replicating agents. Since the mechanisms underlying the development of oral tolerance have not been well defined; it is believed that suppressor T cells ($CD8^+$), cytokines, and other anti-inflammatory cellular products are the principal mediators of oral tolerance. Oral tolerance has been associated with marked downregulation of IL-2, IL-6, IL-8, TNFα, and IFNα, cytokines often involved in proinflammatory immune response (Ernst *et al.*, 1988b). The lack of oral tolerance during naturally acquired infection states is believed to be related to the generation of contrasuppressor T cells, which inhibit suppression of S-IgA production (Manganaro *et al.*, 1994). It may also be influenced by the frequency and dose of orally administered antigens. Thus, it is possible that mucosal immunoprophylaxis utilizing nonreplicating vaccines or soluble proteins may pose a risk for the development of oral tolerance and specific systemic hyporesponsiveness (Manganaro *et al.*, 1994).

One interesting strategy to abrogate the effects of oral tolerance has been the administration of CT or LT with vaccine antigens. By combining purified CT and other protein antigens, either with or without direct conjugation, investigators have demonstrated that CT enhances mucosal and systemic immune responses for IgG and IgA (Elson and Ealding, 1984). CT combined with peptides from SIV has been administered orally and shown to induce strong systemic as well as demonstrable mucosal immunity in nonhuman primates (Lehner *et al.*, 1992). Such approaches support the notion that it may be a useful adjuvant for oral immunization with other peptides. The precise mechanisms for immune enhancing potential of CT remain to be determined. LT is known to possess strong immunoregulatory potential in terms of inhibiting the induction of oral tolerance and adjuvanticity in oral immunization. In addition, it has been shown that oral administration of an immunogenic peptide of LT spanning residues 26–45 of LT-B induces systemic unresponsiveness in BALB/c mice resulting in diminished serum IgG responses. It was also shown that the spleen (SP) $CD4^+$ T cells of tolerized mice failed to proliferate, whereas the Peyer's patches (PP) $CD4^+$ T cells did not generate IL-2 mRNA and the PP $CD4^+$ T cells expressed significant levels of IFNγ IL-2, IL-4, and TGFβ mRNA. Adoptive transfer of LT-B-specific intraepithelial lymphocytes to the tolerant mice abrogated the tolerance. In a related experiment, LT-B-stimulated SP $CD4^+$ T cells from mice expressed significant levels of IFNγ IL-2, IL-4, and IL-6 mRNA. These results indicate that PP $CD4^+$ T cells induce oral tolerance due to systemic T-cell anergy (Takahashi *et al.*, 1995).

In some situations, the recombinant B subunit of CT acts alone as an adjuvant, while in other cases, the alpha subunit of the toxin appears necessary to promote adjuvant effects. CT may facilitate the switch of pre-B cells expressing IgM to more mature IgA B cells. In addition, cholera toxin has been shown to inhibit suppressor T cells *in vitro,* suggesting that it may have a direct effect on the hyporesponsive environment.

B. Changes in Antigen Structure

The luminal environment in the gastrointestinal tract is harsh and is designed to break down environmental macromolecules, dietary antigens, and pathogenic agents in order to minimize the risk of disease. Unprotected microbial or other protein antigens administered orally are highly susceptible to enzyme-induced hydrolysis, which may result in the reduction of the functional antigen mass, loss of critical epitopes necessary for protective immune responses, irreversible conformational changes in available antigens, generation of neoantigens, or exposure of otherwise unacceptable determinants of a microbial agent (Lange *et al.*, 1980; Zhaori *et al.*, 1989;

Abraham *et al.*, 1993). Some of these difficulties can be overcome by developing alternate delivery systems for oral vaccines, as discussed elsewhere in this book.

Nature appears to have intended the intestine to be a relatively hyporesponsive environment in order to protect the host against adverse reactions to food and other environmental antigens. Thus one may anticipate that oral immunization would be associated with a paucity of adverse reactions, particularly of the allergic variety. However, in designing oral vaccines, one of the obvious challenges is to augment an immune response to nonreplicating agents, in such an environment. The techniques designed to circumvent anergy in the intestine could possibly interfere with the intrinsic anergy inducing mechanisms that protect the host from excessive amounts of inflammation. Although modern oral vaccines appear to be quite safe, it is not inconceivable that the induction of immunity against a particular pathogen may lead to an immune response which alters the state of anergy in local, autoreactive T cells. Therefore, as oral immunization with other nonreplicating antigens is applied to man, it is important to consider the possibility that the appropriate combination of genetic and environmental factors may occur and contribute to an adverse response rather than a protective response (Sosroseno, 1995).

It is possible that the induction of immunity to vaccine antigens could also induce a specific response that may be subsequently triggered by food antigens with the appropriate molecular mimicry. For example, celiac disease is a gluten-sensitive enteropathy that is partially genetic and environmental in etiology. Many investigators believe that following sensitization of the host to an environmental antigen, possibly through an infection, the subsequent ingestion of a dietary antigen in various cereal grains activates a local immune response, resulting in villus atrophy and malabsorption (Kagnoff *et al.*, 1989). It would be prudent to consider the potential of oral immunization to similarly sensitize a host to an antigen that cross-reacts with an epitome found in the diet. Other subtle manifestations of an adverse response may be the sensitization of the host to an antigen that is frequently encountered in the environment, particularly in cases where drinking water may often contain pathogens against which one is immunizing. Subsequent introduction of these pathogens via natural infections could trigger immune-mediated alterations in intestinal epithelial cells and nerve or motor function. Recent experimental animal studies have demonstrated a significant increase and altered immune response to dietary macromolecules (ovalbumin) or environmental antigens (ragweed) during active infection in the respiratory syncytial virus in the respiratory tract or rotavirus infection in the intestine (Abraham *et al.*, 1993; Freihorst *et al.*, 1988c).

VI. Concluding Remarks

Immunoprophylaxis by the mucosal route is an important approach to control mucosally acquired infections. The most notable example of the effectiveness of mucosal immunization is the use of live attenuated oral polio vaccines. The ability to induce a balanced systemic and secretory immune response following oral immunization is often determined by the nature of the vaccine antigen (replicating vs nonreplicating), intestinal mucosal microenvironment, the vehicles employed for vaccine delivery, and the potential for induction of oral tolerance. One of the goals of vaccine delivery by the mucosal routes must include approaches to overcome the potential for tolerance that may exist prior to exposure to an antigen, including the presence of anergy that exists in neonates. Abrogation of tolerance is feasible, since tolerance must be reversible so that the host can respond to a surge in antigen during the time of peak antigen load. The role of contrasuppressor pathway which has been described within the lymphoid cell populations of the intestine (Green *et al.*, 1982) remains to be seen. Interestingly, contrasuppressor cells in Peyer's patch can increase antibody responses, and seem to be capable of mediating an isotype-specific response (Suzuki *et al.*, 1986; Ernst *et al.*, 1988a). It is possible that the ability of contrasuppressors to abrogate the suppression of specific responses may allow suppression of less desirable responses to remain in place. (The cytokines produced in response to oral immunization focus their bioactivity on driving in IgA response. This may in part explain why such broadly different immune responses such as the allergic phenomenon like those induced with nematode infections and IgA responses are rarely seen together, even though both are widely believed to be selected by the cytokine profiles secreted by the Th2 subsets of helper T cells.)

The induction of oral tolerance may be potentially detrimental to the successful outcome of mucosal vaccines. A unique approach for the management of autoimmune disorders is the induction of oral tolerance by repeated administrations. The disease states in which oral immunization has been considered for suppression of autoimmune response include rheumatoid arthritis, multiple sclerosis, experimental autoimmune encephalitis, mylitis, uveoretinitis, and diabetes mellitus (Trentham *et al.*, 1993; Weiner *et al.*, 1993; Zhang *et al.*, 1991; Lider *et al.*, 1989; Nussenblatt *et al.*, 1990). In these situations, it may be possible to enhance oral tolerance by increased uptake of the putative etiologic antigens in the Peyer's patches and prolonging antigen presentation in the intestine (Taudorf *et al.*, 1994).

The mechanisms which potentiate mucosal responses or induce oral tolerance are being intensively studied in the context of mucosal immunization for infectious disease and autoimmune disorders, respectively. As a better understanding of the basic mechanism is acquired, it should be possible to manipulate mucosal immunocompetent tissues in the BALT and the GALT to preferentially induce high levels of a protective immune response against infectious agents, and/or to induce specific oral tolerance to reduce the immunologic load in autoimmune and allergic disorders. Professor Besredka would have been proud to note how far the concepts of local immunization have progressed in the past century.

References

Abraham, R., Minor, P., Dunn, G., Modlin, J. F., and Ogra, P. L. (1993). Shedding of virulent poliovirus revertants during immunization with oral poliovirus vaccine after prior immunization with inactivated polio vaccine. *J. Infect. Dis.* **168,** 1105–1109.

Arnon R., Van Regenmortel, M. H. V. (1992). Structural basis of antigenic specificity and design of new vaccines. *FASEB J.* **6,** 3266–3274.

Balk, S. P., Ebert, E. C., Blumenthal, R. L., McDermott, F. V., Wucherpfennig, K. W., Landau, S. B., and Blumberg, R. S. (1991). Oligoclonal expansion and CD1 recognition by human intestinal intra-epithelial lymphocytes. *Science* **253,** 1411–1415.

Belshe, R. B., Anderson, E. L., and Walsh, E. E. (1993). Immunogenicity of purified F glycoprotein of respiratory syncytial virus: Clinical and immune responses to subsequent natural infection in children. *J. Infect. Dis.* **168,** 1024–1029.

Bergmann, K.-C., and Waldman, R. H. (1988). Stimulation of secretory antibody following oral administration of antigen. *Rev. Infect. Dis.* **10,** 939–950.

Besredka, A. (1927). "Local Immunization," p. 7. Williams & Wilkins, Baltimore, Maryland.

Bessen, D., and Fischetti, V. A. (1990). Synthetic peptide vaccine against mucosal colonization by group A streptococci. I. Protection against a heterologous M serotype with shared C repeat region epitopes. *J. Immunol.* **145,** 1251–1256.

Bishop, R. F. (1993). Development of candidate rotavirus vaccines. *Vaccine* **11,** 247–254.

Bland, P. W., and Warren L. G. (1986). Antigen presentation by epithelial cells of the rat small intestine. II Selective induction of suppresor T cells. *Immunology* **58,** 9–14.

Blumberg, R. S., Terhorst, C., Bleicher, P., McDermott, F. V., Allan, C. H., Landau, S. B., Trier, J. S., and Balk, S. P. (1991). Expression of a nonpolymorphic MHC class I-like molecule. CD1d. by human intestinal epithelial cells. *J. Immunol.* **147,** 2518–2524.

Brandtzaeg, P. (1989). Overview of the mucosal immune system. *Curr. Top. Microbiol. Immunol.* **146,** 13–25.

Bromander, A., Holmgren, A., and Lycke, N. (1991). Cholera toxin stimulates IL-1 production and enhances antigen presentation by macrophages *in vitro. J. Immunol.* **146,** 2908–2913.

Challacombe, S. J., and Tomasi, T. B., Jr. (1980). Systemic tolerance and secretory immunity after oral immunization. *J. Exp. Med.* **152,** 1459–1472.

Chan, H. W., Israel, M. A., Garon, C. F., Rowe, W. P., and Martin, M. A. (1979). Molecular cloning of polyoma virus DNA in *Escherichia coli*: Lambda phage vector system. *Science* **203,** 887–892.

Chase, M. W. (1946). Inhibition of experimental drug allergy by prior feeding of the sensitizing agent. *Proc. Soc. Exp. Biol. Med.* **61,** 257–259.

Clements, J. D., Hartzog, N. M., and Lyon, F. L. (1988). Adjuvant activity of *E. coli* heat-labile enterotoxin and effect on the induction of oral tolerance in mice to unrelated protein antigens. *Vaccine* **6,** 269–277.

Cryz, S. J., Jr., Vanprapar, N., Thisyakorn, U., and Olanratnanee (1993). Safety and immunogenicity of *Salmonella typhi* Ty21a vaccine in young Thai children. *Infect. Immun.* **61,** 1149–1151.

Curtiss, R., Kelly, S., and Gulig, P. (1989). Selective delivery of antigens by recombinant bacteria. *Curr. Top. Microbiol. Immunol.* **146,** 35–49.

Czerkinsky, C., Russel, M., Lycke, N., Lindblad, M., and Holmgren, J. (1989). Oral administration of streptococcal antigen coupled to cholera toxin B subunit evokes strong antibody responses in salivary and extramucosal tissues. *Infect. Immun.* **57,** 1072–1077.

Czerkinsky, C., Svennerholm., A-M., and Holmgren, J. (1993). Induction and assessment of immunity at enteromucosal surfaces in humans: Implications for vaccine development. *Clin. Infect. Dis.* **16,** S106–S116.

de Aizpurua, H. J., and Russell-Jones, G. J. (1988). Oral vaccination: Identification of classes of proteins that provide an immune response upon oral feeding. *J. Exp. Med.* **167,** 440–451.

Duncan, C. H. (1916). Autotherapy in ivy poisoning. *N. Y. Med. J.* **104,** 901–902.

Edelman, R., and Levine, M. M. (1986). Summary of an international workshop on typhoid fever. *Rev. Infect. Dis.* **8,** 329–349.

Edwards, K. M., Dupont, W. D., Westrich, M. K., Plummer, W. D., Jr., Palmer, P. S., and Wright, P. F. (1994). A randomized controlled trial of cold-adapted and inactivated vaccines for the prevention of influenza A disease. *J. Infect. Dis.* **169,** 68–76.

Eldridge, J., Gilley, R., Staas, J., Moldoveanu, Z., Meulbroek, J., and Tice, T. (1989). Biodegradable microspheres: Vaccine delivery system for oral immunization. *Curr. Top. Microbiol. Immunol.* **146,** 59–66.

Eldridge, J., Hammond, C., Meulbroek, J,. Staas, J., Gilley, R., and Tice, T. (1990). Controlled vaccine release in the gut-associated lymphoid tissues. I. Orally administered biodegradable microspheres target the Peyer's patches. *J. Controlled Release* **11,** 205–214.

Elson, C. O., and Ealding W. (1984). Cholera toxin feeding did not induce oral tolerance in mice and abrogated oral tolerance to an unrelated protein antigen. *J. Immunol.* **133,** 2892–2897.

Ernst, P. B., Befus, A. D., and Bienenstock, J. (1985). Leukocytes in the intestinal epithelium: An unusual immunological compartment. *Immunol. Today* **6**, 50–55.

Ernst, P. B., Maeba, J., Lee, S.-T., and Paraskevas, F. (1988a). A novel mechanism for the selection of isotype-specific antibody responses: The role of intestinal T cells in the regulation of IgA synthesis by the anti-suppressor circuit. *Immunology* **65**, 59–66.

Ernst, P. B., Scicchitano, R., Underdown, B. J., and Bienenstock, J. (1988b). Oral immunization and tolerance. In "Immunology of the Gastrointestinal Tract and Liver" (M. F. Heyworth and A. L. Jones, eds.), pp. 125–144. Raven, New York.

Freihorst, J., Piedra, P. A., Okamoto, Y., and Ogra, P. L. (1988c). Effect of respiratory syncytial virus infection on the uptake of and immune response to the other inhaled antigens. *Proc. Soc. Exp. Biol. Med.* **188**, 171–197

Freihorst, J., Merrick, J. M., and Ogra, P. L. (1989). Effect of oral immunization with *Pseudomonas aeruginosa* on the development of specific antibacterial immunity in the lungs. *Infect. Immun.* **57**, 235–238.

French, J. M. (1916). Treatment of ivy poisoning. *Clin. Med.* **August,** 753–755.

Green, D. R., Gold, J., Martin S., Gershon, R., and Gershon, R. K. (1982). Microenvironmental immunoregulation: Possible role of contrasuppressor cells in maintaining immune responses in gut-associated lymphoid tissue. *Proc. Natl. Acad. Sci. U.S.A.* **79**, 889–892.

Hackett, J. (1990). *Salmonella*-based vaccines. *Vaccine* **8**, 5–11.

Heshberg, R. M., Eghtesady, P., Sydora, B. Brorson, K., Cheroutre, H., Modlin, R., and Kronenberg, M. (1990). Expression of the thymus leukemia antigen in mouse intestinal epithelium. *Proc. Natl. Acad. Sci. U.S.A.* **87**, 9727–9731.

Holmgren, J. (1991). Mucosal immunity and vaccination. *FEMS Microbiol. Immunol.* **89**, 1–10.

Israel, M. A., Chan, H. W., Rowe, W. P., and Martin, M. A. (1979). Molecular cloning of polyoma virus DNA in *Escherichia coli*: Plasmid vector system. *Science* **203**, 883–887.

Jacobs, W. R., Jr., Snapper, S. B., Lugosi, L., and Bloom, B. R. (1990). Development of BCG as a recombinant vaccine vehicle. *Curr. Top. Microbiol. Immunol.* **155**, 153–160.

Johnson, D. C. (1991). Adenovirus vectors as potential vaccines against herpes simplex virus. *Rev. Infect. Dis.* **13**, S912–916.

Kagnoff, M. F. (1993). Immunology of the intestinal tract. *Gastroenterology* **105**, 1275–1280.

Kagnoff, M. F., Harwood, J. H., Bugawan, T. L., and Erlich, H. A. (1989). Structural analysis of the HLA-DR, -DQ, and -DP alleles on the celiac disease-associated HLA-DR3 (Drw17) haplotype. *Proc. Natl. Acad. Sci. U.S.A.* **86**, 62740–6278.

Keljo D. J., and Hamilton, J. R. (1983). Quantitative determination of macromolecular transport rate across intestinal Peyer's patches. *Am. J. Physiol.* **244**, G637–G644.

Kuno-Sakai, H., Kimura, M., Ohta, K., Shimojima, R., Oh, Y., and Fukumi, H. (1994). Developments in mucosal influenza virus vaccines. *Vaccine* **12**, 1303–1310.

Lange, S., Nygren, H., Svennerholm, A., and Holmgren, J. (1980). Antitoxic cholera immunity in mice: Influence of antigen deposition on antitoxin-containing cells and protective immunity in different parts of the intestine. *Infect. Immun.* **28**, 17–23.

Lefrancois, L. (1991). Extrathymic differentiation of intraepithelial lymphocytes: Generation of a separate and unequal T cell repertoire. *Immunol. Today* **12**, 436–438.

Lefrancois, L., LeCorre, R., Mayo, J., Bluestone, J. A., and Goodman, T. (1990). Extrathymic selection of TCR gamma delta + T cells by class II major histocompatibility complex molecules. *Cell (Cambridge, Mass.)* **63**, 333–340.

Lehner, T., Bergmeier, L., Panagiotidi, C., Tao, L., Brookes, R., Klavinskis, L., Walker, P., Walker, J., Ward, R., Hussain, L., Gearing, A., and Adams, S. (1992). Induction of mucosal and systemic immunity to a recombinant simian immunodeficiency viral protein. *Science* **258**, 1365–1369.

Lehner, T., Tao, L., Panagiotidi, C., Klavinskis, L., Brookes, R., Hussain, L., Meyers, N., Adams, S., Gearing, A., and Bergmeier, L. (1994). Mucosal model of genital immunization in male rhesus macaques with a recombinant simian immunodeficiency virus. *J. Virol.* **68**, 1624–1632.

Levine, M. M., Ferreccio, C., Black, R. E., Tacket, C. O., and Germanier, R. (1989). Chilean Typhoid Committee. Progress in vaccines against typhoid fever. *Rev. Infect. Dis.* **11**, S552–S567.

Lewis, D. J., Gilks, C. F., Ojoo, S., Castello-Branco, L. R., Dougan, G., Evans, M. R., McDermott, S., and Griffin, G. E. (1994). Immune response following oral administration of cholera toxin B subunit to HIV-1-infected UK and Kenyan subjects. *AIDS* **8**, 779–785.

Lider, O., Santos, L. M., Lee, C., Higgins, P., and Weiner, H. (1989). Suppression of experimental autoimmune encephalomyelitis by oral administration of myelin basic protein. II. Suppression of disease and *in vitro* immune response is mediated by antigen-specific CD8 T lymphocytes. *J. Immunol.* **142**, 748–752.

Lycke, N., and Holmgren, J. (1986). Strong adjuvant properties of cholera toxin on gut mucosal immune response to orally presented antigens. *Immunology* **59**, 301–308.

MacDonald, T. T., and Spencer, J. (1988). Evidence that activated mucosal T cells play a role in the pathogenesis of enteropathy in human small intestine. *J. Exp. Med.* **167**, 1341–1349.

McGhee, J., Mestecky, J., Dertzbaugh, M., Eldridge, J. H., Hirasawa, M., and Kiyono, H. (1992). The mucosal immune system from fundamental concepts to vaccine development. *Vaccine* **10**, 75–88.

Mahr, A., and Payne, L. G. (1992). Vaccinia recombinants as vaccine vectors. *Immunobiology* **184**, 126–146.

Manganaro, M., Ogra, P. L., and Ernst, P. B. (1994). Oral immunization: Turning fantasy into reality. *Int. Arch. Allergy Immunol.* **103**, 223–233.

Marshall, J. S., Bienenstock, J., Perdue, M. H., Stanisz, A. M., Stead, R. H., and Ernst, P. B. (1989). Novel cellular interactions and networks involving the intestinal immune system and its microenvironment. *Acta Pathol. Microbiol. Immunol. Scand.* **97**, 383–394.

Mayer, L., and Eisenhardt, D. (1990). Lack of induction of suppresor T cells by intestinal epithelial cells from patients with inflammatory bowel disease. *J. Clin. Invest.* **86,** 1255–1260.

Meitin, C. A., Bender, B. S., and Small, P. A. (1994). Enteric immunization of mice against influenza with recombinant vaccinia. *Proc. Natl. Acad. Sci. U.S.A.* **91,** 11187–11191.

Mestecky, J. (1987). The common mucosal immune system and current strategies for induction of immune responses in external secretions. *J. Clin. Immunol.* **7,** 265–276.

Metchnikoff, E., and Besredka, A. (1911). *Ann. Instit. Pasteur* **March,** 210.

Mirchamsy, H., Hamedi, M., Fateh, G., and Sassani, A. (1994). Oral immunization against diphtheria and tetanus infections by fluid diphtheria and tetanus toxoids. *Vaccine* **12,** 1167–1172.

Moss, B. (1991). Vaccinia virus: A tool for research and vaccine development. *Science* **252,** 1662–1667.

Murphy, B. R. (1993). Use of live attenuated cold-adapted influenza A reassortant virus vaccines in infants, children, young adults, and elderly adults. *Infectious Diseases in Clinical Practice* **2,** 174–181.

Newton, S. M. C., Kotb, M., Poirier, T. P., Stocker, B. A. D., and Beachey, E. H. (1991). Expression and immunogenicity of a streptococcal M protein epitope inserted in *Salmonella flagellin. Infect. Immun.* **59,** 2158–2165.

Nussenblatt, R., Caspi, R., Mahdi, R., Chan, C., Roberge, F., Lider, O., and Weiner, H. (1990). Inhibition of S-antigen induced experimental autoimmune uveoretinitis by oral induction of tolerance with S-antigen. *J. Immunol.* **144,** 1689–1695.

Ogra, P. L., and Karzon, D. T. (1971). Formation and function of poliovirus antibody in different tissues. *Prog. Med. Virol.* **13,** 156–193.

Ogra, P. L., Fishaut, M., and Gallaher, M. R. (1980). Viral vaccination via the mucosal route. *Rev. Infect. Dis.* **2,** 352–369.

Ogra, P. L., Mestecky, J., Lamm, M. E., Strober, W., McGhee, J. R., and Bienenstock, J. (eds). (1994). "Handbook of Mucosal Immunology," pp. 1–766. Academic Press, San Diego.

O'Hagan D., Palin, K., Davis, S., Artursson, P., and Sjoholm, I. (1989). Microparticles as potentially orally active immunological adjuvants. *Vaccine* **7,** 421–424.

Ouellette, A. J., Greco, R. M., James, M., Naftalin, J., and Fallon, J. T. (1991). Class II antigen-associated invariant chain mRNA in mouse small intestine. *Biochem. Biophys. Res. Commun.* **179,** 1642–1648.

Owen, R. L. (1977). Sequential uptake of horseradish peroxidase by lymphoid follicle epithelium of Peyer's patches in the normal unobstructed mouse intestine: An ultrastructural study. *Gastroenterology* **72,** 440–451.

Shahin, R. D., Amsbaugh, D. F., Leef, M. F. (1992). Mucosal immunization with filamentous hemagglutinin protects against *Bordetella pertussis* respiratory infection. *Infect. Immun.* **April,** 1482–1488.

Shalaby, W. S. (1995). Development of oral vaccines to stimulate mucosal and systemic immunity: Barriers and novel strategies. *Clin. Immunol. Immunopathol.* **74,** 127–134.

Shelmire, B. (1941). Cutaneous and systemic reactions observed during oral poison ivy therapy. *J. Allergy* **12,** 252–271.

Slifka, M. A., Shen, H., Matloubian, M., and Jensen, E. R. (1996). Antiviral cytotoxic T-cell memory by vaccination with recombinant listeria monocytogenes. *J. Virol.* **70,** 2902–2910.

Sosroseno, W. (1995). A review of the mechanisms of oral tolerance and immunotherapy. *J. R. Soc. Med.* **88,** 14–17.

Suzuki, K., Kitamura K., Kiyono, H., Kurita, T., Green, D. R., and McGhee, J. R. (1986). Isotype-specific immunoregulation. Evidence for a distinct subset of T contrasuppressor cells for IgA responses in murine Peyer's patches. *J. Exp. Med.* **164,** 501–516.

Tacket, C. O., Losonsky, G., Nataro, J. P., *et al.* (1993). Safety and immunogenicity of live oral cholera vaccine candidate CVD 110, a *ΔoctxA Δzot Δace* derivative of El Tor Ogawa *Vibrio cholerae. J. Infect. Dis.* **168,**1536–1540.

Taguchi T., McGhee, J. R., Coffman, R. L., Beagley, K. W., Eldridge, J. H., Takatsu, K., and Kiyono, H. (1990). Analysis of Th1 and Th2 cells in murine gut-associated tissues. Frequencies of $CD4^+$ and $CD8^+$ cells that secrete IFN gamma and IL-5. *J. Immunol.* **145,** 68–77.

Takahashi, I., Nakagawa, I., Kiyono, H., McGhee, J. R., Clements, J. D., and Hamada, S. (1995). Mucosal T cells induce systemic anergy for oral tolerance. *Biochem. Biophys. Res. Commun.* **206,** 414–420.

Taudorf, E., Moller, C., and Russell, M. W. (1994). Secretory IgA response in oral immunotherapy. Investigation in birch pollinosis. *Allergy* **49,** 760–765.

Tonkonogy, S. L., Mckenzie, D. T., and Swain, S. L. (1989). Regulation of isotype production by IL-4 and IL-5. Effects of lymphokines on Ig production depend on the state of activation of the responding B cells. *J. Immunol.* **142,** 4351–4360.

Tramont, E. C., Boslego, J. W., Chung, R., McChesney, D., Ciak, J., Sadoff, J., Piziak, M., Brinton, C. C., Wood, S., and Bryan, J. (1984). Parenteral gonococcal pilus vaccine. *In* "The pathogenic *Neisseriae*" (G. K. Schoolnik, ed.), pp. 316–322. Proceedings of the Fourth International Symposium, Asilomar, California.

Trentham, D. E., Dynesius-Trentham, R. A., Orav, E., Combitchi, D., Lorenzo, C., Sewell, K., Hafler, D. A., and Weiner, H. L. (1993). Effects of oral administration of type II collagen on rheumatoid arthritis. *Science* **261,** 1727–1730.

Tristram, D. A., Welliver, R. C., Mohar, C. K., Hogerman, D. A., Hildreth, S. W., and Paradiso, P. (1993). Immunogenicity and safety of respiratory syncytial virus subunit vaccine in seropositive children 18–36 months old. *J. Infect. Dis.* **167,** 191–195.

Ulmer, J. B., Donnelly, J. J., Parker, S. E., *et al.* (1993). Heterologous protection against influenza by injection of DNA encoding a viral protein. *Science* **259,** 1745–1749.

Vermillion, D., Ernst, P. B., and Collins, S. M. (1991). T lymphocyte modulation of intestinal muscle function in the *Trichinella*-infected rat. *Gastroenterology* **101,** 31–38.

Wathen, M. W., Brideau, R. J., Thomsen, D. R., and Murphy, B. R. (1989). Characterization of a novel human respiratory syncytial virus chimeric FG glycoprotein expressed using a baculovirus vector. *J. Gen. Virol.* **70,** 2625–2635.

Weiner, H. L., Mackin, G. A., Matsui, M., Orav, E. J., Khoury, S., Dawson, D. M., and Hafler, D. A. (1993). Double blind pilot trial of oral tolerization with myelin antigens in multiple sclerosis. *Science* **259,** 1321–1324.

Wells, H. G., and Osborne, J. B. (1911). The biological reactions of vegetable proteins. *J. Infect. Dis.* **8,** 66–124.

Will, H., Cattaneo, R., Koch, H. G., Darai, G., Schaller, H., Schekllekens, H., van Eerd, P. M., and Deinhardt, F. (1982). Cloned HBV DNA causes hepatitis in chimpanzees. *Nature (London)* **299,** 740–742.

Zhang, Z. J., Davidson, L., Eisenbarth, G., and Weiner, H. L. (1991). Suppression of diabetes in nonobese diabetic mice by oral administration of porcine insulin. *Proc. Natl. Acad. Sci. U.S.A.* **88,** 10252–10256.

Zhaori, G., Sun, M., Faden, H. S., and Ogra, P. L. (1989). Nasopharyngeal secretory antibody response to poliovirus Type 3 virion proteins exhibit different specificities after immunization with live or inactivated poliovirus vaccines. *J. Infect. Dis.* **159,** 1018–1024.

II

Principles of Mucosal Vaccination

2

Application of Basic Principles of Mucosal Immunity to Vaccine Development

HERMAN F. STAATS
Center for AIDS Research
Department of Medicine
Duke University Medical Center
Durham, North Carolina 27710

JERRY R. MCGHEE
Department of Microbiology
Immunobiology Vaccine Center
University of Alabama at Birmingham
Birmingham, Alabama 35294

I. Introduction

The mammalian mucosal immune system is an integrated network of tissues, lymphoid and constitutive cells and effector molecules which protect the host from infection of the mucous membrane surfaces. This signifies a major difference from the peripheral immune system, where lymphoid cells and effector molecules are confined to individual lymph nodes and spleen and intercommunication occurs by cell trafficking through the lymphatic and blood circulation. As you will appreciate in this chapter and throughout this book, the induction of peripheral immune responses does not result in significant mucosal immunity; however, the reverse is not true. Induction of mucosal immune responses can result in protective immunity in the peripheral compartment as well.

The mucosal immune system is anatomically and functionally divided into sites where foreign antigens are encountered and selectively taken up for initiation of immune response, and the more diffuse collection of B and T lymphocytes, differentiated plasma cells, macrophages, and other antigen-presenting cells (APCs), as well as mast cells which compose effector tissues for mucosal immunity. This network is highly integrated and finely regulated and the outcome of mucosal tissue encounters with foreign antigens and pathogens can range from mucosal and serum antibody responses and T-cell-mediated immunity on the one hand to systemic anergy to oral antigen, a response commonly termed mucosal tolerance, on the other. You may ask why the mucosal immune system is separate from the peripheral system and why antigen encounter elicits actual immunity in distant mucosal sites. It would appear that this separation has evolved as a major host defensive mechanism. For example, consider that mucosal surfaces are enormous, approximately 300–400 m^2, and as such require a significant expenditure of lymphoid cell elements for immunity. In this regard, the major antibody isotype in external secretions is immunoglobulin A (IgA) and approximately 40 mg/kg day of IgA is made in mucosal effector tissues, especially in the gastrointestinal (GI) tract (Conley and Delacroix, 1987). When this output of IgA is combined with its synthesis in bone marrow and in peripheral lymphoid tissues, this isotype represents twice the amount of other isotypes combined, including the IgG subclasses, which are produced in higher mammals. In spite of this propensity to produce IgA, the major effector cells in the mucosal immune system are T lymphocytes, of both $CD4^+$ and $CD8^+$ phenotypes, and in some cases can represent up to 80% of the entire cell population. Therefore, this chapter will devote considerable coverage to the multiple roles for regulatory and effector T cells in mucosal immunity.

The use of vaccines that induce protective mucosal immune responses thus becomes attractive when one considers that most infectious agents come in contact with the host at mucosal surfaces. Induction of mucosal immune responses may not only protect the

MUCOSAL VACCINES

TABLE I
Vaccines and Toxoids Licensed in the United States

Vaccine	Type	Route
Adenovirus	Live virus	Oral
Polivirus vaccine, oral (OPV)	Live virus of all three serotypes	Oral
Typhoid (Ty21a oral)	Live bacteria	Oral
Anthrax	Inactivated bacteria	Subcutaneous
BCG	Live bacteria	Intradermal/percutaneous
Cholera	Inactivated bacteria	Subcutaneous or intradermal
Diphtheria–tetanus–perttussis (DTP)	Toxoids and inactivated whole bacteria	Intramuscular
DTP–*Haemophilus influenzae* type b conjugate (DTP–Hib)	Toxoids, inactivated whole bacteria, and bacterial polysaccharide conjugated to protein	Intramuscular
Diphtheria–tetanus–acellular pertussis (DTaP)	Toxoids and inactivated bacterial components	Intramuscular
Hepatitis B	Inactivated viral antigen	Intramuscular
Haemophilus influenzae type B conjugate (Hib)	Bacterial polysaccharide conjugated to protein	Intramuscular
Influenza	Inactivated virus or viral components	Intramuscular
Japanese encephalitis	Inactivated virus	Subcutaneous
Measles	Live virus	Subcutaneous
Measles–mumps–rubella (MMR)	Live virus	Subcutaneous
Meningococcal	Bacterial polysaccharides of serotypes A/C/Y/W-35	Subcutaneous
Mumps	Live virus	Subcutaneous
Pertussis	Inactivated whole bacteria	Intramuscular
Plague	Inactivated bacteria	Intramuscular
Pneumococcal	Bacterial polysaccharides of 23 pneumococcal types	Intramuscular or subcutaneous
Poliovirus vaccine, inactivated (IPV)	Inactivated viruses of all three serotypes	Subcutaneous
Rabies	Inactivated virus	Intramuscular and intradermal
Rubella	Live virus	Subcutaneous
Tetanus	Inactivated toxin (toxoid)	Intramuscular
Tetanus–diphtheria (Td or DT)	Inactivated toxins (toxoids)	Intramuscular or intradermal
Typhoid (parenteral)	Inactivated bacteria	Subcutaneous
Varicella	Live virus	Subcutaneous
Yellow fever	Live virus	Subcutaneous

host from morbidity and mortality due to infection but possibly prevent infection altogether. The Centers for Disease Control (CDC) recommended childhood immunization schedule lists five vaccines that children should receive: (1) hepatitis B, (2) diphtheria–pertussis–tetanus (DPT), (3) *Hemophilus influenzae* type b, (4) poliovirus, and (5) measles–mumps–rubella (MMR) (CDC, 1995). Of those, only the oral poliovirus vaccine is administered by a mucosal route. In fact, of 27 classes of vaccines/toxoids/proteins currently licensed in the United States, only 3 are administered by a mucosal route (Table I) (CDC, 1994). Although parenterally administered vaccines induce protective immune responses, they rarely, if ever, induce mucosal immune responses that may prevent infection at the site of initial contact between the host and infectious agent. This chapter will detail some of the cellular and molecular components of the mucosal immune system of relevance to current mucosal vaccine strategies.

II. Mucosal Immune System Organization

In order to approach the development of mucosal vaccines, it is necessary to appreciate the functional anatomy of the mucosal immune system. Generally, foreign antigens and pathogens are encountered through ingestion or by inhalation and the host has evolved organized lymphoid tissues in these regions which facilitate their uptake. These inductive sites contain B and T lymphocytes which respond, in the presence of appropriate antigen-presenting cells (APC), to the encountered antigen by developing into effector and memory B and T cells. These antigen-specific B- and T-cell populations then emigrate from the inductive environment via lymphatic drainage, circulate through the bloodstream and home to mucosal effector regions. Thus, mucosal effector sites include these more diffuse tissues where antigen-specific T and B lymphocytes ultimately reside and perform their respective functions (i.e., cytokine or antibody synthesis, respectively) to protect mucosal surfaces.

A. Gut-Associated Lymphoreticular Tissue (GALT) as a Major Inductive Site

Mucosal inductive sites of the gastrointestinal (GI) tract include the Peyer's patches (PP), the appendix, and solitary lymphoid nodules which collectively comprise the gut-associated lymphoreticular tissues (GALT), while the tonsils and adenoids, or nasal-associated lymphoreticular tissues (NALT), likely serve as the mucosal inductive sites for the upper respiratory tract and the nasal/oral cavity. The most extensively studied mucosal inductive tissues are the PP of the murine GI tract. The murine PP contains a dome region enriched for B and T lymphocytes, macrophages, and small numbers of plasma cells just below the domed epithelium. Distinct follicles (B-cell zones), which contain germinal centers where significant B-cell division is seen, are located beneath the dome area of the PP. The PP germinal centers are considered to be sites where frequent B-cell switches to IgA and affinity maturation occur and also contain the majority of surface IgA positive ($sIgA^+$) B cells (see Section below) (Lebman *et al.*, 1977; Butcher *et al.*, 1982). However, unlike immune lymph nodes and the spleen in the systemic compartment, plasma cell development of any significance does not occur in the GALT.

All major T-cell subsets are found adjacent to follicles in the T-cell-dependent areas (Table II). The parafollicular PP T cells are mature and >97% of these T cells use the αβ heterodimer form of the T-cell receptor (TCR). Approximately 65% of PP αβ TCR^+ T cells are $CD4^+$,$CD8^-$ and exhibit properties of T helper (Th) cells, including support for IgA responses (Hanson and Brandtzaeg, 1989). Approximately 30% of the αβ TCR^+ T cells in the PP are $CD4^-$,$CD8^+$ T cells; this cell subset has been shown to contain precursors of cytotoxic T lymphocytes (CTLs) (Hanson and Brandtzaeg, 1989; London *et al.*, 1987). Recent studies of the lymphocyte populations associated with the human PP microfold cell (M cell) pockets, the area where lumenal antigen may first be recognized by T and B lymphocytes, have provided evidence for a similar T-cell distribution. M-cell pockets in human PP contain approximately equal numbers of $CD3^+$ T and $CD19^+$/$CD20^+$ B lymphocytes with less frequent numbers of $CD68^+$ macrophages (Farstad *et al.*, 1994). Of the mature T cells at this location, approximately 75% exhibit a T helper cell phenotype.

The surface of the PP is covered by a unique epithelium which contains unique cell types closely associated with lymphoid cells, giving rise to terms such as lymphoepithelium or follicle-associated epithelium (FAE). The FAE is enriched in specialized antigen-sampling cells known as M cells, which exhibit thin extensions around lymphoid cells (Farstad *et al.*, 1994; Bockman and Cooper, 1973; Owen and Jones, 1974; Wolf and Bye, 1984). The thin extensions that almost surround lymphoid cells form an apparent pocket which contains both T and B lymphocytes as well as macrophages (Farstad *et al.*, 1994). The M cells have short microvilli, small cytoplasmic vesicles, and few lysosomes, and are adept at uptake and transport of lumenal antigens, including proteins and particulates such as viruses, bacteria, small parasites, and microspheres (Wolf and Bye, 1984; Ermak *et al.*, 1995). Many investigators involved in this field believe that antigen uptake by M cells does not result in degradation of antigen, but

TABLE II
Major T-Cell Types Associated with the Mucosal Immune System

Tissues	Cell subsets	Functional characteristics
Peyer's patches (PP)	M cells	Antigen sampling from lumen
	$CD3^+$ T cells	
	$CD4^+$, $CD8^-$	T helper cells
	$CD4^-$, $CD8^+$	CTL precursors
	$CD4^-$, $CD8^-$	Double negative, usually express γδ TCR
	$sIgA^+$ B cells	~60% of germinal center B cells
	Accessory cells (Mϕ, B, and dendritic cells)	Ag presentation
Epithelium and lamina propria of small intestine	Epithelial cells	Crypt progenitors produce s.c.
	$CD3^+$ T cells	~60–80% of all cells
	$CD4^+$, $CD8^-$	~60% of T cells
	$CD4^-$, $CD8^+$	~30% of T cells
	$CD4^-$, $CD8^-$	~5%, IEL origin?
	IgA plasma cells	~85% of total plasma cells
	Accessory cells (Mϕ and DC)	Ag presentation

rather in delivery of intact antigen into the underlying lymphoid tissue (Wolf and Bye, 1984). However, findings such as M-cell expression of MHC class II molecules and acidic endosomal–lysosomal compartments suggest that M cells may be involved in antigen processing and presentation as well (Allan *et al.*, 1993). Until M cells can be cultured *in vitro,* the ability of this unique cell type to process and present antigen will remain controversial.

In addition to transportation of lumenal antigens (soluble and particulate), the M cell serves as a portal of entry for pathogens. Invasive strains of *Salmonella typhimurium* initiate murine infection by invading the M cells of the PP (Jones *et al.*, 1994). Although M cells are able to transport lumenal antigen, the fact that noninvasive strains of *S. typhimurium* were unable to penetrate the M cell suggests that the ability of *S. typhimurium* to infect M cells is associated with virulence factors of the bacteria. Reovirus also initiates infection of the murine intestine through the M cell (Wolf *et al.*, 1981). The ability of the reovirus to infect the murine M cell has been associated with the reovirus sigma protein (Nibert *et al.*, 1992). Identification of bacterial and viral virulence factors associated with invasion or infection of PP M cells may provide tools to construct more efficient attenuated bacterial or viral vectors (see below) or target oral vaccines to the inductive environment of the PP.

B. Mucosal Effector Tissues

After the initial exposure to antigen in mucosal inductive sites, mucosal lymphocytes leave the inductive site and home to mucosal effector tissues. Antigen-specific mucosal effector cells include IgA-producing plasma cells as well as B and T lymphocytes. IgA is the primary Ig involved in protection of mucosal surfaces and is locally produced in the gastrointestinal and upper respiratory tracts, nose, middle ear, gall bladder, uterine mucosa, and biliary tree as well as glandular tissues such as salivary, lactating mammary, prostate, and lacrimal glands (Phillips-Quagliata and Lamm, 1994). The observation that antigen-specific secretory IgA (S-IgA) responses may be detected at mucosal surfaces other than the inductive site where antigen uptake initially occurred has led to the use of the phrase "common mucosal immune system." This concept supports the notion that immunization of one mucosal inductive site may induce mucosal immune responses in all mucosal effector tissues.

The lamina propria (LP) region of the GI tract is the mucosal effector tissue most studied. The LP contains T cells with helper functions and CTLs as well as B lymphocytes and the aforementioned plasma cells. Freshly isolated intestinal LP $CD4^+$ T cells contain approximately twofold more IL-5 secreting cells than IFNγ-secreting cells, suggesting that the effector region of the mucosal immune system is biased toward a Th2 phenotype (Taguchi *et al.*, 1990). However, this assumption should be verified by measurement of production of other Th2-type cytokines. Of the antibody secreting cells in the lamina propria region of the murine intestine, IgA secreting cells are present at a frequency nearly 100 times higher than IgG secreting cells and over 20 times more than IgM secreting cells (Mega *et al.*, 1992). The association between IL-5 secreting cells and IgA secreting cells in the lamina propria region seems appropriate when one considers that IL-5 has been shown to enhance IgA synthesis (Strober and Harriman, 1991; Beagley and Elson, 1992; Ramsay and Kohonen-Corish, 1993); however, other cytokines, such as IL-6, which more effectively induces B-cell-terminal differentiation, should also be assessed.

III. Characteristics of Regulatory T Cells in the Mucosal Immune System

It may be useful to the reader to describe the development of regulatory T cells in the mucosal immune system, by simply considering mature T cells which are naive, e.g., which have not yet encountered antigen as precursor T helper (pTh) cells. Note that precursors of Th cells (pTh) normally recognize foreign peptide in association with MHC class II on APCs and express an αβ TCR^+, $CD3^+$, $CD4^+$, $CD8^-$ phenotype. On the other hand, precursor CTLs (pCTLs) express αβ TCR which usually recognize foreign peptide in the context of MHC class I on target cells and normally exhibit a phenotype of $CD3^+$, $CD4^-$, $CD8^+$. Thus, encounter with foreign antigen (peptides) will result in development of effector T cells which either are helper (Th) types for cell-mediated or antibody responses, or which lyse infected target cells (CTLs). Thus, the PP can be considered to be significant reservoirs of pTh cells and pCTLs such that encounter with bacterial or viral pathogens can result in induction of $CD4^+$ Th and $CD8^+$ CTL responses.

A. General Characteristics of Mucosal Th Cells

As Th cells mature in response to foreign antigens, they take on unique characteristics normally manifested by production of distinct cytokine arrays. The naive or pTh cell first produces IL-2 in response to stimuli and develops into a T cell producing multiple cytokines (including IFNγ and IL-4), a stage often termed Th0 (Weinberg *et al.*, 1990; Powers *et al.*, 1988) (Fig. 1). Of great interest has been the finding that the environment and cytokine milieu greatly influences the further differentiation of Th0 cells. For example, stimulation by certain pathogens such as intracellular bacteria lead to the formation of Th1 cells producing IFNγ, IL-2, and tumor necrosis factor beta (TNFβ), and these cells often develop following production of IL-12 by activated macrophages (Hsieh *et al.*, 1993), presumably following ingestion of the particular intracellular pathogen (Fig. 1). There is experimental evidence that secreted IL-12 induces NK cells to produce IFNγ (Kobayashi *et al.*, 1989; Chan *et al.*, 1991), which together with IL-12 triggers Th0 cells to differentiate along the Th1 pathway (Fig. 1). *In vivo*, murine Th1-type immune responses are associated with the development of cell-mediated immune (CMI) responses and B-cell responses characterized by IgG2a synthesis. IFNγ is the major cytokine responsible for IgG2a production in the mouse (Snapper and Paul, 1986). On the other hand, exogenous antigen can also induce a unique $CD4^+$ T-cell subset to produce IL-4 (Seder and Paul, 1994) which can trigger the formation of Th2-type cells (from Th0 cells) which produce IL-4, IL-5, IL-6, IL-9, IL-10, and IL-13 (Seder and Paul, 1994; Mosmann and Coffman, 1989; Coffman *et al.*, 1991) (Fig. 1). This latter array of cytokines is conducive to B-cell switches from sIgM expression to certain IgG subclasses and to IgE (for reviews see Coffman *et al.*, 1988; Finkelman *et al.*, 1990; Esser and Radbruch, 1990). Further, the Th2 cells are considered to be the major helper phenotype for support of IgG1, IgG2b, IgE, and IgA responses in the mouse system.

When freshly isolated, unstimulated PP $CD4^+$ T cells were assayed for the production of IFNγ or IL-5 as an indicator of Th1 or Th2 phenotypes, respectively, equal numbers of IFNγ- and IL-5-secreting cells were detected (approximately 12,000 cytokine secreting cells/10^6 $CD4^+$ T cells) (Taguchi *et al.*, 1990). PP $CD8^+$ T cells were also assayed for the secretion of IFNγ and IL-5 and found to contain comparable but low numbers of cytokine-secreting cells (<1000 cytokine-secreting cells/10^6 $CD8^+$ T cells) (Taguchi *et al.*, 1990). Therefore, the PP inductive environment most likely contains Th0 cells and equal numbers of newly differentiated Th1- and Th2-type cells. However, when *in situ* hybridization was employed, neither IFNγ nor IL-6 mRNA could be detected in the PP of mice but was detected in the lamina propria region (Bao *et al.*, 1993). These differences may be explained by the different techniques used to determine the presence of cytokine mRNA or cytokine secreting cells.

The cytokine secretion profile of anti-CD3 activated PP $CD4^+$ T cells has also been determined. Although the frequency of Th1-like and Th2-like $CD4^+$ T cells in the PP appears to be similar, the assay employed to determine the frequency of Th1- and Th2-like cells (ELISPOT) does not quantify the amount of cytokine produced by each T-cell type. Therefore, even though the frequencies of $CD4^+$ Th1 and Th2 T cells in the PP are comparable, the Th1 cells (or Th2 cells) may produce more cytokine than the other type of cells and bias the PP environment toward Th1 (or Th2). To address this question, PP $CD4^+$ T cells were stimulated with anti-CD3 monoclonal antibody and the concentration of IFNγ, IL-2, IL-3, IL-4, IL-5, and IL-6 released into the culture media was determined and compared to the amount of cytokine produced by activated splenic $CD4^+$ T cells (Tonkonogy and Swain, 1993). For the Th1-type cytokines, PP $CD4^+$ T cells produced similar amounts of IL-2 but lower amounts of IFNγ at the time of peak cytokine production as compared to $CD4^+$ T cells isolated from the spleen. Analysis of the Th2 cytokines IL-4, IL-5, and IL-6 revealed that the PP $CD4^+$ Th cells produced much lower amounts of IL-4 but comparable amounts of IL-5 and IL-6 when compared to spleen $CD4^+$ T cells at the time of peak cytokine production. Therefore, as compared to the systemic lymphoid compartment of the spleen, the mucosal inductive site of the PP produced less IL-4 and IFNγ. The implications of Th-cell subsets producing unique cytokine arrays is discussed in more detail below, in the sections on T-cell regulation of IgA switching and synthesis.

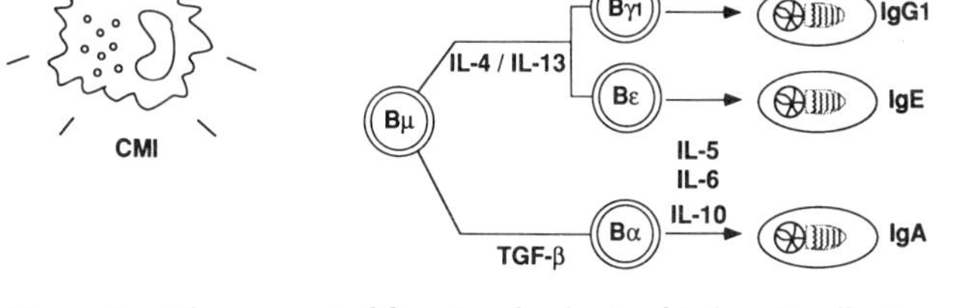

Figure 1. The concept of functional subsets of helper T cells. Precursors of T helper (pTh) cells (naive T cells) respond to vaccine with production of IL-2 which supports autocrine growth. Antigen encounter can result in Th cells producing multiple cytokines, e.g., IFNγ and IL-4 (Th0 cells). The environment in which the vaccine/microbe is present can determine the outcome, e.g., uptake of intracellular microbes by macrophages with production of IL-12 can induce Th cells capable of effective CMI responses (Th1 cells) via production of IFNγ, TNFβ, and IL-2. Other vaccine/APC pathways induce Th2-type responses and their cytokine array can determine the nature of B cell help, e.g., IL-4 for IgG1 and IgE responses and IL-5, IL-6, and IL-10 for mucosal IgA responses.

B. Mucosal CTLs

CTLs have been shown to be important for the elimination of virus-infected cells (Taylor and Askonas, 1986; Yap *et al.*, 1978; Zinkernagel and Doherty, 1979; Zweerink *et al.*, 1977). It is generally accepted that endogenous viral peptide processing that occurs during natural infection is a major pathway for induction of effector CTLs, but CTLs can be induced by immunization with either killed or live influenza virus vaccines (Ennis *et al.*, 1982; Lamb *et al.*, 1987; McMichael and Askonas, 1978; McMichael *et al.*, 1982; Ruby and Ramshaw, 1991; Taylor *et al.*, 1985). Most viral-specific CTLs are $CD4^-$, $CD8^+$ and recognize virus peptides in association with MHC class I expressed on infected target cells (Marrack and Kappler, 1987). Since CTLs have been shown to be important effector cells for the elimination of virus-infected cells, it will be of considerable importance to carefully study antigen-specific CTL responses in mucosa-associated tissues. In this regard, several studies have shown that cell-mediated cytotoxicity, antibody-dependent cytotoxicity, and natural-killer (NK) cell activity can be found in mucosa-associated tissues (Davies and Parrott, 1981; Ernst *et al.*, 1985; Guy-Grand *et al.*, 1978; MacDermott *et al.*, 1980; Nauss *et al.*, 1984; Tagliabue *et al.*, 1981). Furthermore, functional CTLs were also associated with T cells residing in mucosal effector tissues such as the epithelium and LP of the GI tract (Davies and Parrott, 1981; Ernst *et al.*, 1985; Guy-Grand *et al.*, 1978; MacDermott *et al.*, 1980; Nauss *et al.*, 1984; Tagliabue *et al.*, 1981).

Of most relevance to this chapter, it has been shown that oral immunization with viruses can result in the induction of virus-specific CTLs in mucosal inductive sites, e.g., the PP and in other mucosa-associated tissues (Issekutz, 1984; London *et al.*, 1987; Offit and Dudzik, 1989). Oral administration of vaccinia to rats resulted in the induction of virus-specific CTLs in PP and mesenteric lymph nodes (MLN) (Issekutz, 1984). Vaccinia-specific $CD4^-$, $CD8^+$ CTLs were generated in the MLN within 1 week of oral immunization. This finding suggests that after enteric immunization, antigen-stimulated CTLs were disseminated from PP into MLN via the lymphatic drainage (Issekutz, 1984). Furthermore, virus-specific CTLs were also generated in mucosa-associated tissues by oral immunization with reovirus and rotavirus (London *et al.*, 1987; Offit and Dudzik, 1989). A high frequency of virus-specific CTLs was present in the PP as early as 6 days after oral immunization. It should also be noted that oral immunization induced antigen-specific CTLs in systemic tissues such as spleen in addition to mucosa-associated tissues (Offit and Dudzik, 1989). These studies suggest that oral immunization with live virus can induce antigen-specific CTLs in both mucosal inductive and effector tissues for mucosal responses and in systemic lymphoid tissues as well.

It should be emphasized again that oral adjuvants such as cholera toxin also induce mucosal IgA as well as serum IgG and IgA antibody responses (Fig. 2). Thus, both Th-cell-mediated and CTL responses for mucosal and systemic immunity can be induced by oral immunization. Induction of effective mucosal CTL responses to

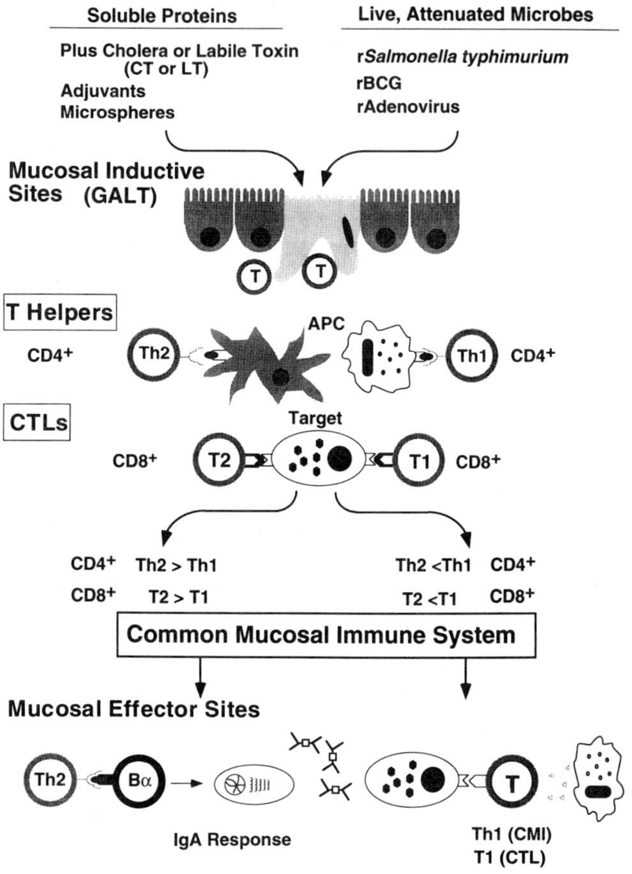

Figure 2. Current mucosal delivery systems, mucosal inductive sites, and the concept of Th1- and Th2-type immune responses. Most mucosal vaccines are given either intranasally or orally, and following uptake in the inductive site, the adjuvant or carrier system can influence the nature of $CD4^+$ Th cell responses, which in turn regulate CMI and the isotype/subclass of mucosal versus serum antibody responses. It is thought that initial induction is followed by homing of Th cell subsets and $sIgA^+$ B cells for ultimate mucosal and systemic antibody synthesis via the CMIS. Reprinted with permission from Academic Press.

virus would be advantageous to the host, because mucosal elimination of virus invasion should be considered a first line of immune defense to prevent subsequent systemic infection. Because the process for induction and function of effector CTLs involves multiple cytokine and cell interactions, we have characterized cytokine-producing CTLs at the single-cell level in humans. We have focused on two mediators, IFNγ and perforin, which are involved in the lysis of virus-infected cells by effector CTLs. In these studies, the cytolytic potential of $CD4^+$, $CD8^-$, and $CD4^-$, $CD8^+$ virus-specific T cells to lyse autologous cells infected with influenza A virus was assessed and a direct correlation between the cytolytic function and production of IFNγ and increased perforin mRNA synthesis was noted (DiFabio *et al.*, 1994).

In this regard, the PBMC of human volunteers who had been immunized with the 1991–1992 standard trivalent inactivated influenza virus vaccine containing A/Beijing/353/89 (H2N2), A/Taiwan/1/86 (N1N1), and B/Panama/45/90 were cultured with influenza virus-infected autologous cells and after 3 or 7 days of culture, T-cell subsets were assessed for IFNγ production by IFNγ-specific ELISPOT and ELISA, whereas IFNγ and perforin mRNA expression was determined by reverse transcriptase-polymerase chain reaction (RT-PCR) (DiFabio *et al.*, 1994). Influenza virus-specific CTL activity was measured in a 4-hr ^{51}Cr release assay. Culture of PBMC with autologous-A/Taiwan influenza (H1N1)-infected target cells resulted in IFNγ spot forming cells (SFC) at 3 days, and the numbers of IFNγ-producing cells in culture were increased after 7 days of incubation. Numbers of IFNγ SFC directly correlated with levels of secreted IFNγ and higher levels were seen in supernatants from 7-day cultures. Separate aliquots of T cells from these cultures were also assessed for virus-specific cytotoxicity, and T cells from 7-day (but not from 3-day) cultures induced high ^{51}Cr release. Analyses indicated a significant direct correlation between cytotoxicity levels, numbers of IFNγ SFC, and levels of IFNγ in culture supernatants (DiFabio *et al.*, 1994).

Studies with purified T-cell subsets showed that elevated IFNγ SFC, IFNγ synthesis, and cytotoxic activity were associated with $CD4^-$, $CD8^+$ T cells but not with the $CD4^+$, $CD8^-$ T-cell subset. When virus-specific T cells were examined for increased production of perforin-specific mRNA, direct correlations were seen for increased production of perforin mRNA, IFNγ SFC, and ^{51}Cr released in target cells incubated with $CD4^-$, $CD8^+$ T cells. These results show that increased IFNγ production, including increased IFNγ mRNA and IFNγ SFC, directly correlates with increased antigen-specific T-cell-mediated cytotoxicity (DiFabio *et al.*, 1994). Thus, assessment of IFNγ SFC may provide an alternative and quantitative means for the assessment of influenza virus-specific CTL in human mucosal effector tissues.

IV. Multiple Roles for T Cells and Cytokines in Mucosal Immunity

A. Early Studies of T-Cell Regulation of IgA Expression

The first direct evidence that T cells regulate IgA synthesis came from a study with PP T cells triggered with the mitogen Con A. Addition of Con A-activated PP T cells to LPS-activated splenic B cells resulted in selective synthesis of IgA. On the other hand, Con A-triggered splenic T cells, when added to LPS-induced B-cell cultures, resulted in suppression of IgA as well as IgM and IgG synthesis (Elson *et al.*, 1979). These results suggested that PP contained T cells which selectively regulate the IgA response, and this novel finding led investigators to determine the cellular basis for regulation by derivation of clonal T-cell populations. Two distinct classes of T-cell clones were subsequently developed from the murine PP, which suggested a role for T cells in B-cell switching to IgA as well as for Th cells that preferentially supported IgA antibody responses.

1. T Switch Cell Clones

One category of T-cell clones induced surface IgM positive ($sIgM^+$) B cells to switch to surface IgA (sIgA) expression (Kawanishi *et al.*, 1983a,b,c), while the second group of Th cells preferentially induced $sIgA^+$ B cells to differentiate into IgA-producing cells (see Helper T-Cell Clones, below). The initial studies with T switch (Tsw) cells used T-cell clones derived by mitogen stimulation and IL-2 supported outgrowth, and when added to $sIgM^+$, $sIgA^-$ B cell cultures resulted in marked increases in $sIgA^+$ cells (Kawanishi *et al.*, 1983a). PP Tsw cells did not induce IgA secretion, even when incubated with $sIgA^+$ B-cell-enriched cultures; however, addition of B-cell growth and differentiation factors readily induced cultures to secrete IgA (Kawanishi *et al.*, 1983b). Additional work showed that Tsw cells were autoreactive and suggested that continued uptake of gut lumenal antigens into the PP resulted in a unique microenvironment for T–B cell interactions and subsequent IgA responses (Kawanishi *et al.*, 1983c). This result suggested that cognate interactions between Tsw cells and B cells were required for induction of the IgA class switch.

Germane to this discussion are other studies with dendritic cells (DC) which reside in T-cell zones of the PP, and which suggested that the DC can influence switching to IgA. For example, coculture of activated T cells and DC from PP with purified $sIgM^+$, $sIgA^-$ B cells resulted in the synthesis of large amounts of IgA, while DC–T cells isolated from spleen were less effective (Spalding *et al.*, 1984). Additional studies showed that DC–T-cell mixtures from PP also induced isotype switching to IgA in a pre-B-cell line, while DC–T-cell mixtures from spleen were without effect (Spalding and Griffin, 1986). Although these studies purported to show that DC was the major cell type promoting B-cell switches to IgA, it remained possible that the PP DC–T-cell mixtures harbored contaminating B cells producing IgA, and thus must await more definitive proof that the DC is directly involved in B-cell switches to IgA.

2. Helper T-Cell Clones for Specific IgA Responses

As already mentioned, clones of antigen-specific PP Th cells were shown to support proliferation and differentiation of $sIgA^+$ B cells into IgA-producing plasma cells (Kiyono *et al.*, 1982, 1984). These Th-cell clones were derived from PP of mice fed sheep erythrocytes (SRBC), and SRBC-specific Th-cell clones could be placed in two categories. The first type supported IgM, IgG1, and high IgA anti-SRBC responses, while the second group preferentially supported only IgA anti-SRBC antibody responses (Kiyono *et al.*, 1982, 1984). The significance of Th-cell clones supporting IgG1 and IgA is not yet fully appreciated; however, it is tempting to suggest that more classical Th2-type cells producing IL-4 would be quite effective helpers for IgG1 responses. Further, it could be speculated that the Th cells which only supported IgA may produce select Th2 cytokines, e.g., IL-5 and IL-6, as suggested by the studies of Tonkonogy and Swain (1993). Additional studies showed that these PP Th-cell clones expressed Fc receptors for IgA (FcαR) (Kiyono *et al.*, 1982), and hybridomas derived from them secreted IgA binding factors (Kiyono *et al.*, 1985), which could help explain their preferential induction of IgA responses. A recent study has provided evidence that the expression of FcαR is often associated with Th2-type but not with Th1-type clones (Sandor *et al.*, 1990). Thus, indirect evidence would suggest that $Fc\alpha R^+$, Th2-type cells support antigen-specific IgG1 and IgA responses. Others have also isolated Th-cell clones specific for keyhole limpet hemocyanin (KLH) from mouse PP, and one of four clones supported KLH-specific IgA responses (Maghazachi and Phillips-Quagliata, 1988). Unfortunately, cytokine profiles of Tsw cells or cloned PP Th cells were not assessed, and thus no conclusions could be drawn as to the role of cytokines for $\mu \rightarrow \alpha$ switches or for preferential help for IgA responses. However, in conjunction with current knowledge of Th1 and Th2 cells as well as their derived cytokines, one could postulate that T cells that are involved in isotype-switching might be TGFβ-producing cells, while Th cells that promote IgA responses may express FcαR and preferentially produce IL-5, IL-6, and IL-10 upon antigen stimulation (see discussion below). Thus, both of the latter groups of Th cells could be Th2-type cells.

3. *Tsw Cells in Humans*

Evidence for Tsw cells in human IgA responses has stemmed from work with malignant T cells from a patient Rac (T_{Rac} cells) who suffered from a mycosis fungoides/Sezary-like syndrome. The T_{Rac} cells induced tonsillar $sIgM^+$ B cells to switch and secrete IgG and IgA (Mayer *et al.*, 1985b). Furthermore, T_{Rac} cells, when added to B-cell cultures obtained from patients with hyper-IgM immunodeficiency, induced eight of nine cultures to secrete IgG and three of nine to produce IgA (Mayer *et al.*, 1985a). T-cell clones have also been obtained from human appendix, and these clones, and their derived culture supernatants, exhibited preferential help for IgA synthesis (Benson and Strober, 1988). Direct evidence was provided that $CD3^+$, $CD4^+$, $CD8^-$, T-cell clones induced $\mu \rightarrow \alpha$ B-cell switches as well as the terminal differentiation of $sIgA^+$ B cells into IgA-producing plasma cells (Benson and Strober, 1988).

B. Coreceptors in Lymphocyte Activation—Relevance to Mucosal Immunity

Specificity in the immune response is determined by the antigen receptor on B and T cells. The B-cell antigen receptor is membrane immunoglobulin (Ig), and following binding to an antigen epitope, the antigen is cross linked and internalized. This signal can result in activation, anergy, or deletion. It is now recognized that the surface Ig (antibody) receptor is associated with a protein complex consisting of Igα and Igβ proteins which contain cytoplasmic domains involved in binding to kinases which lead to signal transduction (for review see Cambier *et al.*, 1994). Likewise, T lymphocytes express heterodimeric receptors of either αβ or γδ chains in association with CD3 protein complex. For $\alpha\beta$ TCR^+ T cells, specific interactions with foreign peptide associated with MHC class II or with class I on either $CD4^+$ or $CD8^+$ T cells, respectively, result in signal transduction pathways mediated in part by cytoplasmic domains of CD3 proteins (for review see Chan *et al.*, 1994). In both cases, interaction of B-cell Ig receptors or of T cells with αβ TCR is insufficient for cell activation, division (proliferation), or terminal differentiation. In other words, delivery of this first signal (antigen-specific) alone often results in T- or B-cell anergy. Thus, a two-signal model of B- and T-lymphocyte activation indicates that the antigen-specific signal and a costimulatory signal are both required (reviewed in Bretscher, 1992).

1. *Costimulation of T Lymphocytes*

The most widely studied coactivation signal for T-cell growth is CD28 (June *et al.*, 1994; Linsley and Ledbetter, 1993; Schwartz, 1992; Allison, 1994), a costimulatory receptor expressed on naive T cells. This costimulatory receptor recognizes one of two similar coreceptors, B7-1 (CD80) or B7-2 (CD86), on antigen-presenting cells (APCs) (Freeman *et al.*, 1989; Azuma *et al.*, 1993; Freeman *et al.*, 1993a,b; Reiser *et al.*, 1992; Boussiotis *et al.*, 1993). Costimulation and signal transduction through the CD28 receptor synergize with αβ TCR–CD3 signaling and result in IL-2 production by pTh cells with subsequent cell division (proliferation). A second costimulatory molecule, CTLA-4, originally thought to be specific for activated $CD8^+$ CTLs, also binds to B7-1. This coreceptor has a higher affinity for B7-1 than does CD28; however, CTLA-4 expression is much lower than is CD28 (Linsley *et al.*, 1992). For example, unlike CD28, CTLA-4 is not expressed on naive $CD4^+$ Th cells and occurs at only 2–3% of the level of CD28 on activated T cells (Linsley *et al.*, 1992). This has led to the assumption that CTLA-4 may be a compensatory receptor for CD28; however, it is equally possible that CD28 and CTLA-4 are differentially expressed on Th1- and Th2-type cells.

Dendritic cells are considered by most experts to

be the initial APC responsible for induction of naive T cells to be antigen-responsive effectors or memory T cells (Metlay *et al.*, 1989; Lassila *et al.*, 1988). The DC expresses B7-1 constitutively, with less B7-2; however, cytokines such as GM-CSF upregulate expression of both receptors (Larsen *et al.*, 1994). Human monocytes express B7-2, but activation by IFNγ results in upregulation of expression of B7-1 (Azuma *et al.*, 1993; Freedman *et al.*, 1991), while in the mouse system IFNγ increases B7-2 and decreases B7-1 expression (Hathcock *et al.*, 1994). Finally, B cells are also effective APCs and IL-4 treatment markedly upregulates both B7-1 and B7-2 expression on B cells (Stack *et al.*, 1994).

As alluded to above, effector Th cells can be subdivided into Th1 and Th2 types based on cytokine secretion patterns, and one possibility for T cell differentiation into subsets could be differences in second signals received by APCs through B7-1 and B7-2 coreceptors. In fact, some evidence revealed that different APC types can selectively trigger either Th1- or Th2-type responses (Weaver *et al.*, 1988; Magilary *et al.*, 1989; Fabry *et al.*, 1993; Fox, 1993; Goodman *et al.*, 1994). Nevertheless, other studies have found that the same APC type functions equally well for Th1- or Th2-type responses (reviewed in Seder and Paul, 1994).

What is clear at this point is that CD28 on T cells is important for activation of T cells for both IL-2 and IL-4 expression (Seder *et al.*, 1994; McKnight *et al.*, 1994); however, anti-CD28 suppressed production of IL-2 and IFNγ (Th1) but was without effect on IL-4 (Th2) production (Tan *et al.*, 1993). Recent studies have directly assessed the role of B7-1 and B7-2 expression on transfected APCs to determine possible effects on T-cell activation and cytokine production (Levine *et al.*, 1995). Interestingly in this study, both B7-1 and B7-2 provided second signals for $CD4^+$ Th1- and Th2-type responses, as well as for cytokine production by $CD8^+$ T cells (Levine *et al.*, 1995). Thus, it would appear that both B7-1 and B7-2 trigger CD28 on T cells for activation, and in this regard mice with disrupted B7-1 gene (knockouts) showed normal immune functions presumably mediated through CD28–B7-2 interactions (Freeman *et al.*, 1993a,b).

In stark contrast to these results, recent studies have presented evidence that B7-1 and B7-2 can play distinct roles in differentiation of Th1- or Th2-type cells (Kuchroo *et al.*, 1995). In this study, which employed the induction of experimental autoimmune encephalitis (EAE) with a proteolipid protein in mice, pretreatment with anti-B7-1 induced Th2-type cells, which were associated with protection from EAE. On the other hand, pretreatment with anti-B7-2 induced Th1-type cells which increased the severity of the EAE-autoimmunity (Kuchroo *et al.*, 1995). Thus, it may be too early to conclude that B7-1 and B7-2 function equally for costimulation of Th1- and Th2-type subsets. It will be of interest to determine if differences in APC expression of B7-1 and B7-2 in mucosal inductive sites regulate Th1- and Th2-type responses to mucosal vaccines.

2. *Costimulation of B Lymphocytes*

An important second receptor of B-cell activation is CD40, a 277-amino acid glycoprotein member of the TNF receptor superfamily (Banchereau *et al.*, 1994). The coreceptor for CD40 is CD40 ligand (CD40L), a 261-amino acid glycoprotein expressed on activated T cells (and other cell types), and is considered a major determinant in direct T–B cell interactions (Banchereau *et al.*, 1994). The most interesting and germane studies relevant to our discussion have been the finding that crosslinking CD40 via cells which express CD40L or which bind anti-CD40 antibody via Fc receptors induces B cells to divide, and in the presence of additional cytokines such as IL-4 can result in generation of long-term B-cell clones (Kansas and Tedder, 1991; Gordon *et al.*, 1988, 1987; Rousset *et al.*, 1991). This model has been most useful in analysis of continuous B-cell clonal growth since the only available B-cell lines had been either tumors or EBV-transformed cells (Banchereau *et al.*, 1994). This recent advance is allowing investigation of the events which occur in response to antigen, presumably leading to the formation of germinal centers (Banchereau *et al.*, 1994). For example, resting B cells activated through CD40 are induced to enter cell cycle and to express CD23, class II MHC, and B7-1 (Banchereau *et al.*, 1994). Addition of IL-4 to this system results in the generation of B cells with a memory phenotype as well as sustained B-cell division (Banchereau *et al.*, 1994). This novel system for clonal B-cell growth has naturally led to studies of B-cell isotype switching including switches to IgA, and this aspect is discussed in a separate section below.

C. Cytokines in Mucosal Immunity

It can be concluded with some confidence that select cytokines can regulate the expression of B-cell Ig isotypes and subclasses as well as influence the maturation of B-cell responses through induction of terminal differentiation into plasma cells. Thus, particular cytokines influence B-cell switching from sIgM, sIgD expression to downstream isotypes including IgG subclasses, IgE and IgA. For B-cell terminal differentiation, IL-6, possibly in combination with other cytokines, appears essential for the continued presence of plasma cells undergoing high-rate secretion of antibodies. Although it is often presumed that isotype switching to IgA, e.g., $\mu \rightarrow \alpha$, occurs in mucosal inductive sites such as PP, and terminal differentiation into plasma cells producing IgA is a major event in effector sites, only indirect evidence is at hand to support these assumptions. In this regard, most studies of $\mu \rightarrow \alpha$ switching have been done with nonmucosal lymphoid cells, e.g., splenic B cells, while *in vitro* studies of B-cell differentiation to IgA synthesis normally employ PP B cells (a mucosal inductive site) to support the idea that this also normally occurs in lamina propria and in exocrine glands, e.g., mucosal effector sites.

1. *Cytokines for B-Cell Switches to IgA*

Isotype switching involves the recombination between DNA segments (switch or S regions) that are located 2 kb 5′ (upstream) of the respective C_H genes, and S regions are composed of multiple repeats of short (~5 bp) sequences. Recombination occurs when upstream and downstream S regions join to form a DNA loop containing the intervening C_H genes which are subsequently deleted. In addition to the IgA isotype switching induced by Tsw cells discussed above, isotype switching can also be induced by cytokines in combination with "non-cognate" activational signals. The best studied example is IL-4-induced switching to IgG1 and IgE in cultures of LPS-stimulated mouse splenic B cells (Isakson *et al.*, 1982; reviewed in Coffman *et al.*, 1988). Cytokine-induced switching is preceded by the induction of germline transcripts corresponding to the immunoglobulin isotype to which the B cell will switch. Thus, IL-4 will induce IgG1 and IgE germline transcripts prior to the expression of either IgG1 or IgE in LPS-stimulated splenic B cells. IFNγ has also been shown to induce isotype switching in mouse splenic B cells to IgG2a (Snapper and Paul, 1987) if LPS is used as the primary stimulus and to IgG3 as well as IgG2a (Snapper *et al.*, 1992) when the stimulus is anti-IgD coupled to dextran.

The most definitive studies to date suggest that transforming growth factor beta (TGFβ) is a major cytokine for B-cell switching to IgA. The first studies showed that addition of TGFβ to LPS-triggered mouse splenic B-cell cultures resulted in switching to IgA, and IgA synthesis was markedly enhanced by IL-2 (Coffman *et al.*, 1989) or IL-5 (Sonada *et al.*, 1989). The effect of TGFβ was on $sIgM^+$, $sIgA^-$ B cells and was not due to selective induction of terminal B-cell differentiation. In an elegant study, it was shown that TGFβ induced sterile Cα germline transcripts (Lebman *et al.*, 1990a,b), an event which clearly preceeds actual switching to IgA.

Subsequent studies showed that TGFβ induced human B cells to switch to either IgA1 or IgA2, and again it was clearly shown that Cα1 and Cα2 germline transcripts preceeded actual switches to IgA1 and IgA2 (Islam *et al.*, 1991). It can be presumed that TGFβ induces $\mu \rightarrow \alpha$ switches in normal physiologic circumstances, since it was shown that $sIgM^+$, $sIgD^+$ B cells triggered through the CD40 ligand were induced to switch to IgA by TGFβ and to secrete IgA in the presence of IL-10 (Defrance *et al.*, 1992; Roussett *et al.*, 1991).

It should be emphasized that all studies to date with TGFβ-induced switches have been done in B-cell cultures stimulated with mitogens or via coreceptor signaling. These studies show that only 2–5% of B cells actually switch to IgA, making it difficult to explain the high rate of switching which normally occurs in PP germinal centers (up to 60%). This point has been addressed recently; McIntyre and associates (1995) showed that TGFβ together with IL-4 and IL-5 induced $sIgA^+$ B cell populations of up to 15–20%. It is unfortunate that the TGFβ gene knockout mouse dies from a generalized lymphoproliferative disease at 3–4 weeks after birth, a fact which makes it difficult to use this mouse to investigate the role of TGFβ in IgA regulation *in vivo*. It should be remembered, however, that prior to studies of TGFβ-induced isotype switching, this cytokine was shown to have profound suppressive effects on the proliferation of both B and T cells, as well as IgA secretion (Kehrl *et al.*, 1986, 1987, 1991), and it is possible that loss of mucosal immunity in these mice contribute to their early death.

2. *Cytokines Regulating IgA Synthesis*

Earlier studies have shown that addition of culture supernatants from DC-T cell clusters, T cell clones, or T-cell hybridomas to cultures of PP or splenic B cells resulted in enhanced secretion of IgA. One factor responsible for this activity was subsequently shown to be IL-5 (Beagley *et al.*, 1987; Coffman *et al.*, 1987; Harriman *et al.*, 1988; Beagley *et al.*, 1988a; Murray *et al.*, 1987; Lebman and Coffman, 1988). Removal of $sIgA^+$ B cells from PP B-cell cultures abrogated the effect of IL-5, demonstrating that the effect of this cytokine was on post-switched IgA committed B cells (Beagley *et al.*, 1988a). When the target B-cell population was PP B cells, no *in vitro* stimulus was required, and IL-4 did not further enhance the effect of IL-5 (Beagley *et al.*, 1987). If splenic B cells were used, these cells first needed to be stimulated with LPS before increased IgA secretion could be shown. Using LPS-stimulated splenic B cells, the IgA-enhancing effect of IL-5 could be further increased by addition of IL-2 or IL-4. Taken together, these results suggest that IL-5 induces $sIgA^+$ B cells which are in cell cycle (blasts) to differentiate into IgA-producing cells. Interestingly, another B-cell population that has been shown to contain precursors of lamina propria IgA B cells, are peritoneal cavity B1 cells (Kroese *et al.*, 1989). This population also contains cells that can be induced by IL-5 to secrete IgA (Beagley *et al.*, 1996).

Human IL-5 is thought to act mainly as an eosinophil differentiation factor and thus may have little effect on B-cell isotype switching and differentiation. It has been reported, however, that human B cells, when stimulated with the bacterium *Branhamella catarrhalis* can be induced by IL-5 to secrete IgA, and also to possibly undergo isotype switching to IgA (Benson *et al.*, 1990). This effect could not be demonstrated using other more conventional B-cell mitogens, a finding which once again demonstrates the important role of the primary *in vitro* activation signal for B-cell switching.

Interleukin-6, when added to PP B cells in the absence of any *in vitro* stimulus, causes a marked increase in IgA secretion with little effect on either IgM or IgG synthesis (Beagley *et al.*, 1989b). In these studies, IL-6 induced two- to threefold more IgA secretion than IL-5 (Beagley *et al.*, 1989b). The removal of $sIgA^+$ B cells abolished the effect of IL-6 demonstrating that this cytokine, like IL-5, also acted on post-switched B cells. In mice where the IL-6 gene has been inactivated (IL-6 knockout) the number of IgA^+ B cells in the lamina propria is markedly reduced and local antibody responses following mucosal challenge with ovalbumin or vaccinia virus are greatly diminished, demonstrating the *in vivo* importance of IL-6 for mucosal IgA responses (Ramsey *et al.*, 1994). B cells isolated from human appendix are also induced to secrete both IgA1 and IgA2 by IL-6 in the absence of any *in vitro* activation (Fujihashi *et al.*, 1991). This effect was also shown in IgA-committed B cells, again demonstrating the importance of IL-6 for terminal differentiation of IgA plasma cells.

V. The Role of Epithelial Cells in Mucosal Immunity

The epithelial cells lining the surface of mucosal tissues subserve a variety of functions including provision of a barrier against potential pathogens from the external environment. In addition to providing a physical barrier, the epithelial cell also appears to play an active role in mucosal immune responses. One very important function which epithelial cells perform in mucosal immune responses is the active transport of polymeric IgA (pIgA) produced in the mucosal and glandular tissues to the mucosal surface. The molecule responsible for transportation of pIgA to mucosal secretions is the polymeric immunoglobulin receptor (pIgR) (Mestecky and McGhee, 1987; Kraehenbuhl and Neutra, 1992). The pIgR is produced by epithelial cells found in secretory glandular tissues and on the mucosal surface of the gastrointestinal and respiratory tracts. The pIgR binds and transports pIgA (and pIgM) through the epithelial cell to the mucosal surface. During transportation through the cell or at the cell surface, the pIgR is cleaved and releases the pIgA into the mucosal secretions. The portion of the pIgR that remains associated with the pIgA is known as secretory component (s.c., see below). Polymeric IgA detected in mucosal secretions that is associated with s.c. is therefore known as secretory IgA (S-IgA).

In addition to the role of transportation of pIgA from the mucosal effector tissues to mucosal secretions, mucosal epithelial cells may play an active role in the induction of mucosal immune responses and systemic unresponsiveness (mucosal tolerance). A number of studies have provided evidence that intestinal epithelial cell lines are able to produce cytokines and express cytokine receptors and adhesion molecules that may affect the induction of mucosal immune responses (McGee *et al.*, 1992, 1993a,b; Bromander *et al.*, 1993; Eckmann *et al.*, 1993; Schürer-Maly *et al.*, 1994; McCormick *et al.*, 1993). The rat intestinal epithelial cell line IEC-6 has been shown to produce IL-6 and treatment of IEC-6 cells with TGFβ enhanced the production of IL-6 (McGee *et al.*, 1992). Additional studies showed that TGFβ and IL-1β act synergistically to enhance IL-6 secretion by IEC-6 cells (McGee *et al.*, 1993a). The mucosal adjuvant cholera toxin (CT) also increased IL-6 production by IEC-6 cells and was able to act synergistically with TGFβ, IL-1β, and tumor necrosis factor α (TNFα) to dramatically increase the production of IL-6 (McGee *et al.*, 1993b). Others have confirmed and expanded upon these studies. The addition of CT to IEC-17 intestinal epithelial cells stimulated IL-1 and IL-6 production (Bromander *et al.*, 1993). Taken together, these results suggest that intestinal epithelial cells may have the ability to produce cytokines that could play a role in the induction of and maintenance of mucosal immune responses and intestinal inflammation.

Human intestinal epithelial cell lines have also been examined for their ability to produce cytokines. Both human intestinal epithelial cell lines and freshly isolated human intestinal epithelial cells have been shown to produce IL-8 (Eckmann *et al.*, 1993; Schürer-Maly *et al.*, 1994). Human intestinal epithelial cell lines also expressed mRNA for IL-1α, IL-1β, IL-10, and TNFα whereas none of the cell lines tested expressed mRNA for IL-2, IL-4, IL-5, IL-6, or IFNγ (Eckmann *et al.*, 1993). Others have shown that the adhesion of *Salmonella typhimurium* to T84 human colonic epithelial cell lines induced the production of IL-8 (McCormick *et al.*, 1993). The adhesion of *Salmonella* to the apical surface of polarized epithelial cells was also associated with an increased transepithelial migration of neutrophils and this transepithelial migration appeared not to be regulated by IL-8 (McCormick *et al.*, 1993).

In addition to the production of cytokines, intestinal epithelial cells lines have been shown to express adhesion molecules necessary for antigen-presenting cells to interact with lymphocytes. Both ICAM-1 and LFA-3 were constitutively expressed at low levels by human intestinal epithelial cells lines and expression of ICAM-1 was enhanced by exposure to the inflammatory cytokines IFNγ, TNFα, IL-1β, and IL-6 (Kvalc *et al.*, 1992). This observation provides support for the finding that rat intestinal epithelial cells were able to present processed antigen to antigen-specific $CD4^+$ T cells (Brandeis *et al.*, 1994). Taken together, the findings that intestinal epithelial cells produce cytokines such as IL-1, IL-6, and IL-8 that express the adhesion molecules ICAM-1 and LFA-3, and are able to present antigen to sensitized T lymphocytes, suggest that intestinal epithelial cells may play an important role in the maintenance of mucosal immune responses in mucosal effector sites. In addition, it is also likely that epithelial cells through APC functions are responsible for some forms of T-cell anergy in mucosal tolerance.

VI. Mucosal Effector Functions for IgA

A. Structure–Function of S-IgA

One major hallmark of the mucosal immune response is the detection of antigen-specific secretory IgA (S-IgA) at mucosal surfaces. In humans, serum IgA is predominantly a monomer while S-IgA is polymeric, usually dimeric (however, trimers, tetramers, and higher MW forms also occur) (Mestecky and McGhee, 1987). In addition to immunoglobulin heavy and light chains, S-IgA contains the peptide J chain (15.6 kDa) and the protein secretory component (s.c.). The J chain is produced by the IgA-producing plasma cell and is associated with polymeric IgA, and appears to enhance the affinity of pIgA for s.c. Epithelial cells found in secretory glandular tissue or on mucosal surfaces of the gastrointestinal and respiratory tracts produce polymeric immunoglobulin receptors (pIgR) (Mestecky and McGhee, 1987). The pIgR is responsible for binding and transportation of polymeric IgA produced by IgA-secreting plasma cells (residing in the lamina propria of mucosal tissues) to the external secretions. The presence of the J chain is essential for pIgA to interact with pIgR; therefore, only polymeric IgA may be transported to mucosal surfaces or into glandular secretions by the pIgR. Polymeric IgA interacts with pIgR at the basolateral surface of $pIgR^+$ epithelial cells, becomes internalized, is transported through the cell, and, after enzymatic cleavage of the pIgR, is released onto the mucosal surfaces as S-IgA. The extracellular region of pIgR that remains associated with the S-IgA is known as s.c. (Mestecky and McGhee, 1987; Kraehenbuhl and Neutra, 1992). In addition to mediating transport across epithelial cells, the presence of s.c. may increase the resistance of S-IgA to proteolytic enyzymes (Brown *et al.*, 1970; Mestecky and McGhee, 1987; Kraehenbuhl and Neutra, 1992). With the estimated daily synthesis of IgA (systemic and secretory) being >66 mg/kg body weight, the daily production of IgA exceeds production of immunoglobulins of all other isotypes combined (Mestecky and McGhee, 1987). The need for a response of such magnitude becomes apparent when one considers that the mucosal surfaces compose the largest area of the body in contact with environmental antigens and potential pathogens and that secretory antibody responses are continually lost through secretion and excretion.

B. Passive Transfer Studies of pIgA in Host Protection

The importance of S-IgA transport across epithelial surfaces to external secretions should be considered when vaccines are being designed to prevent infections that occur at mucosal surfaces. Passive transfer studies in mice using antigen-specific monoclonal IgA have provided evidence that antigen-specific IgA alone was able to protect against intranasal infection with influenza (Renegar and Small, 1991), intestinal infection with *Vibrio cholerae* (Winner *et al.*, 1991; Lee *et al.*, 1994) or *S. typhimurium* (Michetti *et al.*, 1992), as well as gastric infection with *Helicobacter felis* (Czinn *et al.*, 1993) (Table III). Antigen-specific IgA presumably forms immune complexes with the colonizing pathogen and thereby inhibits the interaction of the bacterium with host epithelial cells, a protective mechanism known as immune exclusion (Mestecky and McGhee, 1987). In fact, passive transfer of anti-*S. typhimurium* IgA by the backpack hybridoma system provided protection against oral challenge with virulent organisms but was unable to prevent infection when the organisms were injected intraperitoneally, suggesting that mechanisms for protection at a mucosal surface do not correlate with protection from a systemic challenge (Michetti *et al.*, 1992). This group has also provided evidence that passive transfer of IgA that lead to high titers of serum IgA (indicative of high levels of IgA at the mucosal surfaces) totally prevented infection in three of four mice orally challenged with *S. typhimurium* whereas all animals with low serum IgA titers were infected (Michetti *et al.*, 1992). Therefore, induction of antigen-specific S-IgA responses may provide a means to totally prevent bacterial infections or at least greatly reduce the size of the infectious inoculum at the sites of initial contact between most infectious agents and the host, the mucosal surfaces.

C. Intracellular Functions for pIgA–s.c. Complexes

In addition to immune exclusion, *in vitro* studies with polymeric IgA (pIgA) and $pIgR^+$ epithelial cells have suggested that pIgA may mediate intracellular virus neutralization as well as transportation of immune complexes across epithelial cells (Kaetzel *et al.*, 1991, 1994; Mazanec *et al.*, 1992, 1993), additional functions that would be beneficial in preventing or inhibiting infection

TABLE III
Protection against Infection at Mucosal Surfaces by IgA-Mediated Immune Exclusion

Infectious agent	Route of passive transfer	Route of infection	Outcome of challenge	Reference
Influenza	Intravenous	Intranasally	Protection against homologous virus	Renegar and Small (1991)
Vibrio cholerae	Subcutaneous (backpack hybridoma)	Orally	Protection against lethal challenge	Winner *et al.* (1991)
V. cholerae	Orally 1 hr before challenge	Orally (1 hr after passive transfer)	100-fold reduction in recoverable vibrios	Lee *et al.* (1994)
Salmonella typhimurium	Subcutaneous (backpack hybridoma)	Orally	Prevention of systemic infection	Michetti *et al.* (1992)
Helicobacter felis	Orally with pathogen	Orally	Reduction of bacteria in gastric tissues	Czinn *et al.* (1993)

at mucosal surfaces. Virus-specific polymeric IgA has been shown to neutralize Sendai virus intracellularly in $pIgR^+$ cells (Mazanec *et al.*, 1992). IgA-mediated intracellular virus neutralization required the presence of pIgR on the infected cells (for intracellular transport of IgA) as well as antigen-specific polymeric IgA. Since IgG is not transported by pIgR, anti-Sendai virus IgG was unable to neutralize Sendai virus intracellularly (Mazanec *et al.*, 1992). Another function mediated by polymeric IgA and $pIgR^+$ cells is the transportation of immune complexes across epithelial cells (Kaetzel *et al.*, 1991, 1994; Mazanec *et al.*, 1993). Immune complexes formed with specific antigen and polymeric IgA have been shown to be transported across $pIgR^+$ epithelial cells and released in the same manner as polymeric IgA is transported across $pIgR^-$ epithelial cells (Kaetzel *et al.*, 1991). In additional studies, it was shown that immune complexes containing antigen, antigen-specific monomeric IgA, and IgG could also be transported across epithelial cells in a pIgR-dependent fashion as long as the immune complex contained polymeric IgA (Kaetzel *et al.*, 1994).

Therefore, the induction of S-IgA responses provides at least three means of protecting the host against infection that IgG responses do not. First, antigen-specific S-IgA may be actively transported to the mucosal surfaces by the pIgR, and then combine with infectious organisms and inhibit their interaction with host cells, thereby preventing infection. Second, if a viral pathogen is able to initiate infection at mucosal surfaces, polymeric IgA may reduce the amount of progeny virus released intracellularly, neutralizing the virus in $pIgR^+$ cells. Finally, if infection is initiated at mucosal surfaces, polymeric IgA may form immune complexes with the infectious organism in the lamina propria region and actively transport this across mucosal epithelial cells, thereby reducing the size of the infectious load.

VII. Diverse Antigen Delivery Systems for the Induction of Distinct Mucosal Immune Responses

Oral or intranasal administration of antigen may lead to a state of systemic immune unresponsiveness known as mucosal tolerance. However, the use of mucosal adjuvants such as cholera toxin (CT, see Chapter 4) and the related heat-labile toxin (LT, see Chapter 5) has allowed oral delivery of antigens to induce systemic as well as mucosal immune responses. Other antigen delivery protocols such as attenuated, recombinant bacterial vectors (see Chapters 7 and 9) ISCOMS, and liposomes (see Chapter 13) have permitted oral antigen delivery protocols to escape the induction of mucosal tolerance and induce both mucosal and systemic immune responses. By using different antigen delivery systems that range from soluble proteins with mucosal adjuvants to attenuated, recombinant bacterial and viral vectors, it is not surprising that immune responses with different effector characteristics are induced.

A. T Helper Subsets in Mucosal Immunity to Oral Vaccines

As mentioned earlier, in the mouse, antigen-specific helper T-cell responses may be classified as Th1 or Th2 according to the profile of cytokines produced in response to specific antigen (Mosmann and Coffman, 1989; Coffman *et al.*, 1991). Th1-type responses are characterized by the production of IL-2, IFNγ, and TNFβ. Th1-type cells do not produce IL-4, IL-5, IL-6, or IL-10. In contrast to Th1-type responses, Th2-type responses are characterized by production of IL-4, IL-5,

IL-6, and IL-10 and the lack of production of IL-2, IFNγ, and TNFβ. Th1-type responses are associated with the development of cell-mediated immune responses and enhanced IgG2a responses whereas Th2-type responses support the development of antigen-specific IgG1, IgA, and IgE responses in the absence of cell-mediated immune responses (Mosmann and Coffman, 1989; Coffman *et al.*, 1991; Cher and Mosmann, 1987; Golding, 1991; Mosmann, 1991; Ramsay and Kohonen-Cornish, 1993). It remains to be determined if immune responses to individual antigens will fall into exclusive classification as Th1- or Th2-type. However, it is clear that Th1 and Th2 cells are sensitive to cross-regulation by the opposite cell type. For example, IFNγ produced by Th1 cells inhibits proliferation of Th2 cells and is responsible for an isotype switch from IgM to IgG2a (Snapper and Paul, 1987) while inhibiting isotype switching induced by IL-4 (Gajewski and Fitch, 1988; Golding, 1991). Th2 cells regulate the effects of Th1 cells by secreting IL-10 which inhibits cytokine secretion by Th1 cells, e.g., inhibition of IFNγ secretion, which in turn would decrease IFNγ-mediated inhibition of Th2 cells. Therefore, it is important to determine the antigen-specific cytokine secretion profile as well as the antigen-specific IgG subclass and IgE and IgA profile to fully characterize immune responses induced with mucosal antigen delivery protocols.

IL-4 produced by Th2 cells drives the isotype switch from IgM to IgG1 and IgE (Golding, 1991; Fiorentino *et al.*, 1989; Seder and Paul, 1994). Additionally, the absence of IL-4 is associated with decreased antigen-specific IgG1 levels while antigen-specific IgGa levels increase (Kopf *et al.*, 1993). However, the finding that the absence of the IFNγ receptor was associated with decreased antigen-specific IgA suggests that regulation of IgA responses may be affected by both Th1 and Th2 cells (Schijns *et al.*, 1994). In most cases, careful examination of antigen-specific immunoglobulin isotype and subclass profiles and cytokine secretion profiles of antigen-stimulated cells will allow an immune response to be broadly classified as either Th1- or Th2-type. However, although an immune response may appear to be Th1 or Th2, immune responses are likely to consist of both Th1 and Th2 characteristics as discussed below.

Protection against infectious agents may require immune responses of different Th cell subsets. For example, protection against infectious agents that release toxins but do not invade the host may require production of large amounts of neutralizing antibody responses while protection against invasive infectious agents may require both antibody production and cell-mediated immune responses. Therefore, the careful examination of the immune responses induced by different mucosal delivery protocols is critical.

B. Evidence that Cholera Toxin Promotes Th2-Type Responses

When C57BL/6 mice were orally immunized with 250 μg of tetanus toxoid (TT) and 10 μg of CT at weekly intervals for 3 weeks, fecal IgA and high serum IgG responses were induced (Jackson *et al.*, 1993) (Table IV). This immunization regimen was associated with increased production of IL-4 and IL-5 with only background levels of IL-2 and IFNγ production by PP $CD4^+$ cells cultured *in vitro* with TT, suggesting that this oral immunization protocol induced Th2-type immune responses (Xu-Amano *et al.*, 1993). Further studies with this model revealed that this immunization protocol induced serum IgG responses characterized by high IgG1 titers with low or undetectable IgG2a titers as well as antigen-specific IgE responses (Marinaro *et al.*, 1996). Coadministration of other antigens such as ovalbumin (OVA) and hen egg lysozyme (HEL) with CT using the same immunization schedule gave similar findings. Therefore, oral immunization with soluble proteins TT, OVA, and HEL with CT resulted in the induction of Th2-type responses.

Others have also found that oral immunization of C3H/He, SWR/J, and DBA/1 mice with two doses of 200 μg of the soluble protein HEL and 5–10 μg CT separated by 3 weeks induced antigen-specific IgG (predominantly IgG1), IgA, and IgE responses (Snider *et al.*, 1994). Additionally in this study, systemic challenge of orally immunized mice with HEL led to a fatal anaphylactic reaction due to the high levels of antigen-specific IgE. Oral immunization of C57BL/6 mice with 5 mg keyhole limpet hemocyanin (KLH) and 0.5 μg CT and 10 μg CT-B on three occasions on 10-day intervals resulted in antigen-specific lymphocyte cytokine secretion in both Peyer's patch and lamina propria lymphocyte populations (Wilson *et al.*, 1991). Table IV shows the peak concentration of IL-2, IFNγ , IL-4, and IL-5 in the supernatant of PP lymphocytes (not purified $CD4^+$ T cells) cultured in the presence of KLH for 6 days. Again, the results from this study support the conclusion that oral immunization with soluble protein antigen and CT as an adjuvant induced Th2-type immune responses. The observation that the use of CT as a mucosal adjuvant is associated with increased and potentially dangerous levels of antigen-specific IgE argues against the use of CT as a mucosal adjuvant in humans. However, the recent production of mutant LT that retains mucosal adjuvant properties will be helpful in determining if a molecule with adjuvant activity without the negative side effect of IgE production exists (Douce *et al.*, 1995; Dickinson and Clements, 1995). Toward this end, the use of a mutated form of pertussis toxin (PT) was shown to have mucosal adjuvanticity without the associated elevated IgE responses (Roberts *et al.*, 1995).

TABLE IV
Characteristics of Mucosal Immune Responses after Immunization with Various Mucosal Antigen Delivery Systems

Route of immunization	Mouse strain	Antigen delivery system	Antigen-specific antibody responses					Antigen-specific cytokine secretion profile			
			Fecal IgA	Serum IgG	Serum IgG1	Serum IgG2a	Serum IgE	IL-2	IFNγ	IL-4	IL-5
Oral[a] (Jackson *et al.*, 1993; Marinaro *et al.*, 1995)	C57BL/6	TT + CT	1:128	1:130,000	1:8,192	<1:32	1:3,000	Not detectable	Not detectable	15	35
Oral[a] (Marinaro *et al.*, 1995)	C57BL/6	OVA + CT	1:256	1:130,000	1:6,384	<1:32	1:300	N.D.	N.D.	N.D.	N.D.
Oral[a] (Marinaro *et al.*, 1995)	C57BL/6	HEL + CT	1:64	1:130,000	1:6,384	1:128	1:300	N.D.	N.D.	N.D.	N.D.
Oral (Snider *et al.*, 1994)	C3H/He	HEL + CT	N.D.	N.D.	1:843	1:181	1:100	N.D.	N.D.	N.D.	N.D.
Oral[b] (Wilson *et al.*, 1991)	C57BL/6	KLH + CT, CT-B	N.D.	N.D.	N.D.	N.D.	N.D.	3	3	30	125
Oral[c] (Bourguin *et al.*, 1993)	C57BL/6	TSo + CT	N.D.	N.D.	N.D.	N.D.	N.D.	93.6	4.30	0.16	55
Nasal Reuman *et al.*, 1991)	BALB/C	UV-RSV + CT	N.D.	4.35	0.92	1.85	N.D.	N.D.	N.D.	N.D.	N.D.
Nasal (Roberts *et al.*, 1995)	NIH:S	Frg C + CT	N.D.	3×10^6	50,000	40,000	Not detectable	N.D.	N.D.	N.D.	N.D.
Nasal (Roberts *et al.*, 1995)	NIH:S	Frg C + PT	N.D.	68,642	1,000	300	Not detectable	N.D.	N.D.	N.D.	N.D.
Oral[d] (Yang *et al.*, 1990)	BALB/c	Attenuated *Salmonella*	N.D.	Positive	N.D.	N.D.	N.D.	100	50	<1	N.D.
Nasal (Roberts *et al.*, 1995)	NIH:S	Frg C + Pt-9K/129G	N.D.	625,012	6,000	800	Not detectable	N.D.	N.D.	N.D.	N.D.
Oral (Schödel *et al.*, 1990)	CBA/T6T6	Attenuated *Salmonella*	N.D.	1:163,840	$1:10^4$	$1:10^6$	N.D.	N.D.	N.D.	N.D.	N.D.
Oral[e] (VanCott *et al.*, 1996)	C57BL/6	Attenuated *Salmonella*	1:256	1:262,000	1:256	$>10^5$	Not detectable	1	14	<5	<1

Note. N.D., not determined.

[a]Cytokine results are presented as pg/ml after PP $CD4^+$ lymphocytes were cultured *in vitro* for 6 days with TT-coated latex beads.

[b]Cytokine results are approximate cytokine concentrations in units after PP lymphocytes were cultured with KLH *in vitro* for 6 days.

[c]Cytokine profiles of spleen T lymphocytes cultured with antigen. IL-2 and IL-4 are reported as units/ml; IFNγ is reported as ng/ml; IL-5 is expressed as pg/ml.

[d]Serum IgG was not determined as an endpoint titer but was positive; cytokine responses are reported as units/ml.

[e]Cytokine results are presented as U/ml (for IFNγ and IL-2) or picograms/ml (for IL-4 and IL-5) after 4 days of culture.

In contrast to the results reported above, others have found that oral immunization with a sonicate of *Toxoplasma gondii* and CT resulted in sensitized spleen T lymphocytes that secreted a Th1-type pattern of cytokines after *in vitro* stimulation with antigen (Bourguin *et al.*, 1993). Oral immunization of C57BL/6 mice with 10 mg of *T. gondii* sonicate (TSo) and 10 μg of CT three times at intervals of 10 days resulted in antigen-specific T-lymphocyte proliferation and cytokine secretion *in vitro*. Splenic T cells isolated from mice immunized with TSo plus CT produced increased amounts of IFNγ and IL-2 when compared to T lymphocytes isolated from control mice immunized with TSo or CT only. There was no change in the amount of IL-4 or IL-5 produced by lymphocytes isolated from TSo plus CT immunized mice as compared to lymphocytes from mice immunized with TSo only. The differences between this study and the previous findings may be due to the different nature of the antigen used or the fact that T lymphocytes isolated from the spleen instead of mucosal lymphocytes were examined.

Intranasal immunization is another route of mucosal immunization that is receiving much attention. BALB/c mice intranasally immunized once with UV-inactivated respiratory syncytial virus (UV-RSV) plus 5 μg CT was compared to BALB/c mice intranasally infected with live RSV (Reuman *et al.*, 1991). Both immunization protocols induced serum anti-RSV IgG, lung IgG and IgA, and nasal IgA. When the sera from immunized mice were compared for anti-RSV IgG subclass responses, anti-RSV IgG2a predominated with a titer of 2.02 ($\log_{10}$ reciprocal dilution) in infected mice and a titer of 1.85 in UV-RSV plus CT immunized mice. Mice infected intranasally with RSV had anti-RSV IgG1 serum titers of 1.01 while UV-RSV plus CT immunized mice had serum IgG1 titers of 0.92. Therefore, based on antigen-specific IgG subclass profiles, intranasal immunization with UV-RSV plus CT induced a response characterized by both Th1- and Th2-type responses but biased toward a Th1-type response. The response induced with UV-RSV plus CT was not statistically different from the response induced by RSV infection. Intranasal immunization with the C fragment of tetanus toxoid (Fragment C) with CT as adjuvant resulted in serum antibody responses characterized by comparable IgG1, IgG2a, and IgG2b anti-Frg C titers, suggesting that the use of CT as an adjuvant with Frg C induced a response characterized by both Th1- and Th2-type responses (Roberts *et al.*, 1995). However, when Frg C was administered intranasally with PT or a mutated form of PT known as PT-9K/129G as mucosal adjuvants, anti-Frg C IgG1 predominated suggesting that an immune response biased toward the Th2 type was induced. Direct comparisons between CT and PT or PT-9K/129 in this study are difficult to make due to the fact that the use of CT was associated with a much more potent anti-Frg C IgG response. Further investigation will be needed to determine the role that adjuvants, the vaccine antigen, and the route of immunization play in induction of Th1 and Th2 responses.

The fact that the use of CT as an adjuvant can in some cases be associated with the induction of both Th1 and Th2 responses may be explained by the nature of antigen used for immunization. For example, soluble protein antigens typically induce antigen-specific IgG1 $\gg$ IgG2a, whereas particulate antigen such as virus or bacterial particles induce IgG2a $>$ IgG1 (Golding, 1991). Indeed, the nature of the antigen has been shown to play a role in the type of Th cytokine secretion profiles observed with *in vitro* restimulated spleen cells. Intraperitoneal immunization with OVA induced an antigen-specific immune response characterized by secretion of IL-4, IL-10, and IFNγ in comparable amounts, a response not dominated by Th1 or Th2 (Yang *et al.*, 1993). However, when OVA was polymerized with glutaraldehyde to give OVA with an average molecular weight of 3.5×10^7 and intraperitoneally administered to mice, *in vitro* restimulation of spleen cells with antigen resulted in high levels of IFNγ secretion (~32 units/ml) with low levels of IL-4 and IL-10 (~3 units/ml and ~5 units/ml, respectively). This *in vitro* cytokine secretion profile was associated with the *in vivo* production of IFNγ because *in vivo* administration of anti-IFNγ antibodies resulted in a Th2-like cytokine secretion profile. Therefore, the different Th-type responses observed with the use of CT as an adjuvant may be due to the use of a variety of different antigens. It seems possible that CT is enhancing the immune response that the antigen would normally induce. Further studies with well-characterized antigens are required to determine if CT preferentially induces Th1 or Th2 systemic and mucosa immune responses.

C. Recombinant *Salmonella*-Expressed Proteins Result in Th1-Type Responses

Examination of the antigen-specific IgG subclass profiles and antigen-stimulated, lymphocyte cytokine secretion after oral immunization with attenuated, recombinant *Salmonella* suggests that mucosal immunization with live, attenuated bacterial vectors induces an immune response biased toward a Th1-type response. CBA/T6T6 mice were orally immunized with two doses of attenuated *S. typhimurium* expressing a major surface protein (gp63) from *Leishmania major* at 2-week intervals (Yang *et al.*, 1990). When spleen cells were isolated from these mice and cultured *in vitro* with *L. major* antigen, high levels of IL-2 and IFNγ with undetectable levels of IL-4 were produced, indicating that an antigen-specific Th1-type immune response was induced. Studies by others support this conclusion. Three oral vaccinations of BALB/c mice with an attenuated strain of

Salmonella expressing hepatitis B virus antigens induced a serum anti-HBc IgG response characterized by anti-HBc IgG2a titers of 1 million and IgG1 titers of 10^4 (Schödel *et al.*, 1990). Studies in our group have verified these findings. Oral immunization of C57BL/6 mice with attenuated, recombinant *S. typhimurium* expressing the C fragment of tetanus toxin (VanCott *et al.*, 1996) induced fecal IgA responses (1:256 or greater) as well as serum IgG2a responses ($>10^5$). *In vitro* culture of purified $CD4^+$ T cells isolated from the PP with TT induced the synthesis of IL-2 and IFNγ, but not IL-4 or IL-5. The results from both antigen-induced cytokine secretion profiles and serum antigen-specific IgG subclass profiles suggest that oral immunization with attenuated, recombinant *Salmonella* vectors induces a Th1-type immune response.

With a variety of antigen delivery protocols including ISCOMS, microspheres, liposomes, attenuated viral vectors, bacterial vectors, and soluble protein plus CT as adjuvant being tested for the ability to induce mucosal immune responses after mucosal immunization, careful examination of the immune response is warranted to aid in the design of a mucosal antigen delivery system that induces the desired type of immune response.

VIII. Summary

Mucosal surfaces provide a portal of entry for most infectious viral and bacterial pathogens. The mucosal immune system has evolved to become an elaborate host defense system that is able to protect the host at the mucosal surfaces. Antigen-specific T- and B-cell responses are first initiated at inductive sites of the mucosal immune system (i.e., the PP of the GI tract). Antigen-specific lymphocytes (T and B) then leave the inductive site via the lymphatic system and home to mucosal effector sites such as the lamina propria region of the GI tract; it is at these sites that secretory IgA (S-IgA) antibodies and cytokines from Th cells and CTLs are released in response to specific antigen. Thus, antigen-specific S-IgA, Th cells, and CTLs all play a role in protection of mucosal surfaces. Passive transfer studies with polymeric IgA have provided evidence that the presence of S-IgA alone at mucosal surfaces is able to prevent infection with several infectious agents including influenza, *S. typhimurium*, *V. cholerae*, and *H. felis.*

Mucosal immune responses are intricately regulated by cytokines. TGFβ has been shown to be the major cytokine involved in B-cell switching from surface IgA^- to surface IgA^+ while IL-5 and IL-6 seem to be the major cytokines necessary to enhance secretion of IgA from $sIgA^+$ cells. Intestinal epithelial cells and cell lines have been shown to produce IL-6, suggesting that intestinal epithelial cells may play a role in maintenance of mucosal effector B-cell responses.

Mucosal immunization may induce antigen-specific Th1- or Th2-type responses dependent on the antigen delivery system used. The use of cholera toxin as a mucosal adjuvant with soluble protein antigens predominately induces Th2-type responses, while the use of live vectors such as recombinant, attenuated, *S. typhimurium* induces Th1-type responses. Careful analysis of the type of immune response induced with mucosal immunization protocols is essential for the design of effective mucosal vaccines.

References

Allan, C. H., Mendrick, D. L., and Trier, J. S. (1993). Rat intestinal M cells contain acidic endosomal–lysosomal compartments and express class II major histocompatibility complex determinants. *Gastroenterology* **104,** 698–708.

Allison, J. P. (1994). CD28-B7 interactions in T-cell activation. *Curr. Opin. Immunol.* **6,** 414–419.

Azuma, M., Ito, D., Yagita, H., Okumura, K., Phillips, J. H., Lanier, L. L., and Somoza, C. (1993). B70 antigen is a second ligand for CTLA-4 and CD28. *Nature (London)* **366,** 76–79.

Banchereau, J., Bazan, F., Blanchard, D., Briere, F., Galizzi, J. P., van Kooten, C., Liu, Y. J., Roussett, F., and Saeland, S. (1994). The CD40 antigen and its ligand. *Annu. Rev. Immunol.* **12,** 881–922.

Bao, S., Goldstone, S., and Husband, A. J. (1993). Localization of IFN-γ and IL-6 mRNA in murine intestine by *in situ* hybridization. *Immunology* **80,** 666–670.

Beagley, K. W., and Elson, C. O. (1992). Cells and cytokines in mucosal immunity and inflammation. *Gastroenterology Clinics of North America* **21,** 347–366.

Beagley, K. W., Eldridge, J. H., Kiyono, H., and McGhee, J. R. (1987). The identification of murine Peyer's patch T cell-derived factors which enhance IgA isotype-specific responses. *Adv. Exp. Med. Biol.* **237,** 641–647.

Beagley, K. W., Eldridge, J. H., Kiyono, H., Everson, M. P., Koopman, W. J., Honjo, T., and McGhee, J. R. (1988a). Recombinant murine IL-5 induces high rate IgA synthesis in cycling IgA-positive Peyer's patch B cells. *J. Immunol.* **141,** 2035–2042.

Beagley, K. W., Eldridge, J. H., Lee, F., Kiyono, H., Everson, M. P., Koopman, W. J., Hirano, T., Kishimoto, T., and McGhee, J. R. (1989b). Interleukins and IgA synthesis. Human and murine IL-6 induce high rate IgA secretion in IgA-committed B cells. *J. Exp. Med.* **169,** 2133–2148.

Beagley, K. W., Black, C. A., Dunkley, M. L., and McGhee, J. R. (1996). Regulation of mucosal immunity. *In* "Cytokine Regulation of Humoral Immunity: Basic and Clinical Aspects" (C. M. Snapper, ed.), pp. 391–408. John Wiley and Sons, Ltd.

Benson, E. B., and Strober, W. (1988). Regulation of IgA secretion by T cell clones derived from the human gastrointestinal tract. *J. Immunol.* **140,** 1874–1882.

Benson, E. M., Bertolini, J. N., and Brodtmann, M. E. (1990).

T cell regulation of immunoglobulin isotypes in health and disease. *Pediatr. Infect. Dis. J.* **9,** 525–535.
Bockman, D. E., and Cooper, M. D. (1973). Pinocytosis by epithelium associated with lymphoid follicles in the bursa of Fabricius, appendix and Peyer's patches. An electron microscopic study. *Am. J. Anat.* **136,** 455–477.
Bourguin, I., Chardes, T., and Bout, D. (1993). Oral immunization with *Toxoplasma gondii* antigens in association with cholera toxin induces enhanced protective and cell-mediated, immunity in C57BL/6 mice. *Infect. Immun.* **61,** 2082–2088.
Boussiotis, V. A., Freeman, G. J., Gribben, J. G., Daley, J., Gray, G., and Nadler, L. M. (1993). Activated human B lymphocytes express three CTLA4 counterrreceptors that costimulate T-cell activation. *Proc. Natl. Acad. Sci. U.S.A.* **90,** 11059–11063.
Brandeis, J. M., Sayegh, M. H., Gallon, L., Blumberg, R. S., and Carpenter, C. B. (1994). Rat intestinal epithelial cells present major histocompatibility complex allopeptides to primed T cells. *Gastroenterology* **107,** 1537–1542.
Bretscher, P. (1992). The two-signal model of lymphocyte activation twenty-one years later. *Immunol. Today* **13,** 74–76.
Bromander, A. K., Kjerrulf, M., Holmgren, J., and Lycke, N. (1993). Cholera toxin enhances alloantigen presentation by cultured intestinal epithelial cells. *Scand. J. Immunol.* **37,** 452–458.
Brown, W. R., Newcomb, R. W., and Ishizaka, K. (1970). Proteolytic degradation of exocrine and serum immunoglobulins. *J. Clin. Invest.* **49,** 1374–1380.
Butcher, E. C., Rouse, R. V., Coffman, R. L. Nottenberg, C. N., Hardy, R. R., and Weissman, I. L. (1982). Surface phenotype of Peyer's patches germinal center cells: Implications for the role of germinal centers in B-cell differentiation. *J. Immunol.* **129,** 2698–2707.
Cambier, J. C., Pleimar, C. M., and Clark, M. R. (1994). Signal transduction by the B cell antigen receptor and its coreceptors. *Annu. Rev. Immunol.* **12,** 457–486.
Centers For Disease Control (1994). General recommendations on immunization. Recommendations of the advisory committee on immunization practices (ACIP). *MMWR* **43,** (No. RR-1), 4.
Centers For Disease Control (1995). Recommended childhood immunization schedule—United States, June 16, 1995. *MMWR* **44,** 1–9.
Chan, A. C., Desai, D. L. M., and Weiss, A. (1994). The role of protein tyrosine kinases and protein tyrosine phosphatases in T cell antigen receptor signal transduction *Annu. Rev. Immunol.* **12,** 555–592.
Chan, S. H., Perussia, B., Gupta, J. W., Kobayashi, M., Pospisil, M., Young, H. A., Wolf, S. F., Young, D., Clark, S. C., and Trinchieri, G. (1991). Induction of interferon gamma production by natural killer cell stimulatory factor: Characterization of the responder cells and synergy with other inducers. *J. Exp. Med.* **173,** 869–879.
Cher, D. J., and Mosmann, T. R. (1987). Two types of murine helper T cell clone. II. Delayed-type hypersensitivity is mediated by Th1 clones. *J. Immunol.* **138,** 3688–3694.
Coffman, R. L., Shrader, B., Carty, J., Mosmann, T. R., and Bond, M. W. (1987). A mouse T cell product that preferentially enhances IgA production. I. Biologic characterization. *J. Immunol.* **139,** 3685–3690.
Coffman, R. L., Syemour, B. W. P., Lebman, D. A., Hiraki, D. D., Christiansen, J. A., Shrader, B., Cherwinski, H. M., Saudkoul, H. F. J., Finkelman, F. D., Bond, M. W., and Mosmann, T. R. (1988). The role of helper T Cell products in mouse B cell differentiation and isotype regulation. *Immunol. Rev.* **102,** 5–28.
Coffman, R. L., Lebman, D. A., and Schrader, B. (1989). Transforming growth factor β specifically enhances IgA production by lipopolysaccharide-stimulated murine B lymphocytes. *J. Exp. Med.* **170,** 1039–1044.
Coffman, R. L., Varkila, K., Scott, P., and Chatelain, R. (1991). Role of cytokines in the differentiation of $CD4^+$ T-cell subsets *in vivo*. *Immunol. Rev.* **123,** 189–207.
Conley, M. E., and Delacroix, D. L. (1987). Intravascular and mucosal immunoglobulin A: Two separate but related systems of immune defense? *Ann. Int. Med.* **106,** 892–899.
Czinn, S. J., Cai, A., and Nedrud, J. G. (1993). Protection of germfree mice from infection by *Helicobacter felis* after active oral or passive IgA immunization. *Vaccine* **11,** 637–642.
Davies, M. D. J., and Parrott, D. M. W. (1981). Cytotoxic T Cells in small intestine epithelial, lamina propria and lung lymphocytes. *Immunology* **44,** 367–371.
Defrance, T., Vanbervliet, B., Briére, F., Durand, I., Rousett, F., and Banchereau, J. (1992). Interleukin-10 and transforming growth factor β cooperate to induce anti-CD40-activated naive human B cells to secrete immunoglobulin A. *J. Exp. Med.* **175,** 671–682.
Dickinson, B. L., and Clements, J. D. (1995). Dissociation of *Escherichia coli* heat-labile enterotoxin adjuvanticity from ADP-ribosyltransferase activity. *Infect. Immun.* **63,** 1617–1623.
DiFabio, S., Mbawuike, I. N., Kiyono, H., Fujihashi, K., Couch, R. B., and McGhee, J. R. (1994). Quantitation of human influenza virus-specific cytotoxic T lymphocytes: Correlation of cytotoxicity and increased numbers of IFNγ producing $CD8^+$ T cells. *Int. Immunol.* **6,** 11–19.
Douce, G., Turcotte, C., Cropley, I., Roberts, M., Pizza, M., Domenghini, M., Rappuoli, R., and Dougan, G. (1995). Mutants of *Escherichia coli* heat-labile toxin lacking ADP-ribosyltransferase activity act as nontoxic, mucosal adjuvants. *Proc. Natl. Acad. Sci. U.S.A.* **92,** 1644–1648.
Eckmann, I., Jung, H. C., Schürer-Maly, C., Panja, A., Morzycka-Wroblewska, F., and Kagnoff, M. F. (1993). Differential cytokine expression by human intestinal epithelial cell lines: Regulated expression of interleukin 8. *Gastroenterology* **105,** 1689–1697.
Elson, C. O., Heck, J. A, and Strober, W. (1979). T-cell regulation of murine IgA synthesis. *J. Exp. Med.* **149,** 632–643.
Ennis, F. A., Yi-Hua, Q., and Schild, G. C. (1982). Antibody and cytotoxic T lymphocyte responses of humans to live and inactivated influenza vaccines. *J. Gen. Virol.* **58,** 273–281.
Ermak, T. H., Dougherty, E. P., Bhagat, H. R., Kabok, Z. X., and Pappo, J. (1995). Uptake and transport of copolymer biodegradable microspheres by rabbit Peyer's patch M cells. *Cell Tissue Res.* **279,** 433–436.

Ernst, P. B., Befus, A. D., and Bienenstock, J. (1985). Leukocytes in the intestinal epithelium: An unusual immunological compartment. *Immunol. Today* **6**, 50–55.

Esser, C., and Radbruch, A. (1990). Immunoglobulin class switching: Molecular and cellular analysis. *Annu. Rev. Immunol.* **8**, 717–735.

Fabry, Z., Sandor, M., Gajewski, T. F., Herlein, J. A., Waldschmidt, M. M., Lynch, R. G., and Hart, M. N. (1993). Differential activation of Th1 and Th2 CD4$^+$ cells by murine brain microvessel endothelial cells and smooth muscle/pericytes. *J. Immunol.* **151**, 38–47.

Farstad, I. N., Halstensen, T. S., Fausa, O., and Brandtzaeg, P. (1994). Heterogeneity of M-cell-associated B and T cells in human Peyer's patches. *Immunology* **83**, 457–464.

Finkelman, F. D., Holmes, J., Katona, I. M, Urban, J. F., Beckmann, M. P., Park, L. S., and Paul, W. E. (1990). Lymphokine control of *in vivo* immunoglobulin isotype. *Annu. Rev. Immunol.* **8**, 303–333.

Fiorentino, D. F., Bond, M. W., and Mosmann, T. R. (1989). Two types of mouse T helper cell. IV. Th2 clones secreted a factor that inhibits cytokine production by Th1 clones. *J. Exp. Med.* **170**, 2081–2095.

Fox, B. S. (1993). Antigen presenting cell-derived co-stimulatory signals can selectively regulate IL-2 and IL-4 production from a Th0 cell hybridoma. *Int. Immunol.* **5**, 323–330.

Freedman, A. S., Freeman, G. J., Rhynhart, K., and Nadler, L. M. (1991). Selective induction of B7/BB-1 on interferon-gamma stimulated monocytes: A potential mechanism for amplification of T cell activation through the CD28 pathway. *Cell. Immunol.* **137**, 429–437.

Freeman, G. J., Freedman, A. S., Segil, J. M., Lee, G., Whitman, J. F., and Nadlier, L. M. (1989). B7, A new member of the Ig superfamily with unique expression on activated and neoplastic B cells. *J. Immunol.* **143**, 2714–2722.

Freeman, G. J., Borrielo, F., Hodes, R. J., Reiser, H., Hatchcock, K. S., Laszlo, G., McKnight, A. J., Kim, J., Du, L., Lombard, D. B., Gray, G. S., Nadler, L. M., and Sharpe, A. H. (1993a). Uncovering of functional alternative CTLA-4 counter-receptor in B7-deficient mice. *Science* **262**, 907–909.

Freeman, G. J., Gribben, J. G., Boussiotis, V. A., N. G., J. W., Restivo, V. A., Jr., Lombard, L. A., Gray, G. S., and Nadler, L. M. (1993b). Cloning of B7-2: A CTLA-4 counter-receptor that costimulates human T cell proliferation. *Science* **262**, 909–911.

Fujihashi, K., McGhee, J. R., Lue, C., Beagley, K. W., Taga, T., Hirano, T., Kioshimoto, T., Mestecky, J., and Kiyono, H. (1991). Human appendix B cells naturally express receptors for and respond to interleukin 6 with selective IgA1 and IgA2 synthesis. *J. Clin. Invest.* **88**, 248–252.

Gajewski, T. F., and Fitch, F. W. (1988). Anti-proliferative effect of IFN-γ in immune regulation. I. IFN-γ inhibits the proliferation of Th2 but not Th1 murine helper T lymphocyte clones. *J. Immunol.* **140**, 4245–4252.

Golding, B. (1991). Cytokine regulation of humoral immune responses. *In* "Topics in Vaccine Adjuvant Research," pp. 25–37.

Goodman, R. E., Nestle, F., Naidu, Y. M., Green, J. M., Thompson, C. B., Nickoloff, B. J., and Turka, L. A. (1994). Keratinocyte-derived T cell costimulation induces preferential production of IL-2 and IL-4 but not IFN-gamma. *J. Immunol.* **152**, 5189–5198.

Gordon, J., Millsum, M. J., Guy, G. R., and Ledbetter, J. A. (1987). Synergistic interaction between interleukin 4 and anti-Bp50 (CDw40) revealed in a novel B cell restimulation assay. *Eur. J. Immunol.* **17**, 1535–1538.

Gordon, J., Millsum, M. J., Guy, G. R., and Ledbetter, J. A. (1988). Resting B lymphocytes can be triggered directly through the CDw40 (Bp50) antigen. A comparison with IL-4 mediated signaling. *J. Immunol.* **140**, 1425–1430.

Guy-Grand, D. Y., Griscelli, T. C., and Vassalli, P. (1978). The mouse gut lymphocyte, a novel type of T cell: Nature, origin, and traffic in mice in normal and graft-versus-host conditions. *J. Exp. Med.* **148**, 1661–1677.

Hanson, L. A., and Brandtzaeg, P. (1989). The mucosal defense system. *In* "Immunological Disorders in Infants and Children" (E. R. Stiehm, ed.), p. 16. Saunders, Philadelphia, Pennsylvania.

Harriman, G. R., Kunimoto, D. Y., Elliot, J. F., Paetkau, V., and Strober, W. (1988). The role of IL-5 in IgA B cell differentiation. *J. Immunol.* **140**, 3033–3039.

Hathcock, K. S., Laszlo, G., Pucillo, C., Linsley, P., and Hodes, R. J. (1994). Comparative analysis of B7-1 and B7-2 costimulatory ligands: Expression and function. *J. Exp. Med.* **180**, 631–640.

Hsieh, C. S., Macatonia, S. E., Tripp, C. S., Wolf, S. F., O'Garra, A., and Murphy, K. M. (1993). Development of Th1 CD4$^+$ T cells through IL-12 produced by *Listeria*-induced macrophages. *Science* **260**, 547–549.

Isakson, P. C., Puré, E., Vitetta, E. S., and Krammer, P. H. (1982). T cell derived B cell differentiation factor(s). Effect on the isotype switch of murine B cells. *J. Exp. Med.* **155**, 734–748.

Islam, K. B., Nilsson, L., Sideras, P., Hammastrom, L., and Edvard Smith, C. I. (1991). TGF-β1 induces germ-line transcripts of both IgA subclasses in human B lymphocytes. *Int. Immunol.* **3**, 1099–1106.

Issekutz, T. B. (1984). The response of gut-associated T lymphocytes to intestinal viral immunization. *J. Immunol.* **133**, 2955–2960.

Jackson, R. J., Fujihashi, K., Xu-Amano, J., Kiyono, H., and McGhee, J. R. (1993). Optimizing oral vaccines: Induction of systemic and mucosal B cell and antibody responses to tetanus toxoid by use of cholera toxin as adjuvant. *Infect. Immun.* **61**, 4272–4279.

Jones, B. D., Ghori, N., and Falkow, S. (1994). *Salmonella typhimurium* initiates murine infection by penetrating and destroying the specialized epithelial M cells of the Peyer's patches. *J. Exp. Med.* **180**, 15–23.

June, C. H., Bluestone, J. A., Nadler, L. M., and Thompson, C. B. (1994). The B7 and CD28 receptor families. *Immunol. Today*, **15**, 321–331.

Kaetzel, C. S., Robinson, J. K., Chintalacharuvu, K. R., Vaerman, J. P., and Lamm, M. E. (1991). The polymeric immunoglobulin receptor (secretory component) mediates transport of immune complexes across epithelial cells: A local defense function for IgA. *Proc. Natl. Acad. Sci. U.S.A.* **88**, 8796–8800.

Kaetzel, C. S., Robinson, J. K., and Lamm, M. E. (1994). Epithelial transcytosis of monomeric IgA and IgG cross-linked through antigen to polymeric IgA. A role for monomeric antibodies in the mucosal immune system. *J. Immunol.* **152,** 72–76.

Kansas, G. S., and Tedder, T. F. (1991). Transmembrane signals generated through MHC Class II, CD19, CD20, CD39, and CD40 antigens induce LFA-1-dependent and independent adhesion in human B cells through a tyrosine kinase-dependent pathway. *J. Immunol.* **147,** 4094–4102.

Kawanishi, H., Salzman, L., and Strober, W. (1983a). Mechanisms regulating IgA class-specific immunoglobulin production in murine gut-associated lymphoid tissues I: T cells derived from Peyer's patches that switch sIgM B cells to SIgA B cells *in vitro*. *J. Exp. Med.* **157,** 433–450.

Kawanishi, H., Saltzman, L., and Strober, W. (1983b). Mechanisms regulating IgA class-specific immunoglobulin production in murine gut-associated lymphoid tissues. II: Terminal differentiation of postswitch sIgA-bearing Peyer's patch B cells. *J. Exp. Med.* **158,** 649–669.

Kawanishi, H., Ozato, K., and Strober, W. (1983c). The proliferative response of cloned Peyer's patch switch T-cells to syngeneic and allogenic stimuli. *J. Immunol.* **134,** 3586–3591.

Kehrl, J. H., Roberts, A. B., Wakefield, L. M., Jakowlew, S., Sporn, M. B., and Fauci, A. S. (1986). Transforming growth factor beta is an important immunomodulatory protein for human B lymphocytes. *J. Immunol.* **137,** 3855–3860.

Kehrl, J. H., Wakefield, L. M., Roberts, A. B., Jakowlew, S., Alvarez-Mon, M., Derynck, R. Sporin, M. B., and Fauci, A. S. (1987). Production of transforming growth factor beta by human T lymphocytes and its potential role in the regulation of T cell growth. *J. Exp. Med.* **163,** 1037–1050.

Kehrl, J. H., Thevenin, C., Rieckmann, P., and Fauci, A. S. (1991). Transforming growth factor-beta suppresses human B lymphocyte Ig production by inhibiting synthesis and the switch from the membrane form to the secreted form of Ig mRNA. *J. Immunol.* **146,** 4016–4023.

Kiyono, H., McGhee, J. R., and Mosteller, L. M., *et al.* (1982). Murine Peyer's patch T-cell clones: Characterization of antigen-specific helper T cells for immunoglobulin A responses. *J. Exp. Med.* **156,** 1115–1130.

Kiyono, H., Cooper, M. D., and Kearney, J. F., *et al.* (1984). Isotype-specificity of helper T cell clones: Peyer's patch Th cells preferentially collaborate with mature IgA B cells for IgA responses. *J. Exp. Med.* **159,** 798–811.

Kiyono, H., Mosteller-Barnum, L. M., Pitts, A. M., Williamson, S. I., Michalek, S. M., and McGhee, J. R. (1985). Isotype-specific immunoregulation: IgA binding factors produced by Fcα Receptor$^+$ T cell hybridomas regulate IgA responses. *J. Exp. Med.* **161,** 731–747.

Kobayashi, M., Fitz, L., Ryan, M., Hewick, R. M., Clark, S. C., Chan, S., London, R., Sherman, F., Perussia, B., and Trinchieri, G. (1989). Identification and purification of natural killer cell stimulatory factor (NKSF), a cytokine with multiple biologic effects on human lymphocytes. *J. Exp. Med.* **170,** 827–845.

Kopf, M., Le Gros, G., Bachmann, M., Lamers, M. C., Bluethmann, H., and Köhler, G. (1993). Disruption of the murine IL-4 gene blocks Th2 cytokine responses. *Nature (London)* **362,** 245–248.

Kraehenbuhl, J. P., and Neutra, M. R. (1992). Molecular and cellular basis of immune protection of mucosal surfaces. *Physiol. Rev.* **72,** 853–879.

Kroese, F. G. M., Butcher, E. C., Stall, A. M., Lalor, P. A., Adams, S., and Horzenberg, L. A. (1989). Many of the IgA producing plasma cells in murine gut are derived from self-replenishing precursors in the peritoneal cavity. *Int. Immunol.* **1,** 75–84.

Kuchroo, U. K., Das, M. P., Brown, J. A., Ranger, A. M., Zamvil, S. S., Sobel, R. A., Weiner, H. L., Nabavi, N., and Glimcher, L. H. (1995). B7-1 and B7-2 costimulatory molecules activated differentially the Th1/Th2 developmental pathways: Application to autoimmune disease therapy. *Cell (Cambridge, Mass.)* **80,** 707–718.

Kvalc, D., Krajci, P., and Brandtzaeg, P. (1992). Expression and regulation of adhesion molecules ICAM-1 (CD54) and LFA-3 (CD58) in human intestinal epithelial cell lines. *Scand. J. Immunol.* **35,** 669–676.

Lamb, J. R., McMichael, A. J., and Rothbard, J. B. (1987). T-cell recognition of influenza viral antigens. *Hum. Immunol.* **19,** 79–89.

Larsen, C. P., Ritchie, S. C., Hendrix, R., Linsley, P. S., Hathcock, K. S., Hodes, R. J., Lowry, R. P., and Pearson, T. C. (1994). Regulation of immunostimulatory function and costimulatory molecule (B7-1 and B7-2) expression on murine dendritic cells. *J. Immunol.* **152,** 5208–5219.

Lassila, O., Vainio, O., and Matzinger, P. (1988). Can B cells turn on virgin T cells? *Nature (London),* **334,** 253–255.

Lebman, D. A., Griffin, P. M., and Cebra, J. J. (1977). Relationship between expression of IgA by Peyer's patch cells and functional IgA memory cells. *J. Exp. Med.* **166,** 1405–1418.

Lebman, D. A. and Coffman, R. L. (1988). The effects of IL-4 and IL-5 on the IgA response by murine Peyer's patch B cell subpopulations. *J. Immunol.* **141,** 2050–2056.

Lebman, D. A., Nomura, D. Y., Coffman, R. L., and Lee, F. D. (1990a). Molecular characterization of germ-line immunoglobulin A transcripts produced during transforming growth factor type β-induced isotype switching. *Proc. Natl. Acad. Sci. U.S.A.* **87,** 3962–3966.

Lebman, D. A., Lee, F. D., and Coffman, R. L. (1990b). Mechanism for transforming growth factor β and IL-2 enhancement of IgA expression in lipopolysaccharide-stimulated B cell cultures. *J. Immunol.* **144,** 952–959.

Lee, C. K., Weltzin, R., Soman, G., Georgakopoulos, Houle, D. M., and Monath, T. P. (1994). Oral administration of polymeric immunoglobulin A prevents colonization with *Vibrio cholerae* in neonatal mice. *Infect. Immun.* **62,** 887–891.

Levine, B. L., Ueda, Y., Craighead, N., Huang, M. L., and June, C. H. (1995). CD28 Ligands CD80 (B7-1) and CD86 (B7-2) induce long-term autocrine growth of CD4$^+$ T cells and induce similar patterns of cytokine secretion *in vitro*. *Int. Immunol.* **7,** 891.

Linsley, P. S., and Ledbetter, J. A. (1993). The role of the

CD28 receptor during T cell responses to antigen. *Annu. Rev. Immunol.* **11**, 191–212.

Linsley, P. S., Greene, J. L., Tan, P., Bradshaw, J., Ledbetter, J. A., Anasetti, C., and Damle, N. K. (1992). Co-expression and functional cooperation of CTLA-4 and CD28 on activated T lymphocytes. *J. Exp. Med.* **176**, 1595–1604.

London, S. D., Rubin, D. H., and Cebra, J. J. (1987). Gut mucosal immunization with reovirus serotype 1/L stimulates virus-specific cytotoxic T cell precursors as well as IgA memory cells in Peyer's patches. *J. Exp. Med.* **165**, 830–847.

MacDermott, R. P., Franklin, G. O., Jenkins, K. M., Kodner, I. J., Nash, G. S., and Weinrieb, I. J. (1980). Human intestinal mononuclear cells. 1. Investigation of antibody-dependent, lectin-induced and spontaneous cell-mediated cytotoxic capabilities. *Gastroenterology* **78**, 47–56.

McCormick, B. A., Colgan, S. P., Delp-Archer, C., Miller, S. I., and Madara, J. L. (1993). *Salmonella typhimurium* attachment to human intestinal epithelial monolayers: Transcellular signalling to subepithelial neutrophils. *J. Cell Biol.* **123**, 895–907.

McGee, D. W., Beagley, K. W., Aicher, W. K., and McGhee, J. R. (1992). Transforming growth factor-β enhances interleukin-6 production by intestinal epithelial cells. *Immunology* **77**, 7–12.

McGee, D. W., Beagley, K. W., Aicher, W. K., and McGhee, J. R. (1993a). Transforming growth factor-β and IL-1β act in synergy to enhance IL-6 secretion by the intestinal epithelial cell line, IEC-6. *J. Immunol.* **151**, 970–978.

McGee, D. W., Elson, C. O., and McGhee, J. R. (1993b). Enhancing effect of cholera toxin on interleukin-6 secretion by IEC-6 intestinal epithelial cells: Mode of action and augmenting effect of inflammatory cytokines. *Infect. Immun.* **61**, 4637–4644.

McIntyre, T. M., Kehry, M. R., and Snapper, C. M. (1995). Novel *in vitro* model for high-rate IgA class switching. *J. Immunol.* **154**, 3156–3161.

McKnight, A. J., Perez, V. L., Shea, C. M., Gray, G. S., and Abbas, A. K. (1994). Costimulator dependence of lymphokine secretion by naive and activated $CD4^+$ lymphocytes from TCR transgenic mice. *J. Immunol.* **152**, 5220–5225.

McMichael, A. J., and Askonas, B. (1978). Infuenza virus-specific cytotoxic T cell in man: Induction and properties of the cytotoxic cell. *Eur. J. Immunol.* **8**, 705–711.

McMichael, A. J., Askonas, B. A., Webster, R. G., and Laver, W. G. (1982). Vaccination against influenza. B-cell or T-cell immunity? *Immunol. Today* **3**, 255–260.

Maghazachi, A. L., and Phillips-Quagliata, J. M. (1988). Keyhole limpet hemocyanin-propagated Peyer's Patch T cell clones that help IgA responses. *J. Immunol.* **140**, 3380–3388.

Magilavy, D. B., Fitch, F. W., and Gajewki, T. F. (1989). Murine hepatic accessory cells support the proliferation of Th1 but not Th2 helper T lymphocyte clones. *J. Exp. Med.* **170**, 985–990.

Marinaro, M., Staats, H. F., Hiroi, T., Jackson, R. J., Coste, M., Boyaka, P. N., Okahashi, N., Yamamoto, M., Kiyono, H., Bluethmann, H., Fujihashi, K., and McGhee, J. R. (1995). Mucosal adjuvant effect of cholera toxin in mice results from induction of T helper 2 (Th2) cells and IL-4. *J. Immunol.* **155**, 4621–4629.

Marrack, P., and Kappler, J. (1987). The cell receptor. *Science* **238**, 1073–1079.

Mayer, L., Kwan, S. P., and Thompson C., *et al.* (1985a). Evidence for a defect in "switch" T cells in patients with immunodeficiency and hyperimmunoglobulin M. *N. Engl. J. Med.* **314**, 409–413.

Mayer, L., Postnett, D. N., and Kunkel, H. G. (1985b). Human-malignant T cells capable of inducing an immunoglobulin class switch. *J. Exp. Med.* **161**, 134–144.

Mazanec, M. B., Nedrud, J. G., Kaetzel, C. S., and Lamm, M. E. (1992). Intracellular neutralization of virus by immunoglobulin A antibodies. *Proc. Natl. Acad. Sci. U.S.A.* **89**, 6901–6905.

Mazanec, M. B., Nedrud, J. G., Kaetzel, C. S., and Lamm, M. E. (1993). A three-tiered view of the role IgA in mucosal defense. *Immunol. Today* **14**, 430–435.

Mega, J., McGhee, J. R., and Kiyono, H. (1992). Cytokine- and Ig-producing cells in mucosal effector tissues: Analysis of IL-5- and IFN-γ-producing T cells, T cell receptor expression, and IgA plasma cells from mouse salivary gland-associated tissues. *J. Immunol.* **148**, 2030–2039.

Mestecky, J., and McGhee, J. R. (1987). Immunoglobulin A (IgA): Molecular and cellular interactions involved in IgA biosynthesis and immune response. *Adv. Immunol.* **40**, 153–245.

Metlay, J. P., Pure, E., and Steinman, R. M. (1989). Distinct features of dendritic cells and anti-Ig activated B cells as stimulators of the primary mixed leukocyte reaction. *J. Exp. Med.* **169**, 239–254.

Michetti, P., Mahan, M. J., Slauch, J. M., Mekalanos, J. J., and Neutra, M. R. (1992). Monoclonal secretory immunoglobulin A protects mice against oral challenge with the invasive pathogen *Salmonella typhimurium*. *Infect. Immun.* **60**, 1786–1792.

Mosmann, T. R. (1991). Cytokines: Is there biological meaning? *Curr. Opin. Immunol.* **3**, 311–314.

Mosmann, T. R., and Coffman, R. L. (1989). Th1 and Th2 Cells: Different patterns of lymphokine secretion lead to different functional properties. *Annu. Rev. Immunol.* **7**, 145–173.

Murray, P. D., McKenzie, D. T., Swain, S. L., and Kagnoff, M. F. (1987). Interleukin 5 and interleukin 4 produced by Peyer's patch T cells selectively enhance immunoglobulin A expression. *J. Immunol.* **139**, 2669–2674.

Nauss, K. M., Pavlina, T. M., Kumar, V., and Newberen, P. M. (1984). Functional characteristics of lymphocytes isolated from the rat large intestine. Response to T-cell mitogen and natural killer cell activity. *Gastroenterology* **86**, 468–475.

Nibert, M. L., Furlong, D. B., and Fields, B. N. (1992). Mechanisms of viral pathogenesis. Distinct forms of reoviruses and their roles during replication in cells and host. *J. Clin. Invest.* **88**, 727–734.

Offit, P. A., and Dudzik, K. I. (1989). Rotavirus-specific cytotoxic T lymphocytes appear at the intestinal mucosal surface after rotavirus infection. *J. Virol.* **63**, 3507–3512.

Owen, R. L., and Jones, A. L. (1974). Epithelial cell specialization within human Peyer's patches: An ultrastructural study of intestinal lymphoid follicles. *Gastroenterology* **66,** 189–203.

Phillips-Quagliata, J. M., and Lamm, M. E. (1994). Lymphocyte homing to mucosal effector sites. *In* "Handbook of Mucosal Immunology" (R. Ogra, J. Mestecky, M. Lamm, W. Strober, J. McGhee, and J. Bienestock, eds.), pp. 225–239. Academic Press, San Diego.

Powers, G. D., Abbas, A. K., and Miller, R. A. (1988). Frequencies of IL-2- and IL-4-secreting T Cells in naive and antigen-stimulated lymphocyte populations. *J. Immunol.* **140,** 3352–3357.

Ramsay, A. J., and Kohonen-Corish, M. (1993). Interleukin-5 expressed by a recombinant virus vector enhances specific mucosal IgA responses *in vivo. Eur. J. Immunol.* **23,** 3141–3145.

Ramsay, A. J., Husband, A. J., Ramshaw, I. A., Bao, S., Matthaei, K. I., Koehler, G., and Kopf, M. (1994). The role of interleukin-6 in mucosal IgA antibody responses *in vivo. Science* **264,** 561–563.

Reiser, H., Freeman, G. J., Razi-Wolf, Z., Gimmi, C. D., Beacerraf, B., and Nadlier, L. M. (1992). Murine B7 antigen provides an efficient costimulatory signal for activation of murine T lymphocytes via the T cell receptor/CD3 complex. *Proc. Natl. Acad. Sci. U.S.A.* **89,** 271–275.

Renegar, K. B., and Small, P. A., Jr. (1991). Passive transfer of local immunity to influenza virus infection by IgA antibody. *J. Immunol.* **146,** 1972–1978.

Reuman, P. D., Keely, S. P., and Schiff, G. M. (1991). Similar subclass antibody responses after intranasal immunization with UV-inactivated RSV mixed with cholera toxin or live RSV. *J. Med. Virol.* **35,** 192–197.

Roberts, M., Bacon, A., Rappuoli, R., Pizza, M., Cropley, I., Douce, G., Dougan, G., Marinaro, M., McGhee, J., and Chatfield, S. (1995). A mutant Pertussis toxin molecule that lacks ADP-ribosyltransferase activity, PT-9K/129G, is an effective mucosal adjuvant for intranasally delivered proteins. *Infect. Immun.* **63,** 2100–2108.

Rousset, F., Garcia, E., and Banchereau, J. (1991). Cytokine-induced proliferation and immunoglobulin production of human B lymphocytes triggered through their CD40 antigen. *J. Exp. Med.* **173,** 705–710.

Ruby, J., and Ramshaw, I. (1991). The antiviral activity of immune $CD8^+$ T-cells is dependent on IFN-γ. *Lymphokines Cytokines Res.* **10,** 353–358.

Sandor, M., Gajewski, T., Thorson, J., Kemp, J. D., Fitch, F. W., and Hoover, G. (1990). $CD4^+$ murine T cell clones that express high levels of immunoglobulin binding belong to the interleukin 4-producing T helper cell type 2 subset. *J. Exp. Med.* **171,** 2171–2176.

Schijns, V. E. C. J., Haagmans, B. L., Rijke, E. O., Huang, S., Aguet, M., and Horzinek, M. C. (1994). IFN-γ receptor-deficient mice generate antiviral Th-1 characteristic cytokine profiles but altered antibody responses. *J. Immunol.* **153,** 2029–2037.

Schödel, F., Milich, D. R., and Will, H. (1990). Hepatitis B virus nucleocapsid/pre-S2 fusion proteins expressed in attenuated *Salmonella* for oral vaccination. *J. Immunol.* **145,** 4317–4321.

Schürer-Maly, C.-C., Eckmann, L., Kagnoff, M. F., Falco, M. T., and Maly, F.-E. (1994). Colonic epithelial cell lines as a source of interleukin-8: Stimulation by inflammatory cytokines and bacterial lipopolysaccaride. *Immunology* **81,** 85–91.

Schwartz, R. H. (1992). Costimulation of T lymphocytes: The role of CD28, CTLA-4, and B7/BB1 in Interleukin-2 production and immunotherapy. *Cell (Cambridge, Mass.)* **71,** 1065–1068.

Seder, R. A., and Paul, W. E. (1994). Acquisition of lymphokine-producing phenotype by $CD4^+$ T cells. *J. Allergy Clin. Immunol.* **94,** 1195–1202.

Seder, R. A., Germain, R. N., Linsley, P. S., and Paul, W. E. (1994). CD28-mediated costimulation of interleukin 2 (IL-2) production plays a critical role in T cell priming for IL-4 and interleukin gamma production. *J. Exp. Med.* **179,** 299–304.

Snapper, C. M., and Paul, W. E. (1987). Interferon-gamma and B cell stimulatory factor-1 reciprocally regulate Ig isotype production. *Science* **236,** 944–947.

Snapper, C. M., McIntyre, T. M., Mandler, R., Pecantro, L. M., Finkelman, F. D., Lees, A., and Mond, J. J. (1992). Induction of IgG3 secretion by interferon γ: A model for T cell independent class switching in response to T cell independent type 2 antigens. *J. Exp. Med.* **175,** 1367–1371.

Snider, D. P., Marshall, J. S., Perdue, M. H., and Liang, H. (1994). Production of IgE antibody and allergic sensitization of intestinal and peripheral tissues after oral immunization with protein Ag and cholera toxin. *J. Immunol.* **153,** 647–657.

Sonada, E., Matsumoto, R., Hitoshi, Y., Ishii, T., Sugimoto, M., Araki, S., Tominaga, A., Yamaguchi, N., and Takatsu, K. (1989). Transforming growth factor β induces IgA production and acts additively with interleukin 5 for IgA production. *J. Exp. Med.* **170,** 1415–1420.

Spalding, D. M., and Griffin, J. A. (1986). Different pathways of differentiation of pre-B cell lines are induced by dendritic cells and T cells from different lymphoid tissues. *Cell (Cambridge, Mass.)* **44,** 507–515.

Spalding, D., Williamson, S. I., Koopman, W. J., and McGhee, J. R. (1984). Preferential induction of polyclonal IgA secretion by murine Peyer's patch dendritic cell–T cell mixtures. *J. Exp. Med.* **160,** 941–946.

Stack, R. M., Lenschow, D. J., Gray, G. S., Bluestone, J. A., and Fitch, F. W. (1994). IL-4 treatment of small splenic B cells induces costimulatory molecules B7-1 and B7-2. *J. Immunol.* **152,** 5723–5733.

Strober, W., and Harriman, G. R. (1991). The regulation of IgA B-cell differentiation. *Gastroenterology Clinics of North America* **20,** 473–794.

Tagliabue, A., Luini, W., Soldateschi, D., and Boraschi, D. (1981). Natural killer activity of gut mucosal lymphoid cells in mice. *Eur. J. Immunol.* **11,** 919–922.

Taguchi, T., McGhee, J. R., Coffman, R. L., Beagley, K. W., Eldridge, J. H., Takatsu, K., and Kiyono, H. (1990) Analysis of Th1 and Th2 Cells in murine gut-associated tissues. Frequencies of $CD4^+$ and $CD8^+$ T cells and secrete IFN-γ and IL-5. *J. Immunol.* **145,** 68–77.

Tan, P., Anasetti, C., Hansen, J. A., Melrose, J., Brunvard, M., Bradshaw, J., Ledbetter, J. A., and Linsley, P. S. (1993). Induction of alloantigen-specific hyporesponsiveness in human T lymphocytes by blocking interaction of CD28 with its natural ligand B7/BB1. *J. Exp. Med.* **177,** 165–173.

Taylor, P. M., and Askonas, B. A. (1986). Influenza nucleoprotein specific cytotoxic T cell clones are protective *in vivo*. *Immunology* **58,** 417–420.

Taylor, P. M., Wraith, D. C., and Askonas, B. A. (1985). Control of immune interferon release by cytotoxic T-cell clones specific for influenza. *Immunology* **54,** 607–614.

Tonkonogy, S. L., and Swain, S. L. (1993). Distinct lymphokine production by $CD4^+$ T cells isolated from mucosal and systemic lymphoid organs. *Immunology* **80,** 574–580.

VanCott, J. L., Staats, H. F., Pascual, D. W., Roberts, M., Chatfield, S., Yamamoto, M., Carter, P. B., Kiyono, H., and McGhee, J. R. (1996). Regulation of mucosal and systemic antibody responses by T helper cell subsets, macrophages and derived cytokines following oral immunization with live recombinant *Salmonella. J. Immunol.* **156,** 1504–1514.

Weaver, C. T., Hawrylowicz, C. M., and Unanue, E. R. (1988). T Helper cell subsets require the expression of distinct costimulatory signals by antigen-presenting cells. *Proc. Natl. Acad. Sci. U.S.A.* **85,** 8181–8185.

Weinberg, A. D., English, M., and Swain, S. L. (1990). Distinct regulation of lymphokine production is found in fresh versus *in vitro* primed murine helper T cells. *J. Immunol.* **144,** 1800–1807.

Wilson, A. D., Bailey, M., Williams, N. A., and Stokes, C. R. (1991). The *in vitro* production of cytokines by mucosal lymphocytes immunized by oral administration of keyhole limpet hemocyanin using cholera toxin as an adjuvant. *Eur. J. Immunol.* **21,** 2333–2339.

Winner III, L., Mack, J., Weltzin, R., Mekalanos, J. J., Kraehenbuhl, J. P., and Neutra, M. (1991). New model for analysis of mucosal immunity: Intestinal secretion of specific monoclonal immunoglobulin A from hybridoma tumors protects against *Vibrio cholerae* infection. *Infect. Immun.* **59,** 977–982.

Wolf, J. L., and Bye, W. A. (1984). The membranous epithelial (M) cell and the mucosal immune system. *Annu. Rev. Med.* **35,** 95–112.

Wolf, J. L., Rubin, D. H., Finberg, R., Kaufman, R. S., Sharpe, A. H., Trier, J. S., and Fields, B. N. (1981). Intestinal M cells: A pathway for entry of reovirus into the host. *Science* **212,** 471–472.

Xu-Amano, J., Kiyono, H., Jackson, R. J., Staats, H. F., Fujihashi, K., Burrows, P. D., Elson, C. O., Pillai, S., and McGhee, J. R. (1993). Helper T cell subsets for Immunoglobulin A responses: Oral immunization with tetanus toxoid and cholera toxin as adjuvant selectively induces Th2 cells in mucosa associated tissues. *J. Exp. Med.* **178,** 1309–1320.

Yang, D. M., Fairweather, N., Button, L. L., McMaster, W. R., Kahl, L. P., and Liew, F. Y. (1990). Oral *Salmonella typhimurium* (AroA) vaccine expressing a major leishmanial surface protein (gp63) preferentially induces T helper T cells and protective immunity against leishmaniasis. *J. Immunol.* **145,** 2281–2285.

Yang, X., Gieni, R. S., Mosmann, T. R., and Hayglass, K. T. (1993). Chemically modified antigen preferentially elicits induction of Th1-like cytokine synthesis patterns *in vivo*. *J. Exp. Med.* **178,** 349–353.

Yap, K. L., Ada, G. L, and McKenzie, I. F. C. (1978). Transfer of specific cytotoxic T lymphocytes protects mice inoculated with influenza virus. *Nature (London)* **273,** 238–239.

Zinkernagel, R. M., and Doherty, P. C. (1979). MHC-restricted cytotoxic T cells: Studies on the biological role of polymorphic major transplantation antigens determining T-cell restriction-specificity, function, and responsiveness. *Adv. Immunol.* **27,** 51–177.

Zweerink, H. J., Courtneidge, S. A., Skehel, J. J., Crumpton, M. J., and Askonas, B. A. (1977). Cytotoxic T cells kill influenza virus-infected cells but do not distinguish between serologically distinct type A viruses. *Nature (London)* **267,** 354–356.

3

Antigen Uptake by M Cells for Effective Mucosal Vaccines

MARIAN R. NEUTRA
Department of Pediatrics
Harvard Medical School
Children's Hospital
Boston, Massachusetts 02115

JEAN-PIERRE KRAEHENBUHL
Swiss Institute for Experimental Cancer Research
and Institute of Biochemistry
University of Lausanne
CH-1066 Epalinges, Switzerland

I. Introduction

A. Sampling of Antigens across Epithelial Barriers

Antigens and microorganisms on mucosal surfaces of the oral and nasal cavities, and the gastrointestinal, respiratory and genital tracts, are separated from cells of the mucosal immune system by epithelial barriers. For antigens to be processed and presented to the appropriate lymphocytes and to elicit immune responses, they must be transported across these barriers without compromising the integrity of the epithelium. Epithelial barriers on mucosal surfaces at different sites in the body differ dramatically in their cellular organization, and antigen sampling strategies at diverse mucosal sites are adapted accordingly (Fig. 1). In stratified and pseudostratified epithelia, for example, the mucosal immune system sends motile "scouts," the antigen-processing Langerhans cells, to the outer limit of the epithelium where they may directly contact the outside world and obtain samples to carry back to local or distant organized lymphoid tissues. In simple epithelia whose intercellular spaces are sealed by tight junctions, specialized epithelial M cells deliver samples of foreign material by transepithelial transport from the lumen to organized lymphoid tissues within the mucosa.

B. Application to Mucosal Vaccine Design

Design of effective mucosal vaccines requires information about the cellular and molecular mechanisms that operate during sampling of antigens across mucosal barriers, and about the strategies that pathogens use to exploit these sampling systems. Although transepithelial delivery is a prerequisite, it is only a first step. Mucosal vaccine strategies must also take into account the varying fates of specific macromolecules, particles, and microoganisms after entry into mucosal tissues. For example they may be released at M-cell basolateral surfaces and taken up by intra- or subepithelial antigen presenting cells that function in organized mucosal lymphoid tissues, or they may be carried by Langerhans cells to distant inductive sites. In this chapter we will try to synthesize available information about these early events in the induction of immune responses via mucosal surfaces, and will then consider specific mucosal vaccine strategies in the light of our limited knowledge about these events.

II. Antigen Sampling across Stratified Epithelial Barriers

A. Structural and Functional Barriers Created by Stratified Squamous Epithelia

The stratified, nonkeratinized or parakeratinized epithelia of the oral cavity and vagina consist of multilayered cells that are joined only by desmosomes. Although they lack occluding junctions, these epithelia provide a permeability barrier to most solutes by secretion of a "membrane-coating" glycolipoprotein substance into the nar-

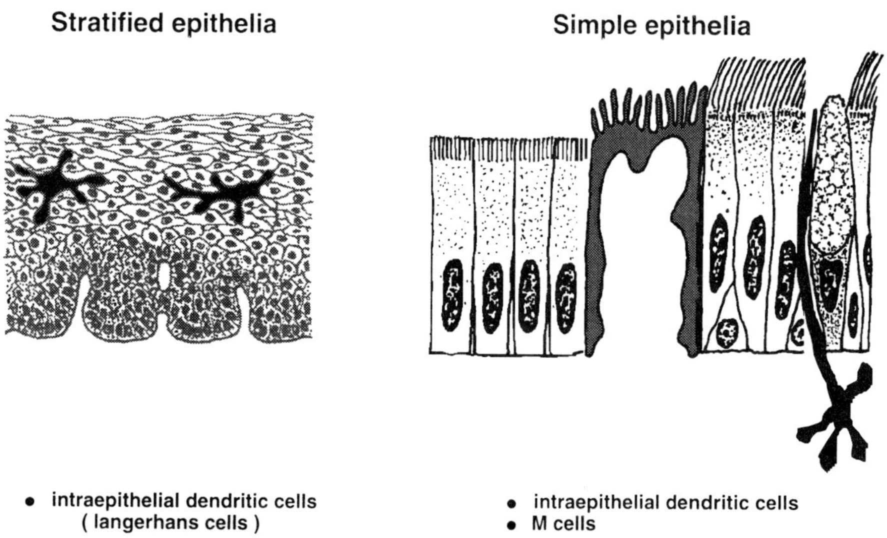

Figure 1. Sampling of antigens at mucosal surfaces is adapted to diverse types of epithelial barriers. Migratory dendritic cells capture antigens throughout the stratified epithelia of the oral cavity and vagina. Simple epithelia of the gastrointestinal tract contain antigen-transporting M cells at specialized local sites. In pseudostratified epithelia of the respiratory tract, both widespread dendritic cells and local M cells function to deliver antigens across the epithelial barrier.

row intercellular spaces of the lower stratified layers. There are many regional variations in the thickness, surface cell phenotypes, and protein expression in stratified squamous epithelia that are determined by interplay of genetic factors with the local environment. In the vagina and exocervix, fluctuations in hormonal signals over the course of the female cycle have dramatic effects on epithelial thickness, endocytic activity of epithelial cells, and turnover of Langerhans cells (Young *et al.*, 1985; Wira *et al.*, 1994). Proteins administered to the luminal surface of the vagina in mice can be taken up by stratified epithelial cells, but such epithelia have no mechanism for directional transcytosis and there is no evidence for vectorial transport across these multicell barriers. It is unlikely that proteins, other macromolecules, or microbes can passively diffuse through the stratified epithelia of the female reproductive tract or the oral cavity. Thus, the immune system obtains samples of intact foreign antigens from these mucosal surfaces through the activities of motile immigrants, the dendritic or Langerhans cells.

B. Role of Dendritic Cells

Dendritic cells are numerous in oral, vaginal, and respiratory epithelia. In the oropharynx, high concentrations of these cells occur in the tonsils (Weinberg *et al.*, 1987), and these could present antigens either locally, in the organized lymphoid tissue of the tonsillar mucosa, or after migration to draining lymph nodes (Okato *et al.*, 1989). Whether the immunological outcome of antigen sampling by dendritic cells and macrophages in organized tonsillar lymphoid tissue differs from the outcome of dendritic cell sampling in the general buccal epithelium is unknown.

The antigen uptake and migratory activities of intraepithelial dendritic (or Langerhans) cells, coupled with their ability to form close associations with T cells (Langhoff and Steinman, 1989), carry a risk of rapid systemic dissemination, particularly of T-cell-tropic viruses that contact mucosal surfaces. Epithelial dendritic cells derived from skin were readily infected after exposure to HIV *in vitro* (Ayehunie *et al.*, 1994; Pope *et al.*, 1994) and comparable cells in intact vaginal tissue of monkeys were found to be infected after mucosal exposure to SIV (Miller *et al.*, 1992a,b). Furthermore, *in vitro* conjugates of dendritic cells and memory T cells showed efficient infection and viral production by the T cells (Ayehunie *et al.*, 1994). Intraepithelial dendritic cells of the vagina are currently thought to be important in transmission of HIV since other transepithelial transport mechanisms such as M cells seem to be absent (Parr and Parr, 1985). Evidence so far predicts that the effectiveness of vaginal vaccines will vary widely, depending on the species, menstrual cycle, and the vaccine or vector used (Parr and Parr, 1994).

III. Antigen Sampling across Simple Epithelia

A. Simple Epithelia Are Semipermeable but Well-Defended

The vast mucosal surfaces of the gastrointestinal tract and airways are lined by a single layer of epithelial cells.

In both systems the epithelial barrier is sealed by tight junctions that are generally effective in excluding peptides and macromolecules with antigenic potential (Madara *et al.*, 1990). The epithelia of the airways, although sealed by tight junctions, have an extensive immune surveillance system similar in some respects to that of stratified epithelia: in upper and lower respiratory tract intraepithelial, dendritic cells form a contiguous network, with up to 700 dendritic cells per mm^2 (Holt *et al.*, 1990). These MHC class II positive cells appear to sample inhaled antigens and migrate rapidly to draining lymph nodes. Their short (average 2 day) residence time in the respiratory mucosa is comparable to that of dendritic cells in the intestinal mucosa (Holt *et al.*, 1994). The bronchi also have an alternative sampling system in the form of lymphoid follicles with overlying epithelium containing M cells (Bienenstock and Clancy, 1994) which share some antigen-transporting characteristics (such as reovirus uptake) with their intestinal counterparts (Morin *et al.*, 1994). However, the relative roles of the dendritic cell network and the organized lymphoid follicles in immune responses to vaccines given by the nasal route are not clear.

Uptake of macromolecules, particulate antigens, and microorganisms across intestinal epithelia can occur only by active transepithelial vesicular transport, and this is restricted by multiple mechanisms including local secretions containing mucins and secretory IgA antibodies (Neutra *et al.*, 1994b), rigid, closely packed microvilli (Mooseker, 1985), and the glycocalyx, a thick (400–500 nm) layer of membrane-anchored glycoproteins (Ito, 1974; Maury *et al.*, 1995). The glycocalyx of enterocytes contains large, negatively charged integral membrane mucin-like molecules (Maury *et al.*, 1995), adsorbed pancreatic enzymes, and stalked glycoprotein enzymes responsible for terminal digestion (Semenza, 1986). It is both a highly degradative microenvironment and a diffusion barrier, impeding the access of macromolecular aggregates, particles, viruses, and bacteria, and preventing direct contact with the microvillus membrane (Amerongen *et al.*, 1991; Apter *et al.*, 1993b; Frey *et al.*, 1996). Although enterocytes can endocytose intact proteins and peptides, most proteins that are taken up are transported to lysosomes. The combined digestive activities of the enterocyte surface and the lysosomes tend to discourage uptake of intact antigens. Nevertheless, enterocytes have been shown to transport small amounts of intact proteins and peptides across the epithelium (Review: Neutra and Kraehenbuhl, 1994), express MHC class I and II (Mayrhofer and Spargo, 1989), and present peptides *in vitro* (Kaiserlian *et al.*, 1989). The role of uptake of antigens by enterocytes in induction of immune responses or immune tolerance *in vivo*, however, is not established.

B. Unique Features of the Follicle-Associated Epithelium (FAE)

The FAE appears to be designed to allow access of antigens and microorganisms to the local epithelial surface and to promote their uptake by transepithelial transport. The cardinal feature of the FAE is the presence of M cells that are joined to their neighbors by tight junctions but provide functional openings in the epithelial barrier through vesicular transport activity (Review: Neutra and Kraehenbuhl, 1992). Restriction of M cells to these sites serves to reduce the inherent risk of transporting foreign material and microbes across the epithelial barrier by assuring immediate exposure to professional phagocytes, other antigen-processing and presenting cells, and the organized inductive machinery of the mucosal immune system.

C. M Cells as Gateways to the Mucosal Immune System

In M cells, unlike most epithelial cells, transepithelial vesicular transport is the major pathway for endocytosed materials (Fig. 2). The M-cell basolateral surface is deeply invaginated to form a large intraepithelial "pocket," a structural modification that shortens the distance from apical to basolateral surface and ensures that transcytosis is rapid and efficient. Transcytosed particles and macromolecules are delivered primarily to the intraepithelial pocket, although we have observed that small

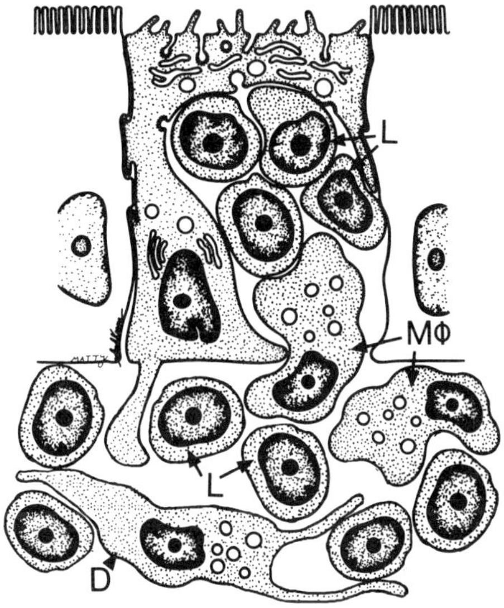

Figure 2. Diagram of an M cell in the follicle-associated epithelium of the intestine. The basolateral surface of the M cell forms an intraepithelial pocket and may send cytoplasmic extensions into the subepithelial tissue. The pocket contains B and T lymphocytes (L) and the occasional macrophage (Mϕ). Under the epithelium are many lymphocytes and macrophages, and a network of dendritic cells (D).

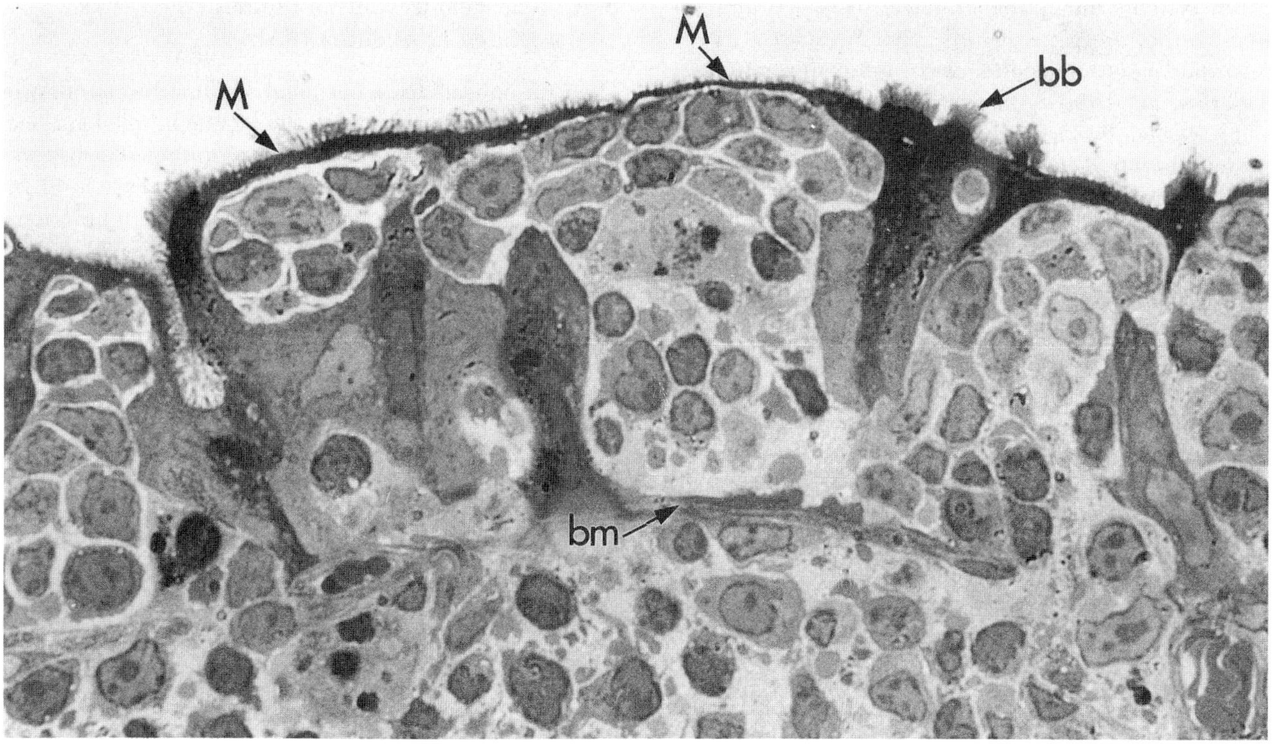

Figure 3. The follicle-associated epithelium in a rabbit Peyer's patch contains many M cells (M), identified by their short, sparse microvilli and thin apical cytoplasm, interspersed with enterocytes, identified by their microvillous brush borders (bb). The intraepithelial pockets formed by contiguous M cells are very large and contain B and T lymphocytes and macrophages (described in Ermak *et al.*, 1990). The basement membrane (bm) is interrupted to accommodate cellular traffic between the intraepithelial pockets and the subepithelial tissue.

amounts of transcytosed lectins can be delivered to lateral and basal surfaces as well (Giannasca *et al.*, 1994). The pocket and its content of immigrant cells allows M cells to be identified in tissue sections.

Multiple types of immigrant cells have been identified in M-cell pockets by immunolabeling of rodent, rabbit, and human Peyer's patches (Ermak and Owen, 1986; Jarry *et al.*, 1989; Ermak *et al.*, 1990; Farstad *et al.*, 1994) (Fig. 3). In all species, both B and T lymphocytes were present along with a small number of macrophages. In mouse, rabbit, and human FAE most of the T cells were $CD4^+$ and none displayed the γ/δ T-cell receptor. In the rabbit, however, some cells were lacking both CD4 and CD8 (Ermak *et al.*, 1990). Human M-cell-associated T cells displayed the marker antigen CD45RO typical of memory cells, although in some specimens naive T cells were observed (Farstad *et al.*, 1994). Most T cells expressed the early activation marker CD69. The B cells, in contrast, expressed the "naive" cell marker CD45RA along with HLA-DR. B memory cells and initial B cell differentiation also may occur here, since the B cells contained IgM plus IgD, or IgM alone, but none had IgG or IgA. Taken together, these observations suggest that T cells can interact with antigen-presenting B cells in the pocket. The fact that the B cells in M cell pockets were phenotypically similar to the subepithelial B cells of the underlying follicle suggested that B-lymphoblast traffic into the M-cell pocket allows continued antigen exposure and extension and diversification of the immune response (Farstad *et al.*, 1994). Much remains to be learned about the complex interactions that occur in the M cell pocket and about the "natural history" of a given epithelial–lymphoid complex over the course of time.

Below the epithelium of the dome lies an extensive network of dendritic cells and macrophages intermingled with $CD4^+$ T and B cells from the underlying follicle (Ermak and Owen 1986; Farstad *et al.*, 1994). These subepithelial cell populations reinforce the idea that M cells serve as gateways to immune inductive sites where endocytosis and killing of incoming pathogens as well as processing, presentation and perhaps storage of antigens occurs. There is very little information available, however, concerning the fates of specific antigens, pathogens and vaccines in the FAE, subepithelial tissue, or follicle. Viruses and bacteria that use the M cell as an invasion route can infect and destroy M cells and local macrophages, as discussed below.

IV. M-Cell Organization and Function

A. The M-Cell Apical Surface

The M-cell apical surface differs from that of intestinal absorptive cells in the increased accessibility of the plasma membrane, especially the apical membrane endocytic domains that function in endocytosis of macromolecules, particles and microbes (Neutra *et al.*, 1988). Most M cells in Peyer's patches lack the highly organized brush border typical of enterocytes, and the distribution of the actin-associated protein villin in M cells is clearly different from that of absorptive cells (Kerneis *et al.*, 1995), reflecting the modified microvillar organization and perhaps the ability to rapidly respond to adherence of microorganisms with ruffling and phagocytosis.

Apical surface components unique to M cells could be useful in M-cell identification and isolation as well as for targeting of vaccines. While enterocyte brush borders have abundant alkaline phosphatase, this enzyme is often (but not always) reduced or absent on M cells (Owen and Bhalla, 1983; Smith *et al.*, 1988). M cells lack the uniform thick glycocalyx seen on enterocytes, but their apical membranes do display abundant glycoconjugates in a cell coat that varies widely in thickness and density (Bye *et al.*, 1984). Recently it has become clear that M cells have specific glycosylation patterns that distinguish them from their epithelial neighbors. In Peyer's patches of BALB/c mice, lectins (UEA I and WBA II) that recognize a range of carbohydrate structures containing α(1-2)-fucose selectively stained all M cells in the FAE (Clark *et al.*, 1993; Falk *et al.*, 1994; Giannasca *et al.*, 1994). Giannasca *et al.* (1994) observed these lectin-binding sites not only on M-cell apical membranes but also on intracellular vesicles and basolateral membranes, including the pocket domain. Lectin staining of M-cell basolateral membranes further revealed that M cells have basal processes that extend 10 μm or more into the underlying lymphoid tissue. If these extensions make direct contact with lymphoid or antigen-presenting cells in the subepithelial tissue, they might play a role in the induction of the unique M-cell phenotype, or in the processing and presentation of antigens after M-cell transport. Lectin labeling also revealed cells with M-cell-like glycosylation patterns on the follicle-facing walls of the lymphoid follicle-associated crypts; these may represent differentiating M cells. Lectin and antibody probes have also revealed variations in the glycosylation patterns of individual M cells within a single FAE. This diversity might expand the possible microbial lectin–M-cell surface carbohydrate interactions of the local M-cell population and allow the M cells to "sample" a wider variety of microorganisms (Giannasca *et al.*, 1994; Neutra *et al.*, 1994a).

It is important to note that glycoconjugates expressed on M cells in other intestinal regions (cecum, appendix, colon, and rectum), in other mouse strains, and in other species are distinct from those in BALB/c mouse Peyer's patches. This finding has been reported in mouse and rabbit (Gebert and Hach, 1993; Falk *et al.*, 1994; Giannasca *et al.*, 1994; Jepson *et al.*, 1993) and has also been observed by us in monkey and human (K. T. Giannasca, P. J. Giannasca, F. Zhou, and M. R. Neutra, unpublished observations). Regional differences in M-cell surfaces must be taken into account when designing mucosal vaccines for region-specific pathogens, and for administration to different mucosal surfaces. For example, lymphoid follicles with M cells are particularly numerous in the distal colonic and rectal mucosa of humans (Langman and Rowland, 1986; O'Leary and Sweeney, 1986) and the surface characteristics of these M cells are relevant to future design of mucosal vaccines against HIV and other sexually transmitted diseases.

B. Endocytosis and Transcytosis

M cells take up macromolecules, particles and microorganisms by adsorptive endocytosis via clathrin-coated pits and vesicles (Neutra *et al.*, 1987; Sicinski *et al.*, 1990), fluid-phase endocytosis (Bockman and Cooper, 1973; Owen, 1977), and phagocytosis involving extension of cellular processes and reorganization of submembrane actin assemblies (Jones *et al.*, 1994; Neutra *et al.*, 1994a). All of these uptake mechanisms result in transport of foreign material into endosomal tubules and vesicles and large multivesicular bodies that lie apically, between the apical membrane and the intraepithelial pocket (Neutra and Kraehenbuhl, 1992). The large vesicles contain the late endosome/lysosome membrane marker lgp120 and generate an acidic internal milieu (Allan *et al.*, 1993). Immunocytochemical analysis revealed the presense of an endosomal protease, cathepsin E in rabbit M cells (Finzi *et al.*, 1993) but the possible presence of other endosomal hydrolases in M-cell transport vesicles has not yet been examined. MHC class II antigens on M-cell membranes have been documented in subpopulations of M cells of some species (Allan *et al.*, 1993). Because of the complexity of these tissues and the lack of an *in vitro* M-cell system, however, it is not yet known to what extent endocytosed materials are degraded during transepithelial transport, or whether M cells participate in the processing and presentation of antigens.

Adherent macromolecules or particles bound to the apical plasma membranes of M cells are efficiently endocytosed or phagocytosed (Neutra *et al.*, 1987). It follows that pathogens or vaccines that can bind selectively to M cells would be most effective in mucosal invasion and induction of mucosal immune responses; this assumption underlies many of the current approaches to vaccine design discussed below. Macromolecules and particles that are endocytosed by M cells can be released at the pocket membrane as rapidly as 10–15 min later. Rapid binding and uptake of polystyrene or latex beads that adhere to M cells (Pappo and Ermak, 1989), along with the lectin binding studies described above, suggest that particles or microorganisms with hydrophobic surfaces as well as those with appropriate lectin-like adhesins could interact with M-cell surfaces. Lectins that fail to recognize mucins and other cells could be highly M-cell-selective, whereas hydrophobic particles would also interact with mucus and the glycocalyx of enterocytes on villi, and this would tend to reduce the efficiency of M-cell uptake.

V. Differentiaton of the FAE and M Cells

At sites of organized mucosal lymphoid tissue such as Peyer's patches, a ring of follicle-associated crypts (FACs) surrounds each lymphoid follicle. A typical FAC contributes cells to a villus on one side and to the dome-shaped FAE on the other. Even deep in the crypt, the epithelium on the wall facing the follicle possesses features that distinguish it from the common absorptive epithelium, such as a total lack of polymeric immunoglobulin receptors (Pappo and Owen, 1988). The origin of M cells, however, has been the subject of debate. On the one hand, there is evidence that M cells represent a distinct lineage that arises from undifferentiated cells in the follicle-associated crypts (Bye *et al.*, 1984). This is supported by the fact that in mice UEA I stains membranes of all Peyer's patch M cells and also stains cells on the wall of the crypt facing the follicle, immediately above the stem cell zone, but not on the opposite crypt wall (Giannasca *et al.*, 1994). In the upper crypt these UEA-positive cells acquired an intraepithelial pocket, a key feature of M cells. In rabbits, M cells are the only epithelial cell type that express the intermediate filament protein vimentin, and vimentin-positive cells appear in the crypts that supply cells to the FAE (Gebert *et al.*, 1992; Jepson *et al.*, 1992). These observations suggest that M cells, like all of the other cell lineages in the intestinal epithelium (Gordon and Hermiston, 1994), are derived from undifferentiated crypt cells and become committed early to the M-cell phenotype. Reconstitution studies in scid mice (Savidge and Smith, 1995), as well as experiments involving injection of Peyer's patch mononuclear cells into normal mucosa (Kerneis *et al.*, 1995), strongly indicate that cell contacts and/or diffusable factors from the subjacent lymphoid follicle act on the epithelium to induce the differentiation of FAE including M cells.

On the other hand, it is also possible that new M cells can be formed rapidly on the surface of the dome, by modification of fully differentiated enterocytes in the FAE. Numbers of M cells increase, for example, after exposure of the rodent Peyer's patch mucosa to the invasive pathogen *Salmonella* (Savidge *et al.*, 1991). Appearance of additional M cells can be rapid (C. Nicoletti, personal communication), and this would rule out the participation of crypt cells. Cells that have both M-cell features (short, irregular microvilli) and enterocyte features (no pocket, low levels of apical membrane enzymes) are observed in the FAE; these features could represent transitional forms (Finzi *et al.*, 1993). Indeed, intestinal epithelial phenotypes arise from common precursors and show considerable plasticity in differentiation pathways (Gordon and Hermiston, 1994). M-cell differentiation may be influenced indirectly by events such as bacterial colonization or invasion that result in epithelial cell signal transduction events (Pace *et al.*, 1993; Eckmann *et al.*, 1995) which in turn invoke influx of subepithelial lymphoid cells. Subepithelial or intraepithelial lymphoid cells could then induce conversion of local enterocytes to the M-cell phenotype, and/or differentiation of M cells in adjacent crypts. Whether live, attenuated vaccine vectors can trigger such events has not been explored.

VI. Interactions of Microorganisms with M Cells

M cell recognition and transport mechanisms carry the risk of infection and disease since they can result in transport of microorganisms that initiate mucosal and/or systemic disease by crossing the epithelial barrier. The exploitation of M-cell transport by viral and bacterial pathogens has been reviewed extensively (Neutra *et al.*, 1994) and will be summarized briefly. The wide range of gram-negative bacteria that bind selectively to M cells includes *Vibrio cholerae* (Owen *et al.*, 1986; Winner *et al.*, 1991; Neutra *et al.*, 1994), some strains of *Escherichia coli* (Inman and Cantey, 1983; Uchida, 1987), *Salmonella typhi* (Kohbata *et al.*, 1986), *Salmonella typhimurium* (Jones *et al.*, 1994), *Shigella flexneri* (Wassef *et al.*, 1989), *Yersinia enterocolitica* (Grutzkau *et al.*, 1990), *Yersinia pseudotuberculosis* (Fujimura *et al.*, 1992), and *Campylobacter jejuni* (Walker *et al.*, 1988). Viruses that use M cells as a route of entry include reovirus (Wolf *et al.*, 1981), poliovirus (Sicinski *et al.*, 1990), and possibly HIV (Amerongen *et al.*, 1991). Due to the lack of stable M-cell culture systems, analysis of microbial–M-cell interactions has been limited to morphological studies. The ultrastructural appearance of various bacterial–M-cell interaction sites suggests that a variety of molecular mechanisms may be at play (Neutra *et al.*, 1994). It is likely that M-cell adherence and uptake involves a sequence of molecular interactions including initial recognition (perhaps via a lectin–carbohydrate interaction) followed by more intimate associations that could require expression of additional bacterial genes, processing of M-cell surface molecules, activation of intracellular signalling pathways, and recruitment of integral or submembrane M-cell proteins to the interaction site.

VII. M Cells and Mucosal Vaccine Strategies

It has been difficult to predict the outcomes of new mucosal immunization strategies in advance because they depend on many factors, including survival or degradation of the vaccine or vector in mucosal environments (such as the digestive tract), interactions with nonspecific mucosal protection mechanisms, efficiency of M-cell uptake, interactions with multiple cells in organized mucosal lymphoid tissues, and spread to distant lymphoid and other organs. In this section we will examine diverse types of mucosal vaccines currently under investigation in light of these factors, with a focus on M-cell transport.

A. Macromolecular Complexes for Enhancement of M-Cell Uptake

1. *Cholera Toxin B Subunit*

Cholera toxin is well-adapted to the GI tract; it is acid-stable, is not bound by mucins, and uses as receptor a glycolipid (ganglioside G_{M1}) present in high concentrations on intestinal epithelial cell surfaces. Cholera toxin tagged with fluorescent rhodamine or visualized with immunoperoxidase histochemistry adhered to both M-cell and enterocyte apical surfaces on both FAE and villi, and was rapidly transported by M cells into underlying lymphoid tissue. The fact that cholera holotoxin is taken up via M cells into Peyer's patches, the sites of T-cell helper responses and B-cell IgA switch, may explain in part its unique effectiveness as a mucosal antigen and adjuvant (Nedrud and Lamm, 1991). CT also interacts with its receptor on enterocytes, is endocytosed and transcytosed across the villus epithelium (Lencer *et al.*, 1995), and can activate signal transduction pathways in villus epithelial as well as subepithelial cells. Thus, both M-cell and enterocyte uptake could be responsible for the complex immunologic effects of CT observed *in vivo*.

CT-B subunit, the nontoxic pentameric portion of the toxin responsible for binding to G_{M1}, was also found to enhance mucosal immune responses when coupled directly to antigen. This response is thought to be due in part to the ability of CT-B to enhance mucosal adherence and uptake (Dertzbaugh and Elson, 1991). In most studies, however, the possible presense of trace amounts of holotoxin was not ruled out, and recently it was demonstrated that antigens coupled to recombinant CT-B (assuring a total absense of holotoxin) induced systemic tolerance (Sun *et al.*, 1994).

To separate the immunologic effects of M-cell uptake from the effects of widespread transport by enterocytes would require a method for targeting of CT or CT-B–antigen complexes exclusively to M cells. EM studies showed that cholera toxin or its B subunit adsorbed to colloidal gold particles lost the ability to bind to enterocyte brush borders (presumably due to the diffusion barrier created by the thick enterocyte glycocalyx) but still adhered to a subpopulation of M cells (Frey *et al.*, 1996). This suggested that adding CT-B to the surfaces of particulate vaccine vectors or carriers (such as copolymer microspheres) would enhance M-cell transport and possibly the uptake of the vaccine by underlying macrophages. Studies in our laboratories have tested this idea by examining the ability of CT-B to adhere to M cells when immobilized on the surfaces of particles of two disparate sizes, 14 nm and 1 μm. Whereas CT-B on 14-nm colloidal gold adhered to M cells, CT-B-coated, fluorescent 1-μm latex microparticles failed to adhere either to enterocytes or to M cells. The inability of 1-μm particles to bind to M cells via the glycolipid receptor was shown to be due to the molecular barrier to large particles provided by the M-cell glycocalyx (Frey *et al.*, 1996). Thus, the M-cell targeting ability of CT-B may be limited to relatively small macromolecular complexes or particles. This has important implications for its use in targeting of oral vaccines to the mucosal immune system.

2. *Lectins*

As described above, M cells display cell-specific complex carbohydrates that could theoretically serve as receptors for mucosal vaccines. Lectins infused into the intestinal or colonic lumens or fed orally to mice showed specific surface labeling of M cells as well as endocytosis of lectin and transport into the M-cell pockets, followed by entry of lectin into subepithelial cells (Giannasca *et al.*, 1994). The uptake of lectin exclusively by M cells suggests that lectins could be conjugated to immunogens and administered as oral or rectal vaccines. The use of lectins for vaccine targeting is complicated by several factors, however. The observed variations in glycosylation patterns among species and among inbred mouse strains suggest that "outbred" humans will show much individual variation. Also, secreted mucins often mimic local epithelial cell surfaces, and mucins would be expected to efficiently bind and eliminate lectin-based vaccines. In addition, certain lectins that bind to enterocyte microvilli cause vesiculation and damage of the brush border (Weinman *et al.*, 1989). Thus lectin–M-cell interaction may be more useful as an experimental tool for elucidating the mechanisms of microbial adherence to M cells (Giannasca *et al.*, 1996).

3. *IgA Immune Complexes*

Although the FAE does not participate in receptor-mediated secretion of IgA, secretory IgA (S-IgA) in the lumen can adhere selectively to the apical membranes of M cells. This was first observed in suckling rabbits as a local accumulation of milk S-IgA on M cells of Peyer's patches, and was thought to play a role in maturation of the mucosal immune system (Roy and Varvayanis, 1987). We subsequently showed that monoclonal IgA or IgA–antigen complexes, as well as polyclonal secretory IgA, adhered to M cells and were transported into the intraepithelial pocket (Weltzin *et al.*, 1989). Uptake of IgA–antigen complexes by M cells could result in repeated uptake of antigen into inductive sites. Antigens complexed with S-IgA might be sampled by intraepithelial or subepithelial antigen-presenting cells to boost an existing secretory immune response to pathogens that have not been effectively cleared from the lumen by S-IgA. Although it seems paradoxical, IgA may serve as a vaccine-targeting strategy.

We have tested this idea using two strategies. IgA-coated liposomes containing ferritin as test antigen were constructed for mucosal immunization via the rectum (Zhou *et al.*, 1995). A colonic/rectal IgA response to liposomal ferritin without IgA was detected when the liposomes were given with free CT as adjuvant. The addition of IgA to the liposome surface enhanced the local rectal/colonic uptake of liposomes into Peyer's patch mucosa and enhanced the secretory immune response to ferritin about fivefold over uncoated liposomes. These results revealed that IgA can enhance the local secretory immune response to antigen in liposomes, apparently by increasing liposome uptake via M cells.

The second strategy was based on the observation that oral administration of secretory IgA can trigger a mucosal immune response against both IgA and secretory component (s.c.). This suggested that it might be possible to use genetically engineered IgA or s.c. to target protective foreign epitopes into mucosal lymphoid tissue. To test this concept we first identified potential insertion sites at the surface of s.c. by mapping the binding site of an anti-s.c. antibody to an exposed loop in the first immunoglogulin-like domain. We then replaced this endogenous epitope with a 10-amino acid linear epitope from the invasin (Ipa B) of *S. flexneri*. The "antigenized" s.c. was recognized by an invasin-specific monoclonal antibody, and when injected intraperitoneally it evoked a systemic immune response that included antibodies against invasin (M. Kaufmann, M. C. Peitsch, A. Phalipon, J. P. Kraehenbuhl, and B. Corthesy, unpublished data). The "antigenized" s.c. was also able to bind dimeric IgA, suggesting that it could be administered mucosally as S-IgA to deliver foreign, protective epitopes to the mucosal immune system.

B. Attenuated Viruses and Viral Vectors

Relatively little is known about selective transport of viruses by M cells or the role of M cells in invasion of viral pathogens. To date, M-cell adherence and transport have been documented for only three viruses, and in no case have the interacting viral and M-cell surface molecules responsible for these interactions been identified. The pathogenic viruses that adhere selectively to M cells could potentially provide information about unique features of the M-cell apical membrane and could be exploited to design M-cell-targeted vaccines.

The best-known example of M-cell-specific adherence and exploitation of M-cell transport is the mouse pathogen, reovirus (Wolf *et al.*, 1981; Bass *et al.*, 1988). Reovirus is well adapted to the degradative intestinal environment; indeed, processing of reovirus by proteases in the intestinal lumen increases viral infectivity through cleavage of the major outer capsid protein sigma 3 and a conformational change resulting in extension of the viral hemagglutinin sigma 1 (Nibert *et al.*, 1991). Studies in our laboratory showed that proteolytic processing of the outer capsid is also required for M-cell adherence (Amerongen *et al.*, 1994) and it follows that either the protease-resistant outer capsid protein μ1c or the extended σ1 protein is used to bind to M cells. It should be noted that reovirus recognizes mouse M cells not only in the Peyer's patches but also in the colon (Owen *et al.*, 1990) and the airways (Morin *et al.*, 1994), and that reovirus binds to rabbit as well as mouse M cells. Although the use of reovirus as a vaccine vector is not practical, the reoviral adhesins, once identified, could potentially serve to design molecular ligands for selective M-cell binding.

Poliovirus, in contrast, has recently been shown to be potentially valuable as a live vaccine vector, as described elsewhere in this book. The molecular structure and pathogenesis of poliovirus in humans show some intriguing parallels with reovirus in mice. For instance, poliovirus enters the body by the oral route, and proliferates in Peyer's patches before spreading systemically (Bodian, 1955). Poliovirus type 1 and the attenuated Sabin strain were shown to selectively adhere to human M cells, and to be taken up in clathrin-coated vesicles (Sicinski *et al.*, 1990). The fact that poliovirus exploits M-cell transport to cross the epithelial barrier greatly enhances its potential importance as an oral vaccine vector for delivery of foreign antigens in humans, either as live recombinant viral particles (Choi *et al.*, 1991) or as inert virus-like particles (Ansardi *et al.*, 1991). Furthermore, poliovirus can stimulate mucosal immune responses after administration via diverse mucosal routes (Ogra and Karzon, 1969). The receptor for poliovirus on neuronal target cell membranes has been identified as a member of the immunoglobulin superfamily, and the cloned gene has been used to create transgenic mice that can be infected by injection of virus (Mendelsohn *et al.*, 1989). Such mice are not infected when challenged orally, however (V. R. Racaniello, personal communication); thus the receptor that poliovirus exploits to adhere to M cells remains unidentified.

C. Attenuated Bacteria and Bacterial Vectors

1. *Vibrio Cholerae*

Among the gram-negative pathogens that adhere to M cells, *V. cholerae* is a particularly attractive candidate for mucosal vaccine strategies since it is efficiently transported by M cells but is not equipped to survive in the mucosa or spread systemically. Within the small intestine, *V. cholerae* express a group of coregulated proteins including adhesins which allow them to adhere to epithelia of the proximal small intestine, pili which stabilize colonies on mucosal surfaces, and cholera toxin which induces secretion of chloride ions from intestinal epithelial cells (Herrington *et al.*, 1988; Miller *et al.*, 1989). We have shown that M-cell transport plays a key role in the induction of specific IgA lymphoblasts in Peyer's patches (Winner *et al.*, 1991; Apter *et al.*, 1993a) and presumably is important in the natural immune response to *Vibrio* and toxin.

Colonization of the small intestinal surface by wild-type *V. cholerae* (which causes toxin-induced diarrhea) is accompanied by M-cell adherence (Owen *et al.*, 1986). However, colonization of the mucosal surface with attenuated vaccine strains can also cause mild symptoms even in the absense of toxin production (Mekalanos, 1992). For optimal immune responses without the attendant reactogenicity, a mutant *Vibrio* that adheres only to M cells would be ideal; this would require a mutant strain unable to colonize enterocytes, but retaining the ability to adhere to M cells. When *V. cholerae* were inoculated into ligated intestinal loops containing Peyer's patches in rabbits or mice, the bacteria were seen to selectively interact with M cells at early times (Owen *et al.*, 1986; Winner *et al.*, 1991). Owen *et al.* (1986) observed that after binding of *V. cholerae* to rabbit M cells, pseudopod-like cell surface processes surrounded the organisms and formed phagocytic vesicles by which *Vibrios* were transported and released into the M-cell pocket. We observed that this process involves close interaction of the bacterial outer membrane with the M-cell apical membrane and assembly of M-cell submembrane actin filaments, suggesting participation of integral membrane components on both sides (Winner *et al.*, 1991; Neutra *et al.*, 1994). These events imply that close contact between *Vibrios* and host cell membranes is a prerquisite for transduction of the intracellular signals responsible for phagocytosis. In contrast, *Vibrios* that adhere to enterocytes on villi remain attached to the periphery of the enterocyte glycocalyx, never make close contact with enterocyte plasma membranes, and do not induce cytoskeletal changes or phagocytosis, but use secreted toxin to induce the epithelial secretory response. Initial adherence to M cells requires live bacteria but does not require live host epithelial cells (Yamamoto *et al.*, 1988; Yamamoto and Yokota, 1989); fixation of host mucosa eliminated the M-cell responses to bacterial binding such as reorganization of apical membrane and cytoskeleton, but still *V. cholerae* adhered to the surfaces of M cells with greater efficiency than to other epithelial cells. This implies that M cells constitutively display surface receptors which are either unique or more accessible than on enterocytes. General colonization of the mucosal surface may increase M-cell adherence and uptake incidentally, by increasing the numbers of *Vibrios* in the local vicinity of Peyer's patches.

2. *Salmonella*

The pathogenesis of *S. typhimurium* in mice following ingestion of bacteria involves the development of initial foci of infection in small intestinal Peyer's patches (Carter and Collins, 1974; Hohmann *et al.*, 1978). *Salmonella typhi* and *S. typhimurium* can also invade directly through the absorptive villus epithelium (Takeuchi, 1967), but it is presumably its ability to rapidly enter and proliferate in organized mucosal lymphoid tissues that makes it a powerful mucosal pathogen and immunogen. M cells show a dramatic response to *Salmonella* infection. Kohbata *et al.* (1986) observed that within 30 min, *S. typhi* selectively adhered to the surfaces of M cells and induced "ballooning" of the M-cell apical surface followed by degeneration and loss of M cells which allowed the bacteria access to the underlying mucosa. *Salmonella typhimurium* produced similar cytopathic effects in mice (Jones *et al.*, 1994) but not in rabbits (Neutra *et al.*, 1994). The probable mechanism of this effect on M cells may be extrapolated from studies utilizing cultured intestinal cell lines in which invasion is accompanied by local cytoplasmic Ca^{2+} spikes, cytoskeletal rearrangements, and membrane ruffling (Bliska *et al.*, 1993; Rosenshine and Finlay, 1993). Invasion of enterocytes occurs later, after entry via M cells, perhaps because processing of brush border surface receptors is required. Uptake of wild type *S. typhi* and *S. typhimurium* leads to the destruction of the M cell itself.

The ability of *S. typhi* to adhere to M cells and to target themselves into Peyer's patches has been exploited in the use of attenuated strains as oral vaccines against typhoid fever (Levine *et al.*, 1990). Various genetically engineered *S. typhi* and *S. typhimurium* strains are currently being developed and tested as vectors for expression of foreign antigens in mucosal inductive sites and other organs, as described elsewhere in this volume. One of the challenges in this strategy has been achieving sufficient attenuation while still preserving M-cell adherence and sufficient proliferation in mucosal cells to provide vigorous and long-lasting immunity.

In a recent study, a live attenuated *Salmonella* vaccine expressing the gene for the core and surface antigens of hepatitis B virus was administered to mice by four different routes: oral, nasal, rectal, and vaginal (Hopkins *et al.*, 1995). By all routes, the vaccine elicited both local and systemic antibody responses against the foreign antigen as well as the vaccine carrier. The attenuated *S. typhimurium* recombinant strain was recovered in the draining lymph nodes, spleen, and mucosa-associated lymphoid tissues. This indicates that *Salmonella* can gain access to inductive sites for mucosal and systemic immune responses across both simple and stratified epithelia. The response after vaginal immunization was correlated with the stage of the estrus cycle and the abundance of Langerhans cells. Thus, it is possible that these immune responses involved interaction of the *Salmonella* vector with intraepithelial dendritic cells in vagina and airways, as well as M cells and antigen-presenting cells in organized mucosal lymphoid tissues of the nasopharynx and GI tract.

3. *Shigella*

Shigella infects cells by adhering to the plasma membrane, inducing phagocytosis, and then disrupting the phagosome membrane to enter the host cell cytoplasm. Once within the cytoplasm the bacteria proliferate, induce assembly of a "tail" of actin filaments, and are extruded in a cytoplasmic process which is phagocytosed by the neighboring cell (Sansonetti, 1991). Studies using polarized monolayers of intestinal enterocytes *in vitro* have shown that *Shigella flexneri* is unable to invade via the apical surfaces of enterocytes (Mounier *et al.*, 1992) but releases chemotactic signals that attract inflammatory cells (Perdomo *et al.*, 1994a). *In vivo*, pathogenic as well as selected nonpathogenic strains of *Shigella* adhered selectively to M cells (Wassef *et al.*, 1989). Transport via M cells allows *Shigella* access to basolateral membranes of both M cells and enterocytes as well as underlying macrophages, all of which may then be invaded (Perdomo *et al.*, 1994b). The resulting release of cytokines and inflammatory response results in shedding of epithelial cells, ulcerations in the FAE, and further entry of bacteria (Perdomo *et al.*, 1994b). In humans, mucosal ulcerations typically found in *Shigella* infections are most frequent in the colon and ileum, sites where lymphoid follicles and M cells are relatively numerous.

Several of the genes and gene products used by *Shigella* to accomplish its elaborate strategy of infection and spread have been identified (Sansonetti, 1991). Attenuated *Shigella* strains lacking key genes are attractive candidates as mucosal vaccines against *Shigella* itself, or as vaccine vectors for targeting expression of foreign antigens to mucosal lymphoid tissues. Such strains should ideally be able to bind to M cells of the ileum or colon, be delivered across the epithelium, and be readily phagocytosed and killed by macrophages either before or after entering the cytoplasm. If they retain the membrane lysin that allows cytoplasmic entry, they should lack the ability to subvert the host cell cytoskeletal machinery for cell–cell spread. Such mutants are currently being designed and are described elsewhere in this volume. A key safety issue for mucosal use of live *Shigella* vaccines may be the possible local release of cytokines and neutrophil chemotactic factors in response to *Shigella* entry, which might cause breakdown of normal epithelial barrier function.

4. *Yersinia*

Certain *Yersinia* species can invade the mammalian intestinal mucosa and cause enteritis and lymphadenitis. The mechanism of attachment of *Yersinia* to intestinal epithelial cells is unknown, but these bacteria bind preferentially to M cells and use the FAE as a route of invasion (Grutzkau *et al.*, 1990). *Yersinia* expresses several virulence factors (Cornelis, 1994), including invasin and the products of the yadA gene, both of which bind to host cell $\beta 1$ integrins (Isberg and Leong, 1988). Although expression of invasin is associated with infection of Peyer's patches (Pepe and Miller, 1993), it is not known whether invasin actually mediates M-cell adherence since integrins are generally confined to the basolateral membrane of epithelial cells (Hynes, 1992). It is possible that invasin interacts with a component of the M-cell membrane, but not via the integrin-binding domain (Bliska *et al.*, 1993). Like *Salmonella*, binding of *Yersinia* to M cells induces apical cytoplasmic disorganization, alteration of the actin network, phagocytosis, and M-cell damage. Studies on cultured cells have shown that *Yersinia*, like *Shigella* and *Salmonella*, injects into the host cell cytoplasm a tyrosine kinase, the YopE protein (Sory and Cornelis, 1994) that activates the host cell kinase pFAK, and small G proteins Rho and Rac, mediators that are capable of inducing cytoskeletal changes (Cornelis, 1994).

Yersinia has been genetically engineered for use as a potential vector for delivery of foreign antigens, including CT and the *Trypanosoma cruzi* CRA gene product, to the mucosal immune system (Sory *et al.*, 1990, 1992; Van Damme *et al.*, 1992). The ability of *Yersinia* to inject antigens fused to YopE into the host cell cytoplasm (Sory and Cornelis, 1994) could theoretically be useful in induction of cellular immune responses. On the other hand, the pathologic effects of *Yersinia* on host cells and its inflammatory effects in the intestinal mucosa may complicate its use as a mucosal vaccine vector.

5. *BCG*

Mycobacteria also exhibit selective M-cell adherence and transcytosis. *Mycobacterium paratuberculosis,* inoculated into ligated ileal loops of calves, entered organized mucosal lymphoid tissues where they accumulated in macrophages (Momotani *et al.*, 1988). An EM study demonstrated that rabbit M cells efficiently transport BCG (Bacillus Calmette-Guerin) into mucosal lymphoid tissue (Fujimura *et al.*, 1986). This is consistent with an early finding in intestinal tuberculosis where lymphoid follicles were identified as the origin of infection. The observed adherence and transport of BCG by M cells lend support to the development of recombinant BCG as a vehicle for expression of foreign antigens in mucosal inductive sites of the respiratory tract (Langermann *et al.*, 1994). Infection of dendritic cells of the lung by BCG (Pancholi *et al.*, 1993) could also play a role. Recent work showing that this vector can serve as an effective vaccine after intranasal delivery is described in another chapter.

VIII. Conclusions

The observations on M-cell biology and the interactions of microorganisms with M cells offered in this chapter are relevant to targeting of attenuated bacterial vaccine strains, live viral and bacterial vectors containing recombinant proteins or genes, and nonliving, particulate immunogens to the mucosal immune system. Information about the specific molecular recognition systems and nonspecific adherence mechanisms that underlie these phenomena is still lacking, however.

In spite of many attempts to rationally design mucosal vaccines that can cross epithelial barriers, much of their development involves trial and error. This is inevitable as long as the mechanisms of M-cell recognition, the nature of the environment on local mucosal surfaces, and the exact fates of specific vaccines, vectors, or foreign gene products in mucosal lymphoid tissue are unknown. Such information will be gained through detailed studies of many specific mucosal vaccines at the tissue, cellular, and molecular levels. As each research group concentrates on its own approach, there will be an increasing need for interlaboratory exchange of materials and head-to-head comparisons of different mucosal vaccines that are designed to elicit protective immune responses.

Acknowledgments

We are grateful to the current and former members of our laboratory that have contributed to the work summarized in this chapter. The authors are supported by NIH Research Grants HD17557 and AI34757 and NIH Center Grant DK34854 to the Harvard Digestive Diseases Center (M.R.N), and Swiss National Science Foundation Grant 31.37155.93 and Swiss League against Cancer Grant 373.89.2 (J.P.K).

References

Allan, C. H., Mendrick, D. L., and Trier, J. S. (1993). Rat intestinal M cells contain acidic endosomal-lysosomal compartments and express Class II major histocompatibility complex determinants. *Gastroenterology* **104,** 698–708.

Amerongen, H. M., Weltzin, R. A., Farnet, C. M., Michetti, P., Haseltine, W. A., and Neutra, M. R. (1991). Transepithelial transport of HIV-1 by intestinal M cells: A mechanism for transmission of AIDS. *J. Acquired Immune Defic. Syndr.* **4,** 760–765.

Amerongen, H. M., Wilson, G. A. R., Fields, B. N., and Neutra, M. R. (1994). Proteolytic processing of reovirus is required for adherence to intestinal M cells. *J. Virol.* **68,** 8428–8432.

Ansardi, D. C., Porter, D. C., and Morrow, C. D. (1991). Coinfection with recombinant vaccinia viruses expressing poliovirus P1 and P3 proteins results in polyprotein processing and formation of empty capsid structures. *J. Virol.* **65,** 2088–2092.

Apter, F. M., Lencer, W. I., Finkelstein, R. A., Mekalanos, J. J., and Neutra, M. R. (1993a). Monoclonal IgA antibodies directed against cholera toxin B subunit prevent the toxin-induced chloride secretory response and block toxin binding to epithelial cells *in vitro. Infect. Immun.* **61,** 5271–5278.

Apter, F. M., Michetti, P., Winner III, L. S., Mack, J. A., Mekalanos, J. J., and Neutra, M. R. (1993b). Analysis of the roles of anti-lipopolysaccharide and anti-cholera toxin IgA antibodies in protection against *Vibrio cholerae* and cholera toxin using monoclonal IgA antibodies *in vivo. Infect. Immun.* **61,** 5279–5285.

Ayehunie, S., Bruzzese, A. M., Groves, R. W., Kupper, T. S., and Langhoff, E. (1994). HIV-1 transmission by mucosal Langerhans cells, blood dendritic cells, and monocytes *in vitro. Regional Immunol.* **6,** 105–111.

Bass, D. M., Trier, J. S., Dambrauskas, R., and Wolf, J. L. (1988). Reovirus type 1 infection of small intestinal epithelium in suckling mice and its effect on M cells. *Lab. Invest.* **55,** 226–235.

Bienenstock, J., and Clancy, R. (1994). Bronchial mucosal lymphoid tissue. *In* "Handbook of Mucosal Immunology." (P. L. Ogra, J. Mestecky, M. E. Lamm, W. Strober, J. R. McGhee, and J. Bienenstock, eds.), pp. 529–538. Academic Press, San Diego.

Bliska, J. B., Galan, J. E., and Falkow, S. (1993). Signal transduction in the mammalian cell during bacterial attachment and entry. *Cell (Cambridge, Mass.)* **73,** 903–920.

Bockman, D. E., and Cooper, M. D. (1973). Pinocytosis by epithelium associated with lymphoid follicles in the bursa of Fabricius, appendix, and Peyer's patches. An electron microscopic study. *Am. J. Anat.* **136,** 455–478.

Bodian, D. (1955). Emerging concept of poliovirus infection. *Science* **122,** 105–108.

Bye, W. A., Allan, C. H., and Trier, J. S. (1984). Structure, distribution and origin of M cells in Peyer's patches of mouse ileum. *Gastroenterology* **86,** 789–801.

Carter, P. B., and Collins, F. M. (1974). The route of enteric infection in normal mice. *J. Exp. Med.* **139,** 1189–1203.

Choi, W. S., Pal-Ghosh, R., and Morrow, C. D. (1991). Expression of human immunodeficiency virus type 1 (HIV-1) gag, pol, and env proteins from chimeric HIV-1-poliovirus minireplicons. *J. Virol.* **65,** 2875–2883.

Clark, M. A., Jepson, M. A., Simmons, N. L., Booth, T. A., and Hirst, B. H. (1993). Differential expression of lectin-binding sites defines mouse intestinal M-cells. *J. Histochem. Cytochem.* **41,** 1679–1687.

Cornelis, G. R. (1994). *Yersinia* pathogenicity factors. *Curr. Top. Microbiol. Immunol.* **192,** 243–263

Dertzbaugh, M. T., and Elson, C. O. (1991). Cholera toxin as a mucosal adjuvant. *In* "Topics in Vaccine Adjuvant Research" (D. R. Spriggs and W. C. Koff, eds.), pp. 119–132. CRC Press, Boca Raton, Florida.

Eckmann, L., Kagnoff, M. F., and Fierer, J. (1995). Intestinal epithelial cells as watchdogs for the natural immune system. *Trends Microbiol.* **3,** 118–120.

Ermak, T. H., and Owen, R. L. (1986). Differential distribution of lymphocytes and accessory cells in mouse Peyer's patches. *Anat. Rec.* **215,** 144–152.

Ermak, T. H., Steger, H. J., and Pappo, J. (1990). Phenotypically distinct subpopulations of T cells in domes and M-cell pockets of rabbit gut-associated lymphoid tissues. *Immunology* **71,** 530–537.

Ermak, T. H., Dougherty, E. P., Bhagat, H. R., Kabok, Z., and Pappo, J. (1995). Uptake and transport of copolymer biodegradable microspheres by rabbit Peyer's patch M cells. *Cell Tissue Res.* **279,** 433–436.

Falk, P., Roth., K. A., and Gordon, J. I. (1994). Lectins are sensitive tools for defining the differentiation programs of epithelial cell lineages in the developing and adult mouse gastrointestinal tract. *Am. J. Physiol.* **266,** G987-G1003.

Farbman, A. I. (1988). The oral cavity. *In* "Cell and Tissue Biology" (L. Weiss, ed.), pp. 573–594. Urban and Schwartzenberg, Baltimore, Maryland.

Farstad, I. N., Halstensen, T. S., Fausa, O., and Brandtzaeg, P. (1994). Heterogeneity of M-cell-associated B and T cells in human Peyer's patches. *Immunology* **83,** 457–464.

Finzi, G., Cornaggia, M., Capella, C., Fiocca, R., Bosi, F., and Solcia, E. (1993). Cathepsin E in follicle associated epithelium of intestine and tonsils: Localization to M cells and possible role in antigen processing. *Histochemistry* **99,** 201–211.

Frey, A., Giannasca, K. T., Weltzin, R., Giannasca, P. J., Reggio, H., Lencer, W. I., and Neutra, M. R. (1996). Role of the glycocalyx in regulating access of microparticles to apical plasma membranes of intestinal epithelial cells: Implications for microbial attachment and oral vaccine targeting. *J. Exp. Med.* (in press).

Fujimura, Y. (1986). Functional morphology of microfold cells (M cells) in Peyer's patches. Phagocytosis and transport of BCG by M cells into rabbit Peyer's patches. *Gastroenterol. Japan* **21,** 325–335.

Fujimura, Y., Kihara, T., and Mine, H. (1992). Membranous cells as a portal of *Yersinia pseudotuberculosis* entry into rabbit ileum. *J. Clin. Electron Microsc.* **25,** 35–45.

Gebert., A., and Hach, G. (1993). Differential binding of lectins to M cells and enterocytes in the rabbit cecum. *Gastroenterology* **105,** 1350–1361.

Gebert, A., Hach, G., and Bartels, H. (1992). Co-localization of vimentin and cytokeratins in M-cells of rabbit gut-associated lymphoid tissue (GALT). *Cell Tissue Res.* **269,** 331–340.

Giannasca, P. J., Giannasca, K. T., Falk, P., Gordon, J. I., and Neutra, M. R. (1994). Regional differences in glycoconjugates of intestinal M cells in mice: Potential targets for mucosal vaccines. *Am. J. Physiol.* **267,** G1108–G1121.

Giannasca, K. T., Giannasca, P. J., and Neutra, M. R. (1996). Adherence of *Salmonella typhimurium* to Caco-2 cells: Identification of a glycoconjugate receptor. *Infect. Immun.* **64,** 135–145.

Gordon, J. I., and Hermiston, M. L. (1994). Differentiation and self-renewal in the mouse gastrointestinal epithelium. *Curr. Opin. Cell. Biol.* **6,** 795–803.

Grutzkau, A., Hanski, C., Hahn, H., and Riecken, E. O. (1990). Involvement of M cells in the bacterial invasion of Peyer's patches: A common mechanism shared by *Yersinia enterocolitica* and other enteroinvasive bacteria. *Gut* **3,** 1011–1015.

Herrington, D.A., Hall, R. H., Losonsky, G., Mekalanos, J. J., Taylor, R. K., and Levine, M. M. (1988). Toxin, toxin-coregulated pili, and the toxR regulon are essential for *Vibrio cholerae* pathogenesis in humans. *J. Exp. Med.* **168,** 1487–1492.

Hohmann, A. W., Schmidt, G., and Rowley, D. (1978). Intestinal colonization and virulence of *Salmonella* in mice. *Infect. Immun.* **22,** 763–770.

Holt, P. G., Schon-Hegrad, M. A., and McMenamin, P. G. (1990). Dendritic cells in the respiratory tract. *Int. Rev. Immunol.* **6,** 139–149.

Holt, P. G., Haining, S., Nelson, D. J., and Sedgwick, J. D. (1994). Origin and steady-state turnover of class II MHC-bearing dendritic cells in the epithelium of the conducting airways. *J. Immunol.* **153,** 256–261.

Hopkins, S., Kraehenbuhl, J. P., Schoedel, F., Potts, A., Peterson, D., De Grandi, P., and Nardelli-Haefliger, D. (1995). A recombinant *Salmonella typhimurium* vaccine induces local immunity by four different routes of immunization. *Infect. Immun.* **63,** 3279–3286.

Hynes, R. O. (1992). Integrins: Versatility, modulation and signalling in cell adhesion. *Cell (Cambridge, Mass.)* **69,** 11–25.

Inman, L. R., and Cantey, J. R. (1993). Specific adherence of *Escherichia coli* (strain RDEC-1) to membranous (M) cells of the Peyer's patch in *Escherichia coli* diarrhea in the rabbit. *J. Clin. Invest.* **71,** 1–8.

Isberg, R.R., and Leong, J.M. (1988). Cultured mammalian cells attach to the invasin protein of *Yersinia pseudotuberculosis. Proc. Natl. Acad. Sci. U.S.A.* **85,** 6682–6686.

Ito, S. (1974). Form and function of the glycocalyx on free cell surfaces. *Philos. Trans. R. Soc. London (Biol.)* **268,** 55–66.

Jarry, A., Robaszkiewicz, M., Brousse, N., and Potet, F. (1989). Immune cells associated with M cells in the follicle-associated epithelium of Peyer's patches in the rat. *Cell Tissue Res.* **225,** 293–298.

Jepson, M. A., Mason, C. M., Bennett, M. K., Simmons, N. L., and Hirst, B. H. (1992). Coexpression of vimentin and cytokeratins in M cells of rabbit intestinal follicle-associated epithelium. *Histochemistry* **24,** 33–39.

Jepson, M. A., Clark, M. A., Simmons, N. L., and Hirst, B. H. (1993). Epithelial M cells in the rabbit caecal lymphoid patch display distinctive surface characteristics. *Histochemistry* **100,** 441–447.

Jones, B. D., Ghori, N., and Falkow, S. (1994). *Salmonella typhimurium* initiates murine infection by penetrating and destroying the specialized epithelial M cells of the Peyer's patches. *J. Exp. Med.* **180,** 15–23.

Kaiserlian, D., Vidal, K., and Revillard, J. P. (1989).Murine enterocytes can present soluble antigen to specific class II-restricted CD4$^+$ T cells. *Eur. J. Immunol.* **19,** 1513–1516.

Kerneis, S., Bogdanova, A., Kraehenbuhl, J. P., and Pringault, E.(1995). Experimental models for the induction of M cells from intestinal cells. *Eur. J. Cell Biol.* Supplement volume ECBO Meeting, Abstract 657.

Kohbata, S., Yokobata, H., and Yabuuchi, E. (1986). Cytopathogenic effect of *Salmonella typhi* GIFU 10007 on M cells of murine ileal Peyer's patches in ligated ileal loops: An ultrastructural study. *Microbiol. Immunol.* **30,** 1225–1237.

Langermann, S., Palaszynski, S., Sadziene, A., Stover, C. K., and Koenig, S. (1994). Systemic and mucosal immunity induced by BCG vector expressing outer-surface protein a of *Borrelia burgdorferi. Nature (London)* **372,** 552–555.

Langhoff, E., and Steinman, R. (1989). Clonal expansion of human T lymphocytes initiated by dendrites. *J. Exp. Med.* **169,** 315–320.

Langman, J. M., and Rowland, R. (1986). The number and distribution of lymphoid follicles in the human large intestine. *J. Anat.* **194,** 189–194.

Lencer, W. I., Moe, S., Rufo, P. A., and Madara, J. L. (1995). Transcytosis of cholera toxin subunits across model human intestinal epithelia. *Proc. Natl. Acad. Sci. U.S.A* **92,** 10094–10098.

Levine, M. M., Hone, D., Tacket, C., Ferreccio, C., and Cryz, S. (1990). Clinical and field trials with attenuated *Salmonella typhi* as live oral vaccines and as "carrier" vaccines. *Res. Microbiol.* **141,** 807–816.

Madara, J. L., Nash, S., Moore, R., and Atisook, K. (1990). Structure and function of the intestinal epithelial barrier in health and disease. *Monogr. Pathol.* **31,** 306–324.

Maury, J., Nicoletti, C., Guzzo-Chambraud, L., and Maroux, S. (1995). The filamentous brush border glycocalyx, a mucin-like marker of enterocyte hyper-polarization. *Eur. J. Biochem.* **228,** 323–331.

Mayrhofer, G., and Spargo, L. D. (1989). Subcellular distribution of class II major histocompatibility antigens in enterocytes of the human and rat small intestine. *Immunol. Cell Biol.* **67,** 25–60.

Mekalanos, J. J. (1992). Bacterial mucosal vaccines. *In* "Genetically Engineered Vaccines" (J. E. Ciardi, J. R. McGhee, J. M. Kieth, eds.), *Adv. Exp. Med. Biol. Vol.* 327. pp. 43–50. Plenum, New York.

Mendelsohn, C. L., Wimmer, E., and Racaniello, V. R. (1989). Cellular receptor for poliovirus: Molecular cloning, nucleotide sequence, and expression of a new member of the immunoglobulin superfamily. *Cell (Cambridge, Mass.)* **56,** 855–865.

Miller, C. J., McChesney, M., and Moore, P. F. (1992a). Langerhans cells, macrophages and lymphocyte subsets in the cervix and vagina of rhesus macaques. *Lab Invest.* **67,** 628–634.

Miller, C. J., Vogel, P., Alexander, N. J., Sutjipto, S., Hendrickx, A. G., and Marx, P. A. (1992b). Localization of SIV in the genital tract of chronically infected female rhesus macaques. *Am. J. Pathol.* **141,** 655–660.

Miller, J. F., Mekalanos, J. J., and Falkow, S. (1989). Coordinate regulation and sensory transduction in the control of bacterial virulence. *Science* **243,** 916–921.

Momotani, E., Whipple, D. L., Thiermann, A. B., and Cheville, N. F. (1988). Role of M cells and macrophages in the entrance of *Mycobacterium paratuberculosis* into domes of ileal Peyer's patches in calves. *Vet. Pathol.* **25,** 131–137.

Mooseker, M. (1985). Organization, chemistry and assembly of the cytoskeletal apparatus of the intestinal brush border. *Anni. Rev. Cell Biol.* **1,** 209–241.

Morin, M. J., Warner, A., and Fields, B. N. (1994). A pathway for entry of reoviruses into the host through M cells of the respiratory tract. *J. Exp. Med.* **180,** 1523–27.

Mounier, J., Vasselon, T., Hellio, R., Lesourdm, M., and Sansonetti, P. J. (1992). *Shigella flexneri* enters human colonic Caco-2 cells through the basolatereal pole. *Infect. Immun.* **60,** 237–248.

Nedrud, J. G., and Lamm, M. E. (1991). Adjuvants and the mucosal immune system. *In* "Topics in Vaccine Adjuvant Research" (D. R. Spriggs and W. C. Koff, eds.), pp. 54–67. CRC Press, Boca Raton, Florida.

Neutra , M. R., and Kraehenbuhl, J. P. (1992). Transepithelial transport and mucosal defence. The role of M cells. *Trends Cell Biol.* **2,** 134–138.

Neutra, M. R., and Kraehenbuhl, J. P. (1994). Cellular and molecular basis for antigen transport in the intestinal epithelium. *In* "Handbook of Mucosal Immunology" (P. L. Ogra, J. Mestecky, M. E. Lamm, W. Strober, J. R. McGhee, and J. Bienenstock, eds.), pp. 27–39. Academic Press, San Diego.

Neutra, M. R., Phillips, T. L., Mayer, E. L., and Fishkind, D. J. (1987). Transport of membrane-bound macromolecules by M cells in follicle-associated epithelium of rabbit Peyer's patch. *Cell Tissue Res.* **247,** 537–546.

Neutra, M. R., Wilson, J. M., Weltzin, R. A., and Kraehenbuhl, J. P. (1988). Membrane domains and macromolecular transport in intestinal epithelial cells. *Am. Rev. Respir. Dis.* **138,** S10-S16.

Neutra, M. R., Giannasca, P. J., Giannasca, K. T., and Kraehenbuhl, J. P. (1994a). M cells and microbial pathogens. *In* "Infections of the GI Tract" (M. J. Blaser, P. D. Smith, J. I. Ravdin, H. B. Greenberg, and R. L. Guerrant, eds.), pp. 163–178. Raven, New York.

Neutra, M.R., Michetti, P., and Kraehenbuhl, J.P. (1994b). Secretory immunoglobulin A: Structure, synthesis, and function. *In* "Physiology of the Gastrointestinal Tract" (L. R. Johnson, ed.) 3rd Ed., Raven, New York.

Nibert, M. L., Furlong, D. B., and Fields, B. N. (1991). Mechanisms of viral pathogenesis. *J. Clin. Invest.* **88,** 727–734.

Ogra, P. L., and Karzon, D. T. (1969). Distribution of poliovirus antibody in serum, nasopharynx and alimentary tract following segmental immunization of lower alimentary tract with poliovaccine. *J. Immunol.* **102,** 1423–1430.

Okato, S., Magari, S., Yamamoto, Y., Sakanaka, M., and Takahashi, H. (1989). An immuno-electron microscopic study on interactions among dendritic cells, macrophages and lymphocytes in the human palatine tonsil. *Arch. Histol. Cytol.* **52,** 231–240.

O'Leary, A. D., and Sweeney, E. C. (1986). Lymphoglandular complexes of the colon: Structure and distribution. *Histopathology* **10,** 267–283.

Owen, R. L. (1977). Sequential uptake of horseradish peroxidase by lymphoid follicle epithelium of Peyer's patches in the normal unobstructed mouse intestine: An ultrastructural study. *Gastroenterology* **72,** 440–451.

Owen, R. L., and Bhalla, D. K. (1983). Cytochemical analysis of alkaline phosphatase and esterase activities and of lectin-binding and anionic sites in rat and mouse Peyer's patch M cells. *Am. J. Anat.* **168,** 199–212.

Owen, R. L., Pierce, N. F., Apple, R. T., and Cray, W. C. J. (1986). M-cell transport of *Vibrio cholerae* from the intestinal lumen into Peyer's patches: A mechanism for antigen sampling and for microbial transepithelial migration. *J. Infect. Dis.* **153,** 1108–1118.

Owen, R. L., Bass, D. M., and Piazza, A. J. (1990). Colonic lymphoid patches. A portal of entry in mice for type 1 reovirus administered anally. *Gastroenterology* **98,** A468.

Pace, J., Hayman, M.J., and Galan, J. E. (1993). Signal transduction and invasion of epithelial cells by *S. typhimurium. Cell (Cambridge, Mass.)* **72,** 505–514.

Pancholi, P., Mirza, A., Schauf, V., Steinman, R. M., and Bhardwaj, N. (1993). Presentation of mycobacterial antigens by human dendritic cells: Lack of transfer from infected macrophages. *Infect. Immun.* **61,** 5326–5332.

Pappo, J., and Ermak, T. H. (1989). Uptake and translocation of fluorescent latex particles by rabbit Peyer's patch follicle epithelium: A quantitative model for M-cell uptake. *Clin. Exp. Immunol.* **76,** 144–148.

Pappo, J., and Owen, R. L. (1988). Absence of secretory component expression by epithelial cells overlying rabbit gut-associated lymphoid tissue. *Gastroenterology* **95,** 1173–1177.

Parr, M. E., and Parr, E. L. (1985). Immunohistochemical localization of immunoglobulins A, G, and M in the mouse female genital tract. *J. Reprod. Fertil.* **74,** 361–370.

Parr, M. E., and Parr, E. L. (1994). Mucosal immunity in the female and male reproductive tracts. *In* "Handbook of Mucosal Immunology." (P. L. Ogra, J. Mestecky, M. E. Lamm, W. Strober, J. R. McGhee, and J. Bienenstock, eds.), pp. 677–690. Academic Press, New York.

Pepe, J. C., and Miller, V. L. (1993). *Yersinia enterocolitica* invasin: A primary role in the initiation of infection. *Proc. Natl. Acad. Sci. U.S.A.* **90,** 6473–6477.

Perdomo, J. J., Gounon, P., and Sansonetti, P. J. (1994a). Polymorphonuclear leukocyte transmigration promotes invasion of colonic epithelial monolayers by *Shigella flexneri. J. Clin. Invest.* **93,** 633–643.

Perdomo, J. J., Cavaillon, J. M., Huerre, M., Ohayon, H., Gounon, P., and Sansonetti, P. J. (1994b). Acute inflammation causes epithelial invasion and mucosal destruction in experimental *Shigellosis. J. Exp. Med.* **180,** 1307–1319.

Pope, M., Betjes, M. G., Romani, N., Hirmand, H., Cameron, P. U., Hoffman, L., Gezelter, S., Schuler, G., and Steinman, R. M. (1994). Conjugates of dendritic cells and memory T lymphocytes from skin facilitate productive infection with HIV-1. *Cell (Cambridge, Mass.)* **78,** 389–398.

Rosenshine, I., and Finlay, B. B. (1993). Exploitation of host signal transduction pathways and cytoskeletal functions by invasive bacteria. *Bioessays* **15,** 17–24.

Roy, M. J., and Varvayanis, M. (1987). Development of dome epithelium in gut-associated lymphoid tissues: Association of IgA with M cells. *Cell Tissue Res.* **248,** 645–651.

Sansonetti, P. J. (1991). Genetic and molecular basis of epithelial cell invasion by *Shigella* species. *Rev Infect. Dis.* **13,** 285–292.

Savidge, T. C., and Smith, M. W. (1995). Evidence that membranous (M) cell genesis is immunoregulated. *In* "Advances in Mucosal Immunology" (J. Mestecky, ed.), pp. 239–241. Plenum, New York.

Savidge, T. C., Smith, M. W., James, P. S., and Aldred, P. (1991). Salmonella-induced M-cell formation in germfree mouse Peyer's patch tissue. *Am. J. Pathol.* **139,** 177–184.

Semenza, G. (1986). Anchoring and biosynthesis of stalked brush border membrane glycoproteins. *Annu. Rev. Cell Bio1.* **2,** 255–314.

Sicinski, P., Rowinski, J., Warchol, J.B., Jarzcabek, Z., Gut, W., Szczygiel, B., Bielecki, K., and Koch, G. (1990). Poliovirus type 1 enters the human host through intestinal M cells. *Gastroenterology* **98,** 56–58.

Smith, M. W., James, P. S., Tivey, D. R., and Brown, D. (1988). Automated histochemical analysis of cell populations in the intact follicle-associated epithelium of the mouse Peyer's patch. *Histochem. J.* **20,** 443–448.

Sory, M. P., and Cornelis, G. R. (1994). Translocation of a hybrid YopE-adenylate cyclase from *Yersinia enterocolitica* into HeLa cells. *Mol. Microbiol.* **14,** 583–594.

Sory, M. P., Hermand, P., Vaerman, J. P., and Cornelis, G. R. (1990). Oral immunization of mice with a live recombinant *Yersinia enterocolitica* 0:9 strain that produces the cholera toxin B subunit. *Infect. Immun.* **58,** 2420–2428.

Sory, M. P., Kaniga, K., Goldenberg, S., and Cornelis, G. R. (1992). Expression of the eukaryotic *Trypanosoma cruzi* CRA gene in *Yersinia enterocolitica* and induction of an immune response against CRA in mice. *Infect. Immun.* **60,** 3830–3836.

Sun, J. B., Holmgren, J., and Czerkinsky, C. (1994). Cholera toxin B subunit: An efficient transmucosal carrier-delivery system for induction of peripheral immunological tolerance. *Proc. Natl. Acad. Sci. U.S.A.* **91,** 10795–10799.

Takeuchi, A. (1967). Electron microscope studies of experimental *Salmonella* infection. I. Penetration into the intestinal epithelium by *Salmonella typhimurium. Am. J. Pathol.* **50,** 109–136.

Uchida, J. (1987). An ultrastructural study on active uptake and transport of bacteria by microfold cells (M cells) to the lymphoid follicles in the rabbit appendix. *J. Clin. Electron Microsc.* **20,** 379–394.

Van Damme, M., Sory, M. P., Biot, T., Vaerman, J. P., and Cornelis, G. R. (1992). Oral immunization against cholera toxin with a live *Yersinia enterocolitica* carrier in mice. *Gastroenterology* **103**, 520–531.

Walker, R. I., Schauder-Chock, E. A., and Parker, J. L. (1988). Selective association and transport of *Campylobacter jejuni* through M cells of rabbit Peyer's patches. *Can. J. Microbiol.* **34**, 1142–1147.

Wassef, J. S., Keren, D. F., and Mailloux, J. L. (1989). Role of M cells in initial antigen uptake and in ulcer formation in the rabbit intestinal loop model of *Shigellosis*. *Infect. Immun.* **57**, 858–863.

Weinberg, D. S., Pinkus, G. S., and Murphy, G. F. (1987). Tonsillar epithelial dendritic cells. Demonstration by lectin binding, immunohistochemical characterization, and ultrastructure. *Lab. Invest.* **56**, 622–628.

Weinman, M. D., Allan, C. H., Trier, J. S., and Hagen, S. J. (1989). Repair of microvilli in the rat small intestine after damage with lectins contained in the red kidney bean. *Gastroenterology* **97**, 1193–1204.

Weltzin, R. A., Lucia Jandris, P., Michetti, P., Fields, B. N., Kraehenbuhl, J. P., and Neutra, M. R. (1989). Binding and transepithelial transport of immunoglobulins by intestinal M cells: Demonstration using monoclonal IgA antibodies against enteric viral proteins. *J. Cell Biol.* **108**, 1673–1685.

Winner III, L., Mack, J., Weltzin, R. A., Mekalanos, J. J., Kraehenbuhl, J. P., and Neutra, M. R. (1991). New model for analysis of mucosal immunity: Intestinal secretion of specific monoclonal immunoglobulin A from hybridoma tumors protects against *Vibrio cholerae* infection. *Infect. Immun.* **59**, 977–982.

Wira, C. R., Richardson, J., and Prabhala, R. (1994). Endocrine regulation of mucosal immunity: Effect of sex hormones and cytokines on the afferent and efferent arms of the immune system in the female reproduction tract. *In* "Handbook of Mucosal Immunology" (P. L. Ogra., J. Mestecky, M. E. Lamm, W. Strober, J. R. McGhee, and J. Bienenstock, eds). pp. 705–718. Academic Press, San Diego.

Wolf, J. L., Rubin, D. H., Finberg, R. S., Kauffman, R. S., Sharpe, A. H., Trier, J. S., and Fields, B. N. (1981). Intestinal M cells: A pathway for entry of reovirus into the host. *Science* **212**, 471–472.

Yamamoto, T., and Yokota, T. (1989). *Vibrio cholerae* O1 adherence to human small intestinal M cells *in vitro*. *J. Infect. Dis.* **160**, 168–169.

Yamamoto, T., Kamano, T., Uchimura, M., Iwanaga, M., and Yokota, T. (1988). *Vibrio cholerae* O1 adherence to villi and lymphoid follicle epithelium: *In vitro* model using formalin-treated human small intestine and correlation between adherence and cell-associated hemagglutinin levels. *Infect. Immun.* **56**, 3241–3250.

Young, W. G., Newcomb, G. M., and Hosking, A. R. (1985). The effect of atrophy, hyperplasia, and keratinization accompanying the estrous cycle on Langerhans cells in mouse vaginal epithelium. *Am. J. Anat.* **174**, 173–186.

Zhou, F., Kraehenbuhl, J. P., and Neutra, M. R. (1995). Mucosal IgA response to rectally administered antigen formulated in IgA-coated liposomes. *Vaccine* **13**, 637–644.

III

Mucosal Modulation for Induction of Effective Immunity

4

Cholera Toxin as a Mucosal Adjuvant

CHARLES O. ELSON
Division of Gastroenterology and Hepatology
Department of Medicine
University of Alabama at Birmingham
Birmingham, Alabama 35294

I. Introduction

Most antigens yield only weak or poor immune responses when given by themselves either parenterally or orally. Thus the generation of an effective immune response usually requires the addition of an adjuvant, which is a substance that enhances immune responses. Adjuvants have been shown to affect virtually every measurable aspect of antibody responses, including the kinetics, duration, quantity, isotype, avidity, and generation of neutralizing or protective antibodies. Adjuvants can also affect the specificity of antibody responses by altering the selection of epitopes to which antibody will be directed (Hui *et al.*, 1991). Some adjuvants can enhance cell-mediated immunity, both delayed hypersensitivity mediated by CD4 cells and cytotoxic lymphocyte responses mediated by CD8 cells. However, the number of adjuvants that stimulate cell-mediated immune responses tend to be lower than the number that stimulate antibody formation.

Although adjuvants have been used empirically for many years, the mechanisms by which they act are not well understood, partly because the adjuvants themselves have been very complex, making such evaluations difficult (Waksman, 1979). Recently, more highly purified molecules have been isolated from traditional adjuvants, such as muramyl dipeptide from mycobacteria and monophosphoryl lipid A from endotoxin. This may simplify the dissection of their effects. Waksman (1979) has made the point that one must define the target cells upon which the adjuvant acts, the distribution of the adjuvant in relation to the location of those target cells, the function of the target cells affected by the adjuvant, and the cellular and molecular mode of action of the adjuvant on the target cells. This information is either rudimentary or nonexistent for most adjuvants. The best understood adjuvants have a multiplicity of effects on immune cells; different adjuvants can have very divergent effects on the same cells. Potential mechanisms of adjuvant activity after systemic administration are shown in Table I. The possible effects of a given adjuvant are complex, may overlap, and are likely to be multiple.

Although many if not all of these mechanisms are likely to apply to mucosal adjuvants as well, there is a profound dearth of data and information on agents with mucosal adjuvanticity despite a great need for such agents. Mucosal immunization is the route of choice for protection from many pathogens but development of effective mucosal vaccines has lagged, in part due to a lack of suitable mucosal adjuvants. Most protein antigens are not only poor immunogens when given mucosally, but induce tolerance instead of immunity. Mucosal adjuvants are needed to overcome this potential outcome of mucosal antigen exposure. Cholera toxin has been shown to enhance the immunogenicity of relatively poor mucosal immunogens when mixed or conjugated together and given orally (Elson and Ealding, 1984a), thus CT and its B subunit have generated a great deal of interest as potential adjuvants for oral vaccines (Elson and Dertzbaugh, 1994). The remainder of this chapter will focus on the remarkable mucosal properties of this molecule. The reader is referred to other chapters in this volume that cover in detail the mucosal immune system, oral immunization, mucosal tolerance and the concept of the common mucosal immune system in which immunization of one mucosal surface also sensitizes other mucosal surfaces at remote sites. This paradigm has formed the basis for one strategy of oral immunization in which the antigen is delivered into the intestine, which has the greatest amount of mucosal lymphoid tissue, to prime the entire mucosal immune system; such priming is then followed by either mucosal or systemic boosting.

TABLE I
General Mechanisms of Adjuvant Action

Prolonged release of antigen over weeks, months
Generation of inflammation, i.e., macrophage (APC) activation
Selective antigen localization in thymic-dependent areas
Increased uptake and presentation of antigen by accessory cells
Alteration of antigen-processing pathway; class I vs class II
Stimulation of T helper cells, nonspecific or specific
Stimulation of increased cytokine production
Stimulation of B-cell isotype switching, proliferation, differentiation
Enhanced maturation of T- and B-cell precursors
Elimination of suppressor cells

Note. Adapted from Waksman (1979).

II. The Molecular and Cellular Biology of Cholera Toxin

The molecular structure of CT has been studied extensively (Betley *et al.*, 1986). It is composed of an A and B subunit (Fig. 1). The toxinogenic A subunit (CT-A) is a 28-kDa protein which is involved in the ADP-ribosylation of the stimulatory Gs protein of adenylate cyclase. The A subunit is post-translationally cleaved into the A1 and A2 peptides, and it is the A1 peptide that has enzymatic activity. Recent crystallographic data on CT and the closely related *Escherichia coli* heat-labile toxin indicate that in both of these enterotoxins the A2 peptide forms an alpha helix that connects the A1 peptide with the binding subunit (Sixma *et al.*, 1991; Zhang *et al.*, 1995a). The B subunit of cholera toxin (CT-B) is a homopentamer of five identical noncovalently-associated subunits (11.6 kDa) that form a ring like structure with a central pore through which the A2 subunit projects (Hol *et al.*, 1995). This structure, which is common to both CT and *E. coli* LT, has been likened to a "ring on a finger." (van Heyningen, 1991) CT-B binds to the monosialoganglioside G_{M1} (Cuatrecasas, 1973), which is present on all nucleated cells, including the surface of intestinal epithelial cells, the primary target of the toxin in nature. CT is endocytosed at the apical border of the enterocyte and in a multistep process the toxin-contain-

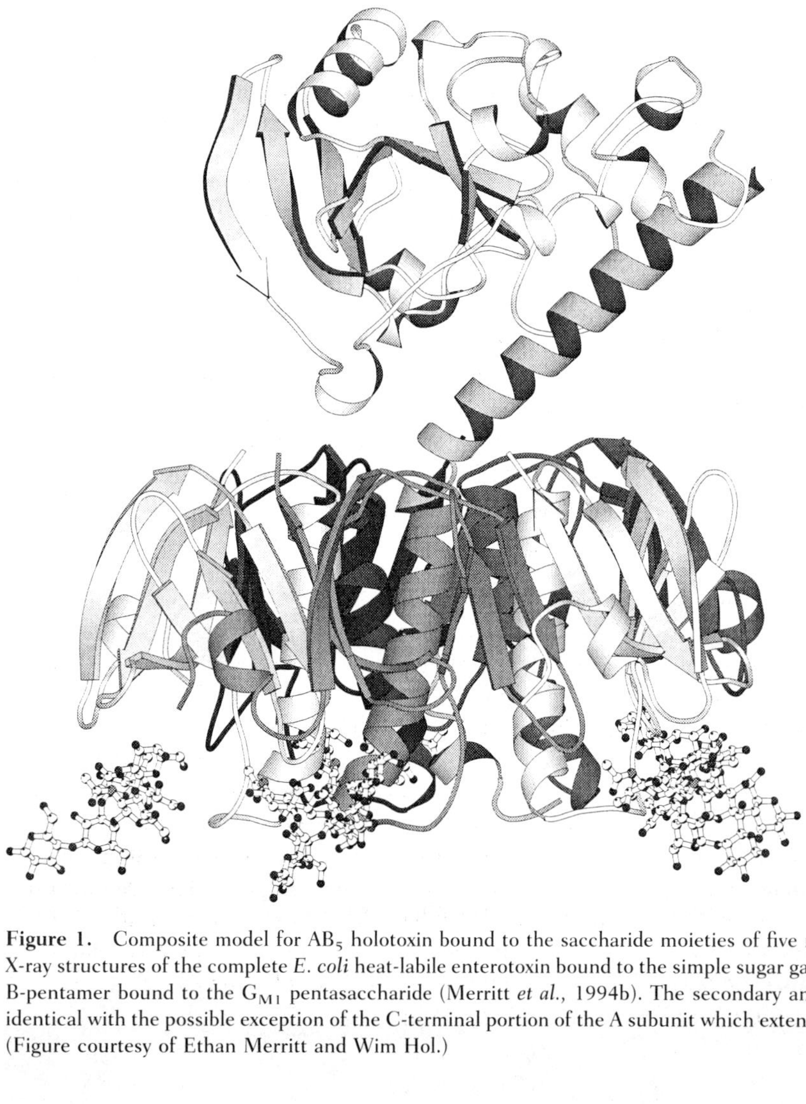

Figure 1. Composite model for AB_5 holotoxin bound to the saccharide moieties of five receptor molecules. This model was derived from the X-ray structures of the complete *E. coli* heat-labile enterotoxin bound to the simple sugar galactose (Merritt *et al.*, 1994a) and of the cholera toxin B-pentamer bound to the G_{M1} pentasaccharide (Merritt *et al.*, 1994b). The secondary and tertiary structures of the two toxins are essentially identical with the possible exception of the C-terminal portion of the A subunit which extends into or through the central pore of the B-pentamer. (Figure courtesy of Ethan Merritt and Wim Hol.)

ing endosomal vesicles transcytose to the basolateral membrane where adenylate cyclase is located (Lencer *et al.*, 1993). The exact cellular location of the interaction between A1 peptide and Gs is unknown. Endocytosis of CT and CT-B occurs also in variety of nonpolar cells, including neurons and lymphocytes, and is likely to be a crucial feature in the effects of the toxin on these cells. Binding of the B subunit to the cell membrane is of course required for endocytosis, but whether other parts of the molecule participate is not yet known. Site-directed mutagenesis is now being utilized to create mutant molecules to define the residues critical to binding, endocytosis, transcytosis, and enzymatic function (Jobling and Holmes, 1991). Such mutants are being tested as well, as mucosal immunogens and adjuvants, as discussed below.

III. Cholera Toxin as a Mucosal Immunogen

CT is one of the most potent mucosal immunogens yet identified (Pierce and Gowans, 1975; Pierce and Cray, 1982), inducing strong intestinal S-IgA responses and plasma IgG responses after oral administration (Elson and Ealding, 1984b). It has been estimated that at the peak of the response up to 5% of all the plasma cells in the intestine are producing antibody to it. Contrary to most protein antigens, feeding CT does not induce oral tolerance for antibody responses (Elson and Ealding, 1984a). Intestinal immunization with CT induces extended memory responses in the mucosa and this presumably applies to immunization at other mucosal sites (Lycke and Holmgren, 1986a). Although generalized mucosal immunization occurs after mucosal immunization, the local immune response is best at the mucosal site that is directly exposed to CT (Pierce and Cray, 1982). Despite these remarkable properties as a mucosal immunogen, the mucosal response to CT follows the "rules" applicable to more conventional protein antigens in that the response is $CD4^+$ T-cell dependent (Hornquist *et al.*, 1991) and requires antigen presentation via class II MHC molecules (Elson and Ealding, 1987). In mice, the response to CT after intestinal immunization is predominately a Th2 response (Xu-Amano *et al.*, 1993). These properties of CT as an oral immunogen (Table II) are summarized here because the same properties seem to extend to antigens for which CT acts as a mucosal adjuvant and are arguably exactly those one would desire for an effective oral vaccine.

Most of the work done with CT has focused on the antibody response and much less is known about the cell mediated immunity or delayed hypersensitivity response to CT. Kay and Ferguson (1989a,b) found that the feeding of CT or its toxoid prior to systemic immunization induced oral tolerance for the DTH response but not for the antibody response to CT. Experiments with cell transfer indicated that this oral tolerance for DTH involved the induction of suppressor cells, but these cells were not further characterized. One can only speculate that these suppressor cells were Th2 cells known to downregulate the Th1 limb of immune responses.

TABLE II
Properties of Cholera Toxin as a Mucosal Immunogen

- Stimulates secretory IgA and serum IgG response
- Does not induce oral tolerance for antibody responses
- Induces extended memory in mucosal tissues
- Local response best at mucosal site in contact with CT
- Restricted by I-A subregion of H-2 major histocompatibility complex
- T-cell dependent

The bulk of the data about CT as a mucosal immunogen comes from studies in rodents. In humans, CT can induce massive diarrhea in doses well tolerated by rodents, but CT-B subunit is well tolerated and immunogenic (Czerkinsky *et al.*, 1991; Quiding *et al.*, 1991). Contrary to mice, where CT is consistently much more immunogenic than CT-B, in humans CT-B can induce levels of serum antibody in volunteers comparable to those found following clinical cholera (Svennerholm *et al.*, 1984). Memory responses as measured by serum antibody occur after immunization with a CT-B containing oral vaccine and persist for years (Jertborn *et al.*, 1988). Antigen-specific T cells have been demonstrated in the peripheral blood after oral immunization with CT-B (Castello-Branco *et al.*, 1994). This CT-B-specific T-cell reactivity is demonstrable for up to 1 year after immunization (Lewis *et al.*, 1993), suggesting prolonged T-cell memory as well. Many of these results parallel those found in rodents, except for the greater mucosal immunogenicity of CT-B relative to CT. More detailed studies are needed concerning the immune response to oral immunization with CT-B, particularly whether it can serve as a mucosal adjuvant in humans.

IV. Cholera Toxin as a Mucosal Adjuvant: General Characteristics

The initial demonstration of CT's adjuvant effects came from studies on whether the feeding of CT resulted in oral tolerance. CT was fed to mice either alone or with the unrelated protein antigen, keyhole limpet hemocyanin (KLH). CT did not induce oral tolerance to itself and when both proteins were fed together, abrogated tolerance to KLH (Elson and Ealding, 1984a). At the same time CT also induced an intestinal sIgA response to KLH which did not occur when KLH was fed alone.

The ability of CT to act as a mucosal adjuvant has since been confirmed by a number of other investigators with a variety of antigens, as shown in Table III. Although many of these are protein antigens, CT has been effective as a mucosal adjuvant for both lipid and carbohydrate types of antigens, as well as for whole viruses, bacteria, and a protozoan! Thus, although the mucosal adjuvant effects of CT may not apply to all antigens, it has shown efficacy with a remarkably broad array of antigen types (Table III).

The ability of CT to act as a mucosal adjuvant depends on a number of parameters (Table IV). In order to induce immunity to the target antigen, CT has to be administered simultaneously with the antigen, and both the antigen and CT must be administered by the same route, i.e., mucosally (Lycke and Holmgren, 1986b). Giving CT by a route different from the antigen is not effective. This suggests that CT acts on mucosal lymphoid tissue in a manner that favors responsiveness to the antigens presented with it. Interestingly, CT does not induce antibody responses to food antigens that would be expected to be present in the intestine at the time of its administration (Nedrud and Sigmund, 1991), nor stimulate polyclonal B cell responses (Jackson *et al.*, 1993). The dose of CT required in mice for the adjuvant effect for most protein antigens ranges between 1 and 10 μg/dose (Lycke and Holmgren, 1986b; Kusnecov *et al.*, 1992) and may vary depending on the antigen involved; although very small amounts of CT sufficed to potentiate the immune response to CT-B, much larger amounts have been used to enhance mucosal responses to viruses. CT induces long-term mucosal and systemic memory B- and T-cell responses to antigens coadministered with it (Vajdy and Lycke, 1993). Although most studies have measured simple enhancement of antibody titers, CT as a mucosal adjuvant has been found to provide protection against challenge with a pathogen in several different systems, e.g., Sendai virus (Nedrud *et al.*, 1987), influenza virus (Tamura *et al.*, 1991), tetanus

TABLE IV

Important Features of Cholera Toxin's Mucosal Adjuvanticity

- Dose: usually microgram amounts
- Route: must be mucosal
- Timing: must be simultaneous with antigen
- Genetics: in mice works best in high responders to CT
- Species: mice, rats, rabbits, ferrets; humans?
- Memory: long-term B-cell and T-cell memory
- Type of antigen: has broad applicability to protein, lipid, carbohydrate antigens
- Antigen form: mixtures, covalent conjugates, molecular chimeras

TABLE III

Antigens with Which CT or CT-B Have Been Effective as Adjuvants

Antigen (adjuvant)	Route	Reference
Proteins		
Keyhole limpet hemocyanin (CT)	p.o.	(Elson and Ealding, 1984a)
Horseradish peroxidase (CT-B)	p.o.	(McKenzie and Halsey, 1984)
Ovalbumin (CT)	p.o.	(Van der Heijden *et al.*, 1991)
Tetanus toxoid (CT)	p.o.	(Jackson *et al.*, 1993)
M protein epitope of group A streptococci (CT-B)	i.n.	(Bessen and Fischetti, 1988)
Antigen I/II *S. mutans* (CT/CT-B)	p.o.	(Czerkinsky *et al.*, 1989; Wu and Russell, 1993)
Protein antigen of *S. mutans* (CT-B)	i.n.	(Takahashi *et al.*, 1990)
Hemagglutinin of influenza virus (CT/CT-B)	p.o., i.n.	(Tamura *et al.*, 1988)
RSV FG glycoprotein (CT/CT-B)	i.n.	(Walsh, 1993)
S. mutans GtfB.1::Pho A fusion protein	p.o.	(Tomasi *et al.*, 1994)
Polysaccharides		
Shigella lipopolysaccharide (CT-B)	p.o.	(Orr *et al.*, 1994)
Dextran–CT-B conjugate (CT)	p.o., i.n.	(Berquist *et al.*, 1995)
P. aeruginosa polysaccharide (CT)	p.o.	(Abraham and Robinson, 1991)
Viruses		
Whole influenza virus (CT)	p.o.	(Chen and Strober, 1990)
Sendai virus (CT)	p.o., i.n.	(Nedrud *et al.*, 1987)
Measles virus (CT-B)	i.n.	(Muller *et al.*, 1995)
Respiratory syncytial virus (RSV)	i.n.	(Reuman *et al.*, 1991)
Bacteria/protozoa		
Helicobacter pylori (CT)	p.o.	(Czinn and Nedrud, 1991)
Toxoplasma gondii (CT)	p.o.	(Bourguin *et al.*, 1991)
Entamoeba histolytica peptide–CT-B fusion protein	p.o.	(Zhang *et al.*, 1995b)

toxin (Jackson *et al.*, 1993), and measles virus (Muller *et al.*, 1995).

The induction of antibody responses by CT is well established. The induction of cellular immune responses or delayed type hypersensitivity (DTH) by CT has not been studied as extensively. As mentioned in the previous section, CT feeding in mice has been found to induce oral tolerance for DTH reactions to CT, perhaps because it seems to generate a predominant type 2 $CD4^+$ T helper response (Kay and Ferguson, 1989a,b). Nevertheless, there are reports of enhanced priming of DTH reactions by CT as a mucosal adjuvant (Kusnecov *et al.*, 1992; Tamura *et al.*, 1995). The intranasal administration of inactivated respiratory syncytial virus plus CT yielded a predominant IgG2a response, a subclass representative of Th1 responses in mice, a result similar to that occurring after infection with the live virus (Reuman *et al.*, 1991). Indeed, some workers have found priming of both Th1 and Th2 cytokines on antigen restimulation *in vitro* after antigen plus CT were given mucosally (Wilson *et al.*, 1991; Vajdy and Lycke, 1993), although others have found priming of Th2 cytokines only (Xu-Amano *et al.*, 1993). Finally, priming of cytotoxic T-cell responses after the feeding of ovalbumin plus CT and/or CT-B as adjuvant has been reported recently (Bowen *et al.*, 1994). These results are consistent with some induction of a cellular immune response by mucosal CT adjuvant, but the duration of this cellular response is unknown.

The adjuvanticity of CT appears to be related to and dependent upon its immunogenicity, e.g., the response of mice to KLH given together with CT orally was significantly higher in H-2 congenic mouse strains that are high responders to CT than in strains that are low responders to CT (Elson, 1992). In addition, mutant CT molecules that lack immunogenicity also lack adjuvanticity and vice versa, as will be discussed below. Although CT generates a strong mucosal and systemic response to itself when coadministered as an adjuvant, preexisting mucosal immunity to CT does not impair its ability to provide mucosal adjuvant activity (Tamura *et al.*, 1989; Wu and Russell, 1994).

CT has been effective as a mucosal adjuvant in mice, rats, rabbits, and ferrets but did not work in one study in chickens (Hoshi *et al.*, 1995). Because CT induces significant diarrhea in humans (Levine *et al.*, 1983), the holotoxin itself cannot be tested orally and it remains unknown whether CT-B or a nontoxic CT mutant will have mucosal adjuvanticity in humans. CT-B containing a trace amount of CT (0.1–5%) has shown mucosal adjuvanticity equivalent to the holotoxin in mice, whether given orally (Wilson *et al.*, 1990; Lee and Chen, 1994) or intranasally (Tamura *et al.*, 1994b). This combination is attractive as a method to reduce the toxicity enough to allow use in humans, particularly with an intranasal route of administration. The incorporation of CT within the lipid particles of multiple emulsions has been found to preserve adjuvanticity while markedly decreasing toxicity and is another possible strategy for translation to humans (Tomasi *et al.*, 1994).

V. Role of CT Subunits in Mucosal Adjuvanticity

Given the dichotomy of function between the two subunits of CT (Fig 1), the role that each plays in CT's mucosal immunogenicity and adjuvanticity has been a subject of continuing interest. McKenzie and Halsey (1984) reported first that horseradish peroxidase (HRP) chemically conjugated to CT-B elicited higher antibody levels in the gut and serum than were observed after feeding either HRP alone or an unconjugated mixture of HRP and CT-B. Since then, the use of CT-B as a vaccine adjuvant has been examined by others with mixed results. In one report, mixtures of KLH and CT-B were unable to stimulate immunity to KLH unless very small doses (<50 ng) of holotoxin were added (Lycke and Holmgren, 1986b); however, KLH conjugated to CT-B was not tested. The use of CT-B conjugates has been reported to be effective in some cases (Bessen and Fischetti, 1988; Tamura *et al.*, 1988), but not in others (Czerkinsky *et al.*, 1989; Liang *et al.*, 1989b). The poor responses that have been observed with CT-B conjugates in some cases may be due to the coupling procedure. The degree of cross-linking and coupling procedure used can significantly affect the immunogenicity of protein conjugates (Verheul *et al.*, 1989). The mucosal route being used could be another important variable in that CT-B has been more effective as a mucosal adjuvant when it has been used for intranasal immunization (Wu and Russell, 1993; Muller *et al.*, 1995), a route discussed below.

Fusion of peptides to CT-B has been accomplished using recombinant gene technology, generating chimeric neoantigens (Sanchez *et al.*, 1988; Dertzbaugh *et al.*, 1990). This approach has been used to test whether CT-B has intrinsic adjuvant activity over and above a control bacterial protein. Thus the same peptide antigen, an immunogenic peptide of glucosyltransferase B of *S. mutans*, was fused either to CT-B or to *E. coli* alkaline phosphatase and purified protein was fed to mice (Dertzbaugh and Elson, 1993a). These studies did demonstrate that CT-B has intrinsic adjuvant activity, but this activity was much less potent than what has been found with the holotoxin in the intestine. The size of the peptide that can be fused to CT-B is effectively restricted to about 20 residues. Peptides or proteins larger than this impair CT-B's ability to fold properly, to bind to G_{M1} ganglioside and to form pentamers, thus abolishing its activity (Dertzbaugh and Elson, 1993b). A solution to this problem was suggested from the crystallographic structure of *E. coli* LT, a closely related molecule (Fig. 1), i.e., the substitution of an antigen for the A1 subunit of CT. This approach was shown to be feasible (Jobling and Holmes, 1992) and the resulting fusion protein containing A2 subunit reassembled with B monomers to form holotoxin-like chimeras. Such a chimera containing a Streptococcal protein adhesin induced strong S-IgA and serum IgG responses when fed to mice (Hajishengallis *et al.*, 1995). This result is again compatible with the notion that the B subunit has intrinsic adjuvant activity.

Information on the role of the A subunit has been conflicting. The consistently higher potency of holotoxin compared to B subunit in mice for both immunogenicity and adjuvanticity suggests an important role for the A subunit. Liang *et al.*, (1989a) concluded that G_{M1} binding but not toxic activity was necessary for the mucosal adjuvanticity of CT- Sendai virus conjugates, based on studies with glutaraldehyde-treated CT. However, very small amounts of residual A subunit may be sufficient and this study does not provide a definitive answer. The opposite conclusion, that the A subunit's ADP-ribosyltransferase activity was crucial to CT's mucosal adjuvanticity, was reached in another study showing deficient mucosal adjuvanticity by recombinant CT-B and by a mutant *E. coli* LT in which a single amino acid substitution had inactivated its enzymatic activity (Lycke *et al.*, 1992). Again, this was not a definitive result.

In order to define the role of the A and B subunits in the immunogenicity and adjuvanticity of CT, mutants of both A and B subunit were generated by site-directed mutagenesis that lacked enzymatic and binding ability, respectively. Holotoxins containing only an A mutant, only a B mutant, or both A and B mutants were compared to wild-type CT for immunogenicity and adjuvanticity in mouse intestine. Each was fed to mice along with tetanus toxoid (TT). Mice receiving wild-type CT had strong responses to both CT and TT. Mice receiving the A mutant or CT-B alone had moderate and weak anti-CT responses, respectively, but no TT response. Mice given the B mutant or the double A and B mutant had no response to either CT or TT (Elson *et al.*, 1995b). These results show clearly that both a functional A and B subunit are required for optimal immunogenicity and adjuvanticity of CT in the intestine. They illustrate also that CT's adjuvanticity appears to be linked to its immunogenicity.

VI. Site of Adjuvant Activity

The requirement for CT to be given at the same time and by the same route as antigen indicates that its adjuvant effect is exerted at the mucosal surface, but the exact site is unknown. The site at which CT acts might be different at various mucosal surfaces with very distinct microenvironments, e.g., the nasal vs the intestinal mucosa. Intranasal immunization using CT or CT-B has been the focus of a number of studies in recent years (Table III). From these studies a number of general conclusions are evident. Most antigen plus CT or CT-B adjuvant combinations that immunize when given into the intestine also do so when given intranasally. In some instances antigen plus CT-B as adjuvant is effective intranasally even though the same combination is ineffective when given into the intestine. The distribution of the response systemically and at various mucosal sites is roughly equivalent when antigen plus adjuvant is given intranasally or orally (Wu and Russell, 1993). Because the dose of CT or CT-B used intranasally is frequently equivalent to that used in the intestine, the ratio of dose to mucosal surface area is much greater with intranasal administration. This may partly explain some of the above differences as well as the apparent lack of genetic restriction of the adjuvant effect with the intranasal route (Hirabayashi *et al.*, 1991) a restriction that is apparent after intragastric administration (Elson, 1992). The nasal mucosa contains organized lymphoid tissue, nasal-associated lymphoreticular tissue or NALT (Kuper *et al.*, 1992), which is analogous to GALT in the intestine, but the exact site of the adjuvant effect of CT or CT-B in nasal mucosa has not been studied.

In regard to the intestine, the current understanding is that the induction of mucosal immune responses occurs in GALT and requires the transport of antigen by specialized M cells into the underlying lymphoid follicles, where antigen processing and presentation to antigen-specific T and B cells occurs. Thus the site of the adjuvant effect of CT presumably occurs in GALT. There is evidence from some recent studies that this is at least one site of CT's adjuvanticity. CT is an effective adjuvant when inserted with antigen into the lipid particles of multiple emulsions and delivered into the gut (Tomasi *et al.*, 1994). Such multiple emulsion particles enter the lymphoid follicles but not the epithelium or lamina propria of the intestine (Hearn, 1995). Gut epithelial cells can act as antigen-presenting cells *in vitro*, although the functional effect of that presentation has been suppression (Bland and Warren, 1986; Mayer *et al.*, 1988). Gut epithelial cells bind the great majority of CT, and in an immunohistochemical light microscopic study, CT was present within epithelial cells as well as within mononuclear cells in the underlying lamina propria (Hansson *et al.*, 1984), indicating that CT can traverse the epithelial layer. CT given into the intestine causes a marked depletion of the cells within the epithelial layer (IEL) and of those in the dome epithelium overlying Peyer's patches (Elson *et al.*, 1995a). This suggests that the CT traversing the epithelium is still able to bind to its receptor on lymphocytes. Although the epithelium and the lamina propria are both potential sites for CT's adjuvanticity, there is only this circumstantial evidence in their favor.

VII. Antigen Uptake across Epithelium or into Lymphoid Follicles

Does CT or its B subunit act on the epithelial layer to increase permeability to macromolecules, thus delivering antigen into the lamina propria and generating an immune response? Lycke and co-workers (1991) addressed this question by placing fluorescein-labeled dextran particles of 3000 Da into the gut lumen along with CT or CT-B and measuring the amount of the former translocating to the peripheral blood as an index of gut permeability. They found an increase in permeability with CT but not CT-B, which seemed to correlate with their relative adjuvant activity, and suggested this as one mechanism explaining the adjuvant activity. However, a number of other observations argue against this idea. For example, there is no polyclonal increase in antibody production in the lamina propria after CT (Jackson *et al.*, 1993), nor is there any increase in antibody responses to food antigens (Nedrud and Sigmund, 1991). CT sequestered within lipid particles of multiple emulsions has excellent adjuvant activity, even though it does not come into contact with the epithelium (Tomasi *et al.*, 1994). Finally, T-cell priming is evident in the Peyer's patches after feeding antigen plus CT (Clarke *et al.*, 1991), which indicates that the adjuvant effect is exerted there, in part if not entirely. There is a report of increased permeability of rabbit nasal mucosa exposed to CT *in vitro* (Gizurarson *et al.*, 1992); the arguments against gut permeability apply to this observation as well.

Might the mucosal adjuvanticity of CT or CT-B be explained by an increased delivery of antigen into intestinal follicles, perhaps related to their ability to bind to mucosa and thus persist in the intestine? Although it is difficult to perceive how this would be a mechanism when antigens are simply mixed with CT or CT-B, this idea has appeal as a mechanism by which CT might potentiate the immune response to fusion chimeras or to antigens to which it is chemically conjugated. There are no data directly addressing this. The form of the resulting antigen might be an important variable, in that colloidal gold particles of 8–12 nm to which CT-B had been conjugated selectively localized to the M cells of the follicle-associated epithelium after being administered into the murine intestine (M. Neutra, personal communication), whereas soluble CT was bound diffusely to the microvillus surface of all enterocytes. Therefore such selective localization of antigen might not pertain to soluble antigen-coupled CT or CT-B.

VIII. Cellular Targets of Adjuvanticity

A. Antigen-Presenting Cells

Little is known about the mechanism of antigen presentation in GALT. CT and other protein antigens must be presented to mucosal T cells in the context of the appropriate class II MHC molecules (Elson and Ealding, 1985). CT and CT-B do not alter macrophage APC antigen uptake or processing *in vitro* (Woogen *et al.*, 1987), nor do they affect macrophage class II MHC expression (Bromander *et al.*, 1991). However, CT has been shown to stimulate the production of IL-1 *in vitro*, an effect that may enhance antigen presentation (Lycke *et al.*, 1989). This stimulation requires microgram amounts of CT, amounts which may not occur *in vivo;* however, Bromander *et al.* (1991) have presented evidence that part of CT's adjuvanticity is due to its potentiation of antigen presentation by enhanced IL-1 production. Although CT-B did not stimulate IL-1 release in the above studies, in other studies low doses of CT-B enhanced primary *in vitro* murine spleen T-cell responses to KLH, due to effects on APCs in these cultures (Hirabayashi *et al.*, 1992). In addition to production of cytokines such as IL-1 and IL-6, cell surface molecules such as B7 on macrophages provide costimulatory signals to T cells that are critical to the induction of immune responses. Thus it is significant that CT in nanogram amounts increases B7 expression and functional activity on macrophages *in vitro* (Y. Cong and C. O. Elson, unpublished data, 1996). If enhanced antigen presentation was an important mechanism of CT's adjuvanticity, one would expect to see evidence of increased T-cell priming in mucosal tissues *in vivo.* Several studies have demonstrated such increased mucosal T-cell priming to antigen when CT was used as an adjuvant, as discussed below. Thus an enhancement of macrophage antigen presentation through increased costimulatory activity seems to be one of the major mechanisms by which CT acts as a mucosal adjuvant (Fig. 2).

Other cells in the intestine might also act as antigen-presenting cells, e.g., dendritic cells, B cells, and epithelial cells. There is little information available on these other APCs relative to CT's adjuvant effects. Epithelial cells are now recognized as an active and important component of the mucosal immune system. They express both class I and class II MHC molecules, produce certain cytokines, and respond to an even wider array of cytokines. CT stimulates the production of IL-6 by the IEC-6 epithelial cell line *in vitro* and such stimulation is synergistically enhanced by the presence of TGFβ, TNFα, or IL-1β in the cultures (McGee *et al.*, 1993a,b). The IEC-17 epithelial cell line showed enhanced alloantigen presentation *in vitro* after treatment with CT, an effect which seemed to be related to in-

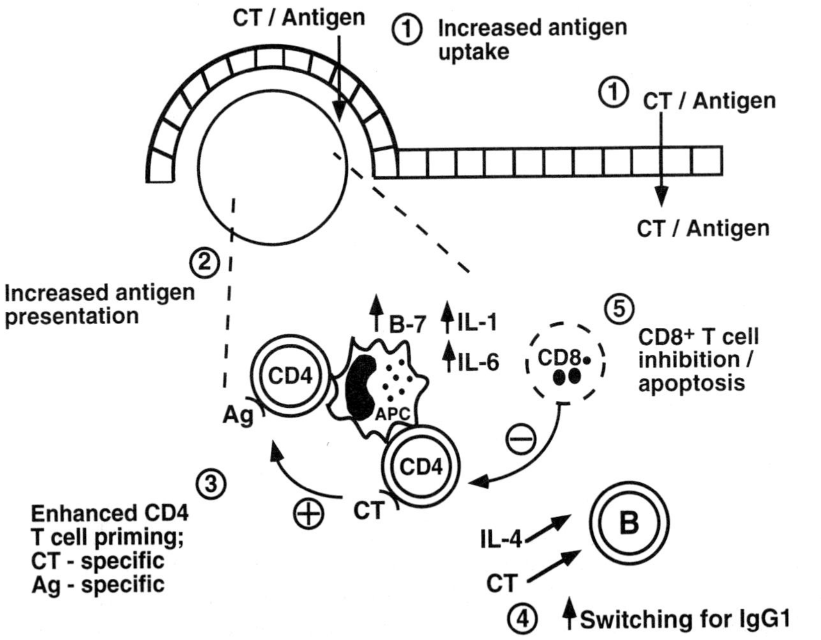

Figure 2. Possible mechanisms of action of CT as a mucosal adjuvant. These include: (1) enhanced uptake of coadministered antigen across either the follicular or the surface epithelial layer. This may apply particularly to conjugates or chimeric molecules. (2) Enhanced antigen presentation within GALT by effects on antigen presenting cells (APC) such as increasing the expression of costimulatory cell surface molecules such as B7 and costimulatory cytokines such as IL-1 and IL-6. This results in (3) enhanced CD4 T-cell priming of T cells specific both for CT/CT-B and for the coadministered antigen. Because immunogenicity and adjuvanticity of CT appear to be linked, the $CD4^+$ T-cell response to CT is shown as providing a positive signal to the $CD4^+$ T-cell specific for the antigen. The cellular and molecular details of this signal are unknown. These primed T cells produce cytokines such as IL-4 that can enhance immunoglobulin constant region heavy-chain gene switching to the IgG1 subclass and (4) CT enhances this effect. Last, (5) CT and CT-B can inhibit lymphocytes in the epithelial layer, particularly $CD8^+$ T cells, that may produce inhibitory cytokines. The inhibition of such cells thus allows and augments the ensuing immune response to antigen.

creased IL-1 and IL-6 production (Bromander *et al.*, 1993). There is no direct evidence that epithelial cells present antigen *in vivo,* but they could influence the process by secreting such cytokines.

B. T Cells

When T-cell antigen receptors are engaged by specific peptide–MHC complexes on APCs and the T cells also receive the proper costimulatory signals, they begin to proliferate and expand exponentially. Clonal expansion of antigen-specific T cells after exposure to antigen *in vivo* can be detected by isolating T cells from tissues, restimulating them with antigen and APCs *in vitro,* and measuring the resulting proliferative response, the release of cytokines, or both. Restimulation of cells with KLH *in vitro* from mice previously fed KLH plus CT as an adjuvant has shown substantial proliferative responses in Peyer's patches, gut lamina propria, mesenteric lymph node, and spleen (Clarke *et al.*, 1991; Hornquist and Lycke, 1993). Similar responses did not occur in mice fed KLH alone. In addition, T cells from these same tissues produced a variety of cytokines when restimulated with KLH. Although the relative quantity of the cytokines secreted varied among tissues, IL-2, IFNγ, IL-4, IL-5, and IL-6 were all produced (Wilson *et al.*, 1990; Clarke *et al.*, 1991; Hornquist and Lycke, 1993). The T cells responding in these cultures were predominately $CD4^+$ (Hornquist and Lycke, 1993). These results indicate that CT as a mucosal adjuvant induces antigen-specific T-cell activation and expansion in both mucosal and systemic lymphoid tissues. Because the direct effects of CT on T cells are very inhibitory, as discussed below, this T-cell priming *in vivo* is not likely to be due to direct effects of CT on T cells but rather indirect effects, e.g., through enhanced APC function and/or downregulation of cells producing inhibitory cytokines (Fig. 2).

Murine $CD4^+$ helper T cells have been subdivided further into Th1 and Th2 subtypes based on the pattern of cytokines that they secrete (Mosmann and Coffman, 1989). The Th1-type helper cells secrete IL-2 and IFNγ whereas Th2-type cells produce IL-4, IL-5, IL-6, IL-10, and IL-13. Several of the Th2 cytokines have been shown to be important in generating IgA responses *in vitro* (Murray *et al.*, 1987; Beagley *et al.*, 1989) and this Th2 subtype may be preferentially expressed in mucosal follicles such as Peyer's patches. In mice the IgG2a subclass antibody response is Th1 dependent, whereas IgG1 and IgE antibody responses are Th2 dependent (Finkelman *et al.*, 1990). The amounts of these antibodies produced during a given immune response can be used as a rough estimate of the proportion of the response that is Th1 vs Th2, although this is not a substitute for direct measurement of the relevant cytokines. The mechanisms by which a given antigen triggers a Th1- or Th2-dominated response are unclear but are being actively investigated. Antigen is one variable in that certain antigens seem to preferentially induce one pathway or the other. This can be critically important relative to host resistance to microbial pathogens, e.g., a Th1 response to an intracellular pathogen is protective whereas a Th2 response is deleterious. Thus it is important to know what effects CT has as a mucosal adjuvant on Th1 vs Th2 responses.

As mentioned above, early after immunization with KLH and CT, both Th1 and Th2 cytokines are detectable in restimulation assays; however, these cytokine phenotypes take time to develop fully. The data on this point are not conclusive, but there seems to be a tendency of CT as adjuvant to preferentially enhance Th2-type responses. The feeding of ovalbumin plus CT to mice primed for (Tamura *et al.*, 1994a) or induced (Snider *et al.*, 1994) IgE responses, the latter being sufficient to result in anaphylaxis after i.p. challenge with ovalbumin. The feeding of tetanus toxoid (TT) plus CT generated TT-specific lamina propria T cells producing Th2 but not Th1 cytokines (Xu-Amano *et al.*, 1993). When CT is added to T-cell clones cultured *in vitro*, it inhibits Th1 clones much more than it does Th2 clones (Gajewski *et al.*, 1990; Munoz *et al.*, 1990). There is a report that the mucosal adjuvanticity of CT is impaired in mice lacking the gene for IL-4 (Vajdy *et al.*, 1995). This is still a very small sampling of antigens and it is unclear whether these antigens themselves trigger a Th2 response that CT simply amplifies. At least with some other antigens CT appears to enhance a Th1 response, e.g., inactivated respiratory syncytial virus (Reuman *et al.*, 1991) and tetanus toxoid fragment C (Roberts *et al.*, 1995) plus CT as adjuvant given intranasally induced a substantial or predominant IgG2a response, respectively. The feeding of OVA plus a mixture of CT-B and CT induced class I MHC-restricted cytotoxic lymphocyte responses to an ovalbumin-transfected cell line (Bowen *et al.*, 1994). Conversely, there is a report that the feeding of small amounts of antigen conjugated to recombinant CT-B induced oral tolerance for Th1-mediated DTH responses (Sun *et al.*, 1994). A wider variety of antigens needs to be tested in order to settle this question, particularly those that preferentially induce Th1 responses.

The feeding of most protein antigens other than CT results in a state of immunologic unresponsiveness or oral tolerance, one mechanism of which is the induction of cells producing suppressive cytokines (Weiner *et al.*, 1994). CT's ability to abrogate oral tolerance to other antigens implies that it is altering the T-cell regulatory environment within the mucosa in a manner that inactivates or inhibits cells producing suppressive cytokines. Both CT and CT-B inhibit murine lymphocyte activation to antigens or mitogens *in vitro* (Woogen *et al.*, 1987). This inhibition requires binding of CT or CT-B to Gm1 ganglioside on the cell surface, but brief pulses lasting only minutes are sufficient. Both CD4 and CD8 T cells are inhibited, although the effect is greater on CD8 cells, probably because they bind more CT (Woogen *et al.*, 1993). Although the signaling events following binding of CT-B to the cell surface are unclear, IL-2 and to a lesser extent IL-2 receptor expression are downregulated and a substantial proportion of the activated T cells undergo apoptosis.This may explain the recent observation that CT given into the mouse intestine causes a marked depletion of intraepithelial lymphocytes in the small intestine as well as cells in the dome epithelium over the Peyer's patches (Elson *et al.*, 1995a). Coincident with these effects CT inhibits the generation of suppressor cells that mediate oral tolerance. In an adoptive transfer system, the feeding of KLH to mice generated suppressor T cells that inhibited both the secretory IgA and plasma IgG response to KLH, but the feeding of both KLH and CT together eliminated this suppression (Elson *et al.*, 1995a). These findings, taken together, support the notion that the perturbation of T cells that produce inhibitory cytokines is an important feature in both the mucosal immunogenicity and adjuvanticity of CT.

C. B Cells

There are many stages of B-cell development that must be traversed before reaching the antibody-secreting plasma cell. The major steps of B-cell development, including isotype commitment or switching, clonal expansion, and terminal differentiation, are all dependent upon and regulated by various cytokines, which act on B cells at defined stages of development (Tesch *et al.*, 1986). For example, the IgE and IgG1 isotype production is preferentially enhanced by IL-4 (Snapper and Paul, 1987), and the IgA isotype by IL-5 (Murray *et al.*, 1987). CT could affect any one or more of these steps. Precisely how CT interacts with B cells and/or with the critical cytokines that regulate them has only just begun to be examined.

CT may possess some pharmacologic activity that drives B cells toward IgA-committed precursors. Lebman *et al.* (1988) have shown that CT given intraduodenally can change the isotype pattern displayed by Peyer's patch B cells primed for an unrelated hapten from IgM to IgG and IgA after antigen-dependent clonal expansion *in vitro*. CT appeared to nonspecifically alter the responsiveness of Peyer's patch B cells to isotype switching signals present in the *in vitro* cultures. This could be due to a direct effect on B cells or could be attributed to the effect CT had on cytokine-mediated signals within the Peyer's patch. CT does have direct effects on B-cell isotype differentiation *in vitro*. CT enhances the effect of both IL-4 and IL-5 on purified B cells stimulated by lipopolysaccharide (LPS) *in vitro* (Lycke and Strober, 1989). In the presence of CT, IL-4 enhanced IgG1-producing B cells three to fourfold, and IL-5 had a similar effect on IgA-producing B cells. This effect of CT was on sIgM+ B cells which is consistent with CT inducing isotype switching in synergy with IL-4. Subsequent analysis demonstrated that CT plus IL-4 increased the expression of germline gamma 1 RNA transcripts, providing direct support for this idea (Lycke *et al.*, 1990). Interestingly, CT plus IL-4 did not have a similar effect on IgA heavy-chain gene transcription. There appear to be two mechanisms involved, an increase in cAMP that causes the increase in the germline IgH gene RNA transcripts, and an enhancement of B-cell differentiation due to CT-B binding to its ligand, Gm1 ganglioside, on the cell surface (Lycke, 1993) (Fig. 2).

Similar to its effects on T cells, CT inhibits B-cell proliferation *in vitro* even though it seems to be predominately stimulatory *in vivo*. Woogen *et. al.* (1987) found that CT inhibited proliferation of purified B cells *in vitro* when they were polyclonally stimulated by either anti-IgM or LPS; CT-B inhibited B cells stimulated by anti-IgM but not by LPS. The inhibition of B-cell proliferation is accompanied by enhancement of differentiation as manifested by an increase in MHC class II expression (Francis *et al.*, 1992). Lycke *et al.* (1989) also found that CT inhibited the B-cell proliferative response to LPS, but observed a mild stimulatory effect on B-cell proliferation relative to the control if the culture period was prolonged to 6 days and low doses of CT were used, although the former condition may not be physiologically relevant. CT is able to stimulate the proliferation of anti-IgM prestimulated human B cells, an effect mediated through increased cAMP (Anastassiou *et al.*, 1992). The effects of CT on B-cell proliferation *in vivo*, particularly after the brief exposures expected there, remain to be determined, but seem predominantly stimulatory. When mice were given influenza virus plus CT as adjuvant the number of B cells producing specific antibody to flu was increased in the Peyer's patches, particularly for IgA (Chen and Strober, 1990). Certainly the large numbers of plasma cells producing anti-CT in the lamina propria following oral immunization with CT, which has been estimated at up to 5% of the total at the peak of the response, indicates that clonal expansion occurs and is vigorous *in vivo*. Just as with T cells, this may well be an indirect effect through the stimulation of cytokines by other cell types.

IX. Summary

Much remains to be learned about the mechanism of both CT's immunogenicity and adjuvanticity, particularly the importance *in vivo* of the multiple effects of CT found *in vitro*. The properties of CT as a mucosal immunogen seem to extend to antigens delivered with it to mucosal surfaces. CT's mucosal adjuvanticity appears to be related to its immunogenicity. Both of its subunits are required. CT has been effective as a mucosal adjuvant with a wide variety of antigen types. The dose, timing, route, antigen type, and genetic background of the host are all important variables. There are indications that the mechanism of CT's adjuvanticity involves multiple aspects of immune induction in the mucosa (Fig. 2), including increased uptake of antigen (with CT-B conjugates or chimeras), enhancement of IL-1 and IL-6 production by APC's, enhancement of T-cell priming; perturbations of regulatory T cells (especially inhibition of cells producing inhibitory cytokines), stimulation of B-cell switching to IgA and IgG, and, possibly, enhancement of B-cell clonal expansion. Different components of these multiple effects may be of more importance for some antigens than for others. CT remains attractive as an adjuvant for mucosal vaccines.

References

Abraham, E., and Robinson, A. (1991). Oral immunization with bacterial polysaccharide and adjuvant enhances antigen-specific pulmonary secretory antibody response and resistance to pneumonia. *Vaccine* **9**, 757–764.

Anastassiou, E. D., Yamada, H., Boumpas, D. T., Tsokos, G. C., Thyphronitis, G., Balow, J., and Mond, J. J. (1992). Cholera toxin promotes the proliferation of anti-mu antibody-prestimulated human B cells. *Cell Immunol* **140**, 237–247.

Beagley, K. W., Eldridge, J. H., Lee, F., Kiyono, H., Everson, M. P., Koopman, W. J., Hirano, T., Kishimoto, T., and McGhee, J. R. (1989). Interleukins and IgA synthesis. Human and murine interleukin 6 induce high rate IgA secretion in IgA-committed B cells. *J. Exp. Med.* **169**, 2133–2148.

Bergquist, C., Lagergard, T., Lindblad, M., and Holmgren, J. (1995). Local and systemic antibody responses to dextran-cholera toxin B subunit conjugates. *Infect Immun* **63**, 2021–2025.

Bessen, D., and Fischetti, V. A. (1988). Influence of intranasal immunization with synthetic peptides corresponding to conserved epitopes of M protein on mucosal colonization by group A streptococci. *Infect Immun* **56**, 2666–2672.

Betley, M., Miller, V., and Mekalanos, J. (1986). Genetics of bacterial enterotoxins. *Annu. Rev. Microbiol.* **40**, 577–605.

Bland, P. W., and Warren, L. G. (1986). Antigen presentation by epithelial cells of the rat small intestine. II. Selective induction of suppressor cells. *Immunology* **58**, 9–14.

Bourguin, I., Chardes, T., Mevelec, M. N., Woodman, J. P., and Bout, D. (1991). Amplification of the secretory IgA response to *Toxoplasma gondii* using cholera toxin. *Fems Microbiol Lett.* **65**, 265–271.

Bowen, J. C., Nair, S. K., Reddy, R., and Rouse, B. T. (1994). Cholera toxin acts as a potent adjuvant for the induction of cytotoxic T-lymphocyte responses with nonreplicating antigens. *Immunology* **81**, 338–342.

Bromander, A., Holmgren, J., and Lycke, N. (1991). Cholera toxin stimulates IL-1 production and enhances antigen presentation by macrophages *in vitro*. *J. Immunol.* **146**, 2908–2914.

Bromander, A. K., Kjerrulf, M., Holmgren, J., and Lycke, N. (1993). Cholera toxin enhances alloantigen presentation by cultured intestinal epithelial cells. *Scand. J. Immunol.* **37**, 452–458.

Castello-Branco, L. R., Griffin, G. E., Poulton, T. A., Dougan, G., and Lewis, D. J. (1994). Characterization of the circulating T cell response after oral immunization of human volunteers with cholera toxin B subunit. *Vaccine* **12**, 65–72.

Chen, K. S., and Strober, W. (1990). Cholera holotoxin and its B subunit enhance Peyer's patch B-cell responses induced by orally administered influenza virus: Disproportionate cholera toxin enhancement of the IgA B-cell response. *Eur. J. Immunol.* **20**, 433–436.

Clarke, C. J., Wilson, A. D., Williams, N. A., and Stokes, C. R. (1991). Mucosal priming of T-lymphocyte responses to fed protein antigens using cholera toxin as an adjuvant. *Immunology* **72**, 323–328.

Cuatrecasas, P. (1973). Gangliosides and membrane receptors for cholera toxin. *Biochemistry* **12**, 3558–3566.

Czerkinsky, C., Russell, M. W., Lycke, N., Lindblad, M., and Holmgren, J. (1989). Oral administration of a streptococcal antigen coupled to cholera toxin B subunit evokes strong antibody responses in salivary glands and extramucosal tissues. *Infect. Immun.* **57**, 1072–1077.

Czerkinsky, C., Svennerholm, A. M., Quiding, M., Jonsson, R., and Holmgren, J. (1991). Antibody-producing cells in peripheral blood and salivary glands after oral cholera vaccination of humans. *Infect. Immun* **59**, 996–1001.

Czinn, S. J., and Nedrud, J. G. (1991). Oral immunization against *Helicobacter pylori*. *Infect. Immun.* **59**, 2359–2363.

Dertzbaugh, M. T., and Elson, C. O. (1993a). Comparative effectiveness of the cholera toxin B subunit and alkaline phosphatase as carriers for oral vaccines. *Infect. Immun.* **61**, 48–55.

Dertzbaugh, M. T., and Elson, C. O. (1993b). Reduction in oral immunogenicity of cholera toxin B subunit by N-terminal peptide addition. *Infect. Immun.* **61**, 384–390.

Dertzbaugh, M. T., Peterson, D. L., and Macrina, F. L. (1990). Cholera toxin B subunit gene fusion: Structural and functional analysis of the chimeric protein. *Infect. Immun.* **58**, 70–79.

Elson, C. O. (1992). Cholera toxin as a mucosal adjuvant: Effects of H-2 major histocompatibility complex and lps genes. *Infect. Immun.* **60**, 2874–2879.

Elson, C. O., and Dertzbaugh, M. T. (1994). Mucosal adjuvants. "Handbook of Mucosal Immunology," pp. 391–401. Academic Press, San Diego.

Elson, C. O., and Ealding, W. (1984a). Cholera toxin feeding did not induce oral tolerance in mice and abrogated oral tolerance to an unrelated protein antigen. *J. Immunol.* **133**, 2892–2897.

Elson, C. O., and Ealding, W. (1984b). Generalized systemic and mucosal immunity in mice after mucosal stimulation with cholera toxin. *J. Immunol.* **132**, 2736–2742.

Elson, C. O., and Ealding, W. (1985). Genetic control of the murine immune response to cholera toxin. *J. Immunol.* **135**, 930–932.

Elson, C. O., and Ealding, W. (1987). Ir gene control of the murine secretory IgA response to cholera toxin. *Eur. J. Immunol.* **17**, 425–428.

Elson, C. O., Holland, S. P., Dertzbaugh, M. T., Cuff, C. F., and Anderson, A. O. (1995a). Morphologic and functional alterations of mucosal T cells by cholera toxin and its B subunit. *J. Immunol.* **154**, 1032–1040.

Elson, C. O., Tomasi, M., Chang, T.-T., Jobling, M. G., and Holmes, R. K. (1995b). Immunogenicity and adjuvanticity of mutant cholera toxin (CT) molecules. *FASEB J.* **9**, A290.

Finkelman, F. D., Holmes, J., Katona, I. M., Urban, J. F. J., Beckmann, M. P., Park, L. S., Schooley, K. A., Coffman, R. L., Mosmann, T. R., and Paul, W. E. (1990). Lymphokine control of *in vivo* immunoglobulin isotype selection. *Annu. Rev. Immunol.* **8**, 303–333.

Francis, M. L., Ryan, J., Jobling, M. G., Holmes, R. K., Moss, J., and Mond, J. J. (1992). Cyclic AMP-independent effects of cholera toxin on B-cell activation. II. Binding of ganglioside GM1 induces B-cell activation. *J. Immunol.* **148**, 1999–2005.

Gajewski, T. F., Schell, S. R., and Fitch, F. W. (1990). Evidence implicating utilization of different T cell receptor-associated signaling pathways by Th1 and Th2 clones. *J. Immunol.* **144**, 4110–4120.

Gizurarson, S., Tamura, S., Aizawa, C., and Kurata, T. (1992). Stimulation of the transepithelial flux of influenza HA vaccine by cholera toxin B subunit. *Vaccine* **10**, 101–106.

Hajishengallis, G., Hollingshead, S. K., Koga, T., and Russell, M. W. (1995). Mucosal immunization with a bacterial protein antigen genetically coupled to cholera toxin A2/B subunits. *J. Immunol.* **154**, 4322–4332.

Hansson, H. A., Lange, S., and Lonnroth, I. (1984). Internalization *in vivo* of cholera toxin in the small intestinal epithelium of the rat. *Acta Pathol. Microbiol. Immunol. Scand. A* **92**, 15–21.

Hearn, T. I. (1995). Murine mucosal and systemic immune responses to antigens delivered by oral infusion in water-in-oil-in-water emulsions containing block copolymer P1005. Emory University, Atlanta, Georgia.

Hirabayashi, Y., Tamura, S. I., Suzuki, Y., Nagamine, T., Aizawa, C., Shimada, K., and Kurata, T. (1991). H-2-unrestricted adjuvant effect of cholera toxin B subunit on murine antibody responses to influenza virus haemagglutinin. *Immunology* **72**, 329–335.

Hirabayashi, Y., Tamura, S. I., Shimada, K., and Kurata, T. (1992). Involvement of antigen-presenting cells in the enhancement of the *in vitro* antibody responses by cholera toxin B subunit. *Immunology* **75**, 493–498.

Hol, W. G. J., Sixma, T. K., and Meritt, E. A. (1995). Structure and function of *E. coli* heat-labile enterotoxin and cholera toxin B pentamer. "Bacterial Toxins and Virulence Factors in Disease." pp. 185–223. Dekker, New York.

Hornquist, E., and Lycke, N. (1993). Cholera toxin adjuvant greatly promotes antigen priming of T cells. *Eur. J. Immunol.* **23**, 2136–2143.

Hornqvist, E., Goldschmidt, T. J., Holmdahl, R., and Lycke, N. (1991). Host defense against cholera toxin is strongly CD4+ T cell dependent. *Infect. Immun.* **59**, 3630–3638.

Hoshi, S., Nakamura, T., Nunoya, T., and Ueda, S. (1995). Induction of protective immunity in chickens orally immunized with inactivated infectious bursal disease virus. *Vaccine* **13**, 245–252.

Hui, G. S. N., Chang, S. P., Gibson, H., Hashimoto, A., Hashiro, C., Barr, P. J., and Kotani, S. (1991). Influence of adjuvants on the antibody specificity to the *Plasmodium falciparum* major merozoite surface protein, gp195. *J. Immunol.* **147**, 3935–3941.

Jackson, R. J., Fujihashi, K., Xu-Amano, J., Kiyono, H., Elson, C. O., and McGhee, J. R. (1993). Optimizing oral vaccines: Induction of systemic and mucosal B-cell and antibody responses to tetanus toxoid by use of cholera toxin as an adjuvant. *Infect. Immun.* **61**, 4272–4279.

Jertborn, M., Svennerholm, A. M., and Holmgren, J. (1988). Five-year immunologic memory in Swedish volunteers after oral cholera vaccination. *J. Infect. Dis.* **157**, 374–377.

Jobling, M. G., and Holmes, R. K. (1991). Analysis of structure and function of the B subunit of cholera toxin by the use of site-directed mutagenesis. *Mol. Microbiol.* **5**, 1755–1767.

Jobling, M. G., and Holmes, R. K. (1992). Fusion proteins containing the A2 domain of cholera toxin assemble with B polypeptides of cholera toxin to form immunoreactive and functional holotoxin-like chimeras. *Infect. Immun.* **60**, 4915–4924.

Kay, R. A., and Ferguson, A. (1989a). The immunological consequences of feeding cholera toxin. I. Feeding cholera toxin suppresses the induction of systemic delayed-type hypersensitivity but not humoral immunity. *Immunology* **66**, 410–415.

Kay, R. A., and Ferguson, A. (1989b). The immunological consequences of feeding cholera toxin. II. Mechanisms responsible for the induction of oral tolerance for DTH. *Immunology* **66**, 416–421.

Kuper, C. F., Koornstra, P. J., Hameleers, D. M., Biewenga, J., Spit, B. J., Duijvestijn, A. M., van, B. V. P. J., and Sminia, T. (1992). The role of nasopharyngeal lymphoid tissue. *Immunol. Today* **13**, 219–224.

Kusnecov, A. W., Cohen, N., and Moynihan, J. (1992). Adjuvant effects of freely ingested cholera toxin on systemic antibody and DTH responses to protein antigen. *Regional Immunology* **4**, 153–161.

Lebman, D. A., Fuhrman, J. A., and Cebra, J. J. (1988). Intraduodenal application of cholera holotoxin increases the potential of clones from Peyer's patch B cells of relevant and unrelated specificities to secrete IgG and IgA. *Regional Immunology* **1**, 32–40.

Lee, A., and Chen, M. (1994). Successful immunization against gastric infection with *Helicobacter* species: Use of a cholera toxin B-subunit-whole-cell vaccine. *Infect. Immun.* **62**, 3594–3597.

Lencer, W. I., de Almeida, J. B., Moe, S., Stow, J. L., Ausiello, D. A., and Madara, J. L. (1993). Entry of cholera toxin into polarized human intestinal epithelial cells. Identification of an early brefeldin A sensitive event required for A1-peptide generation. *J. Clin. Invest.* **92**, 2941–2951.

Levine, M. M., Kaper, J. B., Black, R. E., and Clements, M. L. (1983). New knowledge on pathogenesis of bacterial enteric infections as applied to vaccine development. *Microbiol. Rev.* **47**, 510–550.

Lewis, D. J., Castello, B. L. R., Novotny, P., Dougan, G., Poulton, T. A., and Griffin, G. E. (1993). Circulating cellular immune response to oral immunization of humans with cholera toxin B-subunit. *Vaccine* **11**, 119–121.

Liang, X., Lamm, M. E., and Nedrud, J. G. (1989a). Cholera toxin as a mucosal adjuvant: glutaraldehyde treatment dissociates adjuvanticity from toxicity. *J. Immunol.* **143**, 484–490.

Liang, X. P., Lamm, M. E., and Nedrud, J. G. (1989b). Cholera toxin as a mucosal adjuvant for respiratory antibody responses in mice. *Regional Immunology* **2**, 244–248.

Lycke, N. Y. (1993). Cholera toxin promotes B-cell isotype switching by two different mechanisms. cAMP induction augments germ-line Ig H-chain RNA transcripts whereas membrane ganglioside GM1-receptor binding enhances later events in differentiation. *J. Immunol.* **150**, 4810–4821.

Lycke, N., and Holmgren, J. (1986a). Intestinal mucosal memory and presence of memory cells in lamina propria and Peyer's patches in mice 2 years after oral immunization with cholera toxin. *Scand. J. Immunol.* **23**, 611–616.

Lycke, N., and Holmgren, J. (1986b). Strong adjuvant properties of cholera toxin on gut mucosal immune responses to orally presented antigens. *Immunology* **59**, 301–308.

Lycke, N., and Strober, W. (1989). Cholera toxin promotes B-cell isotype differentiation. *J. Immunol.* **142**, 3781–3787.

Lycke, N., Bromander, A. K., Ekman, L., Karlsson, U., and Holmgren, J. (1989). Cellular basis of immunomodulation by cholera toxin *in vitro* with possible association to the adjuvant function *in vivo*. *J. Immunol.* **142**, 20–27.

Lycke, N., Severinson, E., and Strober, W. (1990). Cholera toxin acts synergistically with IL-4 to promote IgG1 switch differentiation. *J. Immunol.* **145**, 3316–3324.

Lycke, N., Karlsson, U., Sjolander, A., and Magnusson, K. E. (1991). The adjuvant action of cholera toxin is associated with an increased intestinal permeability for luminal antigens. *Scand. J. Immunol.* **33**, 691–698.

Lycke, N., Tsuji, T., and Holmgren, J. (1992). The adjuvant effect of *Vibrio cholerae* and *Escherichia coli* heat-labile enterotoxins is linked to their ADP-ribosyltransferase activity. *Eur. J. Immunol.* **22**, 2277–2281.

McGee, D. W., Beagley, K. W., Aicher, W. K., and McGhee, J. R. (1993a). Transforming growth factor-beta and IL-1 beta act in synergy to enhance IL-6 secretion by the intestinal epithelial cell line, IEC-6. *J. Immunol,* **151**, 970–978.

McGee, D. W., Elson, C. O., and McGhee, J. R. (1993b). Enhancing effect of cholera toxin on interleukin-6 secretion by IEC-6 intestinal epithelial cells: Mode of action and augmenting effect of inflammatory cytokines. *Infect. Immun.* **61**, 4637–4644.

McKenzie, S. J., and Halsey, J. F. (1984). Cholera toxin B subunit as a carrier protein to stimulate a mucosal immune response. *J. Immunol.* **133**, 1818–1824.

Mayer, L., Eisenhardt, D., and Shlien, R. (1988). Selective induction of antigen nonspecific suppressor cells with normal gut epithelium as accessory cells. *Monogr. Allergy* **24**, 78–80.

Merritt, E. A., Sixma, T. K., Kalk, K. H., Van Zanten, B. A. M., and Hol, W. G. J. (1994a). Galactose binding site in *E. coli* heat-labile enterotoxin(LT) and cholera toxin (CT). *Mol. Microbiol.* **13**, 745–753.

Merritt, E. A., Sarfaty, S., van den Akker, F., L'Hoir, C., Martial, J. A., and Hol, W. G. (1994b). Crystal structure of cholera toxin B-pentamer bound to receptor GM1 pentasaccharide. *Protein Sci.* **3**, 166–175.

Mosmann, T. R., and Coffman, R. L. (1989). Th1 and Th2 cells: Different patterns of lymphokine secretion lead to different functional properties. *Annu. Rev. Immunol.* **7**, 145–174.

Muller, C. P., Beauverger, P., Schneider, F., Jung, G., and Brons, N. H. (1995). Cholera toxin B stimulates systemic neutralizing antibodies after intranasal co-immunization with measles virus. *J. Gen. Virol.* **76**, 1371–1380.

Munoz, E., Zubiaga, A. M., Merrow, M., Sauter, N. P., and Huber, B. T. (1990). Cholera toxin discriminates between T helper 1 and 2 cells in T cell receptor-mediated activation: Role of cAMP in T cell proliferation. *J. Exp. Med.* **172**, 95–103.

Murray, P. D., McKenzie, D. T., Swain, S. L., and Kagnoff, M. F. (1987). Interleukin 5 and interleukin 4 produced by Peyer's patch T cells selectively enhance immunoglobulin A expression. *J. Immunol.* **139**, 2669–2674.

Nedrud, J. G., and Sigmund, N. (1991). Cholera toxin as a mucosal adjuvant. III. Antibody responses to nontarget dietary antigens are not increased. *Regional Immunology* **3**, 217–222.

Nedrud, J. G., Liang, X. P., Hague, N., and Lamm, M. E. (1987). Combined oral/nasal immunization protects mice from Sendai virus infection. *J. Immunol.* **139**, 3484–3492.

Orr, N., Arnon, R., Rubin, G., Cohen, D., Bercovier, H., and Lowell, G. H. (1994). Enhancement of anti-*Shigella* lipopolysaccharide (LPS) response by addition of the cholera toxin B subunit to oral and intranasal proteosome-*Shigella flexneri* 2a LPS vaccines. *Infect. Immun.* **62**, 5198–5200.

Pierce, N. F., and Cray, W. C. (1982). Determinants of the localization, magnitude, and duration of a specific mucosal IgA plasma cell response in enterically immunized rats. *J. Immunol.* **128**, 1311–1315.

Pierce, N. F., and Gowans, J. L. (1975). Cellular kinetics of the intestinal immune response to cholera toxoid in rats. *J. Exp. Med.* **142**, 1550–1563.

Quiding, M., Nordstrom, I., Kilander, A., Andersson, G., Hanson, L. A., Holmgren, J., and Czerkinsky, C. (1991). Intestinal immune responses in humans. Oral cholera vaccination induces strong intestinal antibody responses and interferon-gamma production and evokes local immunological memory. *J. Clin. Invest.* **88**, 143–148.

Reuman, P. D., Keely, S. P., and Schiff, G. M. (1991). Similar subclass antibody responses after intranasal immunization with UV-inactivated RSV mixed with cholera toxin or live RSV. *J. Med. Virol,* **35**, 192–197.

Roberts, M., Bacon, A., Rappuoli, R., Pizza, M., Cropley, I., Douce, G., Dougan, G., Marinaro, M., McGhee, J., and Chatfield, S. (1995). A mutant pertussis toxin molecule that lacks ADP-ribosyltransferase activity, PT-9K/129G, is an effective mucosal adjuvant for intranasally delivered proteins. *Infect. Immun.* **63**, 2100–2108.

Sanchez, J., Svennerholm, A. M., and Holmgren, J. (1988). Genetic fusion of a nontoxic heat-stable enterotoxin-related decapeptide antigen to cholera toxin B-subunit. *FEBS Lett.* **241**, 110–114.

Sixma, T. K., Pronk, S. E., Kalk, K. H., Wartna, E. S., van Zanten, B. A. M., Witholt, B., and Hol, W. G. (1991). Crystal structure of a cholera toxin-related heat-labile enterotoxin from *E. coli*. *Nature (London)* **351**, 371–377.

Snapper, C. M., and Paul, W. E. (1987). Interferon-gamma and B-cell stimulatory factor-1 reciprocally regulate Ig isotype production. *Science* **236**, 944–947.

Snider, D. P., Marshall, J. S., Perdue, M. H., and Liang, H. (1994). Production of IgE antibody and allergic sensitization of intestinal and peripheral tissues after oral immunization with protein Ag and cholera toxin. *J. Immunol,* **153**, 647–657.

Sun, J. B., Holmgren, J., and Czerkinsky, C. (1994). Cholera toxin B subunit: An efficient transmucosal carrier-delivery system for induction of peripheral immunological tolerance. *Proc. Natl. Acad. Sci. U.S.A* **91**, 10795–10799.

Svennerholm, A. M., Jertborn, M., Gothefors, L., Karim, A. M. M. M., Sack, D. A., and Holmgren, J. (1984). Mucosal antitoxic and antibacterial immunity after cholera disease and after immunization with a combined B subunit-whole cell vaccine. *J. Infect. Dis.* **149**, 884–893.

Takahashi, I., Okahashi, N., Kanamoto, T., Asakawa, H., and Koga, T. (1990). Intranasal immunization of mice with recombinant protein antigen of serotype c *Streptococcus mutans* and cholera toxin B subunit. *Arch. Oral Biol.* **35**, 475–477.

Tamura, S., Samegai, Y., Kurata, H., Nagamine, T., Aizawa, C., and Kurata, T. (1988). Protection against influenza virus infection by vaccine inoculated intranasally with cholera toxin B subunit. *Vaccine* **6**, 409–413.

Tamura, S., Funato, H., Nagamine, T., Aizawa, C., and Kurata, T. (1989). Effectiveness of cholera toxin B subunit as an adjuvant for nasal influenza vaccination despite pre-existing immunity to CT-B. *Vaccine* **7**, 503–505.

Tamura, S., Funato, H., Hirabayashi, Y., Suzuki, Y., Nagamine, T., Aizawa, C., and Kurata, T. (1991). Cross-protection against influenza A virus infection by passively transferred respiratory tract IgA antibodies to different hemagglutinin molecules. *Eur. J. Immunol.* **21,** 1337–1344.

Tamura, S., Shoji, Y., Hasiguchi, K., Aizawa, C., and Kurata, T. (1994a). Effects of cholera toxin adjuvant on IgE antibody response to orally or nasally administered ovalbumin. *Vaccine* **12,** 1238–1240.

Tamura, S., Yamanaka, A., Shimohara, M., Tomita, T., Komase, K., Tsuda, Y., Suzuki, Y., Nagamine, T., Kawahara, K., and Danbara, H. (1994b). Synergistic action of cholera toxin B subunit (and *Escherichia coli* heat-labile toxin B subunit) and a trace amount of cholera whole toxin as an adjuvant for nasal influenza vaccine. *Vaccine* **12,** 419–426.

Tamura, S., Ishihara, K., Miyata, K., Aizawa, C., and Kurata, T. (1995). Mechanism of enhancement of the immune responses to influenza vaccine with cholera toxin B subunit and a trace amount of holotoxin. *Vaccine* **13,** 339–341.

Tesch, H., Muller, W., and Rajewsky, K. (1986). Lymphokines regulate immunoglobulin isotype expression in an antigen-specific immune response. *J. Immunol.* **136,** 2892–2895.

Tomasi, M., Dertzbaugh, M., Hunter, H., and Elson, C. (1994). Use of multiple emulsions containing cholera toxin (CT) for mucosal immunization. *FASEB J.* **8,** A283.

Vajdy, M., and Lycke, N. (1993). Stimulation of antigen-specific T- and B-cell memory in local as well as systemic lymphoid tissues following oral immunization with cholera toxin adjuvant. *Immunology* **80,** 197–203.

Vajdy, M., Kosco-Vilbois, M. H., Kopf, M., Kohler, G., and Lycke, N. (1995). Impaired mucosal immune responses in interleukin 4-targeted mice. *J. Exp. Med.* **181,** 41–53.

Van der Heijden, P. J., Bianchi, A. T., Dol, M., Pals, J. W., Stok, W., and Bokhout, B. A. (1991). Manipulation of intestinal immune responses against ovalbumin by cholera toxin and its B subunit in mice. *Immunology* **72,** 89–93.

van Heyningen, S. (1991). The ring on a finger. *Nature (London)* **351,** 351.

Verheul, A. F. M., Versteeg, A., DeReuver, M. J., Jansze, M., and Snippe, H. (1989). Modulation of the immune response to pneumococcal type 14 capsular polysaccharide-protein conjugates by the adjuvant quil A depends on the properties of the conjugates. *Infect. Immun.* **57,** 1078–1083.

Waksman, B. H. (1979). Adjuvants and immune regulation by lymphoid cells. *Springer Semin. Immunopathol.* **2,** 5–33.

Walsh, E. E. (1993). Mucosal immunization with a subunit respiratory syncytial virus vaccine in mice. *Vaccine* **11,** 1135–1138.

Weiner, H. L., Friedman, A., Miller, A., Khoury, S. J., al-Sabbagh, A., Santos, L., Sayegh, M., Nussenblatt, R. B., Trentham, D. E., and Hafler, D. A. (1994). Oral tolerance: Immunologic mechanisms and treatment of animal and human organ-specific autoimmune diseases by oral administration of autoantigens. *Annu. Rev. Immunol.* **12,** 809–837.

Wilson, A. D., Clarke, C. J., and Stokes, C. R. (1990). Whole cholera toxin and B subunit act synergistically as an adjuvant for the mucosal immune response of mice to keyhole limpet haemocyanin. *Scand. J. Immunol.* **31,** 443–451.

Wilson, A. D., Bailey, M., Williams, N. A., and Stokes, C. R. (1991). The *in vitro* production of cytokines by mucosal lymphocytes immunized by oral administration of keyhole limpet hemocyanin using cholera toxin as an adjuvant. *Eur. J. Immunol.* **21,** 2333–2339.

Woogen, S. D., Ealding, W., and Elson, C. O. (1987). Inhibition of murine lymphocyte proliferation by the B subunit of cholera toxin. *J. Immunol.* **139,** 3764–3770.

Woogen, S. D., Turo, K., Dieleman, L. A., Beagley, K. W., and Elson, C. O. (1993). Inhibition of murine T cell activation by cholera toxin B subunit is not mediated through the phosphatidylinositol second messenger system. *J. Immunol.* **150,** 3274–3281.

Wu, H. Y., and Russell, M. W. (1993). Induction of mucosal immunity by intranasal application of a streptococcal surface protein antigen with the cholera toxin B subunit. *Infect. Immun.* **61,** 314–322.

Wu, H. Y., and Russell, M. W. (1994). Comparison of systemic and mucosal priming for mucosal immune responses to a bacterial protein antigen given with or coupled to cholera toxin (CT) B subunit, and effects of pre-existing anti-CT immunity. *Vaccine* **12,** 215–222.

Xu-Amano, J., Kiyono, H., Jackson, R. J., Staats, H. F., Fujihashi, K., Burrows, P. D., Elson, C. O., Pillai, S., and McGhee, J. R. (1993). Helper T cell subsets for immunoglobulin A responses: Oral immunization with tetanus toxoid and cholera toxin as adjuvant selectively induces Th2 cells in mucosa associated tissues. *J. Exp. Med.* **178,** 1309–1320.

Zhang, R. G., Scott, D. L., Westbrook, M. L., Nance, S., Spangler, B. D., Shipley, G. G., and Westbrook, E. M. (1995a). The three-dimensional crystal structure of cholera toxin. *J. Mol. Biol.* **251,** 563–573.

Zhang, T., Li, E., and Stanley, S. L., Jr. (1995b). Oral immunization with the dodecapeptide repeat of the serine-rich *Entamoeba histolytica* protein (SREHP) fused to the cholera toxin B subunit induces a mucosal and systemic anti-SREHP antibody response. *Infect. Immun.* **63,** 1349–1355.

5

Use of Escherichia coli *Heat-Labile Enterotoxin as an Oral Adjuvant*

BONNY L. DICKINSON
JOHN D. CLEMENTS
Department of Microbiology and Immunology
Tulane University Medical Center
New Orleans, Louisiana 70112

I. Introduction

Microbial pathogens can infect a host by one of several mechanisms. They may enter through a break in the integument induced by trauma, they may be introduced by vector transmission, or they may interact with a mucosal surface. The majority of human pathogens initiate disease by the last mechanism, i.e., following interaction with mucosal surfaces. Bacterial and viral pathogens that act through this mechanism first make contact with the mucosal surface where they may attach and then colonize or be taken up by specialized absorptive cells (M cells) in the epithelium that overlay Peyer's patches and other lymphoid follicles (Bockman and Cooper, 1973; Owen *et al.*, 1986). Organisms that enter the lymphoid tissues may be readily killed within the lymphoid follicles, thereby provoking a potentially protective immunological response as antigens are delivered to immune cells within the follicles (e.g., *Vibrio cholerae*). Alternatively, pathogenic organisms capable of surviving local defense mechanisms may spread from the follicles and subsequently cause local or systemic disease (i.e., *Salmonella* spp., poliovirus, rotavirus in immunocompromised hosts).

Secretory IgA (S-IgA) antibodies directed against specific virulence determinants of infecting organisms play an important role in overall mucosal immunity. In many cases, it is possible to prevent the initial infection of mucosal surfaces by stimulating production of mucosal S-IgA levels directed against relevant virulence determinants of an infecting organism. Secretory IgA may prevent the initial interaction of the pathogen with the mucosal surface by blocking attachment and/or colonization, neutralizing surface acting toxins, or preventing invasion of the host cells. While extensive research has been conducted to determine the role of cell mediated immunity and serum antibody in protection against infectious agents, less is known about the regulation, induction, and secretion of S-IgA. Parenterally administered inactivated whole-cell and whole-virus preparations are effective at eliciting protective serum IgG and cell-mediated immunity against organisms that have a significant serum phase in their pathogenesis (i.e., *Salmonella typhi*, hepatitis B). However, parenteral vaccines are not effective at eliciting mucosal S-IgA responses and are ineffective against bacteria that interact with mucosal surfaces and do not invade (e.g., *V. cholerae*). There is, however, recent evidence that parenterally administered vaccines may be effective against at least one virus, rotavirus, that interacts primarily with mucosal surfaces (Conner *et al.*, 1993). Protection is presumed to result from transudation of antigen specific IgG onto mucosal surfaces for virus neutralization. Therefore, mechanisms that stimulate both serum and mucosal antibodies are important for the development of effective vaccines.

Oral immunization can be effective for induction of specific S-IgA responses if the antigens are presented to the T and B lymphocytes and accessory cells contained within the Peyer's patches where preferential IgA B-cell development is initiated. The Peyer's patches contain helper T (Th) cells that mediate B-cell isotype switching directly from IgM cells to IgA B cells. The patches also contain T cells that initiate terminal B-cell differentiation. The primed B cells then migrate to the mesenteric lymph nodes and undergo differentiation, enter the thoracic duct and then the general circulation, and subsequently seed all of the mucosal tissues of the body, including the lamina propria of the gut and respiratory tracts. IgA is then produced by mature plasma cells, complexed with membrane-bound secretory component (s.c.), and transported onto the mucosal surface where it is available to interact with invading pathogens (Strober and Jacobs, 1985; Tomasi and Plaut, 1985). The existence of this common mucosal immune system explains in part the potential of live oral vaccines and oral immunization for protection against pathogenic organisms that initiate infection by first interacting with mucosal surfaces.

A number of strategies have been developed for oral immunization, including the use of attenuated mutants of bacteria (i.e., *Salmonella* spp.) as carriers of heterologous antigens (Cárdenas and Clements, 1992; Clements and Cárdenas, 1990; Clements and El-Morshidy, 1984; Clements *et al.*, 1992), encapsulation of antigens into microspheres composed of poly-DL-lactide-glycolide (PGL), protein-like polymer–proteinoids (Santiago *et al.*, 1993), gelatin capsules, and different formulations of liposomes (Alving *et al.*, 1986; Garcon and Six, 1993; Gould-Fogerite and Mannino, 1993), adsorption onto nanoparticles, use of lipophilic immune-stimulating complexes (Mowat and Donachie, 1991), and addition of bacterial products with known adjuvant properties (Clements *et al.*, 1988a; Elson, 1989; Lycke and Holmgren, 1986, 1992). The two bacterial products with the greatest potential to function as oral adjuvants are cholera toxin (CT) produced by various strains of *V. cholerae,* and the heat-labile enterotoxin (LT) produced by some enterotoxigenic strains of *Escherichia coli.* Although LT and CT have many features in common, they are clearly distinct molecules with biochemical and immunologic differences which make them unique (see Section III).

II. Biological and Immunological Properties of Cholera Toxin and LT

The extensive diarrhea of cholera is the result of a potent exo-enterotoxin which causes the activation of adenylate cyclase and a subsequent increase in intracellular levels of cyclic 3′,5′-adenosine monophosphate (cAMP). The cholera enterotoxin is an 84,000-Da polymeric protein composed of two major, noncovalently associated, immunologically distinct regions or domains (cholera-A and cholera-B) (Finkelstein and LoSpalluto, 1969). Of these, the 56,000-Da region, or choleragenoid, is responsible for the binding of the toxin to the host cell membrane receptor, G_{M1} (galactosyl-N-acetylgalactosaminyl-(sialyl)-galactosylglucosyl ceramide), which is found on the surface of essentially all eukaryotic cells. Choleragenoid is composed of five noncovalently associated subunits, while the A region (27,000-Da) is responsible for the diverse biological effects of the toxin.

The relationship of the two subunits of CT with respect to the immunologic properties of the molecule has been a source of considerable debate. On the one hand, CT is an excellent immunogen that provokes the development of both serum and mucosal antitoxin antibody responses when delivered orally. Since cholera patients are known to develop rises in titers of antitoxin antibodies during convalescence from clinical cholera (Finkelstein, 1975), this is not a new finding. One key development concerning the nature of this response was the observation that CT, unlike most other protein antigens, does not induce oral tolerance against itself (Elson and Ealding, 1984a,b). This was also found to be true when just the B subunit was fed to mice, an observation substantiated by the cholera vaccine field trials in Bangladesh in which oral immunization with B subunit combined with killed whole cells gave rise to mucosal as well as systemic antitoxin antibody responses (Svennerholm *et al.*, 1984).

In addition to being a potent oral immunogen, CT has a number of other reported immunologic properties. As indicated above, Elson and Ealding (1984a) observed that orally administered CT does not induce tolerance against itself. Moreover, simultaneous oral administration of CT with a soluble protein antigen, keyhole limpet hemocyanin (KLH), resulted in the development of secretory IgA responses against both CT and KLH and also abrogated the induction of oral tolerance against KLH. These findings were subsequently confirmed and extended by Lycke and Holmgren (1986). The confusion arises when one attempts to define the role of the A and B subunits of CT with respect to the adjuvant properties of the molecule. The following observations, as summarized by Elson (1989), are the basis for that confusion:

- CT does not induce oral tolerance against itself (Elson and Ealding, 1984a).
- CT-B does not induce oral tolerance against itself (Elson and Ealding, 1984a).
- CT can prevent the induction of tolerance against other antigens with which it is simultaneously delivered and also serve as an adjuvant for those antigens (Elson and Ealding, 1984a; Lycke and Holmgren, 1986).
- CT can act as an adjuvant for CT-B (Elson and Ealding, 1984a).
- Heat aggregated CT has little toxicity but is a potent oral immunogen (Pierce *et al.*, 1983).
- CT-B can serve as an immunologic "carrier" in a traditional hapten-carrier configuration (Cebra *et al.*, 1986, McKenzie and Halsey, 1984).

A number of researchers have concluded from these findings that the B subunit must possess some inherent adjuvant activity. The findings of Clements *et al.* (1988) as well as those of Cebra *et al.* (1986), Lycke and Holmgren (1986), and Liang *et al.* (1988) would contradict that conclusion. Cebra *et al.* (1986) demonstrated that purified CT-B was effective at raising the frequency of specific anti-cholera toxin B cells in Peyer's patches when given intraduodenally but, in contrast to CT, did not result in significant numbers of IgA committed B cells. Lycke and Holmgren (1986) compared CT and CT-B for its ability to enhance the gut mucosal immune response to KLH by measuring immunoglobulin-secreting cells in the lamina propria of orally immunized mice. They found no increase in anti-KLH producing cells in response to any dose of B subunit tested in their system. Likewise, Clements *et al.* (1988) examined the ability of LT and LT-B to influence the induction of oral tolerance and serve as an oral adjuvant for soluble protein antigens. In those studies, the binding subunit by itself did not prevent the induction of oral tolerance to simultaneously administered ovalbumin and did not possess oral adjuvant activity. Finally, Liang *et al.* (1988) found no adjuvant effect when CT-B was administered orally in conjunction with inactivated Sendai virus.

Where adjuvant activity has been observed for isolated B subunit, it has typically been for one of two reasons. First, a traditional method of preparing B subunit has been to subject holotoxin to dissociation chromatography by gel filtration in the presence of a dissociating agent (i.e., guanidine HCl or formic acid). The isolated subunits are then pooled and the dissociating agent is removed. B subunit prepared by this technique is invariably contaminated with trace amounts of A subunit such that upon renaturation a small amount of holotoxin is reconstituted. The second reason concerns the definition of an immunologic carrier. Like many other soluble proteins, B subunit can serve as an immunologic vehicle for presentation of antigens to the immune system. If those antigens are sufficiently small as to be poorly immunogenic, they can be made immunogenic in a traditional hapten-carrier configuration. Likewise, there is a "theoretical" immune enhancement associated with B subunit, especially for oral presentation, in that B subunit binds to the surface of epithelial cells and may immobilize an attached antigen for processing by the gut associated lymphoid tissues. The relationships of these events have not been clearly defined for B subunit as a carrier of other antigens, and the use of the term "adjuvant" would seem inappropriate for such an effect.

It is clear that the oral adjuvanticity of the molecule resides in the holotoxin in which B subunit is required for receptor recognition and to facilitate penetration of the A subunit into the cell. The A subunit is also required for adjuvant activity, presumably as a function of its ADP-ribosylating enzymatic activity and ability to increase intracellular levels of cAMP (see Section VI). The B subunit alone may act as a carrier of other antigens in that when conjugated to those antigens they can be immobilized for processing by the gut associated lymphoid tissues. In this capacity it may function as a "depot" adjuvant.

III. Comparison of LT and CT

Although LT and CT have many features in common, these are clearly distinct molecules with biochemical and immunologic differences which make them unique, including a 20% difference in nucleotide and amino acid sequence homology (Dallas and Falkow, 1980). The two toxins have the same subunit number and arrangement, biological mechanism of action, and specific activity in many *in vitro* assays (Clements and Finkelstein, 1979; Clements *et al.*, 1980). There are, however, significant differences between these molecules that influence not only their enterotoxic properties, but also their ability to function as adjuvants. For example, unlike CT produced by *V. cholerae,* LT remains cell-associated and is only released from *E. coli* during cell lysis (Clements and Finkelstein, 1979). CT is secreted from the vibrio as soon as it is synthesized and can be readily identified in, and purified from, culture supernatants. Consequently, in contrast to CT, LT is not fully biologically active when first isolated from the cell. Consistent with the A–B model for bacterial toxins, LT requires proteolysis and disulfide reduction to be fully active. This can best be appreciated by examining the model shown in Fig. 1. One likely scenario is that, in the absence of proteolytic processing, the enzymatically active A_1 moiety is unable to dissociate from the A_2 component and cannot reach its target substrate (adenylate cyclase) on the basolateral surface of the intestinal epithelial cell. This would also be true for CT, but proteases in the culture supernatant,

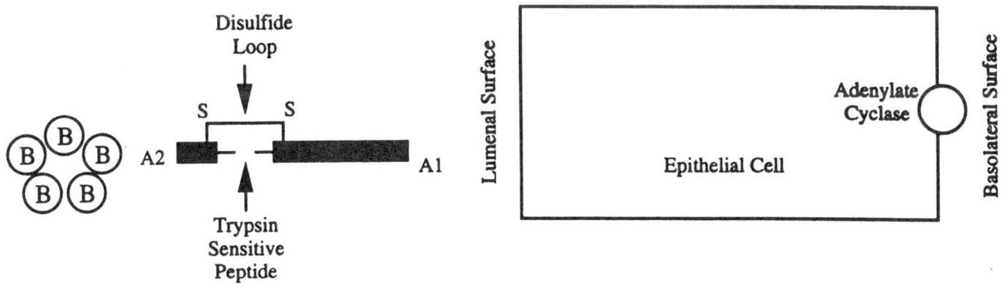

Figure 1. Model of cholera toxin and heat-labile enterotoxin interaction with a polarized intestinal epithelial cell.

to which the toxin is exposed during purification, perform the proteolysis. Since LT is not fully biologically active, it is difficult to identify during purification using *in vitro* biological assays such as the Y-1 adrenal cell assay or permeability factor assay.

This difference in activation of the isolated material results in differences in response thresholds for LT and CT in a variety of biologic systems. However, when LT is exposed to proteolytic enzymes with trypsin-like specificity, the molecule becomes indistinguishable from CT in any biologic assay system. This was demonstrated by Clements and Finkelstein (1979) as shown in Table 1.

In addition to the above reported differences, LT has an unusual affinity for carbohydrate-containing matrices. Specifically, LT, with a molecular weight of 90,000, elutes from Sephadex columns (glucose) with an apparent molecular weight of 45,000 and from Agarose columns (galactose) with an apparent molecular weight of 0. That is, it binds to galactose-containing matrices and can be eluted from those matrices in pure form by application of galactose. LT binds not only to agarose in columns used for purification, but more importantly, to other biological molecules containing galactose, including glycoproteins and lipopolysaccharides. This lectin-like binding property of LT results in a broader receptor distribution on mammalian cells for LT than for CT which binds only to G_{M1} (Angstrom *et al.*, 1994; Clements *et al.*, 1980; Holmgren, 1994). This may account in part for the reported differences in the abilities of these two molecules to induce different helper T lymphocyte responses (McGhee *et al.*, 1993).

The two molecules also have many immunologic differences, as demonstrated by immunodiffusion studies (Clements and Finkelstein, 1978a,b), *in vitro* neutralization studies, and the partial protection against LT-associated *E. coli* diarrhea in volunteers receiving B-subunit whole-cell cholera vaccine (Clemens *et al.*, 1988). Taken together, these findings demonstrate that LT and CT are unique molecules, despite their apparent similarities.

TABLE I
Specific Activity of Purified *E. coli* LT Preparations in Y-1 Adrenal Cells and Rabbit Skin (Permeability Factor) Assays[a]

Toxin	Trypsin treated[b]	Adrenal cells[c] (pg)	Rabbit skin[d] (ng)
LT	−	3320	0.6
LT	+	15.2	0.2
CT	−	3.8	0.2
CT	+	3.8	0.2

[a]Adapted from Clements and Finkelstein (1979).
[b]LT was activated by incubation for 45 min at 37°C in the presence of 0.1 μg of trypsin in a final reaction volume of 100 μl.
[c]Minimum dose (picograms per well) required to produce significant (>50%) cell rounding.
[d]Minimum dose (nanograms per injection) required to produce a 4-mm zone of bluing.

IV. Cellular Targets of Enterotoxin Action

The cellular targets through which CT and LT mediate their adjuvant properties are not known. Clearly, significant efforts have been made to resolve this question (Cebra *et al.*, 1986; Clements *et al.*, 1988; Elson, 1989; Elson and Ealding, 1984a,b). Any proposed mechanism of action must account for an increase in serum and mucosal IgA as well as serum IgG directed against the orally administered antigen. With respect to the B-cell, there are three steps in B-cell differentiation that are likely targets: (1) isotype switching from IgM^+B cells to IgA^+B cells, (2) post-switch IgA B-cell differentiation, and (3) class-specific suppression of S-IgA B-cell terminal differentiation [see Strober and Jacobs (1985) for an overview of the various aspects of cellular differentiation, migration, and function in the mucosal immune system]. Any mechanism invoked to explain the events associated with the adjuvant properties of these molecules will likely involve an increase in intracellular levels of cAMP associated with the ADP-ribosylating activity of the A subunit for the following reasons.

It is well established that cAMP and cAMP-dependent protein kinase A are important mediators in regulation of the immune response (Kammer, 1988). In the T lymphocyte, increasing cAMP has been associated with the induction of suppressor populations, enhancement of suppressor activity, and inhibition of IL-2 production and T-cell proliferation. The effect of increasing cAMP on B lymphocytes is not well characterized and conflicting results are often reported. It is now clear that increasing cAMP blocks the cell-cycle progression of B cells from G_1 to S, thus preventing cellular proliferation. The effect of blockage on antibody production appears to depend upon the milieu in which the B cells are stimulated. In the presence of antigen, IL-1, and cAMP, isolated B lymphocytes increase production of antibody. However, when T cells are added, antibody production is inhibited. Moreover, increasing cAMP in macrophages has been shown to inhibit IL-1 synthesis, at least in some macrophage populations. Clearly, there are a number of potential cellular targets for these bacterially derived adjuvants and the precise mechanism of action remains to be determined. A number of proposed mechanisms are discussed below.

A. Enhanced Luminal Permeability

Lycke *et al.* (1991) have proposed that the adjuvanticity of CT and LT is the result of their ability to stimulate hyperabsorption by the luminal enterocytes of the small intestine, a direct consequence of the ability of these enterotoxins to activate adenylate cyclase and stimulate net ion and water secretion into the lumen. In that study, a permeability marker, fluoresceinated dextran 3000, was administered orally to mice in conjunction with the protein antigen KLH with or without CT or CT-B as adjuvant. At various times after oral inoculation, blood was withdrawn and analyzed spectrophotometrically for the presence of FITC-labeled dextran. An increase in Dextran uptake into the serum was observed only when CT was used as adjuvant and was correlated with an adjuvant effect as evidenced by significant serum anti-KLH antibody responses and an increased number of anti-KLH spot-forming cells in the lamina propria, as determined by ELISPOT analysis. Lycke *et al.* (1991) concluded that the adjuvant effect of CT is associated with the ability of CT to increase gut permeability thereby facilitating access of luminal antigens to the gut mucosal immune system. This effect was attributed to the adenylate cyclase/cAMP activation in that CT-B did not act as an adjuvant for KLH and was unable to increase uptake of the marker. The augmentation of gut permeability was strongest after the first oral inoculation and considerably lower after the second and third inoculations, suggesting a possible anti-toxin effect. The investigators made it clear that the ability of CT to augment the uptake of a "protein" antigen remained to be determined.

Moreover, low-molecular-weight sugars such as dextran are generally nonimmunogenic and are constituents of both host cell glycoproteins and glycoproteins associated with the normal flora; the biological relevance of its enhanced uptake into the general circulation is not clear. In fact, dextran has been found to access the general circulation via two pathways, either by endocytosis–exocytosis of the enterocyte or by a paracellular pathway, the latter of which is thought to be facilitated by CT (Volkheimer and Schulz, 1968). However, if this is a component of the adjuvant mechanism of CT, it would be expected that this increased uptake from lumen to serosa would be discriminatory. In this regard, Nedrud and Sigmund (1991) found that oral immunization with CT does not enhance uptake of dietary antigens. Rather, the adjuvant effect of CT has been found to be restricted to the specific immunogen with which it is coadministered and not to bystander antigens.

B. Selective Induction of a Th2-Mediated Humoral Antibody Response

In contrast to the findings of Lycke *et al.* (1991), Snider *et al.* (1994) found that CT did not lead to an increase of orally administered hen egg lysozyme (HEL) into the peripheral circulation. In that study, mice were orally inoculated with 200 μg of HEL or HEL with CT as adjuvant and their sera was examined for the presence of intact HEL. Coadministration of CT had no effect in that at no point following oral inoculation did the serum HEL levels exceed 200 ng/ml in either group. These investigators demonstrate that CT stimulates antibody production when given orally with HEL, whereas a similar dose of HEL alone does not, and they argue that since there is no difference in the amount of circulating HEL in either case CT must be inducing antibody production by a means other than increased HEL uptake. Hence, when a relatively high-molecular-weight (14,700) immunogenic antigen is used in combination with CT as adjuvant, adjuvanticity cannot be explained simply by increased uptake of antigen from lumen into the general circulation.

In the same study, the authors proposed two distinct mechanisms of adjvanticity. First, the adjuvant effect could be attributed to a combinatorial effect on B cells and T helper cells or on antigen-presenting cells such as macrophages or intestinal epithelial cells themselves. Alternatively, CT may increase antigen uptake into compartments of the intestinal mucosa, such as the lamina propria, and the antigen sequestered there such that estimates of antigen in the general circulation do not reflect the relative amounts of antigen uptake in the presence of CT. This would suggest that antigen in the presence of CT is manipulated differently by the GALT than is antigen administered alone, and that antigen coadministered with CT or LT as adjuvant follows a different course of antigen presentation resulting in the generation of a specific immune response in contrast to antigens processed in the absence of adjuvant.

C. Depletion of $CD8^+$ Intraepithelial Lymphocytes

A recent model for adjuvanticity has been advanced from an evolving understanding of the effects of CT and LT on the induction of oral tolerance. This model proposes that CT and LT abrogate the induction of oral tolerance by depletion of a "suppressor" T-cell population in the GALT. Elson *et al.* (1995) have proposed that adjuvanticity can be explained, in part, by the profound effect of CT on regulatory T cells in the mucosal immune system, specifically, by depleting the $CD8^+$ intraepithelial lymphocyte (IEL) population upon oral administration. In that study, splenic T cells were cultured in the presence of concanavalin A alone, with CT, or with CT-B and the cells were analyzed by flow cytometry for proportions of $CD3^+$, $CD4^+$ and $CD8^+$ T cells. There was a preferential reduction in the $CD8^+$ cell fraction although $CD4^+$ cells were also depleted *in vitro*. Similarly, when $CD4^+$ and $CD8^+$ T-cell subsets were isolated and incubated with phorbol myristic acetate and ionomycin (previously demonstrated to be optimal for mitogenic activity) with and without CT or CT-

B, both subsets were significantly inhibited. There was a consistently greater inhibition of $CD8^+$ T cells than $CD4^+$ T cells as determined by ^{3}H-thymidine incorporation. Importantly, these investigators examined the relevance of this selective depletion *in vivo* using an adoptive transfer model. Mice were immunized with OVA, an irrelevant antigen, or with KLH both with and without CT as adjuvant. Splenic T cells were purified from these donor mice and transferred to a naive population of mice which were then immunized with three doses of KLH at biweekly intervals by i.p. inoculation for the first and last inoculation, and by a single intragastric administration separating the two parenteral immunizations. In the control group receiving T cells from OVA-fed mice there was a strong serum IgG and secretory anti-KLH response, demonstrating that systemic tolerance is an antigen-specific phenomenon. In contrast, the anti-KLH response was significantly reduced in the recipients receiving T cells from the KLH immunized donors, demonstrating that the suppressor T cells in these donors could be transferred to naive donors and tolerize these mice in response to KLH exposure. However, including CT in the oral inoculations inhibited the development of suppressor cells in these mice such that the donor mice produced an anti-KLH response similar to the control group.

These investigators concluded that both CT and CT-B are able to reduce the IEL numbers *in vitro* and therefore suggested that the inhibitory signal to the T cell is not mediated by the adenylate cyclase pathway nor via the phosphatidylinositol system, both of which require the ADP-ribosylating activity of the holotoxin. Rather, they hypothesized that both CT and CT-B are endocytosed and possibly transcytosed by T cells and that this provides the inhibitory signal required for both mucosally induced tolerance and adjuvanticity.

D. Antigen-Specific T-Cell Response Induced by CT as Oral Adjuvant

While CT and LT are physiochemically and immunologically related, they have been found to induce different cytokine profiles *in vitro* and *in vivo* and hence induce different immune responses to coadministered antigens. In this regard, Xu-Amano *et al.* (1994) have extensively analyzed the Th1 and Th2 cell responses following oral immunization with CT. In this study, mice were orally inoculated with CT three times at weekly intervals and sacrificed 1 week after the last immunization. High titers of anti-CT IgG and IgA antibodies were found in serum and fecal extracts, respectively, which correlated with local anti-CT IgA secreting lamina propria lymphocytes (B cells) as determined by a modified ELISPOT. To examine the effect of CT on Th-cell responses during these peak mucosal IgA and serum IgG antibody responses, Peyer's patches (PP) and spleens (SP) were collected from mice and the $CD4^+$ T-cell fractions purified and analyzed for specific cytokine expression. Using an *in vitro* restimulation assay, $CD4^+$ T-cells were incubated with CT-B coated latex microspheres for 1, 3, and 6 days and then analyzed by ELISPOT for IL-2, INFγ, IL-4, and IL-5 secretion. In the CT-immunized mice, high levels of IL-4 and IL-5 SFCs were observed in $CD4^+$ T cells isolated from PP and SP, while IL-2 and IFNγ SFCs were scarce. These findings were confirmed by reverse-transcribed polymerase chain reaction (RT-PCR) of total cellular RNA collected from the $CD4^+$ T-cell fractions of PP and SP cells of immunized mice restimulated *in vitro* with CT-B-coated microspheres. Following restimulation, high levels of IL-4 and IL-5 mRNA were detectable while low to undetectable levels of IL-2 and IFNγ mRNA were observed, indicating that the Th2-type responses induced by oral immunization were due to *de novo* synthesis of cytokines and that the induced cytokine response was due to CT-specific $CD4^+$ T cells, both in the PP and in the SP. These findings are significant in that they suggest Th2 cell regulation of S-IgA responses *in vivo*, and may in part explain how CT acts as an adjuvant. Specifically, Th1 cells secrete IL-2, IFNγ, and TNF-β and are involved in cell-mediated immunity. In contrast, Th2 cells secrete IL-4, IL-5, IL-6, and IL-10 and are most effective in humoral or B-cell responses. Importantly, IL-4 induces isotype switching to IgG1 and IgE while IL-5 and IL-6 stimulate IgA-committed B cells to differentiate into IgA-secreting plasma cells. Thus, it is important to determine if the same antibody and cytokine profiles are initiated when CT is used as an adjuvant for a given antigen. Xu-Amano *et al.* (1993) further investigated the Th-cell subsets induced upon oral immunization with tetanus toxoid as antigen with CT as adjuvant. Similarly, they found that an antigen-specific Th2-type response was generated using similar techniques of restimulation assays with TT-coated microspheres and cytokine specific Northern blots of RT-PCR products from restimulated $CD4^+$ T cells isolated from PP and SP of orally immunized mice.

In contrast to the above findings, Hornquist and Lycke (1993) have observed that CT greatly promotes antigen priming of both Th1 and Th2 cells. In this study, mice were administered a single oral priming of KLH with and without CT as adjuvant. One week later, SP, MLN, PP, and LP T cells were cultured *in vitro* with KLH and peritoneal marcrophages from naive syngeneic mice as APCs and proliferation in response to the recall antigen was determined by incorporation of ^{3}H-thymidine into cellular DNA. CT was found to promote antigen-specific priming of T cells derived from both mucosal tissues (LP and PP) and systemic organs (MLN and SP), in contrast to KLH-primed T cells which responded poorly upon restimulation with KLH. Further, MLN, LP and SP T cells from KLH and CT inoculated mice produced elevated amounts of both Th1 cytokines (IL-2 and INFγ) and Th2 cytokines (IL-4, 5, and 6) upon restimulation compared to KLH-primed mice in which all tested cytokines were low or undetectable. Finally, it was found that KLH-specific $CD8^+$ T cells did not contribute significantly to the CT-enhanced proliferation in that CT did not cause any significant change in the frequencies of either $CD4^+$ or $CD8^+$ T cells in the SP or MLN relative to the distribution observed in KLH primed mice as determined by FACS analysis. Importantly, this study differed from previous studies in that the investigators purposefully separated the antigen primed T cells from CT-exposed APCs, including both macrophages and B cells, prior to reexposure of T cells to recall antigen *in vitro*. This is significant in that previous studies have indicated that CT preferentially induces a Th2 profile upon oral immunization (Clarke *et al.*, 1991; Wilson *et al.*, 1991). Other groups did not separate immune T cells from the primed APCs in their *in vitro* restimulation assays. It is important to note that *in vitro* restimulation assays are useful in determining the effect of CT and LT as adjuvants on single, isolated lymphocyte populations but that this assay system is artificial in the sense that lymphocytes are removed from the immunological milieu in which they were initially primed. Hence, the influence of other antigen-primed cell populations such as B cells, macrophages, dendritic cells, IEL, and epithelial cells on T-cell responses is not present as would be otherwise in a natural *in vivo* situation.

E. Role of Enterocytes in the Adjuvanticity of CT and LT

A role for intestinal epithelial cells in antigen presentation has recently been proposed insofar as they constitute the vast majority of cells in the small intestine. In contrast, M cells overlying the Peyer's patches constitute only a small percentage of cells in the small bowel. Current dogma suggests that the M cells are the predominant antigen-sampling cells of the gut, which pass internalized antigen to the macrophage cells of the Peyer's patches, and the latter serves as the major antigen-presenting cells (APCs) which inititate T- and B-cell priming in response to oral immunization. However, an alternative pathway of antigen uptake and presentation provided by the absorptive epithelial cells of the intestinal mucosa has been suggested by Bromander *et al.* (1993). These investigators analyzed the effect of CT exposure on alloantigen presentation by cultured intestinal epithelial cells. The crypt, small intestinal epithelial cell line, IEC-17, derived from the duodenum of Sprague–Dawley rats was cultured with IFNγ to induce optimal expression of MHC II and in the presence or absence of CT (Quaroni and Isselbacher, 1981). After 48 hr, the IEC-17 cells were washed, treated with mitomycin C, and incubated with histoincompatible spleen cells. Alloantigen-stimulated $CD4^+$ T-cell proliferation was then determined by ^3H-thymidine incorporation. CT enhanced the antigen presentation of IEC-17 cells and this enhancement was not due to an upregulation of MHC II expression, but rather a dose-dependent increase in IL-1 and IL-6 secretion by IEC-17 cells. The data suggest that the potent adjuvanticity of CT may be attributed to its ability to enhance the co-stimulating ability of APCs such as intestinal epithelial cells of the mucosal immune system. However, it was noted that intestinal epithelial cells have only been found to process and present antigens *in vitro* and that whether these cells are capable of functioning as APCs *in vivo* remains to be examined. Two limitations of the above study are the relevance of using a crypt cell line (IEC-17) rather than a non-crypt intestinal cell line, such as Henle-407 cells, and the nature of the antigen that is presented. Specifically, alloantigen presentation is an atypical form of antigen presentation which does not require presentation in the context of self-MHC and therefore, the enhanced "presentation" observed in this study might not accurately reflect the conventional antigen-processing and -presenting capability of intestinal epithelial cells *in vitro*.

V. Mucosal (Oral) Tolerance/ Adjuvant Properties of LT

The demonstration of the adjuvant properties of LT grew out of an investigation of the influence of LT on the development of tolerance to orally administered antigens. As mentioned above, Elson and Ealding (1984a) demonstrated that CT could prevent the induction of tolerance to orally administered KLH when the two were fed simultaneously and that an anti-KLH S-IgA response developed as a consequence of this immunization. These observations were confirmed and extended by Lycke and Holmgren (1986) who also investigated the influence of timing and route of administration on the adjuvant effect, and provided evidence that the adjuvant property is a function of the A subunit. It was not clear whether LT would also influence the induction of oral tolerance or exhibit the adjuvant effects demonstrated for CT, given the observed differences between the two molecules. Consequently, Clements *et al.* (1988) examined a number of parameters, including the effect of LT on oral tolerance to OVA and the role of the two subunits of LT in the observed response, the effect of varying the timing and route of delivery of LT, the effect of prior exposure to OVA on the ability of LT to influence tolerance to OVA, the use of LT as an adjuvant with two unrelated antigens, and the effect of route of immunization on anti-OVA responses. The results obtained from these studies are summarized below:

- Simultaneous administration of LT with OVA was shown to prevent the induction of tolerance to OVA and to increase the serum anti-OVA IgG response 30- to 90-fold over OVA-primed and PBS-primed animals, respectively. This effect was determined to be a function of the enzymatically active A subunit of the toxin since the B subunit alone was unable to influence tolerance induction.
- Animals fed LT with OVA after an initial OVA priming developed a significantly lower serum IgG and mucosal IgA anti-OVA responses than those fed LT with OVA in the initial immunization, indicating that prior exposure to the antigen reduces the effectiveness of LT to influence tolerance and its ability to act as an adjuvant. LT was not able to abrogate tolerance once it had been established. This was also found to be true for CT when animals were preimmunized with OVA prior to oral ovalbumin plus CT and offers some insight into the beneficial observation that antibody responses to non-target dietary antigens are not increased when these adjuvants are used.
- Serum IgG and mucosal IgA responses in animals receiving LT on only a single occasion, that being upon first exposure to antigen, were equivalent to responses after three OVA/LT immunizations indicating that commitment to responsiveness occurs early and upon first exposure to antigen. We also demonstrated that the direction of the response to either predominantly serum IgG or mucosal IgA can be controlled by whether or not a parenteral booster dose is administered.
- Simultaneous administration of LT with two soluble protein antigens results in the development of serum and mucosal antibodies against both antigens if the animal has no prior immunologic experience with either. This was an important finding since one possible application of LT as an adjuvant would be for the development of mucosal antibodies against complex antigens, such as killed bacteria or viruses, where the ability to respond to multiple antigens would be important.

VI. Toward a Practical Adjuvant

Clearly, LT has significant immunoregulatory potential, both as a means of preventing the induction of tolerance to specific antigens and as an adjuvant for orally administered antigens. In addition, LT elicits the production of both serum IgG and mucosal IgA against antigens with which it is delivered. This raises the possibility of an effective immunization program against a variety of pathogens involving the oral administration of killed or attenuated agents or relevant virulence determinants of specific agents. However, this "toxin" can stimulate a net lumenal secretory response when proteolytically cleaved, as by gut proteases, or when administered orally in high enough concentrations. This problem could be resolved if LT could be "detoxified" without diminishing the adjuvant properties of the molecules. In order to appreciate how this might be accomplished, it is necessary to further analyze the mechanism of action of the LT and CT, as well as the structural and functional relationships of these molecules. As indicated previously, both LT and CT are synthesized as multisubunit toxins with A and B components. After the initial interaction of the toxin with the host cell membrane receptor, the B region facilitates the penetration of the A subunit through the cell membrane. On thiol reduction, this A component dissociates into two smaller polypeptide chains. One of these, the A_1 piece, catalyzes the ADP-ribosylation of the stimulatory GTP-binding protein ($G_{S\alpha}$) in the adenylate cyclase enzyme complex on the basolateral surface of the epithelial cell; this results in increasing intracellular levels of cAMP. The resulting increase in cAMP causes secretion of water and electrolytes into the small intestine through interaction with two cAMP-sensitive ion transport mechanisms involving (1) NaCl cotransport across the brush border of villous epithelial cells, and (2) electrogenic Na-dependent Cl secretion by crypt cells (Field, 1980). The A subunit is also the principal moiety associated with immune enhancement by these toxins. This subunit then becomes a likely target for manipulation in order to dissociate the toxic and immunologic functions of the molecules. A recent report by Lycke and Holmgren (1992) makes it clear that alterations that affect the ADP-ribosylating enzymatic activity of the toxin and alter the ability to increase intracellular levels of cAMP also prevent the molecule from functioning as an adjuvant. Consequently, another approach to detoxification was explored.

Both CT and LT are synthesized with a trypsin-sensitive peptide bond that joins the A_1 and A_2 pieces. This peptide bond must be nicked for the molecule to be "toxic." This is also true for diphtheria toxin, the prototypic A–B toxin, and for a variety of other bacterial toxins. If the A_1–A_2 bond is not removed, either by bacterial proteases or by intestinal proteases in the lumen of the bowel, the A_1 piece cannot reach its target on the basolateral surface of the polarized intestinal epithelial cell. In contrast to CT, LT is not fully biologically active when first isolated from the cell. LT also requires proteolysis to be fully active and the proteolytic activation does not occur inside of the bacterium. Therefore, one means of altering the toxicity of the molecule without affecting the ADP-ribosylating enzymatic activity would be to remove by genetic manipulation the trypsin-sensitive amino acids that join the A_1 and A_2 components of the A subunit. If the molecule cannot be cleaved proteolytically, it should not cause net fluid secretion in the bowel (enterotoxicity). It may, however, retain its adjuvant function, especially if adjuvanticity involves interaction of the molecule with nonpolarized lymphoid cells.

Below is the sequence of the disulfide subtended region that separates the A_1 and A_2 pieces. Within this region is a single Arginine residue (*) which is believed to be the site of cleavage necessary to activate the toxic properties of the molecule. Dickinson and Clements (1995) changed this region by site-directed mutagenesis in such a way as to render the molecule insensitive to proteolytic digestion and, consequently, nontoxic. They then characterized this molecule with respect to enzymatic activity, biologic activity, and the ability to function as an oral adjuvant.

						*	
Gly	Cys	Gly	Asn	Ser	Ser	Arg	Thr
GGT	TGT	GGA	AAT	TCA	TCA	AGA	ACA
Ile	Thr	Gly	Asp	Thr	Cys	Asn	
ATT	ACA	GGT	GAT	ACT	TGT	AAT	

A. Construction of $LT_{(R192G)}$

Site-directed mutagenesis can be accomplished by hybridizing to single-stranded DNA a synthetic oligonucleotide which is complementary to the single-stranded template except in a region of mismatch near then center. It is this region that contains the desired nucleotide change or changes. Following hybridization with the single-stranded target DNA, the oligonucleotide is extended with DNA polymerase to create a double-stranded structure. The nick is then sealed with DNA ligase and the duplex structure is transformed into an *Escherichia coli* host. The theoretical yield of mutants using this procedure is 50% due to the semiconservative mode of DNA replication. In practice, the yield is much lower. There are, however, a number of methods available to improve yield and to select for oligonucleotide-directed mutants. The system we employed utilized a second mutagenic oligonucleotide to create altered restriction sites in a double-mutation strategy.

The LT gene has previously been cloned from a human isolate of *E. coli* designated H10407. This subclone consists of a 5.2-kb DNA fragment from the enterotoxin plasmid of H10407 inserted into the *Pst*I site of plasmid pBR322 (Clements *et al.*, 1983). This recombinant plasmid, designated pDF82, has been characterized extensively and expresses LT under control of the native LT promoter. The next step in this process was to place the LT gene under the control of a strong promoter, in this case the *lac* promoter on plasmid pUC18. This was accomplished by isolating the genes for LT-A and LT-B separately and recombining them in a cassette in the vector plasmid. This was an important step because it permitted purification of reasonable quantities of LT and derived mutants for subsequent analysis.

The next step was to substitute another amino acid for Arg (i.e., GGA = Gly replaces AGA = Arg), thus preserving the reading frame while eliminating the proteolytic site. This construction is shown diagramatically in Fig. 2. LT was then purified by agarose affinity chromatography from one mutant (pBD95) which had been confirmed by sequencing. This mutant LT, designated $LT_{(R192G)}$, was then examined by SDS–polyacrylamide gel electrophoresis for modification of the trypsin-sensitive bond. Samples were examined with and without exposure to trypsin and compared with native (unmodified) LT. As predicted, $LT_{(R192G)}$ does not dissociate into A_1 and A_2 when incubated with trypsin, thereby indicating that sensitivity to protease has been removed (not shown). Several predictions were made at this point based upon an understanding of this molecule and the manner in which these alterations would be expected to effect the properties of the molecule.

B. Effect of $LT_{(R192G)}$ on Y-1 Adrenal Cells

The first prediction was that $LT_{(R192G)}$ would not be active in the Y-1 adrenal cell assay. This prediction was based upon previous findings (Clements and Finkelstein, 1979) that un-nicked LT was more than 1000-fold less active in this assay system than was CT and that trypsin treatment activated LT to the same level of biological activity as CT in this assay. The residual activity of LT observed in this assay in the absence of trypsin activation was presumed to be a function of some residual protease activity which could not be accounted for. For instance, trypsin is used in the process of subculturing Y-1 adrenal cells. It was therefore assumed that LT that could not be nicked would be completely inactive in the Y-1 adrenal cell assay. The finding that $LT_{(R192G)}$ retained a basal level of activity in the Y-1 adrenal cell assay even though it could not be proteolytically processed was therefore unexpected. As shown in Table II, CT and native LT treated with trypsin have the same level of activity (15 pg) on Y-1 adrenal cells. By contrast, $LT_{(R192G)}$ (48,000 pg) was >1000-fold less active than CT or native LT and could not be activated by trypsin. The residual basal activity undoubtedly reflects a different and heretofore unknown pathway of adrenal cell activation compared to that requiring separation of the A_1–A_2 linkage.

C. ADP-ribosylating Enzymatic Activity of $LT_{(R192G)}$

The next prediction was that $LT_{(R192G)}$ would retain its ADP-ribosylating enzymatic activity since this mutation

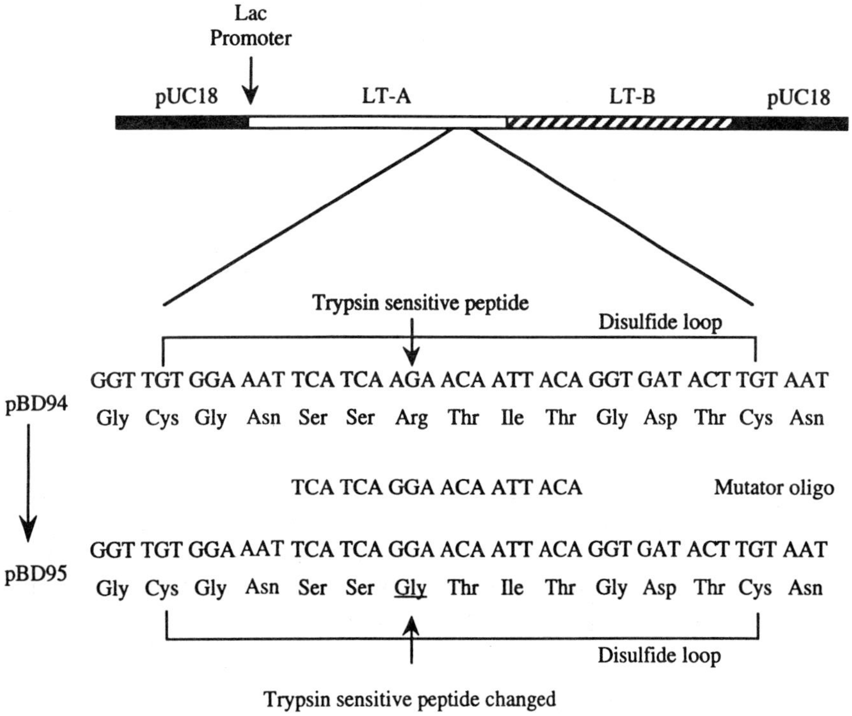

Figure 2. Schematic diagram of the plasmid pBD94, which encodes both subunits A and B of LT under control of the *lac* promoter. Plasmid pBD95 contains the single base substitution in amino acid residue 192 of subunit A, coding for Gly rather that Arg, which preserves the reading frame but eliminates the proteolytic site. The amino acid sequence corresponding to the region of trypsin sensitivity and the site of amino acid change Arg 192–Gly 192 is shown (from Dickinson and Clements, 1995).

TABLE II
Mouse Y-1 Adrenal Cell Activity of CT, Native LT, and $LT_{(R192G)}$[a]

Toxin	Trypsin activated[b]	Specific activity[c]
Cholera toxin	−	15
LT	+	15
$LT_{(R192G)}$	−	48,800
$LT_{(R192G)}$	+	48,800

[a]From Dickinson and Clements (1995).

[b]LT and $LT_{(R192G)}$ were activated by incubation for 45 min at 37°C in the presence of 0.1 μg of trypsin in a final reaction volume of 100 μl.

[c]Minimum dose (picograms per well) required to produce significant (>50%) cell rounding.

does not alter the enzymatic site of the A_1 moiety. In order to examine this property, the NAD-agmatine ADP-ribosyltransferase assay (Moss *et al.*, 1993) was employed. CT produces a dose-dependent increase in the levels of ADP-ribosylagmatine, a function of the ADP-ribosyltransferase activity of this molecule. As shown in Table III, $LT_{(R192G)}$ lacked any detectable ADP-ribosylating enzymatic activity, with or without trypsin activation, even though the enzymatic site had not been altered and the molecule retained a basal level of activity in the Y-1 adrenal cell assay.

D. Adjuvant Activity of $LT_{(R192G)}$

In order to examine the adjuvant activity of $LT_{(R192G)}$ the following experiment was performed. Three groups of BALB/c mice were immunized. Animals were inoculated intragastrically with a blunt tipped feeding needle (Popper & Sons, Inc., New Hyde Park, NY). On Day 0, each group was immunized orally as follows: Group A received 0.5 ml of PBS containing 5 mg of OVA, Group B received 0.5 ml of PBS containing 5 mg of OVA and 25 μg of native LT, and Group C received 0.5 ml of PBS containing 5 mg of OVA and 25 μg of $LT_{(R192G)}$. Each regimen was administered again on Days 7 and 14. On Day 21, all animals were boosted i.p. with 1 μg of OVA in 20% Maalox. One week after the i.p. inoculation animals were sacrificed and assayed for serum IgG and mucosal IgA antibodies directed against OVA and LT by ELISA.

Reagents and antisera for the ELISA were obtained from Sigma Chemical Co. Samples for ELISA were serially diluted in phosphate buffered saline (pH

TABLE III
ADP-Ribosyltransferase Activity of CT, Native LT, and $LT_{(R192G)}$[a]

Experiment:	1	2	3	4	Mean ± SEM
No toxin	ND	9.12	5.63	14.17	9.64 ± 2.48
1 μg CT	ND	17.81	17.60	25.75	20.39 ± 2.68
10 μg CT	ND	107.32	111.28	104.04	107.55 ± 2.09
100 μg CT	351.55	361.73	308.09	ND	340.46 ± 16.45
100 μg LT	17.32	14.48	13.86	ND	15.22 ± 1.07
100 μg LT + trypsin	164.10	189.89	152.96	ND	168.98 ± 10.94
100 μg $LT_{(R192G)}$	14.58	12.34	9.30	ND	12.07 ± 1.53
100 μg $LT_{(R192G)}$ + trypsin	14.73	8.90	10.47	ND	11.37 ± 1.74

Note. ND, not done; data are expressed as fmol min^{-1}.
[a]From Dickinson and Clements (1995).

7.2)–0.05% Tween-20 (PBS–TWEEN). For anti-LT determinations, microtiter plates were precoated with 1.5 μg per well of mixed gangliosides (Type III), then with 1 μg per well of purified LT. Anti-OVA was determined on microtiter plates precoated with 10 μg per well of OVA. Serum anti-LT and anti-OVA were determined with rabbit antiserum against mouse IgG conjugated to alkaline phosphatase. Mucosal anti-LT and anti-OVA IgA were assayed with goat antiserum against mouse IgA [alpha-chain specific] followed by rabbit antiserum against goat IgG conjugated to alkaline phosphatase. Reactions were stopped with 3 N NaOH. Values for IgG and IgA were determined from a standard curve with purified mouse myeloma proteins (MOPC 315, γA(IgAλ2); MOPC 21, γG1: Litton Bionetics, Inc., Charleston, SC).

As shown in Fig. 3, animals primed orally with OVA and LT developed a significantly higher serum IgG anti-OVA response following subsequent parenteral immunization with OVA than those primed with OVA alone and subsequently immunized parenterally with OVA (no detectable anti-OVA response) (Student *t* test, $P = 0.031$). Significantly, animals primed orally with OVA and $LT_{(R192G)}$ also developed a significantly higher serum IgG anti-OVA response following subsequent parenteral immunization with OVA than those primed with OVA alone and subsequently immunized parenterally with OVA (no detectable anti-OVA response) (Student *t* test, $P = 0.0007$).

Similar results were obtained when anti-OVA IgA responses were compared within the same groups of animals. Also shown in Fig. 3, animals primed orally with OVA and LT developed a significantly higher mucosal IgA anti-OVA response following subsequent parenteral immunization with OVA than those primed with OVA alone and subsequently immunized parenterally with OVA (no detectable anti-OVA response) (Student *t* test, $P = 0.0131$). As above, animals primed orally with OVA and $LT_{(R192G)}$ also developed a significantly higher mucosal IgA anti-OVA response following subsequent parenteral immunization with OVA than those primed

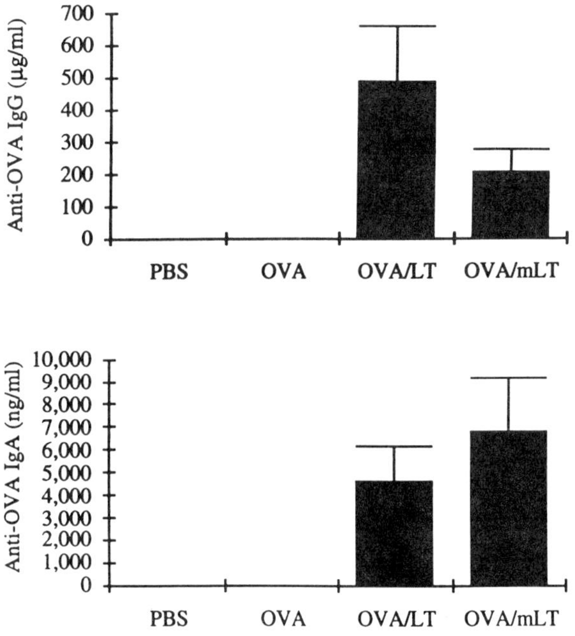

Figure 3. Ability of $LT_{(R192G)}$ to act as an immunological adjuvant. Mice were primed orally with PBS, OVA, or OVA in combination with $LT_{(R192G)}$ at weekly intervals as indicated. Animals were boosted i.p. with OVA and serum anti-OVA IgG and mucosal anti-OVA IgA were determined by ELISA. Bars represent mean ± SEM antibody response in each group 1 week after boost. Each group contained eight mice (from Dickinson and Clements, 1995).

with OVA alone and subsequently immunized parenterally with OVA (no detectable anti-OVA response) (Student *T* test, $P = 0.0189$).

The abilities of LT and $LT_{(R192G)}$ to elicit an anti-LT antibody response in these same animals were also compared. This was important in that it would provide an indication of whether the mutant LT was able to prevent induction of tolerance to itself in addition to functioning as an adjuvant for other proteins. As shown in Fig. 4, animals primed orally with OVA and LT developed a significantly higher serum IgG anti-LT response

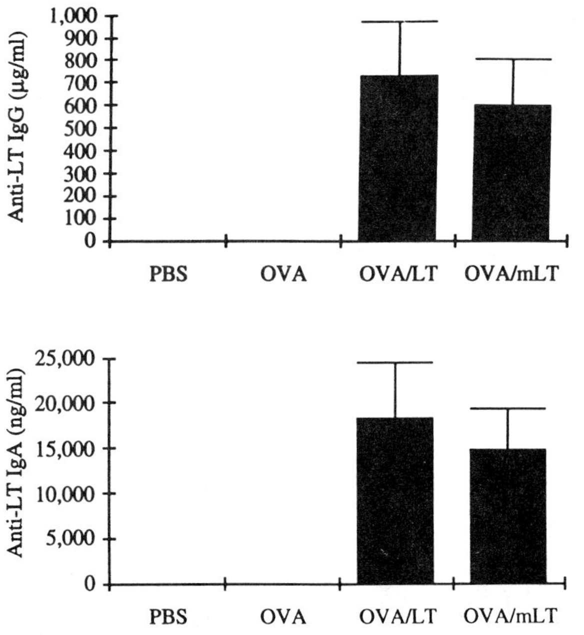

Figure 4. Ability of $LT_{(R192G)}$ to prevent induction of oral tolerance to LT. Mice were primed orally with PBS, OVA, or OVA in combination with $LT_{(R192G)}$ at weekly intervals as indicated. Animals were boosted i.p. with OVA and serum anti-LT IgG and mucosal anti-LT IgA were determined by ELISA. Bars represent mean ± SEM antibody response in each group 1 week after boost. Each group contained eight mice (from Dickinson and Clements, 1995).

following subsequent parenteral immunization with OVA than those primed with OVA alone and subsequently immunized parenterally with OVA (no detectable anti-LT response) (Student t test, $P = 0.0005$). Animals primed orally with OVA and $LT_{(R192G)}$ also developed a significantly higher serum IgG anti-LT response following subsequent parenteral immunization with OVA than those primed with OVA alone and subsequently immunized parenterally with OVA (no detectable anti-LT response) (Student t test, $P = 0.0026$).

Similar results were obtained when anti-LT IgA responses were compared within the same groups of animals. Also shown in Fig. 4B, animals primed orally with OVA and LT developed a significantly higher mucosal IgA anti-LT response following subsequent parenteral immunization with OVA than those primed with OVA alone and subsequently immunized parenterally with OVA (no detectable anti-LT response) (Student t test, $P = 0.0047$). As above, animals primed orally with OVA and $LT_{(R192G)}$ also developed a significantly higher mucosal IgA anti-LT response following subsequent parenteral immunization with OVA than those primed with OVA alone and subsequently immunized parenterally with OVA (no detectable anti-LT response) (Student t test, $P = 0.0323$).

VII. Summary

Both LT and CT have significant immunoregulatory potential, not only as a means of preventing the induction of tolerance but also as adjuvants for orally administered antigens. This raises the possibility of an effective immunization program against a variety of pathogens involving the oral administration of killed or attenuated agents or relevant virulence determinants of specific agents in conjunction with LT or CT. However, the fact that these "toxins" can stimulate a net lumenal secretory response may prevent their use. This problem could be resolved if the molecules could be detoxified without diminishing their adjuvant properties. A number of attempts have been made to alter the toxicity of LT or CT using site-directed mutagenesis to change amino acids associated with the crevice where NAD binding and catalysis are thought to occur. Both Glu 112 and Ser 61, which share a side-chain hydrogen bond, are important for catalysis while the side chain for Arg 7 forms the binding cleft. Replacement of any of these amino acids by site-directed mutagenesis has been shown to alter ADP-ribosyltransferase activity with a corresponding loss of toxicity in a variety of biological assay systems. In addition, it has been shown that exchanging Lys for Glu 112 removes not only ADP-ribosylating enzymatic activity, but cAMP activation and adjuvant activity as well. A logical conclusion is that ADP-ribosylation and induction of cAMP are essential for the adjuvant activity of these molecules.

The mutant $LT_{(R192G)}$ differed from those previously reported in that the mutation in $LT_{(R192G)}$ affects A_1–A_2 cleavage and not the putative NAD-catalytic site. In a model in which the cellular target is located on the basolateral surface of polarized intestinal epithelial cells, the inability to dissociate A_1 from A_2 could prevent access to the substrate adenylate cyclase, thereby reducing or eliminating cAMP accumulation and the ensuing events associated with secretion. In nonpolarized lymphoid tissues this would presumably not be the case and adjuvant activity would not be affected. On the other hand, single amino acid changes in the catalytic site may have undetermined conformational effects which influence adjuvanticity in addition to ADP-ribosyltransferase activity, but the two may not, in fact, be the same.

$LT_{(R192G)}$ retained the ability to act as a mucosal adjuvant, increasing the serum IgG and mucosal IgA responses to coadministered antigen (OVA) beyond that achieved with administration of that antigen alone. Further, $LT_{(R192G)}$ prevented the induction of tolerance to that antigen and did not induce tolerance against itself as demonstrated by the presence of significant serum anti-LT IgG and mucosal anti-LT IgA antibodies in immunized mice. This is an important finding because it provides a means of inducing the production of antibodies directed against both A and B subunits of LT and CT without the associated toxicity of the holotoxin. In addition to its potential use as an adjuvant for unrelated antigens, use of this nontoxic adjuvant as one component of a whole-cell/toxoid vaccine against cholera-related enteropathies should provide more epitopes for induction of neutralizing antibodies as well as adjuvant activity not associated with B subunit alone. Furthermore this mutant LT provides for the first time a model system in which to examine the role of proteolytic processing with respect to the enterotoxic and immunologic properties of ADP-ribosylating toxins both *in vitro* and *in vivo*.

Acknowledgments

This work was supported by Office of Naval Research Grant N00014–92-J-1980. B.J.D. is a recipient of a Department of Defense Augmentation Award for Science & Engineering Research Training (ASSERT), Grant N00014–93–1-1071.

References

Alving, C. R., Richards, R. L., Moss, J., Alving, L. I., Clements, J. D., Shiba, T., Kotan, S., Wirtz, R. A., and Hockmeyer, W. T. (1986). Effectiveness of liposomes as potential carriers for vaccines. Applications to cholera toxin and human malaria sporozoite antigen. *Vaccine* **4**, 166–172.

Angstrom, J., Teneberg, S., and Karlsson, K. A. (1994). Delineation and comparison of ganglioside-binding epitopes for the toxins of *Vibrio cholerae, Escherichia coli,* and *Clostridium tetani:* Evidence for overlapping epitopes. *Proc. Natl. Acad. Sci. U.S.A.* **91**, 11859–11863.

Bockman, D. E., and Cooper, M. D. (1973). Pinocytosis by epithelium associated with lymphoid follicles in the bursa of Fabricius, appendix and Peyer's patches. An electron microscopic study. *Am. J. Anat.* **136**, 455–477.

Bromander, A. K., Kjerrulf, M., Holmgren, J., and Lycke, N. (1993). Cholera toxin enhances alloantigen presentation by cultured intestinal epithelial cells. *Scand. J. Immunol.* **37**, 452–458.

Cárdenas, L., and Clements, J. D. (1992). Oral immunization using live attenuated *Salmonella* spp. as carriers of foreign antigens. *Clin. Microbiol. Rev.* **5**, 328–342.

Cebra, J. J., Fuhrman, J. A., Lebman, D. A., and London, S. D. (1986). Effective gut mucosal stimulation of IgA-committed B-cells by antigen. *In* "Vaccines 86: New Approaches to Immunization. Developing Vaccines against Parasitic, Bacterial, and Viral Diseases" (F. Brown, R. M. Channok, and R. A. Lerner, eds.), pp. 129–133. Cold Spring Harbor Laboratory, Cold Spring Harbor, New York.

Clarke, C. J., Wilson, A. D., Williams, N. A., and Stokes, C. R. (1991). Mucosal priming of T-lymphocyte responses to fed protein antigens using cholera toxin as an adjuvant. *Immunology* **72**, 323–328.

Clemens, J. D., Sack, D. A., Harris, J. R., Chakraborty, J., Neogy, P. K., Stanton, B. F., Huda, N., Khan, M. U., Kay, B. A., Khan, M. R., Ansaruzzanan, M., Yunus, M., Rao, R., Svennerholm, A., and Holmgren, J. (1988b). Cross protection by B subunit–whole cell cholera vaccine against diarrhea associated with heat-labile toxin-producing enterotoxigenic *Escherichia coli:* Results of a large-scale field trial. *J. Infect. Dis.* **158**, 372–377.

Clements, J. D., and Cárdenas, L. (1990). Vaccines against enterotoxigenic bacterial pathogens based on hybrid *Salmonella* that express heterologous antigens. *Res. Microbiol.* **141**, 981–993.

Clements, J. D., and El-Morshidy, S. (1984). Construction of a potential live oral bivalent vaccine for typhoid fever and cholera- *Escherichia coli*-related diarrheas. *Infect. Immun.* **46**, 564–569.

Clements, J. D., and Finkelstein, R. A. (1978a). Demonstration of shared and unique immunological determinants in enterotoxins from *Vibrio cholerae* and *Escherichia coli. Infect. Immun.* **22**, 709–713.

Clements, J. D., and Finkelstein, R. A. (1978b). Immunological cross- reactivity between a heat-labile enterotoxin(s) of *Escherichia coli* and subunits of *Vibrio cholerae* enterotoxin. *Infect. Immun.* **21**, 1036–1039.

Clements, J. D., and Finkelstein, R. A. (1979). Isolation and characterization of homogeneous heat-labile enterotoxins with high specific activity from *Escherichia coli* cultures. *Infect. Immun.* **24**, 760–769.

Clements, J. D., Yancey, R. J., and Finkelstein, R. A. (1980). Properties of homogeneous heat-labile enterotoxin from *Escherichia coli* cultures. *Infect. Immun.* **24**, 91–97.

Clements, J. D., Flint, D. C., Engert, R. F., and Klipstein, F. A. (1983). Cloning and molecular characterization of the B subunit of *Escherichia coli* heat-labile enterotoxin. *Infect. Immun.* **40**, 653–658.

Clements, J. D., Hartzog, N. M., and Lyon, F. L. (1988). Adjuvant activity of *Escherichia coli* heat-labile enterotoxin and effect on the induction of oral tolerance in mice to unrelated protein antigens. *Vaccine* **6**, 269–277.

Clements, J. D., Bao, J. X., and Cárdenas, L. (1992). Use of attenuated bacteria as live oral vaccine vectors. *In* "Recombinant DNA Vaccines: Rationale and Strategy" (R. E. Isaacson, ed.), pp. 293–321. Decker, New York.

Conner, M. E., Crawford, S. E., Barone, C., and Estes, M. K. (1993). Rotavirus vaccine administered parenterally induces protective immunity. *J. Virol.* **67**, 6633–6641.

Dallas, W. S., and Falkow, S. (1980). Amino acid sequence homology between cholera toxin and *Escherichia coli* heat-labile toxin. *Nature (London)* **288**, 499–501.

Dickinson, B. L., and Clements, J. D. (1995). Dissociation of *Escherichia coli* heat-labile enterotoxin adjuvanticity from ADP-ribosyltransferase activity. *Infect. Immun.* **63**, 1617–1623.

Elson, C. O. (1989). Cholera toxin and its subunits as potential oral adjuvants. *Immunol. Today* **146**, 29–33.

Elson, C. O., and Ealding, W. (1984a). Cholera toxin feeding did not induce oral tolerance in mice and abrogated oral tolerance to an unrelated protein antigen. *J. Immunol.* **133,** 2892–2897.

Elson, C. O., and Ealding, W. (1984b). Generalized systemic and mucosal immunity in mice after mucosal stimulation with cholera toxin. *J. Immunol.* **132,** 2736–2741.

Elson, C. O., Holland, S. P., Dertzbaugh, M. T., Cuff, C. F., and Anderson, A. O. (1995). Morphologic and functional alterations of mucosal T cells by cholera toxin and its B subunit. *J. Immunol.* **154,** 1032–1040.

Field, M. (1980). Regulation of small intestinal ion transport by cyclic nucleotides and calcium. *In* "Secretory Diarrhea" (M. Field, J. S. Fordtran, and S. G. Schultz, eds.), pp. 21–30. Waverly Press, Baltimore, Maryland.

Finkelstein, R. A. (1975). Immunology of cholera. *Curr. Top. Microbiol. Immunol.* **69,** 137–196.

Finkelstein, R. A., and LoSpalluto, J. J. (1969). Pathogenesis of experimental cholera: Preparation and isolation of choleragen and choleragenoid. *J. Exp. Med.* **130,** 185–202.

Garcon, N. M. J., and Six, H. R. (1993). Universal vaccine carrier. Liposomes that provide T-dependent help to weak antigens. *J. Immunol.* **146,** 3697–3702.

Gould-Fogerite, S., and Mannino, R. J. (1993). Targeted fusogenic proteoliposomes: Functional reconstitution of membrane proteins through protein-cochleate intermediates. *In* "Liposome Technology, Interaction of Liposomes with the Biological Milieu" (G. Gregoriadis, ed.), 2nd Ed., Vol. 3, pp. 261–176. CRC Press, Boca Raton, Florida.

Holmgren, J. (1994). Receptors for cholera toxin and *Escherichia coli* heat-labile enterotoxin revisited. *Prog. Brain Res.* **101,** 163–177.

Hornquist, E., and Lycke, N. (1993). Cholera toxin adjuvant greatly promotes antigen priming of T-cells. *Eur. J. Immunol.* **23,** 2136–2143.

Kammer, G. M. (1988). The adenylate cyclase-cAMP-protein kinase A pathway and regulation of the immune response. *Immunol. Today* **9,** 222–229.

Liang, X., Lamm, M. E., and Nedrud, J. G. (1988). Oral administration of cholera toxin-Sendai virus conjugate potentiates gut and respiratory immunity against Sendai virus. *J. Immunol.* **141,** 1495–1501.

Lycke, N., and Holmgren, J. (1986). Strong adjuvant properties of cholera toxin on gut mucosal immune responses to orally presented antigens. *Immunology* **59,** 301–308.

Lycke, N., and Holmgren, J. (1992). The adjuvant effect of *Vibrio cholerae* and *Escherichia coli* heat-labile enterotoxins is linked to their ADP-ribosyltransferase activity. *Eur. J. Immunol.* **22,** 2277–2281.

Lycke, N., Karlsson, U., Sjolander, A., and Magnusson, K. E. (1991). The adjuvant effect of cholera toxin is associated with an increased intestinal permeability for luminal antigen. *Scand. J. Immunol.* **33,** 691–698.

McGhee, J. R., Marinaro, M., Takahashi, I., Jackson, R. J., Clements, J., Staats, H. F., Bost, K. L., and Kiyono, H. (1993). Vaccines for mucosal immunity: Unique delivery systems and immune response analyses for Th1/Th2 cells and IgE/IgA B cells. Abstracts of the 29th U.S.–Japan Joint Conference on Cholera.

McKenzie, S. J., and Halsey, J. F. (1984). Cholera toxin B subunit as a carrier protein to stimulate a mucosal immune response. *J. Immunol.* **133,** 1818–1824.

Moss, J., Stanley, S. J., Vaughan, M., and Tsuji, T. (1993). Interaction of ADP-ribosylation factor with *Escherichia coli* enterotoxin that contains an inactivating lysine 112 substitution. *J. Biol. Chem.* **268,** 6383–6387.

Mowat, A. M., and Donachie, A. M. (1991). ISCOMS—a novel strategy for mucosal immunization. *Immunol. Today* **12,** 383–385.

Nedrud, J., and Sigmund, N. (1991). Cholera toxin as a mucosal adjuvant. III: Antibody responses to nontarget dietary antigens are not increased. *Regional Immunology* **3,** 217–222.

Owen, R. L., Pierce, N. F., Apple, R. T., and Cray, J. W. C. (1986). M cell transport of *Vibrio cholerae* from the intestinal lumen into Peyer's patches: a mechanism for antigen sampling and for microbial transepithelial migration. *J. Infect. Dis.* **153,** 1108–1118.

Pierce, N. F., Cray, W. C., Jr., Sacci, J. B., Jr., Craig, J. P., Germanier, R., and Fürer, E. (1983). Procholeragenoid: A safe and effective antigen for oral immunization against experimental cholera. *Infect. Immun.* **40,** 1112–1118.

Quaroni, A., and Isselbacher, K. (1981). Cytotoxic effects and metabolism of benzo(a)pyrene and 7, 12-diamethylbenzene(a)anthrazene in duodenal and ileal epithelial cell cultures. *J. Natl. Cancer Inst.* **67,** 1353–1359.

Santiago, N., Milstein, S., Rivera, T., Garcia, W., Zaidl, T., Hong, H., and Bucher, D. (1993). Oral immunization of rats with proteinoid microspheres encapsulating influenza virus antigens. *Pharm. Res.* **10,** 1243–1247.

Snider, D. P., Marshall, J. S., Perdue, M. H., and Liang, H. (1994). Production of IgE antibody and allergic sensitization of intestinal and peripheral tissues after oral immunization with protein Ag and cholera toxin. *J. Immunol.* **153,** 647–657.

Strober, W., and Jacobs, D. (1985). Cellular differentiation, migration, and function in the mucosal immune system. *In* "Advances in Host Defense Mechanisms. Volume 4. Mucosal Immunity" (J. I. Gallin and A. S. Fauci, eds.), pp. 1–30. Raven, New York.

Svennerholm, A.-M., Jertborn, M., Gothefors, L., Karim, A. M., Sack, D. A., and Holmgren, J. (1984). Local and systemic antibody responses and immunological memory in humans after cholera disease and after immunization with a combined B subunit-whole cell vaccine. *J. Infect. Dis.* **149,** 884–893.

Tomasi, T. B., and Plaut, A. G. (1985). Cellular differentiation, migration, and function in the mucosal immune system. *In* "Advances in Host Defense Mechanisms. Volume 4. Mucosal Immunity" (J. I. Gallin and A. S. Fauci, eds.), pp. 36–61. Raven, New York.

Volkheimer, G., and Schulz, F. H. (1968). The phenomenon of persorption. *Digestion.* **1,** 213–218.

Wilson, A. D., Bailey, M., Williams, N. A., and Stokes, C. R. (1991). The *in vitro* production of cytokines by mucosal lymphocytes immunized by oral administration of keyhole limpet hemocyanin using cholera toxin as an adjuvant. *Eur. J. Immunol.* **21,** 2333–2339.

Xu-Amano, J., Jackson, R. J., Staats, H. F., Fujihashi, K., Kiyono, H., Burrows, P. D., Elson, C. O., Pillai, S., and

McGhee, J. R. (1993). Helper T cell subsets for immunoglobulin A responses: Oral immunization with tetanus toxoic and cholera toxin as adjuvant selectively induces Th2 cells in mucosal-associated tissues. *J. Exp. Med.* **178,** 1309–1320.

Xu-Amano, J., Jackson, R. J., Fujihashi, K., Kiyono, H., Staats, H. F., and McGhee, J. R. (1994). Helper Th1 and Th2 cell responses following mucosal or systemic immunization with cholera toxin. *Vaccine* **12,** 903–911.

6

Consideration of Mucosally Induced Tolerance in Vaccine Development

HIROSHI KIYONO
Immunobiology Vaccine Center
University of Alabama at Birmingham
Birmingham, Alabama 35294;
and Department of Mucosal Immunology
Research Institute for Microbial Diseases
Osaka University
Suita City, Osaka 565, Japan

CECIL CZERKINSKY
Department of Medical Microbiology
University of Göteborg
Göteborg, S-413 46, Sweden

I. Introduction

For the development of mucosal vaccines, several advantages can be pointed out over classical parenteral immunization. From a practical standpoint, oral immunization is less stressful for vaccine recipients and does not require professional skill to administer the antigen. Delivery of vaccine via the intestinal epithelium is safer in comparison to systemic injection since the former route of immunization uses a form of routine physiological movement, namely ingestion. Further, oral immunization can induce antigen-specific responses in both mucosal and systemic immune compartments, while the injection of antigen generally results in the induction of only systemic immune responses. Since the majority of mucosal surfaces consist of sites where pathogens enter the host, it is essential to induce effective mucosal immunity in addition to classical systemic immunity. A major form of protection at mucosal surface areas is provided by antibodies of secretory IgA (S-IgA) isotype (Hanson and Brandtzaeg, 1989; Mestecky and McGhee, 1987). Thus, external secretions of approximately 80% of antibodies in humans and over 90% in mice are of the IgA isotype, and are unique in terms of regulation of synthesis and transport through epithelial cells. The induction of S-IgA antibody responses to protein vaccine is totally dependent on cognate help provided by $CD4^+$ Th cells via their respective cytokines (McGhee and Kiyono, 1993).

Investigations of cytokine synthesis by murine and human Th cell clones have provided direct evidence that $CD4^+$ Th cells are divided into two distinct subsets according to the profile of cytokine production, namely Th1 and Th2 cells (Mosmann and Coffman, 1989; Romagnani, 1994). In particular, an array of cytokines including IL-2, IFNγ and TNFβ is produced by Th1 cells, while IL-4, IL-5, IL-6, and IL-10 were secreted by Th2 cells. The outcome of antigen-specific immune responses following vaccination is manipulated and regulated by interactions among these Th subsets, B cells, and antigen-presenting cells (APC) via the respective cytokines, including those of Th1- and Th2-type cytokines. Collective studies since 1987 have shown that two Th2-cell-derived cytokines, e.g., IL-5 and IL-6, are of particular importance for inducing surface IgA-positive ($sIgA^+$) B cells to differentiate into IgA plasma cells (Beagley *et al.*, 1988, 1989; Coffman *et al.*, 1987; Fujihashi *et al.*, 1991; Harriman *et al.*, 1987; Lebman and Coffman, 1988; Matsumoto *et al.*, 1989; Murray *et al.*, 1987). In this regard, IL-6 induced high rates of IgA synthesis in cultures containing mucosal B cells from both mice (Beagley *et al.*, 1989) and humans (Fujihashi *et al.*, 1991). More recently, it was shown that mice with targeted disruption of the IL-6 gene resulted in a defi-

MUCOSAL VACCINES

ciency of IgA plasma cells in mucosa-associated tissues and restoration of mucosal IgA was accomplished by introduction of a vector producing recombinant IL-6 (Ramsay *et al.*, 1994). In contrast, it was recently shown that the mucosal immune system was intact in IL-$6^{-/-}$ mice including those of the induction of antigen-specific IgA response (Bromonder *et al.*, 1996). Also, IL-10 has been shown to be an important cytokine for IgA synthesis especially in humans (Briére *et al.*, 1994; DeFrance *et al.*, 1992). Thus, Th2 cytokines including IL-5, IL-6, and IL-10 are essential soluble factors for the generation of antigen-specific IgA B-cell responses. Although these findings emphasize the importance of Th2-type responses for the induction of IgA production, one must also realize that cytokines produced by Th1-type cells, e.g., IL-2, can synergistically enhance the effect of these Th2 cytokines on IgA B-cell responses. Thus, IL-2 has been shown to support some IgA synthesis in LPS-stimulated or IL-5-cocultured B cells (Coffman *et al.*, 1987; Murray *et al.*, 1985).

Mucosal immunization is a beneficial system employed to induce antigen-specific S-IgA and serum IgG immune responses when an optimal mucosal modulator and/or vectors are utilized. However, oral immunization with large doses or multiple spaced, lower doses of free protein antigen can also elicit distinct and opposite immune responses in mucosa-associated and systemic lymphoid tissues. For example, oral administration of large amounts of ragweed antigen or of *Streptococcus mutans* cell-wall antigen resulted in the induction of antigen-specific IgA responses in the mucosal compartment, while unresponsiveness to the same antigen was evident in the systemic immune system (Challacombe and Tomasi, 1980). Further, soluble protein antigens including ovalbumin (OVA), keyhole-limpet hemocyanin (KLH), γ-globulin or casein, as well as heterologous erythrocytes, have all been shown to induce systemic unresponsiveness in both humoral and cell-mediated immunity (Carr *et al.*, 1987; Elson and Ealding, 1984a,b; Gesualdo *et al.*, 1990; Hachimura *et al.*, 1994; Kagnoff, 1978; Lamont *et al.*, 1988; Mowat, 1987; Mowat *et al.*, 1988; Peng *et al.*, 1990; Vives *et al.*, 1980). It was also demonstrated that oral immunization of mice with sheep red blood cells (SRBC) for extended periods resulted in the induction of SRBC-specific unresponsiveness in the systemic immune compartment (Kiyono *et al.*, 1982; Michalek *et al.*, 1982; Wannemuehler *et al.*, 1982). These studies provided suggestive evidence that $CD4^+$ and $CD8^+$ T-cell subsets which reside in the mucosa-associated and systemic lymphoid tissues are involved in the regulation of IgA responses and systemic unresponsiveness, respectively. These immunologically unique responses, where systemic unresponsiveness to orally administered antigen was induced in the presence of mucosal IgA responses, have been termed mucosal tolerance (Tomasi, 1980).

For the development of effective vaccines which can provide two layers of protective immunity in both mucosal and systemic compartments, one might wish to avoid development of oral tolerance to mucosal vaccines. However, the concept of oral tolerance can be applied to the prevention of diseases caused by systemic immunological disorders such as autoimmune disease and allergy. In this chapter, recent developments in the induction of oral tolerance are discussed in order to better understand the molecular and cellular mechanisms of this unique immunological phenomenon for the mucosal and parenteral immune system. Further, possible applications of oral tolerance to prevention and treatment of disease are summarized as well.

II. Mucosal Immune System for Vaccines and Mucosally Induced Tolerance

A. Mucosal Vaccines

Immune responses expressed in mucosal tissues are typified by S-IgA, the predominant Ig class in human external secretions (and by far the most abundant class of antibodies in this species), and the best known entity providing specific immune protection for mucosal tissues (Brandtzaeg, 1995; Hanson and Brandtzaeg, 1989; Mestecky and McGhee, 1987). S-IgA antibodies provide "immune exclusion" of bacterial and viral pathogens, bacterial toxins, and other potentially harmful molecules, and have also been reported to directly neutralize a number of viruses, to mediate antibody-dependent cell-mediated cytotoxicity (in cooperation with macrophages, lymphocytes, and eosinophils), and to interfere with the utilization of growth factors for bacterial pathogens in the mucosal environment (Childers *et al.*, 1989; McGhee and Mestecky, 1993). Interestingly, S-IgA not only functions well in external secretions but also can express its antimicrobial properties within the epithelial cell, which is the very same cell that transports newly formed IgA molecules from the subepithelial lymphoid compartment to the external side of a mucosal tissue (Brandtzaeg and Kaetzel, 1994). Furthermore, being devoid of complement-activating properties and relatively inefficient as opsonins, S-IgA represents a unique type of noninflammatory specific immune effector molecule. Based on the concept of a common mucosal immune system through which a fraction of IgA-committed B cells recruited in the gut, e.g., by ingestion of antigen, can disseminate immunity not only in the intestine but also to other mucosal and glandular tissues (see Chapter 2), there is currently much interest in the possibility of developing oral vaccines against, e.g., infections in the buccal, ocular, respiratory, and genital mucosae.

It is now almost axiomatic that in order to be efficacious, vaccines against mucosal infections must stimulate the mucosal immune system, and that this goal is usually more effectively achieved by administering immunogens via the mucosal route (e.g., oral immunization) rather than parenterally. Further, an optimal dose of mucosal immunization can lead to the induction of systemic immune response as well. However, stimulation of mucosal immune responses by, e.g., the oral consumption, inhalation, or topical deposition of most nonviable antigens is often inefficient, requiring multiple administrations of large (milligram to gram) quantities of immunogens and yielding, if any, modest and short-lasting antibody responses. It has thus been widely assumed that only live vaccines would efficiently stimulate a mucosal immune response. The use of live attenuated recombinant bacteria and viruses which can be genetically engineered to express unrelated antigens is being advocated since natural infection with live microorganisms is known to induce persistent and strong immune responses in both mucosal and systemic compartments (see Chapters 7–11).

Alternative strategies of antigen delivery include liposomes, biodegradable microspheres such as copolymers of poly-DL-lactide-co-glycolide-, polyphosphacenes, polyalginates, and cellulose starch with incorporated or surface-adsorbed antigens (see Chapters 12 and 13); however, their preparation generally requires relatively large amounts of antigens and/or harsh chemical treatments which can result in potential denaturation of vaccine antigens. Mucosal lectin-like molecules endowed with immunostimulatory properties (or mucosal modulators), such as cholera toxin (CT), the most potent mucosal immunogen and adjuvant known so far, and its analog *Escherichia coli* heat-labile enterotoxin (LT), when coadministered with either unconjugated or conjugated antigens have been shown to promote mucosal and systemic antibody responses. This is primarily due to the ability of CT to bind avidly to G_{M1} ganglioside on cell surfaces including epithelial M cells, a property ascribed to its B subunit, and to another extent the adjuvant properties of the toxin which appear to require the ADP-ribosylating action of the enterotoxic A subunit (Holmgren *et al.*, 1993). Several formulations based on chemical coupling or genetic fusion of CT-B with selected antigens or nucleotides are now being evaluated as potential vaccines (see Chapters 4 and 5).

B. Mucosal Tolerance

Mucosal uptake of antigen has far more ensuing consequences than systemic intake for the development of immune responsiveness. Mucosal uptake can induce not only S-IgA antibody responses in various mucosal tissues, but also, and often, systemic responses, or even both. Induction of both types of responses could be advantageous to protect the host from colonization by mucosal pathogens and from pathogenic systemic responses. However, mucosal administration of antigens is in fact a long-recognized method of inducing peripheral tolerance (Wells, 1911). The phenomenon, often referred to as "oral tolerance" (because initially documented by the effect of oral administration of antigen: Tomasi, 1980), is characterized by the fact that animals fed with large quantities of a protein antigen become refractory or have diminished capability to develop an immune response when reexposed to that very same Ag introduced by the systemic route (e.g., by injection) (Tomasi, 1980; Mowat, 1994). This phenomenon is an important natural physiological mechanism whereby the host avoids development of DTH reactions to many ingested food proteins and other antigens (Mowat, 1987). Depending on the dose of antigen administered, anergy of antigen-specific T cells and/or expansion of cells producing immunosuppressive cytokines (IL-4, IL-10 and TGFβ) may result in decreased T-cell immune responsiveness. It is interesting to note that the latter scenario involves cytokines that are also known to upregulate IgA production (Czerkinsky and Holmgren, 1995) and is thus compatible with the observation that secretory immune responses and systemic tolerance may develop concomitantly (Challacombe and Tomasi, 1980; Tomasi, 1980). Because tolerance can be transferred by both serum and cells from tolerized animals, it is possible that humoral antibodies (IgG and IgA? idiotype antibody? immune complex?), circulating undegraded antigens or tolerogenic fragments and cytokines may act synergistically to confer T-cell unresponsiveness (Mowat, 1994). Since it is exquisitely specific of the antigen initially ingested or inhaled, and thus does not influence the development of systemic immune responses against other antigens, its manipulation has become an increasingly attractive strategy for preventing and possibly treating illnesses associated with or resulting from the development of untoward immunological reactions against specific antigens encountered or expressed (autoantigens) in nonmucosal tissues.

III. Protein Vaccine Diphtheria Toxoid (DT) Induces Mucosal Tolerance

Oral administration of antigen using appropriate mucosal modulators and/or mucosal delivery vehicles is considered to be an effective immunization regimen to induce mucosal IgA and systemic IgG immune responses. However, this route of immunization can also induce systemic unresponsiveness dependent on the dose of antigen and frequency of administration. In order to understand the mechanisms of induction of antigen-specific responses and unresponsiveness following oral administration, protein vaccine DT was given via the oral route for different periods (Fujihashi *et al.*, manuscript in preparation). BALB/c mice (8–12 weeks old) were immunized with 250 μg of DT by gastric intubation on either 6 or 12 occasions at 3 to 4-day intervals. Mice were then give 10 μg of antigen intravenously 1 week after the last oral dose of vaccine. Seven days later, serum and fecal extracts were obtained and assessed for isotype and levels of DT-specific antibodies (Fig. 1). Further, mononuclear cells were isolated from the spleen and intestinal lamina propria of these orally immunized mice. These cells were then subjected to isotype- and antigen-specific ELISPOT assays for the assessment of antibody producing cells in both mucosal and systemic compartments (Fig. 1).

Comparison of DT-specific serum antibody responses between the two groups of mice that received oral DT either 6 or 12 times revealed that high levels of DT-specific serum IgM, IgG and IgA responses were only seen in the former group following systemic challenge with DT (Fujihashi *et al.*, manuscript in preparation). In contrast, DT-specific systemic unresponsiveness was induced in mice given DT orally in 12 spaced doses (Table I). This observation indicated that prolonged oral administration of protein vaccine antigen induces systemic suppression while an optimal regimen and dose of oral antigen application resulted in DT-specific serum antibody responses. Analysis of DT-specific IgG subclass responses in mice optimally immunized with DT via the oral route showed predominantly IgG1 subclass. Further, antigen-specific IgA responses were also induced in mucosal-associated tissues since fecal extracts from the same mice contained DT-specific IgA antibodies. According to the pattern of antigen-specific antibody responses, one can suggest that Th2-type responses are induced in both systemic and mucosal immune compartments following an optimal oral immunization. Taken together, these observations revealed that systemic unresponsiveness was induced following oral administration of DT 12 times, while a more optimal schedule of 6 oral immunizations induced an appropriate systemic antibody response (Fujihashi *et al.*, manuscript in preparation).

TABLE I

Induction of Mucosal Responses and Systemic Unresponsiveness by Oral Vaccine

Characteristics of DT-specific immune responses		Oral administration of DT	
Site	Isotype and subclasses	6 times	12 times
Systemic compartment	Serum IgG	+++	—
	γ1	+++	—
	γ2a	—	—
	γ2b	—	—
	γ3	—	—
	Splenic IgG AFC	+++	—
Mucosal compartment	Fecal IgA	++	++
	Intestinal IgA AFC	++	++

Since antigen-specific unresponsiveness was induced in the blood circulation of mice orally immunized with DT for 12 times, it was important to assess whether antigen-specific IgA responses were maintained in these mice. When fecal extracts from mice orally immunized with DT 6 or 12 times were examined by ELISA, approximately the same levels of brisk DT-specific IgA responses were seen in both groups of mice (Table I). These findings demonstrated that oral immunization with DT 6 or 12 times induced antigen-specific IgA responses in the mucosal compartment. However, prolonged oral administration of DT resulted in the induction of systemic unresponsiveness in the presence of DT-specific mucosal IgA responses.

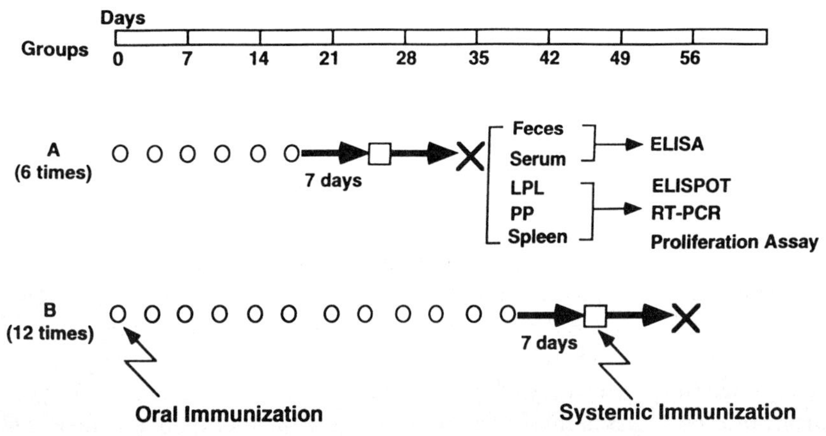

Figure 1. Immunization schedule for the induction of oral tolerance.

In order to ensure that DT-specific IgA responses were induced in mucosa-associated tissues of orally tolerized mice, DT-specific antibody producing cells were enumerated by isotype- and antigen-specific ELISPOT assay. Single-cell suspensions were obtained from intestinal lamina propria (LP) and spleen (SP) of mice orally immunized with 250 μg of DT 12 times as examples of mucosa-associated and systemic compartments, respectively. High numbers of DT-specific IgA antibody forming cells (AFC) were found only in intestinal LP of orally tolerized mice. In contrast, SP did not contain DT-specific AFC (Table I). These findings provide additional supportive evidence that DT-specific unresponsiveness was seen only in the peripheral immune system of orally tolerized mice, while antigen-specific IgA responses were maintained in the mucosal compartment (Fujihashi *et al.*, manuscript in preparation).

IV. Cholera Toxin B Subunit as Transmucosal Carrier–Delivery System for Induction of Systemic Tolerance

It has been widely assumed that only molecules with known mucosa-binding properties can induce local and systemic immune responses when administered by a mucosal routes; such as the oral route, without inducing systemic immunological tolerance (De Aizpurua and Russell-Jones, 1988). A notable example is CT, one of the most potent mucosal immunogens known (Elson and Ealding, 1984a), which, when administered simultaneously with an unrelated antigen by the oral route, can also prevent induction of systemic immunological tolerance to the coadministered antigen (Elson and Ealding, 1984b). Thus, mucosal administration of antigens coupled to mucosa-binding molecules such as CT or its mucosa-binding fragment CT-B subunit, has been proposed as a strategy to induce local and systemic immune responses rather than systemic tolerance (McKenzie and Halsey, 1984; Nedrud *et al.*, 1987; Czerkinsky *et al.*, 1989). Some years ago, CT and its B subunit (CT-B) attracted interest not only as potent mucosal immunogens and efficient carrier molecules for oral delivery of foreign protein antigens, but also as agents capable of abrogating oral tolerance when coadministered with various antigens/tolerogens (Elson and Ealding, 1984b). However, it was recently suspected that the tolerance-breaking properties attributed to both CT and CT-B might be selective for CT and thus, with regard to CT-B, may be explained by low yet significant levels of contamination by the toxin moiety of commercial CT-B preparations used in previous studies. Consistent with this hypothesis, it was observed that physical coupling of an antigen to recombinantly produced CT-B which was inherently uncontaminated with the toxin led to effects contrary to those reported previously; when given by various mucosal (oral, intranasal, vaginal, rectal) routes in the absence of CT adjuvant, CT-B induced a strong mucosal IgA immune response to itself as well as to conjugated antigens in the gastrointestinal (GI) tract, but instead of abrogating systemic tolerance to itself and to the conjugated antigen, it enhanced tolerance profoundly (Sun *et al.*, 1994). Based on this unexpected finding and on the results of recent experiments with several soluble protein antigens (γ-globulins, myelin basic protein, collagen type II, insulin), haptens, and particulate antigens (red blood cells, allogeneic thymocytes), it was suggested that such a mucosal delivery system based on coupling antigens to a mucosa-binding, nontoxic carrier molecule may be extremely advantageous for inducing peripheral tolerance (Czerkinsky and Holmgren, 1995).

The validity of this concept has been exemplified by the use of recombinant CT-B as a mucosa-binding molecule, and of SRBC as antigen/tolerogen in a murine system. This antigen was chosen as a model since it is one of the best characterized oral tolerogens with regard to both antibody formation and cell-mediated immune reactions (Kagnoff, 1980; Kiyono *et al.*, 1980, 1982; Mattingly and Waksman, 1978), the latter reactions being typified by the classical delayed type hypersensitivity (DTH) reaction. Both types of immune reactions have been implicated in the development of autoimmune diseases, allergic reactions, acute graft rejection, and a number of chronic inflammatory conditions. The effects of oral administration of CT-B/SRBC on the development of systemic serum antibody responses and DTH reactions to systemically administered antigens can be summarized as follows. Oral administration of a single dose of CT-B/SRBC suppressed *in vitro* antigen-induced proliferative responses of T cells, *in vivo* DTH reactivity to SRBC, and, although to a lower extent, serum antibody responses (Sun *et al.*, 1994). In the case of DTH reactivity, both early (2–4 hr) and late (24–48 hr) responses were either abrogated or considerably reduced (Table II). In contrast, daily consecutive administration of unconjugated SRBC for 20 to 30 days was required to suppress antibody responses and DTH reactivity to levels comparable to those obtained after feeding a single dose of CT-B-conjugated antigen. With respect to DTH reactivity, only late (24–48 hr) reactions were suppressed with no apparent effect on the early component (Table II). The latter observation is especially important since it suggests that the suppressive effects of oral administration of antigens coupled to CT-B involve mechanisms that appear to be distinct from those implicated in conventional regimens of oral tolerance induction.

Most importantly, this new strategy could be employed to suppress cellular responses even in animals

TABLE II

Prevention of Early and Late Delayed-Type Hypersensitivity (DTH) Reactions by Oral Administration of Sheep Red Blood Cells (SRBC) Coupled to the B Subunit of Cholera Toxin (CT-B)

	SRBC-specific DTH reaction (thickness increment $\times 10^{-3}$ cm)		
Oral tolerogen	Number of doses	2 hr	48 hr
SRBC-CT-B	1	0	2
SRBC-CT-B	1	9	36
SRBC	1	13	32
SRBC	10	11	24
SRBC	20	10	2
Saline		8	38

Note. Mice were fed a single dose of SRBC-CT-B, SRBC alone, or saline which was given 1 to 8 weeks before a primary systemic immunization with SRBC injected in the left rear footpad. Five days after this injection, the right rear footpad was challenged so as to elicit a DTH reaction. The intensity of DTH reactions elicited in mice fed SRBC alone was comparable to that recorded in control mice fed saline only. In contrast, DTH reactions recorded in mice fed SRBC conjugated to the mucosa-binding molecule CT-B were considerably decreased, at all times recorded. Thus, 2–4 hr after challenge with SRBC [that is, at a time corresponding to the early peak of DTH responses seen in control (saline fed only) animals], footpad swelling was absent in mice previously fed a single dose of SRBC-CT-B. Furthermore, the late DTH response which in mice peaks around 24 hr postchallenge was significantly decreased as compared to saline-fed control animals as well as to animals fed SRBC alone. Mice were fed single or daily consecutive doses of SRBC-CT-B or SRBC. One week after the last oral administration, animals were primed and challenged as above by systemic injections of SRBC in the left footpad followed 5 days later by the right footpad. It was found that the daily oral administration of SRBC for 3–4 weeks was required to suppress the 24-hr DTH reactions to a level comparable to that achieved by a single administration of SRBC conjugated to CT-B. As many as 20 consecutive feedings with SRBC over a 4-week period had no effect on the development of the early phase (2–4 hr) of the DTH response, in contrast to the situation seen with animals fed a single dose of SRBC conjugated to CT-B who failed to develop an early DTH response.

TABLE III

Inhibition of Early and Late DTH Reactions by Oral Administration of Sheep Red Blood Cells (SRBC) Coupled to the B Subunit of Cholera Toxin (CT-B) in Immune Mice

	SRBC-specific DTH reaction (thickness increment $\times 10^{-3}$ cm)	
Oral tolerogen	2 hr	48 hr
SRBC-CT-B	0	0
SRBC-CT-B + CT	20	57
SRBC	19	22
Saline	24	33

Note. SRBC were first injected in the left rear footpad of mice to induce a state of primary system immunity. Four days later, animals were fed a single oral dose of SRBC conjugated to CT-B with or without free CT, SRBC alone, or saline. Two days after the latter feeding, animals were given a second injection of SRBC in the right footpad to elicit DTH reactions. The latter DTH responses were monitored at various times after this secondary systemic immunization. Whereas mice fed SRBC alone developed DTH responses indistinguishable from those seen in control animals fed only saline, mice fed SRBC conjugated to CT-B had considerably reduced early and late DTH responses to SRBC.

previously sensitized at systemic sites. Thus, when mice were first sensitized systemically (by footpad injection) with SRBC and then fed a single dose of CT-B/SRBC, these animals failed to develop early as well as late DTH reactivity to a subsequent systemic challenge with SRBC (Table III). In contrast, mice fed the same dose of unconjugated SRBC displayed normal skin DTH reactivity to SRBC (Table III). Further, adding as little as 100 ng to 1 μg of intact CT to the oral CT-B/SRBC conjugate abrogated the tolerogenic effects of the conjugated antigen (Table III). The initial finding using the CT-B/SRBC conjugate has now been extended to other antigens, including allogeneic thymocytes, a number of soluble protein antigens such as selected autoantigens, and also haptenic compounds. In all instances, single or double mucosal (oral or intranasal) administrations of CT-B-conjugated antigens were effective at doses 100- to 1000-fold lower than those of corresponding antigens required or known to induce similar levels of inhibition of late DTH responses. Furthermore, overexpression systems have been developed to allow large scale production of CT-B preparations amenable to simple chemical coupling procedures, thereby facilitating the preparation of tolerogenic conjugates.

V. Mechanisms of Oral Tolerance: Role of αβ and γδ T Cells

In the late 1970s and early 1980s, mucosal immunologists had already made attempts to investigate the possible mechanisms of oral tolerance at a time when the immune system was not characterized at the molecular and cellular levels. Although several possible mechanisms (e.g., B-cell tolerance, anti-idiotypic antibody, antigen intestinal processing event for tolerogen and APC) have been shown to involve induction of oral tolerance (Mowat, 1994), the most compelling evidence to date suggests that T lymphocytes are the major cell type involved in the induction of oral tolerance. In earlier work, it was shown that systemic unresponsiveness was induced by adoptive transfer of T cells from rats fed orally with bovine serum albumin (Thomas and Parrott, 1974). Subsequently, a large number of studies demonstrated that oral immunization of protein antigen induces CD4$^+$ T cells in mucosal associated tissues which support IgA responses, while suppressor T cells were induced in systemic compartments such as spleen which downregulate antigen-specific IgM, IgG, and IgE responses (Kagnoff, 1980; Kiyono *et al.*, 1980, 1982; Mattingly and Waksman, 1978; Mowat *et al.*, 1988; Ngan and Kind, 1978; Richman *et al.*, 1981). For example, oral feeding of OVA to mice led to the generation of Th cells supporting IgA responses and suppressor T cells for IgG and IgE responses in gut-associated lymphoreticular tissues (GALT) (Mattingly and Waksman, 1978; Ngan and Kind, 1978; Richman *et al.*, 1981). Further, the former T cells for IgA responses remained in Peyer's patches (PP), while the suppressor T cells migrated into the systemic compartment (e.g., SP). These observations were considered to be logical explanations for cellular mechanisms of oral tolerance where PP derived CD4$^+$ Th cells support IgA responses, while SP T suppressor cells induce systemic unresponsiveness (Fig. 2). However, it is now generally agreed that a functional suppressor mechanism has existed for the downregulation of the immune response, but the nature and properties of these suppressor T cells are now disputed.

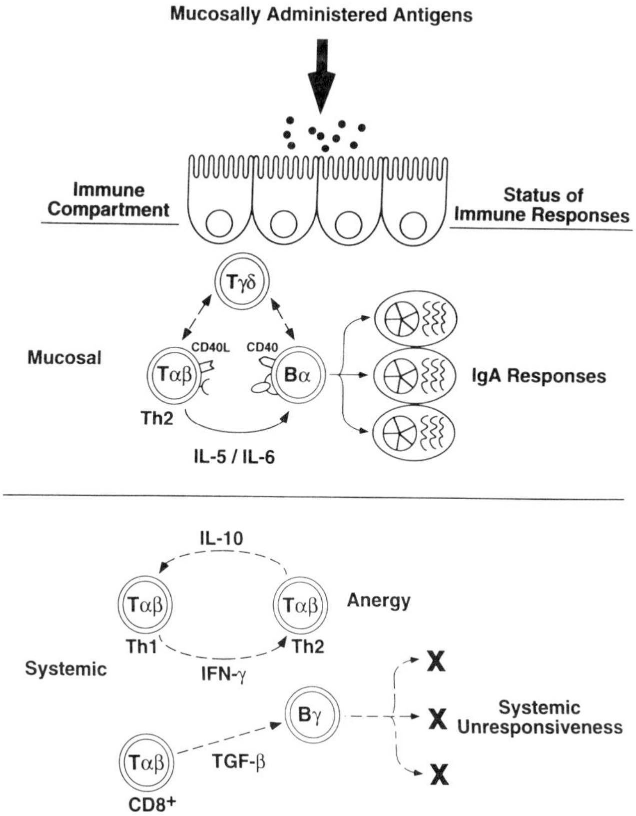

Figure 2. Mucosally administered antigens induce both S-IgA response and peripheral tolerance.

A. αβ T-Cell-Mediated Systemic Unresponsiveness following Oral Feeding

T lymphocytes are divided into two groups based on the usage of two heterodimer chains forming T-cell receptor (TCR) for the recognition of processed peptides on grooves of MHC class II expressed on APC. This includes αβ and γδ TCR bearing T cells. Classical effector T cells include CD4$^+$ Th cells and CD8$^+$ cytototoxic T lymphocytes (CTLs) which express αβ TCR for the detection of processed foreign peptide presented by MHC class II and I restriction, respectively. Considering the past and recent studies concerning cellular and molecular mechanisms of oral tolerance, αβ T cells were involved in the downregulation of systemic immune responses to orally administered antigens (Table IV). Further, current dogma suggests that the status of oral tolerance can be explained by clonal anergy and/or deletion of T cells, and active suppression by T cells via the secretion of inhibitory cytokines (Friedman and Weiner, 1994; Garside *et al.*, 1995; Gregerson *et al.*, 1993; Hirahara *et al.*, 1995; Melamed and Friedman, 1993, 1994; Miller *et al.*, 1992; Whitacre, *et al.*, 1991). Low doses of oral antigen favor the latter form of inhibition, while high doses of feeding induce clonal anergy of immunocompetent T cells (Friedman and Weiner, 1994; Garside *et al.*, 1995; Gregerson *et al.*, 1993; Hirahara *et*

TABLE IV
Possible Role of αβ and γδ T Cells in Mucosal Tolerance

T-cell subsets	Function of T cells for oral tolerance	
	Systemic	Mucosal
αβ T cells	(1) Anergy (2) Cross-regulation by Th1 and Th2 cells (3) Suppression (4) Clonal detection	Th2-type CD4$^+$ T Cells for IgA$^+$ B Cells
γδ T cells	Inhibition of IgE responses	Maintenance for IgA responses
Status of immune response	Inhibition of Ag-specific CMI and B-cell responses	Antigen-specific IgA responses

al., 1995). These two forms of oral tolerance are not mutually exclusive and may occur simultaneously following oral administration of antigens.

1. T-Cell Anergy

A condition of "anergy" is defined as a state of T-cell unresponsiveness characterized by the lack of proliferation and IL-2 synthesis and diminished IL-2R expression (Schwartz, 1990). This state can be reversed by preculturing of cells with IL-2 (DeSilva *et al.*, 1991). Anergy has recently been demonstrated in one condition of oral tolerance where a large dose of protein antigen induced anergy in OVA-specific T cells which did not respond to the antigen by proliferation, IL-2 synthesis, or IL-2R expression (Melamed and Friedman, 1993). Further, oral administration of myelin basic protein (MBP) diminished IL-2 and IFNγ synthesis (Whitacre *et al.*, 1991). These findings suggested that Th1-type T cells may be susceptible to the induction of anergy after oral feeding. To this end, it has been shown that Th1-type cells appear to be more sensitive to the induction of tolerance *in vitro* than Th2-type cells (Williams *et al.*, 1990). Recent *in vivo* evidence has demonstrated that Th1 cells are likely to be anergized in oral tolerance (Melamed and Friedman, 1994). Further, in order to identify which lymphocyte compartment (e.g., $CD4^+$ vs $CD8^+$ T cells) preferentially mediates the induction of oral tolerance, cell transfer experiments were recently performed using SCID and *nu/nu* mice (Hirahara *et al.*, 1995). Adoptive transfer of splenic lymphocytes from orally tolerized mice with bovine α-casein resulted in the induction of tolerance in these immunocompromised mice. Further, it was shown that oral tolerance was induced by anergized $CD4^+$ but not $CD8^+$ T cells. Taken together, a form of oral tolerance can be achieved by the induction of anergic $CD4^+$ T cells in the systemic compartment.

2. Cross-Regulation by Th1 and Th2 Cells via Cytokines

It has been suggested that the induction of tolerance can be explained by dysregulation of homeostasis between Th1 and Th2-type cells. For example, preferential activation of Th2 cells may lead to downregulation of Th1 cell-mediated CMI responses by Th2 cytokines such as IL-4 and IL-10 (Burstein and Abbas, 1993). In addition, and as described above, Th1 type cells are much more sensitive to anergy induction following oral administration of protein antigens (Table IV). These findings suggest the possibility that oral tolerance is associated with selective downregulation of Th1 cells by Th2 cells via respective cytokines in the systemic immune compartment. This possibility is consistent with the fact that oral tolerance has more profound effects on Th1-regulated CMI responses than on Th2 cell-mediated humoral responses. However, recent studies have shown that feeding of high doses of OVA inhibited production of both Th1 (IL-2 and IFNγ) and Th2 (IL-4, IL-5, and IL-10) cytokines which accompanied the reduction of IFNγ and IL-4-dependent antigen-specific IgG2a and IgG1 antibody responses, respectively (Garside *et al.*, 1995). These findings indicated that both subsets of Th cells are equally involved in the induction of oral tolerance (Table IV and Fig. 2).

3. Suppression

As summarized above, many past studies have demonstrated that a form of suppression is an important element of oral tolerance. Recent reports have provided evidence that inhibitory cytokine producing $CD8^+$ T cells are induced in oral tolerance (Weiner *et al.*, 1994). Oral administration of MBP generated TGFβ-secreting $CD8^+$ T cells (Lider *et al.*, 1989; Miller *et al.*, 1992, 1993) (Table IV). These $CD8^+$ T cells can inhibit antigen-specific immune responses both *in vivo* and *in vitro*. These TGFβ-producing $CD8^+$ T cells were initially induced in GALT since these cells were found in PP 24–48 hr following oral administration of MBP (Weiner *et al.*, 1994). It is possible that these GALT originated TGFβ-producing $CD8^+$ T cells migrate to systemic sites and then mediate active suppression (Fig. 2). Further, these TGFβ-producing regulatory T cells were shown to be involved by standard suppression. The cells from MBP-fed animals suppressed OVA responses when they were stimulated with fed antigen (Miller *et al.*, 1991). In an analogous manner, cells from OVA-administered animals inhibited MBP responses upon restimulation with the fed antigen. Induction of this active suppression has been shown to be dependent upon antigen dosage and frequency of feeding (e.g., low-dose oral tolerance) (Freidman and Weiner, 1994).

B. Mucosal γδ T Cells Maintain IgA Responses in Oral Tolerance

In order to maintain opposite immune responses (e.g., systemic unresponsiveness and mucosal IgA response) to orally administered antigens, one should consider that a subset of regulatory T cells in mucosa-associated tissues may play an important role in maintenance of antigen-specific IgA responses in the presence of systemic unresponsiveness (Table IV). It has been shown that mucosal immune compartments such as the intestinal epithelium contain large numbers of γδ T cells in addition to αβ T cells (reviewed in Kiyono and McGhee, 1994). Further, the lamina propria region of small intestine also contains γδ T cells (Aicher *et al.*, 1992). Since these γδ T cells are localized in the mucosa-associated tissues, it was logical to hypothesize that mucosal γδ T cells may involve maintenance of antigen-specific IgA responses in the presence of systemic unresponsiveness following oral administration of antigens.

To directly test this possibility, $CD3^+$ T cells from

intestinal intraepithelial lymphocytes (IELs) of mice orally immunized with SRBC were separated into γδ and αβ T cells. When purified γδ and αβ T cells were adoptively transferred to mice orally tolerized with SRBC, a conversion of systemic unresponsiveness to IgM, IgG, and IgA anti-SRBC responses was achieved in mice that received γδ but not αβ T cells (Fujihashi *et al.*, 1990, 1992). A more recent study has also demonstrated that γδ T cells isolated from mucosa-associated tissues of mice orally immunized with peptide vaccine (e.g., LT-B) exhibited similar activity where intraepithelial γδ T cells from LT-B-fed mice with oral tolerance abrogated systemic unresponsiveness following adoptive transfer to syngeneic mice orally tolerized with the same antigen (Takahashi *et al.*, 1995). Taken together, mucosal γδ T cells could be an important regulatory mechanism for the maintenance of an appropriate immunological homeostasis between local IgA responses and systemic unresponsiveness in oral tolerance (Fig. 2).

Mutant mice lacking γδ T cells have been produced by introducing germ-line mutations in the TCRγ-chain gene (Itohara *et al.*, 1993). These TCRγ-chain-deleted mice could be useful models to elucidate the exact role of γδ T cells for the induction and regulation of mucosal IgA immune responses. Thus, a recent study has taken advantage of these unique $TCR\gamma^{-/-}$ mice in order to determine the role of γδ T cells in mucosal immunity (Fujihashi *et al.*, 1996). If mucosal γδ T cells are involved in the induction of IgA B-cell responses, one might expect alterations in the mucosal immune system of these TCRγ gene disrupted mice.

The initial experiment was aimed at an examination of the possible effects of TCRγ gene disruption by characterizing the total number of IgM, IgG, and IgA producing cells in systemic and mucosal-associated tissues, and levels of IgM, IgG, and IgA titers in serum and fecal extracts obtained from $TCR\gamma^{-/-}$ mice. When the frequencies of Ig-producing cells were compared between SP of $TCR\gamma^{-/-}$ mice and their background strains [(129 × B6)F2], essentially identical numbers of IgM and IgG-producing cells were seen. However, the numbers of IgA-secreting cells in mucosa-associated tissues such as intestinal LP and PP of $TCR\gamma^{-/-}$ mice were significantly lower than control background mice (Fujihashi *et al.*, 1996). These observations were further confirmed by the assessment of antibodies in serum and fecal extracts of $TCR\gamma^{-/-}$ mice. The levels of IgA were reduced by approximately 40% in fecal extracts obtained from $TCR\gamma^{-/-}$ mice when compared with normal background mice. In addition, serum IgA titers in $TCR\gamma^{-/-}$ mice were also reduced. These results suggested that the depletion of γδ T cells resulted in the reduction of IgA synthesis but did not affect IgM and IgG isotypes. These findings further support the notion that mucosal γδ T cells can involve regulation of $CD4^+$ αβ T-cell dependent IgA B-cell responses (Fig. 2). Further, mucosal γδ T cells could be key regulatory T cells for the maintenance of the IgA immune response in the presence of systemic unresponsiveness (e.g., oral tolerance).

VI. Clinical Application of Oral Tolerance

Mucosally induced immunological tolerance has earlier been proposed as a strategy to prevent or reduce the intensity of allergic reactions to chemical drugs (Chase, 1946), soluble protein antigens, and particulate antigens (Thomas and Parrott, 1974; Mattingly and Waksman, 1978), and to reduce or suppress immune responses against self antigens (Bitar and Whitacre, 1988; Higgins and Weiner, 1988; Thompson and Staines, 1986; Nagler-Anderson *et al.*, 1986). As a result, it has been possible to delay the onset and/or to decrease the intensity of experimentally induced autoimmune diseases in a variety of animal systems by mucosal deposition of autoantigens onto the intestinal (by feeding) or the respiratory mucosa (by aerosolization or intranasal instillation of antigens). Pilot clinical trials of oral tolerance have recently been conducted in patients with autoimmune diseases and promising clinical applications have been reported (Weiner *et al.*, 1994). Much in the same way, oral administration of antigens had earlier been proposed to prevent and/or treat allergic reactions to common allergens such as house dust components or substances present in grass pollen (Rebien *et al.*, 1982; Wortmann, 1977). Although the above examples indicate that oral tolerance offers promise for inducing specific immunologic tolerance, its therapeutic potential remains limited by practical problems. Indeed, large quantities of antigens (e.g., mg to kg) are required to induce systemic unresponsiveness in experimental animals as well as humans by the oral route. To overcome this practical disadvantage, mucosal delivery of CT-B-conjugated autoantigen was recently applied to an experimental autoimmune animal model in order to examine the possible clinical application.

It was recently shown that a single dose of oral CT-B subunit conjugated to myelin basic protein (MBP) prevents experimental autoimmune encephalomyelitis (EAE) in Lewis rats (Sun *et al.*, 1995). Animals were injected in the hind footpad with MBP plus Freund's complete adjuvant after being pretreated with different antigens by the oral route. Animals who were fed saline, or an irrelevant antigen coupled to CT-B subunit, or repeated moderate doses of MBP all developed EAE disease with severe paralysis. In contrast, rats fed repeatedly with a high dose of MBP antigen (5 × 1 mg) or with a single low (25 μg) dose of CT-B subunit-coupled MBP remained healthy. The clinical picture was in complete accordance with the presence or absence of inflammation in the central nervous system as judged by histopathology (Sun *et al.*, 1995). It thus appears that by using CT-B subunit-coupled MBP (CT-B-MBP) one can both reduce the number of doses and dramatically decrease the amount of antigen needed for preventing this autoimmune disease which has many similarities with multiple sclerosis in humans. Analyses of cytokine production after *in vitro* stimulation of lymph node cells from CT-B-MBP-treated animals with MBP have disclosed that oral administration of CT-B-conjugated MBP leads to profound downregulation of IL-2 production and concurrent upregulation of IFNγ secretion. The latter finding is in sharp contrast with the effect of feeding repeated large doses (5×1 mg) of unconjugated MBP which resulted in the suppression of both IL-2 and IFNγ production, suggesting again that CT-B exerts unique immunomodulating properties on peripheral T-cell responses to coadministered antigens.

The efficiency of this strategy of tolerance induction was also demonstrated in a murine model of collagen-induced arthritis. DBA mice having inhaled as little as 25 μg of collagen type II chemically coupled to CT-B given 1 week after disease induction (by intracutaneous injection of collagen type II in Freund's adjuvant) showed considerably delayed (by approximately 30 days) onset of arthritis and had decreased disease severity (joint swelling and errosiveness) as compared to animals given comparable doses of unconjugated collagen type II or CT-B alone (Tarkowski *et al.*, 1996). More recently, using the NOD mouse model of spontaneous autoimmune diabetes, it was also shown that a single oral dose of insulin conjugated to CT-B could protect animals against diabetes. In adoptive transfer experiments, T cell-enriched spleen cells from animals fed CT-B-insulin were shown to suppress autoimmune diabetes when cotransferred with syngeneic diabetogenic T cells (Thivolet *et al.*, 1996). Furthermore, coupling thymocytes to CT-B and feeding this conjugate to mice resulted in the significantly prolonged the survival of transplanted hearts in allogeneic mouse recipients. Again, the effect was superior to that obtained by feeding the cells alone (Sun *et al.*, 1995). Based on these new findings, it may be possible to use CT-B subunit as a mucosal carrier delivery system for inducing specific systemic T-cell tolerization. Although this new toleration principle is still in the early stages of animal experimentation, it may lead to the development of safe, medical immunotherapeutic agents in selected autoimmune and DTH-type diseases.

Acknowledgments

We gratefully acknowledge the active contributions of Drs. Kohtaro Fujihashi and Jerry R. McGhee (UAB) and Drs. Thomas Olsson, Charles Thivolet, Andrej Tarkowski and Jan Holmgren (Göteborg). The studies summarized here were supported in part by NIH Grants AI 35932, AI 18958, AI 35544, and DE 09873 and Contract AI 15128, grants from Ministry of Health and Welfare, Asahi Chemical Co., Ltd. (Japan), the Swedish Medical Research Council and the Institut National de la Santé et de la Recherche Médicale (France). We also thank Ms. Sheila D. Shaw and Ms. Wendy Jackson for the preparation of this chapter.

References

Aicher, W. K., Fujihashi, K., Yamamoto, M., Kiyono, H., Pitts, A. M., and McGhee, J. R. (1992). Effects of the lpr/lpr mutation on T and B cell populations in the lamina propria of the small intestine, a mucosal effector site. *Int. Immunol.* **4**, 959–968.

Beagley, K. W., Eldridge, J. H., Kiyono, H., Everson, M. P., Koopman, W. J., Honjo, T., and McGhee, J. R. (1988). Recombinant murine IL-5 induces high rate IgA synthesis in cycling IgA-positive Peyer's patch B cells. *J. Immunol.* **141**, 2035–2042.

Beagley, K. W., Eldridge, J. H., Lee, F., Kiyono, H., Everson, M. P., Koopman, W. J., Hirano, T., Kishimoto, T., and McGhee, J. R. (1989). Interleukins and IgA synthesis. Human and murine interleukin 6 induce high rate IgA secretion in IgA-committed B cells. *J. Exp. Med.* **169**, 2133–2148.

Brandtzaeg, P. (1995). Basic mechanisms of mucosal immunity. A major adaptive defense system. *Immunologists* **3**, 89–96.

Brandtzaeg, P., and Kaetzel, C. S. (1994). Epithelial and hepatobiliary transport of polymeric immunoglobulins. *In* "Handbook of Mucosal Immunology" (P. L. Ogra, J. Mestekcy, M. E. Lamm, W. Strober, J. R. McGhee, and J. Bienenstock, eds.), pp. 113–126, Academic Press, San Diego.

Bitar, D. M., and Whitacre, C. C. (1988). Suppression of experimental autoimmune encephalomyelitis by the oral administration of myelin basic protein. *Cell. Immunol.* **112**, 364–370.

Briére, F., Brindon, J.-M., Chevet, D., Souillet, G., Bienvenu, F., Guret, C., Martinez-Valdez, H., and Banchereau, J. (1994). Interleukin 10 induces B lymphocytes from IgA-deficient patients to secrete IgA. *J. Clin. Invest.* **94**, 97–104.

Bromander, A. K., Ekman, L., Kopf, M., Nedrud, J. G., and Lycke, N. Y. (1996). IL-6 deficient mice exhibit normal mucosal IgA responses to local immunizations and *Helicobacter felis* infection. *J. Immunol.* **156**, 4290–4297.

Burstein, H. J., and Abbas, A. K. (1993). *In vivo* role of interleukin 4 in T cell tolerance induced by aqueous protein antigen. *J. Exp. Med.* **177**, 457–463.

Carr, R., Forsyth, S., and Sadi, D. (1987). Abnormal responses to ingested substances in murine systemic lupus erythematosus: Apparent effect of a casein-free diet on the development of systemic lupus erythematosus in NZB/W mice. *J. Rheum.* **14**, 158–165.

Challacombe, S. J., and Tomasi, T. B., Jr. (1980). Systemic

tolerance and secretory immunity after oral immunization. *J. Exp. Med.* **152,** 1459–1472.

Chase, M. W. (1946). Inhibition of experimental drug allergy by prior feeding of the sensitilizing agent. *Proc. Soc. Exp. Biol.* **61,** 257–259.

Childers, N. K., Bruce, M. G., and McGhee, J. R. (1989). Molecular mechanisms of immunoglobulin A defense. *Annu. Rev. Microbiol.* **43,** 503–536.

Coffman, R. L., Shrader, B., Carty, J., Mosmann, T. R., and Bond, M. W. (1987). A mouse T cell product that preferentially enhances IgA production. I. Biologic characterization. *J. Immunol.* **139,** 3685–3690.

Czerkinsky, C., and Holmgren, J. (1995). The mucosal immune system and prospects for anti-infectious and anti-inflammatory vaccines. *Immunologists* **3,** 97–103.

Czerkinsky, C., Russell, M. W., Lycke, N., Lindblad, M., and Holmgren, J. (1989). Oral administration of a streptococcal antigen coupled to cholera toxin B subunit evokes strong antibody responses in salivary glands and extramucosal tissues. *Infect. Immun.* **57,** 1072–1077.

De Aizpurua, H. J., and Russell-Jones, G. J. (1988). Oral vaccination. Identification of classes of proteins that provoke an immune response upon oral feeding. *J. Exp. Med.* **167,** 440–451.

DeFrance, T., Vanbervliet, B., Briére, F., Durand, I., Rousset, F., and Banchereau, J. (1992). Interleukin 10 and transforming growth factor-β cooperate to induce anti-CD40 activated naive human B cells to secrete immunoglobulin A. *J. Exp. Med.* **175,** 671–682.

DeSilva, D. R., Urdahl, K. B., and Jenkins, M. K. (1991). Clonal anergy is induced *in vitro* by T cell receptor occupancy in the absence of proliferation. *J. Immunol.* **147,** 3261–3267.

Elson, C. O., and Ealding, W. (1984a). Generalized systemic and mucosal immunity in mice after mucosal stimulation with cholera toxin. *J. Immunol.* **132,** 2736–2741.

Elson, C. O., and Ealding, W. (1984b). Cholera toxin feeding did not induce oral tolerance in mice and abrogated oral tolerance to an unrelated protein antigen. *J. Immunol.* **133,** 2892–2897.

Friedman, A., and Weiner, H. L. (1994). Induction of anergy or active suppression following oral tolerance is determined by antigen dosage. *Proc. Natl. Acad. Sci. U.S.A* **91,** 6688–6692.

Fujihashi, K., Taguchi, T., McGhee, J. R., Eldridge, J. H., Bruce, M. G., Green, D. R., Singh, B., and Kiyono, H. (1990). Regulatory function for murine intraepithelial lymphocytes. Two subsets of $CD3^+$, T cell receptor-1^+ intraepithelial lymphocyte T cells abrogate oral tolerance. *J. Immunol.* **145,** 2010–2019.

Fujihashi, K., McGhee, J. R., Lue, C., Beagley, K. W., Taga, T., Hirano, T., Kishimoto, T., Mestecky, J., and Kiyono, H. (1991). Human appendix B cells naturally express receptors for and respond to interleukin 6 with selective IgA1 and IgA2 synthesis. *J. Clin. Invest.* **88,** 248–252.

Fujihashi, K., Taguchi, T., Aicher, W. A., McGhee, J. R., Bluestone, J. A., Eldridge, J. H., and Kiyono, H. (1992). Immunoregulatory functions for murine intraepithelial lymphocytes: γ/δ T cell receptor-positive (TCR^+) T cells abrogate oral tolerance, while α/β TCR^+ T cells provide B cell help. *J. Exp. Med.* **175,** 695–707.

Fujihashi, K., McGhee, J. R., Kweon, M., Cooper, M. D., Tonegawa, S., Takahashi, I., Hiroi, T., Mestecky, J., and Kiyono, H. (1996). γ/δ T cell-deficient mice have impaired mucosal immunoglobulin A responses. *J. Exp. Med.* **183,** 1929–1935.

Garside, P., Steel, M., Worthey, E. A., Satoskar, A., Alexander, J., Bleuthmann, H., Liew, F. Y., and Mowat, A. McI. (1995). T helper 2 cells are subject to high dose oral tolerance and are not essential for its induction. *J. Immunol.* **154,** 5649–5655.

Gesualdo, L., Lamm, M. E., and Emancipator, S. N. (1990). Defective oral tolerance promotes nephritogenisis in experimental IgA nephropathy induced by oral immunization. *J. Immunol.* **145,** 3684–3691.

Gregerson, D. S., Obritsch, W. F., and Donoso, L. A. (1993). Oral tolerance in experimental autoimmune unveoretintits. Distinct mechanisms of resistance are induced by low dose vs. high dose feeding protocols. *J. Immunol.* **151,** 5751–5761.

Hachimura, S., Fujikawa, Y., EnoZmoto, A., Kim, S.-M., Ametani, A., and Kaminogaa, S. (1994). Differential inhibition of T and B cell responses to individual antigenic determinants in orally tolerized mice. *Int. Immunol.***6,** 1791–1797.

Hanson, L. A., and Brandtzaeg, P. (1989). The mucosal defense system. *In* "Immunobiological Disorders in Infants and Children" (E. R. Stiehm ed.), pp. 116–155 Saunders, Philadelphia, Pennsylvania.

Harriman, G. R., Kunimoto, D. Y., Elliott, J. F., Paetkau, V., and Strober, W. (1988). The role of IL-5 in IgA B cell differentiation. *J. Immunol.* **140,** 3033–3039.

Higgins, P. J., and Weiner, H. L. (1988). Suppression of experimental autoimmune encephalomyelitis by oral administration of myelin basic protein and its fragments. *J. Immunol.* **140,** 440–445.

Hirahara, K., Hisatsune, T., Nishijima, K., Kato, H., Shiho, O., and Kaminogawa, S. (1995). $CD4^+$ T cells anergized by high dose feeding establish oral tolerance to antibody responses when transferred in SCID and nude mice. *J. Immunol.* **154,** 6238–6245.

Holmgren, J., Lycke, N., and Czerkinsky, C. (1993). Cholera toxin and cholera B subunit as oral-mucosal adjuvant and antigen vector systems. *Vaccine* **11,** 1179–1184.

Itohara, S., Mombaerts, P., Lafaille, J., Iacomini, J., Nelson, A., Farr, A., and Tonegawa, S. (1993). T cell receptor g gene mutant mice: Independent generation of αβ T cells and programmed rearrangements of γδ TCR gene. *Cell (Cambridge, Mass.)* **72,** 337–348.

Kagnoff, M. F. (1978). Effects of antigen-feeding on intestinal and systemic immune responses. III. Antigen-specific serum-mediated suppression of humoral antibody responses after antigen feeding. *Cell. Immunol.* **40,** 186–203.

Kagnoff, M. F. (1980). Effects of antigen-feeding on intestinal and systemic immune responses. IV. Similarity between the suppressor factor in mice after erythrocyte-lysate injection and erythrocyte feeding. *Gastroenterology* **79,** 54–61.

Kiyono, H., and McGhee, J. R. (1994). Mucosal immunology:

Intraepithelial lymphocytes. *Adv. Host Def. Mech.* **9**, 1–194.

Kiyono, H., Babb, J. L., Michalek, S. M., and McGhee, J. R. (1980). Cellular basis for elevated IgA response in C3H/HeJ mice. *J. Immunol.* **125**, 732–737.

Kiyono, H., McGhee, J. R., Wannemuehler, M. J., and Michalek, S. M. (1982). Lack of oral tolerance in C3H/HeJ mice. *J. Exp. Med.* **155**, 605–610.

Lamont, A. G., Bruce, M. G., Watret, K. C., and Ferguson, A. (1988). Suppression of an established DTH response to ovalbumin in mice by feeding antigen after immunization. *Immunology* **64**, 135–139.

Lebman, D. A., and Coffman, R. A. (1988). The effects of IL-4 and IL-5 on the IgA response by murine Peyer's patch B cell subpopulations. *J. Immunol.* **141**, 2050–2056.

Lider, O., Santos, L. M. B., Lee, C. S. Y., Higgins, P. J., and Weiner, H. L. (1989). Suppression of experimental autoimmune encephalomyelitis by oral administration of myelin basic protein II. Suppression of disease and *in vitro* immune responses is mediated by antigen-specific $CD8^+$ T lymphocytes. *J. Immunol.* **142**, 748–752.

McGhee, J. R., and Kiyono, H. (1993). New perspectives in vaccine development: Mucosal immunity to infections. *Infect. Agents Dis.* **2**, 55–73.

McGhee, J. R., and Mestecky, J. (1993). Mucosal vaccines: Areas arising. *Mucosal Immunol. Update* **1**, 1–17.

McKenzie, S. J., and Halsey, J. F. (1984). Cholera toxin B subunit as a carrier protein to stimulate a mucosal immune response. *J. Immunol.* **133**, 1818–1824.

Matsumoto, R., Matsumoto, M., Mita, S., Hitoshi, Y., Ando, M., Araki, S., Yamaguchi, N., Tominaga, A., and Takatsu, K. (1989). Interleukin 5 induces maturation but not class switching of surface IgA-positive B cells into IgA-secreting cells. *Immunology* **66**, 32–38.

Mattingly, J. A., and Waksman, B. H. (1978). Immunologic suppression after oral administration of sheep erythrocytes and their systemic migration. *J. Immunol.* **121**, 1878–1883.

Melamed, D., and Friedman, A. (1993). Direct evidence for anergy in T lymphocytes tolerized by oral administration of ovalbumin. *Eur. J. Immunol.* **23**, 935–942.

Melamed, D., and Friedman, A. (1994). *In vivo* tolerization of Th1 lymphocyte following a single feeding with ovalbumin: Anergy in the absence of suppression. *Eur. J. Immunol.* **24**, 1974–1981.

Mestecky, J., and McGhee, J. R. (1987). Immunoglobulin A (IgA): Molecular and cellular interactions involved in IgA biosynthesis and immune response. *Adv. Immunol.* **40**, 153–245.

Michalek, S. M., Kiyono, H., Wannemuehler, M. J., Mosteller, L. M., and McGhee, J. R. (1982). Lipopolysaccharide (LPS) regulation of the immune responses: LPS influence on oral tolerance induction. *J. Immunol.* **128**, 1992–1998.

Miller, A., Lider, O., and Weiner, H. L. (1991). Antigen-drive bystander suppression following oral administration of antigens. *J. Exp. Med.* **174**, 791–798.

Miller, A., Lider, A., Roberts, A. B., Sporn, M. B., and Weiner, H. L. (1992). Suppressor T cells generated by oral tolerization to myelin basic protein suppress both *in vitro* and *in vivo* immune responses by the release of transforming growth factor β after antigen-specific triggering. *Proc. Natl. Acad. Sci. U.S.A.* **89**, 421–425.

Miller, A., Al-Sabbagh, A., Santos, L. M. B., Prabhu-Das, M., and Weiner, H. L. (1993). Epitopes of myelin basic protein (MBP) that trigger TGF-β release after oral tolerization are distinct from encephalitogenie epitopes and mediate epitope-driven bystander suppression. *J. Immunol.* **151**, 7307–7315.

Mosmann, T. R., and Coffman, R. L. (1989). Th1 and Th2 cells: Different patterns of lymphokine secretion lead to different functional properties. *Annu. Rev. Immunol.* **7**, 145–173.

Mowat, A. M. (1987). The regulation of immune responses to diettary protein antigens. *Immunol. Today* **8**, 93–98.

Mowat, A. M. (1994). Oral tolerance and regulation of immunity to dietary antigens. *In* "Handbook of Mucosal Immunology" (P. L. Ogra, J. Mestecky, M. E. Lamm, W. Strober, J. R. McGhee, and J. Bienenstock, eds.), pp. 185–201. Academic Press, San Diego.

Mowat, A. M., Lamont, A. G., and Parrott, D. M. (1988). Suppressor T cells, antigen presenting cells and the role of I–J restriction in oral tolerance to ovalbumin. *Immunology* **64**, 141–145.

Murray, P. D., Swain, S. L., and Kagnoff, M. F. (1985). Regulation of the IgM and IgA anti-dextran B1355 response: Synergy between IFN-γ, BCG-II and IL-2. *J. Immunol.* **135**, 4015–4020.

Murray, P. D., McKenzie, D. T., Swain, S. L., and Kagnoff, M. F. (1987). Interleukin 5 and interleukin 4 produced by Peyer's patch T cells selectively enhance immunoglobulin A expression. *J. Immunol.* **139**, 2669–2674.

Nagler-Anderson, C., Bober, L. A., Robinson, M. E., Siskind, G. W., and Thorbecke, G. J. (1986). Suppression of type II collagen-induced arthritis by intragastric administration of soluble type II collagen. *Proc. Natl. Acad. Sci. U.S.A.* **83**, 7443–7446.

Nedrud, J. G., Liang, X., Hague, N., and Lamm, M. E. (1987). Combined oral/nasal immunization protects mice from Sendai virus infection. *J. Immunol.* **139**, 3484–3492.

Ngan, J., and Kind, L. S. (1978). Suppressor T cells for IgE and IgG in Peyer's patches of mice made tolerant by the oral administration of ovalbumin. *J. Immunol.* **120**, 861–865.

Peng, H.-J., Turner, M. W., and Strobel, S. (1990). The generation of a "tolerogen" after the ingestion of ovalbumin is time-dependent and unrelated to serum levels of immunoreactive antigen. *Clin. Exp. Immunol.* **81**, 510–515.

Ramsay, A. J., Husband, A. J., Ramshaw, I. A., Bao, S., Matthaei, K. I., Koehler, G., and Kopf, M. (1994). The role of interleukin-6 in mucosal IgA antibody responses *in vivo*. *Science* **264**, 561–563.

Rebien, W., Puttonen, E., Maasch, H. J., Stix, E., and Wahn, U. (1982). Clinical and immunological response to oral and subcutaneous immunotherapy with grass pollen extracts. A prospective study. *Eur. J. Pediatry* **138**, 341–344.

Richman, L. K., Graeff, A. S., Yarchoan, R., and Strober, W. (1981). Simultaneous induction of antigen-specific IgA helper T cells and IgG suppressor T cells in the murine Peyer's patch after protein feeding. *J. Immunol.* **126**, 2079–2083.

Romagnani, S. (1994). Lymphokine production by human T cells in disease states. *Annu. Rev. Immunol.* **12,** 227–257.

Schwartz, R. H. (1990). A cell culture model for T lymphocyte clonal anergy. *Science* **248,** 1349–1356.

Sun, J. B., Holmgren, J., and Czerkinsky, C. (1994). Cholera toxin B subunit: An efficient transmucosal delivery system for induction of peripheral tolerance. *Proc. Natl. Acad. Sci. U.S.A.* **91,** 10795–10799.

Sun, J. B., *et al.*, (1995).

Takahashi, I., Nakagawa, I., Kiyono, H., McGhee, J. R., Clements, J. D., and Hamada, S. (1995). Mucosal T cells induce systemic anergy for oral tolerance. *Biochem. Biophys. Res. Commun.* **206,** 414–420.

Tarkowski (1966). Manuscript in preparation.

Thivolet (1996). Manuscript in preparation.

Thomas, H. C., and Parrott, D. M. W. (1974). The induction of tolerance to a soluble protein antigen by oral administration. *Immunology* **27,** 631–639.

Thompson, H. S. G., and Staines, N. A. (1986). Gastric administration of type II collagen delays the onset and severity of collagen-induced arthritis in rats. *Clin. Exp. Immunol.* **64,** 581–586.

Tomasi, T. B., Jr. (1980). Oral tolerance. *Transplantation* **29,** 353–356.

Vives, J., Parks, D. E., and Weigle, W. O. (1980). Immunologic unresponsiveness after gastric administration of human γ-globulin: Antigen requirements and cellular parameters. *J. Immunol.* **125,** 1811–1816.

Wannemuehler, M. J., Kiyono, H., Babb, J. L., Michalek, S. M., and McGhee, J. R. (1982). Lipopolysaccharide (LPS) regulation of the immune response: LPS converts germfree mice to sensitivity to oral tolerance induction. *J. Immunol.* **129,** 959–965.

Weiner, H. L., Friedman, A., Miller, A., Khoury, S. J., Al-Sabbagh, A., Santos, L., Sayegh, M., Nussenblatt, R. B., Trentham, D. E., and Hafler, D. A. (1994). Oral tolerance: Immunologic mechanisms and treatment of animal and human organ-specific autoimmune diseases by oral administration of autoantigens. *Annu. Rev. Immunol.* **12,** 809–837.

Wells, H. (1911). Studies on the chemistry of anaphylaxis III. Experiments with isolated proteins, especially those of hen's egg. *J. Infect. Dis.* **9,** 147–151.

Whitacre, C. C., Gienapp, I. E., Orosz, C. G., and Bitar, D. M. (1991). Oral tolerance in experimental autoimmune encephalomyelitis. III. Evidence for clonal anergy. *J. Immunol.* **147,** 2155–2163.

Williams, M. E., Lichtman, A. H., and Abbas, A. K. (1990). Anti-CD3 antibody induces unresponsiveness to IL-2 in Th1 clones but not in Th2 clones. *J. Immunol.* **144,** 1208–1214.

Wortmann, F. (1977). Oral hyposensitization of children with pollinosis or house-dust asthma. *Allergol. Immunopathol.* **5,** 15–26.

IV

Current and New Approaches for Mucosal Vaccine Delivery

7

Attenuated Salmonella *as Vectors for Oral Immunization*

TERESA A. DOGGETT
PETER K. BROWN
Department of Biology
Washington University
St. Louis, Missouri 63130

The ability to generate attenuated strains of *Salmonella* that are capable of inducing protective immunity against salmonellosis has led many researchers to investigate their potential as vehicles for the expression and delivery of heterologous antigens to the immune system. Both *Escherichia coli* and a number of *Salmonella* spp have been developed that are capable of expressing potentially protective antigens from a wide variety of animal and human pathogens. Immunization with these recombinant bacteria can result in the induction of both humoral and cell-mediated immune responses to the antigen being expressed and, in some instances, protection against the pathogen and the host bacterium. Perhaps one of the most attractive aspects of utilizing recombinant *Salmonella* is that as an enteric pathogen it can be used to express antigenic epitopes from other organisms that colonize mucosal surfaces. To prevent reversion of the strain back to a virulent form, the attenuating mutations should be deletions of one or more genes which are stable and cannot be complemented by host functions. In addition, the attenuating characteristics should be inherent properties of the strain, and not dependent on the hosts functioning immune system. The ideal vaccine candidate should be avirulent, highly immunogenic, easy to grow, and relatively cheap to manufacture. Since vaccines may be needed in areas which have poor facilities for growth and maintenance of bacteria, they will probably be produced in a lyophilized form.

I. Attenuated *Salmonella* for Use as Live Oral Vaccines

Salmonella is one of the best studied organisms genetically, and a wide variety of genetic tools are available for its manipulation. This has resulted in the development of numerous *Salmonella* strains which have attenuating mutations in different genes. These mutations can be grouped into three basic categories: mutations in (1) biosynthetic genes, (2) regulatory genes, and (3) genes involved in virulence.

A. Biosynthetic Mutants

Deletion (Δ) of a number of biosynthetic genes has been shown to attenuate *Salmonella* spp., including *galE*, and various genes for aromatic amino acid and purine biosynthesis. Mutations in the *galE* gene of *Salmonella typhimurium* and *Salmonella dublin* render these strains avirulent and immunogenic in mice (Germanier and Furer, 1971; Nnalue and Stocker, 1987). The *galE* gene encodes UDP-galactose-4-epimerase, which is involved in the interconversion of UDP-glucose and UDP-galactose. UDP-galactose is a substrate for synthesis of the core and O-antigen of lipopolysaccharide (LPS), and *galE* mutants exhibit a rough phenotype when grown in the absence of exogenous galactose. However, growth of *galE* mutants in low levels of galactose results in a smooth phenotype, while high concentrations of galactose cause lysis, presumably due to accumulation of toxic levels of galactose-1-phosphate (Adhya, 1987). It is not known whether attenuation is due to galactose sensitivity or to the avirulence of a rough phenotype *in vivo*.

One of the first successful attenuated *Salmonella* strains produced was a *galE* mutant of *Salmonella typhi* Ty2, acheived by treating the virulent wild-type strain with nitrosoguanidine, a potent mutagen (Germanier and Furer, 1975). The resulting strain, Ty21a, is a *galE* mutant lacking the Vi antigen, and is avirulent and highly immunogenic when administered to mice. In addition, Ty21a provided long-lasting immunity against *S. typhi* when administered orally to human volunteers

MUCOSAL VACCINES

(Edelman and Levine, 1986; Levine *et al.*, 1987; Murphy *et al.*, 1991; Wahdan *et al.*, 1982). However, a defined *galE via* (Vi antigen-negative) mutant of *S. typhi* Ty2 is still capable of causing typhoid fever in humans, indicating that strain Ty21a carries at least one other attenuating mutation (Hone *et al.*, 1988).

Attenuation of *Salmonella spp.* by the deletion of genes for aromatic amino acid biosynthesis was discovered and developed by Stocker and colleagues (Hoiseth and Stocker, 1981). *Salmonella* strains carrying mutations in the genes *aroA, aroC,* and *aroD* are both attenuated and highly immunogenic (Hone *et al.*, 1991; Hoiseth and Stocker, 1981; Miller *et al.*, 1991). All three genes encode enzymes that are essential for the synthesis of chorismate, which is an intermediate in the synthesis of aromatic amino acids, 2,3-dihydroxybenzoic acid, and *p*-aminobenzoic acid (pABA). 2,3-dihydroxybenzoic acid and pABA, which are not available in mammalian cells, are precursors of enterochelin (an iron chelator) and folic acid, respectively (Pittard, 1987). Since mutants of *Salmonella* that are impaired in their ability to transport iron retain their virulence, it is likely that avirulence of *aro* mutants is due to their inability to synthesize pABA (Benjamin *et al.*, 1985).

Several *aroA* mutants of *S. typhimurium, S. enteritidis,* and *S. dublin* have been shown to have reduced virulence and protect against wild-type oral challenge in mice and other animals (Alderton *et al.*, 1991; Brennan *et al.*, 1994; Cooper *et al.*, 1992, 1994; Hoiseth and Stocker, 1981; Mukkur *et al.*, 1991; Smith *et al.*, 1993). In addition, single *aroC* or *aroD* mutants of *S. typhimurium* and *S. typhi* have reduced virulence in mice (Hone *et al.*, 1991; Miller *et al.*, 1989), and *S. typhi* strains carrying these mutations have reduced virulence in humans (Tacket *et al.*, 1992).

Ideally, live attenuated *Salmonella* vaccines should possess at least two separate mutations that independently attenuate the strain to reduce the risk of reversion to a virulent phenotype. An *aroA, aroD* double mutant of *S. typhimurium* was shown to be attenuated in 7-day-old calves following oral inoculation and provided protection from oral challenge with the wild-type strain (Jones *et al.*, 1991). Double mutants of *S. typhi* harboring deletions in *aroA* and *aroC* or *aroC* and *aroD* are attenuated and immunogenic in mice (Chatfield *et al.*, 1992b; Hone *et al.*, 1991; Jones *et al.*, 1991). *S. typhi* Ty2 carrying a deletion in *aroC* and *aroD* is nonfebrile when tested in human volunteers, and stimulates specific IgA secreting gut derived lymphocytes in 100% of vaccinees (Tacket *et al.*, 1992). *S. typhi* strain ISP1820 carrying an *aroC aroD* mutation has been tested in humans and found to be immunogenic, although it was found to induce a mild vaccinemia and fever in a few subjects (Tacket *et al.*, 1992).

Mutants in other biosynthetic pathway genes such as *purA, purE,* and *asd* have been less successful as vaccine strains (O'Callaghan *et al.*, 1988). The enzymes encoded by the *purA* and *purE* genes are necessary for purine synthesis, while the *asd* gene product is involved in peptidoglycan and lysine biosynthesis. *S. typhimurium* strains carrying deletions in *purA, asd,* or *purA aroA* double mutants are totally attenuated, but are poorly immunogenic, while *purE* mutants are poorly attenuated (O'Callaghan *et al.*, 1988). Therefore, purine mutants are of limited use in vaccine development. However, immunization with Δ*asd S. typhimurium* mutants does induce a secretory immune response.

B. Regulatory Mutants

An alternative method to attenuate *Salmonella* is to construct strains carrying mutations in genes which regulate important biosynthetic processes and/or virulence factors. Deletion of central regulators renders a pathogen unable to activate a number of metabolic and virulence functions, and is therefore an effective means of attenuation.

Salmonella strains carrying a deletion of the *phoP* gene are highly attenuated and highly immunogenic (Galan and Curtiss, 1989). The *phoP* and *phoQ* genes encode proteins which make up a two component regulatory system involved in the regulation of acid phosphatases, and the genes necessary for survival in the macrophage (Fields *et al.*, 1989; Galan and Curtiss, 1989; Miller *et al.*, 1989, 1993). Orally administered *phoP* mutants are reduced in their ability to survive in the intestinal tract, and are rarely found in the liver or spleen, presumably due to their inability to survive attack from phagocytic cells in the GALT, mesenteric lymph nodes, liver, and spleen.

Mutants of *Salmonella* carrying deletions in the genes *cya* and *crp* have been shown to be avirulent and immunogenic in a number of animal species (Coe and Wood, 1992; Curtiss *et al.*, 1988; Curtiss and Kelly, 1987; Fields *et al.*, 1989; Galan and Curtiss, 1989; Hassan and Curtiss, 1994a; Hassan *et al.*, 1993; Miller *et al.*, 1989, 1993; Tacket *et al.*, 1992) The *cya* gene encodes adenylate cyclase which is involved in the synthesis of cAMP, and *crp* encodes the cAMP receptor protein which complexes with cAMP to form the cAMP–CRP global regulatory complex. The cAMP–CRP complex regulates expression of proteins involved in the transport and breakdown of carbohydrates and amino acids, and in the synthesis of fimbriae, OmpA, glycogen, hydrogen sulfide production, and flagella formation. Deletion of both *cya* and *crp* ensures that even in the presence of exogenous cAMP, the wild-type phenotype is not restored.

Salmonella choleraesuis and *S. typhimurium* strains carrying deletions of the *cya* and *crp* genes exhibit a diminished ability to reach the mesenteric lymph nodes and spleen. Mice orally immunized with these mutants are resistant to oral challenge with the respective wild-type strains (Curtiss and Kelly, 1987; Kelly *et al.*, 1992). Oral immunization of chickens at 2 and 4 weeks with a Δ*cya* Δ*crp* mutant of *S. typhimurium* also resulted in protection against challenge from other group B, D and E *Salmonella* (Hassan and Curtiss, 1994a). Recent studies have also shown that Δ*cya* Δ*crp* mutants of *S. typhimurium* are impaired in their ability to cause lymphocyte depletion in the bursa of Fabricius of chickens, and are therefore less likely to enter the carrier state (Hassan and Curtiss, 1994b).

C. Virulence Mutants

A number of virulence factors have been identified in *Salmonella* spp., mutations which may be candidates for attenuating live vaccine strains. While studying the effect of *cya crp* deletions on the virulence of *S. cholerasuis* in mice, Kelly *et al.* (1992) found that mutants carrying deletions that extend beyond the *crp* gene to *cysG* were less virulent and afforded more complete protection against challenge than a Δ*cya* Δ*crp* double mutant, indicating that an additional attenuating allele had been deleted. The new allele was designated *cdt* (colonization of deep tissue), and mutants in this allele are defective in their ability to colonize the liver and spleen. The *cdt* locus maps between *argD* and *cysG*, but a *cdt* single mutant has yet to be tested to establish whether *cdt* alone attenuates *Salmonella* (Bollen *et al.*, 1995)

The virulence plasmid is essential for infection by *S. typhimurium, S. dublin, S. enteritidis, S. choleraesuis,* and *S. gallinarum;* loss of the plasmid in any of these strains renders them avirulent (Gulig, 1990). Plasmid-cured derivatives of *S. typhimurium, S. dublin,* and *S. enteritidis* protect mice against oral challenge from the wild-type strain (Fierer *et al.*, 1988; Nakamura *et al.*, 1985). A plasmid-cured derivative of *S. gallinarum* has been shown to partially protect from challenge by the parent strain following intramuscular innoculation (Barrow, 1990).

Derivatives of *S. typhimurium* carrying mutations in the *htrA* gene are highly attenuated and provide significant protection against oral challenge in mice (Chatfield *et al.*, 1992c). The *htrA* gene encodes a stress-induced polypeptide, and mutants exhibit sensitivity to redox cycling reagents such as menedione and hydrogen peroxide. *S. typhimurium htrA* mutants give a level of protection similar to *aroA, aroC* mutants, but exhibit a reduced ability to persist in tissues; *S. typhimurium htrA, aroA* double mutants persist at even lower levels but still afford significant protection against oral challenge in mice. The inability to persist in tissues is an ideal property for human vaccines where tolerance criteria are much greater.

II. Vectors for the Expression of Foreign Epitopes

In addition to providing protection against *Salmonella* infection, live attenuated *Salmonella* have the potential to be used as delivery systems for expressing foreign proteins from pathogens of viral, parasitic, and bacterial origin. Replicons that are commonly used in *E. coli* such as ColE1, R6K, p15A, and pSC101 all operate in *Salmonella* spp., and therefore represent a wide variety of vector systems into which foreign genes can be cloned and expressed. One of the major problems associated with expression of foreign epitopes is the stability of foreign DNA within *Salmonella* during infection of the animal. Plasmids encoding antibiotic resistance and carrying foreign genes tend to be lost by segregation following growth of the *Salmonella* in the animal since there is no selection for the plasmid.

To increase plasmid stability, balanced-lethal host-vector systems have been developed where plasmid vectors carry biosynthetic markers such as *asd, thyA,* or *purA,* which are stably maintained in *Salmonella* strains carrying chromosomal deletions of the respective genes (Fulginiti *et al.*, 1992; Morona *et al.*, 1991; Nakayama *et al.*, 1988). An alternative approach is to integrate the gene for the foreign antigen into the *Salmonella* chromosome (Cárdenas and Clements, 1993; Hone *et al.*, 1989). This method, however, restricts the level of expression of the foreign protein, and humoral and mucosal antibody levels tend to be greater for antigens expressed from plasmids (Cárdenas and Clements, 1993). Another alternative method to stabilize strains and/or plasmids encoding heterologous antigens is to use promoters which are activated *in vivo.* For example, promoters for nitrate reductase *nirB* (Chatfield *et al.*, 1992a) and aerobactin (Su *et al.*, 1992b) are induced under anaerobiosis and limiting iron, respectively; both conditions are thought to be encountered in animal tissue. Recently, a number of genes have been identified which are activated in response to the host (Slauch *et al.*, 1994). The promoters from these genes may facilitate the development of better *in vivo* expression systems.

Current evidence suggests that a good mucosal response to an expressed foreign antigen is dependent on high expression of the protein (Wick *et al.*, 1994), which can be obtained using strong promoters such as P_{lpp}, P_{tac}, and P_{trc} (Hone *et al.*, 1994). However, high expression of some foreign proteins may be deleterious to the *Salmonella* strain. Ideally, the foreign protein should be maximally expressed in the animal, but tightly controlled *in vitro* to allow easy genetic manipulation of the construct. Ervin *et al.* (1993) constructed a virulence plasmid cured derivative of a Δ*asd S. typhimurium* strain in which the foreign gene (*lacZ*) is expressed from a P_{trc} promoter on an *asd*-containing plasmid. The P_{trc}

promoter is repressed by lacI^q carried on a second, incompatible plasmid which is lost by segregation *in vivo*, and the P_{trc} promoter is subsequently derepressed, resulting in expression *in vivo*. Recently, Tijhaar *et al.* (1994) described a vector in which the foreign gene is expressed from a strong promoter (P_L) that is flanked by inverted repeats. The promoter's orientation is changed randomly by an invertase encoded by the vector, and the strain containing the plasmid thus has a subpopulation which does not express the foreign gene, and is therefore stable. However, nonexpressing bacteria will segregate expressing bacteria, and the antigen is continuously presented to the immune system. Using the B subunit of cholera toxin (CtxB) as a model antigen, the vector was stably maintained and induced CtxB specific IgA and IgG in mice following oral immunization.

An alternative to expressing full-length foreign genes in *Salmonella* is to insert antigen epitopes into carrier proteins that are readily expressed in *Salmonella*. Examples of carrier proteins that have been employed successfully to express epitopes include flagellin, the structural subunit of flagella, the periplasmic maltose binding protein MalE, and the outer membrane proteins OmpA and LamB (Hayes *et al.*, 1991; Newton *et al.*, 1989; Schorr *et al.*, 1991; Stocker and Newton, 1994).

III. Expression of Heterologous Antigens by Attenuated *Salmonella*

Salmonella are being used to express an increasing number of antigens from a variety of human and animal pathogens, including virulence antigens from bacteria, viruses, and protozoans. Expression of these heterologous antigens has resulted in the induction of both humoral and cell-mediated immune responses to purified recombinant antigen and, in some instances, to the organism from which the gene was cloned.

A. Antigens of Bacterial Origin

The first report of the use of an avirulent *Salmonella* sp. as a carrier for a heterologous antigen was the expression of the *Shigella sonnei* O-antigen (O-Ag) in the human vaccine *S. typhi* Ty21a, a *galE* mutant, and resulted in the coexpression of both somatic antigens of *S. typhi* and the *S. sonnei* O-Ag (Formal *et al.*, 1981). Mice immunized either intraperitoneally or subcutaneously with this recombinant *S. typhi* strain could be protected against challenge with either *S. typhi* or *S. sonnei*. This vaccine strain has also been shown to be safe when orally administered to human volunteers and to protect against dysentery (Van de Verg *et al.*, 1990). In addition, the appearance of *S. sonnei* specific IgA antibody secreting cells (ASC) in the blood was also noted. Mice immunized with *galE S. typhi* expressing the *Shigella flexneri* 2a O-Ag were protected against challenge with *S. flexneri* but not *S. typhi* (Baron *et al.*, 1987). In each case, growth conditions of the recombinant *S. typhi* were the same; however, Baron *et al.* (1987) suggested that the lack of protection against *S. typhi* may be due to interference by the *S. flexneri* O-Ag being expressed by the recombinant *S. typhi*. This may be alleviated, in part, by altering the growth conditions of these *galE* hybrids, as demonstrated by Forrest and LaBrooy (1991). If they grew their *S. typhi*/*Vibrio cholerae* O-Ag hybrid in growth media devoid of galactose, there was an increase in the amount of cholera O-Ag expressed by *S. typhi*, which accordingly resulted in an increase in anti-cholera IgA titers in the intestinal secretions of immunized subjects.

A number of pathogenic antigens of a different *E. coli* have been expressed in a variety of *Salmonella* vaccine strains. One of these is the heat-labile toxin B subunit (LT-B) which is analogous to the cholera toxin B subunit (CT-B) of *V. cholerae*. Clements and El-Morshidy (1984) were the first to introduce a recombinant plasmid encoding the LT-B gene into *S. typhi* Ty21a which could induce antitoxin antibodies when injected intraperitoneally into mice. Oral immunization of mice with an *aroA* mutant of *S. dublin* expressing LT-B resulted in the appearance of *Salmonella* LPS-specific and LT-B-specific neutralizing antibodies in intestinal washes (Clements *et al.*, 1986). Similar results were observed by Maskell *et al.* (1987) following immunization with an *aroA S. typhimurium* mutant expressing LT-B. Fulginiti *et al.* (1992) have also used *aroA purA* mutants of *S. typhimurium* and *S. typhi* to stably express LT-B on a *purA*-complementing plasmid, thus eliminating the need for antibiotic selection markers. As an alternative to the expression of a cloned gene product from a plasmid, Cárdenas and Clements (1993) generated a *galE* mutant of *S. typhimurium* in which the LT-B gene had been incorporated into the chromosome. One of the problems with this method is the reduction of recombinant protein expressed. In a comparative study they observed that anti-LT-B antibodies were only detected in mice immunized with *S. typhimurium* that expressed LT-B from a recombinant plasmid, but required the presence of ampicillin for stability.

With current interest in both CT-B and LT-B, which have potent adjuvant effects when administered perorally, recent research has been geared toward developing vectors that express LT-B alone or as a fusion with another antigen. One of the first descriptions of an LT-B fusion protein was that of Clements and Cárdenas (1990) where they constructed a LT-B/heat-stable toxin (ST) fusion. Jagusztyn-Krynicka *et al.* (1993) have also constructed LT-B fusions using the surface protein antigen A (SpaA) and dextranase antigens from oral streptococci. These fusions were only stable in *S. typhimurium* in vectors with a p15a origin and varied in stability *in vitro.* Other hybrid vaccines are also being developed which express fusion proteins such as the Shiga toxin B subunit (Stx-B) with either haemolysin A (Su *et al.*, 1992a) or LamB protein (Su *et al.*, 1992b) of *E. coli.* These fusion proteins could be localized to either the cytoplasm or the surface of *Salmonella* harboring the recombinant plasmids. Oral immunization of mice with *S. typhimurium aroA* mutants expressing these fusion proteins resulted in a significant humoral and mucosal immune response to Stx-B which appeared to be independent of the location of the fusion. Since the adjuvant effect of LT and CT is derived from the presence of the toxic A subunit, F. Sebastiani and Curtiss (personal communication, 1995) have generated LT-A/LT-B constructs which have single amino acid substitutions in the A subunit that should maintain the adjuvant effect but remove the toxic effect. These constructs will soon be evaluated in mice for toxicity and induction of immune responses.

A continuing problem both in the Western world and in developing countries is the occurence of tetanus. The immunogenic fragment of tetanus toxin, fragment C, is believed to be involved in the binding of the toxin to cell receptors prior to internalization. A single oral immunization of mice with a *S. typhimurium aroA* mutant expressing fragment C resulted in partial protection against a lethal challenge with tetanus toxin; however, mice that received two oral immunizations 28 days apart were completely protected (Fairweather *et al.*, 1990). One of the problems with this construct is that it contains the *lacI* gene and *tac* promotor which repressed the production of fragment C *in vivo* thereby effectively reducing the amount of antigen being expressed. To overcome this problem, two alternative systems have been developed; one utilizes the expression of fragment C from the anaerobically inducible *nirB* promoter in an *aroA aroD S. typhimurium* strain (Chatfield *et al.*, 1992a), and the other incorporates the fragment C gene sequence into the chromosome of an *aroA aroC S. typhi* Ty2 strain (Chatfield *et al.*, 1992b). Using the *nirB* expression system high levels of circulating anti-tetanus antibodies could be detected after a single oral dose together with protection against lethal challenge with toxin. No experimental data are available for the *S. typhi* strain; however, lower levels of expression were observed *in vitro* and may be a problem in inducing protective immunity to tetanus toxin.

Dental caries and periodontal diseases are associated with microorganisms that are present in the oral cavity, and potential immunogenic and protective antigens from these microbes have been defined and expressed in attenuated *Salmonella.* Among these are the hemagglutinin of *Porphyromonas gingivalis,* which is believed to aid in the colonization of the host and enhance the virulence of this bacterium (Dusek *et al.*, 1993), and the SpaA (Curtiss *et al.*, 1988; Doggett *et al.*, 1993) and dextranase (Jagusztyn-Krynicka *et al.*, 1993) antigens from oral streptococci using the balanced-lethal host-vector system for the stable expression of the cloned gene products (Nakayama *et al.*, 1988). Goldschmidt and Curtiss (1990) identified a major antigenic epitope of the SpaA protein and constructs have been generated with single or multiple tandem repeats of this region. Oral immunization of mice with Δ*cya* Δ*crp* Δ*asd S. typhimurium* χ4072 containing the plasmid pYA2905 with multiple tandem repeats of the SpaA epitope resulted in significant serum and salivary anti-SpaA response (Doggett *et al.*, 1993). Similar results were obtained when rats were immunized orally with two doses of χ4072(pYA2905), and could be enhanced if a booster immunization was given (Redman *et al.*, 1994). As suggested earlier, the induction of immune responses to heterologous antigens appears to be dependent upon the quantity of antigen expressed by recombinant *Salmonella.* High-level expression using high copy number vectors can be deleterious, however, this can be overcome by expressing multimers of the cloned gene product.

The recombinant *Salmonella* system is now being used for the expression of protective antigens from animal pathogens, such as BCSP31, a 31-kDa protein from *Brucella abortus,* an organism that infects cattle and causes abortion. Mice immunized with Δ*cya* Δ*crp* Δ*asd S. typhimurium* expressing BCSP31 developed both serum and intestinal antibody responses to BCSP31 after two oral immunizations with recombinant *Salmonella* (Stabel *et al.*, 1990). This same protein has also been expressed in an attenuated Δ*cya* Δ[*crp-cdt*] *Salmonella choleraesuis* mutant with the same results (Stabel *et al.*, 1993). Interestingly, if this same recombinant *S. choleraesuis* was used to orally immunize swine the converse results were observed; that is, there was no induction of either serum or intestinal antibody responses to BCSP31, but significant DTH responses to both the cloned protein and *S. choleraesuis* were detected.

Also of economic importance is the diarrheal disease of neonatal pigs (scours) which can cause considerable loss in commercial pig farms. *E. coli* that infect swine and other domestic animals express the fimbrial antigen K88 which enables the bacteria to adhere to the mucosal epithelium. Antibodies directed against K88, derived from maternal milk of K88-immunized sows, have been shown to protect suckling pigs against enteropathogenic *E. coli* (Nagi *et al.*, 1978). The gene encoding the K88 fimbrial antigen has been successfully expressed in both *galE* (Stevenson and Manning, 1985) and *aroA* (Dougan *et al.*, 1986) mutants of *S. typhimurium.* In both cases systemic anti-K88 antibodies were detected in mice orally immunized with the *Salmonella* mutant expressing K88 fimbriae. In addition, mucosal anti-K88 antibodies were detected in mice immunized with the *galE* mutant. Hone *et al.* (1989) integrated the K88 gene into the chromosome of a *galE* mutant of *S. typhimurium* and, unlike other studies, observed production of antibodies against the expressed antigen in immunized mice. Morona *et al.* (1994) have generated a *thyA* mutant of the *galE S. typhimurium* G30 to express the ETEC fimbrial antigens K88 or K99. Plasmids that encoded either K88 or K99 had a nonantibiotic selection marker, ThyA$^+$, which complemented the *thyA* mutation. Oral immunization of 4- to 6-month-old pigs resulted in the production of significant serum anti-K88 and anti-K99 antibody titers and a booster immunization resulted in titers equivalent to those observed following intramuscular injection with killed organisms.

Some of the earliest reports of heterologus antigen expression involved *aroA S. typhimurium* vaccine strains that expressed β-galactosidase which is not normally expressed by *Salmonella.* Intravenous immunization with this recombinant *Salmonella* induced both humoral and cellular (DTH) responses to the cloned gene product (Brown *et al.*, 1987) and was one of the first methods to demonstrate that an intracellular recombinant protein was capable of inducing cell-mediated immunity. The *aroA S. typhimurium* SL3261 has also been used to express the *caf1* gene of *Yersinia pestis,* which encodes the F1 antigen which is believed to confer resistance to phagocytosis in this pathogen. Intragastric or intravenous immunization with recombinant *Salmonella* expressing *caf1* resulted in significant protection against challenge with a virulent strain of *Y. pestis* and was correlated with the induction of high anti-*Yersinia* IgG titers in the serum and a F1 specific T-cell response (Oyston *et al.*, 1995).

Some of the most attractive features of recombinant *Salmonella* vaccines are that they are potentially less expensive and may be more efficient systems of vaccination than those currently available. One such case is the development of a vaccine against *B. pertussis.* The filamentous hemagglutinin (FHA) of *B. pertussis* is protective and yet nontoxic (Kimura *et al.*, 1990), and both full-length and truncated forms have been expressed in an *aroA* mutant of *S. dublin* (Molina and Parker, 1990). Oral immunization of mice with *S. dublin* expressing the truncated FHA protein resulted in moderate serum anti-FHA IgG and intestinal IgA titers. Since *B. pertussis* invades the respiratory mucosa it would be more desirable to induce S-IgA responses in the respiratory tract. To this end, Walker *et al.* (1992) expressed a S1 subunit of the pertussis toxin in *aroA* mutants of *S. typhimurium* and *S. typhi* Ty21a which are more suitable delivery vehicles than *S. dublin.* Oral immunization with either of these *Salmonella* expressing the S1 subunit resulted in serum anti-S1 IgG titers equivalent to those detected after i.p. immunization as well as anti-S1 IgA titers in lung washes.

Antigens from intracellular bacteria such as *Francisella tularensis* and *Mycobacterium leprae* need to induce cell-mediated immune responses to the pathogen from which they are derived. Since it has been shown that both CD4$^+$ and CD8$^+$ T-cell responses can be elicited against antigens expressed by recombinant *Salmonella,* genes for potentially protective T-cell antigens from bacteria have been cloned with the ultimate goal of being expressed in attenuated *Salmonella.* The lipoprotein TUL4 of *F. tularensis* has been expressed in the *Δcya Δcrp Δasd S. typhimurium* vaccine strain χ4072 (Sjöstedt *et al.*, 1992). Both a serum antibody and a T-cell response were generated against the TUL4 protein expressed by χ4072. Antibodies raised against TUL4 recognized two overlapping peptides within aa 86–116 of the TUL4 protein. More importantly this response was affected by the haplotype of the mouse strain. This is an important consideration when using inbred mouse strains since the response to LT-B and CT-B has also been shown to be haplotype-restricted (Elson and Ealding, 1985).

There has been increasing interest in targeting mucosal responses in the female reproductive tract against pathogens such as *Neisseria gonorrhoeae. N. gonorrhoeae* only infects humans and at present there is no vaccine available. Several gonococcal antigens are potential candidates in the development of such a vaccine but the porin protein Por has been examined with respect to expression in recombinant *Salmonella.* Elkins *et al.* (1994) have expressed the *por* gene both on a plasmid and intergrated into the chromosome of attenuated *Salmonella.* Although they used different *S. typhimurium* mutants to express the Por protein, their results were in accord with other reports in that a higher level of expression was observed when the *por* gene was encoded on a plasmid as compared to incorporation into the chromosome.

B. Antigens of Viral Origin

Recombinant *Salmonella* have also been used successfully to express a number of viral antigens with the induction of both humoral and cell-mediated responses to the heterologous antigen. Tite *et al.* (1990a) were able to express the nucleoprotein (NP) of influenza A virus in an *aroA S. typhimurium.* They then orally immunized mice with NP-expressing *S. typhimurium* and were able to show anti-viral antibodies in the serum and an *in vitro* CD4$^+$ T-cell proliferative response of spleen cells isolated from immunized animals (Tite *et al.*, 1990b). Proliferation of these CD4$^+$ T cells, which could be inhibited by the addition of anti-CD4 monoclonal antibodies, was accompanied by the production of IFNγ and IL-2. Protection against challenge with influenza virus was also demonstrable if the mice received an intranasal boost prior to challenge. Brett *et al.* (1993)

further examined the $CD4^+$ induction of NP-specific T-cells following immunization with recombinant *Salmonella*. Both human monocytes and a monocytic cell line (THP-1) were found to present several different NP epitopes to human $CD4^+$ class-II restricted T lymphocytes but were unable to present NP to class-I restricted T cells when infected with either NP-expressing *S. typhimurium* or recombinant NP. The reverse was true when macrophages or THP-1 cells were infected with live influenza virus. An epitope of the hemagglutinin (HA^{91-108}) of influenza virus has been cloned into the flagella of an *aroA S. dublin* (McEwen *et al.*, 1992), thus allowing the HA epitope to be expressed at the surface of the *Salmonella*. Oral immunization with recombinant *S. dublin* expressing the HA epitope in flagella resulted in significant anti-epitope IgA titers in lung washes but low levels of HA-specific serum IgG. These results, however, may be due in part to the choice of the *Salmonella* strain rather than the expression system itself.

Considerable effort has been focused on the generation of a vaccine to hepatitis B virus (HBV) which continues to be a major public health problem. Schödel and colleagues have reported the expression of several hybrid HBV constructs that contain portions of the small envelope protein (pre-S1 and -S2) and the nucleocapsid in *Salmonella* (Schödel *et al.*, 1991, 1994). Translation products of this hybrid construct self-assemble to form 27-nm particles (Schödel *et al.*, 1992) and are highly immunogenic when administered in recombinant *aroA S. typhimurium* and *S. dublin* mutants via the oral route (Schödel *et al.*, 1990). Significant serum anti-pre-S IgG titers were elicited in mice immunized with a single oral dose of *Δcya Δcrp Δasd S. typhimurium* mutants (Schödel *et al.*, 1994), however, booster immunizations were required to induce antibody titers equivalent to those detected in previous studies with *Δcya Δcrp S.typhimurium*. This system is currently being investigated for its potential to express other antigenic epitopes within the HBV particles (A. Nayak 1996, personal communication).

With the demonstration of the appearance of antigen-specific antibodies at mucosal sites distant to the site of antigenic stimulation, and that the reproductive tract is part of this common mucosal network, it is not surprising that attention has turned to the expression of possible protective epitopes of HIV in recombinant *Salmonella*. It has been demonstrated that the major neutralization epitope is located in the V3 loop, a variable domain of the gp120 component of gp160 that includes residues 307–330 (Javaherian *et al.*, 1989) and contains T-cell epitopes (Takahashi *et al.*, 1989). Hofnung *et al.* (1988) succeeded in expressing V3 loop residues 293–343 as a fusion within "permissive" sites of two envelope proteins, MalE and LamB, of *E. coli* and could thus be expressed within the periplasm or on the cell surface of *Salmonella*, respectively. Only the MalE-V3 loop hybrid, however, was found to be stably expressed by *aroA S. typhimurium* (Charbit *et al.*, 1993). Intravenous immunization of BALB/c mice with *Salmonella* expressing the MalE-V3 fusion resulted in the production of serum anti-HIV1 envelope antibodies and purified MalE-V3 hybrid protein was capable of stimulating V3 loop-specific T-cell proliferative responses both *in vivo* and *in vitro*.

Other viral epitopes have been expressed in recombinant *Salmonella*, including the C-terminal domain of gB1 of the herpes simplex virus (Childress and Clements, 1988). Herpes simplex virus types 1 and 2 are the cause of several clinical syndromes including genital herpes, neonatal herpes, eczema, and acute gingivostomatitis. A portion of the envelope (E) protein of the dengue virus, which contains several neutralizing epitopes, has been cloned into an *aroA* mutant of *S. typhimurium* but the plasmid carrying this gene was unstable *in vitro* and further experimentation is required (Cohen *et al.*, 1990).

C. Antigens of Protozoan Origin

Malaria is still a major health problem; although programs are in effect to control the spread of malaria, a more effective approach would be the development of an anti-malarial vaccine. Although protection against *Plasmodium* sp. is mediated, in part, by induction of humoral response to immunodominant epitope repeats of the circumsporozoite protein (CSP), recent evidence indicates that the induction of cell-mediated immunity alone may be protective. Immunization of mice with radiation attenuated sporozoites resulted in the proliferation of $CD8^+$ T cells and protection, which could be eliminated by *in vivo* depletion of these cells (Schofield *et al.*, 1987; Weiss *et al.*, 1988). Sadoff *et al.* (1988) were able to demonstrate the induction of protective cell-mediated immunity following oral immunization of mice with an attenuated *S. typhimurium* expressing the CSP of *Plasmodium berghei*. Later studies were able to show that this immunity was also mediated through the induction of specific $CD8^+$ T lymphocytes (CTL) directed against amino acids 242–253 of the CSP (Aggarwal *et al.*, 1990). $CD8^+$ CTL were also induced to CS peptide aa 371–390 of *P. falciparum*, which is identical to the target of CTL induced by immunization with sporozoites. More recently the *csp* gene of *P. falciparum* encoding amino acids 21–398 has been integrated into the chromosome of an *aroA aroD S. typhi* (Gonzalez *et al.*, 1994). In human trial, volunteers received two oral immunizations with attenuated *S. typhi* expressing the CSP. One volunteer developed anti-sporozoite antibodies, another developed antibodies to a peptide of the CS protein (containing residues 309–345) and the third developed a CSP-specific $CD8^+$ CTL response. This, as the authors point out, is probably the first report that demonstrates that an attenuated S. *typhi* expressing heterologous antigens is able to induce a humoral and CTL response to that antigen. However, since other studies using chromosomal integration have shown a reduced level of expression of the cloned antigen, a more consistent response may be induced using a plasmid expresion systems such as PurA$^+$, Thy$^+$, or Asd$^+$ vectors (discussed earlier) that do not require antibiotic markers.

Schistosomiasis is also a major problem in developing countries where human infection causes a chronic debilitating disease and infection of cattle can result in a considerable economic loss. The 28-kDa glutathione S-transferase (P28) from *Schistosoma mansoni* has been investigated for its potential in developing a vaccine against schistosomiasis. Genetic fusions of tetanus toxin fragment C and P28 (Khan *et al.*, 1994a) or a P28 peptide (aa 115–131) (Khan et al., 1994b) have been constructed and expressed in *aroA* S. *typhimurium*. Intravenous immunization with live *Salmonella* expressing the fusion proteins resulted in the induction of antibodies to both fragment C and P28 or P28 peptide. Antibody responses to the P28 peptide were greatly increased when the level of peptide produced was increased either by using a high copy number vector or by fusions using an eight-tandem repeat of the peptide. This eight-peptide repeat has also been expressed as a fusion with fragment C of TT (Chabalgoity *et al.*, 1995) in *aroA* S. *typhiuurium* under the control of the *nirB* promoter. Mice that had previously been immunized with TT were subsequently immunized intravenously with *Salmonella* expressing P28/fragment C and significant anti-fragment C titers were detected, as well as an enhanced response to the P28 peptide. This is an interesting observation, but it is important to note that the iv route of immunization was used and should be repeated using oral immunization with these recombinant *Salmonella*.

A number of antigens from other protozoan parasites have also been expressed in recombinant *Salmonella*, including the gp63 gene of *Leishmania major* (Yang *et al.*, 1990). CBA mice orally immunized with an *aroA* S. *typhimuirum* expressing gp63 developed both antibody and T cell proliferative responses to *L. major*. These activated T cells were mainly CD4$^+$ and secreted IL-2 and IFNγ but no IL-4. Mice also developed a significant level of protection against challenge with *L. major*. Another protozoan which causes debilitating disease in infected humans is the intestinal parasite *Entamoeba histolytica*. The serine-rich *E. histolytica* protein (SREHP) is a surface antigen recognized by sera from patients recovering from amoebiasis. SRHEP has been expressed as a fusion with MalE in a *Δcya Δcrp Δasd* S. *typhimurium* χ3987 (Cieslak *et al.*, 1993) and is currently being investigated for the induction of protective immunity against amoebiasis.

IV. Use of *Salmonella* for Expression of Novel Antigens

The mucosal immune network is distinct from the systemic component of the host's immune surveillance equipment and can be divided into separate and discrete sites: the inductive site where antigens are recognized and processed and the effector sites where differentiation and proliferation occur in response to an antigen (Kagnoff, 1993; McGhee *et al.*, 1989; McGhee and Kiyono, 1994; Mestecky *et al.*, 1988). Mucosal immune responses are characterized by the secretion of secretory IgA (S-IgA) from B cells at effector sites. Activated sIgA$^+$ B cells are driven to produce S-IgA by IL-5 and IL-6, cytokines preferentially secreted by Th2 cells which occur at a higher frequency at these sites. On the other hand, Th1 cells which produce IL-2, IFNγ and TNFβ are involved in cell-mediated immunity and these are preferentially located at inductive sites. It is with this in mind that a number of strategies have been developed that would optimize the response to antigens presented at mucosal surfaces by recombinant *Salmonella*.

One such strategy is the coexpression of adjuvants such as LT-B (discussed earlier); the other is the expression of cytokines by recombinant *Salmonella*. It has now become apparent that the involvement of cytokines at the mucosal surface is an important function of the host reaction to an invading pathogen. One of the first cytokines to be expressed in a S. *typhimurium* background was human IL-1ß as a model system for therapeutic administration of IL-1 (Carrier *et al.*, 1992). Tocci and colleagues (1987) were the first to express fully active recombinant human IL-1β in *E. coli*. IL-1β is expressed as a soluble protein by S. *typhimurium* as in eukaryotic cells, a key consideration when utilizing this system. Mice immunized with S. *typhimurium* expressing IL-1β were significantly protected against 825 rad of γ-irradiation 10 days after immunization, whereas control mice that received PBS died 12 days postirradiation. Carrier *et al.* (1992) calculated that the dose of recombinant *Salmonella* expressed approximately as 75 ng of IL-1β, a dose which in itself is not capable of protection against radiation-induced mortality. In another study, Denich and colleagues (1993) used a S. *typhimurium aroA* strain to express murine IL-4 using a high-level expression vector, pOmpAmIL-4. *Salmonella* expressing IL-4 were able to colonize mice to a greater degree than the parent strain and were more able to withstand macrophage killing. This would seem to indicate that the expression of IL-4 by *Salmonella* confers an advantage with respect to survival. IL-5 and IL-6 have been successfully expressed in a recombinant vaccinia virus and recombinant fowlpox virus in conjunction with the HA glycoprotein of influenza virus (Ramsay *et al.*, 1994).

Intranasal immunization of mice with these vectors resulted in elevated IgA titers in the lungs that were four times higher than those elicited with control viruses.

Another novel approach for the use of recombinant *Salmonella* is the development of contraceptive vaccines. Several gamete-specific antigens, such as the sperm antigens SP10 (Herr *et al.*, 1990) and lactate dehydrogenase LDH-C4 (Goldberg, 1977) and the oocyte antigen ZP3 (Ringuette *et al.*, 1988), are currently being investigated for their expression in recombinant *Salmonella*. In particular SP10 can be expressed at a high level by *Δcya Δcrp Δasd S. typhimurium* and significant antibody titers can be detected in the serum and vaginal secretions of BALB/c mice after a single oral immunization (Srinivasan *et al.*, 1995). The 15-aa peptide of ZP3 that encodes the T- and B-cell epitope (Rhim *et al.*, 1992) has been expressed as a fusion protein with LT-B in recombinant *Salmonella*. (T. A. Doggett 1996, unpublished data). This 14-kDa fusion protein remains within the cytoplasm of the host *Salmonella* and reacts with both anti-porcine LT antisera and the anti-ZP3 monoclonal IE-10 (East *et al.*, 1985). Mice immunized either perorally or intravaginally with a *Δcya Δcrp Δasd S. typhimurium* expressing the ZP3/LT-B fusion resulted in detectable anti-LT-B S-IgA and IgG titers in vaginal secretions (T. A. Doggett 1996, unpublished data). The presence of IgG anti-LT-B antibodies in vaginal wash samples may be a result of sequestering from the blood (Tjokronegro and Sirisinha, 1975), although no serum titers were detected.

V. Concluding Remarks

The use of recombinant *Salmonella* for the expression of heterologous antigens and the development of vaccines offers many exciting possibilities. It has, however, been demonstrated that there are many pitfalls to the expression of such antigens, such as stability of recombinant plasmids, level of antigen expression and correct presentation of the expressed antigen to the immune system. Earlier concerns were voiced about the placement of antigens expressed by recombinant *Salmonella*, in regard to whether antigens would be recognized and processed more efficiently if expressed within the periplasmic or cytoplasmic compartments or on the surface of the bacteria or even secreted. Researchers have used various methods to investigate these questions and in many instances have obtained contradicting results. In the end, it may come down to finding the correct method for the optimum presentation for each antigen, whether it be intracellular or extracellullar. One of the more intriguing directions in recombinant vaccine development is the coexpression of antigen and a specific cytokine to enhance or direct specific types of immune responses. It will be interesting to see which data become available concerning the coexpression of cytokines that are important in the modulation and control of mucosal immune responses in particular; we believe that this is probably one of the major directions of future research.

Acknowledgments

We thank M. Wilmes-Riesenberg, B. Morrow, J. Srinivasan, and A. Honeyman for their critical review of the manuscript. Research conducted by T.D. is supported by Grant CSA-94-129 from the contraceptive Research and Development Program, the Eastern Virginia Medical School (DPE-3044-19-00-2015-00), and a grant from Bristol-Myers Squibb.

References

Adhya, S. (1987). The galactose operon. *In* "*Escherichia coli* and *Salmonella typhimurium*: Cellular and Molecular Biology" (F. C. Neidhardt, ed.), Vol. 2, pp. 1503–1512. American Society for Microbiology, Washington, D.C.

Aggarwal, A., Kumar, S., Jaffe, R., Hone, D., Gross, M., and Sadoff, J. (1990). Oral *Salmonella*: Malaria circumsporozoite recombinants induce specific $CD8^+$ cytotoxic T cells. *J. Exp. Med.* **172,** 1083–1090.

Alderton, M. R., Fahey, K. J., and Coloe, P. J. (1991). Humoral responses and salmonellosis protection in chickens given a vitamin-dependent *Salmonella typhimurium* mutant. *Avian Dis.* **35,** 435–442.

Baron, L. S., Kopecko, D. J., Formal, S. B., Seid, R., Guerry, P., and Powell, C. (1987). Introduction of *Shigella flexneri* 2a type and group antigen genes into oral typhoid vaccine strain *Salmonella typhi* Ty21a. *Infect. Immun.* **55,** 2797–2801.

Barrow, P. A. (1990). Immunity to experimental fowl typhoid in chickens induced by a virulence plasmid-cured derivative of *Salmonella gallinarum*. *Infect. Immun.* **58,** 2283–2288.

Benjamin, W. H., Jr., Turnbough, C. L., Jr., Posey, B. S., and Briles, D. E. (1985). The ability of *Salmonella typhimurium* to produce the siderophore enterobactin is not a virulence factor in mouse typhoid. *Infect. Immun.* **50,** 392–397.

Bollen, W. S., Burns-Keliher, L., and Curtiss III, R. (1995). Molecular analysis of the *cdt* gene in *Salmonella typhimurium* UK-1. B299, p. 217. American Society for Microbiology, Washington, D.C.

Brennan, F. R., Oliver, J. J., and Baird, G. D. (1994). Differences in the immune responses of mice and sheep to an aromatic-dependent mutant of *Salmonella typhimurium*. *J. Med. Microbiol.* **41,** 20–28.

Brett, S. J., Rhodes, J., Liew, F. Y., and Tite, J. P. (1993). Comparison of antigen presentation of influenza A nucleoprotein expressed in attenuated AroA-*Salmonella ty-*

phimurium with that of live virus. *J. Immunol.* **150,** 2869–2884.

Brown, A., Hormeache, C. E., Demarco de Hormeache, R., Winther, M., Dougan, G., Maskell, D. J., and Stocker, B. A. D. (1987). An attenuated *aroA Salmonella typhimurium* vaccine strain elicits humoral and cellular immunity to cloned β-galactosidase in mice. *J. Infect. Dis.* **155,** 86–92.

Cárdenas, L., and Clements, J. D. (1993). Stability, immunogenicity and expression of foreign antigens in bacterial vaccine vectors. *Vaccine* **11,** 126–135.

Carrier, M. J., Chatfield, S. N., Dougan, G., Nowicka, U. T., O'Callaghan, D., Beesley, J. E., Milano, S., Cillari, E., and Liew, F. Y. (1992). Expression of human IL-1 beta in *Salmonella typhimurium.* A model system for the delivery of recombinant therapeutic proteins *in vivo. J. Immunol.* **148,** 1176–1181.

Chabalgoity, J. A., Villareal-Ramos, B., Khan, A. C. M., Chatfield, S. N., DeMarco de Hormaeche, R., and Hormaeche, C. E. (1995). Influence of preimmunization with tetanus toxoid on immune responses to tetanus toxin fragment C-guest antigen fusions in a *Salmonella* vaccine carrier. *Infect. Immun.* **63,** 2564–2569.

Charbit, A., Martineau, P., Ronco, J., Leclerc, C., Lo-Man, R., Michel, V., O'Callaghan, D., and Hofnung, M. (1993). Expression and immunogenicity of the V3 loop from the envelope of human immunodeficiency virus type 1 in an attenuated *aroA* strain of *Salmonella typhimurium* upon genetic coupling to two *Escherichia coli* carrier proteins. *Vaccine* **11,** 1221–1228.

Chatfield, S. N., Charles, I. G., Makoff, A. J., Oxer, M. D., Dougan, G., Pickard, D., Slater, D., and Fairweather, N. F. (1992a). Use of the *nirB* promoter to direct the stable expression of heterologus antigens in *Salmonella* oral vaccine strains: Development of a single-dose oral tetanus vaccine. *Bio/Technology* **10,** 888–892.

Chatfield, S. N., Fairweather, N., Charles, I., Pickard, D., Levine, M., Hone, D., Posada, M., Strugnell, R. A., and Dougan, G. (1992b). Construction of a genetically defined *Salmonella typhi* Ty2 *aroA, aroC* mutant for the engineering of a candidate oral typhoid-tetanus vaccine. *Vaccine* **10,** 53–60.

Chatfield, S. N., Strahan, K., Pickard, D., Charles, I.G., Hormaeche, C.E. and Dougan, G. (1992c). Evaluation of *Salmonella typhimurium* strains harbouring defined mutations in *htrA* and *aroA* in the murine salmonellosis model. *Microbial Pathogen.* **12,** 145–151.

Childress, A. M., and Clements, J. D. (1988). Construction of a chimeric plasmid expressing glycoprotien B (gB) of herpes simples virus type 1 and heat-labile enterotoxin (LT-B) of *Escherichia coli.* S-6, p. 316. American Society for Microbiology, Washington, D.C.

Cieslak, P. R., Zhang, T., and Stanley, S., Jr. (1993). Expression of a recombinant *Entamoeba histolytica* antigen in a *Salmonella typhimurium* vaccine strain. *Vaccine* **11,** 773–776.

Clements, J. D., and Cardenas, L. (1990). Vaccines against enterotoxigenic bacterial pathogens based on hybrid *Salmonella* that express heterologous antigens. *Res. Microbiol.* **141,** 981–993.

Clements, J. D., and El-Morshidy, S. (1984). Construction of a potential live oral bivalent vaccine for typhoid fever and cholera-*Escherichia coli*-related diarrheas. *Infect. Immun.* **46,** 564–569.

Clements, J. D., Lyon, F. L., Lowe, K. L., Farrand, A. L., and El-Morshidy, S. (1986). Oral immunization of mice with attenuated *Salmonella enteriditis* containing a recombinant plasmid which codes for production of the B subunit of heat-labile *Escherichia coli* enterotoxin. *Infect. Immun.* **53,** 685–692.

Coe, N. E., and Wood, R. L. (1992). The effect of exposure to a Δ*cya* Δ*crp* mutant of *Salmonella typhimurium* on the subsequent colonization of swine by the wild-type parent strain. *Vet. Microbiol.* **31,** 207–220.

Cohen, S., Powell, C. J., Dubois, D. R., Hartman, A., Summers, P. L., and Eckels, K. H. (1990). Expression of the envelope antigen of dengue virus in vaccine strains of *Salmonella. Res. Microbiol.* **141,** 855–858.

Cooper, G. L., Venables, L. M., Nicholas, R. A., Cullen, G. A., and Hormaeche, C. E. (1992). Vaccination of chickens with chicken-derived *Salmonella enteritidis* phage type 4 *aroA* live oral *Salmonella* vaccines. *Vaccine* **10,** 247–254.

Cooper, G. L., Venables, L. M., Woodward, M. J., and Hormaeche, C. E. (1994). Vaccination of chickens with strain CVL30, a genetically defined *Salmonella enteritidis aroA* live oral vaccine candidate. *Infect. Immun.* **62,** 4747–4754.

Curtiss III, R., and Kelly, S. M. (1987). *Salmonella typhimurium* deletion mutants lacking adenylate cyclase and cyclic AMP receptor protein are avirulent and immunogenic. *Infect. Immun.* **55,** 3035–3043.

Curtiss, R., Goldschmidt, R. M., Fletchall, N. B., and Kelly, S. M. (1988). Avirulent *Salmonella typhimurium* Δ*cya* Δ*crp* oral vaccine strains expressing a streptococcal colonization and virulence antigen. *Vaccine* **6,** 155–160.

Denich, K., Borlin, P., O'Hanley, P. D., Howard, M., and Heath, A. W. (1993). Expression of the murine interleukin-4 gene in an attenuated *aroA* strain of *Salmonella typhimurium*: Persistence and immune response in BALB/c mice and susceptibility to macrophage killing. *Infect. Immun.* **61,** 4818–4827.

Doggett, T. A., Jagusztyn-Krynicka, E. K., and Curtiss III, R. (1993). Immune responses to *Streptococcus sobrinus* surface protein antigen A expressed by recombinant *Salmonella typhimurium. Infect. Immun.* **61,** 1859–1866.

Dougan, G., Sellwood, R., Maskell, D., Sweney, K., Liew, F. Y., Beesley, J., and Hormaeche, C. E. (1986). *In vivo* properties of a cloned K88 adherence antigen determinant. *Infect. Immun.* **52,** 344–347.

Dusek, D. M., Progulske-Fox, A., Whitlock, J., and Brown, T. A. (1993). Isolation and characterization of a cloned *Porphyromonas gingivalis* hemagglutinin from an avirulent strain of *Salmonella typhimurium. Infect. Immun.* **61,** 940–946.

East, I. J., Gulyas, B. J., and Dean, J. (1985). Monoclonal antibodies to the murine zona pellucida protein with sperm receptor activity: Effects on fertilization and early development. *Dev. Biol.* **109,** 268–273.

Edelman, R., and Levine, M. M. (1986). Summary of an international workshop on typhoid fever. *Rev. Infect. Dis.* **8**, 329–349.

Elkins, C., Carbonetti, N. H., Coimbre, A. J., Thomas, C. E., and Sparling, P. F. (1994). Cloning and constitutive expression of structural genes encoding gonococcal porin protein in *Escherichia coli* and attenuated *Salmonella typhimurium* vaccine strains. *Gene* **138**, 43–50.

Elson, C. O., and Ealding, W. (1985). Genetic control of the murine immune response to cholera toxin. *J. Immunol.* **135**, 930–932.

Ervin, S. E., Small, P., Jr., and Gulig, P. A. (1993). Use of incompatible plasmids to control expression of antigen by *Salmonella typhimurium* and analysis of immunogenicity in mice. *Microbial Pathogen.* **15**, 93–101.

Fairweather, N. F., Chatfield, S. N., Makoff, A. J., Strugnell, R. A., Bester, J., Maskell, D. J., and Dougan, G. (1990). Oral vaccination of mice against tetanus by use of a live attenuated *Salmonella* carrier. *Infect. Immun.* **58**, 1323–1326.

Fields, P., Groisman, E., and Heffron, F. (1989). A *Salmonella* locus that controls resistance to microbicidal proteins from phagocytic cells. *Science* **243**, 1059–1062.

Fierer, J., Chikami, L., Hatlen, E., Heffernan, E. J., and Guiney, D. (1988). Active immunization with LD842, a plasmid-cured strain of *S. dublin*, protects mice against group D and group B *Salmonella* infection. *J. Infect. Dis.* **158**, 460–463.

Formal, S. B., Baron, L. S., Kopecko, D. J., Washington, O., Powell, C., and Life, C. A. (1981). Construction of a potential bivalent vaccine strain: Introduction of *Shigella sonnei* form 1 antigen genes into the *galE Salmonella typhi* Ty21a typhoid vaccine strain. *Infect. Immun.* **34**, 746–750.

Forrest, B. D., and LaBrooy, J. T. (1991). *In vivo* evidence of immunological masking of the *Vibrio cholerae* O antigen of a hybrid *Salmonella typhi* Ty21a-*Vibrio cholerae* oral vaccine in humans [published erratum appears in *Vaccine* 1991 Dec.; 9(12):915]. *Vaccine* **9**, 515–520.

Fulginiti, J., Brey, R., and Anilionis, A. (1992). *purA* complementation as a means to deliver foreign antigens in vaccine strains of *Salmonella*. E-24, p. 48. American Society for Microbiology, New Orleans.

Galan, G., and Curtiss III, R. (1989). Virulence and vaccine potential of *phoP* mutants of *Salmonella typhimurium*. *Microbial Pathogen.* **6**, 433–443.

Germanier, R., and Furer, E. (1971). Immunity in experimental Salmonellosis. II. Basis for the virulence and protective capacity of *galE* mutants of *Salmonella typhimurium*. *Infect. Immun.* **4**, 663–673.

Germanier, R., and Furer, E. (1975). Isolation and characterization of *galE* mutant Ty21a of *Salmonella typhi*: A candidate strain for a live, oral typhoid vaccine. *J. Infect. Dis.* **131**, 553–558.

Goldberg, E. (1977). Isozymes in tests and spermatozoa. *In* "Isozymes: Current Topics in Biological and Medical Research" (M. C. Ratazzi, J. G. Scandalios, and G. S. Whitt, eds.), Vol. 1, pp. 79–84. Alan R. Liss, New York.

Goldschmidt, R. M., and Curtiss III, R. (1990). Cross-reactivity between the immunodominant determinant of the antigen I component of the *Streptococcus sobrinus* SpaA protein and surface antigens of other members of the *Streptococcus mutans* group. *Infect. Immun.* **58**, 2276–2282.

Gonzalez, C., Hone, D., Noriega, F. R., Tacket, C. O., Davis, J. R., Losonsky, G., Nataro, J. P., Hoffman, S., Malik, A., Nardin, E., Sztein, M. B., Heppner, D. G., Fouts, T. R., Isibasi, A., and Levine, M. M. (1994). *Salmonella typhi* vaccine strain CVD 908 expressing the circumsporozoite protein of *Plasmodium falciparum*: Strain construction and safety and immunogenicity in humans. *J. Infect. Dis.* **169**, 927–931.

Gulig, P. A. (1990). Virulence plasmids of *Salmonella typhimurium* and other Salmonellae. *Microbial Pathogen.* **8**, 3–11.

Hassan, J. O., Porter, S. B., and Curtiss III, R. (1993). Effect of infective dose on humoral immune responses and colonization in chickens experimentally infected with *Salmonella typhimurium*. *Avian Dis.* **37**, 19–26.

Hassan, J. O., and Curtiss III, R. (1994a). Development and evaluation of an experimental vaccination program using a live avirulent *Salmonella typhimurium* strain to protect immunized chickens against challenge with homologous and heterologous *Salmonella* serotypes. *Infect. Immun.* **62**, 5519–5527.

Hassan, J. O., and Curtiss III, R. (1994b). Virulent *Salmonella typhimurium*-induced lymphocyte depletion and immunosuppression in chickens. *Infect. Immun.* **62**, 2027–2036.

Hayes, L. J., Conlan, J. W., Everson, J. S., Ward, M. E., and Clarke, I. N. (1991). *Chlamydia trachomatis* major outer membrane protein epitopes expressed as fusions with LamB in an attenuated *aroA* strain of *Salmonella typhimurium;* their application as potential immunogens. *J. Gen. Microbiol.* **137**, 1557–1564.

Herr, J. C., Flickinger, C. J., Homyk, M., Klotz, K., and John, E. (1990). Biochemical and morphological characterization of the intra-acrosomal antigen SP-10 from human sperm. *Biol. Reprod.* **42**, 181–185.

Hofnung, M., Bedoulle, H., Boulain, J.-C., Clément, J.-M., Charbit, A., and Duplay, P. (1988). Genetic approaches to the study and the use proteins: Random point mutations and random linker insertions. *Bull. Inst. Pasteur* **86**, 95–101.

Hoiseth, S. K., and Stocker, B. A. D. (1981). Aromatic-dependent *Salmonella typhimurium* are nonvirulent and effective as live vaccines. *Nature (London)* **291**, 238–239.

Hone, D. M., Attridge, S. R., Forrest, B., Morona, R., Daniels, D., LaBrooy, J. T., Bartholomeusz, R. C. A., Shearman, D. J. C., and Hackett, J. (1988). A *galE* via (Vi antigen-negative) mutant of *Salmonella typhi* Ty2 retains virulence in humans. *Infect. Immun.* **56**, 1326–1333.

Hone, D., Attridge, S., van den Bosch, L., and Hackett, J. (1989). A chromosomal intergration system for stabilization of heterologous genes in *Salmonella* based vaccine strains. *Microbial Pathogen.* **156**, 167–174.

Hone, D. M., Harris, A. M., Chatfield, S., Dougan, G., and Levine, M. M. (1991). Construction of genetically defined double *aro* mutants of *Salmonella typhi*. *Vaccine* **9**, 810–816.

Hone, D. M., Lewis, G. K., Beier, M., Harris, A., McDaniels, T., and Fouts, T. R. (1994). Expression of human immunodeficiency virus antigens in an attenuated *Salmonella typhi* vector vaccine. (Review). *Dev. Biol. Standard.* **82,** 159–162.

Jagusztyn-Krynicka, E. K., Clark-Curtiss, J. E., and Curtiss III, R. (1993). *Escherichia coli* heat-labile toxin subunit B fusions with *Streptococcus sobrinus* antigens expressed by *Salmonella typhimurium* oral vaccine strains: Importance of the linker for antigenicity and biological activities of the hybrid proteins. *Infect. Immun.* **61,** 1004–1015.

Javaherian, K., Langlois, A. J., McDanal, C., Ross, K. L., Eckler, L. I., and Jellis, C. L. (1989). Principal neutralizing domain of the human immunodeficiency virus type 1 envelope protein. *Proc. Natl. Acad. Sci. U.S.A.* **86,** 6768–6773.

Jones, P. W., Dougan, G., Hayward, C., MacKenzie, N., Collins, P., and Chatfield, S. N. (1991). Oral vaccination of calves against experimental salmonellosis using a double *aro* mutant of *Salmonella typhimurium. Vaccine* **9,** 29–34.

Kagnoff, M. F. (1993). Immunology of the intestinal tract. (Review). *Gastroenterology* **105,** 1275–1280.

Kelly, S. M., Bosecker, B. A., and Curtiss III, R. (1992). Characterization and protective properties of attenuated mutants of *Salmonella choleraesuis. Infect. Immun.* **60,** 4881–4890.

Khan, C. M. A., Villareal-Ramos, B., Pierce, R. J., Riveau, G., Demarco de Hormaeches, R., McNeill, H., Ali, T., Fairweather, N., Chatfield, S., Capron, A., Dougan, G., and Hormaeche, C. E. (1994a). Construction, expression and immunogenicity of the *Schistosoma mansoni* P28 glutathione S-transferase as a genetic fusion to tetanus toxin fragment C an a live *Aro* attenuated vaccine strain of *Salmonella. Proc. Natl. Acad. Sci. U.S.A.* **91,** 11261–11265.

Khan, C. M. A., Villareal-Ramos, B., Pierce, R. J., Riveau, G., Demarco de Hormaeches, R., McNeill, H., Ali, T., Fairweather, N., Chatfield, S., Capron, A., Dougan, G., and Hormaeche, C. E. (1994b). Construction, expression and immunogenicity of multiple tandem copies of the *Schistosoma mansoni* peptides 115–131 of the P28 glutathione S-transferase expressed as C-terminal fusions to tetanus toxin fragment C in a live *Aro*-attenuated vaccine strain of *Salmonella. J. Immunol.* **153,** 5634–5642.

Kimura, A., Mountzouros, K. T., Relman, D. A., Falkow, S., and Cowell, J. L. (1990). *Bordatella pertussis* filamentous hemagglutinin: Evaluation as a protective antigen and colonization factor in a mouse respiratory infection model. *Infect. Immun.* **58,** 7–16.

Levine, M. M., Black, R. E., Ferreccio, C., and Germanier, R. (1987). Chilean Typhoid Committee. Large-scale field trial of Ty21a live oral typhoid vaccine in enteric-coated capsule formulation. *Lancet* **2,** 1049–1052.

McGhee, J. R., Mestecky, J., Elson, C. O., and Kiyono, H. (1989). Regulation of IgA synthesis and immune response by T cells and interleukins. *J. Clin. Immunol.* **9,** 175–199.

McGhee, J. R., and Kiyono, H. (1994). Effective mucosal immunity. Current concepts for vaccine delivery and immune response analysis. (Review). *Int. J. Tech. Assess. Health Care* **10,** 93–106.

McEwen, J., Levi, R., Horwitz, R. J., and Arnon, R. (1992). Synthetic recombinant vaccine expressing influenza haemagglutinin epitope in *Salmonella* flagellin leads to partial protection in mice. *Vaccine* **10,** 405–411.

Maskell, D., Sweeney, K., O'Callaghan, D., Hormeache, C. E., Liwe, F. Y., and Dougan, G. (1987). *Salmonella typhimurium aroA* mutants as carriers of the *Escherichia coli* heat-labile enterotoxin B subunit to the murine secretory and systemic immune systems. *Microbial Pathogen.* **2,** 211–221.

Mestecky, J., McGhee, J. R., and Elson, C. O. (1988). Intestinal IgA system. *Immunol. Allergy Clinics N. Am.* **8,** 349–368.

Miller, I. A., Chatfield, S., Dougan, G., DeSilva, L., Joysey, H., and Hormaeche, C. H. (1989). Bacteriophage P22 as a vehicle for transducing gene banks between smooth strains of *Salmonella typhimurium:* Use in identifying a role for *aroD* in attenuating virulent *Salmonella* strains. *Mol. Gen. Genet.* **215,** 312–316.

Miller, S. I., Kukrak, A. M., and Mekalanos, J. J. (1989). A two-component regulatory system (*phoP phoQ*) controls *Salmonella typhimurium* virulence. *Proc. Natl. Acad. Sci. U.S.A.* **86,** 5054–5058.

Miller, S. I., Loomis, W. P., Alpuche-Aranda, C., Behlau, I., and Hohmann, E. (1993). The *PhoP* virulence regulon and live oral *Salmonella* vaccines. *Vaccine* **11,** 122–125.

Molina, N. C., and Parker, C. D. (1990). Murine antibody response to oral infection with live *aroA* recombinant *Salmonella dublin* vaccine strains expressing filamentous haemagglutinin antigen from *Bordatella pertussis. Infect. Immun.* **58,** 2523–2528.

Morona, R., Yeadon, J., Considine, A., Morona, J. K., and Manning, P. A. (1991). Construction of plasmid vectors with a non-antibiotic selection system based on the *Escherichia coli thyA*+ gene: Application to cholera vaccine development. *Gene* **107,** 139–144.

Morona, R., Morona, J. K., Considine, A., Hackett, J. A., van den Bosch, L., Beyer, L., and Attridge, S. R. (1994). Construction of K88- and K99-expressing clones of *Salmonella typhimurium* G30: Immunogenicity following oral administration to pigs. *Vaccine* **12,** 513–517.

Mukkur, T. K., Stocker, B. A., and Walker, K. H. (1991). Genetic manipulation of *Salmonella* serotype *Bovismorbificans* to aromatic-dependence and evaluation of its vaccine potential in mice. *J. Med. Microbiol.* **34,** 57–62.

Murphy, J. R., Grez, L., Schlesinger, L., Ferreccio, C., Baqar, S., Munoz, C., Wasserman, S. S., Losonsky, G., Olson, J. G., and Levine, M. M. (1991). Immunogenicity of *Salmonella typhi* Ty21a vaccine for young children. *Infect. Immun.* **59,** 4291–4293.

Nagi, L. K., Walker, P. D., Bhogal, B. S., and MacKenzie, T. (1978). Evaluation of *Escherichia coli* vaccines against experimental colibacillus. *Res. Vet. Sci.* **24,** 39–45.

Nakamura, M., Sato, S., Ohya, T., Suzuki, S., Ikeda, S., and Koeda, T. (1985). Plasmid-cured *Salmonella enteritidis* AL1192 as a candidate for live vaccines. *Infect. Immun.* **50,** 586–587.

Nakayama, K., Kelly, S. M., and Curtiss III, R. (1988). Construction of an Asd^{+} expression-cloning vector: stable maintenance and high level expression of cloned genes in a *Salmonella* vaccine strain. *Bio/Technology* **6**, 693–697.

Newton, S. M., Jacob, C. O., and Stocker, B. A. D. (1989). Immune response to cholera toxin epitope inserted in *Salmonella* flagellin. *Science* **244**, 70–72.

Nnalue, N. A., and Stocker, B. A. D. (1987). Tests of the virulence and live-vaccine efficacy of auxotrophic and *galE* derivatives of *Salmonella cholerasuis. Infect. Immun.* **55**, 955–962.

O'Callaghan, D., Maskell, D., Liew, F. Y., Easman, C. S. F., and Dougan, G. (1988). Characteriation of aromatic- and purine-dependent *Salmonella typhimurium:* Attenuation, persistence and ability to induce protective immunity in BALB/c mice. *Infect. Immun.* **56**, 419–423.

Oyston, P. C. F., Williamson, E. D., Leary, S. E. C., Eley, S. M., Griffin, K. F., and Titball, R. W. (1995). Immunization with live recombinant *Salmonella typhimurium aroA* producing F1 antigen protects against plague. *Infect. Immun.* **63**, 563–568.

Pittard, A. J. (1987). Biosynthesis of the aromatic amino acids. *In* "*Escherichia coli* and *Salmonella typhimurium*: Cellular and Molecular Biology" (F. C. Neidhardt, ed.), Vol. 1, pp. 368–394. American Society for Microbiology, Washington, D.C.

Ramsay, A. J., Leong, K.-H., Boyle, D., Ruby, J., and Ramshaw, I. A. (1994). Enhancement of mucosal IgA responses by interleukins 5 and 6 encoded in recombinant vaccine vectors. *Reprod. Fertil. Dev.* **6**, 389–392.

Redman, T. K., Harmon, C. C., and Michalek, S. M. (1994). Oral immunization with recombinant *Salmonella typhimurium* expressing surface protein antigen A of *Streptococcus sobrinus:* Persistence and induction of humoral responses in rats. *Infect. Immun.* **62**, 3162–3171.

Rhim, S. H., Millar, S. E., Robey, F., Luo, A.-M., Lou, Y.-H., Yule, T., Allen, P., Dean, J., and Tung, K. S. K. (1992). Autoimmune disease of the ovary induced by a ZP3 peptide from the mouse zona pellucida. *J. Clin. Invest.* **89**, 28–35.

Ringuette, M. J., Chamberlain, M. E., Baur, A. W., Sobieski, D. A., and Dean, J. (1988). Molecular analysis of cDNA coding fro ZP3, a sperm binding protein of the mouse zona pellucida. *Dev. Biol.* **127**, 287–293.

Sadoff, J. C., Ripley Ballou, W., Baron, L. S., Majarian, W. R., Brey, R. N., Hockmeyer, W. T., Young, J. F., Cryz, S. J., Ou, J., Lowell, G. H., and Chulay, J. D. (1988). Oral *Salmonella typhimurium* vaccine expressing circumsporozoite protein protects against malaria. *Science* **242**, 336–338.

Schödel, F., Milich, D. R., and Will, H. (1990). Hepatitis B viruls nucleocapsid/pre-S2 fusion proteins expressed in attenuated *Salmonella* for oral vaccination. *J. Immunol.* **145**, 4317–4321.

Schödel, F., Will, H., Johansson, S., Sanchez, J., and Holmgren, J. (1991). Synthesis in *Vibrio cholerae* and secretion of hepatitis B virus antigens fused to *Escherichia coli* heat-labile enterotoxin subunit B. *Gene* **99**, 255–259.

Schödel, F., Moriarty, A. M., Peterson, D. L., Zheng, J., Hughes, J. L., H., W., Leturcq, D. J., McGhee, J. R., and Milich, D. R. (1992). The position of heterologous epitopes inserted in hepatitis B virus core particles determines their immunogenicity. *J. Virol.* **66**, 106–112.

Schödel, F., Kelly, S. M., Peterson, D. L., Milich, D. R., and Curtiss III, R. (1994). Hybrid hepatitis B virus core-pre-S proteins synthesized in avirulent *Salmonella typhimurium* and *Salmonella typhi* for oral vaccination. *Infect. Immun.* **62**, 1669–1676.

Schofield, L., Villaquiran, R., Ferreira, A., Schellekens, H., Nussenzweig, R. S., and Nussenzweig, V. (1987). Interferon, $CD8^+$ T cells and antibodies are required for immunity to malaria sporozoites. *Nature (London)* **330**, 664–665.

Schorr, J., Knapp, B., Hundt, E., Kupper, H. A., and Amann, E. (1991). Surface expression of malarial antigens in *Salmonella typhimurium-* induction of serum antibody-response upon oral vaccination of mice. *Vaccine* **9**, 675.

Sjöstedt, A., Sandström, G., and Tärnvik, A. (1992). Humoral and cell-mediated immunity in mice to a 17-kilodalton lipoprotein of *Francisella tularensis* expressed by *Salmonella typhimurium. Infect. Immun.* **60**, 2855–2862.

Slauch, J. M., Mahan, M. J., and Mekalanos, J. J. (1994). *In vivo* expression technology for selection of bacterial genes specifically induced in host tissues. (Review). *In* "Methods in Enzymology" (V. L. Clark and P. M. Bavoil, eds.), Vol. 235, pp. 481–492. Academic Press, San Diego.

Smith, B. P., Dilling, G. W., Da Roden, L., and Stocker, B. A. (1993). Vaccination of calves with orally administered aromatic-dependent *Salmonella dublin. Am. J. Vet. Res.* **54**, 1249–1255.

Srinivasan, J., Tinge, S., Wright, R., Herr, J. C., and Curtiss III, R. (1995). Oral immunization with attenuated *Salmonella* expressing human sperm antigen induces antibodies in serum and the reproductive tract. *Biol. Reprod.* **53**, 462–471.

Stabel, T. J., Mayfield, J. E., Tabatabai, L. B., and Wannemeuhler, M. J. (1990). Oral immunization of mice with attenuated *Salmonella typhimurium* containing a recombinant plasmid which codes for production of a 31-kilodalton protein of *Brucella abortus. Infect. Immun.* **58**, 2048–2055.

Stabel, T. J., Mayfield, J. E., Morfitt, D. C., and Wannemuehler, M. J. (1993). Oral immunization of mice and swine with an attenuated *Salmonella choleraesuis* [Δ*cya*-12 Δ(*crp-cdt*)19] mutant containing a recombinant plasmid. *Infect. Immun.* **61**, 610–618.

Stevenson, G., and Manning, P. (1985). Galactose epimeraseless (*galE*) mutant G30 of *Salmonella typhimurium* is a good potential carrier of fimbrial antigens. *FEMS Microbiol. Lett.* **28**, 317–321.

Stocker, B. A., and Newton, S. M. (1994). Immune responses to epitopes inserted in *Salmonella* flagellin. (Review). *Int. Rev. Immunol.* **11**, 167–178.

Su, G. F., Brahmbhatt, H. N., L. V., Wehland, J., and Timmis, K. N. (1992a). Extracellular export of Shiga toxin B-subunit/haemolysin A (C-terminus) fusion protein expressed in *Salmonella typhimurium aroA*-mutant and stimulation of B-subunit specific antibody responses in mice. *Microbial Pathogen.* **13**, 465–476.

Su, G. F., Brahmbhatt, H. N., Wehland, J., Rohde, M., and Timmis, K. N. (1992b). Construction of stable LamB-

Shiga toxin B subunit hybrids: Analysis of expression in *Salmonella typhimurium aroA* strains and stimulation of B subunit-specific mucosal and serum antibody responses. *Infect. Immun.* **60,** 3345–3359.

Tacket, C. O., Hone, D. M., Curtiss III, R., Kelly, S. M., Losonsky, G., Guers, L., Harris, A. M., Edelman, R., and Levine, M. M. (1992). Comparison of the safety and immunogenicity of Δ*aroC* Δ*aroD* and Δ*cya* Δ*crp Salmonella typhi* strains in adult volunteers. *Infect. Immun.* **60,** 536–541.

Takahashi, H., Merli, S., Putney, S. D., Houghteen, R., Moss, B., Germain, R. N., and Berzofsky, J. A. (1989). A single amino acid interchange yields reciprocal CTL specificity for HIV-1 gp 160. *Science* **246,** 118–121.

Tijhaar, E. J., Zheng-Xin, Y., Karlas, J. A., Meyer, T. F., Stukart, M. J., Osterhaus, A. D., and Mooi, F. R. (1994). Construction and evaluation of an expression vector allowing the stable expression of foreign antigens in a *Salmonella typhimurium* vaccine strain. *Vaccine* **12,** 1004–1011.

Tite, J. P., Hughes-Jenkins, C. M., O'Callaghan, D., Dougan, D., Russel, S. M., Gao, X.-M., and Liew, F. Y. (1990a). Anti-viral immunity induced by recombinant influenza A virus: II. Protection from influenza infections and mechanism of protection. *Immunology* **71,** 202–207.

Tite, J. P., Gao, X.-M., Hughes-Jenkins, C. M., Lipscombe, M., O'Callaghan, D., Dougan, G., and Liew, F. Y. (1990b). Anti-viral immunity induced by recombinant nucleoprotein of influenza A virus. III. Delivery of recombinant nucleoprotein to the immune system using attenuated *Salmonella typhimurium* as a live carrier. *Immunology* **70,** 540–546.

Tjokronegro, A., and Sirisinha, S. (1975). Quantitative analysis of immunoglobulins and albumin in secretions of female reproductive tract. *Fertil. Steril.* **26,** 413–417.

Tocci, M. J., Hutchinson, N. I., Cameron, P. M., Kirk, D. E., Norman, D. J., Chin, J., Rupp, E. A., Limjuco, G. A., Boniila-Argudo, V. M., and Schmidt, J. A. (1987). Expression in *Escherichia coli* of fully active recombinant IL-1β: Comparison with native IL-1β. *J. Immunol.* **138,** 1109–1115.

Van de Verg, L., Herrington, D. A., Murphy, J. R., Wasserman, S. S., Formal, S. B., and Levine, M. M. (1990). Specific immunoglobulin A-secreting cells in peripheral blood of humans following oral immunization with a bivalent *Salmonella typhi–Shigella sonnei* vaccine or infection by pathogenic *S. sonnei. Infect. Immun.* **58,** 2002–2004.

Wahdan, M. H., Serie, C., Cerisier, Y., Sallam, S., and Germanier, R. (1982). A controlled field trial of live *Salmonella typhi* strain Ty21a oral vaccine against typhoid: Three-year results. *J. Infect. Dis.* **145,** 292–295.

Walker, M. J., Rohde, M., Timmis, K. N., and Guzman, C. A. (1992). Specific lung mucosal and systemic immune responses after oral immunization of mice with *Salmonella typhimurium aroA, Salmonella typhi* Ty21a, and invasive *Escherichia coli* expressing recombinant pertussis toxin S1 subunit. *Infect. Immun.* **60,** 4260–4268.

Weiss, W. R., Sedegah, M., Beaudoin, R. L., Miller, L. H., and Good, M. F. (1988). $CD8^+$ T cells (cytotoxic/suppressor) are required for protection in mice immunized with malaria sporozoites. *Proc. Natl. Acad. Sci. U.S.A.* **85,** 573–577.

Wick, M. J., Harding, C. V., Normark, S. J., and Pfeifer, J. D. (1994). Parameters that influence the efficiency of processing antigenic epitopes expressed in *Salmonella typhimurium. Infect. Immun.* **62,** 4542–4548.

Yang, D. M., Fairweather, N., Button, L. L., McMaster, W. R., Kahl, L. P., and Liew, F. Y. (1990). Oral *Salmonella typhimurium* (AroA-) vaccine expressing a major leishmanial surface protein (gp63) preferentially induces T helper 1 cells and protective immunity against leishmaniasis. *J. Immunol.* **145,** 2281–2285.

8

Prospects for Induction of Mucosal Immunity by DNA Vaccines

JEFFREY B. ULMER
JOHN J. DONNELLY
JOHN W. SHIVER
MARGARET A. LIU
Department of Virus and Cell Biology
Merck Research Laboratories
West Point, Pennsylvania 19486

I. Introduction

The expression of heterologous proteins *in vivo* can be achieved by several means, including the administration of recombinant or attenuated pathogens, replicating DNA vectors, mRNA, and nonreplicating plasmid DNA (for review see Donnelly *et al.*, 1995a). The application of this concept to induce immune responses for the purposes of vaccination, in the form of attenuated live viruses, has been used successfully for many years (e.g., vaccinia virus for smallpox). The advantages of expressing antigens in the host rather than administering antigens such as inactivated viruses, recombinant proteins, or peptides include: (i) circumventing potential loss of antigenicity by the inactivation process (e.g., chemical cross-linking), (ii) synthesis of proteins with conformation and post-translational modification similar or identical to native antigens, (iii) intracellular antigen-processing and presentation by MHC class I molecules leading to the induction of cytotoxic T lymphocyte (CTL) responses, and (iv) allowing for MHC determinant selection.

The most recent approach to applying protein expression systems to vaccines is nonreplicating plasmid DNA vectors. This technique was inspired by observations that administration of plasmid DNA could result in expression of the encoded gene *in situ,* such as the use of calcium phosphate-precipitated DNA (Benvenisty and Reshef, 1986), expression of reporter genes in myocytes after intramuscular (i.m.) injection of "naked" DNA (i.e., plasmid DNA in saline) (Wolff *et al.*, 1990), and transfection of dermal and epidermal cells of the skin by particle bombardment of DNA-coated gold particles (Williams *et al.*, 1991) (see also Figs. 1 and 2). Subsequently, administration of DNA *in vivo* was demonstrated to induce antibody responses against human growth hormone (Tang *et al.*, 1992) and cell-mediated immunity (CMI) leading to cross-strain protection against influenza (Ulmer *et al.*, 1993). Shortly thereafter, antibody responses and/or protection were shown to be induced by DNA vaccines against several viral antigens (Wang *et al.*, 1993; Robinson *et al.*, 1993; Cox *et al.*, 1993; Davis *et al.*, 1993; Montgomery *et al.*, 1993; Xiang *et al.*, 1994; Sedegah *et al.*, 1994). These observations have spawned a new approach to vaccinology, with an accumulation of preclinical efficacy data that suggests potential utility in humans.

In this chapter, the types of immune responses induced by DNA vaccines and data concerning the basic mechanisms involved (e.g., DNA uptake, protein expression, and antigen presentation) will be presented. In addition, the prospects of this technology for mucosal immunity will be discussed.

II. Immune Responses Induced by DNA Vaccines

A. Humoral Immune Responses

DNA vaccines have been shown to induce high-titer serum antibodies to a variety of different antigens, including viral, bacterial, eukaryotic, and tumor-associated proteins. For example, DNA constructs encoding viral proteins such as influenza hemagglutinin (HA) (Ulmer *et al.*, 1994; Fynan *et al.*, 1993; Donnelly *et al.*, 1995b), HIV envelope protein (Wang *et al.*, 1993, Shiver *et al.*, 1995), bovine herpesvirus glycoproteins (Cox *et*

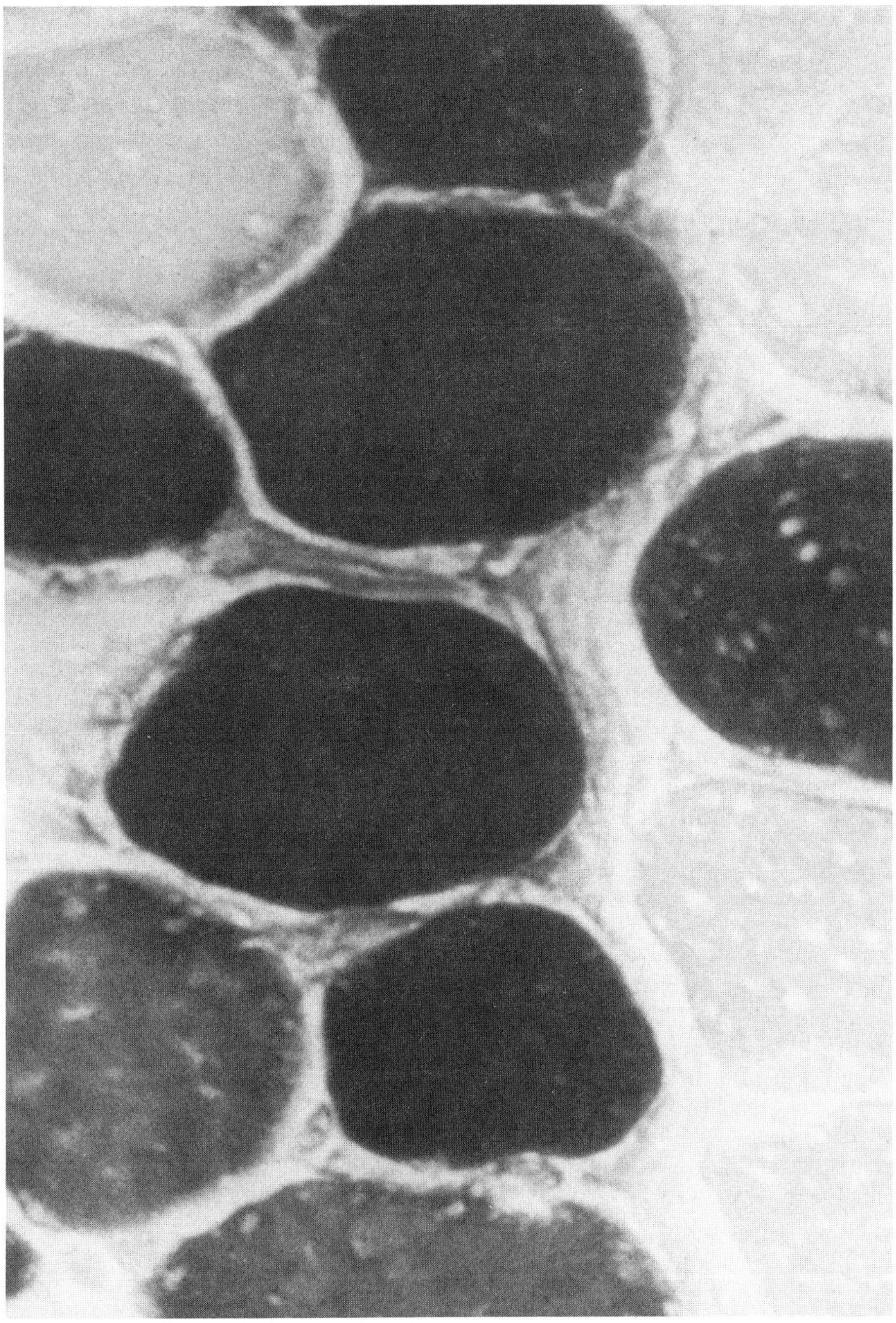

Figure 1. Expression of a reporter protein in myocytes after i.m. injection of DNA. Mice were injected into the tibialis anterior muscle with DNA encoding β-galactosidase and necropsied for protein expression in tissue sections. Expression is seen in several myocytes in this cross-section (micrograph courtesy of Dr. H. Davis, Loeb Medical Research Institute, Ottawa).

al., 1993), rabies virus glycoprotein (Xiang *et al.*, 1994), hepatitis B surface antigen (Davis *et al.*, 1993), and papillomavirus capsid protein (Donnelly *et al.*, 1996) have generated humoral immune responses in mice, rabbits, ferrets, or monkeys. Antibodies against antigens from other types of pathogens such as malaria circumsporozoite protein (Sedegah *et al.*, 1994) and *Mycobacterium tuberculosis* antigen 85 (Ulmer *et al.*, 1996a) have also been generated after DNA injection. In addition, genes encoding eukaryotic proteins, such as human growth hormone (Tang *et al.*, 1992), idiotypic immunoglobulins (Hawkins *et al.*, 1993), and carcinoembryonic antigen (Conry *et al.*, 1994) have been used in DNA vaccines to induce antibodies. All these proteins contain signal sequences that allow them to be transported to the cell surface via the secretory pathway, whereupon they are

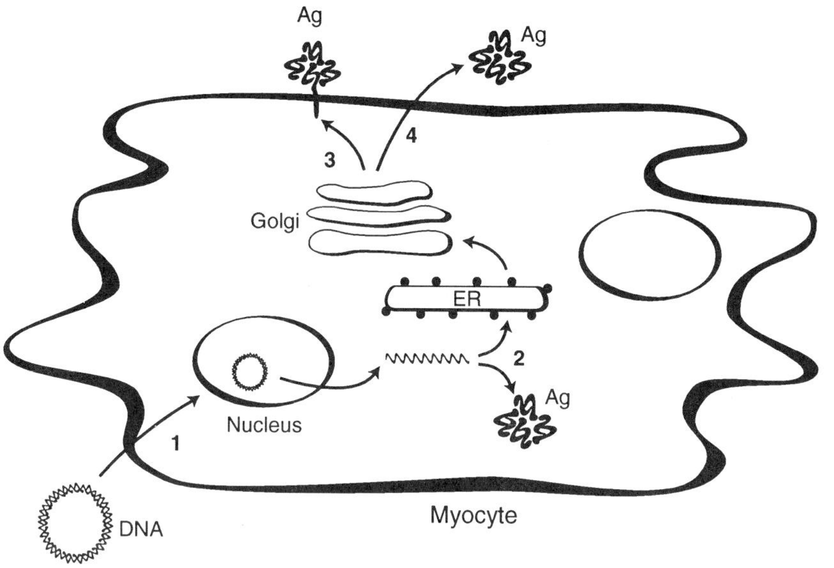

Figure 2. Expression of antigens in muscle cells after DNA vaccination. Intramuscular injection of plasmid DNA results in the deposition of DNA in the extracellular spaces of the muscle. Uptake by muscle cells is mediated by a poorly defined mechanism that may involve endocytosis and subsequent delivery to the cytoplasm and nucleus (step 1). Thereafter, the DNA is thought to be maintained as a nonreplicating, extrachromosomal plasmid (Wolff *et al.*, 1992; Nichols *et al.*, 1995). Transfection of muscle cells *in vivo* after injection of DNA has been achieved for various types of proteins, including cytoplasmic (step 2), membrane (step 3), and secreted (step 4) proteins.

accessible for induction of B-cell responses. However, other proteins not destined for secretion, such as influenza nucleoprotein (NP), can also induce humoral immune responses (Ulmer *et al.*, 1993; Yankauckas *et al.*, 1993). The generation of neutralizing or protective antibodies most likely requires the presence of conformational antigenic epitopes. In the case of influenza HA, this would require trimerization in the endoplasmic reticulum for efficient folding and intracellular transport of HA to the cell surface (Wiley *et al.*, 1977). The hypothesis that DNA vaccines induce relevant humoral immune responses is supported by the following observations: (i) transfection of cells with influenza HA DNA *in vitro* resulted in cell surface expression of HA capable of binding red blood cells (D. L. Montgomery, A. Friedman, J. J. Donnelly, and M. A. Liu, 1995, unpublished observations), (ii) virus-neutralizing antibodies against HIV envelope protein (Wang *et al.*, 1993) and hemagglutination-inhibiting antibodies against influenza HA (see Fig. 3) (Ulmer *et al.*, 1994; Donnelly *et al.*, 1995b) have been detected, and (iii) protective efficacy based on humoral immunity can be generated (Cox *et al.*, 1993; Ulmer *et al.*, 1994).

The duration of humoral immune responses after DNA vaccination has been shown to be long-term in some species. Antibodies have persisted in mice for up to 6 months to 2 years after injection of influenza NP (Yankauckas *et al.*, 1993), influenza HA (Deck *et al.*, 1996), hepatitis B surface antigen (Michel *et al.*, 1995), HIV gp120 (Shiver *et al.*, 1995), and papillomavirus L1 capsid protein (Donnelly *et al.*, 1996c) DNA. In nonhuman primates, anti-HA antibodies were detected for at least 18 weeks after DNA injection, with peak titer and duration equivalent to or better than those induced by conventional inactivated virus vaccines (Donnelly *et*

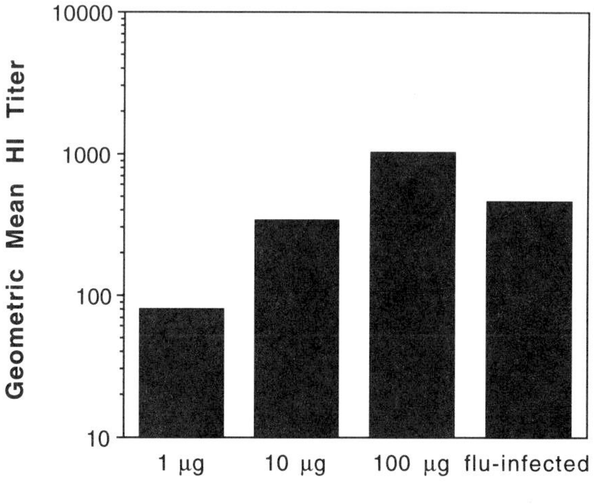

Figure 3. Hemagglutination inhibiting (HI) antibody titers in HA DNA-vaccinated mice. BALB/c mice were injected with HA DNA at doses of 1, 10, and 100 µg three times at 3-week intervals. Serum samples were collected 9 weeks after the first inoculation and tested for HI antibodies. Data are represented as geometric mean reciprocal HI titer, where $n = 15$. As a positive control, HI titers were determined for convalescent immune mice infected with influenza virus (A/PR/8/34). Reprinted from Ulmer *et al.*, *Vaccine* **12,** 1541–1544, 1994, with kind permission from Butterworth-Heinemann journals (Elsevier Science Ltd., The Boulevard, Langford Lane, Kidlington OX5 1GB, UK).

al., 1995b). The immunoglobulin isotype profile induced by NP and HA DNA in mice was predominantly IgG2a with lesser amounts of IgG2b and IgG1 and very little IgG3 (Ulmer *et al.*, 1994). In addition to IgG, IgM and IgA antibodies against HA were detected in sera (Deck *et al.*, 1996).

Certain types of DNA expression vectors (e.g., *Vaccinia*) can induce humoral immune responses against the vaccine vector itself, which can limit the effectiveness of subsequent vaccinations with that vector (Cooney *et al.*, 1991). Naked DNA is not considered to be immunogenic in this respect. Anti-DNA antibodies are not readily elicited unless DNA is denatured, complexed with a protein carrier, and coinjected with an adjuvant (Gilkeson *et al.*, 1993). Injection of plasmid DNA expression vectors in mice and nonhuman primates has not induced detectable anti-DNA antibodies (Jiao *et al.*, 1992; Xiang *et al.*, 1994; J. B. Ulmer, C. M. DeWitt, and M. A. Liu, 1995, unpublished observations).

B. Cell-Mediated Immune Responses

Expression of proteins in some host cells allows for antigen processing and presentation by MHC class I molecules, and leads to the generation of CTL. This is in contrast to inactivated virus vaccines, which in general are not processed in this way and, therefore, primarily elicit antibody responses. The ability of DNA vaccines to induce CTL responses was first demonstrated using influenza NP (Ulmer *et al.*, 1993) (see also Fig. 4). This antigen is a conserved, internal protein of the virus and a target for cross-reactive CTL (Wraith *et al.*, 1987). The NP DNA induced CTL in mice, as demonstrated using both concanavalin A/IL-2-activated and antigen-restimulated spleen cells. Furthermore, mice were protected from a cross-strain, lethal challenge with influenza virus (Ulmer *et al.*, 1993, 1994). Cell-mediated immunity induced by DNA encoding influenza NP or matrix protein likely also played a role in protection of ferrets, as measured by reductions in virus shedding in nasal secretions (Donnelly *et al.*, 1995a). DNA-induced CTL have now been demonstrated for rabies virus glycoprotein (Xiang *et al.*, 1994), malaria circumsporozoite protein (Sedegah *et al.*, 1994), lymphocytic choriomeningitis virus NP (Pedroz Martins *et al.*, 1995; Yokoyama *et al.*, 1995; Zarozinski *et al.*, 1995), HIV envelope protein (Wang *et al.*, 1994; Shiver *et al.*, 1995), human factor IX (Katsumi *et al.*, 1994), and MHC class I (Geissler *et al.*, 1994, Plautz *et al.*, 1994; Hui *et al.*, 1994). In some cases, CTL responses have been detected for 1–2 years after immunization (Yankauckas *et al.*, 1993; Raz *et al.*, 1994; Ulmer *et al.*, 1996b).

DNA vaccines also induced strong lymphoproliferative responses against rabies virus glycoprotein (Xiang *et al.*, 1994), HIV envelope protein (Wang *et al.*, 1993; Shiver *et al.*, 1995), carcinoembryonic antigen (Conry *et al.*, 1994), human T-cell lymphotrophic virus envelope protein (Agadjanyan *et al.*, 1994), *M. tuberculosis* antigen 85 (Ulmer *et al.*, 1996a), and influenza NP and HA (J. B. Ulmer, R. R. Deck, and M. A. Liu, 1995, unpublished observations). When measured, the cytokine profile secreted from antigen-restimulated spleen cells was predominated by IL-2 and interferon-γ (Xiang *et al.*, 1994; Xu and Liew, 1994; Shiver *et al.*, 1995; Ulmer *et al.*, 1996; J. B. Ulmer, R. R. Deck, and M. A. Liu, 1995, unpublished observations), which is indicative of a Th1-like helper T-cell response.

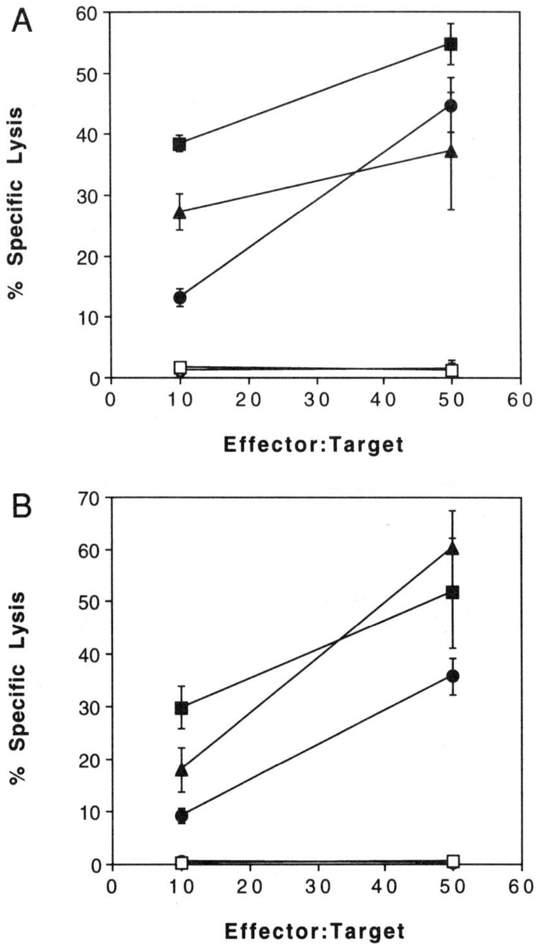

Figure 4. Cytotoxic T-lymphocytes in NP DNA-vaccinated mice. BALB/c mice were injected with NP DNA at doses of 1, 10, and 100 μg (solid triangles, squares, and circles, respectively) three times at 3-week intervals. As negative controls, mice injected with blank vector without gene insert (open circles) at 100 μg or uninjected mice (open squares) were also tested. Spleens were taken 17 weeks after the first inoculation. P815 target cells were either infected with influenza virus (A/Victoria/73) (A) or pulsed with NP peptide (B). Data are represented as percentage specific lysis versus effort:target ratios, where *n* = 3. Reprinted from *Ulmer et al.*, *Vaccine* **12**, 1541–1544, 1994, with kind permission from Butterworth-Heinemann journals (Elsevier Science Ltd., The Boulevard, Langford Lane, Kidlington OX5 1GB, UK).

The mechanisms by which CTL are induced after i.m. DNA vaccination are not yet known. Myocytes are transfected after i.m. injection but their role in the induction of CMI, if any, has not been elucidated. Figure 5 illustrates some possible means of inducing CTL after DNA vaccination. Injected plasmid DNA may transfect antigen presenting cells (APCs) that are resident in the muscle at the time of injection, have infiltrated the muscle after injection, or are at distant sites to which DNA has been carried by the circulation or lymphatics (Fig. 5B). However, PCR analysis of tissues after DNA injection has not detected plasmid DNA anywhere outside of the injected muscle, including regional lymph nodes (Nichols *et al.*, 1995). Furthermore, transplantation of NP-expressing myoblasts into naive syngeneic mice resulted in the generation of CTL and protective immunity, suggesting that transfection of APCs may not be necessary for the induction of CTL after DNA injection (Ulmer *et al.*, 1996c). Hence, antigen expression in myocytes after i.m. injection of DNA may lead to the generation of CTL. This could be a result of antigen presentation by myocytes themselves (Fig. 5A) or transfer of antigen from myocytes to APCs (Fig. 5C). The low-level expression of MHC class I and the lack of detectable levels of costimulatory molecules, such as B7, by muscle cells suggests that they may not be capable of functioning as APCs. However, the recent discovery of IL-15 and its high levels of expression in skeletal muscle cells (Grabstein *et al.*, 1994) suggests that muscle cells may not be as immunologically inert as once thought. The best explanation for antigen presentation after DNA vaccination may involve transfer of antigen from transfected muscle cells to professional APCs, since tumor antigens are thought to be transfered from

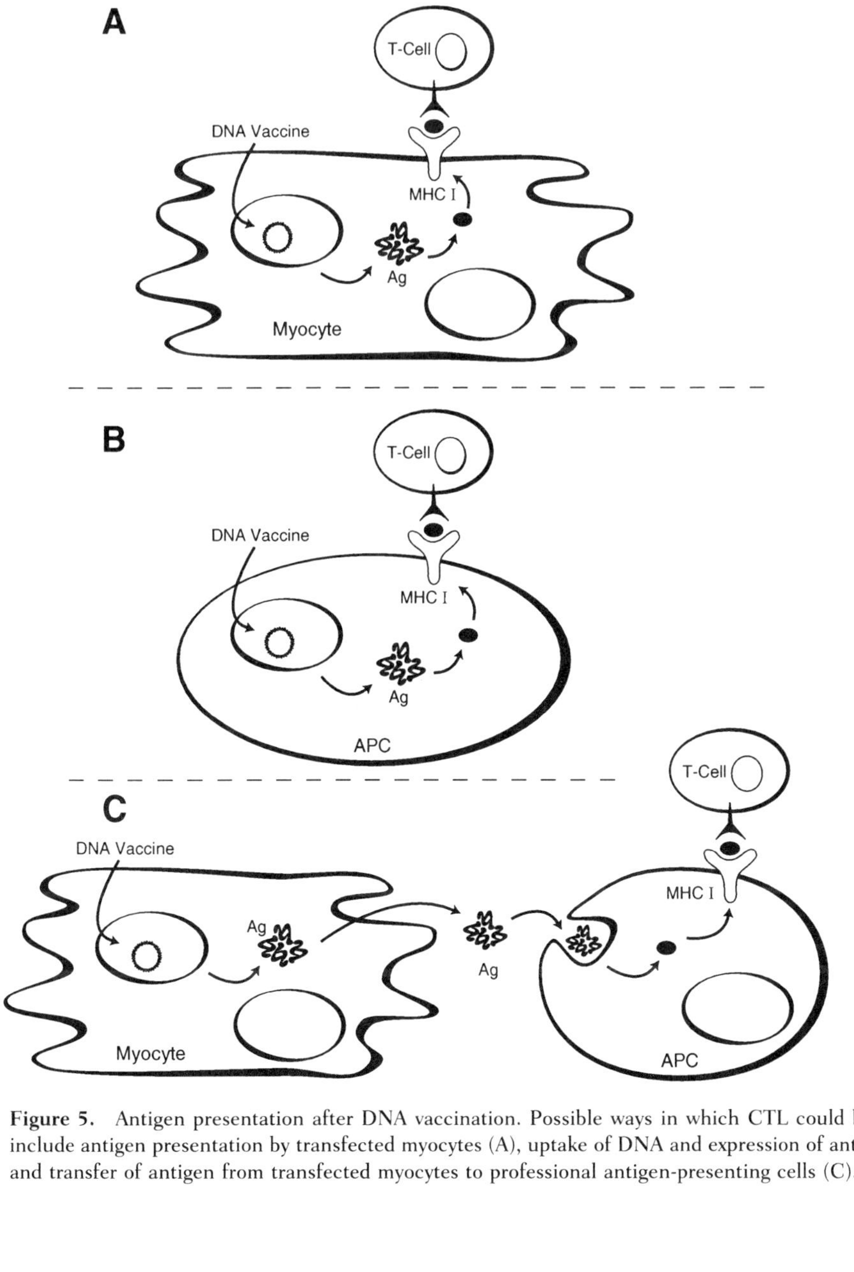

Figure 5. Antigen presentation after DNA vaccination. Possible ways in which CTL could be induced after i.m. injection of DNA vaccines include antigen presentation by transfected myocytes (A), uptake of DNA and expression of antigen by professional antigen-presenting cells (B), and transfer of antigen from transfected myocytes to professional antigen-presenting cells (C).

tumor cells in this way (Huang *et al.*, 1994) and our data indicate that NP CTL can be induced after transfer of NP from tranfected myoblasts *in vivo* (Ulmer *et al.*, 1996c). Transfer of antigen from myocytes to APCs could be mediated by secretion from transfected cells. In the case of influenza NP, high-titer antibodies were induced by DNA vaccination (Ulmer *et al.*, 1993; Yankauckas *et al.*, 1993), indicating that while NP does not have a signal sequence it was nevertheless secreted or excreted from transfected cells. However, the mere presence of extracellular NP in the muscle is not sufficient to induce CTL or protection, as demonstrated after i.m. injection of NP protein (Donnelly *et al.*, 1994). Therefore, DNA vaccination may stimulate the immune system to process exogenous antigen differently than after injection of protein. Certain types of bone marrow-derived APCs have the capability of presenting exogenous antigens in the context of MHC class I (Rock *et al.*, 1993). These cells have been implicated in the presentation of tumor-associated antigens in the induction of anti-tumor CTL (Huang *et al.*, 1994) and may play a role in the generation of DNA vaccine-induced CTL.

III. Antigen Expression at Mucosal Sites

The induction of mucosal immune responses by vaccination generally requires delivery of antigen to mucosal inductive sites, such as Peyer's patches of the gastrointestinal tract. This can be accomplished by complexing antigen to molecules that target such sites (e.g., cholera toxin or *Escherichia coli* heat-labile enterotoxin), by incorporating antigens into phagocytosable particles, or by recombinant organisms that can be administered to mucosal surfaces. In the latter case, the antigen of interest is expressed by the organism inside or in the vicinity of M cells present on the surface of Peyer's patches. For example, *Salmonella typhi* expresses adhesive proteins that targets it to M cells, and attenuated forms of this pathogen have been used as vaccines to express heterologous antigens and induce mucosal immune responses (for review see McGhee and Kiyono, 1993). Similarly, recombinant BCG-expressing antigens of *Borrelia burgdorferi* induced mucosal IgA antibodies when administered intranasally (Langermann *et al.*, 1994). Viral vectors, such as vaccinia, adenovirus, and herpes simplex virus, have also been studied as potential expression systems for the induction of mucosal immune responses (Gallichan *et al.*, 1993). The potential advantage of using live mucosal vaccines over other types is that, in some cases, colonization of the host can lead to persistent expression of antigen and, therefore, provide a longer antigen stimulus. In support of this hypothesis, prolonged exposure to antigen at mucosal surfaces resulted in more rapid and stronger immune responses compared to those after bolus administration (Bloom and Rowley, 1979). Some drawbacks of using recombinant organisms to achieve antigen expression *in vivo* are: (i) the need for potentially complex genetic engineering to attenuate the pathogen and construct the vaccine, (ii) limitations in the size of the gene insert, (iii) risk of reversion to virulence, and (iv) induction of immune responses against the vector itself, which could limit the utility of subsequent immunizations.

IV. Delivery of DNA to Mucosal Sites

The success and general applicability of using plasmid DNA expression vectors to transfect cells *in vivo* leading to the induction of humoral and cell-mediated immune responses suggest that this approach may also be appropriate for generating mucosal immunity. One report has demonstrated that intranasal administration of DNA-encoding influenza HA resulted in protection from virus challenge (Fynan *et al.*, 1993). However, the utility of naked DNA for mucosal vaccination may be limited by the lability of DNA in tissue fluids. The *in vivo* half-life of injected plasmid DNA is minutes (Lew *et al.*, 1995; Kawabata *et al.*, 1995). Therefore, it is likely that a barrier must be placed between DNA vaccines and extracellular digestive enzymes if effective mucosal delivery is to be achieved. In addition, it is not known whether or not plasmid DNA would effectively target epithelial cells lining mucosal surfaces. While i.m. injection of naked DNA results in uptake by myocytes, transfection of epithelial cells may not occur efficiently. However, successful transfection of airway epithelial cells has been detected after aerosol delivery of DNA/cationic lipid complexes (Stribling *et al.*, 1992; Canonico *et al.*, 1994). The formulation consisted of a cationic lipid (e.g., DOTMA) and a neutral lipid (DOPE). Using the same DNA/cationic lipid formulation, several other types of cells including lung, spleen, lymph nodes, and lymphocytes were transfected after subcutaneous (s.c.) and intraperitoneal (i.p.) injection (Zhu *et al.*, 1993; Philip *et al.*, 1993). In addition, cells of the stomach, colon, liver, and pancreas were transfected using DNA/cationic lipids (Schmid *et al.*, 1994). These results suggest that cationic lipids facilitated DNA uptake via a nonspecific mechanism or a physiologic pathway present on various cell types. In either case, mucosal delivery of DNA in this way can potentially transfect many cell types. In addition to potential facilitation of cellular uptake, cationic lipids may also protect DNA from degradation. For example, *in vitro* studies have shown that DNA/cationic lipids have longer half-lives than DNA alone (Puyal *et al.*, 1995). This approach of formulating DNA with cationic lipids is presently being tested for gene therapy. The cystic fibrosis transmembrane conductance regulator (CFTR) gene has been delivered to epithelial cells by intranasal administration in rats (Logan *et al.*, 1995) and human clinical trials are underway (Caplen *et al.*, 1995). Because of the successful transfection of mucosal surfaces by DNA-encoding reporter genes and CFTR formulated with cationic lipids, this technique holds promise as a means of delivering genes encoding antigens to the mucosa for potential induction of immune responses.

Parenteral administration of DNA vaccines induces strong systemic humoral and cell-mediated immune responses but has not resulted in the generation of detectable mucosal immune responses. For certain mucosal pathogens, such as influenza virus, transudation of serum antibodies occurs via discontinuities of the epithelial barrier as a consequence of infection, and can provide some protection from disease in the absence of preexisting mucosal immunity. However, local mucosal immunity against influenza virus can also be protective and is mediated by IgA (Renegar and Small, 1991a,b). Therefore, in certain instances, it may be desirable to design a vaccine that could induce both mucosal and systemic immune responses. In theory, this could be achieved by DNA vaccines. Because different types of cells may be transfected by mucosal administration of DNA/cationic lipids (or other delivery system), both local and systemic immune responses may be induced. In support of this possibility is the observation that a recombinant BCG induced local IgA and serum IgG antibodies against a heterologous antigen (Langermann *et al.*, 1994) and a recombinant *Salmonella* vector given orally induced cell-mediated immunity (Aggarwal *et al.*, 1990). Alternatively, a combination of parenteral and mucosal delivery could elicit the spectrum of immune responses. This approach has been tested in several systems, using parenteral priming followed by mucosal boosting (Keren *et al.*, 1988) and vice versa (Forrest *et al.*, 1992).

V. Summary

Induction of mucosal immune responses by expression of antigens *in vivo* via attenuated and recombinant organisms has been demonstrated in a number of systems. Because of possible long-term expression of antigens after colonization by some organisms, this approach may induce stronger and longer-lived immune responses than do subunit or inactivated vaccines. Since DNA vaccines likewise have the potential for long-lived expression of antigens *in vivo,* it is possible that such mucosal responses could also be induced by mucosal delivery of plasmid DNA. The relative simplicity of DNA vaccines compared to recombinant organisms and the repeated use of DNA vaccines without generation of neutralizing immune responses against the vaccine vector itself make DNA vaccination an attractive prospect for inducing mucosal immunity.

References

Agadjanyan, M. G., Wang, B., Ugen, K. E., Villafana, T., Merva, M., Petrushina, I., Williams, W. V., and Weiner, D. B. (1994). DNA inoculation with an HTLV-1 envelope DNA construct elicits immune responses in rabbits. *In* "Vaccines 94" (F. Brown, R. M. Chanock, M. S. Ginsberg, and R. A. Lerner, eds.), pp. 47–53. Cold Spring Harbor Laboratory, Cold Spring Harbor, New York.

Aggarwal, A., Kumar, S., Jaffe, R., Hone, D., Gross, M., and Sadoff, J. (1990). Oral *Salmonella*: Malaria circumsporoxoite recombinants induce specific $CD8^+$ cytotoxic T cells. *J. Exp. Med.* **172,** 1083–1090.

Benvenisty, N., and Reshef, L. (1986). Direct introduction of genes into rats and expression of the genes. *Proc. Natl. Acad. Sci. U.S.A.* **83,** 9551–9555.

Bloom, L., and Rowley, D. (1979). Persistence in the mouse gut as an important factor in oral immunogenicity of strains of *V. cholerae. Aust. J. Exp. Biol. Med. Sci.* **57,** 313–323.

Canonico, A. E., Conary, J. T., Meyrick, B. O., and Brigham, K. L. (1994). Aerosol and intravenous transfection of human α1-antitrypsin gene to lungs of rabbits. *Am. J. Respir. Cell Mol. Biol.* **10,** 24–29.

Caplen, N. T., Alton, E. W. F. W., Middleton, P. G., Dorin, J. R., Stevenson, B. J., Gao, X., Durham, S. R., Jeffrey, P. K., Hodson, M. E., Coutelle, C., Huang, L., Porteus, D. J., Williamson, R., and Geddes, D. M. (1995). Liposome-mediated CFTR gene transfer to the nasal epithelium of patients with cystic fibrosis. *Nature Med.* **1,** 39–46.

Conry, R. M., LoBuglio, L. F., Kantor, J., Schlom, J., Loechel, F., Moore, S. E., Sumeral, L. A., Barlow, D. L., Abrams, S., and Curiel, D. T. (1994). Immune response to a carcinoembryonic antigen polynucleotide vaccine. *Cancer Res.* **54,** 1164–1168.

Cooney, E. L., Collier, A. C., Greenberg, P. D., Coombs, R. R. W., Zarling, J. C., Arditti, D. E., Hoffman, M. C., Hu, S. L., and Corey, L. (1991). Safety of and immunological response to a recombinant vaccinia virus vaccine expressing HIV envelope glycoprotein. *Lancet* **337,** 567–572.

Cox, G. J. M., Zamb, T. J., and Babiuk, L. A. (1993). Bovine Herpesvirus 1: Immune responses in mice and cattle injected with plasmid DNA. *J. Virol.* **67,** 5664–5668.

Davis, H. L., Michel, M.-L., and Whalen, R. G. (1993). DNA-based immunization induces continuous secretion of hepatitis B surface antigen and high levels of circulating antibody. *Hum. Mol. Genet.* **2,** 1847–1851.

Deck, R. R., DeWitt, C. M., Donnelly, J. J., Lui, M. A., and Ulmer, J. B. (1996). Characterization of humoral immune responses induced by an influenza DNA vaccine. *Vaccine,* in press.

Donnelly, J. J., Ulmer, J. B., and Liu, M. A. (1994). Immunization with DNA. *J. Immunol. Meth.* **176,** 145—152.

Donnelly, J. J., Ulmer, J. B., and Liu, M. A. (1995a). Recombinant vaccines: Technology and applications. *Exp. Opin. Ther. Patents* **5,** 211–217.

Donnelly, J. J., Friedman, A., Martinez, D., Montgomery, D. L., Shiver, J. W., Motzel. S., Ulmer, J. B., and Liu, M. A. (1995b). Efficacy of a prototype clinical DNA vaccine: Enhanced protection against antigenic drift in influenza virus. *Nature Med.* **1,** 583–587.

Donnelly, J. J., Martinez, D., Jansen, K., Montgomery, D., and Liu, M. A. (1996). Protection against papillomavirus with a polynucleotide vaccines. *J. Infect. Dis.* **713,** 314–320.

Forrest, B. D., Labrooy, J. T., Dearlove, C. E., and Sheearman, D. J. C. (1992). Effect of parenteral immunization on the intestinal immune response to *Salmonella typhi* Ty21a. *Infect. Immun.* **60,** 465–471.

Fynan, E. F., Webster, R. G., Fuller, D. H., Haynes, J. R., Santoro, J. C., and Robinson, H. L. (1993). DNA vaccines: Protective immunizations by parenteral, mucosal, and gene-gun inoculations. *Proc. Nat. Acad. Sci. U.S.A.* **90,** 11478–11482.

Gallichan, W.S., Johnson, D.C., Graham, F.L., and Rosenthal, K.L. (1993). Mucosal immunity and protection after intranasal immunization with recombinant adenovirus expressing Herpes simplex virus glycoprotein B. *J. Infect. Dis.* **168,** 622–629.

Geissler, E. K., Wang, J., Fechner, J. H., Burlingham, W. J., and Knechtle, S. J. (1993). Immunity to MHC Class I antigen following direct DNA transfer into skeletal muscle. *J. Immunol.* **152,** 413–421.

Gilkeson, G. S., Ruiz, P., Howell, D., Lefkowith, J. B., and Pisetsky, D. S. (1993). Induction of immune mediated glomerulonephritis in normal mice immunized with bacterial DNA. *Clin. Immunopathol.* **68,** 283–292.

Grabstein, K. H., Eisenman, J., Shanebeck, K., Rauch, C., Srinivasan, S., Fung, V., Beers, C., Richardson, J., Schoenborn, M. A., Ahdieh, M., Johnson, L., Alderson, M. R., Watson, J. D., Anderson, D. M., and Giri, J. G. (1994). Cloning of a T cell growth factor that interacts with the β chain of the interleukin-2 receptor. *Science* **264,** 961–965.

Hawkins, R. E., Winter, G., Hamblin, T. J., Stevenson, F. K., and Russell, S. J. (1993). A genetic approach to idiotypic vaccination. *J. Immunother.* **14,** 273–278.

Huang, A. Y. C., Golumbek, P., Ahmadzadeh, M., Jaffee, E., Pardoll, D., and Levitsky, H. (1994). Role of bone marrow-derived cells in presenting MHC class I-restricted tumor antigens. *Science* **264,** 961–965.

Hui, K. M., Sabapathy, T. K., Oei, A., and Chia, T. F. (1994). Generation of alloreactive cytotoxic T lymphocytes by particle bombardment-mediated gene transfer. *J. Immunol. Methods* **171,** 147–155.

Jiao, S., Williams, P., Berg, R. K., Hodgeman, B. A., Liu, L., Repetto, G., and Wolff, J. A. (1992). Direct gene transfer into nonhuman primate myofibers *in vivo*. *Hum. Gene Ther.* **3,** 21–33.

Katsumi, A., Emi, N., Abe, A., Hasegawa, Y., Ito, M., and Saito, H. (1994). Humoral and cellular immunity to an encoded protein induced by direct DNA injection. *Hum. Gene Ther.* **5,** 1335–1339.

Kawabata, K., Takakura, Y., and Hashida, M. (1995). The fate of plasmid DNA after intravenous injection in mice: Involvement of scavenger receptors in its hepatic uptake. *Pharm. Res.* **12,** 825–830.

Keren, D. F., McDonald, R. A., and Carey, J. L. (1988). Combined parenteral and oral immunization results in an enhanced mucosal immunoglobulin A response to *Shigella flexneri*. *Infect. Immun.* **56,** 910–915.

Langermann, S., Palaszynski, S., Sadziene, A., Stover, C. K., and Koenig, S. (1994). Systemic and mucosal immunity induced by BCG vector expressing outer-surface protein A of Borrelia burgdorferi. *Nature (London)* **372,** 552–555.

Lew, D., Parker, S. E., Latimer, T., Abai, A. M., Kuwahara-Rundell, A., Doh, S. G., Yang, Z.-Y., LaFace, D., Gromkowski, S. H., Nabel, G. J., Manthorpe, M., and Norman, J. (1995). Cancer gene therapy using plasmid DNA: Pharmacokinetic study of DNA following injection in mice. *Hum. Gene Ther.* **6,** 553–564.

Logan, J. J., Bebok, Z., Walker, L. C., Peng, S., Felgner, P. L., Siegal, G. P., Frizzell, R. A., Dong, J., Howard, M., Matalon, S., Lindsey, J. R., DuVall, M., and Sorscher, E. J. (1995). Cationic lipids for reporter gene and CFTR transfer to rat pulmonary epithelium. *Gene Ther.* **2,** 38–49.

McGhee, J. R., and Kiyono, H. (1993). New perspectives in vaccine development: Mucosal immunity to infections. *Infect. Agents Dis.* **2,** 55–73.

Michel, M.-L., Davis, H. L., Schleef, M., Mancini, M., Tiollais, P., and Whalen, R. G. (1995). DNA-mediated immunization to the hepatitis B surface antigen in mice: Aspects of the humoral response mimice hepatitis B viral infection in humans. *Proc. Natl. Acad. Sci. U.S.A.* **92,** 5307–5311.

Montgomery, D. L., Shiver, J. W., Leander, K. R., Perry, H. C., Friedman, A., Martinez, D., Ulmer, J. B., Donnelly, J. J., and Liu, M. A. (1993). Heterologous and homologous protection against influenza A by DNA vaccination: Optimization of vectors. *DNA Cell Biol.* **12,** 777–783.

Nichols, W. W., Manam, S., and Ledwith, B. (1995). Potential DNA vaccine integration into host cell genome. *Ann. N.Y. Acad. Sci.* **772,** 30–39.

Pedroz Martins, L., Lau, L. L., Asano, M. S., and Ahmed, R. (1995). DNA vaccination against persistent viral infection. *J. Virol.* **69,** 2574–2582.

Philip, R., Liggitt, D., Philip, M., Dazin, P., and Debs, R. (1993). *In vivo* gene delivery: Efficient transfection of T lymphocytes in adult mice. *J. Biol. Chem.* **268,** 16087–16090.

Plautz, G. E., Yang, Z.-Y., Wu, B.-Y., Gao, X., Huang, L., and Nabel, G. J. (1993). Immunotherapy of malignancy by *in vivo* gene transfer into tumors. *Proc. Natl. Acad. Sci. U.S.A.* **90,** 4645–4649.

Puyal, C., Milhaud, P., Bienvenue, A., and Philippot, J. R. (1995). A new cationic liposome encapsulating genetic material. A potential delivery system for polynucleotides. *Eur. J. Biochem.* **228,** 697–703.

Raz, E., Carson, D. A., Parker, S. E., Parr, T. B., Abai, A. M., Aichinger, G., Gromkowski, S. H., Singh, M., Lew, D., Yankauckas, M. E., Baird, S. M., and Rhodes, G. R. (1994). Intradermal gene immunization: The possible role of DNA uptake in the induction of cellular immunity to viruses. *Proc. Natl. Acad. Sci. U.S.A.* **91,** 9519–9523.

Renegar, K. B., and Small, P. A. (1991a). Passive transfer of local immunity to influenza virus infection by IgA antibody. *J. Immunol.* **146,** 1972–1978.

Renegar, K. B., and Small, P. A. (1991b). Immunoglobulin A mediation of murine nasal anti-influenza virus immunity. *J. Virol.* **65,** 2146–2148.

Robinson, H. L., Hunt, L. A., Webster, R. G. (1993). Protection against a lethal influenza virus challenge by immunization with a haemagglutinin-expressing plasmid DNA. *Vaccine* **11,** 957–960.

Rock, K. L., Rothstein, L., Gamble, S., and Fleischacker, C. (1993). Characterization of antigen-presenting cells that present exogenous antigens in association with class I MHC molecules. *J. Immunol.* **150,** 438–446.

Schmid, R. M., Weidenbach, H., Draenert, G. F., Lerch, M. M., Liptay, S., Schorr, J., Beckh, K. H., and Adler, G. (1994). Liposome mediated *in vivo* gene transfer into different tissues of the gastrointestinal tract. *Acta. Gastroenterol.* **32,** 665–670.

Sedegah, M., Hedstrom, R., Hobart, P., and Hoffman, S. L. (1994). Protection against malaria by immunization with circumsporozoite protein plasmid DNA. *Proc. Natl. Acad. Sci. U.S.A.* **91,** 9866–9870.

Shiver, J. W., Davies, M., Perry, H. C., and Liu, M. A. (1995). Cytotoxic T lymphocyte and helper T cell responses following HIV polynucleotide vaccination. *Ann. N.Y. Acad. Sci.* **772,** 198–211.

Stribling, R., Brunette, E., Liggitt, D., Gaensler, K., and Debs, R. (1992). Aerosol gene delivery *in vivo*. *Proc. Natl. Acad. Sci. U.S.A.* **89,** 11277–11281.

Tang, D. C., Devit, M., and Johnston, S. A. (1992). Genetic immunization is a simple method for eliciting an immune response. *Nature (London)* **356,** 152–154.

Ulmer, J. B., Donnelly, J. J., Parker, S. E., Rhodes, G. H., Felgner, P. L., Dwarki, V. J., Gromkowski, S. H., Deck, R. R., DeWitt, C. M., Friedman, A., Hawe, L. A., Leander, K. R., Martinez, D., Perry, H. C., Shiver, J. W., Montgomery, D. L., and Liu, M. A. (1993). Heterologous protection against influenza by injection of DNA encoding a viral protein. *Science* **259,** 1745–1749.

Ulmer, J. B., Deck, R. R., DeWitt, C. M., Friedman, A., Donnelly, J. J., and Liu, M. A. (1994). Protective immunity by intramuscular injection of low doses of influenza virus DNA vaccines. *Vaccine* **12,** 1541–1544.

Ulmer, J. B., Liu, M. A., Montgomery, D. L., Denis, O., Yawman, A. M., Drowart, A., Lozes, E., Vandenbussche, P., Van Vooren, J.-P., DeWitt, C. M., Deck, R. R., Content, J., and Huygen, K. (1996a). Immunogenicity and efficacy of a Tuberculosis DNA vaccine. *In* "Vaccines 96" (F. Brown, R. M. Chanock, M. S. Ginsberg, and R. A. Lerner, eds.), pp. 39–43. Cold Spring Harbor Laboratory, Cold Spring Harbor, New York.

Ulmer, J. B., Deck, R. R., Yawman, A., Friedman, A., DeWitt, C. M., Martinez, D., Montgomery, D. L., Donnelly, J. J., and Liu, M. A. (1996b). DNA vaccines for bacteria and viruses. *Adv. Exp. Med. Biol.* **397,** 49–53.

Ulmer, J. B., Deck, R. R., DeWitt, C. M., Donnelly, J. J., and Liu, M. A. (1996c). Generation of MHC class I-restricted cytotoxic T lymphocytes by expression of a viral protein in muscle cells: Antigen presentation by nonmuscle cells. *Immunol.* in press.

Wang, B., Ugen, K. E., Srikantan, V., Agadjanyan, M. G., Dang, K., Refaeli, Y., Sato, A. I., Boyer, J., Williams, W. V., and Weiner, D. B. (1993). Gene inoculation generates immune responses against human immunodeficiency virus type 1. *Proc. Natl. Acad. Sci. U.S.A.* **90,** 4156–4160.

Wang, B., Merva, M., Dang, K., Ugen, K. E., Boyer, J., Williams, W. V., and Weiner, D. B. (1994). DNA inoculation induces protective *in vivo* immune responses against cellular challenge with HIV-1 antigen-expressing cells. *AIDS Res. Hum. Retroviruses* **10,** S35-S41.

Wiley, D. C., Skehel, J. J., and Waterfield, M. D. (1977). Evidence from studies with a cross-linking reagent that the haemagglutinin of influenza virus is a trimer. *Virology* **79,** 446–448.

Williams, R. S., Johnston, S. A., Riedy, M., Devit, M. J., McElligott, S. G., and Sanford, J. C. (1991). Introduction of foreign genes into tissues of living mice by DNA-coated microprojectiles. *Proc. Natl. Acad. Sci. U.S.A.* **88,** 2726–2730.

Wolff, J. A., Malone, R. W., Williams, P., Chong, W., Acsadi, G., Jani, A., and Felgner, P.L. (1990). Direct gene transfer into mouse muscle *in vivo*. *Science* **247,** 1465–1468.

Wolff, J. A., Ludtke, J. J., Acsadi, G., Williams, P., and Jani, A. (1992). Long-term persistence of plasmid DNA and foreign gene expression in mouse muscle. *Hum. Mol. Gen.* **1,** 363–369.

Wraith, D. C., Vessey, A. E., and Askonas, B. A. (1987). Purified influenza virus nucleoprotein protects mice from lethal infection. *J. Gen. Virol.* **68,** 433–440.

Xiang, Z. Q., Spitalnik, S., Tran, M., Wunner, W. H., Cheng, J., and Ertl, H. C. J. (1994) Vaccination with a plasmid vector carrying the rabies virus glycoprotein gene induces protective immunity against rabies virus. *Virology* **199,** 132–140.

Xu, D., and Liew, F. Y. (1995). Protection against leishmaniasis by injection of DNA encoding a major surface glycoprotein, gp63, of *L. major*. *Immunology* **84,** 173–176.

Yankauckas, M. A., Morrow, J. E., Parker, S. E., Abai, A., Rhodes, G. H., Dwarki, V. J., and Gromkowski, S. H. (1993). Long-term anti-nucleoprotein cellular and humoral immunity is induced by intramuscular injection of plasmid DNA containing gene. *DNA Cell Biol.* **12,** 771–776.

Yokoyama, M., Zhang, J., and Whitton, J. L. (1995). DNA immunization confers protection against lethal lymphocytic choriomeningitis virus infection. *J. Virol.* **69,** 2684–2688.

Zarozinski, C. C., Fynan, E. F., Selin, L. K., Robinson, H. L., and Welsh, R. M. (1995). Protective CTL-dependent immunity and enhanced immunopathology in mice immunized by particle bombardment with DNA encoding an internal virion protein. *J. Immunol.* **154,** 4010–4017.

Zhu, N., Liggitt, D., Liu, Y., and Debs, R. (1993). Systemic gene expression after intravenous DNA delivery into adult mice. *Science* **261,** 209–211.

9

Recombinant BCG as Vector for Mucosal Immunity

Solomon Langermann
Department of Mucosal Immunity and Vaccines
MedImmune, Inc.
Gaithersburg, Maryland 20878

I. Introduction

The ultimate aim of any vaccine is the production of long-term protective immune responses against a pathogen. These responses include systemic humoral antibodies which neutralize invasive microorganisms and cytotoxic T cells which destroy intracellular pathogens (Hilleman, 1993). Since most bacteria and viruses initiate infections at mucosal surfaces where secretory IgA (S-IgA) antibodies are thought to play an important role in prevention of microbial attachment and colonization, there may be an added advantage for vaccines that stimulate long-lasting secretory immunity against pathogens (Brandtzaeg, 1989; Childers *et al.*, 1989; Holmgren *et al.*, 1992; Krahenbuhl and Neutra, 1992; McGhee *et al.*, 1992; McGhee and Kiyono, 1993) in addition to functional humoral antibodies. Whereas systemic, humoral, and cell-mediated immunity can be induced by parenteral immunization, a prerequisite for the generation of S-IgA antibodies is that antigens be delivered at mucosal sites (Mestecky, 1987; Brandtzaeg, 1992; Kiyono *et al.*, 1992). This requires the transport of antigen from the mucosal surface, across the epithelium into organized lymphoid tissue, where it can be taken up and processed by cells of the mucosal immune system.

Mucosal delivery of antigens is conducted by specialized cells called M (microfold) cells present in epithelium overlying lymphoid follicles present throughout mucosal surfaces in the colon, rectum, genitourinary tract, bronchial-associated lymphoid tissue (BALT), and nasopharyngeal-associated lymphoid tissue (NALT) (Brandtzaeg, 1984; Ermack and Owen, 1986; Brandtzaeg, 1987; Neutra *et al.*, 1987; Sminia *et al.*, 1989; Owen *et al.*, 1991; Bernstein, 1992; Kuper *et al.*, 1992). M cells conduct active transepithelial transport of luminal contents, including microorganisms, from the apical to basolateral surface of mucosal tissue (Trier, 1991; Neutra and Krahenbuhl, 1992). This property of M cells can be exploited in vaccine development with live recombinant microorganisms expressing foreign antigens, since these organisms will be handled similarly to invading pathogens (Wassef *et al.*, 1989; Childers *et al.*, 1990; Sicinski *et al.*, 1990; Langermann and Amerongen, 1993).

BCG, a live attenuated strain of *Mycobacterium bovis,* qualifies as an excellent candidate for mucosal delivery of antigens. Previously, BCG has been shown to bind to M cells in the gut whereupon the organisms are endocytosed and delivered to intraepithelial spaces containing lymphocytes and macrophages (Fujimura, 1986; Momotani *et al.*, 1988). Since the BCG bacterium can accommodate large pieces of exogenous DNA and can express foreign genes efficiently (Jacobs *et al.*, 1987, 1990; Snapper *et al.*, 1988; Stover *et al.*, 1991), it could serve as a carrier to stimulate mucosal immune responses to a wide spectrum of foreign antigens.

Earlier experiments showed that mucosally administered (oral) BCG traversed mucosal linings and could be found systemically within a short period of time. However, these studies provided no data on the capacity for mucosal immunization to elicit systemic or mucosal immune responses either to BCG itself or to cloned antigens expressed in BCG. More recently, studies utilizing recombinant BCG (rBCG) expressing foreign proteins from bacteria have demonstrated that a single mucosal immunization is a powerful method for inducing a long-term systemic, protective IgG response, as well as a S-IgA response against a target pathogen (Langermann *et al.*, 1994a). These recombinant BCG strains will be described in greater detail below.

Studies with rBCG have shown that intranasal (i.n.) delivery is a more effective route of mucosal immunization than oral delivery. The mucosal IgA response to foreign antigens induced by intranasal (i.n.) delivery of rBCG is disseminated throughout the mucosal immune system, including the respiratory, gastrointestinal (GI), and urogenital tracts (Langermann *et al.*, 1994a), thus supporting the notion of a common mucosal immune system (Mestecky, 1987; Brandtzaeg, 1992; McGhee *et al.*, 1992). Intranasal delivery of rBCG, as opposed to parenteral or oral delivery, induces discrete foci of lymphocytic infiltrates in the NALT and lungs, as well as the gut-associated lymphoid tissue (GALT) of immunized mice. The appearance and persistence of these lymphoid aggregates correlates with the development of secretory immunity (Langermann *et al.*, 1994a).

II. Background on BCG

A. Safety of BCG as a Vaccine Delivery Vehicle

BCG, which has been used for many years as an antituberculosis vaccine, is the most widely administered safe, live human vaccine. It has been given to over three billion people worldwide since 1948, with a low incidence of serious complications ($0.19/10^6$) (Stover *et al.*, 1995). Because of its safety record, it is also suitable for immunization of young children and infants. Hence BCG should prove to be a safe and effective live vaccine delivery system in humans as well (Bloom, 1989; Fine, 1988).

The most frequent, albeit rare, adverse reaction to systemic (intradermal) vaccination with BCG is suppurative lymphadentitis (Lugosi, 1992). However, it has been shown in studies conducted with a number of different BCG strains used as tuberculosis vaccines that this reactogenicity can be attributed to two factors relating to growth conditions of the BCG organisms: (i) homogeneity of the bacterial suspension, and (ii) viability of the final vaccine preparation. Whereas the conventional static growth of BCG yields a nondispersed, low-viability preparation that induces this severe reactogenicity at the site of injection, the growth conditions that we and others have used, employing roller bottles, yields well-dispersed cultures of high viability. Such growth conditions result in high immunogenicity without the associated clinical complications (Langermann *et al.*, 1994b; Stover *et al.*, 1993; Gheorgiu *et al.*, 1988).

More recently, with the emergence of AIDS, there has been some concern about disseminated disease with BCG and other live vaccine vectors (e.g., vaccinia) in immunocompromised hosts (Weltman and Rose, 1993). However, the number of case reports suggesting a link between disseminated BCG and HIV infections is small, despite the fact that many HIV-infected individuals have been vaccinated with BCG (Braun and Cauthen, 1992; Reichman, 1988, 1989). Nonetheless, more extensive, case-controlled studies are required before drawing any conclusions about the actual risk of disseminated BCG disease in immunocompromised individuals.

In terms of safety issues related to mucosal delivery of BCG it should be noted that BCG was given as an oral vaccine until 1976. Oral administration of BCG was discontinued because of a *relatively* high incidence of local lymphadenitis in tonsillar tissue of newborns taking the vaccine. However, these vaccine preparations were also the nondispersed, low-viability lots associated with severe reactogenicity as described above. Furthermore, the oral doses administered were 100-fold higher than the doses given intradermally in order to ensure delivery of sufficient BCG to the gastrointestinal tract (Gaudier and Gernez-Rieux, 1962; Schwarting, 1948).

In preclinical studies, *intranasal* delivery of well-dispersed, highly viable cultures of BCG has been studied extensively in mice and guinea pigs to evaluate any untoward effects. While i.n. immunization has resulted in strong, long-lasting systemic and mucosal immune responses in both species of animals, there has been no evidence of fibrosis or granuloma formation in either the upper or lower respiratory tract or in the spleen (Langermann *et al.*, 1994a).

B. Adjuvant Properties and *in Vivo* Persistence of BCG

BCG offers unique advantages as a vaccine delivery vehicle. It produces sensitization (from 5 to 50 years) to tuberculoproteins. It has strong adjuvant properties in both animals and man. The adjuvant properties are thought to be associated with its cell wall components as well as its potential for sustained boosting due to persistent replication within the host. Whether persistent replication within the host is a prerequisite for long-term immunity is not clear.

Following systemic immunization, BCG is taken up by macrophages whereupon the intracellular BCG disseminate to a variety of organs, including the liver and spleen, and establish foci of infection. The duration of long-term *in vivo* replication and persistence in humans is not entirely clear. However, persistence studies with both nonrecombinant and recombinant BCG have been done in a number of animal models. Vaccination studies performed at MedImmune have shown that both nonrecombinant and recombinant BCG persist in the livers, spleens, and lungs of mice at least 3 to 4 months following systemic immunization. Furthermore, analysis of rBCG from 60-day intervals showed that the rBCG retained the capacity to express the appropriate foreign antigens *in vivo* (Hanson *et al.*, 1995). Studies in guinea pigs with the same rBCG strains yielded similar results (S. Langermann, D. N. McMurray, S. W. Phaler, and S. R. Palaszynski, 1994, unpublished results).

While the beneficial effect of *in vivo* persistence on the host's immune response to foreign antigens expressed by rBCG is obvious from a vaccine delivery standpoint, this benefit must be counterbalanced by the concern for potential disseminated disease in vaccinees who may become immunocompromised. More recent studies have focused on the development of defined auxotrophic mutants of BCG to further attenuate this bacterium (Hanson *et al.*, 1995). The hope would be that such strains would retain the advantages of providing a good vaccine delivery system with potent adjuvant properties, but with limited persistence in the host. Studies with such auxotrophic mutants should also shed light on the issue of whether persistence of replication is required to sustain immunity to foreign antigens expressed in BCG, or if merely delivering the foreign antigen with the immunostimulatory BCG vehicle is sufficient.

III. rBCG as a Vaccine Delivery Vehicle: Expressing Foreign Proteins on the Surface of BCG

The model protein which was used in a number of studies to evaluate immune responses to cloned antigens in BCG is the outer surface protein (OspA) antigen of *Borrelia burgdorferi,* the causative agent of Lyme disease. OspA is a bacterial lipoprotein amenable to membrane translocation (Dunn, *et al.*, 1990), which has been shown to elicit protective antibody responses in the mouse model for Lyme borreliosis (Fikrig, *et al.*, 1990, 1992). For many of these primary studies addressing the utility of BCG as a vaccine vehicle, an *osp*A gene segment excluding the 5′ region encoding the N-terminal signal peptide was cloned into rBCG vectors to generate chimeric ospA gene fusions which express OspA in rBCG as a surface lipoprotein or a cytoplasmic protein respectively (Stover *et al.*, 1993). In these rBCG vectors, signal peptides derived from mycobacterial lipoproteins direct export and surface expression of the recombinant OspA lipoprotein in BCG. During post-translational processing of the cloned gene product, the export signal is removed and the target antigen is anchored in the bacterial membrane via a covalent N-terminal lipid tail allowing for expression of the foreign antigen as a lipoprotein on the surface of the rBCG. Surface expression of foreign antigens in BCG offers at least two advantages over cytoplasmically expressed recombinant proteins: (1) the surface-expressed antigen may be more readily processed by antigen-presenting cells, and (2) since it is a lipoprotein, the antigenicity of the recombinant protein is greatly enhanced in terms of its ability to stimulate B cells as well as CTLs (Brandt, *et al.*, 1990; Chamberlain *et al.*, 1989; Melchers, *et al.*, 1975).

Initial experiments to assess humoral antibody responses to OspA after intraperitoneal (IP) immunizations of BALB/c mice with the rBCG-OspA lipoprotein vaccine demonstrated that this recombinant vaccine elicited higher titer anti-OspA responses that were protective in a mouse model for Lyme borreliosis. These protective responses were also seen in mice that were otherwise low responders to purified preparations of OspA protein (Stover *et al.*, 1993). Furthermore, anti-OspA responses elicited by rBCG-OspA lipoprotein vaccines resulted from immunization with rBCG that were expressing OspA at only 5–10 ng per 10^6 rBCG (vaccine inoculum). In contrast, immunization of mice with such small amounts of purified lipid-acylated OspA alone or together with a variety of adjuvants did not result in comparable anti-OspA titers, nor did it afford protection in the challenge model.

IV. rBCG as a Mucosal Vaccine Delivery Vehicle for the Upper Respiratory Tract

A. rBCG-OspA as a Model Vaccine to Assess Mucosal Immune Responses

Although mucosal immune responses may not be relevant to protection against Lyme disease, the well-characterized "model" rBCG-OspA vaccine described above was tested for its ability to elicit antibody responses in mice following mucosal immunization. A single intranasal immunization with 10^8 cfu of rBCG-OspA resulted in a prolonged (greater than 2 years) protective systemic IgG response in mice (Langermann *et al.*, 1994b; Langermann, 1996). Lower doses of rBCG (10^6 and 10^5 cfu) induced similar long-term systemic immune responses. Intranasal immunization also yielded a S-IgA response to OspA which was disseminated throughout the mucosal immune system, including the respiratory, gastrointestinal, and urogenital tracts. In addition, intranasal immunization induced a pronounced, organized lymphocytic infiltrate in the proximal NALT as well as in the BALT and GALT. The appearance and persistence of lymphoid aggregates in NALT and BALT correlated with the secretory immune response.

Culturing of spleen and lung tissue from intranasally immunized mice showed that BCG rapidly disseminated to these organs following immunization. Furthermore, isolation and characterization of plasmids from rBCG-OspA isolated and grown from these tissues demonstrated that the rBCG continued to express recombinant protein at least 3–4 months following immunization. While the persistence of rBCG replication in spleen and lung tissue may account in part for the prolonged immunogenicity induced by rBCG, it would not explain why local IgA responses are induced only in lungs of mice immunized intranasally, since rBCG were found in lungs of mice immunized IP as well (Hanson *et al.*, 1995). One possibility is that, similar to GALT, NALT serves as an inductive site for priming of antigen-specific IgA-producing cells which then migrate to mucosal sites via mucosal addressins (Fig. 1). Whether the NALT serves as the inductive site for priming of IgA producing cells by rBCG remains to be determined.

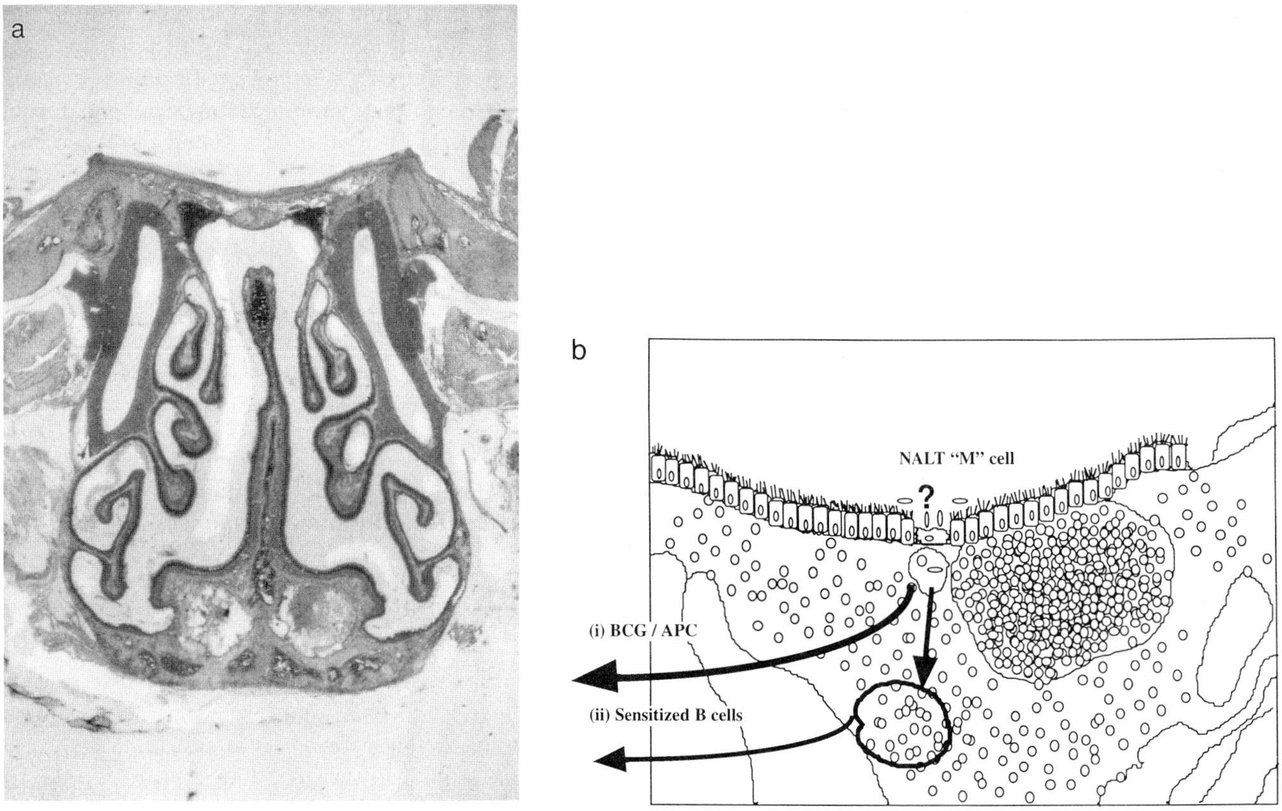

Figure 1. (a) Mouse nasopharyngeal-associated lymphoid tissue (NALT) section stained with hematoxylin and eosin; cross-section through mouse nasal passages, at the level of the ecto- and endoturbinates revealing bipolar distribution of nasopharyngeal lymphoid tissue (NALT; arrows). Magnification ×20. (b) Hypothetical diagram to explain induction of local and systemic immunity to rBCG vaccines following intranasal delivery. The induction of organized lymphoid aggregates in NALT and at distal mucosal effector sites suggests a role for NALT in the generation of systemic and secretory responses against inhaled vaccines/antigens. Presumably BCG enter the NALT via "M cells" in the epithelium overlying lymphoid follicles (Kuper *et al.*, 1992), whereupon they are taken up by macrophages/antigen-presenting cells (APC) that migrate in and out of the underlying lymphoid tissue. At this point it is uncertain whether the appearance of lymphocytic foci in NALT and in distal tissues, which correlates temporally with the induction of a local immune response, is due to: (i) uptake of BCG by APC followed by dissemination of BCG to distal tissues or (ii) stimulation of antigen-specific lymphocytes in the nasal mucosa followed by recirculation and homing back to the NALT as well as to distal mucosal tissues.

B. Assessing Mucosal Immune Responses to rBCG Vaccines Expressing Antigens from the Mucosal Pathogens *Streptococcus pneumoniae* and Uropathogenic *Escherichia coli*

Systemic IgG and S-IgA responses can also be engendered against other foreign antigens in BCG such as the Pneumococcal surface protein A (PspA) from *Streptococcus pneumoniae* (Briles *et al.*, 1988; McDaniel *et al.*, 1986), following intranasal delivery. In the case of the rBCG-PspA vaccines, booster immunization were required at 17 to 20 weeks post-primary immunization to induce protective antibody levels in the mice, as was the case with systemic administration of the same vaccines (Langermann *et al.*, 1994b).

Additional studies with the rBCG-PspA vaccines further demonstrated that: (1) humoral antibody responses to PspA engendered by a primary mucosal immunization with the rBCG-PspA could be boosted either by a secondary mucosal immunization with the same rBCG-PspA vaccine or by systemic vaccination with either rBCG-PspA or purified PspA protein alone. This demonstrated that mucosal immunization with a live recombinant BCG vector did not tolerize the host to subsequent vaccination with the same type of vector-based vaccines. Furthermore, the fact that the antibody response induced by primary immunization with rBCG-PspA was boosted with purified PspA suggested that rBCG vaccines delivered mucosally induced strong B-cell responses against the cloned antigen. Thus, prolonged responses to antigens cloned into rBCG cannot be explained by long-term replication of the rBCG alone.

Preliminary experiments with the rBCG-PspA suggested that mucosal delivery of these vaccines protected against systemic challenge with virulent *S. pneumoniae* utilizing a well-characterized IP challenge model in mice (Langermann *et al.*, 1994b). While this confirmed results seen with systemically administered rBCG-PspA vaccines, and demonstrated that intranasal delivery of rBCG vaccines elicits protective IgG responses in mice, these studies did not convey any information on the ability of mucosally administered rBCG vaccines to protect against true mucosal infections.

In order to test whether mucosal vaccination with rBCG vaccines will protect against infection with mucosal pathogens *in vivo,* in an appropriate animal model for mucosal colonization, recent efforts have focused on cloning surface adhesins such as PapG and FimH (Lindberg *et al.*, 1984, 1986, 1987; Maurer and Orndorff, 1987; Abraham *et al.*, 1987; Hanson and Brinton, 1988) from uropathogenic *Escherichia coli* into rBCG (Fig. 2). The majority of uropathogenic strains of *E. coli* assemble adhesive surface organelles called type 1 pili and/or Pap pili which allow the bacteria to bind to bladder or kidney epithelium (Schaeffer *et al.*, 1979; Leffler and Svanborg-Eden, 1980; Ofek *et al.*, 1981; Vaisanen *et al.*, 1981; Roberts *et al.*, 1994). The FimH and PapG adhesins are components of distinct tip fibrillae substructures that are joined to the ends of thicker type 1 or Pap rods, respectively (Kuehn *et al.*, 1992; Hultgren *et al.*, 1993; Jones *et al.*, 1995). FimH mediates microbial attachment with stereochemical specificity to mannose receptors distributed throughout the human bladder mucosal epithelium, whereas PapG mediates binding to globoside receptors in the kidney. Both FimH and PapG have been cloned into BCG as surface-expressed, chimeric lipoproteins (Fig. 2). The immune responses to these adhesin proteins expressed in BCG following intranasal delivery of these rBCG vaccines are currently under investigation (Langermann *et*

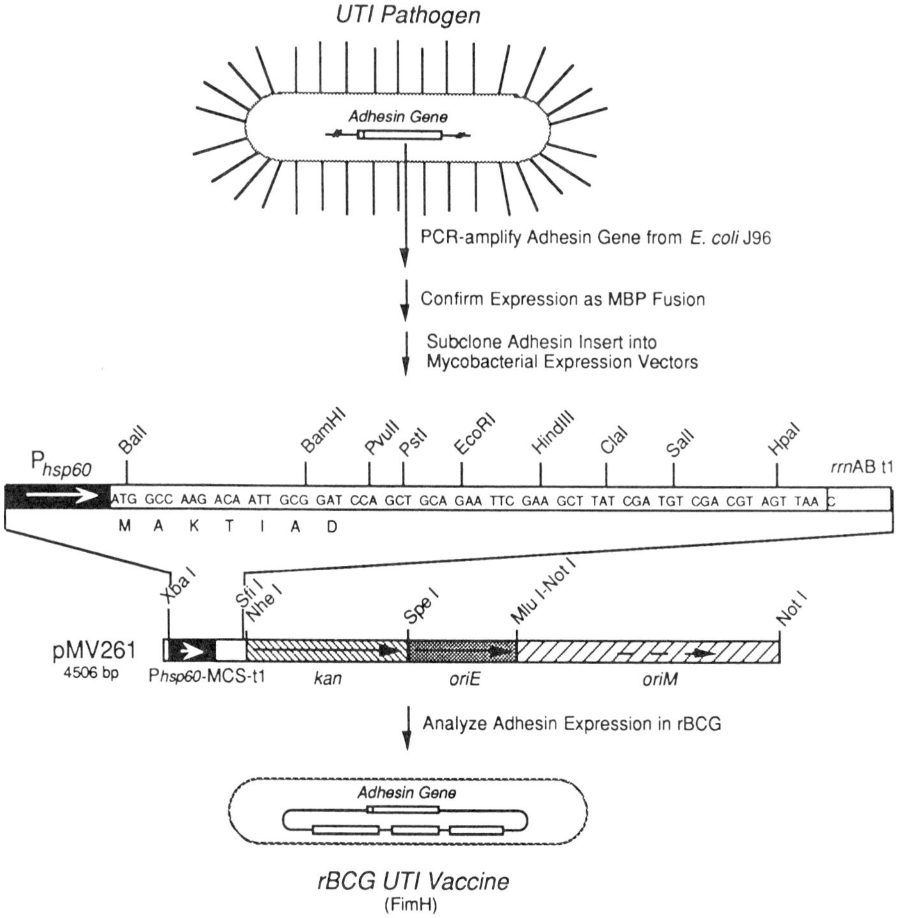

Figure 2. Expression of pilus adhesins in rBCG (rBCG-FimH/ rBCG-PapGII). Using genomic DNA extracted from the *E. coli* cystitis or pyelonephritis isolates, DNA encoding the FimH and PapGII adhesin were amplified by polymerase chain reaction (PCR) with primers based on the sequence reported for *fimH* (Klemm and Christiansen, 1987) or papG (Lindberg *et al.*, 1984). Only the amino-terminal sequence encoding the receptor-binding domain of the mature proteins was utilized. PCR primers incorporated synthetic restriction sites to facilitate cloning. Inserts were initially screened for expression as fusions with the *E. coli* maltose-binding protein using a derivative (pGMALc) of a commercially available maltose-binding protein fusion expression vector modified to have a multiple cloning site identical to that in the mycobacterial (rBCG) translational fusion vectors. Inserts were then subcloned into rBCG vectors expressing foreign antigens as fusions with cytoplasmic (i.e., pMV261, see Fig. 1 or export/ membrane localization leaders (pMV2619) (Langermann *et al.*, 1994a). Expression of these chimeric adhesins was verified by immunoblotting with adhesin-specific antisera.

al., unpublished data). Furthermore, the protective efficacy of secretory antibody raised against the rBCG-PapG and rBCG-FimH vaccines adhesins will be tested in intraurethral challenge models for cystitis and pyelonephritis in mice (Aronson *et al.*, 1979; O'Hanley *et al.*, 1985; Liao *et al.*, 1991).

V. Conclusions

Substantial efforts have been made in vaccine development toward the identification of protective antigens for a wide variety of infectious diseases. Although significant progress has been made, at least two basic problems associated with general vaccine development still exist: (i) the safe, low-cost production and purification of antigens from a pathogen in sufficient quantities for vaccine studies; (ii) the delivery of this antigen in a suitable adjuvant to promote protective immune responses. Additionally, there is the problem of designing appropriate vaccine delivery vehicles to engender mucosal immune responses pathogens. One approach to all of these problems has been the development of live recombinant vaccines. Live recombinant vaccines such as BCG have the advantage of expressing the desired antigen *in vivo,* at low cost, and in the context of a natural delivery system. Furthermore, BCG which binds to M cells in the mucosal epithelium can be utilized to target antigens to the mucosal epithelium to engender mucosal as well as systemic immunity. To date, it has been shown that inoculation with live recombinant BCG (rBCG) expressing a number of diverse recombinant target antigens results in long-lasting humoral, cellular, and mucosal immune responses to the recombinant antigen in several animal model systems and protects against a variety of systemic infections. It remains to be determined whether the ability to induce long-lasting secretory immunity with rBCG correlates with protection against mucosal challenge.

References

Abraham, S. N., Goguen, J. D., Sun, D., Klemm, P., and Beachey, E. H. (1987). Identification of two ancillary subunits of *Escherichia coli* type 1 fimbriae by using antibodies against synthetic oligopeptides of *fim* gene products. *J. Bacteriol.* **169,** 5530–5536.

Aronson, M., Medalia, O., Schori, L. Mirelman, D., Sharon, N., and Ofek, I. (1979). Prevention of colonization of the urinary tract of mice with *Escherichia coli* by blocking of bacterial adherence with methyl α-D-mannopyranoside. *J. Infect. Dis.* **139,** 329–332.

Bernstein, J. M. (1992). Mucosal immunology of the upper respiratory tract. *Respiration* **59,** (Suppl. 1), 3–13.

Bloom, B. R. (1989). Vaccines for the third world. *Nature (London)* **342,** 115–120.

Brandt, M. E., Riley, B. S., Radolf, J., and Norgard, M. V. (1990). Immunogenic integral membrane proteins of *Borrelia burgdorferi* are lipoproteins. *Infect. Immun.* **58,** 983–991.

Brandtzaeg, P. (1984). Immune functions of human nasal mucosa and tonsils in health and disease. *In* "Immunology of the Lung and Upper Respiratory Tract" (J. Bienenstock, ed.), pp. 28–95. McGraw-Hill, New York.

Brandtzaeg, P. (1987). Immune functions and immunopathology of palatine and nasopharyngeal tonsils. *In* "Imunology of the Ear" (J. M. Bernstein and P. L. Ogra, eds.), pp. 63–106. Raven, New York.

Brandtzaeg, P. (1989). Overview of the mucosal immune system. *Curr. Top. Microbiol. Immunol.* **146,** 13–25.

Brandtzaeg, P. (1992). Humoral immune response patterns of human mucosae: Induction and relation to bacterial respiratory trace infections. *J. Infect. Dis.* **165** (Suppl. 1), S167–S176.

Braun, M. M., and Cauthen, G. (1992). Relationship of the human immunodeficiency virus epidemic to pediatric tuberculosis and Bacillus Calmette–Guerin immunization. *Pediatr. Infect. Dis.* **11,** 220–227.

Briles, D. E., Yother, J., and McDaniel, L. S. (1988). Role of Pneumococcal surface protein A in the virulence of *Streptococcus pneumoniae. Rev. Infect. Dis.* **10,** S372–S374.

Chamberlain, N. R., Brandt, M. E., Erwin, A. L., Radolf, J. D., and Norgard, M. V. (1989). Major integral membrane proteins immunigens of *Treponema pallidum* are proteolipids. *Infect. Immun.* **57,** 2872–2877.

Childers, N. K., Bruce, M. G., and McGhee, J. R. (1989). Molecular mechanisms of immunoglobulin A defense. *Annu. Rev. Microbiol.* **43,** 503–536.

Childers, N. K., Denys, F. R., McGee, N. F., and Michalek, S. M. (1990). Ultrastructural study of liposome uptake by M cells of rat Peyer's patch: An oral vaccine system for delivery of purified antigen. *Regional Immunology* **3,** 8–16.

Dunn, J. J., Lade, B. N., and Barbour, A. G. (1990). Outer surface protein A (OspA) from the Lyme disease spirochete, *Borrelia burgdorferi:* High level expression and purification of a soluble recombinant form of OspA. *Protein Expression Purif.* **1,** 159–168.

Ermak, T. H., and Owen, R. L. (1986). Differential distribution of lymphocytes and accessory cells in mouse Peyer's patches. *Anat. Rec.* **215,** 144–152.

Fikrig, E., Barthold, S. W., Kantor, F. S., and Flavell, R. (1990). Protection of mice against the Lyme disease agent by immunizing with recombinant OspA. *Science* **250,** 553–556.

Fikrig, E., Barthold, S. W., Marcantonio, N., Deponte, K., Kantor, F. S., and Flavell, R. (1992). Roles of OspA, OspB, and flagellin in protective immunity to *Lyme borreliosis* in laboratory mice. *Infect. Immun.* **60,** 657–661.

Fine, P. E. M. (1988). BCG vaccination against tuberculosis and leprosy. *Br. Med. Bull.* **44,** 691–703.

Fujimura, Y. (1986). Functional morphology of microfold cells (M cells) in Peyer's Patches—Phagocytosis and transport of BCG by M cells into rabbit Peyer's patches. *Gasteroenterol. Jpn.* **21,** 325–335.

Gaudier, B., and Gernez-Rieux, C. (1962). Etude experimentale de la vitalite du BCG au cours de la traverse gastro-intestinale chez des enfants non allergiques vaccines par voie digestive. *Ann. Inst. Pasteur* **13,** 77–87.

Gheorghiu, M., Lagrange, P. H., and Fillastre, C. (1988). The stability and immunogenicity of a dispersed-grown freeze-dried Pasteur BCG vaccine. *J. Biol. Stand.* **16,** 15–26.

Hanson, M. S., and Brinton, C. C. (1988). Identification and characterization of *E. coli* type-1 pilus tip adhesion protein. *Nature (London)* **332,** 265–268.

Hanson, M. S., Bansal, G. P., Langermann, S., Stover, C. K., and Orme, I. (1995). Efficacy and safety of live recombinant BCG vaccines. *Dev. Biol. Standard.* **84,** 229–236.

Hilleman, M. R. (1993). Paper presented at the International Symposium on Recombinant Vectors in Vaccine Development, Albany, New York, 23 May 1993 (Nucleic Acids Technologies Foundation, sponsored by IABS, FDA, USDA/APHIS, and NIAID/NIH).

Holmgren, J., Czerkinsky, C., Lycke, N., and Svennerholm, A.-M. (1992). Mucosal immunity: Implications for vaccine development. *Immunobiology* **184,** 157–179.

Hultgren, S. J., Abraham, S., Caparon, M., Falk, P., St. Geme III, J. W., and Normark, S. (1993). Pilus and nonpilus bacterial adhesins: Assembly and function in cell recognition. *Cell (Cambridge, Mass.)* **73,** 887–901.

Jacobs, W. R., Jr., Tuckman, M., and Bloom, B. R (1987). Introduction of foreign DNA into mycobacteria using a shuttle plasmid. *Nature (London)* **327,** 532–535.

Jacobs, W. R., Jr., Snapper, S. B., Lugosi, L., and Bloom, B. R. (1990). Development of BCG as a recombinant vaccine delivery vehicle. *Curr. Top. Microbiol. Immunol.* **155,** 153–160.

Jones, C. H., Pinkner, J. S., Roth, R., Heuser, J., Nicholes, A. V., Abraham, S. N., and Hultgren, S. J. (1995). FimH adhesin of type 1 pili is assembled into a fibrillar tip structure in the *Enterobacteriacae. Proc. Natl. Acad. Sci. U.S.A.* **92,** 2081–2085.

Kiyono, H., Bienenstock, J., McGhee, J. R., and Ernst, P. B. (1992). The mucosal immune system: Features of inductive and effector sites to consider in mucosal immunization and vaccine development. *Regional Immunol.* **4,** 54–62.

Klemm, P., and Christensen, G. (1987). Three *fim* genes required for the regulation of length and mediation of adhesion of *Escherichia coli* isolate. *Infect. Immun.* **33,** 933–938.

Krahenbuhl, J. P., and Neutra, M. R. (1992). Molecular and cellular basis of immune protection of mucosal surfaces. *Physiol. Rev.* **72,** 853–880.

Kuehn, M. J., Neuser, J., Normark, S., and Hultgren, S. J. (1992). P pil in uropathogenic *E. coli* are composite fibres with distinct fibrillar adhesive tips. *Nature (London)* **356,** 252–255.

Kuper, C. F., Koornsta, P. J., Hameleers, D. M. H., Biewenga, J., Spit, B. J., Duijvestijn, A. M., van Breda Vriesman, P. J. C., and Sminia, T. (1992). The role of nasopharyngeal lymphoid tissue. *Immunol. Today* **13,** 219–225.

Langermann, S. (1996). New approaches to mucosal immunization. *Seminars in Gastrointestinal Disease* **7,** 12–18.

Langermann, S., and Amerongen, H. M. (1993). Antigen transport by intestinal M cells. *Curr. Opin. Gastroentroenterol.* **8,** 983–987.

Langermann, S., Palaszynski, S., Sadzienne, A., Stover, C. K., and Koenig, S. (1994a). Systemic and mucosal immunity induced by BCG vector expressing outer surface protein A of *Borrelia burgdorferi. Nature (London)* **372,** 552–555.

Langermann, S., Palaszynski, S. R., Burlein, J. E., Koenig, S., Hanson, M. S., Briles, D. E., and Stover, C. K. (1994b). Protective humoral response against pneumococcal infection in mice elicited by recombinant Bacille Calmette–Guerin vaccines expressing pneumococcal surface protein A. *J. Exp. Med.* **180,** 2277–2286.

Leffler, H., and Svanborg-Eden, C. (1980). Chemical identification of a glycosphinfolipid receptor for *Escherichia coli* attaching to human urinary tract epithelial cells and agglutinating human erythrocytes. *FEMS Microbiol. Lett.* **8,** 127–134.

Liao, J., Tomochika, K.-I., Watanabe, S., and Kanemasa, Y. (1991). Establishment of a mouse model of cystitis and roles of type 1 fimbriated *Escherichia coli* in its pathogenesis. *Microbiol. Immunol.* **36,** 243–256.

Lindberg, F. P., Lund, B., and Normark, S. (1984). Genes of pyelonephritic *E. coli* required for digalactoside specific agglutination of human cells. *EMBO J.* **3,** 1167–1173.

Lindberg, F., Lund, B., and Normark, S. (1986). Gene products specifying adhesion of uropathogenic *Escherichia coli* are minor components of pili. *Proc. Natl. Acad. Sci. U.S.A.* **83,** 1891–1895.

Lindberg, F., Lund, B., Johansson, L., and Normark, S. (1987). Localization of the receptor binding protein at the tip of the bacterial pilus. *Nature (London)* **328,** 84–87.

Lugosi, L. (1992). Theoretical and methodological aspects of BCG vaccine from the discovery of Calmette and Guerin to molecular biology. A review. *Tubercle and Lung Disease* **73,** 252–261.

McDaniel, L. S., Scott, Widenhofer, K., Carroll, J., and Briles, D. E. (1986). Analysis of a surface protein of *Streptococcus pneumoniae* recognized by protective monoclonal antibodies. *Microbial Pathogen.* **1,** 519–531.

McGhee, J. R., and Kiyono, H. (1993). New perspectives in vaccine development: Mucosal immunity to infections. *Infect. Agents Dis.* **2,** 55–73.

McGhee, Mestecky, J., Dertzbaugh, M. T., Eldridge, J. H., Hirasawa, M., and Kiyono, H. (1992). The mucosal immune system: From fundamental concepts to vaccine development. *Vaccine* **10,** 75–88.

Mauer, L., and Orndorff, P. E. (1987). Identification and characterization of genes determining receptor binding and pilus length of *Escherichia coli* type 1 pili. *J. Bacteriol.* **169,** 640–645.

Melchers, F., Braun, V., and Galanos, C. (1975). The lipoprotein of the outer membrane of *Escherichia coli:* A B-lymphocyte mitogen. *J. Exp. Med.* **142,** 473–982.

Mestecky, J. (1987). The common mucosal immune system and current strategies for induction of immune responses in external secretions. *J. Clin. Immunol.* **7,** 265–276.

Momotani, E., Whipple, D. L., Thiermann, A. B., and Cheville, N. F. (1988). Role of M cells and macrophages in the entrance of *Mycobacterium paratuberculosis* into domes of ileal Peyer's patches in calves. *Vet. Pathol.* **25,** 131–137.

Neutra, M. R., and Krahenbuhl, J. P. (1992). Transepithelial transport and mucosal defense: The role of M cells. *Trends Cell Biol.* **2,** 134–138.

Neutra, M. R., Phillips, T. L., Mayer, E. L., and Fishkind, D. J. (1987). Transport of membrane-bound macromolecules by cells in follicle-associated epithelium of rabbit Peyer's patches. *Cell Tissue Res.* **247,** 537–546.

O'Hanley, P., Lark, D., Falkow, S., and Schoolnik, G. (1985). Molecular basis of *Escherichia coli* colonization of upper urinary tract in BALB/c Mice. *J. Clin. Invest.* **75,** 347–360.

Ofek, I., Mosek, A., and Sharon, N. (1981). Mannose-specific adherence of *Escherichia coli* freshly excreted in the urine of patients with acute urinary tract infections and of isolates subcultured from the infected urine. *Infect. Immun.* **34,** 708–714.

Owen, R. L., Piazza, A. J., and Ermak, T. H. (1991). Ultrastructural and cytoarchitectural features of lymphoreticular organs in the colon and rectum of adult BALB/c mice. *Am. J. Anat.* **190,** 10–18.

Reichman, L. B. (1988). HIV infection—a new face of tuberculosis. *Bull. Int. Union Tubercle Lung Dis.* **63,** 19–24.

Reichman, L. B. (1989). Why hasan't BCG proved dangerous in HIV-infected patients? (letter) *JAMA, J. Am. Med. Assoc.* **261,** 3246.

Roberts, J. A., Marklund, B.-I., Ilver, D., Haslam, D., Kaack, M. B., Baskin, G., Louis, M., Möllby, R., Winberg, J., and Normark, S. (1994). The Gal(al-4)Gal-specific tip adhesin of *Escherichia coli* P-fimbriae is needed for pyelonephritis to occur in the normal urinary tract. *Proc. Natl. Acad. Sci. U.S.A.* **91,** 11889–11893.

Schaeffer, A. J., Amundsen, S. K., and Scnidt, L. N. (1979). Adherence of *Escherichia coli* to human urinary tract epithelial cells. *Infect. Immun.* **24,** 753–758.

Schwarting, V. M. (1948). The action of gastric contents on tubercle bacilli. *Am. Rev. Tuberc.* **58,** 213–128.

Sicinski, P., Rowinski, J., Warchol, J. B., Jarzacbek, Z., Gut, W., Szczygiel, B., Bielecki, K., and Koch, G. (1990). Poliovirus type 1 enters the human host through intestinal M cells. *Gastroenterology* **98,** 56–58.

Sminia, T., van der Brugge-Gamelkoorn, G. J., and Jeurissen, S. H. M. (1989). Structure and function of bronchus-associated lymphoid tissue (BALT). *Crit. Rev. Immunol.* **9,** 119–150.

Snapper, S. B., Lugosi, L., Jekkel, A., Melton, R. E., Kieser, T., Bloom, B. R., and Jacobs, W. R., Jr. (1998). Lysogeny and transformation in Mycobacteria: Stable expression of foreign genes. *Proc. Natl. Acad. Sci. U.S.A.* **85,** 6987–6991.

Stover, C. K., de la Cruz, V. F., Fuerst, T. R., Burlein, J. E., Benson, L. A., Bennett, L. T., Bansal, G. P., Young, J. F., Lee, M. H., Hatfull, G. F., Snapper, S. B., Barlett, R. G., Jacobs, W. R., Jr., and Bloom, B. R. (1991). New use of BCG for recombinant vaccines. *Nature (London)* **351,** 456–460.

Stover, C. K., Bansal, G. P., Hanson, M. S., Burlein, J. E., Palaszynski, S. R., Young, J. R., Koenig, S., Young, D. B., Sadziene, A., and Barbour, A. (1993). Protective immunity elicited by recombinant BCG expressing OspA lipoprotein: A candidate lyme disease vaccine. *J. Exp. Med.* **178,** 197–209.

Stover, C. K., Hanson, M. S., and Langermann, S. (1995). Recombinant BCG vaccines and the development of mycobacterial molecular biology. *In* "Tuberculosis" (W. Rom and S. Garay, eds.), pp. 911–925. Little, Brown, and Co., New York.

Trier, J. S. (1991). Structure and function of intestinal M cells. *Gastroenterology Clinics of North America* **20,** 531–547.

Vaisanen, V., Tallgren, L., Makela, P., *et al.* (1981). Mannose resistance hemagglutination and P antigen recognition are characteristics of *Escherichia coli* causing primary pyelonephritis. *Lancet* **2,** 1366–1369.

Wassef, J. S., Keren, D. F., and Mailloux, J. L. (1989). Role of M cells in initial antigen uptake and in ulcer formation in the rabbit intestinal loop model of shigellosis. *Infect. Immun.* **57,** 858–863.

Weltman, A. C., and Rose, D. N. (1993). The safety of Bacille Calmette–Guerin vaccination in HIV infection and AIDS. *AIDS* **7,** 149–157.

10

Poliovirus Replicons as a Vector for Mucosal Vaccines

CASEY D. MORROW
ZINA MOLDOVEANU
MARIE J. ANDERSON
DONNA C. PORTER
Department of Microbiology
University of Alabama at Birmingham
Birmingham, Alabama 35294

I. Introduction

In order for a vaccine targeted to the mucosal immune system to be effective, the antigens must be delivered to immunoreactive sites such as the small intestine, nasaopharynx, genital tract, or rectum where discrete lymphoid follicles are found (Mestecky, 1988; McGhee and Mestecky, 1992; Ogra and Ogra, 1973). In accordance with the concept of a common mucosal immune system, antigen stimulation at a mucosal site can generate large numbers of plasma cell precursors which may migrate to particular mucosal sites, resulting in the appearance of antibodies in the corresponding secretions (Mestecky and McGhee, 1987). Although vaccine strategies designed to stimulate the mucosal immune system have clear advantages, the practical aspects of an efficient delivery of antigens to the inductive sites present a formidable challenge. For example, the harsh environment of the stomach and upper small intestine (i.e., low pH), and the presence of proteolytic enzymes, precludes the oral administration of many antigens (Mestecky, 1988). Therefore, numerous methods to protect antigens have been investigated. Included in this approach are the use of biodegradable protective shells (e.g. microspheres, enteric coating of antigens) and liposomes (Michalek *et al.*, 1989; Eldridge *et al.*, 1989; Moldoveanu *et al.*, 1993). In recent years viruses such as vaccinia have received considerable attention as vaccine vectors (Moss, 1990, 1991; Mackett *et al.*, 1985). We have taken a different approach and have developed the RNA virus poliovirus as a vaccine vector. Poliovirus is attractive for use as a mucosal vaccine because of several inherent properties of the virus. The natural transmission of poliovirus is by the fecal–oral route and thus the virus is stable to the harsh environment of the gastrointestinal tract (Horstmann, *et al.*, 1959). The attenuated strains of poliovirus have been utilized to develop a safe and effective oral vaccine which can be given to infants (Sabin and Boulger, 1973). The virus can be delivered not only by the oral but also by the nasal route to stimulate both systemic and mucosal antibodies to poliovirus (Sanders and Cramblett, 1974; Hanson *et al.*, 1984; Ogra and Karzon, 1971; Ogra *et al.*, 1968; Ogra, 1984). Finally, the generation of a cell-mediated immune response to poliovirus has been demonstrated in orally vaccinated volunteers (Simmons *et al.*, 1993; Graham *et al.*, 1993).

The development of a recombinant vaccine vector based on poliovirus has been facilitated because of the immense knowledge available about the virus. The complete viral RNA genome has been sequenced and the viral proteins identified (Kitamura *et al.*, 1981; Racaniello and Baltimore, 1981a). An infectious cDNA of the viral genome has been generated making it possible to manipulate the virus genetically (Racaniello and Baltimore, 1981b; Semler *et al.*, 1984). The three dimensional structure of the complete virus is known and the major antigenic epitopes have been identified on the molecular level (Hogle *et al.*, 1985). The receptor that poliovirus utilizes to gain entry into the cells has been cloned and the nucleic acid sequence has been determined (Mendelsohn *et al.*, 1989; Ren and Racaniello, 1992). Transgenic mice have been generated which express the receptor and are susceptible to poliovirus infection (Ren and Racaniello, 1992; Ren *et al.*, 1990). Therefore, the vast information available about poliovirus makes it an ideal target for the development of vectors able to deliver antigens to the mucosal sites.

In this chapter, we will summarize the salient features of the biology of the poliovirus genome as a framework for our efforts to develop poliovirus as a vector to express foreign genes. Ongoing studies on the immu-

MUCOSAL VACCINES

nogenicity of some of the recombinant poliovirus genomes which express foreign proteins will also be presented.

II. The Poliovirus Genome

Poliovirus is a member of the family of *Picornaviridae*. This virus family includes members that infect not only humans but also a wide variety of experimental animals (porcine, bovine, and avian) (Rueckert, 1990). Poliovirus is classified as an enterovirus because of its fecal–oral transmission route (Rueckert, 1990). Included with poliovirus, as enteroviruses, are members of the Coxsackieviruses and echoviruses. Hepatitis A virus, in spite of its transmission via a fecal–oral route, is classified separately because the genome structure differs from that of the other enteroviruses. Another more prominent member of the picornavirus family is the agent of the common cold, human rhinovirus. Although the genome organization of human rhinovirus is similar to that of poliovirus, the inherent features of this virus with regard to the transmission route, sensitivity to low pH, and optimum replication temperature at 34°C distinguish rhinovirus from enteroviruses (Rueckert, 1990).

The hallmark of all picornaviruses is that they are plus-stranded RNA viruses whose genome is approximately 7400 nucleotides in length including a polyadenylated 3′ end (Kitamura *et al.*, 1981; Racaniello and Baltimore, 1991a). The 5′ end of the RNAs have a small covalently attached viral protein, VPg (Wimmer, 1982). The architecture of the poliovirus genome contains many interesting features. The genome contains a long 5' nontranslated region of 743 nucleotides which functions as an internal ribosome entry site (IRES) to promote the initiation of the translation of the viral RNA (Pelletier and Sonenberg, 1988). An open reading frame of 2207 consecutive triplets spans over 89% of the nucleotide sequence and encodes a single long-viral protein. The mature viral proteins arise by a proteolytic cascade which occurs predominately at glutamine–glycine amino acid pairs and is mediated by the viral-encoded proteinase $3C^{pro}$ (Hanecak *et al.*, 1982, 1984; Nicklin *et al.*, 1987; Harris *et al.*, 1990; Palmenberg, 1990). A fusion of the $3C^{pro}$ and $3D^{pol}$, the viral RNA-dependent RNA polymerase, also has proteolytic activity; the 3CD protease functions mainly to process the capsids from the poliovirus polyprotein (Ypma-Wong and Semler, 1987; Ypma-Wong *et al.*, 1988; Jore *et al.*, 1988) (see Fig. 1).

The poliovirus genome has been arbitrarily divided into three regions: P1, P2, and P3 (Rueckert and Wimmer, 1994) (Fig. 1). The viral capsid proteins are encoded within a polyprotein designated as P1. A second viral protease, 2A, autocatalytically cleaves the viral polyprotein during translation to release the P1 protein (Toyoda *et al.*, 1986). Three viral proteins are encoded within the P1 region, VP0, VP3, and VP1, which are released by the viral protease, 3CD. Once the P1 protein has been processed by the viral protease, the process of poliovirus assembly begins. VP0, VP3, and VP1 interact to form a structure known as a 5S capsid protomer (Putnak and Phillips, 1981; Rueckert, 1990; Koch and Koch, 1985; Hellen and Wimmer, 1992). Twelve 5S protomers assemble into a 14S pentamer; 5 14S pentamers assemble into a 75S empty capsid or provirion structure. Previous studies from our laboratory have shown that the process of poliovirus assembly will occur *in vivo* in the absence of genomic RNA (Ansardi *et al.*, 1991). At some point during the virus life cycle, the capsid protein interacts with the viral RNA genome. In the presence of genomic RNA, a final maturation cleavage occurs in which the VP0 protein is cleaved to VP2 and VP4 on encapsidation (Arnold *et al.*, 1987; Jacobson *et al.*, 1970; Jacobson and Baltimore, 1968; Rueckert, 1990).

The P2 and P3 regions of the viral genome encode proteins required for replication of the genomic RNA. Encoded within the P3 region are the viral protease, $3C^{pro}$, and the viral RNA-dependent RNA polymerase, $3D^{pol}$, which is the enzyme responsible for the synthesis for the poliovirus RNA genome (Wimmer *et al.*, 1993). During replication, the genomic plus strand RNA is first copied to a complementary minus strand; only low levels of minus strand are actually found in poliovirus infected cells. The minus strand serves as a template for the synthesis of plus strand RNA molecules (Harris *et al.*, 1990). Poliovirus replication is asymmetric in that many more plus strand molecules are synthesized than minus strands. The plus strand RNA molecules can serve as a template for the synthesis of new minus-strand RNAs, undergoing translation to produce new viral proteins or become encapsidated. The mechanism by which poliovirus regulates the production and distribution of plus strand RNA molecules is unknown (Wimmer *et al.*, 1987, 1993).

III. Development of Poliovirus as an Expression Vector

The serial passage of poliovirus *in vitro* at a high multiplicity of infection results in the generation, in some cases, of poliovirus genomes referred to as defective interfering genomes (DIs). Many times, the DI genomes replicate and become the predominant species in the stocks of poliovirus (Cole *et al.*, 1971; Kajigaya *et al.*, 1985; Kuge *et al.*, 1986). Previous studies have described the molecular cloning and sequencing of poliovirus DI genomes (Hagino-Yamagishi and Nomoto,

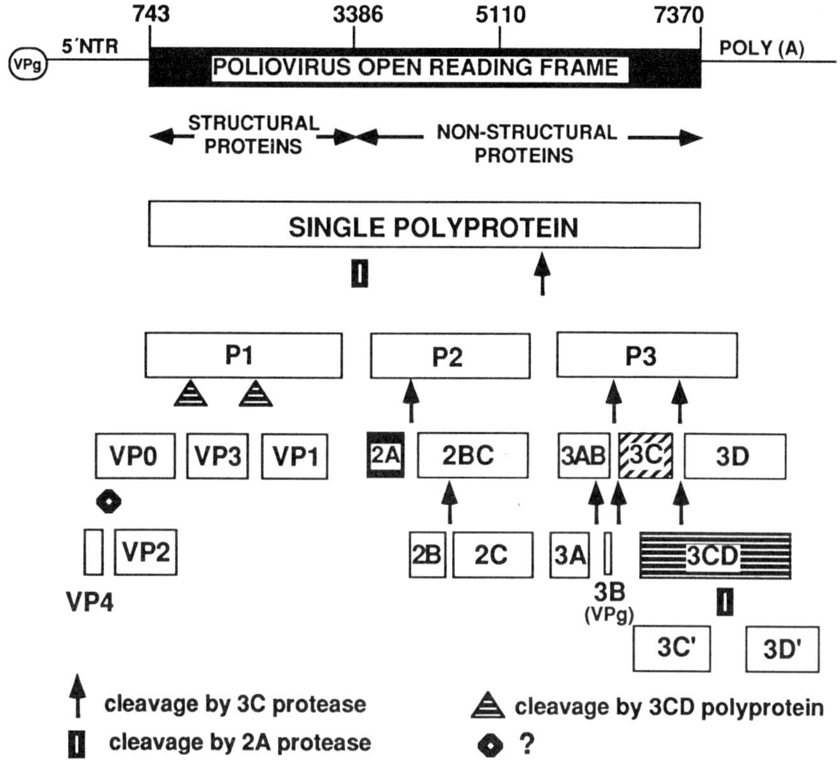

Figure 1. Poliovirus genome organization and cascade of polyprotein processing. The poliovirus RNA genome is a single-stranded plus-sense molecule that is approximately 7500 base pairs in length. The 5′ end of the RNA molecule is covalently attached to a small protein, VPg, and the 3′ end contains a genetically encoded poly A tract. The first 742 nucleotides of the 5′ end of the genome compose the nontranslated region which contains sequences necessary for the internal ribosome entry site (IRES). Poliovirus genomes contain a single long open reading frame which encodes a 2209-amino acid polyprotein precursor. Viral encoded proteases 2A and 3C catalyze cleavages of the polyprotein to form an individual viral protein. The 3CD polyprotein catalyzes a cleavage of the P1 capsid precursor to VP0, VP3, and VP1. The 2A protease catalyzes cleavage between the P1 and P2 regions of the viral polyprotein. The final cleavage event occurs at an asparagine–serine amino acid pair on the interior of the virion resulting in the cleavage of VP0 to VP2 and VP4.

1989). One of the unifying features of all the DIs of poliovirus was that the genomes contained deletions within the capsid (P1) genes so that the translational reading frame was maintained between the remaining capsid proteins and the P2 and P3 region genes. Therefore, all of the defective genomes of poliovirus maintain the capacity for self replication. The DIs are propagated from cell to cell by "stealing" the capsid proteins (P1) from poliovirus.

The availability of an infectious poliovirus cDNA (Racaniello and Baltimore, 1981b; Semler *et al.*, 1984) has prompted further investigation into the regions of the poliovirus genome that can be deleted without compromising the replication capacity of the RNA. These RNA molecules, which retain the property for self-replication when introduced into cells, are referred to as "replicons." Early studies by Kaplan and Racaniello described poliovirus replicons which contained deletions that encompassed the majority of the P1 region (Kaplan and Racaniello, 1988). Taking advantage of these initial observations, previous studies from this laboratory have described poliovirus replicons which contain fragments of up to 1.5 kb of the HIV-1 *gag, pol,* or *env* genes (Choi *et al.*, 1991). The foreign genes were inserted so the translational reading frame was maintained between the remaining capsid proteins and the P2- and P3-region proteins. Transfection of these RNAs into cells resulted in the replication of these genomes as well as the expression of the foreign protein as a fusion protein with the flanking capsid proteins.

In more recent studies, we have further modified the poliovirus cDNA to accommodate much larger genes for expression of proteins which retain native features (Porter *et al.*, 1995). In these vectors, we have deleted the complete P1 region of poliovirus. A replicon was constructed which contained the complete gene for HIV-1 *gag* (approximately 1.5 kb). Transfection of this replicon into cells resulted in the production of the HIV-1 Gag precursor protein, $Pr55^{gag}$. Analysis of the supernatant of cells infected with this replicon using electron microscopy revealed the presence of virus-like particles that had a size and morphology consistent with that of immature HIV-l Gag particles (Porter *et al.*, 1996). Although the replicon with the HIV-1*gag* gene substituted for the complete P1 gene was replication competent and could be encapsidated, we have found that inclusion of the VP4 coding region increases the titer of the encapsidated replicons after serial passage. In order to express proteins in their native form in the replicon which contains the VP4 coding region, we have inserted a cleavage site for the 2A proteinase that will release the foreign protein at the amino and carboxy termini. The cleavage site consists of nine amino acids, two of which include a tyrosine–glycine amino acid pair. The proteolytic processing by 2A results in the expression of a foreign protein which has minimal sequence changes at the amino terminus (one or two amino acids) and an additional eight amino acids at the carboxy terminus (Fig. 2). Using this replicon, we have expressed a wide array of proteins including HIV and SIV *gag* and *pol* genes, SIV *nef* genes, carcinoembryonic antigen, HER2/neu oncogene, firefly luciferase, β-galactosidase, and the C fragment of tetanus toxin.

Although we have expressed a diverse array of foreign proteins including enzymes, from replicons, we initially encountered difficulties with the expression of genes encoding glycoproteins. Previous studies from this and other laboratories have shown that poliovirus genomes which contain a gene encoding a signal sequence were not replication competent (Alexander *et al.*, 1994; Lu *et al.*, 1995; M. J. Anderson, D. C. Porter, and C. D. Morrow, unpublished, 1996). Although the exact reasons for this are unclear, we speculate that the targeting of the poliovirus polyprotein into the endoplasmic reticulum (ER) by the signal sequence might preclude the correct proteolytic processing by the poliovirus proteases. In recent studies, we have found that replicons which contain the first 200 nucleotides of the VP4 coding sequence, followed by the gene encoding the signal sequence and extracellular domain of the glycoprotein, were replication competent. Following proteolytic processing to expose the signal sequence, the expressed protein was translocated into the ER where it was glycosylated and ultimately secreted from the cell (Anderson *et al.*, 1996). The results of our studies demonstrate that it is possible to express a wide variety of foreign genes including genes encoding glycosylated proteins, using the poliovirus replicon system.

Since the replicons do not encode capsid proteins, they do not have the capacity to spread from cell to cell. Defective interfering genomes of poliovirus are propagated from cell to cell because they have the capacity to utilize the capsid proteins expressed by a coinfecting wild-type genome. The results of the characterization of the defective genomes established that the poliovirus capsid protein, P1, can be provided *in trans* to the viral genomes. We have taken advantage of this feature to develop a complementation system in which we can supply the capsid proteins of poliovirus *in trans* to encapsidate the replicon RNA (Fig. 3), (Porter *et al.*, 1995; Ansardi *et al.*, 1993; Morrow *et al.*, 1994). For our studies we use a recombinant vaccinia virus, VV-P1 which expresses the poliovirus P1 capsid precursor protein. To encapsidate our replicons, we transfect the replicon RNA into cells previously infected with VV-P1. The $3C^{pro}$ protease (in the form of the 3CD protein) expressed from the replicon processes the P1 protein expressed from the VV-P1, resulting in initiation of the assembly cascade for poliovirus and ultimately leading to the encapsidation of the replicon RNA. After cell lysis, the encapsidated replicons can be isolated by centrifugation and used to reinfect new cells. To derive large stocks, the encapsidated replicons are passaged in the presence of VV-P1 for multiple serial passages; in some cases, we have propagated the encapsidated replicons for 30–40 serial passages. No wild-type poliovirus has been detected in the passages, indicating that no recombination occurred between the replicon and the P1 RNA (Porter and Morrow, unpublished). Using an assay developed in this laboratory, we estimate that the levels of encapsidated replicons can reach $10^7$to 10^8 infectious units of replicon per milliliter after extended serial passage; under these same experimental conditions, it is possible to propagate poliovirus at 10^8 pfu per milliliter. The designation of infectious units per milliliter correlates with that of plaque-forming units per

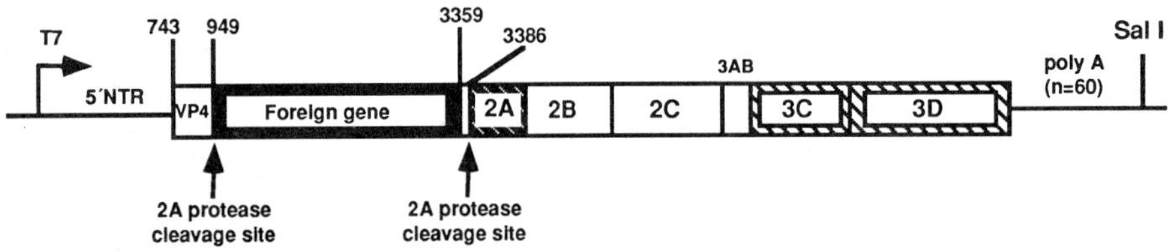

Figure 2. A poliovirus replicon. A cDNA containing the complete poliovirus genome was modified to insert restriction sites at nucleotides 949 and 3359. The exact details for the construction of this cDNA can be found in Porter *et al.* (1995). The plasmid which contains a promoter for the T7 RNA polymerase is linearized using the restriction enzyme *SalI,* followed by transfection of the *in vitro*-transcribed RNA into cells. The replicon RNA encodes the viral proteins required for replication of the RNA genome (e.g., $3D^{pol}$). Following the translation of the RNA genome, the foreign protein is released from the polyprotein as a fusion protein with the poliovirus VP4 protein. We have engineered a consensus cleavage site for the 2A protease at the carboxy terminus of VP4 such that the released foreign protein contains minimal amino acid changes at the amino and carboxy terminus.

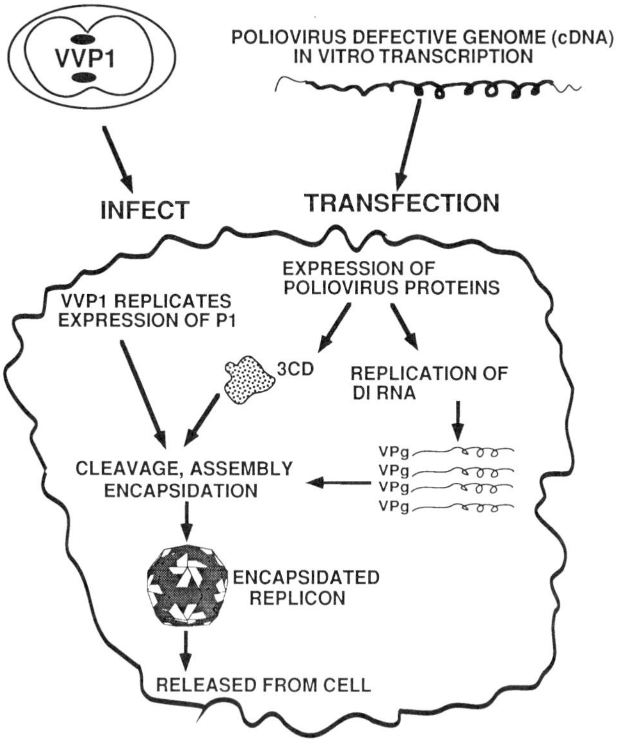

Figure 3. Encapsidation of poliovirus replicons. For the encapsidation of poliovirus replicons, the RNA derived from *in vitro* transcription of a poliovirus replicon cDNA is transfected into cells which have been infected previously with a vaccinia virus, VV-P1, which expresses the poliovirus capsid precursor protein P1. The replication of the replicon RNA results in the production of a viral protease 3CD which processes the P1 protein expressed from VV-P1 into VP0, VP3, and VP1. The processed capsid proteins assemble into subviral intermediates. The replicated replicon RNA is then encapsidated. The encapsidated replicon is released from the cell. To derive stocks, these cells are first infected with VV-P1 followed by infection with the encapsidated replicon. This procedure is repeated for 20 serial passages, to derive high titer stocks of the encapsidated replicon (approximately 10^7 infectious units of replicon per milliliter).

milliliter found with wild-type poliovirus (Porter and Morrow, unpublished). Using conventional ultracentrifugation techniques, the replicons can be concentrated to levels of 10^8 to 10^9 infectious units per milliliter.

In summary, we have developed methodologies for the construction and characterization of poliovirus RNA molecules which contain foreign genes substituted for the capsid genes. Using a complementation system developed in this laboratory, we can encapsidate these genomes into poliovirions. The infection of cells with an encapsidated replicon results in a single round of replication in which the replicon RNA undergoes amplification and expression of the foreign protein. Since the replicon does not encode the capsid proteins, it does not have the capacity to spread from cell to cell. Thus, the encapsidated replicons lack the capacity to infect neighboring cells, but retain many of the inherent biological and physiochemical features of poliovirus.

IV. Immunological Studies

The analysis of the immunogenicity of the encapsidated replicons containing foreign genes has proved challenging. Some of this is due to the fact that the natural hosts for poliovirus are humans. However, it has been known for some time that the type 2 Lansing strain of poliovirus can be adapted for growth in laboratory mice by serial passage through the brain (Armstrong, 1939). Although the infection process does not exactly mimic vaccine in the human host, intracerebral injection of the type 2 Lansing strain of poliovirus into BALB/C mice results in paralysis and death (La Monica *et al.*, 1986). For our initial analysis of the immunogenicity of the replicons, we took advantage of the fact that the type 2 Lansing stain of poliovirus has some capacity to infect mice. For these studies, we have passaged the replicons which express the capsid (p24) region of HIV-l Gag in the presence of poliovirus type 2 Lansing. During serial passage, the encapsidated replicons are maintained within the stock of type 2 Lansing poliovirus. We estimate in these stocks that the titer of the type 2 Lansing was approximately 10^7 plaque forming units per milliliter and the replicon was approximately 10^6 infectious particles per milliliter.

We have utilized this stock of encapsidated replicons to immunize BALB/c mice by three different routes: intramuscular, intrarectal, and intragastric. The details for the immunization procedures as well as the analysis of the anti-poliovirus and anti-HIV Gag responses can be found in a recent publication (Moldoveanu *et al.*, 1995). The mice were immunized twice, 4 weeks apart, via the same routes. The analysis of the anti-poliovirus antibody responses revealed that serum antibodies to poliovirus were present in mice receiving replicons by the intramuscular route, but not by intrarectal or intragastric routes. Analysis of saliva and feces from the same mice revealed that IgA anti-poliovirus antibodies were present in mice given the replicons by all three immunization routes. We also analyzed the above-mentioned samples for antibodies against HIV-1 Gag. It is important to note that the replicons must enter and replicate in the animals in order to express the HIV-1 Gag protein that will be recognized by the immunocompetent cells. The analysis of sera and secretions revealed that the immunized animals had antibodies against HIV-1 Gag. Higher titers of anti-HIV-1 Gag antibodies were found in sera of mice immunized intramuscularly compared with mice given the replicon/poliovirus type 2 Lansing by the intragastric route. The analysis of secretions for anti-HIV-1 Gag antibodies revealed that saliva and feces of mice given the replicon/

poliovirus type 2 Lansing by the three different routes contained specific antibodies of IgA isotype with higher levels in mice receiving replicon/poliovirus type 2 Lansing intragastrically. Based on these studies, we concluded that the replicons were immunogenic when given in combination with poliovirus and were able to induce a systemic as well as mucosal immune response.

The studies on poliovirus pathogenesis were greatly facilitated during the last several years with the identification and cloning of the human receptor for poliovirus (Mendlesohn *et al.*, 1989). Although the function of the poliovirus receptor in cells is presently unknown, the receptor has several characteristics of an immunoglobulin-like molecule and has been classified in the immunoglobulin superfamily (Mendlesohn *et al.*, 1989). Transgenic mice have been constructed which express the receptor for poliovirus (Ren and Racaniello, 1992). Infection of these mice via the intramuscular, intracerebral, or even intraperitoneal routes with wild type poliovirus results in infection, paralysis, and death. However, it has not been possible to demonstrate paralysis when the wild-type virus was given to the mice via intragastric or any other mucosal route.

We have exploited the poliovirus receptor transgenic mice to analyze the immune response generated by intramuscular administration of the replicons alone, that is, without infectious poliovirus. For these studies, we have utilized replicons which express regions of the HIV-1 Gag and envelope (Moldoveanu *et al.*, 1995) or, in a separate study, the gene encoding the carcinoembryonic antigen (Ansardi *et al.*, 1994). To test the immunogenicity of these replicons, we utilized intramuscular injection followed by the measurement of serum antibody against the foreign protein. The results of our studies established that after the third injection of encapsidated replicons, a clear serum antibody response was observed against HIV-1 Gag or envelope proteins. The antibody response to poliovirus has a profile similar to that observed for the recombinant antigen (Fig. 4). Therefore, the results of these studies demonstrate that it is possible to administer intramuscularly the encapsidated replicons alone and induce an antibody response against the vector (poliovirus) and the expressed protein (HIV-1 Gag).

Recently, we have evaluated different routes of in-

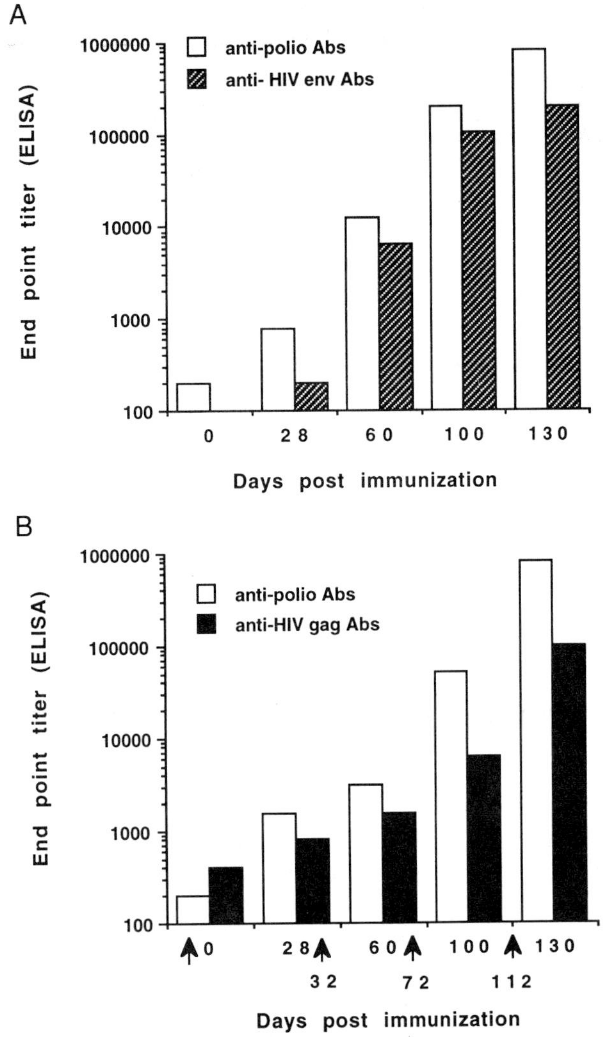

Figure 4. Serum antibody response to replicons. Antibodies induced in transgenic mice after immunization with encapsidated replicons expressing HIV-1 Gag or envelope. Transgenic mice were immunized intramuscularly four times (denoted by arrow) at monthly intervals with approximately 10^6 infectious units of encapsidated poliovirus replicon, expressing HIV-1 envelope (A) or Gag (B); 28 days after each injection, the collected serum (pool of four or five mice) was analyzed for specific antibodies against poliovirus type 1, as well as HIV-1 Gag or envelope antigens. The results are expressed as endpoint titer.

TABLE I

Susceptibility of Transgenic Mice to Poliovirus Infection

Mouse group	Route of administration	Remarks
1	Systemic (intratongue)	All five mice died in 7 days.
2	Systemic (intraperitoneal)	Four mice died in 8 days; one survivor had immune response at 10 days postinfection (serum end-point titer ELISA: 102,400 vs preimmune 3200).
3	Systemic [intramuscular (thigh)]	All mice showed signs of paralysis at 3 days, and died at 5 days postinfection.
4	Intragastric	All mice survived with no sign of sickness. Immune responses were measured in sera and secretions.
5	Intranasal	
6	Intrarectal	

Note. Poliovirus type I (Mahoney) was administered to Tg mice at a dose of 10^7 pfu/mouse by the indicated route.

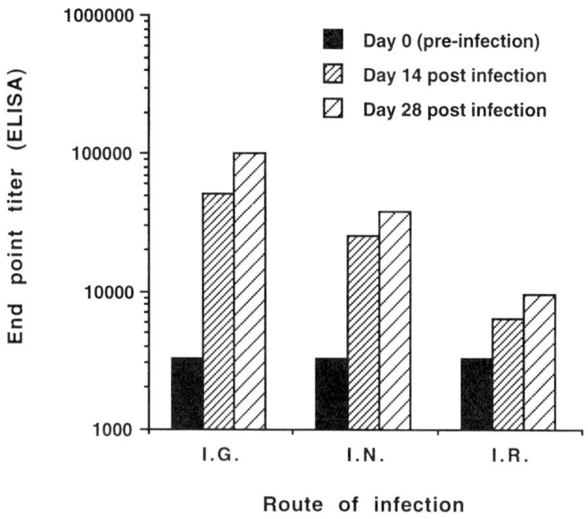

Figure 5. Antibodies in sera of mice given poliovirus type 1 Mahoney. Antibodies against poliovirus type 1 (Mahoney), in sera of transgenic mice infected with 10^7 pfu of poliovirus by various mucosal routes: intragastric (I.G.), intranasal (I.N.), or intrarectal (I.R.). Serum anti-poliovirus antibodies were measured 14 and 28 days postinfection. The ELISA results are presented as end point titer.

fection of the transgenic mice with wild type poliovirus type 1 for the capacity to generate an anti-poliovirus antibody response. For these studies, we have utilized intramuscular, intraperitoneal, intragastric, intrarectal, and intranasal inoculations. We have found that intramuscular as well as intraperitoneal injection with wild-type poliovirus results in paralysis and death of the transgenic mice, while administration by the intranasal, intragastric, or intrarectal routes does not exhibit paralysis (Table I). In the surviving mice, the antibody response to poliovirus in the serum as well as secretions was measured. A serum antibody response to poliovirus was evident in the mice given the virus via the intragastric or intranasal route; no clear response was seen in the serum of the mice given poliovirus by the intrarectal route (Fig. 5). More importantly, IgA anti-poliovirus antibodies in saliva, feces, and vaginal washes were detected in mice given the virus via the intragastric or intranasal routes (Fig. 6). Taken together, the results of these studies demonstrate that it is feasible to stimulate an immune response in the transgenic mice when poliovirus is given by these alternative mucosal routes. Fur-

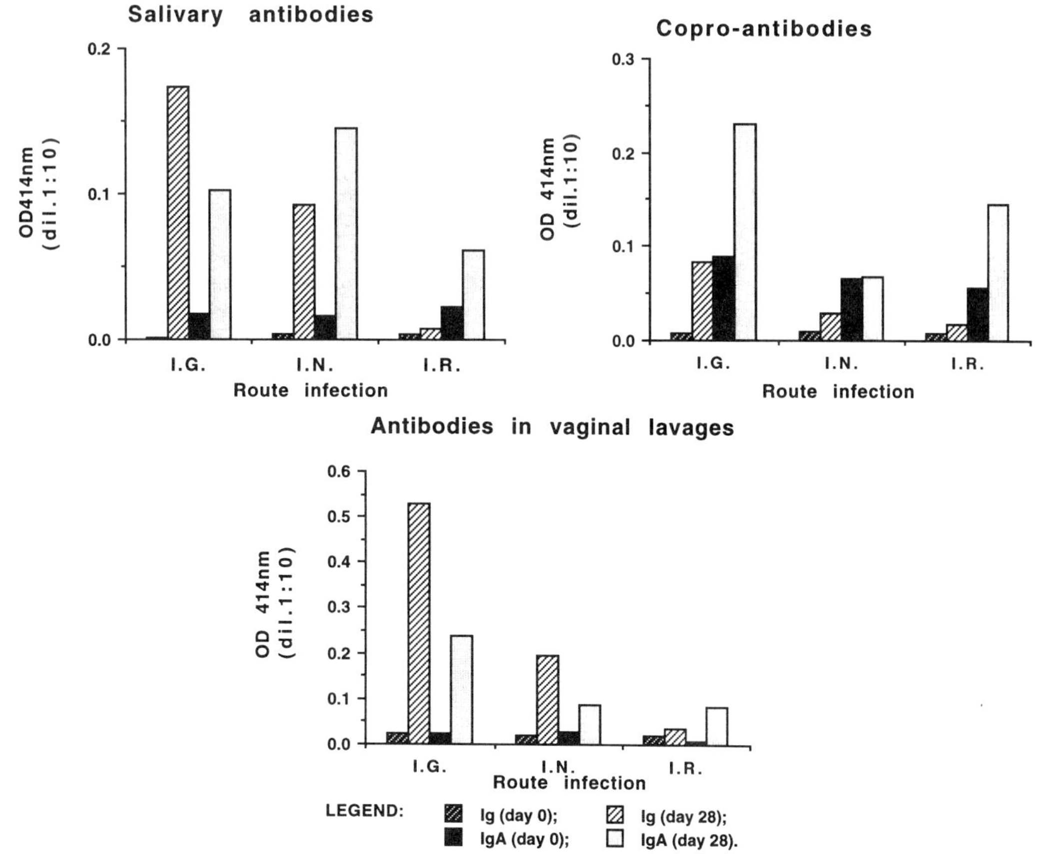

Figure 6. Anti-poliovirus antibodies in secretions of mice given poliovirus type 1 Mahoney. The IgA anti-poliovirus type 1 antibodies were analyzed in the saliva, feces (copro-antibodies), and vaginal washes of infected mice as previously described (I.G., intragastric; I.N., intranasal; I.R., intrarectal). The levels of poliovirus specific antibody (total Ig and IgA) in secretions were measured by solid-phase ELISA (Moldoveanu *et al.*, 1995). The data are presented as the OD^{414nm} at a fixed dilution (1:10) of samples.

ther studies will analyze the immune response induced by the encapsidated replicons passaged in the presence of poliovirus given via these mucosal routes. We anticipate that it will be possible to evaluate the capacity of the replicons to stimulate mucosal immunity using this system.

V. Perspectives

In this review we have described our studies on the development and characterization of an expression system based on poliovirus. For these studies, we have made use of the fact that we can delete regions of the poliovirus genome corresponding to the capsids to substitute foreign genes. To date, we have expressed a wide array of genes including those for HIV and SIV *gag* and *env*, SIV-*nef*, carcinoembryonic antigen, HER2/neu oncogene, β-galactosidase, firefly luciferase, and tetanus toxin C fragment. We have found that complementation of these defective genomes with the poliovirus capsid protein *in trans* results in the encapsidation of these replicons. Utilizing serial passage in the presence of a vaccinia virus, VV-P1, which provides the poliovirus capsid protein *in trans,* results in the establishment of stocks of these encapsidated replicons. We have demonstrated that these replicons are immunogenic when given in combination with poliovirus via several different routes. In addition, the encapsidated replicons alone are immunogenic when given intramuscularly to transgenic mice which contain the receptor for poliovirus. Current studies are exploring different methods and routes to deliver these encapsidated replicons to the transgenic mice. Preliminary results indicate that it might be possible to deliver these replicons via the intragastric or intranasal routes to stimulate specific antibody responses in secretions. Future studies will be directed at further characterizing the humoral and cellular immune responses, as well as developing different methods for administration of the encapsidated replicons.

Acknowledgments

MIA was supported by NIH Training Grant AI 07150. This research was supported by a grant from the Pediatric AIDS Foundations (50449-l5-PG), a National Cooperative Vaccine Development grant (AI28147), and a grant from the NIH (AI 25005) to C.D.M.

References

Alexander, L., Lu, H. H., Gromeier, M., and Wimmer, E. (1994). Strategies for inducing and evaluation mucosal immunity. *AIDS Res. Hum. Retroviruses.* **10,** S57–S66.

Anderson, M. J., Porter D. C., Fultz, P. N., and Morrow, C. D. (1996). Poliovirus replicons that express the Gag or the envelope surface protein of simian immunodeficiency virus SIV_{smm} PBJ14. *Virology* **219,** 140–149.

Ansardi, D. C., Porter, D. C., and Morrow, C. D. (1991). Coinfection with recombinant vaccinia virus expressing poliovirus P1 and P3 proteins results in polyprotein processing and formation of empty capsid structures. *J. Virol.* **65,** 2088–2092.

Ansardi, D. C., Porter D. C., and Morrow, C. D. (1993). Complementation of a poliovirus defective genome by a recombinant vaccinia virus which provides poliovirus P1 capsid precursor in *trans. J. Virol.* **67,** 3684–3690.

Ansardi, D.C., Z. Moldoveanu, D.C. Porter, D.E. Walker, Conry, A.F. LoBuglio, S. McPherson and C.D. Morrow. (1994). Characterization of poliovirus replicons encoding carcinoembryonic antigen. *Cancer Res.,* **54,** 6359–6364.

Armstrong, C. (1939). The experimental transmission of poliomyelitis to the Eastern cotton rat, *Sigmodon hispiders. Public Health Rep.* **54,** 1719–1721.

Arnold, E., Luo, M., Vriend, G., Rossman, M. G., Palmenberg, A. C., Parks, G. D., Nicklin, M. J. H., and Wimmer, E. (1987). Implications of the picornavirus capsid structure for polyprotein processing. *Proc. Natl. Acad. Sci. U.S.A.* **84,** 21–25.

Choi, W. S., Pal-Ghosh, R., and Morrow, C. D. (1991). Expression of human immunodeficiency virus type 1 (HIV-1) *gag, pol,* and *env* proteins from chimeric HIV-1-poliovirus minireplicons. *J. Virol.* **65,** 2875–2883.

Cole, C. N., Smoler, D., Wimmer, E., and Baltimore, D. (1971). Defective interfering particles of poliovirus. I. Isolation and physical properties. *J. Virol.* **7,** 478–485.

Eldridge, J. H., Gilley, R. M., Staas, J. K., Moldoveanu, Z., Meulbroek, J. A., and Tice, T. R. (1989). Biodegradable microspheres: Vaccine delivery system for oral immunization. *Curr. Top. Microbiol. Immun.* **146,** 59–66.

Graham, S., Wang, E.C.Y., Jenkins, O., and Borysiewicz, L. K. (1993). Analysis of the human T-cell response to picornaviruses: Identification of T-cell epitopes close to B-cell epitopes in poliovirus. *J. Virol.* **67,** 1627–1637.

Hagino-Yamagishi, K., and Nomoto, A. (1989). *In vitro* construction of poliovirus defective interfering particles. *J. Virol.* **63,** 5386–5392.

Hanecak, R., Semler, B. L., Anderson, C. W., and Wimmer, E. (1982). Proteolytic processing of poliovirus polypeptides: Antibodies to polypeptide P3–7c inhibit cleavage of glutamine–glycine pairs. *Proc. Natl. Acad. Sci.* U.S.A. **79,** 3973–3977.

Hanecak, R., Semler, B. L., Ariga, H., Anderson, C. W., Wimmer, E. (1984). Expression of a cloned gene segment of poliovirus in *E. coli*: Evidence for autocatalytic production of the viral proteinase. Cell (*Cambridge, Mass.*) **37,** 1063–1073.

Hanson, L. A., Carlsson, B., Jalil, F., Lindblad, B. S., Khan, S. R., and van Wezel, A. L. (1984). Different secretory IgA antibody responses after immunization with inactivated and live poliovirus vaccines. *Rev. Infect. Dis.* **6,** S356–S360.

Harris, K. S., Hellen, C. U. T., and Wimmer, E. (1990). Proteolytic processing in the replication of picornaviruses. *Semin. Virol.* **1**, 323–333.

Hellen, C. U. T., and Wimmer, E. (1992). The role of proteolytic processing in the morphogenesis of virus particles. *Experientia* **48**, 201–215.

Hogle, J. M., Chow, M., and Filman, D. F. (1985). Three-dimensional structure of poliovirus at 2.9 A resolution. Science **229**, 1358–1365.

Horstmann, D. M., Niederman, I. C., and Paul, J. R. (1959). Attenuated type I poliovirus disease: Capacity to infect and spread from "vaccinees" within institutional populations. *JAMA, J. Am. Med. Assoc.* **170**, 1–8.

Jacobson, M. F., and Baltimore, D. (1968). Morphogenesis of poliovirus. I. Association of the viral RNA with the coat protein. *J. Mol. Biol.* **33**, 369–378.

Jacobson, M. F., Asso, J., and Baltimore, D. (1970). Further evidence on the formation of poliovirus. *J. Mol. Biol.* **49**, 657–669.

Jore, J., Degues, B., Jackson, J., Pouwels, P. H., and Enger-Valk, B. (1988). Poliovirus protein 3CD is the active protease for processing of the precursor protein P1 *in vitro*. *J. Gen. Virol.* **69**, 1627–1636.

Kajigaya, S., Arakawa, H., Kuge, S., Koi, T., Imura, N., and Nomoto, A. (1985). Isolation and characterization of defective-interfering particles of poliovirus Sabin 1 strain. *Virology* **142**, 307–316.

Kaplan, G., and Racaniello, V. R. (1988). Construction and characterization of poliovirus subgenomic replicons. *J. Virol.* **62**, 1687–1696.

Kitamura, N., Semler, B. L., Rothberg, P. G., Larsen, G. R., Adler, C. J., Dorner, A. J., Emini, E. A., Hanecak, R., Lee, J. J., van der Werf, S., Anderson, C. W., and Wimmer, E. (1981). Primary structure, gene organization and polypeptide expression of poliovirus RNA. *Nature (London)* **291**, 547–553.

Koch, F., and Koch, G. (1985). "The Molecular Biology of Poliovirus." Springer-Verlag, Vienna.

Kuge, S., Saito, I., and Nomoto, A. (1986). Primary structure of poliovirus defective-interfering particle genomes and possible generation mechanisms of the particles. *J. Mol. Biol.* **192**, 473–487.

La Monica, N., Meriam, C., and Racaniello, V. R. (1986). Mapping of sequences required for mouse neurovirulence of poliovirus type 2 Lansing. *J. Virol.* **57**, 515–525.

Lu, H.-H., Alexander, L., and Wimmer, E. (1995). Construction and genetic analysis of dicistronic polioviruses containing open reading frames for epitopes of human immunodeficiency virus type 1 gp120. *J. Virol.* **69**, 4797–4806.

McGhee, J. R., and Mestecky, J. (1992). The mucosal immune system in HIV infection and prospects for mucosal immunity to AIDS. *AIDS Res. Rev.* **2**, 289–312.

Mackett, M., Smith, G. L., and Moss, B. (1985). The construction and characterization of vaccinia virus recombinants expressing foreign genes. *In* "Cloning," D. M. Glover, ed., Vol. 2, pp. 191–212. IRL Press, Oxford.

Mendelsohn, C., Wimmer, E., and Racaniello, V. R. (1989). Cellular receptor for poliovirus: Molecular cloning, nucleotide sequence and expression of a new member of the immunoglobulin superfamily. *Cell (Cambridge, Mass.)* **56**, 855–865.

Mestecky, J. (1988). The common mucosal immune system and current strategies for induction of immune responses in external secretions. *J. Clin. Immunol.* **7**, 265–276.

Mestecky, J., and McGhee, J. R. (1987). Immunoglobulin A (IgA): Molecular and cellular interactions involved in IgA biosynthesis and immune response. *Adv. Immunol.* **40**, 153–245.

Michalek, S. M., Childers, N. K., Katz, J., Denys, F. R., Berry, A. K., Eldridge, J. H., McGhee, J. R., and Curtiss III, R. (1989). Liposomes and oral adjuvants. *Curr. Top. Microbiol. Immun.* **146**, 51–58.

Moldoveanu, Z., Novak, M., Hunag, W.-Q., Gilley, T. M., Staas, J. K., Schafer, D., Compans, R. W., and Mestecky, J. (1993). Oral immunization with influenza virus in biodegradable microspheres. *J. Infect. Dis.* **167**, 84–90.

Moldoveanu, Z., Porter, D. C., Lu, A., McPherson, S., and Morrow, C. D. (1995). Immune responses induced by administration of encapsidated poliovirus replicons which express HIV-1 gag and envelope proteins. *Vaccine* **13**, 1013–1022.

Morrow, C. D., Porter, D. C., Ansardi, D. A., Moldoveanu, Z., and Fultz, P. N. (1994). New approaches for mucosal vaccines for AIDS: Encapsidation and serial passage of poliovirus replicons that express HIV-1 proteins upon infection. *AIDS Res. Hum. Retroviruses* **10**, (Suppl. 2) S61–S66.

Moss, B. (1990). Poxvividae and their replication. *In* "Virology" (B. N. Fields *et al.*, eds.), 2nd Ed. Raven, New York.

Moss, B. (1991). Vaccinia virus: A tool for research and vaccine development. Science. **252**, 1662–1667.

Nicklin, M. J. H., Krausslich, H. G., Toyoda, H., Dunn, J. J., and Wimmer E. (1987). Poliovirus polypeptide precursors: Expression *in vitro* and processing by exogenous 3C and 2A proteinases. *Proc. Natl. Acad. Sci. U.S.A.* **84**, 4002–4006.

Ogra, P. L. (1984). Mucosal immune response to poliovirus vaccines in childhood. *Rev. Infect. Dis.* **6**, S361–S368.

Ogra, P. L., and Karzon, D. T. (1971). Formation and function of poliovirus antibody in different tissues. *Prog. Med. Virol.* **13**, 156–193.

Ogra, P. L., Karzon, D. T., Righthand, F., and MacGillivray, M. (1968). Immunoglobulin response in serum and secretions after immunization with live and inactivated poliovaccine and natural infection. *N. Engl. J. Med.* **279**, 893–900.

Ogra, P. L., and Ogra, S. S. (1973). Local antibody response to poliovaccine in the human female genital tract. *J. Immunol.* **110**, 1307–1311.

Palmenberg, A. C. (1990). Proteolytic processing of picornaviral polyprotein. *Annu Rev. Microbiol.* **44**, 603–623.

Pelletier, J., and Sonenberg, N. (1988). Internal initiation of translation of eukaryotic mRNA directed by a sequence from poliovirus RNA. *Nature (London)* **334**, 32–35.

Porter, D. C., Ansardi, D. C., Choi, W. S., and Morrow C. D. (1993). Encapsidation of genetically engineered poliovirus minireplicons which express human immunodeficiency virus type 1 gag and pol proteins upon infection. *J. Virol.* **67**, 3712–3719.

Porter, D. C., Ansardi, D. C., and Morrow, C. D. (1995).

Encapsidation of poliovirus replicons encoding the complete human immunodeficiency virus type 1 *gag* gene using a complementation system which provides the P1 capsid protein *in trans*. *J. Virol.* **69**, 1548–1555.

Porter, D. C., Melsen, L. R., Compans, R. W., and Morrow, C. D. (1996). Release of virus-like particles from cells infected with poliovirus replicons which express HIV-1 Gag. *J. Virol.* **70**, 2643–2649.

Putnak, J. R., and Phillips, B. A. (1981). Picornaviral structure and assembly. *Microbiol. Rev.* **45**, 287–315.

Racaniello, V. R., and Baltimore, D. (1981a). Molecular cloning of poliovirus DNA and determination of the complete nucleotide sequence of the viral genome. *Proc. Natl. Acad. Sci. U.S.A.* **78**, 4887–4891.

Racaniello, V. R., and Baltimore, D. (1981b). Cloned poliovirus complementary DNA is infectious in mammalian cells. *Science* **214**, 916–919.

Ren, R., and Racaniello, V. R. (1992). Poliovirus spreads from muscle to the central nervous system by neural pathways. *J. Infect. Dis.* **166**, 747–752.

Ren, R., Constantini, F. C., Gorgacz, E. J., Lee, J. J., and Racaniello, V. R. (1990). Transgenic mice expressing a human poliovirus receptor: A new model for poliomyelitis. *Cell (Cambridge, Mass.)* **63**, 353–362.

Rueckert, R. R. (1990). Picornaviridae and their replication. "Virology" (B. M. Fields *et al.*, eds.), 2nd Ed., pp. 507–548. Raven, New York.

Rueckert, R., and Wimmer, E. (1984). Systematic nomenclature for picornavirus proteins. *J. Virol.* **50**, 957–959.

Sabin, A. B., and Boulger, L. R. (1973). History of Sabin attenuated poliovirus oral live vaccine strains. *J. Biol. Stand.* **1**, 115–118.

Sanders, D. Y. and Cramlett, H. G. (1974). Antibody titers to polioviruses in patients ten years after immunization with Sabin vaccine. *J. Pediatr.* **84**, 406–408.

Semler, B. L., Dorner, A. J., and Wimmer, E. (1984). Production of infectious poliovirus from cloned cDNA is dramatically increased by SV40 transcription and replication signals. *Nucleic Acids Res.* **12**, 5123–5141.

Simmons, J., Kutubuddin, M., and Chow, M. (1993). Characterization of poliovirus-specific T lymphocytes in the peripheral blood of Sabin-vaccinated humans. *J. Virol.* **67**, 1262–1268.

Toyoda, H., Nicklin, M. J. H., Murray, M. G., Anderson, C. W., Dunn, J. J., Studier, F. W., and Wimmer, E. (1986). A second virus-encoded proteinase involved in proteolytic processing of poliovirus polyprotein. *Cell (Cambridge, Mass.)* **45**, 761–770.

Wimmer, E. (1982). Genome-linked proteins of viruses. *Cell (Cambridge, Mass.)* **28**, 199–201.

Wimmer, E., Kuhn, R. J., Pincus, S., Yang, C.-F., Toyoda, H., Nicklin, M. J. H., and Takeda, N. (1987). Molecular events leading to picornavirus genome replication. *J. Cell Sci.* **7**(Suppl.), 251–276.

Wimmer, E., Hellen, C. U. T., and Cao, X. (1993). Genetics of poliovirus. *Annu. Rev. Genet.* **27**, 353–436.

Ypma-Wong, M. F., and Semler, B. (1987). Processing determinants required for *in vitro* cleavage of the poliovirus P1 precursor to capsid proteins. *J. Virol.* **61**, 3181–3189.

Ypma-Wong, M. F., Dewalt, P. G., Johnson, V. H., Lamb, J. G., and Semler, B. L. (1988). Protein 3CD is the major poliovirus proteinase responsible for cleavage of the P1 capsid precursor. *Virology* **166**, 265–270.

11

Recombinant Adenoviruses as Vectors for Mucosal Immunity

KENNETH L. ROSENTHAL
KAREN F.T. COPELAND
W. SCOTT GALLICHAN
Molecular Virology and Immunology Program
Departments of Pathology and Biology
McMaster University
Hamilton, Ontario L8N 3Z5, Canada

I. Introduction

In recent years, adenovirus (Ad) vectors have been used for the expression of foreign genes in mammalian cells (Berkner, 1992; Graham and Prevec, 1991), and have been studied as recombinant vaccine vectors (Graham and Prevec, 1992; Imler, 1995) and, more recently, as gene transfer vectors for gene therapy (Siegfried, 1993; Trapnell, 1993; Kozarsky and Wilson, 1993; Bramson *et al.*, 1995a). A number of properties make the Ad system a good candidate for each of these applications, not the least of which is the extensive body of information regarding their structure and biology that has been gained through their use as a model system for studying all aspects of gene expression and DNA replication. This has led to the establishment of straightforward methods to construct recombinant adenovirus vectors. Adenoviruses have sufficiently high cloning capacity to accomodate most foreign DNA sequences. Once generated, adenovirus recombinants are stable, can be grown to high titers, and are easily purified. Adenovirus vectors can be rendered replication-defective, which will contribute to their safe application. Both replicating and quiescent cells can be infected with adenoviruses, which can deliver DNA with high efficency both *in vitro* and *in vivo*. As a live vaccine candidate, adenoviruses have an established and proven track record. Ad vaccines based on serotypes 4 and 7 have proven safe and effective when administered to millions of military recruits over the last 30 years. Most importantly for their application as mucosal vaccines, adenoviruses can be administered mucosally. Indeed, oral administration with enteric-coated capsules containing both lyophilized serotypes produces an asymptomatic intestinal infection inducing protection against Ad-induced acute respiratory disease. These properties have contributed to the interest in recombinant Ads as potential live mucosal vaccines.

II. Adenoviruses and Their Molecular Biology

Human adenoviruses were first isolated over four decades ago by Rowe *et al.*, (1953) as a transmissible agent responsible for the degeneration of primary cultures of tonsil and adenoidal tissues. Since then, over 47 distinct human adenovirus serotypes have been identified. These have been classified into six subgroups (A–F) based on a number of biological, chemical, immunological, and structural criteria (Ginsberg, 1984; Straus, 1984; Horwitz, 1990a). The best characterized serotypes to date have been Ad2 and Ad5 (subgroup C), Ad7 (subgroup B), and Ad 12 (subgroup A). Ad12 was the first serotype reported to have the potential to induce tumors in newborn rodents (Trentin *et al.*, 1962; Huebner *et al.*, 1962), but Ads have never been linked to naturally occurring malignancies in any animal and surveys of human tumours have failed to find any virus-specific sequences (Gilden *et al.*, 1970; McAllister *et al.*, 1972; Mackey *et al.*, 1976; Graham 1984).

The various Ad serotypes can infect and replicate at a number of locations in the body including the upper respiratory tract, the gastrointestinal tract, the eye, and the urinary bladder (Straus, 1984; Horwitz, 1990b). Only about one-third of the serotypes are associated with disease in humans while most infections are subclinical. Infection with adenovirus usually results in mild respiratory illness with symptoms including rhinorrhea, nasal congestion, sneezing, or pharyngoconjunctivitis characterized by fever, sore throat, and conjunctivitis (Horwitz, 1990b). The pathogenesis and pathology of the various Ad serotypes have been reviewed by Horwitz (1990b).

Adenoviruses are nonenveloped, icosahedral viruses containing a linear double-stranded DNA as their genome. The virus life cycle is divided into two phases, early and late, corresponding to events before and after the initiation of viral DNA replication (reviewed in Horwitz, 1990a). In early infection, transcription from the early (E) regions E1a, E1b, E2-4, results in the generation of over 30 messages. Late gene expression occurs at approximately 8 hr postinfection, generates most of the viral structural proteins, and is largely driven by the major late promoter (MLP).

The E1a region encodes gene products which mediate transactivation of viral and cellular genes (Jones and Shenk, 1978; Berk *et al.*, 1979; Nevins *et al.*, 1981, 1982), transformation of cells in culture (Branton *et al.*, 1985; Whyte *et al.*, 1988) and cellular DNA synthesis and mitosis (Zerler *et al.*, 1987; Bellett *et al.*, 1989; Howe *et al.*, 1990; Howe and Bayley, 1992). In addition, E1a and E1b gene products are necessary for high-efficiency transformation of rodent cells (Graham, 1984; Branton *et al.*, 1985; McLorie *et al.*, 1991). The E2 region of Ad encodes proteins required for viral replication, while E4 gene products (Falgout and Ketner, 1987) are necessary for the transition from early to late expression (reviewed in Berkner, 1988).

Proteins encoded by the E3 region appear to play an important role in evasion of host cell-mediated immune responses *in vivo* (reviewed in Wold and Gooding, 1991; Mullbacher, 1992). This is supported by the fact that although the E3 region is dispensable for growth *in vitro* (Anderson *et al.*, 1976; Berker and Sharp, 1983), it is maintained in natural isolates. The gp19K protein, encoded by the E3, noncovalently associates with the heavy chain of class I major histocompatibility complex (MHC) molecules and blocks transport of class I antigens to the cell surface (Andersson *et al.*, 1985; Burgert and Kvist, 1985, 1987; Cox *et al.*, 1991; Lippe *et al.*, 1991). This decreases the efficiency of viral antigen presentation and recognition by cytotoxic T lymphocytes (CTL). In addition, the E3 14.7K and 10.4/14.5K Ad proteins protect infected mouse and human cells against lysis by tumor necrosis factor (TNF) (Gooding *et al.*, 1988, 1990, 1991).

Adenoviruses have a restricted host range and do not replicate to the same extent in all cells. Human Ads grow well in most human epithelial cells and in some human fibroblast cell lines which are permissive for replication, but can exhibit poor or nonpermissive replication in other cell types, such as human peripheral blood lymphocytes (Horvath and Weber, 1988), African green monkey (Klessig, 1984), rhesus macaque, mouse, and canine cells (Graham and Prevec, 1992). Although adenoviruses cannot undergo fully permissive replication in all cell types, they are still able to infect a wide variety of cells, both dividing and quiescent (Graham and Prevec, 1992).

III. Construction of Recombinant Adenovirus Vectors

The ease of manipulation of Ad combined with well-characterized methods for generating Ad recombinants (Graham and Prevec, 1991), has helped to define Ad as an attractive gene delivery system. The construction of Ad recombinants involves the introduction of foreign DNA sequences into the adenovirus genome. Ad virions can package up to 105% of the wild-type genome (Bett *et al.*, 1993), which represents 2 kb of additional foreign DNA. Three regions of the Ad genome have been used to accept insertions of foreign DNA, the E1 and E3 regions and a region between E4 and the right inverted terminal repeat (ITR) (reviewed in Graham and Prevec, 1991, 1992). In order to insert larger fragments, compensating deletions must be made in the Ad genome. The two regions most commonly deleted to accommodate larger inserts are E1 and E3. Deletion of the E1 region produces conditional helper-independent viruses that must be grown in complementing 293 cells which contain and express the left end of the Ad genome (Graham *et al.*, 1977). Up to 3 kb can be deleted from E1 with a replacement insertion of 5 kb of foreign DNA. The deletion cannot, however, include coding sequences for protein IX, a structural protein required for the packaging of full-length virus (Ghosh-Choudhury *et al.*, 1987). Foreign genes inserted in the E1 deletion must be driven by a promoter introduced as part of the insert. Further, the level of expression obtained from inserts in the E1 region can be dependent on the orientation of the insert. Generally, higher levels of expression can be obtained when inserts are oriented so that transcription is E1 parallel (Hitt *et al.*, 1995). Xu *et al.* (1995) investigated the expression of a rotavirus antigen, VP7sc, under the control of a variety of commonly used promoters carried in E1-substituted cell Ad vectors in both permissive and nonpermissive cells. Their results clearly indicated that in the absence of virus replication, gene cassette orientation and the choice of promoter were critical to the level and kinetics of expression of VP7sc (Xu *et al.*, 1995). Significant differences in the efficiency of expression were also observed in cells from different species. These results have important implications for construction and testing of replication-deficient E1-substituted Ad recombinants.

In contrast, the E3 region is not required for viral replication *in vitro* (Klessig, 1984; Anderson *et al.*,

1976; Berkner and Sharp, 1983) and can be deleted to generate nonconditional helper-independent viruses that can replicate in any normally permissive cells (Berkner and Sharp, 1983). Generally, in the E3 region, 1.9 kb can be deleted and replaced with 4 kb of foreign DNA. Although the SV40 promoter was introduced as part of the expression cassette in many early replication-competent vectors with inserts in the E3 region, inclusion of heterologous promoters is not required with inserts in the left-to-right orientation, since expression is efficiently driven by the upstream major late promoter (MLP) or E3 promoters (Morin *et al.*, 1987; Graham and Prevec, 1992). Recombinant Ad systems have recently been constructed in which both E1 and E3 regions are deleted and may be replaced by up to 8.3 kb of DNA to create an additional class of conditional helper-independent viruses (Bett *et al.*, 1994).

A number of strategies have been developed to construct Ad vectors which all involve the manipulation of subgenomic fragments of the Ad genome (reviewed in Berkner, 1988, 1992; Graham and Prevec, 1991, 1995). Strategies currently used involve recombination between two plasmids which together contain sequences composing the entire Ad genome but are noninfectious separately. A number of plasmid systems have been developed for rescuing inserts into E1 (McGrory *et al.*, 1988) or E3 (Ghosh-Choudhury *et al.*, 1986; Mittal *et al.*, 1993). The steps involved in rescuing foreign inserts into Ad are basically the same for all the above-mentioned systems. Briefly, the gene of interest plus appropriate regulatory sequences are first introduced into a shuttle plasmid containing a subsegment of the viral genome. This shuttle plasmid will contain either right or left end viral sequences with appropriate deletions and cloning sites into which the foreign gene can be inserted. The next step involves cotransfection of the recombinant plasmid into mammalian cells, usually 293 cells, with overlapping viral DNA sequences that can reconstitute an infectious viral genome. Recombinant virus is then generated through recombination between the cotransfected plasmids or plasmid and viral DNA in the recipient cells. Methods to construct Ad recombinants have recently been reviewed by Graham and Prevec (1995) and Hitt *et al.* (1995).

IV. Adenovirus as a Vaccine Vector

In addition to the extensive understanding of the structure and biology of adenoviruses there are other features that make Ad vectors an excellent system for the expression of foreign genes, especially for use as recombinant viral vaccines. As described above, relatively straightforward methods to construct recombinant Ads are well established that can accommodate inserts of up to 8.3 kb, a size which should accommodate most genes along with regulatory sequences. Further, high-level expression can be obtained from inserts in both proliferating and quiescent cells, and the virus infects cells from a variety of animals including human and other primates, canine, bovine, and rodent. High-titered stocks can be readily and inexpensively produced. Ad recombinants also appear to be stable, with no subsequent loss or rearrangement during successive rounds of replication.

Recombinant Ads have also proven effective in inducing both humoral and cell-mediated immune responses to their expressed antigens in vaccinated animals and, in many cases, to protect the animals from lethal challenge (Berkner, 1992; Imler, 1995). The greater majority of these constructs have substituted the E3 region of Ad with foreign genes. These include glycoproteins of vesicular stomatitis virus (VSV) (Prevec *et al.*, 1989), rabies virus (Prevec *et al.*, 1990; Charlton *et al.*, 1992), herpes simplex virus (HSV) (McDermott *et al.*, 1989a; Zheng *et al.*, 1993), and hepatitis B virus (HBV) (Morin *et al.*, 1987; Levrero *et al.*, 1991). Vectors expressing VSV or rabies glycoprotein raised high levels of virus-neutralizing antibody in mice and induced protection from challenge with VSV given intravenously (iv) (Prevec *et al.*, 1989) or rabies virus intracerebrally (Prevec *et al.*, 1990). Two of four rhesus macaque monkeys given two subcutaneous inoculations of a vector containing human immunodeficiency virus type 1 (HIV-1) p24 in the E3 region developed measurable levels of serum anti-p24 antibodies (Prevec *et al.*, 1991). Recombinant Ad4, 5, and 7 vectors expressing either HIV envelope glycoprotein (gp120) or *gag* genes in E3 were found to be immunogenic in chimpanzees immunized by the oral and intranasal routes, inducing low-titer neutralizing antibodies, secretory IgA antibodies, and T-cell responses (Lubeck *et al.*, 1994; Natuk *et al.*, 1993).

A replication-defective Ad5 recombinant containing the gene for tick-born encephalitis virus (TBEV) nonstructural protein (NS1) in E1 under the control of the HCMV promoter was able to induce a good antibody response to the protein in mice and protect them from challenge with TBEV (Jacobs *et al.*, 1992). A similar E1 replacement vector containing measles virus nucleocapsid protein driven by the HCMV promoter was shown to induce good humoral and MHC class I-restricted antigen-specific cytotoxic T lymphocyte (CTL) responses and protection against challenge with measles virus in i.p.-immunized mice (Fooks *et al.*, 1995).

The success obtained in expressing foreign genes in recombinant adenoviruses, the extensive use and documented safety of Ad4 and Ad7 as human vaccines, the numerous examples of efficient elicitation of both humoral and cell-mediated immune responses, and particularly the demonstration of the development of mucosal immunity (Gallichan *et al.*, 1993) by adenovirus vectors indicate that this system may have potential application in the production of safe, effective, recombinant vaccines for protection against a variety of mucosally/sexually transmitted viruses.

V. Induction of Mucosal Immunity by Adenoviruses

Adenoviruses have proven to be excellent mucosal vaccine vectors. Unattenuated adenovirus type 4 and 7 vaccines have been administered orally in enteric-coated capsules to millions of U.S. and Canadian military recruits and have proven effective in preventing adenovirus-induced acute respiratory disease without evidence of adverse reactions (Top *et al.*, 1971a; Top, 1975; Chaloner-Larsson *et al.*, 1986). When Ad4 and Ad7 were orally administered, 70–82% of the vaccinees given Ad4 developed neutralizing antibodies (Chanock *et al.*, 1966), while individuals given a placebo were susceptible to infection (Edmonston *et al.*, 1966). Oral type 1, 2, and 5 Ad vaccines have also been evaluated and shown to be safe in volunteers during a clinical trial (Schwartz *et al.*, 1974). Evidence that recombinant adenovirus vectors target mucosal tissues was obtained by the transfer of normal copies of both the human cystic fibrosis transmembrane conductance regulator gene and the α1-antitrypsin gene to airway epithelium of cotton rats (Rosenfeld *et al.*, 1991, 1992). In order to acheive effective immunity against mucosally and sexually transmitted viruses, such as HSV or HIV, it may be necessary to immunize mucosal surfaces.

Previously, we used a replication-competent recombinant Ad vector, designated AdgB8, that produced high-level expression of herpes simplex virus type 1 (HSV-1) glycoprotein B (gB) (Johnson *et al.*, 1988) to demonstrate that gB was a major target recognized by murine H-2^b-restricted anti-HSV CTL (Witmer *et al.*, 1990). Indeed, we went on to use recombinant adenoviruses containing truncations and deletions of the gB gene to help identify a major epitope of gB recognized by anti-HSV CTL (Hanke *et al.*, 1991). Further, McDermott *et al.* (1989a) demonstrated that a single intraperitoneal (i.p.) inoculation of mice with recombinant Ad capable of expressing HSV-1 gB protected mice from a lethal systemic challenge with HSV-2. Since a major advantage of adenovirus-based vaccines is their utility as mucosal immunogens and since gB is a major target for both neutralizing antibodies and anti-HSV CTL, we set out to examine the induction of mucosal immune responses using this vector and to determine its ability to protect against a mucosal HSV infection.

Our initial studies compared different routes of administration of recombinant adenovirus expressing HSVgB. Interestingly, we demonstrated that intranasal (i.n.) immunization of mice with AdgB8 induced both serum anti-HSVgB IgG and secretory IgA in lung and nasal washes, whereas i.p. immunization did not elicit mucosal anti-HSVgB IgA (Gallichan *et al.*, 1993). IgA is an important component of the mucosal immune system (McGhee and Mestecky, 1990; McDermott and Bienenstock, 1979; Bienenstock and Befus, 1980; Phillips-Quagliata *et al.*, 1983; Butcher, 1988). In several animal models, the presence of specific IgA after mucosal immunization correlated with protection against mucosal virus challenge (Moldoveanu *et al.*, 1993; Meitin *et al.*, 1991; Nedrud *et al.*, 1986).

Cytotoxic T lymphocytes also play a central role in controlling the spread and severity of HSV infections (Larsen *et al.*, 1983; Sethi *et al.*, 1983; Wildy and Gell, 1985; Nash *et al.*, 1987) and may contribute significantly to local protection and clearance of virus. McDermott *et al.* (1989b) demonstrated that upon adoptive transfer, murine genital lymph node CTL, generated against an attenuated strain of HSV-2, preferentially migrated into genital tissue and provided resistance against genital infection with HSV-2. These results emphasize the importance of local mucosal T-cell responses in protection against HSV infection. In our study, splenic anti-HSV cytotoxic T lymphocytes (CTL) were generated after intranasal (i.n.) and i.p. immunization; however, there was a time-dependent decrease in the anti-HSV CTL activity from spleens of i.n.-immunized mice. Anti-HSV CTL were also present in the mediastinal lymph nodes that drain the lung after i.n. but not i.p. AdgB8 immunization (Gallichan *et al.*, 1993). Further, mice immunized i.n. with AdgB8 were protected against heterologous i.n. challenge with HSV-2, and this protection lasted longer than that of i.p.-immunized mice (Gallichan *et al.*, 1993). These results indicate that mucosal (i.n.) immunization with a recombinant adenovirus induced mucosal and systemic immune responses and provided long-term protection from mucosally transmitted virus.

We have extended these results and demonstrated that i.n. immunization of female mice with AdgB8 induced anti-HSVgB IgA and IgG in vaginal washes, whereas i.p. immunization only induced IgG, which appeared to be serum derived (Gallichan and Rosenthal, 1995). Interestingly, intravaginal (ivag) immunization with AdgB8 resulted in little or no anti-HSVgB IgA and only low levels of specific IgG in vaginal washes. Additionally, ivag boosting with AdgB8 did not significantly alter the serum or vaginal wash antibody responses in i.n.- or i.p.-immunized mice. These results indicate that i.n. immunization of mice with a recombinant adenovirus is an effective method for inducing specific immune responses at local and distant mucosal surfaces. Furthermore, it indicates that i.n. administration of Ad vectors expressing immunogenic antigens should serve as excellent vaccine candidates for STDs such as HSV or HIV. Indeed, one key property of an "ideal" AIDS vaccine includes a candidate that will induce local immunity in the genital tract.

More recently, we examined the effect of the estrous cycle on the titers of anti-HSVgB IgG and IgA in vaginal washes following i.n. immunization with AdgB8 (Gallichan and Rosenthal, 1996a). Interestingly, absolute titers of anti-HSVgB IgG and IgA were found to vary inversely with each other over the estrous cycle. Anti-gB IgG was detected at relatively high levels in vaginal washes during diestrus compared to estrus. In contrast, anti-gB IgA was found at relatively high levels during estrus compared to diestrus. Furthermore, we found that naive mice were only susceptible to intravaginal HSV-2 infection during diestrus (Gallichan and Rosenthal, 1996a). These results reflect the changes that occur in the female reproductive tract during the course of the estrous cycle. During estrus, or at the time of mating, the female genital tract is subjected to numerous pathogens (Parr and Parr, 1994; Tristram and Ogra, 1994; Profet, 1993). During this period specific IgA titers in vaginal washes were relatively high. Two hormonally controlled factors contribute to increased IgA levels: increased migration of plasma cells to the genital tract during estrus (McDermott *et al.*, 1980; Rachman *et al.*, 1983) and an increase in production of secretory component (s.c.) in the uterine epithelium (Parr and Parr, 1994; Wira *et al.*, 1994). The relative decrease in IgG during estrus is likely due, in part, to architectural changes in the epithelium of the vagina. These results have important implications for the development and evaluation of mucosal vaccines designed against sexually transmitted pathogens. In light of our observations, it is clear that the induction of both IgG and IgA in mucosal secretions is a requirement that vaccines will have to meet in order to maintain a blanket of humoral immunity in the female genital tract over the course of the reproductive cycle. Furthermore, evaluation of humoral immunity in the genital tract should take into account the fluctuations in the levels of immunity as a function of the estrous or menstrual cycle.

The induction and maintenance of long-term CTL memory at mucosal surfaces may be a critical component of protection against mucosal pathogens and is one goal toward development of effective mucosal vaccines. As mentioned above, we previously demonstrated that i.n. immunization with AdgB8 induced longer-term protection from mucosal challenge with heterologous HSV-2 than i.p. AdgB8 immunization (Gallichan *et al.*, 1993). Most recently, we functionally evaluated short- and long-term CTL memory in systemic- and mucosal-associated lymphoid tissue following mucosal or systemic AdgB8 immunization (Gallichan and Rosenthal, 1996b). Our results indicate that shortly after AdgB8 immunization, mice were able to mount anti-HSV-2 CTL memory responses in the systemic- and mucosal-associated lymphoid tissues regardless of the route of inoculation. In contrast, several months after immunization, CTL memory was compartmentalized to mucosal or systemic tissues dependent on the route of immunization. Thus, mice immunized i.n. maintained memory responses in the respiratory- and genital-associated lymphoid tissues, but had no significant anti-HSV CTL memory in the systemic immune system. Conversely, systemic immunization resulted in the long-term maintenance of CTL memory in systemic tissues, but not in mucosal-associated lymphoid tissues. Our results indicate that T-cell memory, when examined functionally, has both an early and late phase and that the generation and maintenance of long-term T-cell memory is dependent on the route of immunization. To our knowledge, this is the first functional demonstration of long-term antigen-specific CTL memory in local and distant mucosal tissues following i.n. immunization. Development of successful vaccines against mucosal pathogens, such as HSV and HIV, will require the induction of long-term mucosal immune responses. Following intranasal immunization, the ability of recombinant Ads to induce specific mucosal humoral responses and the long-term maintenance of anti-HSV CTL in respiratory and genital tissues suggest that these vectors may serve as excellent mucosal vaccines. Finally, our results have important implications with regard to the evaluation of vaccines since only after several months did the memory CTL responses compartmentalize to mucosal or systemic tissues. Thus, the time of assessment following vaccination may affect detection of CTL activity; further, the functional evaluation of memory CTL against mucosal pathogens should be based on assessment of CTL in mucosal-associated lymphoid tissues and not in the spleen.

The importance of intranasal immunization with recombinant adenoviruses has been confirmed in a number of studies. Comparison of intranasal and intraduodenal administration of Ad5 recombinants expressing respiratory syncytial virus (RSV) F protein demonstrated that only the i.n. route provided complete protection (Collins *et al.*, 1990). Natuk *et al.* (1993) demonstrated anti-HIV antibody responses in the vaginal fluids of chimpanzees following oral or i.n. immunization with adenovirus type 4-, 5-, and 7-vectored vaccines expressing either HIV *env* or *gag*-protease genes. In particular, i.n. immunization appeared to induce the highest antibody responses. Intravenous, intraperitoneal, and intranasal routes of administration of a recombinant Ad expressing rotavirus VP7sc were also compared, and efficient protection against rotavirus-induced diarrhea in mice was demonstrated with a single dose of recombinant virus given intranasally (Both *et al.*, 1993). These results may not be surprising, since the Chinese were practicing a method of preventing smallpox which involved drying a smallpox lesion on cotton and then placing the material up the nostril of an uninfected individual long before Jenner introduced cowpox vaccination in the late 1700s (Silverstein and Miller, 1989).

Further, the nasopharyngeal-associated lymphoid tissue (NALT) is known to be very sensitive to antigenic stimulation (Kuper *et al.*, 1992).

In addition to supporting the efficacy of i.n. immunization with recombinant Ad vectors, the study by Both et al. (1993) is interesting because it demonstrated that a single dose of Ad5 capable of expressing rotavirus VP7sc given i.n. to naive female mice, who were subsequently mated, was sufficient to induce immunity that could be transferred passively to protect suckling neonates. Rotavirus is a major cause of severe acute gastritis in children worldwide. These results demonstrate a novel application of the ability of recombinant adenoviruses to induce mucosal immunity and passive protection of offspring.

Recently, a phase I clinical trial of a recombinant Ad7 vector expressing hepatitis B surface antigen (HBsAg) was reported (Tacket *et al.*, 1992); 10^7 plaque-forming units (pfu) of a replication-competent Ad-HBsAg was administered orally in enteric coated capsules to three volunteers, while three other volunteers received 10^6 pfu of Ad7. Recipients of the recombinant virus shed less vaccine virus in stool for a shorter period of time and had a lower anti-Ad7 antibody titer than recipients of wild-type Ad7. Interestingly, however, no antibodies against HBsAg were induced (Tacket *et al.*, 1992). This was surprising since the same vector was able to induce protection in chimpanzees (Lubeck *et al.*, 1989). It is possible that this Ad recombinant replicated poorly in the human gut or did not adequately express the HBsAg. These results emphasize the fact that there is a great deal to learn about adenovirus-based vaccines.

VI. Advances in Adenovirus Vector Methodology and Future Directions

The degree of success of a particular recombinant Ad in vaccine trials is influenced at many levels, including the mode of vaccine delivery and subsequent challenge as well as the animal system used. At the level of construct development, several improvements to vector methodology have been described recently. HSV-1 glycoprotein D (gD) contains a linear neutralizing epitope in the amino acid residues 8–23 (Cohen *et al.*, 1984). Zheng et al. (1993) constructed and determined the immunogenicity of Ad5 recombinants containing and expressing from one to four tandem repeats of this epitope. Interestingly, the mean antibody titer induced by a single i.p. inoculation of the Ad vector increased with the number of epitope repeats expressed by the recombinant. Recombinant vectors expressing four tandem repeats of the linear neutralizing epitope of HSV-1gD were as effective in antibody induction and protection as an adenovirus containing and expressing the entire gD protein. The expression of tandem repeats of appropriate epitopes by adenovirus vectors may provide improved immunogenicity in candidate vaccines and in some instances may provide safer and more efficient vaccination.

One of the advantages of adenovirus recombinants as vaccines is that they can be used without adjuvants. Nevertheless, we are now aware that immune responses involve interactions by a complex network of distinct cell types and cytokines. Indeed, cytokines can profoundly influence the nature of immune responses. With regard to mucosal immune responses, cytokines expressed by type 2 helper T cells (Th2 cells) have been implicated as being important in the development of isotype specific antibody responses (Taguchi *et al.*, 1990). *In vitro* studies have shown that Th2 cytokines, interleukin 5 and 6, can both enhance IgA production (Beagley *et al.*, 1988, 1989; Schoenbeck *et al.*, 1989; Kunimoto *et al.*, 1989). In order to determine the relevance of these cytokines on mucosal immune responses *in vivo,* independent Ad vectors capable of expressing IL-5 and IL-6 (Braciak *et al.*, 1993) were constructed. Intranasal or intratracheal administration of AdIL-6 was shown to lead to highly compartmentalized expression of IL-6 within the lung and bronchus of treated mice (Xing *et al.*, 1994). Recently, in a collaborative study (Braciak *et al.*, 1996), it was shown that i.n. inoculation of recombinant Ad5 vectors expressing either IL-5 or IL-6 markedly increased specific anti-adenovirus IgA recovered in lung lavage fluid. In addition, simultaneous expression of both cytokines following coinoculation resulted in synergistic enhancement of anti-Ad5 IgA recovered in lung lavage fluid. Seven days following i.n. AdIL-6 treatment the lungs of rodents were found to contain a significant lymphocytic infiltrate consisting largely of $CD3^+$ $CD8^+$ T cells (Xing *et al.*, 1994). In light of this, we are currently investigating the effect of these recombinant Ad cytokine vectors on mucosal anti-adenovirus CTL responses in the lung. These results support the relevant role of IL-5 and IL-6 in mucosal immune responses and suggest that incorporation of these cytokines into recombinant Ad vectors may enhance protective immunity. It is interesting to note that an Ad vector expressing the hepatitis B virus surface antigen (HBsAg) gene in E4 and IL-6 in E3 was recently described (Lindley *et al.*, 1994).

Transfer of specific cytokine genes to tumor cells *in vitro* can reduce their tumorigenicity *in vivo* and effectively vaccinate animals against further challenge with unmodified tumor cells. Recently, transduction of tumor cells *in vitro* with a recombinant Ad vector expressing IL-2, in a murine transgenic breast cancer model, reduced tumorigenicity of the tumor cells and prolonged survival (Addison *et al.*, 1995). More importantly, when these viruses were injected directly into tumors *in vivo,* they induced tumor regression that was associated with protection against further challenge with unmodified tumor cells (Addison *et al.*, 1995). These findings suggest that Ad vectors expressing cytokines may form the basis for highly effective immunotherapies of human cancers.

The choice of E1 versus E3 deletions in recombinant Ad constructions may also be influenced at different levels. However, a novel system was recently described in which Ad vectors containing deletions in both E1 and E3 can accept up to 8.3 kb of foreign DNA (Bett *et al.*, 1994). Using this system, two foreign genes, each under the control of a promoter, were rescued in tandem, representing 7.8 kb of foreign DNA. The level of expression of each rescued gene was similar to that observed for Ad containing only one of the foreign genes. This approach may provide for enhanced expression of a foreign gene. For example, the enhanced accumulation of HIV-1 glycoprotein transcripts may be permitted by the coexpression of an accompanying HIV-1 rev gene (Cheng *et al.*, 1992). More recently, this system was used to construct recombinant Ad vectors containing and capable of expressing a heterodimeric cytokine, IL-12 (Bramson *et al.*, 1995b). IL-12 is a heterodimeric cytokine that is important in the development of cellular immunity. A double Ad vector was constructed containing the p35 subunit cDNA of IL-12 in E1 and the cDNA for p40 in E3. Biologically active IL-12 was produced *in vitro.* Further, mice infected with these vectors displayed dose-dependent increases in serum IL-12 levels and increases in splenic and lung NK cell activity. This vector may be useful to modulate cellular immunity *in vivo.* Increased understanding of Ad at the molecular level may in the future provide unique cloning strategies and vector methodology to improve gene expression and the safety and efficacy of candidate Ad vaccines.

VII. Summary

Adenovirus vectors have already joined the arsenal of the new age of genetic medicine. They are being used for expression of foreign genes in cells, as recombinant vaccine vectors, and as gene transfer vectors for gene therapy and immunotherapy. An ideal vaccine vector should readily admit insertion of foreign DNA sequences, be nonpathogenic, and be capable of eliciting protective immunity to foreign antigens or pathogens in the host. Adenoviruses have many advantages as vaccine vectors. Methods to construct replication-competent and -defective Ad vectors are well established, and new methods are being developed. Adenoviruses are stable and have a high enough cloning capacity to accommodate most cDNAs. They can be grown to high titers and be easily purified. Also, high-level expression can be obtained from inserts in both replicating and quiescent cells and the virus infects cells from a variety of animals including humans and other primates, canines, bovines, and rodents. Ad recombinants also appear to be stable, with no sequence loss or rearrangement during successive rounds of replication. Adenovirus vectors have also proven effective in inducing both humoral and T-cell-mediated immune responses to their expressed antigens in vaccinated animals and in many cases have elicited protection from lethal challenge. Most importantly, adenoviruses are natural mucosal immunogens with a proven track record as safe and effective vaccines in humans against acute respiratory disease. Our studies in a murine model demonstrate that mucosal (intranasal) immunization with recombinant adenoviruses capable of expressing herpes simplex virus glycoprotein B (AdgB) induced both systemic and mucosal humoral and T-cell-mediated immune responses and long-term protection from heterologous mucosal virus challenge. Although we did not determine the mechanism of protective immunity, intranasal, but not systemic, immunization induced specific anti-HSVgB IgA in the local respiratory tract and at distant genital mucosal surfaces. Similarly, mucosal immunization induced specific anti-HSV cytotoxic T lymphocytes (CTL) in mucosal-associated lymphoid tissue, whereas systemic immunization did not, and the induction of long-term memory CTL in mucosal-associated lymphoid tissues was dependent on the route of immunization. Collectively, our results bode well for the ability of Ad vectors to induce mucosal immunity and protection. Nevertheless, the study and application of live recombinant viral vectors as mucosal vaccines is still in its infancy. Indeed, although numerous studies have been performed that test the efficacy of recombinant viral vaccines to protect animals after mucosal immunization, these studies have not critically examined the induction of mucosal immune responses or the mechanism of protection. Although they are presumably safer, we have little information concerning the ability of replication-defective E1 vectors to induce strong mucosal immune responses. More studies concerning the effects of prior exposure to adenovirus on its immunogenicity need to be conducted. Also, production of replication-defective adenoviruses will require the establishment of new complementation cells lines.

Today, we continue to face the challenges of respiratory, enteric, and sexually transmitted pathogens. Some of these are well known, others, like human immunodeficiency virus (HIV), are relatively newly emergent, and still others, such as *Mycobacterium tuberculosis,* are old pathogens with a new lease on life. Although much remains to be determined, recombinant adenoviruses currently represent one of the most promising systems to achieve mucosal immunity and protection from mucosally transmitted pathogens.

Acknowledgments

The studies concerning the ability of recombinant adenovirus vectors to induce mucosal immune responses to HSV glycoprotein B (AdgB) were supported in part by grants from the Medical Research Council (MRC) of Canada. K.F.T.C. is supported by a Postdoctoral Fellowship Award from the National Health Research Development Program (NHRDP) of Health Canada. K.L.R. is the recipient of a Canadian Industrial Research Award from the Canadian Foundation for AIDS Reserach (CanFAR).

References

Addison, C. L., Braciak, T., Ralston, R., Muller, W. J., Gauldie, J., and Graham, F. L. (1995). Intratumoral injection of an adenovirus expressing interleukin 2 induces regression and immunity in a murine breast cancer model. *Proc. Natl. Acad. Sci. U.S.A.* **92,** 8522–8526.

Anderson, C.W., Lewis, J.B., Baum, P.R., and Gesteland, R.F. (1976) Simian virus 40-specific polypeptides in $Ad2^+$ ND1- and $Ad2^+$ ND4-infected cells. *J. Virol.* **18,** 685–692.

Andersson, M., Paabo, S., Nilsson, T., and Peterson, P. A. (1985). Impaired intracellular transport of class I MHC antigens as a possible means for adenovirus to evade immune surveillance. *Cell (Cambridge, Mass.)* **43,** 215–222.

Beagley, K.W., Eldridge, J.H., Kiyono, H., Everson, M.P., Koopman, W.J., Honjo, T., and McGhee, J.R. (1988). Recombinant murine IL-5 induces high rate IgA synthesis in cycling IgA-positive Peyer's patch B cells. *J. Immunol.* **141,** 2035–2042.

Beagley, K.W., Eldridge, J.H., Lee, F., Kiyono, H., Everson, M.P., Koopman, W.J., Hirano, T., Kishimoto, T., and McGhee, J.R. (1989). Interleukins and IgA synthesis. Human and murine interleukin 6 induce high rate IgA secretion in IgA-committed B cells. *J. Exp. Med.* **169,** 2133–2148.

Bellett, A. J. D., Jackson, P., David, E. T., Bennett, E. J., and Cronin, B. (1989). Functions of the two adenovirus early E1A products and their conserved domains in cell cycle alteration, actin reorganization, and gene activation in rat cells. *J. Virol.* **63,** 303–310.

Berk, A. J., Lee, F., Harrison, T., Williams, J., and Sharp, P. A. (1979). A pre-early adenovirus 5 gene product regulates synthesis of early virus messenger RNAs. *Cell (Cambridge, Mass.)* **17,** 935–944.

Berkner, K. L. (1988). Development of adenovirus vectors for the expression of heterologous genes. *BioTechniques* **6,** 616–629.

Berkner, K. L. (1992). Expression of heterologous sequences in adenoviral vectors. *Curr. Top. Microbiol. Immunol.* **158,** 39–66.

Berkner, K. L., and Sharp, P. A. (1983). Generation of adenovirus by transfection of plasmids. *Nucleic Acids Res.* **11,** 6003–6020.

Bett, A. J., Prevec, L., and Graham, F. L. (1993). Packaging capacity and stability of human adenovirus type 5 vectors. *J. Virol.* **67,** 5911–5921.

Bett, A. J., Haddara, W., Prevec, L., and Graham, F. L. (1994). An efficient and flexible system for construction of adenovirus vectors with insertions or deletions in early regions 1 and 3. *Proc. Natl. Acad. Sci. U.S.A.* **91,** 8802–8806.

Bienenstock, J., and Befus, A. D. (1980). Mucosal immunology. *Immunology* **41,** 249–270.

Both, G. W., Lockett, L. J., Janardhana, V., Edwards, S. J., Bellamy, A. R., Graham, F. L., Prevec, L., and Andrew, M. E. (1993). Protective immunity to rotavirus-induced diarrhoea is passively transfered to newborn mice from naive dams vaccinated with a single dose of a recombinant adenovirus expressing rotavirus VP7sc. *Virology* **193,** 940–950.

Braciak, T. A., Mittal, S. K., Graham, F. L., Richards, C. D., and Gauldie, J. (1993). Construction of recombinant human type 5 adenoviruses expressing rodent IL-6 genes: An approach to investigate *in vivo* cytokine function. *J. Immunol.* **151,** 5145–5153.

Braciak, T. A., Gallichan, W. S., Graham, F. L., Richards, C. D., Ramsay, A. J., Rosenthal, K. L., and Gauldie, J. (1996). Recombinant human adenovirus vectors expressing interleukin 5 and 6 synergistically enhance mucosal IgA responses in the lung. *J. Immunol.,* in press.

Bramson, J. L., Graham, F. L., and Gauldie, J. (1995). The use of adenoviral vectors for gene therapy and gene transfer *in vivo*. *Curr. Opin. Biotechnol.* **6,** 590–595.

Bramson, J. L., Hitt, M., Gallichan, W. S., Rosenthal, K. L., Gauldie, J., and Graham, F. L. (1996). Construction of a double recombinant adenovirus vector expressing a heterodimeric cytokine: *In vitro* and *in vivo* production of biologically active interleukin 12. *Hum. Gene Ther.* **7,** 333–342.

Branton, P.E., Bayley, S.T., and Graham, F.T. (1985). Transformation by human adenoviruses. *Biochim. Biophys. Acta* **780,** 67–94.

Burgert, H.-G., and Kvist, S. (1985). An adenovirus type 2 glycoprotein blocks cell surface expression of human histocompatibility class I antigens. *Cell (Cambridge, Mass.)* **41,** 987–997.

Burgert, H.-G., and Kvist, S. (1987). The E3/19K protein of adenovirus type 2 binds to the domains of histocompatibility antigens required for CTL recognition. *EMBO J.* **6,** 2019–2026.

Butcher, E. C. (1988). Lymphocyte migration and mucosal immunity. *In* "Lymphocyte Migration and Mucosal Immunity" (M. F. Heyworth and A. L. Jones, eds.), pp. 93–103. Raven, New York.

Chaloner-Larsson, G., Contreras, G., Furesz, J., Boucher, D. W., Krepps, D., Humphreys, G. R., and Mohanna, S. M. (1986). Immunization of Canadian armed forces personnel with live type 4 and type 7 adenovirus vaccines. *Can. J. Public Health* **77,** 367–370.

Chanock, R. M., Ludwig, W., Heubner, R. J., Cate, T. R., and Chu, L. W. (1966). Immunization by selective infection with type 4 adenovirus grown in human diploid tissue culture. *JAMA, J. Am. Med. Assoc.* **195,** 445–452.

Charlton, K. M., Artois, M., Prevec, L., Campbell, J. B., Casey, G. A., Wandeler, A. I., and Armstrong, J. (1992). Oral rabies vaccination of skunks and foxes with a recombinant human adenovirus vaccine. *Arch. Virol.* **123**, 169–179.

Cheng, S.-M., Lee, S. G., Ronchetti-Blume, M., Virk, K. P., Mizutani, S., Eichberg, J. W., Davis, A., Hung, P. P., Hirsch, V. M., Chanock, R. M., Purcell, R. H., and Johnson, P. R. (1992). Coexpression of the simian immunodeficiency virus *env* and *rev* proteins by a recombinant human adenovirus host range mutant. *J. Virol.* **66**, 6721–6727.

Cohen, G. H., Dietzschold, B., Ponce de Leon, M., Long, D., Golub, E., Varrichoi, A., Pereira, L., and Eisenberg, R. J. (1984). Localization and synthesis of an antigenic determinant of herpes simplex virus glycoprotein D that stimulates the production of neutralizing antibody. *J. Virol.* **49**, 102–108.

Collins, P. L., Prince, G. A., Camargo, E., Purcell, R. H., Chanock, R. M., Murphy, B. R., Davis, A. R., Lubeck, M. D., Mizutani, S., and Hung, P. P. (1990). Evaluation of the protective efficacy of recombinant vaccinia viruses and adenoviruses that express respiratory syncytial virus glycoproteins. *In* "Vaccines: Modern Approaches to New Vaccines Including Prevention of AIDS" (F. Brown, R. M. Chanock, H. Ginsberg, and R. A. Lerner, eds.), pp. 79–84. Cold Spring Harbor Laboratory, Cold Spring Harbor, New York.

Cox, J. H., Benniink, J. R., and Yewdell, J. W. (1991). Retention of adenovirus E19 glycoprotein in the endoplasmic reticulum is essential to its ability to block antigen presentation. *J. Exp. Med.* **174**, 1629–1637.

Edmonston, W. P., Purcell, R. H., Gundelfinger, B. F., Love, J. W. P., Ludwig, L., and Chanock, R. M. (1966). Immunization by selective infection with type 4 adenovirus grown in human diploid tissue culture. *JAMA, J. Am. Med. Assoc.* **195**, 453–459.

Falgout, B., and Ketner, G. (1987). Adenovirus early region 4 is required for efficient virus particle assembly. *J. Virol.* **61**, 3759–3768.

Fooks, A. R., Schadeck, E., Liebert, U. G., Dowsett, A. B., Rima, B. K., Steward, M., Stephenson, J. R., and Wilkinson, G. W. G. (1995). High-level expression of the measles virus nucleocapsid protein by using a replication-deficient adenovirus vector: Induction of an MHC-1-restricted CTL response and protection in a murine model. *Virology* **210**, 456–465.

Gallichan, W. S., and Rosenthal, K. L. (1995). Specific secretory immune responses in the female genital tract following intranasal immunization with a recombinant adenovirus expressing glycoprotein B of herpes simplex virus. *Vaccine* **13**, 1589–1595.

Gallichan, W. S., and Rosenthal, K. L. (1996a). Humoral immunity and protection against herpes simplex virus type 2 infection in the genital tract of intranasally immunized female mice. Submitted.

Gallichan, W. S., and Rosenthal, K. L. (1996b). Long-lived cytotoxic T lymphocyte memory in mucosal tissues following mucosal but not systemic immunization. Submitted.

Gallichan, W. S., Johnson, D. C., Graham, F. L., and Rosenthal, K. L. (1993). Mucosal immunity and protection after intranasal immunization with recombinant adenovirus expressing herpes simplex virus glycoprotein B. *J. Infect. Dis.* **68**, 622–629.

Ghosh-Choudhury, G., Haj-Ahmad, Y., Brinkley, P., Rudy, J., and Graham, F. L. (1986). Human adenvirus cloning vectors based on bacterial plasmids. *Gene* **50**, 161–171.

Ghosh-Choudhury, G., Haj-Ahmad, Y., and Graham, F. L. (1987). Protein IX, a minor component of the human adenovirus capsid, is essential for the packaging of full length genomes. *EMBO J.* **6**, 1733–1739.

Gilden, R. Z., Kern, J., Lee, Y. K., Rapp, F., Melnick, J. L., Riggs, J. L., Lennette, E. H., Zbar, B., Rapp, H. J., Turner, H. C., and Huebner, R. J. (1970). Serologic surveys of human caner patients for antibodies to adenovirus T antigens. *Am. J. Epidemiol.* **91**, 500–509.

Ginsberg, H. S. (ed.) (1984). "The Adenoviruses." Plenum, New York.

Gooding, L. R., Elmore, L. W., Tollefson, A. E., Brady, H. A., and Wold, W. S. M. (1988). A 14,700 MW protein from the E3 region of adenovirus inhibits cytolysis by tumor necrosis factor. *Cell (Cambridge, Mass.)* **53**, 341–346.

Gooding, L. R., Sofola, I. O., Tollefson, A. E., Duerksen-Hughes, P., and Wold, W. S. M. (1990). The adenovirus E3–14.7K protein is a general inhibitor of tumour necrosis factor-mediated cytolysis. *J. Immunol.* **145**, 3080–3086.

Gooding, L. R., Ranheim, T. S., Tollefson, A. E., Aquino, L., Duerksen-Hughes, P., Horton, T. M., and Wold, W. S. M. (1991). The 10,400- and 14,500-dalton proteins encoded by region E3 of adenovirus function together to protect many but not all mouse cell lines against lysis by tumour necrosis factor. *J. Virol.* **65**, 4114–4123.

Graham, F. L. (1984). Transformation by and oncogenicity of human adenoviruses. *In* "The Adenoviruses" (H. Ginsberg, ed.), pp. 339–398. Plenum, New York.

Graham, F. L., and Prevec, L. (1991). Manipulation of adenovirus vectors. *In* "Methods in Molecular Biology: Gene Tranfer and Expression Protocols" (E. J. Murray, ed.), Vol. 7, pp. 109–129. Humana Press, Totowa, New Jersey.

Graham, F. L., and Prevec, L. (1992). Adenovirus-based expression vectors and recombinant vaccines. *In* "Vaccines: New Approaches to Immunological Problems" (R. W. Ellis, ed.), pp. 363–390. Butterworth-Heinemann, Boston.

Graham, F. L., and Prevec, L. (1995). Methods for construction of adenovirus vectors. *Mol. Biotechnol.* **3**, 207–220.

Graham, F. L., Smiley, J., Russell, W. C., and Nairn, R. (1977). Characteristics of a human cell line transformed by DNA from human adenovirus 5. *J. Gen. Virol.* **36**, 59–72.

Hanke, T., Graham, F. L., Rosenthal, K. L., and Johnson, D. C. (1991). Identification of an immunodominant cytotoxic T-lymphocyte recognition site in glycoprotein B of herpes simplex virus by using recombinant adenovirus vectors and synthetic peptides. *J. Virol.* **65**, 1177–1186.

Hitt, M., Bett, A. J., Addison, C., Prevec, L., and Graham, F. L. (1995). Techniques for human adenovirus vector construction and characterization. *In* "Methods in Molecular Genetics, Volume 7. Molecular Virology Tech-

niques Part B" (K. W. Adolph, ed.), in press. Academic Press, San Diego.
Horvath, J., and Weber, J. M. (1988). Nonpermissivity of human peripheral blood lymphocytes to adenovirus type 2 infection. *J. Virol.* **62,** 341–345.
Horwitz, M. S. (1990a). Adenoviridae and their replication. *In* "Virology" (B. N. Fields and D. M. Knipe, eds.), pp. 1679–1721. Raven, New York.
Horwitz, M. S. (1990b). Adenoviruses. *In* "Virology" (B. N. Fields and D. M. Knipe, eds.), pp. 1723–1740. Raven, New York.
Howe, J. A., and Bayley, S. T. (1992). Effects of Ad5 E1A mutant viruses on the cell cycle in relation to the binding of cellular proteins including the retinoblastoma protein and cyclin A. *Virology* **186,** 15–24.
Howe, J. A., Mymryk, J. S., Egan, C., Branton, P. E. and Bayley, S. T. (1990). Retinoblastoma growth suppressor and a 300-kDa protein appear to regulate cellular DNA synthesis. *Proc. Natl. Acad. Sci. U.S.A.* **87,** 5883–5887.
Huebner, R. J., Rowe, W. P., and Lane, W. T. (1962). Oncogenic effects in hamsters of human adenovirus types 12 and 18. *Proc. Natl. Acad. Sci. U.S.A.* **48,** 2051–2058.
Imler, J.-L. (1995). Adenovirus vectors as recombinant viral vaccines. *Vaccine* **13,** 1143–1151.
Jacobs, S. C., Stephenson, J. R., and Wilkinson, G. W. G. (1992). High-level expression of the tick-borne encephalitis virus NS1 protein by using an adenovirus-based vector: Protection elicited in a murine model. *J. Virol.* **66,** 2086–2095.
Johnson, D. C., Ghosh-Choudhury, G., Smiley, J. R., Fallis, L., and Graham, F. L. (1988). Abundant expression of herpes simplex virus glycoprotein gB using an adenovirus vector. *Virology* **164,** 1–14.
Jones, N., and Shenk, T. (1978). Isolation of deletion and substitution mutants of adenovirus type 5. *Cell (Cambridge, Mass.)* **13,** 181–188.
Klessig, D. F. (1984). Adenovirus-simian virus 40 interactions. *In* "The Adenoviruses" (H. Ginsberg, ed.), pp. 399–449. Plenum, New York.
Kozarsky, K. F., and Wilson, J. M. (1993). Gene therapy: Adenovirus vectors. *Curr. Opin. in Genet. Dev.* **3,** 499–503.
Kunimoto, D. Y., Nordan, R. P., and Strober, W. (1989). IL-6 is a potent cofactor of IL-1 in IgM synthesis and of IL-5 in IgA synthesis. *J. Immunol.* **143,** 2230–2235.
Kuper, C. F., Koornstra, P. J., Hameleers, D. M. H., Biewenga, J., Spit, B. J., Duijvestijn, A. M., van Breda Vriesman, P. J. C., and Sminia, T. (1992). The role of nasopharyngeal lymphoid tissue. *Immunol. Today* **13,** 219–224.
Larsen, H. S., Russel, R. G., and Rouse, B. T. (1983). Recovery from lethal herpes simplex virus type 1 infection is mediated by cytotoxic T lymphocytes. *Infect. Immun.* **41,** 197–204.
Levrero, M., Barban, V., Manteca, S., Ballay, A., Balsamo, C., Avantagiatti, M. L., Natoli, G., Skellekens, H. Tiollais, P., and Perricaudet, M. (1991). Defective and nondefective adenovirus vectors for expressing foreign genes *in vitro* and *in vivo*. *Gene* **101,** 195–202.
Lindley, T., Virk, K. P., Ronchetti-Blume, M., Goldberg, K., Lee, S.-W., Eichberg, J. W., Hung, P. P., and Cheng, S.-M. (1994). Construction and characterization of adenovirus co-expressing hepatitis B virus surface antigen and interleukin-6. *Gene* **138,** 165–170.
Lippe, R., Luke, E., Kuah, Y. T., Lomas, C., and Jefferies, W. A. (1991). Adenovirus infection inhibits the phosphorylation of major histocompatibility complex class I proteins. *J. Exp. Med.* **174,** 1159–1166.
Lubeck, M. D., Davis, A. R., Chengalvala, M., Natuk, R. J., Morin, J. E., Molnar-Kimber, K., Mason, B. B., Bhat, B. M., Mizutani, S., Hung, P. P., and Purcell, R. H. (1989). Immunogenicity and efficacy testing in chimpanzees of an oral hepatitis B vaccine based on live recombinant adenovirus. *Proc. Natl. Acad. Sci. U.S.A.* **86,** 6763–6767.
Lubeck, M. D., Natuk, R. J., Chengalvala, M., Chanda, P. K., Murthy, K. K., Murthy, S., Mizutani, S., Lee, S. G., and Wade, M. S. (1994). Immunogenicity of recombinant adenovirus-human immunodeficiency virus vaccines in chimpanzees following intranasal administration. *AIDS Res. Hum. Retroviruses* **10,** 1443–1449.
McAllister, R. M., Gilden, R. V., and Green, M. (1972). Adenoviruses in human cancer. *Lancet* **1,** 831–833.
McDermott, M. R., and Bienenstock, J. (1979). Evidence for a common mucosal system. I. Migration of B immunoblasts into intestinal, respiratory, and genital tissues. *J. Immunol.* **122,** 1892–1898.
McDermott, M. R., Clark, D. A., and Bienenstock, J. (1980). Evidence for a common mucosal immunologic system. II. Influence of the estrous cycle on B immunoblast migration into genital and intestinal tissues. *J. Immunol.* **124,** 2536–2539.
McDermott, M. R., Graham, F. L., Hanke, T., and Johnson, D. C. (1989a). Protection of mice against lethal challenge with herpes simplex virus by vaccination with an adenovirus vector expressing HSV glycoprotein B. *Virology* **169,** 244–247.
McDermott, M. R., Goldsmith, C. H., Rosenthal, K. L., and Brais, L. J. (1989b). T lymphocytes in genital lymph nodes protect mice from intravaginal infection with herpes simplex virus type 2. *J. Infect. Dis.* **159,** 460–466.
McGhee, J. R., and Mestecky, J. (1990). In defense of mucosal surfaces: Development of novel vaccines for IgA responses protective at the portals of entry of microbial pathogens. *Infect. Dis. Clin. North Am.* **4,** 315–341.
McGrory, W. J., Bautista, D. S., and Graham, F. L. (1988). A simple technique for the rescue of early region 1 mutations into infectious human adenovirus type 5. *Virology* **163,** 614–617.
McLorie, W., McGlade, C. J., Takayesu, D., and Branton, P. E. (1991). Individual adenovirus E1B proteins induce transformation independently but by additive pathways. *J. Gen. Virol.* **72,** 1467–1471.
Mackey, J. K., Rigden, P. M., and Green, M. (1976). Do highly oncogenic group A human adenoviruses cause human cancer? Analysis of human tumors for adenovirus 12 transforming DNA sequences. *Proc. Natl. Acad. Sci. U.S.A.* **73,** 4657–4661.
Meitin, C. A., Bender, B. S., Small, P. A., Jr. (1991). Influenza immunization: Intranasal live vaccinia recombinant contrasted with parenteral inactivated vaccine. *Vaccine* **9,** 751–756.
Mittal, S. K., McDermott, M. R., Johnson, D. C., Prevec, L.,

and Graham, F. L. (1993). Monitoring foreign gene expression by a human adenovirus based vector using the firefly luciferase as a reporter gene. *Virus Res.* **28,** 67–90.

Moldoveanu, Z., Novak, M., Huang, W. Q., Gilley, R. M., Staas, J. K., Schafer, D., Compans, R. W., and Mestecky, J. (1993). Oral immunization with influenza virus in biodegradable microspheres. *J. Infect. Dis.* **167,** 84–90.

Morin, J. E., Lubeck, M. D., Barton, J. E., Conley, A. J., Davis, A. R., and Hung, P. P. (1987). Recombinant adenovirus induces response to hepatitis B virus surface antigen in hamsters. *Proc. Natl. Acad. Sci. U.S.A.* **84,** 4626–4630.

Mullbacher, A. (1992). Viral escape from immune recognition: Multiple strategies of adenovirus. *Immunol. Cell Biol.* **70,** 59–63.

Nash, A. A., Jayasuriya, A., Phelan, J., Cobbold, S. P., Waldmann, H., and Prospero, T. (1987). Different roles for $L3T4^+$ and $Lyt2^+$ T cell subsets in the control of an acute herpes simplex virus infection of the skin and nervous system. *J. Gen. Virol.* **68,** 825–833.

Natuk, R. J., Lubeck, M. D., Chanda, P. K., Chengalvala, M., Wade, M. S., Murthy, S. C. S., Wilhelm, J., Vernon, S. K., Dheer, S. K., Mizutani, S., Lee, S.-G., Murthy, K. K., Eichberg, J., Davis, A. R., and Hung, P. P. (1993). Immunogenicity of recombinant human adenovirus-human immunodeficiency virus vaccines in chimpanzees. *AIDS Res. Human Retroviruses* **9,** 395–404.

Nedrud, J. G., Liang, X., Hague, N., and Lamm, M. E. (1986). Combined oral/nasal immunization protects mice from Sendai virus infection. *J. Immunol.* **139,** 3484–3492.

Nevins, J. R. (1981). Mechanism of activation of early viral transcription by the adenovirus E1A gene product. *Cell (Cambridge, Mass.)* **26,** 213–220.

Nevins, J. R. (1982). Induction of the synthesis of a 70,000 dalton mammalian heat shock protein by the adenovirus E1A gene product. *Cell (Cambridge, Mass.)* **29,** 913–919.

Parr, M.B., and Parr, E.L. (1994). Mucosal immunity in the female and male reproductive tract. *In* "Handbook of Mucosal Immunology" (P.L. Ogra, W. Strober, J. Mestecky, J.R. McGhee, M.E. Lamm, and J. Bienenstock, eds.), pp. 677–689. Academic Press, San Diego.

Phillips-Quagliata, J. M., Roux, M., Arny, E., Kelly-Hatfield, P., McWilliams, M., and Lamm, M. E. (1983). Migration and regulation of B cells in the mucosal immune system. *Ann. N.Y. Acad. Sci.* **409,** 194–203.

Prevec, L., Schneider, M., Rosenthal, K. L., Belbeck, L. W., Derbyshire, J. B., and Graham, F. L. (1989). Use of human adenovirus-based vectors for antigen expression in animals. *J. Gen. Virol.* **70,** 429–434.

Prevec, L., Campbell, J. B., Christie, B. S., Belbeck, L. and Graham, F. L. (1990). A recombinant human adenovirus vaccine against rabies. *J. Infect. Dis.* **161,** 27–30.

Prevec, L., Christie, B. S., Laurie, K. E., Bailey (Smith), M. M., Graham, F. L., and Rosenthal, K. L. (1991). Immune response to HIV-1 *gag* antigens induced by recombinant adenovirus vectors in mice and rhesus macaque monkeys. *J. Acquired Immune Defic. Syndr.* **4,** 568–576.

Profet, M. (1993). Menstruation as a defense against pathogens transported by sperm. *Q. Rev. Biol.* **68,** 335–386.

Rachman, F., Casimiri, V., Psychoyos, A., and Bernard, O. (1983). Immunoglobulins in the mouse uterus during the oestrous cycle. *J. Reprod. Fertil.* **69,** 17–21.

Rosenfeld, M. A., Siegfried, W., Yoshimura, K., Yoneyama, K., Fukayama, M., Stier, L. E., Paakko, P. K., Gilardi, P., Stratford-Perricaudet, L. D., Perricaudet, M., Jallet, S., Pavirani, A., Lecoq, J.-P., and Crystal, R. G. (1991). Adenovirus-mediated transfer of a recombinant α1-antitrypsin gene to the lung epithelium *in vivo*. *Science* **252,** 431–434.

Rosenfeld, M. A., Yoshimura, Y., Trapnell, B. C., Yoneyama, K., Rosenthal, E. R., Dalemans, W., Fukayama, M., Bargon, J., Stier, L. E., Stratford-Perricaudet, L., Perricaudet, M., Guggino, W. B., Pavirani, A., Lecoq, J.-P., and Crystal, R. G. (1992). *In vivo* transfer of the human cystic fibrosis transmembrane conductance regulator gene to the airway epithelium. *Cell (Cambridge, Mass.)* **68,** 143–155.

Rowe, W. P., Huebner, R. J., Gillmore, L. K., Parrott, R. H., and Ward, T. G. (1953). Isolation of a cytogenic agent from human adenoids undergoing spontaneous degeneration in tissue culture. *Proc. Soc. Exp. Biol. Med.* **84,** 570–579.

Schoenbeck, S., McKenzie, D. T., and Kagnoff, M. F. (1989). Interleukin 5 is a differentiation factor for IgA B cells. *Eur. J. Immunol.* **19,** 965–969.

Schwartz, A. R., Togo, Y., and Hornick, R. B. (1974). Clinical evaluation of live, oral types 1, 2 and 5 adenovirus vaccines. *Am. Rev. Respir. Dis.* **109,** 233–238.

Sethi, K. K., Omata, Y., and Schneweis, K. E. (1983). Protection of mice from fatal herpes simplex virus type 1 infection by adoptive transfer of cloned virus-specific and H-2-restricted cytotoxic T lymphocytes. *J. Gen. Virol.* **64,** 443–447.

Siegfreid, W. (1993). Perspectives in gene therapy with recombinant adenoviruses. *Exp. Clin. Endocrinol.* **101,** 7–11.

Silverstein, A. M., and Miller, G. (1989). History of immunology. The Royal Experiment on Immunity: 1721–1722. *Cell. Immunol.* **61,** 437–447.

Straus, S. E. (1984). Adenovirus infections in humans. *In* "The Adenoviruses" (H. Ginsberg, ed.), pp. 451–498. Plenum, New York.

Tacket, C. O., Losonsky, G., Lubeck, M. D., Davis, A. R., Mizutani, S., Horwith, G., Hung, P. P., Edelman, R., and Levine, M. M. (1992). Initial safety and immunogenicity studies of oral recombinant adenohepatitis B vaccine. *Vaccine* **10,** 673–676.

Taguchi, T., McGhee, J. R., Coffman, R. L., Beagley, K. W., Eldridge, J. H., Takatsu, K., and Kiyono, H. (1990). Analysis of Th1 and Th2 cells in murine gut-associated tissues. Frequencies of CD4 and CD8 T cells that secrete IFN-gamma and IL-5. *J. Immunol.* **145,** 68–77.

Top, F. H., Jr. (1975). Control of adenovirus acute respiratory disease in U.S. army trainees. *Yale J. Biol. Med.* **48,** 185–195.

Top, F. H., Jr., Grossman, R. A., Barelloni, P. J., Segal, H. E., Dudding, B. A., Russell, P. K., and Buesher, E. L.

(1971a). Immunization with live types 7 and 4 adenovirus vaccines. I. Safety, infectivity, antigenicity, and potency of adenovirus type 7 vaccine in humans. *J. Infect. Dis.* **124,** 148–154.

Top, F. H., Jr., Buesher, E. L., Bancroft, W. H., and Russell, P. K. (1971b). Immunization with live types 7 and 4 adenovirus vaccines. II. Antibody response and protective effect against acute respiratory disease due to adenovirus type 7. *J. Infect. Dis.* **124,** 155–160.

Trapnell, B.C. (1993). Adenoviral vectors for gene transfer. *Adv. Drug Rev.* **12,** 185–199.

Trentin, J. J., Yabe, Y., and Taylor, G. (1962). The quest for human cancer viruses. *Science* **137,** 835–841.

Tristram, D. A., and Ogra, P. L. (1994). Genital tract infection: Implications in the prevention of maternal and fetal disease. *In* "Handbook of Mucosal Immunology" (P. L. Ogra, W. Strober, J. Mestecky, J. R. McGhee, M. E. Lamm, and J. Bienenstock, eds.), pp.729–744. Academic Press, San Diego.

Whyte, P., Ruley, H. E., and Harlow, E. (1988). Two regions of the adenovirus early region 1A proteins are required for transformation. *J. Virol.* **62,** 257–265.

Wildy, P., and Gell, P. G. H. (1985). The host response to herpes simplex virus. *Br. Med. Bull.* **41,** 86–91.

Wira, C. R., Richardson, J., and Prabhala, R. (1994). Endocrine regulation of mucosal immunity: Effect of sex hormones and cytokines on the afferent and efferent arms of the immune system in the female reproductive tract. *In* "Handbook of Mucosal Immunology" (P.L. Ogra, W. Strober, J. Mestecky, J.R. McGhee, M.E. Lamm and J. Bienenstock, eds.), pp. 705–718. Academic Press, San Diego.

Witmer, L. A., Rosenthal, K. L., Graham, F. L., Friedman, H. M., Yee, A., and Johnson, D. C. (1990). Cytotoxic T lymphocytes specific for herpes simplex virus (HSV) studied using adenovirus vectors expressing HSV glycoproteins. *J. Gen. Virol.* **71,** 387–396.

Wold, W. S. M., and Gooding, L. R. (1991). Region E3 of adenovirus: A cassette of genes involved in host immunosurveillance and virus–cell interactions. *Virology* **184,** 1–8.

Xing, Z., Braciak, T. A., Jordana, M., Croitoru, K., Graham, F. L., and Gauldie, J. (1994). Adenovirus-mediated cytokine gene transfer at tissue sites: Overexpression of IL-6 induces lymphocytic hyperplasia in the lung. *J. Immunol.* **153,** 4059–4069.

Xu, Z. Z., Krougliak, V., Prevec, L., Graham, F. L., and Both, G. W. (1995). Investigation of promoter function in humans and animal cells infected with human recombinant adenoviruses expressing rotavirus antigen VP7sc. *J. Gen. Virol.* **76,** 1971–1980.

Zerler, B., Roberts, R. J., Mathews, M. B., and Moran, E. (1987). Different functional domains of the adenovirus E1A gene are involved in regulation of host cell cycle products. *Mol. Cell. Biol.* **7,** 821–829.

Zheng, B., Graham, F. L., Johnson, D. C., Hanke, T., McDermott, M. R., and Prevec, L. (1993). Immunogenicity in mice of tandem repeats of an epitope from herpes simplex gD protein when expressed by recombinant adeno virus vectors. *Vaccine* **11,** 1191–1198.

12

Poly(lactide-co-glycolide) Microencapsulation of Vaccines for Mucosal Immunization

JACQUELINE D. DUNCAN
RICHARD M. GILLEY
Pharmaceutical Formulations Department
Southern Research Institute
Birmingham, Alabama 35205

DENNIS P. SCHAFER
Zynaxis, Inc.
Malvern, Pennsylvania 19355

ZINA MOLDOVEANU
JIRI F. MESTECKY
Department of Microbiology
University of Alabama at Birmingham
Birmingham, Alabama 35294

I. Introduction

A. Background

Microencapsulation technology found its first commercial application in 1957 when carbonless paper was developed using liquid ink trapped in fragile microcapsules that were adhered to the back of paper (Green and Schleicher, 1957). It has since been improved and adapted to a variety of other applications including *in vivo* delivery of bioactive agents such as polypeptides, proteins, and viruses. Simply defined, microencapsulation involves the coating of a substance with a protective material, usually a polymer, such that small particles of less than about 1 mm are formed. Terms commonly used to describe the microencapsulated substance include core material, active agent, internal phase, and fill. Terms used to describe the protective coating material that forms the microcapsule include membrane, shell, and wall. The small particles produced by microencapsulation processes are described by several different terms. Generally when the core material is surrounded by a continuous wall or outer shell the structure is called a *microcapsule*. If, on the other hand, the particle consists of a monolithic matrix of the coating material, with the core material randomly dispersed throughout this matrix, the structure is generally called a *microsphere* (Figs. 1 and 2). Such usage is not consistent throughout the literature. In this chapter, we will deal principally with microencapsulation processes that produce *microspheres,* and we will refer to the resulting structures more often by this term.

B. Methods of Microencapsulation

For preparation of vaccine microspheres, the coating material used to form the microspheres is usually a biodegradable polymer. Vaccine microspheres must be produced under relatively mild conditions to protect the encapsulated antigen agent from harm, and the microencapsulation process should be selected based on the properties of the active ingredient as well as the polymer. Methods used to microencapsulate bioactive agents include polymer–polymer phase separation techniques, such as complex coacervation and polymer–polymer incompatibility (Green and Schleicher, 1957); spray drying (Masters, 1976); air-suspension coating techniques, such as pan coating and Wurster coating (Hall and Pondell, 1980; Deasy, 1988); ionic gelation (Lim and Sun, 1980); and emulsion methods, such as

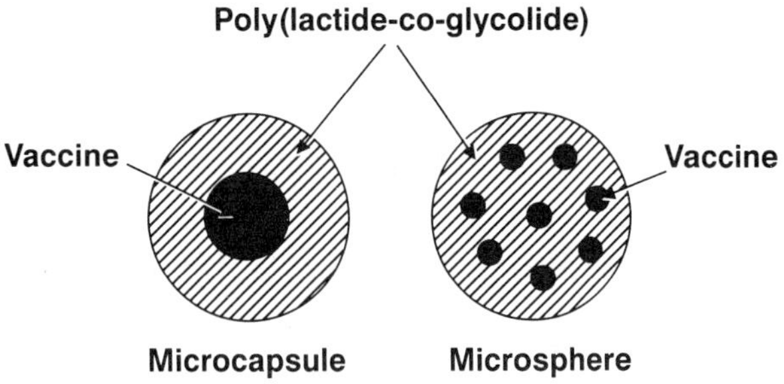

Figure 1. Internal structure of controlled-release particles. Adapted from Tice and Cowsar (1984).

solvent evaporation and solvent extraction (Cowsar *et al.*, 1985).

To date emulsion methods have been used most commonly to make vaccine microspheres, so a brief description of these methods is in order. In one vessel the polymer selected as the encapsulating material is put into solution, usually with an organic solvent. Into this solution, the core material is dissolved (if soluble in the same solvent), suspended (if particulate in nature), or emulsified (if in the form of an aqueous solution or suspension). The contents of this first vessel are then emulsified into water in a second vessel, using agitation and appropriate emulsifying aids. The polymer droplets of this emulsion (an "oil-in-water" emulsion) contain the active ingredient and harden into microspheres as the solvent is removed by evaporation or extraction techniques. The resulting microspheres are then collected and dried by filtration, centrifugation, lyophilization, or a combination of these. The microspheres produced are spherical and can range from ≤1 μm to as large as 2 to 3 mm, and the final product is a free-flowing powder. Emulsion methods have been used commonly to make vaccine microspheres for a simple reason: they are the most practical current methods for producing microspheres using poly(DL-lactide-co-glycolide) (DL-PLG) that are small enough to inject (≤150 μm, approximately) or to be taken up by macrophages and M cells (≤10 μm, approximately). In practice, the choice of polymer is most often the starting point in working out microencapsulation methods, and vaccinologists have turned first to DL-PLG polymers largely due to their safety, their history of successful use in humans, and their ready availability. These polymers, which have been widely used and studied for drug delivery applications have now been studied for a broad variety of vaccine delivery applications (Gilligan and Po, 1991;

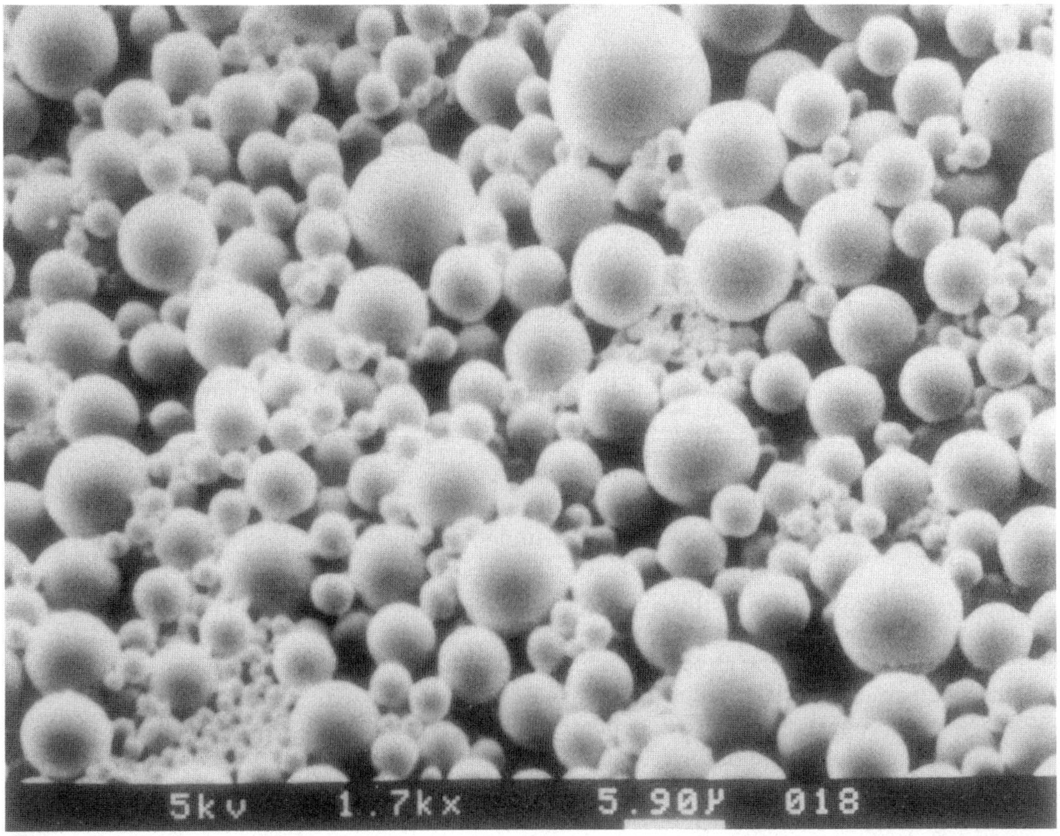

Figure 2. Scanning electron micrograph of poly(DL-lactide-*co*-glycolide) influenza vaccine containing microspheres. Size range: 1–10 μm. Courtesy of Secretech, Inc. (Birmingham, AL).

O'Hagan, 1992; McGhee *et al.*, 1992; Wilding *et al.*, 1994; Morris *et al.*, 1994; Walker, 1994; Brannon-Peppas, 1995; Shallaby, 1995). The remainder of this chapter will focus principally on vaccine microspheres made with this polymer using emulsion methods.

II. Characteristics of DL-PLG Microspheres

A. Biocompatibility and Safety: Controlled Release

Biodegradable polymers such as DL-PLG are of interest for controlled release of drugs and vaccines because they exhibit low toxicity and can be reabsorbed by the body, thus avoiding the need for surgical removal of the delivery device. Many advantages of these polymers have already been described (Heller, 1984; Baker, 1987; Hsieh, 1988). DL-PLG has a history of safe use in man, and has been approved by the U.S. Food and Drug Administration for use as resorbable sutures, in surgical implants, and recently in controlled-release drug-delivery systems (Wise *et al.*, 1979; Langer, 1990). Experimental studies have addressed the encapsulation of anti-cancer agents in DL-PLG microspheres by solvent evaporation methods (Wada *et al.*, 1988a,b). Aclacinomycin, adriamycin, and cisplatin are anti-cancer agents that could produce dose-limiting side effects such as nausea, vomiting, and anorexia. Controlled-release formulations offer the potential of reducing drug toxicity and thereby allowing higher dosing. Lewis *et al.* (1980) investigated the sustained release of antibiotics such as ampicillin, gentamicin, polymyxin B, and chloramphenicol from biodegradable microspheres. Due to short drug half-life, large daily doses of these antibiotics can be required to keep circulatory or tissue concentration at therapeutic levels. Sustained-release formulations could reduce the total daily dose needed. Examples of anti-inflammatory agents microencapsulated with DL-PLG are methylprednisolone and hydrocortisone (Leelarassama *et al.*, 1986; Tice *et al.*, 1985). Controlled-release formulations of steroids are intended for the treatment of inflammatory diseases such as arthritis. More recently, bioactive agents such as vaccines have been microencapsulated with DL-PLG and protective efficacy has been demonstrated (Marx *et al.*, 1993; Moldoveanu *et al.*, 1993; Ray *et al.*, 1993), as further discussed below.

B. Biodegradation

Biodegradation of DL-PLG has been well studied (Holland *et al.*, 1986; Lewis, 1990). It occurs by bulk erosion via simple hydrolysis of the polymer's ester linkages to yield two natural body constituents, lactic acid and glycolic acid, which are eliminated from the body through the Krebs cycle, primarily as carbon dioxide and in urine. The rate of hydrolysis has been an important consideration in regard to drug release, for it has been determined that water uptake increases as the glycolide ratio in the copolymer increases, thereby changing the rate of biodegradation (Miller *et al.*, 1977; Gilding and Reed, 1979). Degradation rates of several copolymers of lactide/glycolide are presented in Table I. Active ingredient is released from DL-PLG microspheres as a result both of diffusion through matrix pores and of matrix degradation and eventual collapse. Diffusion is typically slow *in vivo* because the polymers remain in their glassy state at 37°C. Therefore, matrix degradation is usually the rate-controlling step for *in vivo* release from the microspheres, and one of the advantages of the DL-PLG microsphere delivery system is the ability to control the rate at which the active ingredient is released.

C. Pulsed Release

For vaccines, this ability to vary the release kinetics of microspheres enables the design of delivery systems that release antigen in a pattern selected to optimize the immune response after a single administration. One important advantage of this approach could be a reduction in mass immunization costs; examples of vaccines that could benefit are diphtheria, tetanus, pertussis (DTP), polio, and hepatitis B (Aguado and Lambert, 1992). One promising strategy for vaccine delivery would be to produce a pulsed release of antigen analogous to primary and booster immunizations. Eldridge *et al.* (1993) demonstrated in a series of studies that this could be accomplished either by blending batches of vaccine microspheres prepared with different copolymer ratios, or by blending batches of vaccine microspheres having two distinct size distributions. His studies showed that microspheres less than 10 μm in diameter apparently were phagocytized by macrophages, released antigen rapidly as a result, and produced an immune response faster than microspheres of the same copolymer ratio that

TABLE I
Biodegradation of Lactide/Glycolide Polymers

Polymer	Approximate time for biodegradation (months)[a]
Poly(L-lactide)	18–24
Poly(DL-lactide)	12–16
Poly(glycolide)	2–4
50:50 (DL-lactide-*co*-glycolide)	2
85:15 (DL-lactide-*co*-glycolide)	5
90:10 (DL-lactide-*co*-caprolactone)	2

Note. Adapted from Lewis (1990).
[a] Biodegradation times vary depending on implant surface area, porosity, and molecular weight.

were too large to be phagocytized. Based on these findings, Eldridge demonstrated in further experiments that the desired release kinetics for boosting immune responses could be achieved by using a blend of microsphere batches, all less than 10 μm in diameter but prepared with DL-PLGs having different lactide to glycolide ratios. The resulting immune response, after a single administration, was biphasic and exhibited primary as well as secondary components.

Other investigators have subsequently demonstrated pulsed release of antigens by DL-PLG microspheres. Cleland *et al.* (1994) microencapsulated the HIV-1 subunit antigen, MN rgp 120, with DL-PLG in formulations designed to yield an *in vivo* auto-boost at 1-, 2-, 3-, and 4 to 6 months. Yan *et al.* (1995) demonstrated that DL-PLG microspheres incorporating ricin toxoid (RT) could produce both protracted and pulsed release, thereby reducing the need for multiple doses as well as the time required to induce complete protection against lethal aerosol-borne ricin challenge. The release rate of RT encapsulated in DL-PLG microparticles was controlled by polymer selection and by varying the preparation procedures. McGee *et al.* (1995) also showed that by manipulation and optimization of polymer, microsphere size, and microsphere loading levels, controlled release of entrapped protein could be achieved, including even zero-order release. The microspheres for this work were prepared by a modified phase-separation method that is potentially useful for microencapsulation of bioactive agents. If these initial results are successfully extended, DL-PLG microspheres represent a promising approach to reducing the cost and complexity of immunization programs by reducing the number of doses that must be administered.

D. Immunopotentiation

The need for safe and effective adjuvants has grown as vaccinologists have explored the use of novel immunogens, such as proteins expressed in vectors, subunit vaccines, and synthetic peptides, many of which are weakly immunogenic. A variety of adjuvants are currently being investigated, such as muramyl dipeptides (Azuma *et al.*, 1976; Chedid *et al.*, 1976), detoxified lipopolysaccharides (Ribi *et al.*, 1984), aluminum compounds (Wardlaw and Aprile, 1966), liposomes (Allison and Gregoriadis, 1974), and oil emulsions (Herbert, 1968). Despite a large body of recent work, aluminum hydroxide and aluminum phosphate are currently the only adjuvants approved for use in humans, and additional safe and effective adjuvants are needed.

The mechanisms by which DL-PLG microspheres potentiate the immune response have not been clearly elucidated, but a number of investigations have reported clear enhancement of immune responses by microspheres (Eldridge *et al.*, 1991a,b, 1992, 1993). Eldridge determined that subcutaneous (s.c.) injection of a toxoid vaccine of staphylococcal enterotoxin B (SEB) encapsulated in 1- to 10-μm DL-PLG microspheres stimulated a circulating immunoglobin G (IgG) antitoxin response in mice that was 500-fold greater than the response induced by an optimal dose of nonencapsulated SEB toxoid (Fig. 3). Eldridge also determined that it was necessary for the antigen to be contained within the microspheres to potentiate an antibody response by immunizing mice with SEB toxoid alone, toxoid within microspheres, and a mixture of toxoid and empty microspheres. Toxoid delivered inside the microspheres induced a significantly potentiated IgG antitoxin response

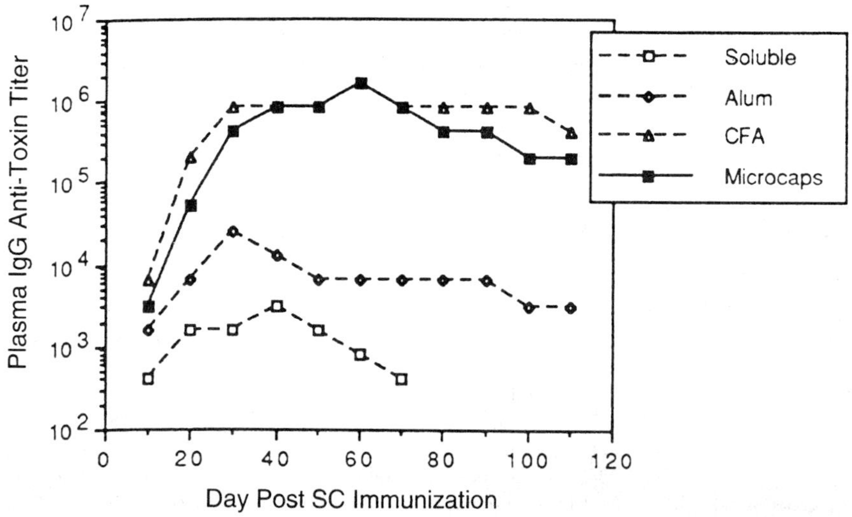

Figure 3. Enhancement of the antibody response to SEB toxin through immunization with microencapsulated SEB toxoid. Groups of six mice were subcutaneously immunized with 50 μg of SEB toxoid in PBS, precipitated on alum, emulsified in CFA, or encapsulated in 1- to 10-μm microspheres [50:50 DL-PLG; 1.76% (wt/wt) SEB toxoid]. Plasma samples were obtained at 10-day intervals, and the IgG, antitoxin titer was determined by endpoint titration in an RIA with solid-phase-adsorbed SEB toxin. Adapted from Eldridge *et al.* (1991b).

TABLE II
IgG Anti-SEB Toxin Antibody Elicited by Administration of Microencapsulated SEB Toxoid or Free SEB Toxoid as a Mixture with Empty Microspheres

	Plasma IgG antitoxin titer[a]			
Immunogen form	Day 10	Day 25	Day 35	Day 50
Toxoid[b]	400	3,200	1,600	400
Toxoid in microspheres[c]	3200	102,400	409,800	1,638,400
Toxoid plus emply microspheres[d]	100	1,600	1,600	50

Note. Adapted from Eldridge *et al.* (1991b).
[a]Titer determined by endpoint titration in an RIA with solid-phase-adsorbed SEB toxin.
[b]SEB toxoid (50 μg) in 0.5 ml of PBS injected subcutaneously.
[c]Microspheres (2.8 mg) [50:50 DL-PLG; 1- to 10-μm diameter; 1.76% (wt/wt) SEB toxoid] containing 50 μg of SEB toxoid in 0.5 ml of PBS injected subcutaneously.
[d]SEB toxoid (50 μg) plus 2.8 mg of placebo microspheres (50:50 DL-PLG; 1- to 8-μm diameter) in 0.5 ml of PBS injected subcutaneously.

in serum when compared with either free toxoid or the mixture of free antigen and empty microspheres (Table II). In these experiments, microsphere size also had a profound effect on the degree to which the response was potentiated and the kinetics of the response: 10 μg of SEB toxoid in microspheres ≤ 10 μm in diameter stimulated a more rapid and stronger serum IgG antitoxin response in mice after s.c. injection than did the same dose of toxoid in 10- to 110-μm microspheres (Fig. 4).

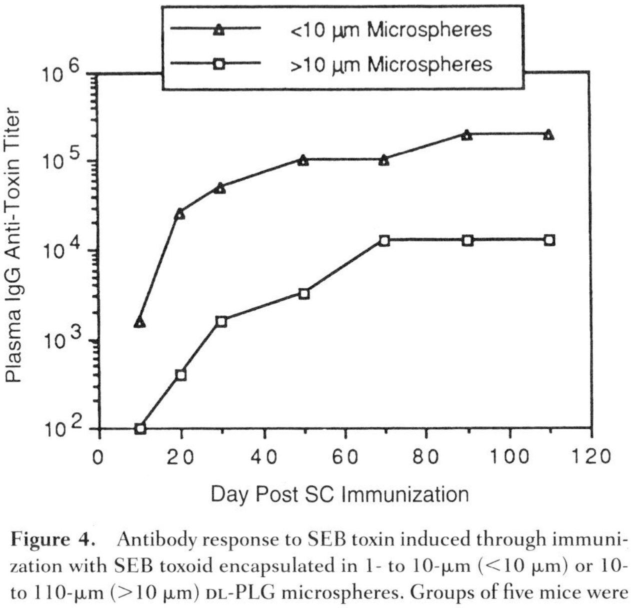

Figure 4. Antibody response to SEB toxin induced through immunization with SEB toxoid encapsulated in 1- to 10-μm (<10 μm) or 10- to 110-μm (>10 μm) DL-PLG microspheres. Groups of five mice were subcutaneously immunized with 10 μg of SEB toxoid encapsulated in 1- to 10-μm [85:15 DL-PLG; 0.65% (wt/wt) SEB toxoid] or 10- to 110-μm [85:15 DL-PLG; 1.03% (wt/wt) SEB toxoid] microspheres. Plasma samples were obtained at 10-day intervals, and the IgG antitoxin titer was determined by endpoint titration in an RIA with solid-phase-adsorbed SEB toxin.

The authors concluded that microspheres smaller than 10 μm in diameter may be phagocytized and transported by macrophages into the draining lymph nodes, whereas larger microspheres localize antigen at the site of injection releasing it slowly by porous diffusion until the microspheres degrade via bulk hydrolysis and begin to fragment. Because the immunopotentiating effect of the microspheres larger than 10 μm may be produced by the phagocytized fragments, it would be diminished to the extent that antigen is lost or degraded prior to microsphere collapse.

Other investigators have demonstrated that systemically as well as mucosally administered microspheres containing antigen can enhance an immune response. Moldoveanu *et al.* (1989, 1993) examined the immune response to an influenza virus vaccine encapsulated in DL-PLG microspheres less than 10 μm in diameter, concluding that systemic immunization with microencapsulated influenza vaccine potentiates the plasma hemagglutination inhibition titer, and that oral boosting with encapsulated vaccine is particularly effective in the induction of salivary immunoglobulin A (IgA) anti-influenza antibodies. O'Hagan *et al.* (1991a,b) entrapped ovalbumin (OVA) in DL-PLG microspheres and demonstrated that the primary and secondary IgG antibody responses obtained in mice with OVA microspheres compared favorably to that obtained with OVA emulsified in complete Freund's adjuvant by both the intraperitoneal (i.p.) and s.c. routes of injection. Microspheres with entrapped OVA were also prepared using two different DL-PLGs with different rates of degradation and were orally administered to two groups of mice. Both groups showed enhanced serum IgG and salivary IgA antibody responses in comparison to mice immunized with soluble OVA, but the level of response induced depended on the polymer used to prepare the microspheres. Challacombe *et al.* (1992) immunized groups of mice orally with either DL-PLG microspheres containing OVA or OVA solution only. After primary and secondary immunizations, the serum IgG and salivary IgA antibodies detected were significantly greater in the group receiving microencapsulated OVA than in the group receiving free OVA, supporting the conclusion that DL-PLG microspheres can function as potent antigen delivery systems enhancing both mucosal and systemic immune responses.

E. Microsphere Uptake via Peyer's Patches

Because the vast majority of infectious disease agents are first encountered through the body's mucosal surfaces, including many such as human immunodeficiency virus (HIV) for which effective vaccines are not available, the induction of mucosal immunity has become a central theme of vaccine development. Experimental evidence emphasizes the need for secretory IgA at mucosal sites to achieve protection at mucosal surfaces and the need for mucosal immunization strategies to induce such protection (Mestecky and McGhee, 1987; Bergmann and Waldman, 1988). Considering that the gastrointestinal (GI) tract contains the largest mass of mucosal tissue in the body, and that it is an organ rich in lymphoid tissue, oral delivery of vaccines has been widely pursued by investigators seeking to induce effective mucosal immunity. The efficient targeting of antigen to Peyer's patches (PP), which play a crucial role in the induction and regulation of secretory immune responses, has become a major issue in vaccine development. Since pioneering work by Eldridge *et al.* (1989) demonstrated the feasibility of delivering antigen to PP in microspheres, microencapsulation has been explored extensively as a method to achieve this goal. The following section of this chapter reviews the full range of vaccines for which microspheres have been employed to induce mucosal immunity. Because the mechanisms of gastrointestinal transport of particulates and their exploitation for vaccine strategies have been reviewed elsewhere (O'Hagan, 1994), these mechanisms are only briefly summarized here. Emphasis is placed on the central issue for vaccinologists, which is how microsphere composition, morphology, and other characteristics might be manipulated to control immune responses.

A considerable body of literature supports the uptake of microparticulate matter from the GI tract (e.g., Pappo and Ermak, 1989; Jani *et al.*, 1989; Jepson *et al.*, 1993a; Howard *et al.*, 1993). Evidence shows that microparticles are taken up via endocytic mechanisms by M cells, which are specialized epithelial cells on the surface of PP and are responsible for transporting antigens into the PP (Owen and Ermak, 1990). While the phenomenon of particulate transport across the GI surface via PP is well established, it nonetheless appears to be a highly variable phenomenon, and vaccinologists must come to grips with this variability in order to fully exploit the phenomenon. Hodges *et al.* (1995) demonstrated absorption of 2-μm latex particles by all parts of the rat intestine but determined that the preferred site of absorption was in the proximal segment of the intestine via the villous tissue adjacent to PP. Maximum uptake occurred at 0.5 hr after dosing. Jepson *et al.* (1993b) compared uptake of DL-PLG and polystyrene microspheres in the rabbit, and determined that binding of DL-PLG microspheres to the follicle-associated epithelium was an order of magnitude lower for DL-PLG than for polystyrene microspheres of equivalent size. Although DL-PLG microspheres were not bound to the M-cell surface as effectively as polystyrene microspheres, a high proportion of those that bound were transcytosed. Ermak *et al.* (1995) also demonstrated M-cell absorption of DL-PLG microspheres and their subsequent transport into the PP of rabbits.

The fate of microparticles following uptake via the PP has been determined by several investigators to be size dependent. After histological studies in mice using fluorescent-labeled microspheres, Eldridge *et al.* (1989) concluded: that microparticles ≤10 μm are taken up by PP and transported to the T- and B-cell zones of those tissues; that microspheres ≤5 μm are ingested by macrophages in PP and transported to mesenteric lymph nodes (MLN) and spleen, where the released antigen may stimulate production of systemic immune responses; and that microspheres ≥5 μm remain trapped in the PP where they may provide a sustained release of antigen to induce mucosal immune responses. Ebel (1990) similarly determined that 2.65-μm particles were present in the spleen following uptake, but 9.13-μm particles were not. Jani *et al.* (1990) identified 0.1-μm particles and smaller in the MLN, spleen, liver, blood, and bone marrow, but failed to find particles 0.5 μm and larger in the blood and bone marrow and could not detect 3-μm particles in the liver or spleen.

A number of studies have explicitly addressed the efficiency of particle uptake via the PP. Eldridge *et al.* (1990) prepared microspheres of comparable size from various polymers and determined that after oral administration to mice microspheres made of polystyrene,poly(methyl methacrylate), poly(hydroxybutyrate), poly(DL-lactide), poly(L-lactide), and DL-PLG, all hydrophobic polymers, were absorbed into the PP; whereas microspheres prepared from cellulosics were poorly ab-

TABLE III

Targeted Absorption of 1- to 10-μm Microspheres with Various Excipients by the Peyer's Patches of the Gut-Associated Lymphoid Tissues Following Oral Administration

Microsphere excipient	Biodegradable	Absorption by the Peyer's patch[a]
Poly(styrene)	No	Very good[b]
Poly(methyl methacrylate)	No	Very good
Poly(hydroxybutyrate)	Yes	Very good
Poly(DL-lactide)	Yes	Good
Poly(L-lactide)	Yes	Good
85:15 Poly(DL-lactide-*co*-glycolide)	Yes	Good
50:50 Poly(DL-lactide-*co*-glycolide)	Yes	Good
Cellulose acetate hydrogen phthalate	No	None
Cellulose triacetate	No	None
Ethyl cellulose	No	None

Note. Adapted from Eldridge *et al.* (1991b).

[a]Mice were administered 0.5 mL of a suspension containing 20 mg of coumarin-containing microspheres into the stomach with the aid of an animal feeding needle. Forty-eight hours after administering the microspheres, 3 representative Peyer's patches were removed and serial sectioned at 5 μm intervals.

[b]The results denote the efficiency of absorption by the Peyer's patches of the microspheres composed of various excipients where *very good* is 1000 to 1500, *good* is 200 to 1000, and *none* is <10 microspheres observed when all the sections from three Peyer's patches were viewed with a fluorescence microscope.

sorbed (Table III). Studies involving nanoparticles have suggested that particle uptake is size dependent, with smaller particles gaining access to all tissues more rapidly (Jani *et al.*, 1990, 1992; Hillery *et al.*, 1994; Couvreur *et al.*, 1995). Studies attempting to quantify the efficiency of uptake have produced conflicting results. A number of investigators have reported uptake efficiencies approximating 0.01% of an administered dose (Jenkins *et al.*, 1994; Ebel, 1990), while other investigators have reported uptake efficiencies several orders of magnitude greater. Alpar *et al.* (1989) reported 39% of a dose of 1.1-μm polystyrene microparticles were absorbed in rats after 45 min, while Jani *et al.* (1990) reported that 34% of a dose of 0.05-μm polystyrene particles and 5% of a dose of 1-μm particles were absorbed. Although these results are conflicting, even at efficiencies of 0.01% or lower, sizeable numbers of microparticles containing antigen can reach PP and, as reviewed in the following section of this chapter, produce mucosal immune responses.

III. Microencapsulated Vaccines for Mucosal Immunization

A. Studies of Model Antigens

Ingestion of soluble antigens, or particulate antigens such as viruses that can be broken down in the gastrointestinal environment, generally results in the induction of low levels of serum or mucosal antibodies due to poor absorption of undigested antigens from the intestinal tract and their enzymatic degradation. To overcome this problem experimentally, high doses of soluble antigens have been given by the oral route. In some species such as mice, rats, and guinea pigs, this treatment may result in the induction of *oral tolerance,* defined as systemic unresponsiveness to antigens given first by the oral route (Mowat, 1994). Therefore, optimal dosage of an antigen in a given species must be considered in order to achieve a mucosal and systemic response while avoiding tolerance or alternatively to induce the state of oral tolerance. Incorporation of antigens into biodegradable microparticles offers clear advantages for inducing an immune response by the oral route. Incorporated antigens are protected from proteolytic digestion by stomach acid and gastrointestinal enzymes, and biologically active antigens have been recovered from solubilized microspheres (Sharif *et al.*, 1995). To the extent that smaller doses can be administered, the potential problem of induction of oral tolerance may be avoided.

Several studies of well-characterized model antigens such as OVA, bovine serum albumin (BSA), and keyhole limpet hemocyanin (KLH) have explored the range of humoral as well as cellular immune responses that can be induced by microencapsulated antigens in mouse models. Generally, a single oral immunization with OVA in microspheres did not induce high titers of specific antibodies in sera or external secretions. However, boosting with microencapsulated OVA resulted in significantly higher levels of both serum and secretory antibodies than were induced by repeated immunization with soluble OVA (O'Hagan *et al.*, 1993a, 1994; Challacombe *et al.*, 1992; Maloy *et al.*, 1994). Furthermore, cell-mediated immunity, determined *in vitro* by T-cell proliferation and IL-2 release, was also induced (O'Hagan *et al.*, 1993a; Maloy *et al.*, 1994). In some experiments, cytotoxic T cells (CTL) specific to OVA were also detected in spleen cells of animals immunized systemically or orally with microencapsulated OVA (Maloy *et al.*, 1994). s.c. immunization with microencapsulated OVA also primed for delayed-type hypersensitivity (Maloy *et al.*, 1994). In all cases, multiple oral immunizations were required for the induction of systemic and especially mucosal, humoral, and cellular immune responses.

B. Studies of Vaccine Antigens

Investigators have incorporated a variety of vaccine antigens into microspheres for experimental purposes or to address specific problems of vaccine development. Some of the major published studies that are representative of this growing body of work are summarized below, with attention given first to soluble antigens followed by viruses.

1. *Staphylococcal Enterotoxin B (SEB)*

SEB was the first biologically active antigen used in extensive studies of immunogenicity after DL-PLG microencapsulation (Eldridge *et al.*, 1989, 1991a,b). The superior immunogenicity of microsphere-incorporated versus free SEB-toxoid was demonstrated by systemic i.p. or mucosal (oral or intratracheal) routes of immunization. Systemic responses were dominated by high titers of IgG anti-SEB. When a mixture of small (1- to 10-μm) and large (20- to 50-μm) microspheres was injected simultaneously, both primary and secondary immune responses overlapped and high levels of antibodies were maintained for an extended time. To induce mucosal responses manifested by the concurrent presence of IgA antibodies in several external secretions (saliva, gut, and lung washings), either three oral doses or systemic priming followed by oral or intratracheal (i.t.) boosting were employed. In addition to secretory antibodies, serum IgM, IgA, and IgG antibodies were also induced. The antigenic integrity of microencapsulated SEB was preserved, and enhanced levels of toxin-neutralizing antibodies were measured (Eldridge *et al.*, 1991b). Analogous results were obtained in a rhesus monkey model (Tseng *et al.*, 1995). Animals immunized by combined intramuscular (i.m.) and subsequent i.t. routes survived a challenge with a lethal dose of SEB in an aerosolized form. This protection was correlated with specific antibody levels both in circulation and in respiratory tract-secretions. Furthermore, SEB-reactive T cells were also stimulated, as evidenced by SEB-induced proliferation of T cells from peripheral blood.

2. Escherichia coli *Antigens*

A rabbit diarrhea model was employed to determine the efficacy of oral immunization with microencapsulated pili of *Escherichia coli* RDEC-1 (McQueen *et al.*, 1993). When given intraduodenally to rabbits, the adhesion antigen AF/R1 incorporated into DL-PLG microparticles induced biliary IgA antibodies against AF/R1 and antigen-driven proliferation of spleen cells. No side effects were observed. Moreover, when challenged with infectious RDEC-1, all immunized animals remained in good health, presumably due to the impaired attachment of bacteria to caecal epithelium. Purified enterotoxigenic *E. coli* (ETEC) fimbrial antigen, CFA/I, was incorporated into DL-PLG microspheres of 10- to 200-μm diameter (mean 27 μm) (Edelman *et al.*, 1993). Intragastric intubation of rabbits with microencapsulated antigen induced a strong serum IgG anti-CFA/I response compared with rabbits receiving the CFA/I alone. CFA-specific IgA fecal antibodies were also detected in one of the three rabbits fed the microencapsulated antigen. No challenge was performed to determine the anti-colonization effect. ETEC antigens consisting of colonization factor antigen II (CFA/II), containing two component antigens CS1 and CS3, were also incorporated into DL-PLG microspheres of 5 to 10 μm in diameter and administered intraduodenally to rabbits (Reid *et al.*, 1993). Spleen cells secreting antibodies against CFA/II and *in vitro* proliferation of PP cells cultured with CFA/II were detected in the immunized animals.

In further studies by this group, microencapsulated ETEC antigens were administered to 10 healthy human volunteers by intestinal intubation (Tacket *et al.*, 1994). One week after administering the last of the four vaccine doses, antibody-secreting cells of IgA isotype against CS3 were detected in the peripheral blood of 5 volunteers, 3 of them having also ASC against CS1. Additionally, jejunal S-IgA against CFA/II was measured in 5 vaccinees. When the 10 vaccinees were challenged with infectious *E. coli* 2 months after the first dose, those 3 who had developed the highest titers of S-IgA and the highest ASC counts were protected. None of the 10 unimmunized volunteers were protected.

3. *Cholera Toxin B (CT-B) Subunit*

Almeida *et al.* (1992) immunized mice by the oral route with CT-B adsorbed onto small DL-PLG microspheres. Four doses were given, on Days 1, 2, 3, and 28, and CT-B adsorbed to microspheres induced higher serum IgG responses than free CT-B. In an analogous study (O'Hagan *et al.*, 1993a), spleens and MLN of mice orally immunized with CT-B entrapped in microspheres displayed significant numbers of antibody-secreting cells. Free CT-B does not induce such cells. The addition of small amounts of cholera toxin remarkably increased both the numbers of antibody-secreting cells and the serum anti-CT antibody levels. A subsequent study by the same authors (O'Hagan *et al.*, 1995) further improved the immunogenicity of CT-B in DL-PLG microspheres. The antigenic integrity and the ability of CT-B to bind to G_{M1} ganglioside were not impaired by the microencapsulation procedure.

4. *Tetanus Toxoid (TT)*

TT incorporated into or adsorbed to DL-PLG microspheres has been used for systemic or mucosal immunization of animals in several studies (Almeida *et al.*, 1993; Alpar *et al.*, 1994; Jackson *et al.*, 1994). Intranasal (i.n.) immunization of guinea pigs with TT adsorbed to microparticles enhanced the systemic IgG responses when compared to free TT (Almeida *et al.*, 1993); even higher titers of anti-TT antibodies were achieved by boosting 5 weeks after the priming dose. In a subsequent study, considerably higher i.n. doses of TT appeared to be required to achieve similar levels of serum antibodies (Alpar *et al.*, 1994). Oral immunization with TT adsorbed to DL-PLG microspheres was ineffective for the induction of serum or mucosal antibodies. Jackson *et al.* (1994) confirmed this finding in studies performed in mice. However, two oral boostings with TT incorporated *into* DL-PLG microspheres resulted in high levels of serum IgG antibodies and low or immeasurable titers of IgA and IgM antibodies to TT. When coadministered with TT microspheres, CT further enhanced the level of serum anti-TT antibodies, and after the third oral immunization also induced mucosal IgA responses. Thus, in animal models CT can serve as an adjuvant when coadministered with microspheres.

5. Bordetella Pertussis

Intranasal immunization of mice with filamentous hemagglutinin (FHA) from *B. pertussis* incorporated into microspheres resulted in the induction of serum IgG and lung fluid IgG and IgA responses (Cahill *et al.*, 1995). The magnitude of these responses was similar for animals immunized i.n. with either soluble or microencapsulated FHA. *In vitro* proliferative responses of spleen cells were detected in both groups of animals as well, and spleen cells also secreted IL-2, suggesting the preferential induction of Th1 responses. Sera from immunized animals significantly inhibited *in vitro* binding of *B. pertussis* to HeLa cells; *in vivo,* immunized mice displayed a rapid clearance from lungs when challenged with live *B. pertussis.* In a parallel study Shahin *et al.* (1995) used microencapsulated pertussis toxoid, pertactin, and FHA for parenteral or i.n. immunization of mice. All three antigens retained their immunogenicity after microencapsulation and induced vigorous IgG and IgA responses in respiratory tract secretions. Furthermore, i.n. immunization with microencapsulated, but not unencapsulated, antigen significantly reduced experimental pertussis infection upon challenge. These results suggest that immunization with microencapsulated antigens from *B pertussis* by the mucosal route induces both humoral and cellular protective immune responses. Further studies in other species should follow soon to explore this promising approach for future vaccination of humans.

6. *HIV Antigen*

A synthetic branched peptide containing the main neutralizing domain of the V3 loop of HIV-1 has been incorporated into microparticles prepared from two different DL-PLG copolymers and from poly(DL-lactide), resulting in microspheres similar in size (~1 μm) and peptide incorporation (McGee *et al.*, 1994). Each of these microsphere preparations was administered to a single baboon as a series of one systemic and three oral doses over 4 days. Two other baboons were s.c. immunized twice with the peptide adsorbed onto alum, 4 weeks apart. V3 peptide-specific IgG antibody titers and HIV neutralization were superior in sera obtained from baboons immunized with the microencapsulated antigen.

7. *Ricin Toxoid (RT)*

RT incorporated into DL-PLG microspheres induced serum IgG2a when given i.n. and IgG2a/IgA when given orally (Yan *et al.*, 1995; Kende *et al.*, 1995). By each route, serum responses thus induced were higher than for RT given in an aqueous solution. All animals were protected from a lethal dose of ricin given by aerosol.

8. *Allergens*

Studies reported to date have not addressed the quantitative and qualitative aspects of immune responses to allergens such as those isolated from house dust mites (*Dermatophagoides pteronyssinus*). However, the properties of allergens obtained from this species and entrapped into DL-PLG microspheres were not significantly altered by their microencapsulation as evaluated by physicochemical (isoelectric focusing) and immunological (radioallergosorbent test, RAST) techniques (Sharif *et al.*, 1995). These results suggest that allergens incorporated into microspheres might be suitable candidates for oral immunotherapy.

9. *Sperm Antigen*

Oral immunization of rats with three doses of recombinant fox sperm antigen incorporated into DL-PLG microspheres resulted in the induction of antigen-specific IgA secreting cells in the intestine (Muir *et al.*, 1994). Although levels of specific antibodies were not measured in sera or mucosal secretions, microencapsulated sperm antigen remained immunogenic as evidenced by IgA cellular responses.

10. *Influenza Virus*

DL-PLG microspheres were employed as a vaccine delivery system for parenteral and oral immunization with influenza virus (Moldoveanu *et al.*, 1989, 1993). Mice immunized either orally or s.c. with formalin-inactivated influenza virus in microspheres produced levels of specific antibodies in serum and in saliva that were higher and longer-lasting than did animals given equal doses of free antigen by the same routes. The serum and salivary levels of anti-influenza antibodies, measured by ELISA and hemagglutination-inhibition assays, could be boosted by oral immunization with encapsulated antigen, and oral-boosting protocols provided complete protection to animals challenged with live virus by nasal instillation.

11. *Simian Immunodeficiency Virus (SIV)*

Whole formalin-inactivated SIV particles incorporated into DL-PLG microspheres were administered to rhesus macaques by i.m. injection, followed by gastric intubation or i.t. installation. This is the first report of an immunization protocol providing protection against a vaginal challenge with SIV designed to mimic the heterosexual route of HIV transmission (Marx *et al.*, 1993). Oral immunization alone was not protective, but three of the four systemically primed and mucosally boosted monkeys remained protected even after a second vaginal challenge with infectious SIV.

12. *Parainfluenza Virus*

Human parainfluenza virus type 3 (PI3) was incorporated into DL-PLG microspheres and administered to hamsters by i.p., intragastric, and i.n. routes (Ray *et al.*, 1993). Following immunization, antibodies specific to viral surface glycoproteins and able to neutralize virus infectivity *in vitro* were measured in hamster sera. On challenge with live virus by the nasal route, i.p. immunized hamsters had significantly lower virus titers in the respiratory tract than unimmunized controls, demonstrating that the microencapsulated parainfluenza virus can confer protection against infection.

13. *Rotavirus*

Because rotavirus is a leading cause of gastroenteritis in infants and young children, an effective rotavirus vaccine is one of the priority targets of the Children's Vaccine Initiative. Due to its instability in an acidic milieu, the live, attenuated rotavirus strains currently undergoing human tests as oral vaccines lose efficacy when administered without buffering of gastric acid. Microspheres composed of water-soluble anionic polymers and amines were tested for their capacity to improve vaccine performance (Offit *et al.*, 1994). Infectious bovine rotavirus (WC3) was entrapped in microspheres made of sodium alginate and spermine hydrochloride, or sodium chondroitin sulfate and spermine hydrochloride. After oral inoculation of mice, more rotavirus was measured in PP in animals immunized with microencapsulated virus than with the free virus, as determined by indirect immunofluorescence. Following both oral and parenteral immunization of mice, virus-specific immune responses were enhanced in sera and in intestinal lavages of animals immunized with microencapsulated virus compared to free virus. In a subsequent study (Khoury *et al.*, 1995), oral immunization of mice with microencapsulated, noninfectious simian rotavirus increased the number of IgA-secreting cells in the small intestinal lamina propria and the quantities of virus-specific IgA in the intestinal fragment culture compared to animals immunized with free virus.

C. Routes of Mucosal Immunization

The studies described above have tested a number of immunization protocols and routes, including mucosal immunization of both the gastrointestinal and respiratory tract. Oral immunization with microencapsulated antigens induced both mucosal and systemic immune responses and protection against challenge in some of these studies. The results lend support to a position held for many years by mucosal immunologists, that oral immunization is an important alternate route for vaccinologists to consider, particularly when mucosal protection is a target. These studies clearly establish the value of microencapsulation as a means to improve immunization results achieved by the oral route. For some vaccines examined (e.g., SIV or *B. pertussis*) the respiratory route appeared to be more effective, a finding that would surprise some immunologists. This may be due to more efficient absorption of antigens by this route or to a lessened degree of antigen degradation in the respiratory tract. The animal species used, frequency of immunization, and type of antigen may be of importance in the induction of protective immune responses, and these factors have not yet been adequately studied in relation to immunization route. The effectiveness of intrarectal or intravaginal immunization with antigens microencapsulated in DL-PLG remains to be explored.

IV. Future Directions

The body of work accomplished in the field of microencapsulated vaccines is now substantial and confirms that microspheres hold promise as a tool for vaccine formulation and delivery. In the work done to date, two clear themes have emerged that suggest directions in which microencapsulation technology needs improvement to better suit the needs of vaccinologists: first, the need to better protect antigens both during encapsulation and storage thereafter; and second, the need to improve the efficiency with which microspheres deliver their contents. Although still preliminary, work is already underway to address these themes in at least four areas: (1) exploration of alternative polymers for microencapsulation; (2) improvement of microencapsulation processes to better protect antigens; (3) improved control and optimization of microsphere size; and (4) modification of microsphere surface chemistry.

DL-PLG has dominated the first generation of work in this field for reasons that, while entirely valid and compelling, are in the end principally pragmatic. The polymers are readily available from commercial sources, they do work for this purpose, and microencapsulation methods successful for vaccines could with some ingenuity be adapted from methods previously used to encapsulate various drugs. Early studies suggested that other polymers might work better (Eldridge *et al.*, 1990) and numerous other polymers have now been tested. As reviewed above, rotavirus has been encapsulated in alginate-based microspheres and has shown an enhanced virus-specific humoral immune response following oral immunization in mice (Khoury *et al.*, 1995). One advantage of this system is that it is water-based, involving no organic solvents to denature the antigen during the encapsulation process. Polyphosphazene polymers have also been used to prepare antigen- containing microspheres for mucosal immunization (Payne *et al.*, 1995). These polymers appear to be relatively nontoxic and are water soluble, alleviating the need for organic solvents, although they are unfortunately not biodegradable. Polyacrylamide (O'Hagan *et al.*, 1989a) and poly(butyl-2-cyanoacrylate) (O'Hagan *et al.*, 1989b) microparticles containing OVA have been used to boost rats orally following an i.p. prime. Another polymer being examined is polymethyl methacrylate (Kreuter, 1995). With this approach, nanoparticles are produced and antigens are either incorporated into the particles or adsorbed onto the surface. Degradable starch microparticles containing a glycoprotein fragment from the influenza virus have been used to intravaginally immunize sheep (O'Hagan *et al.*, 1993b). Agarose beads have been used to immunize rats intrabronchially against *Bordetella pertussis* (Parton *et al.*, 1994). Finally, "proteinoid" microspheres containing both HA-NA and M1 antigens of influenza virus type A have been prepared from natural amino acids and induced a measurable serum IgG response following a single oral immunization (Santiago *et al.*, 1995). Microspheres made of a variety of other polymers, both synthetic and natural, have been studied for other drug delivery applications and could be investigated for the mucosal delivery of vaccines. These include polyvinylpyrrolidone, polyvinyl alcohol, polyacrylic acid, polyanhydrides, poly-ortho esters, albumin, gelatin, dextran, and chitosan.

Much of the work with alternate polymers has been inspired by concerns that the organic solvents used to fabricate DL-PLG microspheres will damage sensitive bioactive materials such as vaccine antigens. A second approach to this problem has been to modify DL-PLG microencapsulation methods to better protect antigens during microsphere fabrication or even, in the case of certain antigens such as TT, during storage and *in vivo* dissolution of the spheres. Unfortunately, most such method improvements are treated as trade secrets and remain unpublished, but the authors are aware of significant progress in antigen stabilization, improvements in emulsion methods to sequester antigens from polymer and solvent during fabrication; improvements in processing speed to minimize the time during which antigens are stressed; and progress toward fabricating DL-PLG microspheres in the absence of organic solvents or even loading them in an aqueous environment after fabrication.

While protection of antigen has been a key concern, improvement of the efficiency with which microspheres are absorbed into tissues of the immune system, whether PP in the GI tract or other tissues by other immunization routes, is equally important if this field is to flourish. The most common point estimate of microsphere uptake by PP after oral immunization in studies reviewed above has been 0.01% of the administered dose, a less than impressive finding. That protective immune responses have been demonstrated in other studies using such delivery systems is a tribute to the potency of PP as an immune inductive tissue, not to the efficiency of current microsphere systems. Some experimentation with alternate polymers has been motivated by these considerations. Other work that is underway to improve uptake efficiency focuses on microsphere size and on the surface chemistry of the spheres.

While no firm conclusions can be drawn from the early studies of the relations between microsphere size, rate of uptake, and biodistribution after uptake reviewed above, these studies do suggest that uptake may be improved by optimizing size. Moreover, microencapsulators appear to be improving their ability to control size—an impression of the authors that at this point is not yet clearly reflected in the literature. At least one study has extended the exploration of size beyond histology and cytology to the measurement of immune responses as an end-point. Uchida and Goto (1994) reported that 4-μm DL-PLG microspheres containing OVA induced higher levels of anti-OVA antibodies after oral administration to mice than microspheres that were either smaller (1.3 μm) or larger (7.5 to 14 μm) in diameter. Clearly, further studies of this nature are required, particularly in species with GI tracts more closely approximating the human, before useful generalizations can emerge.

A final approach to improving microsphere efficiency is to alter the surface chemistry of microspheres, whether made with DL-PLG or with other polymers. Based on the uptake studies reviewed above, several goals might be to increase the hydrophobicity of microsphere surfaces, to adhere receptor-specific or nonspecific attachment factors to microsphere surfaces, and to coat microspheres with surfactants, for example, or with other polymers that impart desired characteristics. Again, more work is underway in these areas than has yet been reported in the literature, but at least one relevant line of investigation has begun to be reported. CT-B, which binds to G_{M1} ganglioside and is a potent mucosal adjuvant, has been successfully adsorbed to the surface of DL-PLG microspheres in one study (Almeida *et al.*, 1992) and the coadministration of whole CT with microspheres has been shown in another study to enhance immune responses to TT incorporated into the microspheres (Jackson *et al.*, 1994). While neither accomplishment may represent a practical solution by itself, these studies suggest that approaches to surface modification of microspheres may bear fruit in the future.

The body of accomplishments in microencapsulated vaccines that has been reviewed in this chapter is a tribute to the successful collaboration of practitioners from two previously unacquainted fields: polymer chemistry and mucosal immunology. Work in this field has moved well beyond initial explorations of a novel phenomenon, as evidenced by the number of vaccine candidates that are moving into human testing, with the literature reporting at least one candidate having completed a preliminary human trial (Tacket *et al.*, 1994). For the field to reach its full potential, and for the vaccines it produces to contribute their full value to medical practice and public health programs, the successful collaborations already in place must be deepened and extended to yield further improvements of this promising technology.

Acknowledgments

The authors express their gratitude to Kim McCain, Sandra Benoit, Melissa Hubbard, Mary Pullen, Richard Remy, Ann Billingsley, and Dale Stringfellow from Southern Research Institute for their time and assistance in the preparation of this chapter.

References

Aguado, M. T., and Lambert, P. H. (1992). Controlled-release vaccines-biodegradable polylactide/polyglycolide (PL/PG) microspheres as antigen vehicles. *Immunobiology* **184**, 113–125.

Allison, A. C., and Gregoriadis, G. (1974). Liposomes as immunologic adjuvants. *Nature (London)* **252**, 252.

Almeida, A. J., Alpar, H. O., and Brown, R. W. (1993). Immune response to nasal delivery of antigenically intact tetanus toxoid associated with poly(L-lactic acid) microspheres in rats, rabbits, and guinea pigs. *J. Pharm. Pharmacol.* **45,** 198–203.

Almeida, A. J., Alpar, H. O., Williamson, D., and Brown, M. R. W. (1992). Poly(Lactic Acid) microspheres as immunological adjuvants for orally delivered cholera toxin B subunit. *Biochem. Soc. Trans.* **20,** 316S.

Alpar, H. O., Field, W. N., Hyde, R., and Lewis, D. A. (1989). The transport of microspheres from the gastrointestinal tract to inflammatory air pouches in the rat. *J. Pharm. Pharmacol.* **41,** 194–196.

Alpar, H. O., Almeida, A. J., Brown, M. R. W., and Williamson, E. D. (1994). Immune responses to mucosally administered tetanus toxoid in biodegradable PLA microspheres. *Proc. Int. Symp. Control. Rel. Bioact. Mater.* **21,** 867–868.

Azuma, T., Sugimura, K., Taniyama, T., Yamawaki, M., Yamamura, Y., Kusumoto, S., Okada, S., and Shiba, T. (1976). Adjuvant activity of mycobacterial fractions: Immunological properties of synthetic *N*-acetylmuramyl dipeptide and related compounds. *Infect. Immun.* **14,** 18–27.

Baker, R. (1987). "Controlled Release of Biologically Active Materials" (R. Baker, ed.), Wiley, New York.

Bergmann, K. C., and Waldman, R. H. (1988). Stimulation of secretory antibody following oral administration of antigen. *Rev. Infect. Dis.* **10,** 939–950.

Brannon-Peppas, L. (1995). Recent advances on the use of biodegradable microparticles and nanoparticles in controlled drug delivery. *Int. J. Pharm.* **116,** 1–9.

Cahill, E. S., O'Hagan, D. T., Illum, L., Barnard, A., Mills, K. H. G., and Redhead, K. (1995). Immune responses and protection against *Bordetella pertussis* infection after intranasal immunization of mice with filamentous hemagglutinin in solution or incorporated in biodegradable microparticles. *Vaccine* **13,** 455–462.

Challacombe, S. J., Rahman, D., Jeffery, H., Davis, S. S., and O'Hagan, D. T. (1992). Enhanced secretory IgA and systemic IgG antibody responses after oral immunization with biodegradable microparticles containing antigen. *Immunology* **76,** 164–168.

Chedid, L., Audibert, F., Lefrancier, P., Choay, J., and Lederer, E. (1976). Modulation of the immune response by a synthetic adjuvant and analogues. *Proc. Natl. Acad. Sci. U.S.A.* **73,** 2472–2475.

Cleland, J. L., Powell, M. F., Lim A., Barron, L., Berman, P. W., Eastman, D. J., Nunberg, J. H., Wrin, T., and Vennari, J. C. (1994). Development of a single shot subunit vaccine for HIV-1. *AIDS Res. Hum. Retroviruses* **10,** S2, S21–S26.

Couvreur, P., Dubernet, C., and Puisieux, F. (1995). Controlled drug delivery with nanoparticles: Current possibilities and future trends. *Eur. J. Pharmacol. Biopharmacol.* **41,** 2–13.

Cowsar, D. R., Tice, T. R., Gilley, R. M., and English J. P. (1985). Poly (lactide-co-glycolide) microcapsules for controlled release of steroids. *In* "Methods in Enzymology" (K. J. Widder and R. Green, eds.), Vol. 112, pp. 101–116. Academic Press, Orlando, Florida.

Deasy, P. B. (1988). Microencapsulation of drugs by pan and air suspension techniques. *Crit. Rev. Ther. Drug Carrier Syst.* **S(2),** 99–139.

Ebel, J. P. (1990). A method for quantifying particle absorption from the small intestine of the mouse. *Pharm. Res.* **7,** 848.

Edelman, R., Russell, R. G., Losonsky, G., Tall, B. D., Tacket, C. O., Levine, M. M., and Lewis, D. H. (1993). Immunization of rabbits with enterotoxigenic *Escherichia coli* colonization factor antigen (CFA/I) encapsulated in biodegradable microspheres of poly(lactide-co-glycilide). *Vaccine* **11,** 155–158.

Eldridge, J. H., Gilley, R. M., Staas, J. K., Moldoveanu, Z., Meulbroek, J. A., and Tice, T. R. (1989). Biodegradable microspheres: Vaccine delivery system for oral immunization. *Curr. Top. Microbiol. Immunol.* **146,** 59–66.

Eldridge, J. H., Hammond, C. J., Meulbroek, J. A., Staas, J. K., Gilley, R. M., and Tice, T. R. (1990). Controlled vaccine release in the gut-associated lymphoid tissues. I. Orally administered biodegradable microspheres target the Peyer's patches. *J. Controlled Release* **11,** 205–214.

Eldridge, J. H., Staas, J. K., Meulbroek, J. A., McGhee, J. R., Tice, T. R., and Gilley, R. M. (1991a). Biodegradable microspheres as a vaccine delivery system. *Mol. Immunol.* **28,** 287–294.

Eldridge, J. H., Staas, J. K., Meulbroek, J. A., Tice, T. R., and Gilley, R. M. (1991b). Biodegradable and biocompatible poly(DL-lactide-co-glycolide) microspheres as an adjuvant for staphylococcal enterotoxin B toxoid which enhance the level of toxin-neutralizing antibodies. *Infect. Immun.* **59,** 2978–2985.

Eldridge, J. H., Staas, J. K., Tice, T. R., and Gilley, R. M. (1992). Biodegradable poly(DL-lactide-co-glycolide) microspheres. *Res. Immunol.* **143,** 557–563.

Eldridge, J. H., Staas, J. K., Dexiang Chen, Marx, P. A., Tice, T. R., and Gilley, R. M. (1993). New advances in vaccine delivery systems. *Semin. Hematol.* **30,** (Suppl. 4), 16–25.

Ermak, T. H., Dougherty, E. P., Bhagat, H. R., Kabok, Z., and Pappo, J. (1995). Uptake and transport of copolymer biodegradable microspheres by rabbit Peyer-patch M-cells. *Cell Tissue Res.* **279,** 433–436.

Gilding, D. K., and Reed, A. M. (1979). Biodegradable polymers for use in surgery: Poly(glycolic)/poly(lactic acid) homo- and copolymers: 1. *Polymers* **20,** 1459.

Gilligan, C. A., and Li Wan Po, A. (1991). Oral vaccines: Design and Delivery. *Int. J. Pharm.* **75,** 1–24.

Green, B. K., and Schleicher, L. (July 1957). U.S. Patent 2,800,457.

Hall, H. S., and Pondell, R. E. (1980). The Wurster Process. *In* "Controlled Release Technologies: Methods, Theory, and Applications" (A. F. Kydonieus, ed.), Vol. 2, pp. 133–154. CRC Press, Boca Raton, Florida.

Heller, J. (1984). Bioerodible systems. *In* "Medical Applications of Controlled Release" (R. S. Langer and D. L. Wise, eds.), Vol. 1, pp. 70–98. CRC Press, Boca Raton, Florida.

Herbert, W. J. (1968). The mode of action of mineral oil emulsion adjuvants on antibody production in mice. *Immunology* **14,** 301–318.

Hillery, A. M., Jani, P. U., and Florence, A. T. (1994). Comparative, quantitative study of lymphoid and non-lymphoid uptake of 60-nm polystyrene particles. *Journal of Drug Targeting* **2**, 151–156.

Hodges, G. M., Carr, E. A., Hassard, R. A., and Carr, K. E. (1995). Uptake and translocation of microparticles in small-intestine—Morphology and quantification of particle distribution. *Dig. Dis. Sci.* **40**, 967–975.

Holland, S. J., Tighe, B. J., and Gould, P. L. (1986). Polymers for biodegradable medical devices, I. The potential of polyesters as controlled macromolecular release systems. *J. Controlled Release* **4**, 155.

Howard, K. A., Thomas, N. W., Davis, S. S., and O'Hagan, D. T. (1993). Microparticulate uptake into intestinal lymphoid tissue—As a route for delivery of oral vaccines. *Proc. Int. Symp. Control. Rel. Bioact. Mater.* **20**, 296–297.

Hsieh, D. S. T. (1988). "Controlled Release Systems: Fabrication Technology," Vol. 2. CRC Press, Boca Raton, Florida.

Jackson, R. J., Staats, H. F., Xu-Amano, J., Takahashi, I., Kiyono, H., Hudson, M. E., Gilley, R. M., Chatfield, S. N., and McGhee, J. R. (1994). Oral vaccine models: Multiple delivery systems employing tetanus toxoid. Microbial pathogenesis and immune response. *Ann. N.Y. Acad. Sci.* **730**, 217–234.

Jani, P., Halbert, G. W., Langridge, J., and Florence, A. T. (1989). The uptake and translocation of latex nanospheres and microspheres after oral administration to rats. *J. Pharm. Pharmacol.* **41**, 809–812.

Jani, P., Halbert, G. W., Langridge, J., and Florence, A. T. (1990). Nanoparticle uptake by the rat gastrointestinal mucosa: Quantitation and particle size dependency. *J. Pharm. Pharmacol.* **42**, 821–826.

Jani, P. U., Florence, A. T., and McCarthy, D. E. (1992). Further histological evidence of the gastrointestinal absorption of polystyrene nanospheres in the rat. *Int. J. Pharm.* **84**, 245–252.

Jenkins, P. G., Howard, K. A., Blackhall, N. W., Thomas, N. W., Davis, S. S., and O'Hagan, D. T. (1994). Microparticulate absorption from the rat intestine. *J. Controlled Release* **29**, 339–350.

Jepson, M. A., Simmons, N. L., Savidge, T. C., James, P. S., and Hirst, B. H. (1993a). Selective binding and transcytosis of latex microspheres by rabbit intestinal M cells. *Cell Tissue Res.* **271**, 399–405.

Jepson, M. A., Simmons, N. L., O'Hagan, D. T., and Hirst, B. H. (1993b). Comparison of poly(DL-lactide-co-glycolide) and polystyrene microsphere targeting to intestinal M cells. *Journal of Drug Targeting* **1**, 245–249.

Kende, M., Yan, C., Rill, W., Malli, R., Naseem, H., Hewetson, J., and Tammariello, R. (1995). Oral delivery of ricin toxoid (RT) vaccine in microspheres stimulates protective IgA and IgG2a antibodies. *Proc. Int. Symp. Control. Rel. Bioact. Mater.* **22**, 200–201.

Khoury, C. A., Moser, C. A., Speaker, T. J., and Offit, P. A. (1995). Oral inoculation of mice with low doses of microencapsulated, noninfectious rotavirus induces virus-specific antibodies in gut-associated lymphoid tissues. *J. Infect. Dis.* **172**, 870–874.

Kreuter, J. (1995). Nanoparticles as adjuvants for vaccines. *In* "Vaccine Design the Subunit and Adjuvant Approach" (M.F. Powell and M.J. Newman, eds.), Vol. 19, pp. 463–472. Plenum, New York and London.

Langer, R. (1990). New methods of drug delivery. *Science* **249**, 1527–1533.

Leelarasamee, N., Howard, S. A., Malanga, C. J., Cuzzi, L. A., Hogan, T. F., Kandzari, S. J., and Ma, J. K. (1986). Kinetics of drug release from polylactic acid–hydrocortisone microcapsules, *J. Microencapsulation* **3**, 171–179.

Lewis, D. H. (1990). Controlled release of bioactive agents from lactide/gycolide polymers. *In* "Biodegradable Polymers as Drug Delivery Systems" (M. Chasin and R. Langer, eds.), pp. 1–41. Dekker, New York.

Lewis, D. H., Dappert, T. O., Meyers, W. E., Pritchett, G., and Suling, W. J. (1980). Sustained release of antibiotics from biodegradable microcapsules. *Proc. Int. Symp. Control. Rel. Bioact. Mater.* **7**, 129.

Lim, F., and Sun, A. M. (1980). Microencapsulated islets as bioartificial endocrine pancreas. *Science* **210**, 908–910.

McGhee, J. R., Mestecky, J., Dertzbaugh, M. T., Eldridge, J. H., Hirasawa, M., and Kiyono, H. (1992). The mucosal immune system: From fundamental concepts to vaccine development. *Vaccine* **10**, 75–88.

McGee, J. P., Koff, W. C., Wang, C. Y., Potts, B., Kennedy, R. C., and O'Hagan, D. T. (1994). Controlled release microparticles with an entrapped branched V3 peptide from HIV-1: Assesment of immunogenicity in baboons. *Proc. Int. Symp. Control. Rel. Bioact. Mater.* **21**, 871–872.

McGee, J. P., Stanley, S. D., and O'Hagan, D. T. (1995). Zero order release of protein from poly(DL-lactide-co-glycolide) microparticles prepared using a modified phase separation technique. *J. Controlled Release* **34**, 77–86.

McQueen, C. E., Boedeker, E. C., Reid, R., Jarboe, D., Wolf, M., Le, M., and Brown, W. R. (1993). Pili in microspheres protect rabbits from diarrhea induced by *Escherichia coli* strain RDEC-1. *Vaccine* **11**, 201–206.

Maloy, K. J., Donachie, A. M., O'Hagan, D. T., and Mowat, A. MI. (1994). Induction of mucosal and systemic immune responses by immunization with ovalbumin entrapped in poly(lactide-co-glycolide) microparticles. *Immunology* **81**, 661–667.

Marx, P. A., Compans, R. W., Gettie, A., Staas, J. K., Gilley, R. M., Mulligan, M. J., Yamshchikov, G. V., Chen, D., and Eldridge, J. H. (1993). Protection against vaginal SIV transmission with microencapsulated vaccine. *Science* **260**, 1323–1327.

Masters, K. (1976). "Spray Drying," 2nd Ed. Wiley, New York.

Mestecky, J., and McGhee, J. R. (1987). Immunoglobulin A (IgA): Molecular and cellular interactions involved in IgA biosynthesis and immune response. *Adv. Immunol.* **40**, 153–245.

Miller, R. A., Brady, J. M., and Cutright, D. W. (1977). Degradation rates of oral resorbable implants (polylactates and polyglycolates): Rate modification with changes in PLA/PGA copolymer ratios. *J. Biomed. Mater. Res.* **11**, 711.

Moldoveanu, Z., Staas, J. K., Gilley, R. M., Ray, R., Compans, R. W., Eldridge, J. H., Tice, T. R., and Mestecky, J. (1989). Immune responses to influenza virus in orally and systemically immunized mice. *Curr. Top. Microbiol. Immunol.* **146**, 91–99.

Moldoveanu, Z., Novak, M., Huang W.-Q, Gilley, R. M., Staas, J. K., Schafer, D., Compans, R. W., and Mestecky, J. (1993). Oral immunization with influenza virus in biodegradable microspheres. *J. Infect. Dis.* **167,** 84–90.

Morris, W., Steinhoff, M. C., and Russell, P. K. (1994). Potential of polymer microencapsulation technology for vaccine innovation. *Vaccine* **12,** 5–11.

Mowat, A., M.I. (1994). Oral tolerance and regulation of immunity to dietary antigens. *In* "Handbook of Mucosal Immunology" (P.L. Ogra, J. Mestecky, M.E. Lamm, W. Strober, J.R. McGhee, and J. Bienenstock, eds.), pp. 185–201. Academic Press, San Diego.

Muir, W., Husband, A. J., Gipps, E. M., and Bradley, M. P. (1994). Induction of specific IgA responses in rats after oral vaccination with biodegradable microspheres containing a recombinant protein. *Immunol. Lett.* **42,** 203–207.

Offit, P. A., Khoury, C. A., Moser, C. A., Clark, H. F., Kim, J. E., and Speaker, T. J. (1994). Enhancement of rotavirus immunogenicity by microencapsulation. *Virology* **203,** 134–143.

O'Hagan, D. T. (1992). Oral delivery of vaccines. *Clin. Pharmacokinet.* **22,** 1–10.

O'Hagan, D. T. (1994). Microparticles as oral vaccines. *In* "Novel Delivery Systems for Oral Vaccines" (D.T. O'Hagan ed.), pp. 175–205. CRC Press, Boca Raton, Florida.

O'Hagan, D. T., Palin, K. J., and Davis, S. S. (1989a). Poly(butyl-2-cyanoacrylate) particles as adjuvants for oral immunization. *Vaccine* **7,** 213–216.

O'Hagan, D. T., Palin, K. J, Davis, S. S., Artursson, P., and Sjoholm, I. (1989b). Microparticles as potentially orally active immunological adjuvants. *Vaccine* **7,** 421–424.

O'Hagan, D. T., Jeffery, H., Roberts, M. J. J., McGee, J. P., and Davis, S. S. (1991a). Controlled release microparticles for vaccine development. *Vaccine* **9,** 768–771.

O'Hagan, D. T., Rahman, D., McGee, J. P., Jeffery, H., Davies, M. C., Williams, P., and Davis, S. S. (1991b). Biodegradable microparticles as controlled release antigen delivery systems. *Immunology* **73,** 239–242.

O'Hagan, D. T., McGee, J. P., Holmgren, J., Mowat, A. MCl., Donachie, A. M., Mills, K. H. G., Gaisford, W., Rahman, D., and Challacombe, S.J. (1993a). Biodegradable microparticles for oral immunization. *Vaccine* **11,** 149–154.

O'Hagan, D. T., Rafferty, D., Wharton, S., and Illum, L. (1993b). Intravaginal immunization in sheep using a bioadhesive microsphere antigen delivery system. *Vaccine* **11,** 660–664.

O'Hagan, D.T., Rahman, D., Jeffery, H., Sharif, S., and Challacombe, S.J. (1994). Controlled release microparticles for oral immunization. *Int. J. Pharm.* **108,** 133–139.

O'Hagan, D. T., McGee, J. P., Lindblad, M., and Holmgren, J. (1995). Cholera toxin B subunit (CT-B) entrapped in microparticles shows comparable immunogenicity to CT-B mixed with whole cholera toxin following oral immunization. *Int. J. Pharm.* **119,** 251–255.

Owen, R. L., and Ermak, T. H. (1990). Structural specializations for antigen uptake and processing in the digestive tract. *Springer Semin. Immunopathol.* **12,** 139.

Pappo, J., and Ermak, T. H. (1989). Uptake and translocation of fluorescent latex particles by rabbit Peyer patch follicle epithelium: A quantitative model for M cell uptake. *Clin. Exp. Immunol.* **76,** 144–148.

Parton, R., Hall, E., and Wardlaw, A. C. (1994). Responses to *Bordetella pertussis* mutant strains and to vaccination in the coughing rat model of pertussis. *J. Med. Microbiol* **40,** 307–312.

Payne, L. G., Jenkins, S. A., Andrianov, A., and Roberts, B. E. (1995). Water-soluble phosphazene polymers for parenteral and mucosal vaccine delivery. *In* "Vaccine Design the Subunit and Adjuvant Approach" (M. F. Powell and M. J. Newman, eds.), Vol. 20, pp. 473–493. Plenum, New York and London.

Ray, R., Novak, M., Duncan, J. D., Matsuoka, Y., and Compans, R. W. (1993). Microencapsulated human parainfluenza virus induces a protective immune response. *J. Infect. Dis.* **167,** 752–755.

Reid, R. H., Boedeker, E. C., McQueen, C. E., Davis, D., Tseng, L. Y., Kodak, J., Sau, K., Wilhelmsen, C. L., Nellore, R., Dalal, P., and Bhagat, H. R. (1993). Preclinical evaluation of microencapsulated CFA/II oral vaccine against enterotoxigenic *Escherichia coli. Vaccine* **11,** 159–167.

Ribi, E., Cantrell, J. L., Takayama, K., Qureshi, N., Peterson, J., and Ribi, H. O. (1984). Lipid A and immunotherapy. *Rev. Infect. Dis.* **6,** 567–572.

Santiago, N., Haas, S., and Baughman, R. A. (1995). Vehicles for oral immunization. *In* "Vaccine Design the Subunit and Adjuvant Approach" (M.F. Powell and M.J. Newman, eds.), Vol. 17, pp. 413–438. Plenum, New York and London.

Shahin, R., Leef, M., Eldridge, J., Hudson, M., and Gilley, R. (1995). Adjuvanticity and protective immunity elicited by *Bordetella pertussis* antigens encapsulated in poly(DL-lactide-co-glycolide) microspheres. *Infect. Immun.* **63,** 1195–1200.

Shalaby, W. S. W. (1995). Development of oral vaccines to stimulate mucosal and systemic immunity: Barriers and novel strategies. *Clin. Immunol. Immunopathol.* **74,** 127–134.

Sharif, S., Wheeler, A. W., and O'Hagan, D. T. (1995). Biodegradable microparticles as a delivery system for the allergens of dermatophagoides pteronyssinus (house dust mite): I. Preparation and characterization of microparticles. *Int. J. Pharm.* **119,** 239–246.

Tacket, C. O., Reid, R. H., Boedeker, E. C., Losonsky, G., Nataro, J. P., Bhagat, H., and Edelman, R. (1994). Enteral immunization and challenge of volunteers given enterotoxigenic *Escherichia coli* CFA/II encapsulated in biodegradable microspheres. *Vaccine* **12,** 1270–1274.

Tice, T. R., and Cowsar, D. R. (1984). Biodegradable controlled-release parenteral systems. *Pharmacol. Technol.,* 26.

Tice, T. R., Lewis, D. H., Cowsar, D. R., and Beck, L. R. (1985). U. S. Patent 4,542,025.

Tseng, J., Komisar, J. L., Trout, R. N., Hunt, R. E., Yok-Jen Chen, J., Johnson, A. J., Pitt, L., and Ruble, D. L. (1995). Humoral immunity to aerosolized staphylococcal enterotoxin B (ETB), a superantigen, in monkeys vaccinated with SEB toxoid-containing microspheres. *Infect. Immun.* **63**, 2880–2885.

Uchida, T., and Goto, S. (1994). Oral delivery of poly(lactide-co-glycolide) microspheres containing ovalbumin as vaccine formulation: Particle size study. *Biol. Pharm. Bull.* **17**, 1272–1276.

Wada, R., Hyon, S. H., Ikada, Y., Nakao, Y., Yoshikawa, H., and Muranishi, S. (1988a). Lactic acid oligomer microspheres containing an anticancer agent for selective lymphatic delivery: I. *In vitro* studies. *J. Bioact. Compat. Polym.* **3**, 126–136.

Wada, R., Tabata, Y., Hyon, S. H., and Ikada, Y. (1988b). Preparation of poly(lactic acid) microspheres containing anti-cancer drugs. *Bull. Inst. Chem. Res., Kyoto Univ.* **66**, 241–150.

Walker, R. I. (1994). New strategies for using mucosal vaccination to achieve more effective immunization. *Vaccine* **12**, 387–400.

Wardlaw, A. C., and Aprile, M. A. (1966). Field trials of aluminum adjuvant vaccines and toxoids: A review. *Symp. Ser. Immunobiol. Stand.* **6**, 257–261.

Wilding, I. R., Davis, S. S., and O'Hagan, D. T. (1994). Optimizing gastrointestinal delivery of drugs. *Baillieres Clinical Gastroenterology* **8**, 255–270.

Wise, D. L., Fellmann, T. D. Sanderson, J. E., and Wentworth, R. L. (1979). Lactic/glycolic acid polymers. *In* "Drug Carriers in Biology and Medicine" (G. Gregoriadis, ed.), Chap. 12. Academic Press, London.

Yan, C. H., Rill, W. L., Malli, R., Hewetson, J., Tammariello R., and Kende, M. (1995). Dependence of ricin toxoid vaccine efficacy on the structure of poly(lactide-co-glycolide) microparticle carriers. *Vaccine* **13**, 645–651.

13

ISCOMs, Liposomes, and Oil-Based Vaccine Delivery Systems

MAURIZIO TOMASI
Laboratorio di Biologia Cellulare
Istituto Superiore di Sanita'
00161 Rome, Italy

THOMAS L. HEARN
Division of Laboratory Systems
Public Health Practice Program Office
Centers for Disease Control and Prevention
Atlanta, Georgia 30333

I. Introduction

In ancient medicine, it was often observed that those who survived the plague acquired protection from the same disease. Only with the advent of the Contemporary Era was this previous observation translated into practical medicine. Interestingly, in the same year (1796) that Jenner discovered that a mild infection of cowpox disease can protect against a more deadly disease, Hahnemann published the theoretic basis of homeopathic medicine. That is, he hypothesized that a disease can be cured by inducing the symptoms of that disease. Although both scientists had similar ideas, the success of the Jenner approach from a theoretical viewpoint does not need any further comment. This recounting of an important finding in medical science emphasizes the subtle line joining traditional observations to current vaccinology. The first point is that good vaccines are, more often than not, discovered and introduced in advance of knowledge about their mechanism of action. The second point is that vaccine efficacy may be associated with mild disease symptoms. The realization that we can induce full protection from disease without triggering any disease symptoms is a very recent achievement in vaccine development. Detoxified toxins such as diphtheria, tetanus, and recently pertussis toxin, which have been obtained by using the cDNA techniques, are examples.

The development of new vaccines does not seem to parallel the enormous achievements in other areas of modern medicine. If the number of available therapeutic medications (about 1000) is compared with the number of vaccines (about 30), one might conclude that vaccine research is lagging. What must be considered in the equation, however, is that the introduction of every new vaccine has a tremendous, broadly beneficial impact on public health. Because of this benefit to populations, vaccine research has high priority for funding by major health organizations such as the World Health Organization.

Even though the mechanisms of action of investigational vaccines are not always known in advance of their entry into the public, safety factors are well-characterized. Because vaccines are targeted for use in healthy populations, strict rules of investigation and expensive clinical trials are required before any new vaccine is released into the market. The safety of a vaccine is an essential prerequisite.

Cost, ease of use, and the route of immunization are also important in the design of vaccines. The ideal vaccine is one that can be administered orally, is multivalent, and can be safely administered in the first suckling period. Oral immunization is preferable on a practical basis because no special expertise or equipment is needed for administering the vaccine. On a scientific basis oral immunization may be preferable because protection is conferred at the portal level through which the majority of pathogens enter. Moreover, mucosal immunity has the unique property of extending to mucosa and lymphoid tissues distal to the site of immunization (Mestecky, 1987; James, 1993).

While it is feasible to develop an oral vaccine for a disease requiring systemic protection like diphtheria and tetanus, developing a parentally administered vaccine for mucosal protection is often difficult. The mucosal immune system has its own structure and its own working rules, and is only partially superimposable on the rules governing the systemic immune system. Studies in humans and experimental animals demonstrated the induction of mucosal immunity at distant mucosal sites, such as tears, saliva, and genital secretion, following oral immunization (Bergmann and Waldman, 1986). After lymphocytes in mucosal tissue have been induced to proliferate into effector and memory cells by mucosal antigen presenting cells (APCs) at the antigen sampling sites, they migrate and home in distant tissues. There the lymphocytes become antibody secreting cells, cytotoxic lymphocytes, and memory cells (Chin *et al.*, 1991). This explains why the induction of mucosal lymphoid tissue extends throughout the entire organism while systemic immunity tends to remain compartmentally confined.

The mucosal immune system responds to immunogenic challenges in a different way than the systemic one. Peripheral antibody production can be stimulated in the mucosal immune system but just as importantly antibody production can be depressed. This phenomenon, called oral tolerance, plays a pivotal role in regulating the entire immune system. The lymphoid tissue of the gastrointestinal tract is constantly challenged, both in number and in type, by large amounts of antigens. Not only do samples of food come in contact with the gut associated lymphoid tissue (GALT) but so do a variety of microorganisms that are layered in the intestinal lumen. Some microorganisms, for example *Helicobacter pylori,* live for years without causing problems, then suddenly become pathogenic. The GALT responds in different ways according to the antigen and to the context of antigen presentation. Tolerance, anergy, and immunostimulation are the three pathways which antigens may encounter in GALT. The pathway chosen appears to be resolved in a relatively short time. Knowledge of the mechanisms underlying pathway selection and the events in the pathway are poorly understood. Nevertheless, reproducible experimental models have been developed where induction of tolerance is obtained and in other experimental models where a protective immune response is obtained. One reliable model for studying oral tolerance is to feed mice ovalbumin (Mowat, 1994), while a reproducible model for promoting a strong local immune response is to co-feed mice antigen and cholera toxin (Dertzbaugh and Elson, 1991). The strong side effects of cholera toxin limits, if not precludes, its use in humans. Unfortunately it is these toxic side effects that seem to promote adjuvanticity (Lycke *et al.*, 1992). This observation seems to suggest that in order to mount an immune response, some yet unknown biological stimulus is likely involved. The induction of tolerance also probably needs some specific stimulus, but this is a matter of current research, is not based on solid data, and is therefore only a speculative hypothesis. Answering important questions about antibody production and tolerance is the subject of much research and the answers are essential for optimal design of vaccines and immunotherapeutics.

In the field of oral vaccines the use of live attenuated strains has shown some accomplishments. Polio myelitis vaccine is the best example of a successful live-attenuated oral vaccine (Hogle *et al.*, 1985). The live-attenuated strain differs from the wild type by one amino acid residue; it is not pathogenic; and it still confers full protection. The advantages of using live-attenuated vaccines are that the attenuated forms share with the pathogen the same processing pathway and the same endogenous pathway of antigen presentation. As a consequence, the desired immunoprotective response is induced. In other cases, such as human immunodeficiency virus (HIV), the live-attenuated vaccine approach does not seem at all practical. An alternative approach is to challenge the GALT with antigen associated with specific carriers, with and without immune adjuvant.

An essential task that a delivery system must accomplish is to allow the antigen to be transported through the M cells to the microenvironment of organized lymphoid tissue. A good delivery system carries the antigen intact through the full repertoire of degrading conditions (acidic pH, proteases, bile acids, etc.), transports the antigen into the lamina propria, and releases the antigen to M cells which will present the last obstacle to the underlying core of the Peyer's patches. Getting to the Peyer's patches is a prerequisite for generating a protective immune response, but presentation of an antigen *per se* does not guarantee induction.

Several lines of evidence suggest that to obtain the proper immune response the antigen processing and presentation *in vivo* must occur in the proper microenvironment (Janeway, 1992). In the last few years the knowledge has emerged that inducing full protection depends on achieving the right balance between a Th1 or Th2 response pattern. Whether a predominant Th1 or Th2 immunoresponse pattern is elicited, it appears to be determined by the microbial components delivered with the antigen and not by the antigen epitopes alone. In other words, the adjuvant used may influence the antibody idiotypes and cellular responses. Rook and Stanford discuss this hypothesis in a review of therapeutic vaccine design (Rook and Stanford, 1995). An important component of antiviral protection appears to involve the specific recognition of the infected cell surface by the $CD8^+$ T-lymphocytes, which is brought about by MHC class I peptide presentation. Many findings indicate that the antigen peptide–MHC class I complex assembles in the cytoplasm compartment (Germain, 1986). Therefore, an optimal antigen delivery system which evokes an antiviral response must transport the antigenic protein into the cytoplasm. The ability to overcome the membrane barrier without provoking serious damage to the cell is typical of envelope virus (White *et al.*, 1983). For example, influenza and parainfluenza viruses are able to fuse with cell membranes enabling them to directly reach the cytoplasmic compartment. It seems reasonable, therefore, that an effective delivery system for a viral vaccine should reproduce at least part of the functions of a viral envelope. It also seems reasonable that a synthetic or subunit vaccine formulation should mimic to some extent the structure of the pathogen.

This chapter is devoted to research of lipid-based delivery systems. With lipid-based delivery systems numerous copies of the antigen may be either located inside or associated with the external surface of the delivery systems; the systems may contain adjuvants or have adjuvant properties themselves, and the systems may contain immune modulators. The lipid-based delivery systems discussed in this review are immunostimulating complexes (ISCOMs), liposomes, and oil-based emulsions. Although all of these systems are similar in that they are all primarily lipid in nature, they are quite different from each other in structure, size, and activity.

II. Immunostimulating Complexes

A. Structural Properties and Preparation Procedure

In 1974 Dalsgaard observed that saponin, a complex glycoside widely distributed in plants, possessed adjuvant activity. Saponin is the active component of a variety of lipid mixtures known as ISCOMs which associate with protein antigens (Morein *et al.*, 1984). The more widely used ISCOM formulation contains Quil A (a saponin extract from *Quillaja saponaria* Molina bark), cholesterol, and phospholipids (see also the reviews of Mowat and Donachie, 1991; Morein, 1990; Kersten and Crommelin, 1995).

The saponins are surfactants with a hydrophilic moiety, composed of a variable number (8–10) of monosaccharides covalently linked with a steroid or triterpene (as in the case of Quil A). The amphiphatic structure allows the formation of a lipid matrix and the association directly with proteins having a hydrophobic portion available (Morein, 1990). Figure 1 shows the typical cage-like matrix obtained by electron microscopy for Quil A and cholesterol (Ozel *et al.*, 1989).

The preparation of ISCOMs requires adding the different components in a precise sequence. Proteins previously solubilized in nonionic detergents are supplemented with Quil A, cholesterol and phosphatidylcholine are added, and finally the ISCOMs matrix is assembled under dialysis or gradient centrifugation (Lovgren and Morein, 1988). Several copies of antigens may be incorporated in a single ISCOM matrix.

The spontaneous association with transmembrane proteins favors ISCOMs as carriers for viral antigens, particularly those which constitute the external surface of envelope virus (for example, influenza and fusion protein of respiratory syncytial virus). However, ISCOMs may also be constituted with soluble proteins like bovine serum albumin (BSA) and ovalbumin (OVA) after expo-

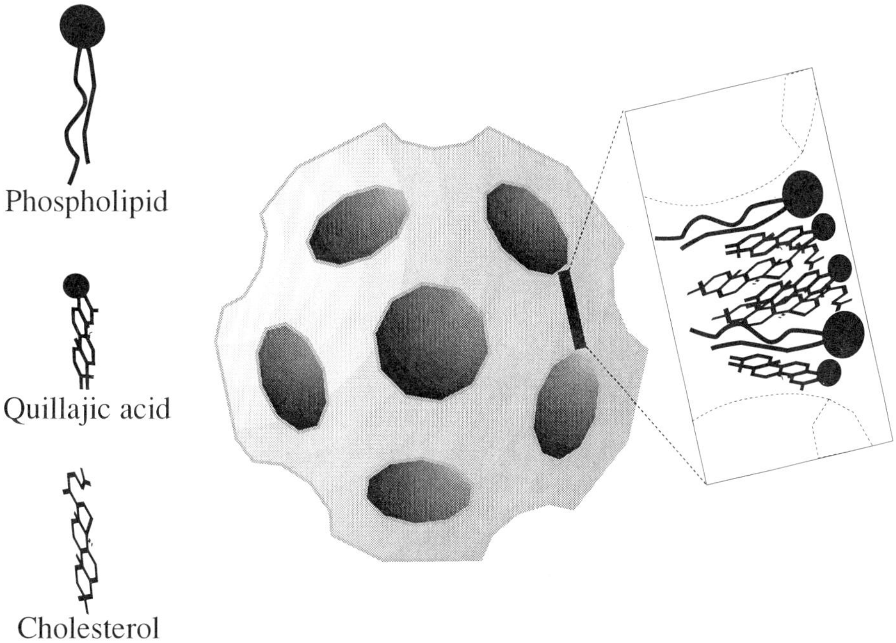

Figure 1. Graphic representation of an empty ISCOM particle, inferred from the review of Kersten and Crommelin (1995). The insert depicts a hypothetical arrangement of phospholipids, cholesterol, and quillajic acid.

sure of hydrophobic regions under acidic pH (Newman *et al.*, 1992), with bacterial polysaccharides (White *et al.*, 1991), or by addition of a hydrophobic tail with palmitic acid as in the case of p24 of feline immunodeficiency virus (FIV) and HIV. Another strategic use of ISCOMs is to chemically conjugate soluble peptides bearing reactive cysteine residues (Larsson *et al.*, 1993).

B. ISCOMs as Adjuvant Carriers

Many studies of ISCOM systems have been performed in mice using influenza virus. Several parameters of this vaccine model have been evaluated. They are: serum antibody response distributed by subclass and isotype (Lovgren, 1988), the efficacy of influenza formulation (Lovgren *et al.*, 1990), immune response to oral versus parenteral immunization (Ghazi *et al.*, 1995), targeting to immunocompetent cells (Watson *et al.*, 1989), internalization process by professional antigen presenting cells (Morein *et al.*, 1994), and the high immunogenic response of bacterial, parasitic, and other soluble proteins and peptides after incorporation into the saponin-lipid matrix, e.g., toxoplasmosis (Claassen and Osterhaus, 1992) and Epstein-Barr virus-induced tumors (Larsson *et al.*, 1993), human cytomegalovirus (Britt *et al.*, 1995), and mixtures of antigens from herpes simplex virus type 1 and influenza A virus (Ghazi *et al.*, 1995). The ability of saponins to potentiate the immune response in parenteral immunization is even higher than that elicited using complete Freund's adjuvant (Takahashi *et al.*, 1990). Furthermore, immunization with ISCOMs produced cell-mediated immunity and systemic delayed-type hypersensitivity (DTH) reactions (Mowat and Donachie, 1991; Villacres-Eriksson *et al.*, 1992) which are typical signs of a Th1-like response (Phillips and Emili, 1992). One of the most striking properties of ISCOMs is the ability to induce an HIV-1 dependent cytotoxic T-lymphocyte (CTL) response (Takahashi *et al.*, 1990).

Because of the success in generating humoral and cell mediated responses against viruses administered in ISCOMs, much research now explores the potential of ISCOMs as vaccine vehicles and adjuvants for use against HIV infection. For example, one study describes that intramuscular immunization of macaques with HIV-2 ISCOM vaccines provided protective immunity (Putkonen *et al.*, 1994). Only 50% protection against simian immunodeficiency virus (SIV) grown in simian cells was obtained when 120 macaques were immunized with ISCOMs and muramyl dipeptide (MDP) containing SIV grown in human cells. The adjuvant made by combining monophosphoryl lipid A, trealose dimycolate, and cell-wall skeleton from BCG, named RIBI, was not protective at all (The European Concerted Action on Macaque Models for AIDS Research, 1995). Not all studies of ISCOMs as vaccine carriers are as promising, however. A recent paper reports that macaques vaccinated with ISCOMs containing antigens from SIV-mac32 are not protected from SIV infection (Hulskotte *et al.*, 1995).

Intranasal inoculations with ISCOMs have also been successful. In a study of murine responses to the influenza virus, protective immunity was achieved with as little as one intranasal administration of virus envelope proteins in ISCOMs (Lovgren *et al.*, 1990). However, other studies showed that the IgA levels induced by the intranasal route were not fully protective and that the IgA levels dramatically decreased after 7 weeks (Ben-Ahmeida *et al.*, 1993). The authors stress that intramuscular injection elicited protection only when the influenza virus infection occurs in the lower respiratory tract, whereas viral infection in the upper level of the respiratory tract can be prevented only by immunization with a live influenza vaccine which appears to be able to induce the production of secretory IgA response (Ben-Ahmeida *et al.*, 1992). Similar results were obtained against a lung infection with respiratory syncytial virus (RSV). In this case, the intramuscular immunization was also more effective than intranasal immunization (Hancock *et al.*, 1995). The data showed that the induction of $CD8^+$ T-cell response was quite similar to that obtained by experimental infection. Further, similar results were obtained in studies where a comparison between the intravaginal immunization route and pelvic presacral space was performed (Thapar *et al.*, 1991). Once again, nonmucosal immunization with ISCOMs seems to be more effective in promoting a CTL response. Therefore, the current interpretation on efficacy of the intramuscular immunization with ISCOMs seems related to their ability to elicit a CTL response and not to the IgG level.

ISCOMs have also been shown to be capable of inducing antibody responses after oral immunization (Mowat *et al.*, 1991), which is not surprising since saponins alone had been previously reported to be effective oral adjuvants for associated antigens (Chavali and Campbell, 1987). Local protective immunization was confirmed in mice models using influenza A virus nucleoprotein (NP) incorporated into ISCOMs, but the findings indicated that the effective immunization site was the mucous membrane of the oropharyngeal cavity. Intragastric infusion did not give comparable protection (Scheepers and Becht, 1994).

C. Mechanism of Action and Side Effects

Several studies investigating the mechanism of action of ISCOMs have been reviewed (Morein *et al.*, 1994). These studies suggest that the ISCOM is a potent enhancer of antigen presentation. Murine peritoneal macrophages can internalize up to 55% of deposited ISCOM containing influenza virus antigen. Under the same conditions micelles bearing the antigen and of about the same size—40 nm—were internalized between 30- and 70-fold less than the ISCOM. Probably the most important property uniquely elicited by ISCOMs is, as mentioned above, the ability to induce a $CD8^+$ T-cell response. This response appears to be directed by the ISCOM and not by the incorporated antigen. In fact, the OVA–ISCOM matrix promotes a specific CTL to the antigenic peptide of the OVA (Heeg *et al.*, 1991; Newman *et al.*, 1992). Since a CTL response requires MHC I presentation and the MHC-I–antigen complex is assembled in the cytoplasm (Germain, 1986), one simple interpretation for the CTL response is that ISCOMs fuse with the membrane and facilitate transport of antigen into the cytoplasm compartment. The nonspecific fusogenic ability of ISCOMS may explain the strong CTL response.

Although it is well known that saponins and Quil A elicit strong hemolytic and cytolytic activity when parenterally injected (even at very low doses), they are not toxic when orally administered to animals. Because ISCOMs are currently being used in parenteral vaccine formulations even for inducing immune protection at the mucosal level, it may be worthwhile to consider up-to-date information about side effects that have been associated with parenteral vaccine administration.

In a study comparing 24 different adjuvants, a dose of 50 μg of Quil A mixed with 125 μg cholesterol and 125 μg l-α-phosphatidyl ethanolamine was lethal to 100% of subcutaneously injected mice (Stieneker *et al.*, 1995). This would appear to tremendously limit the use of ISCOMS in humans, especially when proposing a parenteral route of administration. As a consequence, much effort has been devoted to isolating a fraction of Quil A that retains adjuvanticity but avoids toxicity. The highly purified fraction OS-21 seems to retain adjuvant activity with very low toxicity (Kensil *et al.*, 1991). It is interesting that among 22 different components of Quil A extract, one fraction lacked both toxicity and adjuvanticity. So far, we do not know why this fraction, rather similar to the other active molecules, is devoid of any activity. In human trials 100 μg of OS-21 appears to be the maximum tolerated dose that provides the highest adjuvant activity (Livingston *et al.*, 1994).

III. Liposomes

A. Liposomes as a Biological Membrane Model

The delivery system which most closely parallels nature is the liposome delivery system. Liposomes can be made from a large number of lipid mixtures provided they, to some extent, reproduce the lipid composition of biologic cell membranes. Because of the close structural similarity between liposomes and cell membranes, liposomes have been used primarily as a model system for studying biological membranes. Liposomes afford a versatile way to mimic the external surface of mammalian cells (Ifversen *et al.*, 1995; Auland *et al.*, 1994), parasite (Fries *et al.*, 1992) and bacterial cytoplasm membranes (Elkins *et al.*, 1994), and viral envelopes (Bui *et al.*, 1994; de Haan *et al.*, 1995). In addition, transmembrane proteins and other membrane components may be incorporated directly into the lipid bilayer.

Although the process of reconstituting the membrane proteins involves loss of asymmetric distribution between the outer and inner sides of the membrane vesicles, the resulting liposomes may elicit the function of the reconstituted protein, for example, reconstituting the viral envelope glycoproteins into liposomes. The liposomes acquire the binding and fusogenic activities of the virus (Dallocchio *et al.*, 1995). Reconstituting the viral envelope glycoproteins into liposomes contributes significantly to the immunogenicity of the viral glycoproteins (Gregoriadis *et al.*, 1992). The possibility that the liposomes may be associated with other antigens and adjuvants has been extensively studied and reviewed (Alving, 1991, 1994, 1995; Alving and Wassef, 1994; Gregoriadis, 1990, 1994; Van Rooijen, 1993; Michalek *et al.*, 1992; Kersten and Crommelin, 1995). Coating the liposome surface with various antigens has also been explored (Leserman *et al.*, 1980; Loughrey *et al.*, 1990, 1993; Zhou *et al.*, 1995). Recently a method has been developed to conjugate cholera toxin and its B subunit to the liposomal external surface. Because the liposomes specifically are able to bind to the ganglioside G_{M1}, the system appears promising as a mucosal delivery system (Harokopakis *et al.*, 1995).

B. Preparation and Structural Properties

Liposomes are aqueous suspensions of spheroid vesicles which are phospholipids organized in bilayer structures (Michalek *et al.*, 1992). For water-soluble antigens, the simplest way to prepare liposomes for vaccine research consists of rapidly mixing dissolved antigen with a dehydrated lipid mixture. The most common liposome vaccine composition is dipalmitoyl phosphatidylcholine, cholesterol, diacetylphosphate, and antigen (Michalek *et al.*, 1989; Childers *et al.*, 1987). Following the aforementioned preparation procedure results in the formation of multilamellar vesicles (MLV), having an onion-like structure with an average size of 3–5 nm (Fig. 2a). Extensive sonification of MLV produces the small unilamellar vesicles (SULV) (Fig. 2b). Extrusion of MLV through polycarbonate membranes results in a more stable and homogeneous preparation (Hope *et al.*, 1985). In order to obtain large unilamellar vesicles and to incorporate transmembrane proteins, alternative procedures have been developed (Szoda and Papahadjopoulos, 1980; Zumbuehl and Weder, 1981). The antigen

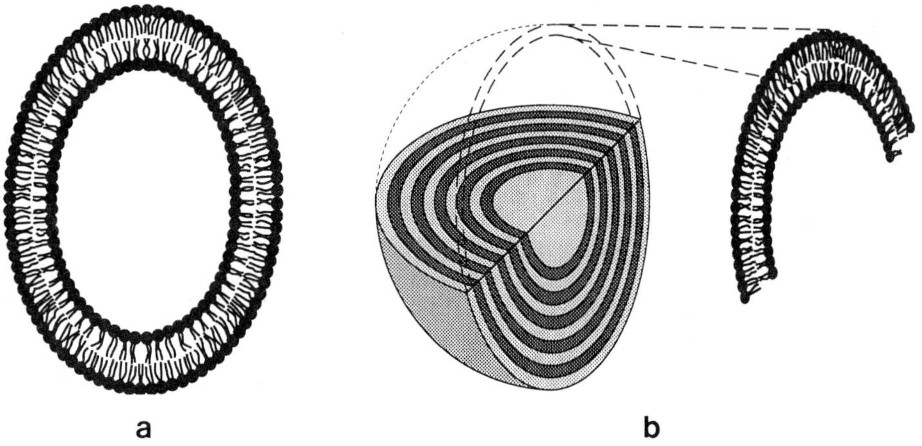

Figure 2. Schematic drawing of liposomes: (a) cross-sectional picture of unilamellar liposomes; (b) cross-section view of a multilamellar liposome particle.

entrapment efficiency is affected by the antigen hydrophilicity and by the preparation procedure employed. By using the water-soluble antigen method, the MLV may entrap up to 90% of a hydrophilic antigen, while with the detergent dialysis method antigen trapping may be as low as 0.2–5.0%. On the other hand, with the detergent dialysis method, 90% of a hydrophobic protein can be entrapped within the liposome.

C. Immunological Properties

Liposomes are much like ISCOMs in that they provide protection for incorporated antigens and a means for concentrating subunit protein antigens into small spheres for delivery to lymphoid tissue. Liposomes have been used mostly for systemic immunizations, but more recently have also been used as oral vaccine vehicles (Michalek *et al.*, 1992; Jackson *et al.*, 1990). Even though liposomes are relatively fragile, they are still sufficiently stable when injected into the intestinal lumen to enhance delivery of antigen to the antigen presentation pathway. Changing of the liposomes' lipid composition in order to enhance their carrier ability has been a matter of intensive investigation since the work of the Kinsky group (Yasuda *et al.*, 1977). This topic has recently been reviewed (Kersten and Crommelin, 1995). Phosphatidylserine renders a negative charge to the surface of the liposome and enhances uptake into Peyer's patches after luminal administration (Aramaki *et al.*, 1993).

Cationic lipids may also play a role in antigen presentation (Latif and Bachhawat, 1984; Walker *et al.*, 1992). In the late 1970s there was much thought of using liposomes as specific drug carriers. However, *in vivo* studies showed that tissue macrophages were preferential targets for the liposomes (Ellens *et al.*, 1981). This, along with many other reports, brought attention to liposomes as a candidate for the vaccine delivery system (Alving and Wassef, 1994; Gregoriadis, 1990). At the mucosal level liposomes have been tested in animal models by administration through both the oral route (Pierce and Sacci, 1984; Childers *et al.*, 1987; Jackson *et al.*, 1990) and the intranasal route (Abraham, 1992; Aramaki *et al.*, 1993; de Haan *et al.*, 1995). Comparison of the efficiency of the two routes for inducing long-lasting local immune response appears to favor the intranasal route.

A possible mechanism whereby liposomes may act on the immune system is their ability to deliver antigen preferentially to macrophages. It is known that macrophages possess an efficient machinery for taking up cellular debris and a wide variety of particles. Thus, they are often referred to as professional phagocytes (Dal Monte and Szoka, 1989). When dichloro-methylene-diphosphonate was included in liposomes, an extensive macrophage depletion was observed after the liposome was intravenously administered (Claassen *et al.*, 1987). The inclusion within the liposomal formula of substances such as lipid A, which affects the specific stimulation of the macrophages APC function, may further help the adjuvant activity of the liposomes (Fries *et al.*, 1992; Alving, 1993; Ravindranath *et al.*, 1994). An effective protection was achieved in mice against *Klebsiella pneumonia* septicemia by liposomes including muraminyl peptide and interferon gamma (ten Hagen *et al.*, 1995). The data lead to the conclusion that effective protection was not caused entirely by activating the resident macrophages. Probably the concommitant release of interferon gamma affects the lymphoid tissue in a more complex pattern. The fact that the efficacy of the liposome formulations are strongly affected by the molecules associated with them may also be important for the mucosal vaccine delivery.

IV. Oil-Based Delivery Systems

A. Multiple Emulsions

Emulsions are used widely to incorporate water into oil. An emulsion has chemical and physical characteristics totally different from its components, such as a high viscosity, which renders the emulsion a useful tool in various fields. Manufacturing, cosmetic, food, and pharmaceutical industries have developed a large number of products based on water-in-oil emulsions (w/o). In immunology, the Freund adjuvant is extensively employed in animal experimentation. The Freund adjuvant (FA) formulation is based on mineral oil (Freund, 1951), and when parenterally injected it produces extensive side effects; thus, its utilization in humans is unlikely. As alternatives to FA, several combinations of adjuvants and biodegradable oil were tested. First squalene, a metabolic precursor in cholesterol synthesis, has been demonstrated to be a suitable oil matrix, and has been included in some formulas. Other formulas have used squalane, the saturated form of squalene. Detox is a mixture containing monophosphoryl lipid A, cell-wall combination of a synthetic muramyl dipeptide analog, pluronic polymer, and squalane (Allison and Byars, 1990). A more elaborate emulsion, but conversely more practical and quite efficient as parenteral adjuvant, contains emulsifiers and nonionic block copolymers (Bennett *et al.*, 1992). The detergents dissolve the emulsion in water and a water-in-oil-in-water (w/o/w) multiple emulsion (ME) is obtained. An ME is a heterogeneous mixture of stable, discrete, oil, and water phases stabilized by emulsifiers. The inner most aqueous phase can consist of either single or multiple vesicles encapsulated by a thick lipid layer with emulsifier at the interface (Fig. 3). Key to the stability of the w/o emulsions and their ability to act as surface active agents is the hydrophile to lipophile balance (HLB) of the emulsifying agent. Since surface active agents preferentially localize at the interface of the oil and water phases, the desired characteristic is that they have a HLB that reduces surface-free energy at the interface promoting the integrity and stability of the formed vesicles.

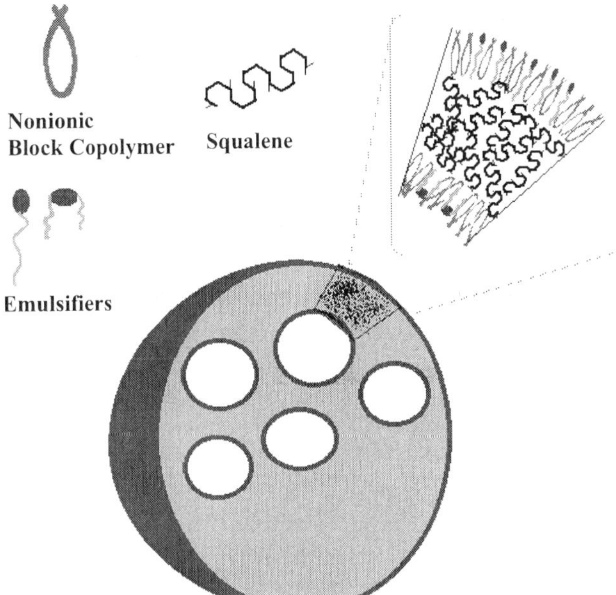

Figure 3. Schematic drawing representing the oil particle of a w/o/w emulsion containing water phase.

B. Nonionic Block Copolymer

For nonionic surface active agents a range of HLBs for applications from w/o emulsifiers to detergents and solubilizers has been published (Adamson, 1982). The nonionic block copolymers and the surfactants exhibiting adjuvant activity that have HLBs less than two are generally considered spreading agents (Hunter *et al.*, 1981). The nonionic block copolymers examined in oral vaccine research have typically consisted of polymers of polyoxypropylene (POP), which is hydrophobic, and polyoxyethylene (POE), which is hydrophilic. In previous research, a correlation has been shown between the ability of copolymers of this particular construct to promote retention of macromolecules on the surface of oil drops and their activities as adjuvants (Hunter *et al.*, 1981). Nonionic copolymers of various lengths of POP and POE and of varying ratios of POP to POE have been constructed and evaluated as adjuvants in oil-in-water emulsions containing the antigen trinitrophenyl conjugated to OVA (TNP–OVA) (Hunter *et al.*, 1981) and in oil-in-water emulsions containing malaria peptides (Kalish *et al.*, 1991). The results were that copolymers with hydrophobe molecular weights less than 3000 Da and those which were greater than 10% hydrophile were not effective adjuvants. In contrast, copolymers with POP (hydrophobe) molecular weights of 3250 to 10,000 Da and percentages of POE (hydrophile) of 10 to 4% were shown to have adjuvant activity. All produced high levels of IgGl. However, those with smaller molecular weights also tended to induce strong IgG3 responses while those with higher molecular weights strongly induced IgG2b and IgG2a responses.

C. Immunological Properties

Features which make ME with nonionic block copolymer attractive as vaccine vehicles are: they are readily produced using standard laboratory procedures; stringent preparation conditions such as organic solvents, heat, high shear force, or other denaturing procedures are not required; they can be frozen and are stable for many months refrigerated; antigen in ME resides in saline vesicles within particles that protect it from the digestive enzymes of the intestine; ME have proven to be effective vehicles for delivering particles to Peyer's patches and for inducing systemic and intestinal mucosal immune responses (Hearn, 1994); and they have not been toxic to laboratory animals in oral vaccine experiments.

High-titer, long-lasting mucosal and systemic antibodies were induced in mice using ME containing antigen and nonionic block copolymer P1005 and cholera toxin (CT) (Tomasi *et al.*, 1996). Once incorporated in the ME, CT decreases its toxicity more than 200 times. Immunologic responses from antigens orally infused in ME vary. The magnitude of the mucosal and systemic antibody responses after oral infusions has been shown to be dependent on the antigen, antigen concentration, number of oral infusions administered, copolymer dose, and the boosting regimen (Hearn, 1994). However, ME may also enhance oral tolerance. Experiments showed that mice orally immunized and boosted subcutaneously within 2 weeks of the last oral dose developed tolerance (unpublished findings of R. L. Hunter and M. R. Olsen, 1995; Elson *et al.*, 1996). Tolerance was not induced when oral immunizations were followed more than 2 months later by subcutaneous boosting. In fact, subcutaneously injecting mice with TNP–HEA in ME months after oral infusions demonstrated high anamnestic mucosal and systemic antibody responses to both TNP and HEA.

While the mechanism of action is not clear, it has been shown that oral infusions of ME containing P1005 and titanium dioxide particles, but no antigen, stimulate a rapid influx of lymphocytes into Peyer's patch follicle-associated epithelium (Hearn, 1994) without apparent toxic changes in the epithelium and lymphoid tissue. ME appeared to increase the rate and quantity of particles transported from the gut into Peyer's patches. Infusions of ME resulted in hypertrophy of Peyer's patches. Antigens orally infused in ME stimulated cellular changes in Peyer's patches similar to those seen in lymph nodes from parenterally immunized mice. In addition, ME appears to protect the entrapped antigen from digestion in the gut before reaching the Peyer's patches (Tomasi *et al.*, 1996).

V. Concluding Remarks

Although oral vaccination using a subunit formulation based on the lipid delivery system is still under development, this line of research has shown enormous progress, in terms of both new knowledge and technical achievements. A good adjuvant for parenteral immunization does not necessarily work with mucosal immunizations. While lipid systems appear capable of delivering their content to the lymphoid tissue, their effectiveness varies according to the route and the vaccination protocol. In this respect, vaccination by the oral route must be viewed with extreme caution since the antigen feeding may result in inducing oral tolerance. In other words, although antigen delivery may be quite efficient, antigen must be associated with the right adjuvant molecule. In this respect, ISCOMs represent the most paradoxical case. On one hand, they are able to induce proliferation of antigen-specific MHC I-restricted $CD8^+$ CTL after parenteral immunization, and in turn may protect against a virus infection even when virus enters at the mucosal level. On the other hand, ISCOMs are the less efficient carrier systems because they form stable complexes only with amphiphatic molecules such as viral envelope glycoproteins. Therefore, their application is strictly related to their adjuvant activity. Unfortunately, their adjuvanticity parallels their toxicity. With parenteral immunization some toxicity occurs but adjuvant activity is maximum. When toxicity is absent, as in the case of the oral route, immune response is poor (Ghazi *et al.*, 1995). While the intranasal route appears to be very promising, additional studies are required to develop a suitable protocol for human trials. Intramuscular immunization, in mice, seems to have an advantage over intranasal immunization and particularly over oral immunization in terms of reliability and long-lasting protection. The side effects seen in humans with doses of over 50–100 μg pose a risk *versus* benefit problem.

Because the biologic properties of liposomes are strikingly dependent on lipid content, and because even small differences in lipid content appear to make large differences in their biologic properties, experimental data have had poor reproducibility. A common cause of the variability in lipid structure is the spontaneous degradation of lipids due to their reaction with oxygen.

Although studies in animal models have provided encouraging results, the stability of liposome preparations during storage remains limited. In addition, problems in the gut, where it has been reported that liposomes are not stable, are not taken up by epithelial cells, and do not promote absorption of entrapped drugs, must be overcome (Chiang and Weiner, 1987).

At this time, ME containing block copolymers appears to be a good oral vehicle to deliver antigens to GALT. The ME system seems to protect entrapped antigen from the digestive conditions present in the intestinal lumen. This is probably due to the thickness of the lipidic wall separating the internal water-soluble antigen from the lumen. However, the presence of additional adjuvants such as CT seems necessary to guarantee a high protective response at the intestinal mucosa level. Without CT in the ME formulation, oral tolerance may be induced. Therefore, much additional work must be done to increase understanding of the immunological determinants when ME are used as vaccine vehicles, and hence to increase the predictability of the immune response.

Acknowledgments

We thank Dr. Charles O. Elson and Dr. Robert L. Hunter for their generous technical and scientific contributions, Ms. Marianne Simon for her technical editing, Ms. Charlene Beach for editing and preparing the manuscript, and Mr. Curiano' Cosimo Marino for producing the graphics for the figures.

References

Abraham, E. (1992). Intranasal immunization with bacterial polysaccharide containing liposomes enhances antigen-specific pulmonary secretory antibody response. *Vaccine* **10,** 461–468.

Adamson, A. W. (1982). "Physical Chemistry of Surfaces." Wiley, New York.

Allison, A. C., and Byars, N. E. (1990). Adjuvant formulations and their mode of action. *Semin. Immunol.* **2,** 369–374.

Alving, C. R. (1991). Liposomes as carriers of antigens and adjuvants. *J. Immunol. Methods* **140,** 1–13.

Alving, C. R. (1993). Lipopolysaccharide, lipid A, and liposomes containing lipid A as immunologic adjuvants. *Immunobiology* **187,** 430–446.

Alving, C. R. (1994). Liposomes as vehicles for vaccines. *In* "Handbook of Natural Toxins Volume 8: Microbial Toxins" (B. Igleviski, M. Vaughan, A. T. Tu, and J. Moss, eds.), Dekker, New York.

Alving, C. R. (1995). Liposomal vaccines: Clinical status and immunological presentation for humoral and cellular immunity. *Ann. N.Y. Acad. Sci.* **754,** 143–152.

Alving, C. R., and Wassef, N. M. (1994). Cytotoxic T lymphocytes induced by liposomal antigens: Mechanisms of immunological presentation. *AIDS Res. Hum. Retroviruses* **10**(Suppl. 2), S91–S94.

Aramaki, Y., Tomizawa, H., Hara, T., Yachi, K., Kikuchi, H., and Tsuchiya, S. (1993). Stability of liposomes *in vitro* and their uptake by rat Peyer's patches following oral administration. *Pharm. Res.* **10,** 1228–1231.

Auland, M. E., Roufogalis, B. D., Devaux, P. F., and Zachowski, A. (1994). Reconstitution of ATP-dependent aminophospholipid translocation in proteoliposomes. *Proc. Natl. Acad. Sci. U.S.A.* **91,** 10938–10942.

Ben-Ahmeida, E. T., Jennings, R., Erturk, M., and Potter, C. W. (1992). The IgA and subclass IgG responses and protection in mice immunised with influenza antigens administered as ISCOMs, with FCA, ALH or as infectious virus. *Arch. Virol.* **125,** 71–86.

Ben-Ahmeida, E. T. S., Gregoriadis, G., Potter, C. W., and Jennings, R. (1993). Immunopotentiation of local and systemic humoral immune responses by ISCOMS, liposomes and FCA: Role in protection against influenza A in mice. *Vaccine* **11,** 1302–1309.

Bennett, B., Check, I. J. , Olsen, M. R., and Hunter, R. L. (1992). A comparison of commercially available adjuvants for use in research. *J. Immunol. Methods* **153,** 31–40.

Bergmann, K. C., and Waldman, R. H. (1986). Stimulation of secretary antibody following oral administration of antigen. *Rev. Infect. Dis.* **10,** 939–950.

Britt, W., Fay, J., Sealr, J., and Kensil, C. (1995). Formulation of an immunogenic human cytomegalovirus vaccine: responses in mice. *J. Infect. Dis.* **171,** 18–25.

Bui, T., Dykers, T., Hu, S. L., Faltynek, C. R., and Ho, R. J. (1994). Effect of MPT-PE liposomes and interleukin-7 on induction of antibody and cell-mediated immune responses to a recombinant HIV-envelope protein. *J. Acquired Immun. Defic. Syndr.* **7,** 799–806.

Chavali, S. R., and Campbell, J. B. (1987). Adjuvant effects of orally administered saponins on humoral and cellular immune responses in mice. *Immunobiology* **174,** 347–359.

Chiang, C. M., and Weiner, N. (1987). Gastrointestinal uptake of liposomes. I. *In vitro* and *in situ* studies. *Int. J. Pharm.* **37,** 75–83.

Childers, N. K., Michalek, S. M., Denys, F., and McGhee, J. R. (1987). Characterization of liposomes for oral vaccines. *Adv. Exp. Med. Biol.* **216B,** 1771–1780.

Chin, Y. H., Cai, J., and Hieselaar, T. (1991). Lymphocyte migration into mucosal lymphoid tissues: Mechanism and modulation. *Immunol. Res.* **10,** 271–278.

Claassen, E., Kors, N., and van Rooijen, N. (1987). Immunomodulation with liposomes: The immune response elicited by liposomes with entrapped dichloromethylene-diphosphonate and surface-associated antigen or hapten. *Immunology* **60,** 509–515.

Claassen, I., and Osterhaus, A. (1992). The ISCOM structure as an immune-enhancing moiety experience with viral systems. *Res. Immunol.* **143,** 531–541.

Dallocchio, F., Tomasi, M., and Bellini, T. (1995). Activation of the Sendai virus fusion protein by receptor binding. *Biochem. Biophys. Res. Commun.* **208,** 36–41.

Dal Monte, P. D., and Szoka, F. C. (1989). Effect of liposomes encapsulation on antigen presentation *in vitro*. Comparison of presentation by peritoneal macrophages and B cell tumors. *J. Immunol.* **142,** 1437–1443.

Dalsgaard, K. (1974). Saponin adjuvants: III. Isolation of a substance from *Quillaja saponaria* Molina with adjuvant activity in foot-and-mouth disease vaccines. *Arch. Gesamte. Virusforsch.* **44,** 243–254.

de Haan, A., Renegar, K. B., Small, P. A., Jr., and Wilschutt, J. (1995). Induction of a secretory IgA response in the murine female urogenital tract by immunization of the lungs with liposome-supplemented viral subunit antigen. *Vaccine* **13,** 613–616.

Dertzbaugh, M. T., and Elson, C. O. (1991). Cholera toxin as a mucosal adjuvant. *In* "Topics in Vaccine Adjuvant Research" (D. Spriggs and W. Koff, eds.), pp. 119–132. CRC Press, Boca Raton, Florida.

Elkins, C., Barkley, K. B., Carbonetti, N. H., Coimbre A. J., and Sparling, P. F. (1994). Immunobiology of purified recombinant outer membrane porin protein I of *Neisseria gonorrhoeae. Mol. Microbiol.* **14,** 1059–1075.

Ellens, H., Morselt, H., and Scherphof, G. (1981). *In vivo* fate of large unilamellar sphingomyelin–cholesterol liposomes after intraperitoneal and intravenous injection into rats. *Biochim. Biophys. Acta* **674,** 10–18.

Elson, C. O., Tomasi, M., Dertzbaugh, M. T., Thaggard, G., Hunter, R. L., and Weaver C. (1996). Oral antigen delivery via a multiple emulsion system enhances oral tolerance. *Proc. N.Y. Acad. Sci.* in press.

Fries, L. F., Gordon, D. M., Richards, R. L., Egan, J. E., Hollingdale, M. R., Gross, M., Silverman, C., and Alving, C. R. (1992). Liposomal malaria vaccine in humans: A safe and potent adjuvant strategy. *Proc. Natl. Acad. Sci. U.S.A.* **89,** 358–362.

Freund, J. (1951). The effect of paraffin oil and mycobacteria on antibody formation and sensitization. *Am. J. Clin. Pathol.* **21,** 645–657.

Germain, R. N. (1986). Immunology. The ins and outs of antigen processing and presentation. *Nature (London)* **322,** 687–689.

Ghazi, H. O., Potter, C. W., Smith, T. L., and Jennings, R. (1995). Comparative antibody response and protection in mice immunised by oral or parenteral routes with influenza virus subunit antigens in aqueous form or incorporated into ISCOMS. *J. Med. Microbiol.* **42,** 53–61.

Ghazi, H. O., Erturk, M., Stannard, L. M., Faulkner, M., Potter, C. W., and Jennings, R. (1995). Immunogenicity of influenza and HSV-1 mixed antigen ISCOMs in mice. *Arch. Virol.* **140,** 1015–1031.

Gregoriadis, G. (1990). Immunological adjuvants: A role for liposomes. *Immunol. Today* **11,** 89–97.

Gregoriadis, G. (1994). The immunological adjuvant and vaccine carrier properties of liposomes. *J. Drug Targeting* **2,** 351–356.

Gregoriadis, G., Tan, L., Ben-Ahmeida, E. T., and Jennings, R. (1992). Liposomes enhance the immunogenicity of reconstituted influenza virus A/PR/8 envelopes and the formation of protective antibody by influenza virus A/Sichuan/87 (H3N2) surface antigen. *Vaccine* **10,** 747–753.

Hancock, G. E., Speelman, D. J., Frenchick, P. J., Mineo-Kuhn, M. M., Baggs, R. B., and Hahn, D. J. (1995). Formulation of the purified fusion protein of respiratory syncytial virus with the saponin QS-21 induces protective immune responses in BALB/c mice that are similar to those generated by experimental infection. *Vaccine* **13,** 391–400.

Harokopakis, E., Childers, N. K., Michalek, S. M., Zhang, S. S., and Tomasi, M. (1995). Conjugation of cholera toxin or its B subunit to liposomes for targeted delivery of antigens. *J. Immunol. Methods* **185,** 31–42.

Hearn, T.L. (1994). Murine mucosal and systemic immune responses to antigens delivered by oral infusion in water-in-oil-in-water emulsions containing nonionic block copolymer P1005. Unpublished Ph.D. Dissertation, Emory University, Atlanta, Georgia.

Heeg, K., Kuon, W., and Wagner, H. (1991). Vaccination of class I major histocompatibility complex (MHC)-restricted murine $CD8^+$ cytotoxic T lymphocytes towards soluble antigens: Immunostimulating-ovalbumin complexes enter the class I MHC-restricted antigen pathway and allow sensitization against the immunodominant peptide. *Eur. J. Immunol.* **21,** 1523–1527.

Hogle, J. M., Chow, M., and Filman, D. J. (1985). Three dimensional structure of poliovirus at 2.9 A resolution. *Science* **229,** 1358–1365.

Hope, M. J., Bally, M. B., Webb, G., and Cullis, P. R. (1985). Production of large unilamellar vesicles by a rapid extrusion procedure. Characterization of size distribution, trapped volume and ability to maintain a membrane potential. *Biochim. Biophys. Acta* **812,** 55–65.

Hulskotte, E. G., Geretti, A. M ., Siebelink, K. H., van Amerongen, G., Cranage, M. P., Rud, E. W., Norley, S. G., de Vries, P., and Osterhaus, A. D. (1995). Vaccine-induced virus-neutralizing antibodies and cytotoxic T cells do not protect macaques from experimental infection with simian immunodeficiency virus SIVmac32H (J5). *J. Virol.* **69,** 6289–6296.

Hunter, R. L., Strickland, F., and Kezdy, F. (1981). The adjuvant activity of nonionic block polymer surfactants I. The role of hydrophile–lipophile balance. *J. Immunol.* **127,** 1244–1250.

Ifversen, P., Martensson, C., Danielsson, L., Ingvar, C., Carlsson, R., and Borrebaeck, C. A. (1995). Induction of primary antigen-specific immune responses in SCID-hu-PBL by coupled T-B epitopes. *Immunology* **84,** 111–116.

Jackson, S., Mestecky, J., Childers, N. K., and Michalek, S. M. (1990). Liposomes containing anti-idiotypic antibodies: An oral vaccine to induce protective secretory immune responses specific for pathogens of mucosal surfaces. *Infect. Immun.* **58,** 1932–1936.

James, S. P. (1993). The gastrointestinal mucosal immune system. *Dig. Dis.* **11,** 146–156.

Janeway, C. A., Jr. (1992). The immune system evolved to discriminate infectious nonself from non-infection self. *Immun. Today* **13,** 11–16.

Kalish, M. L., Check, I. J., and Hunter, R. L. (1991). Murine IgG isotype responses to the *Plasmodium cynomolgi* circumsporozoite peptide $(NAGG)_5$. I. effects of carrier, copolymer adjuvants, and lipopolysaccharide on isotype selection. *J. Immunol.* **146,** 3583–3590.

Kensil, C. R., Patel, C.; Lennick, M., and Marciani, D. (1991). Separation and characterization of saponins with adjuvant activity from *Quillaja saponaria* Molina cortex. *J. Immunol.* **146,** 431–437.

Kersten, G. F., and Crommelin, D. J. (1995). Liposomes and ISCOMs as vaccine formulations. *Biochim. Biophys. Acta* **1241,** 117–138.

Larsson, M., Lovgren, K., and Morein, B. (1993). Immunopotentiation of synthetic oligopeptides by chemical conjugation to ISCOMS. *J. Immunol. Methods* **162,** 257–260.

Latif, N., and Bachhawat, B. K. (1984). The effect of surface charges of liposomes in immunopotentiation. *Biosci. Rep.* **4,** 99–107.

Leserman, L. D., Barbet J., Kourilsky, F., and Weinstein, J. N. (1980). Targeting to cells of fluorescent liposomes covalently coupled with monoclonal antibody or protein A. *Nature (London)* **288,** 602–604.

Livingston, P. O., Adiuri, S., Heliing, F., Yao, T.-J., Kensil, O. R., Newman, M. J., and Marciani, O. (1994). Phase I trial of immunological adjuvant QS-21 with a GM2 ganglioside-keyhole limpet haemocyanin conjugate vaccine in patients with malignant melanoma. *Vaccine* **12,** 1275–1280.

Loughrey, H. C., Choi, L. S., Cullis, P. R., and Bally, M. B. (1990). Optimized procedures for the coupling of proteins to liposomes. *J. Immunol. Methods* **132,** 25–35.

Loughrey, H. C., Choi, I. S., Wong, W. F., Cullis, P. R., and Bally, M. B. (1993). Preparation of streptavidin-liposomes for use in ligand specific targeting applications. *In* "Liposome Technology" (G. Gregoriadis, ed.), Vol. 3, 2nd Ed., p. 163. CRC Press, Boca Raton, Florida.

Lovgren, K. (1988). The serum antibody response distributed in subclasses and isotypes after intranasal and subcutaneous immunization with influenza virus immunostimulating complexes. *Scand. J, Immunol.* **27**, 241–245.

Lovgren, K., and Morein, B. (1988). The requirement of lipids for the formation of immunostimulating complexes (ISCOMs). *Biotechnol. Appl. Biochem.* **10**, 161–172.

Lovgren, K., Kaberg, H., and Morein, B. (1990). An experimental influenza subunit vaccine (ISCOM): Induction of protective immunity to challenge infection in mice after intranasal or subcutaneous administration. *Clin. Exp. Immunol.* **82**, 435–439.

Lycke, N., Tsuji, T., and Holmgren, J. (1992). The adjuvant effect of *Vibrio cholerae* and *E. coli* heat labile enterotoxins is linked to the ability to stimulate cAMP. *Eur. J. Immunol.* **22**, 2277–2281.

Mestecky, J. (1987). The common mucosal immune system and current strategies for induction of immune responses in external secretions. *J. Clin. Immunol.* **7**, 265–276.

Michalek, S. M., Childers, N. K., Katz, J., Denys, F. R., Berry, A. K., Eldridge, J. H., McGhee, J. R., and Curtiss, R. (1989). Liposomes as oral adjuvants. *Curr. Top. Microbiol. Immunol.* **146**, 51–62.

Michalek, S. M., Childers, N. K., Katz, J., Dertzbaugh, M., Zhang, S., Russell, M. W., Macrina, F. L., Jackson, S. and Mestecky, J. (1992). Liposomes and conjugate vaccines for antigen delivery and induction of mucosal immune responses. *Adv. Exp. Med. Biol.* **327**, 191–198.

Morein, B. (1990). The ISCOM: An immunostimulating system. *Immunol. Lett.* **25**, 281–283.

Morein, B., Sundquist, B., Hoglund, S., Dalsgaard, K., and Osterhaus, A. (1984). ISCOM, a novel structure for antigenic presentation of membrane proteins from enveloped viruses. *Nature (London)* **308**, 457–460.

Morein, B., Villacres-Eriksson, M., Akerblom, L., Ronnberg, B., Lovgren, K., and Sjolander, A. (1994). Mechanism behind the immune response induced by immunostimulating complexes. *AIDS Res. Hum. Retroviruses* **10**(Suppl. 2), S109–S114.

Mowat, A. M. (1994). Oral tolerance and regulation of immunity to dietary antigens. *In* "Handbook of Mucosal Immunology"(P. L. Ogra *et al.*, eds.), pp. 185–201. Academic Press, New York.

Mowat, A. M., and Donachie, A. M. (1991). ISCOMS—a novel strategy for mucosal immunization. *Immunol. Today* **12**, 383–385.

Mowat, A. M., Donachie, A. M., Reid, G., and Jarrett, O. (1991). Immune-stimulating complexes containing Quil A and protein antigen prime class I MHC-restricted T lymphocytes *in vivo* and are immunogenic by the oral route. *Immunology* **72**, 317–322.

Newman, M. J., Wu, J. Y., Gardner, B. H., Munroe, K, J., Leombruno, D., Recchia, J., Kensil, C. R., and Coughlin, R. T. (1992). Saponin adjuvant induction of ovalbumin-specific $CD8^+$ cytotoxic T-lymphocyte responses. *J. Immunol.* **148**, 2357–2362.

Ozel, M., Hoglund, S., Gelderblom, H. R., and Morein, B. (1989). Quaternary structure of the immunostimulating complex (iscom). *J. Ultrastruct. Mol. Struct Res.* **102**, 240–248.

Phillips, N. C., and Emili, A. (1992). Enhanced antibody response to liposome-associated protein antigens: Preferential stimulation IgG2a/b production. *Vaccine* **10**, 151–158.

Pierce, N. F., and Sacci, J. B., Jr. (1984). Enhanced mucosal priming by cholera toxin and procholeragenoid with a lipoidal amine adjuvant (avridine) delivered in liposomes. *Infect. Immun.* **44**, 469–473.

Putkonen, P., Siorling, E., Akerblom, L., Thorstensson, R., Lovgren, K., Benthin, L., Chiodi, F., Morein, B., Biberfield, G., Norrby, E., and Wigzell, H. (1994). Long-standing protection of macaques against cell-free HIV-2 with a HIV-2 iscom vaccine. *J. Acquired Immun. Defic. Syndr.* **7**, 551–559.

Ravindranath, M. H., Morton, D. L., and Irie, R. F. (1994). Attachment of monophosphoryl lipid A (MPL) to cells and liposomes augments antibody response to membrane-bound gangliosides. *J. Autoimmun.* **7**, 803–816.

Rook, G. A., and Stanford, J. L. (1995). Adjuvant, endocrines and conserved epitopes; factors to consider when designing a therapeutic vaccine. *Int. J. Immunopharmacol.* **17**, 91–102.

Scheepers, K., and Becht, H. (1994). Protection of mice against an influenza virus infection by oral vaccination with viral nucleoprotein incorporated into immunostimulating complexes. *Med. Microbiol. Irnmunol.* **183**, 265–278.

Schultz, N., Oratz, R., Chen, D., Zeleniuch-Jacquotte A., Abeles, G., and Bystryn, J. C. (1995). Effect of DETOX as an adjuvant for melanoma vaccine. *Vaccine* **13**, 503–508.

Stieneker, F., Kersten, G., van Bloois, L., Crommelin, D. J. A., Hem, S. L., Lower, J., and Kreuter, J. (1995). Comparison of 24 different adjuvants for inactivated HIV-2 split whole virus as antigen in mice. Induction of titres of binding antibodies and toxicity of the formulations. *Vaccine* **13**, 45–53.

Szoda, F., Jr., and Papahadjopoulos, D. (1980). Comparative properties and methods of preparation of lipid vesicles (liposomes). *Annu. Rev. Biophys. Bioeng.* **9**, 467–508.

Takahashi, H., Takeshita, T., Morein, B., Putney, S., Germain, R. N., and Berzofky, J. (1990). Induction of $CD8^+$ cytotoxic T cells by immunization with purified HIV-1 envelope protein in ISCOMS. *Nature (London)* **344**, 873–875.

ten Hagen, T.L., van Vianen W., and Bakker-Woudenberg, I.A. (1995). Modulation of nonspecific antimicrobial resistance of mice to *Klebsiella pneumoniae* septicemia by liposome-encapsulated muramyl tripeptide phosphatidylethanolamine and interferon-gamma alone or combined. *J. Infect. Dis.* **171**, 385–392.

Thapar, M. A., Parr, E. L., Bozzola, J. J., and Parr, M. B. (1991). Secretory immune responses in the mouse vagina after parenteral or intravaginal immunization with an immunostimulating complex (ISCOM). *Vaccine* **9**, 129–133.

The European Concerted Action on Macaque Models for AIDS Research (1995). Protection of macaques against simian immunodeficiency virus infection with inactivated vaccines: Comparison of adjuvants, doses and challenge viruses. *Vaccine* **13**, 295–300.

Tomasi, M., Dertzbaugh, M. T., Hunter, R. L., and Elson, C. O. (1996). The use of multiple emulsion system containing non-ionic block copolymers and cholera toxin for oral immunization. Submitted.

Van Rooijen, N. (1993). Immunoadjuvant activities of liposomes: two different macrophage-mediated mechanisms. *Vaccine* **11**, 1170–1176.

Villacres-Eriksson, M., Bergstrom-Mollaoglu, M., Kaberg, H., and Morein, B. (1992). Involvement of interleukin and interferon-gamma in the immune response induced by influenza virus iscoms. *Scand. J. Immunol.* **36**, 421–426.

Walker, C., Selby, M., Erickson, A., Cataldo, D., Valensi, J. P., and Van Nest, G. (1992). Cationic lipids direct a viral glycoprotein into the class I major histocompatibility complex antigen-presentation pathway. *Proc. Natl. Acad. Sci. U.S.A.* **89**, 7915–7918.

Watson, D. L., Lovgren, K., Watson, N. A., Fossum, C., and Morein, B. (1989). Inflammatory response and antigen localization following immunization with influenza virus ISCOM. *Inflammation* **13**, 641–649.

White, A., Cloutier, P., and Coughlin, R. (1991). A purified saponin acts as an adjuvant for T-independent antigen. *In* "Immunobiology of Proteins and Peptides. Human Immunodeficiency Virus, Antibody Immunoconjugates, Bacterial Vaccines and Immunomodulators" (M. Z. Atassi, ed.), pp. 207–210. Plenum, New York.

White, J., Kielian, M., and Helenius, A. (1983). Membrane fusion proteins of enveloped virus. *Rev. Biophys.* **16**, 151–195.

Yasuda, T., Dancey, G. F., and Kinsky, S. C. (1977). Immunogenicity of liposomal model membranes in mice: Dependence on phospholipid composition. *Proc. Natl. Acad. Sci. U.S.A.* **74**, 1234–1236.

Zhou, F., Kraehenbuhl, J. P., and Neutra, M. R. (1995). Mucosal IgA response to rectally administrated antigen formulated in IgA-coated liposomes. *Vaccine* **13**, 637–644.

Zumbuehl, O., and Weder, H. G. (1981). Liposomes of controllable size in the range of 40 to 180 nm by defined dialysis of lipid/detergent mixed micelles. *Biochim. Biophys. Acta* **640**, 252–262.

14

Passive Immunity for Protection against Mucosal Infections and Vaccination for Dental Caries

SHIGEYUKI HAMADA
Department of Oral Microbiology
Osaka University Faculty of Dentistry
Suita, Osaka 565, Japan

YOSHIKATSU KODAMA
Immunology Research Institute in Gifu
Sano, Gifu 501–11, Japan

I. Introduction

A variety of innate and acquired defense mechanisms exist that protect the host from potential pathogenic microorganisms. The outcome of a particular infection depends on interactions between the virulent capability of the pathogen to evade and damage the host as well as the degree of adaptive immune responses in the host. The adaptive immune response is quiescent until stimulated by immunizing events, usually infections. Vaccination is the intentional process that can stimulate adaptive resistance in the host by enhancing humoral immune responses. Since a variety of microbial infections occur at the mucosa or penetrate through mucosal surfaces of the body, induction of antibodies in the mucosa is desirable in vaccinations. Since it is frequently difficult to induce sufficient immunoglobulin levels for protecting the host following current immunization procedures, passive immunization may be considered as an alternative measure for controlling infectious diseases in humans and animals. Use of egg yolk antibodies from hens immunized by specific virulence factors or microorganisms may provide a novel approach to the control of infectious disease; this approach is reviewed in this chapter.

II. Concept of Passive Immunity

A. Basic Aspects of Passive Immunity

Empirical observations of the transfer of immunity from mother to offsprings represent perhaps the first observation for passive antibody protection. The factors conferring immunity not produced by the infants or the fetus could be provided by the mother who possessed antibodies directed against microbes present in her environment (Goldman *et al.*, 1985). It is now well known that IgG alone among the five immunoglobulin classes is actively transported across the placenta. This property provides passive immunity to the newborn baby. The IgG molecules are degraded with a half-life of about 1 month, which accounts for the decrease in the serum IgG concentration in the newborn over the first 3 months after birth. During the first 6 months of life, the rate of newly synthesized IgG by the infants overcomes the decrease of the IgG passively derived from the mother. IgM in infants reaches adult levels by 9 month of age; however, other immunoglobulins, i.e., IgA, IgE, and IgD, are not clearly demonstrated in the serum of infants (Lydyard and Grossi, 1989).

The first successful demonstration of passive immunity can be attributed to von Behring and Kitasato (1890). They clearly demonstrated that immunity to diphtheria and tetanus could be transferred passively to naive mice by the antisera produced in rabbits. This discovery revolutionized the concept of humoral immunity, revealing that serum antibodies were the active entity for protecting the host from infectious and/or toxemic diseases. Thus, recipient animals which had serum antitoxin antibodies became resistant to the challenge with the culture filtrate of *Corynebacterium diphtheriae* or *Clostridium tetani,* which contained an otherwise lethal dose of diphtheria or tetanus toxin, respectively. Their pioneering approach revealed that serum antibodies played a pivotal role in host defense against virulence factors of infectious agents. Passive immunization can confer immunity in the host very quickly. This prin-

MUCOSAL VACCINES

ciple is practically applied to the treatment or prophylaxis of venoms from snake or spider bites, from tetanus toxin, or from the rabies virus that may result in otherwise lethal consequences (Renegar and Small, 1994).

B. Naturally Occurring Passive Immunity

Evidence indicates that colostrum and mother's milk sustain and even augment the protection of infants against infections in humans and in experimental animals prior to the development of gastrointestinal (GI) tract immunity. Epidemiological surveys also revealed that breast-fed infants induced fewer intestinal infections and hospital admissions than non-breast-fed control subjects (Goldman *et al.*, 1985). The class of immunoglobulins in milk and colostrum may vary with the animal species. In humans, secretory IgA (S-IgA) is the major antibody isotype found in milk and colostrum; however, the concentrations of IgG and IgM are as high as 600 mg/liter in colostrum and 50 mg/liter in milk (Mehta *et al.*, 1989). S-IgA is resistant to proteinases and gastric acid and remains active in the intestinal tract of infants. Thus, S-IgA and most probably other components in milk and colostrum provide local passive immunity in the urinary and intestinal tracts (Haneberg, 1974; Prentice, 1987; Glass *et al.*, 1983; Rolfe and Song, 1995).

In ungulates, the major antibody in their colostrum is IgG; however, during lactation, the concentration of S-IgA markedly increases, which of course is the opposite for levels of S-IgA in human colostrum and milk. For example, piglets receive almost all of their maternal antibody contribution from colostrum (i.e., IgG) during the first 24 hr after birth. Thus, piglets at birth obtain IgG from the colostrum of the dam, which is absorbed by the intestinal mucosa for up to 34 hr and is then transported to the circulation of the suckling pig (Yokoyama *et al.*, 1993). In calves, absorption of colostral antibodies is limited to the first few hours of life (Besser and Gay, 1994). Rodents, on the other hand, can actively take up IgG for about 2 weeks, and their protection may be supported either by the direct action of the milk suckled or by the maternal antibody being adsorbed into the blood stream and secretions of the offspring, or both (Shope and Schiemann, 1991). In summary, the mother's colostrum is an effective means by which the offspring can acquire passive immunity to infectious agents which are encountered from the environment.

III. Experimental Approach for Mucosal Passive Immunization against Infections

A. Use of Specific Antibodies for Passive Immunization

Relatively large quantities of antibodies specific for targeted pathogenic microorganisms are required in order to accomplish passive transfer of systemic and local immunity. For this purpose, antibodies elaborated in other individuals of the same animal species or in some cases in other animal species are prepared from various sources. Polymeric antibodies have been isolated from serum, milk, and colostrum of immunized animals as well as egg yolks from immunized hens. Monospecific antibodies can be easily obtained from these sources if a highly purified antigen from a pathogen is used as an immunogen together with appropriate adjuvant. In addition to obtaining preformed antibodies from live animals or humans, antibodies can be prepared from culture supernatants of hybridoma cells producing monoclonal antibodies (mAb). Theoretically, mAbs can be continuously obtained without sacrificing animals, and is a good source for use in passive immunity (Zimmerman *et al.*, 1985).

There are various methods commonly used for preparation and purification of antibodies, mainly IgG, from serum of immunized animals or humans (Motin *et al.*, 1994; Wong *et al.*, 1994). Nonpurified antibody preparations can be used successfully for passive immunization; however, in most cases, antibodies are purified to various degrees by using salt precipitation, ion exchange column chromatography, and/or gel filtration (Marchalonis and Warr, 1982). Some examples of antibody-containing preparations other than antiserum for testing efficacy of passive immunization are summarized below.

1. *Saliva and Mucosal Surface Wash*

As has been suggested, S-IgA at the mucosal tissue surface may protect from colonization and invasion by pathogenic organisms. However, unlike serum antibodies it is not easy to prepare S-IgA in sufficient quantity to use for passive immunity.

Human saliva is but one of the sources used for this purpose. Pooled saliva cleared by ultracentrifugation can be applied to jacalin (a lectin with specificity for human IgA1)-immobilized agarose columns and eluted with melibiose solution (0.1 *M*), dialyzed, and concentrated. This unpure preparation is purified from a saliva sample containing S-IgA by passage over glutardialdehyde glass beads coupled with a protein antigen, which can be eluted with glycine-HCl buffer (0.1 *M*, pH 2.1), dialyzed, and concentrated. This preparation may be recognized as monospecific, purified salivary S-IgA. It was found that an affinity-purified S-IgA protected against group A streptococcal infection under conditions where serum derived IgG was not effective (Bessen and Fischetti, 1988).

Body fluids bathing the mucosal surfaces can be obtained by washing the surfaces with buffered saline. The nasal cavity and the upper respiratory tract from immunized mice were flushed with balanced salt solution as a source of mucosal antibodies (Tamura *et al.*, 1991). The washings were next concentrated, and applied to a protein G–Sepharose column. The effluent could be further loaded on the affinity column using tresyl-activated Sepharose 4B coupled with goat anti-mouse α chain. IgA was eluted with an alkaline buffer, the pH neutralized and the column effluent concentrated. The purified IgA contained 20% monomeric and 80% polymeric IgA as revealed by fractionation profile on Sephacryl S-300 HR column. Intranasal administration of the purified IgA from respiratory tract washings of mice immunized with influenza A virus hemagglutinin (HA) protected mice from challenge with live influenza A virus.

2. *Colostrum and Milk Antibodies*

Bovine milk immunoglobulins given orally/passively have been shown to prevent infections by GI tract pathogenic microorganisms. Immunoglobulin concentrates were prepared from the colostrum of dairy cows immunized with a specific pathogen. The cows were vaccinated by intracutaneous and/or intramuscular injections with a vaccine at appropriate intervals until calving. Hyperimmune colostrum on the first 3 days (typically 5–10 liters/cow/day) after calving was collected, and fat was removed by a cream separator. Colostral nonfat milk which had been pasteurized could be used for oral passive administration to subjects. After casein was removed from the colostral nonfat milk, immunoglobulins were purified by salt fractionation and column chromatography. Both IgG and IgA were found to exhibit anti-pathogen activities (Michalek *et al.*, 1987; Ebina *et al.*, 1990; Petschow and Talbott, 1994).

3. *Hen Egg Yolk Antibodies*

Hen egg yolk is another good source of IgG antibody for passive immunization (Bartz *et al.*, 1980; Yolken *et al.*, 1988; Ikemori *et al.*, 1992). Hens immunized intramuscularly or intradermally with adjuvant produce IgM and IgG antibodies in serum. Serum IgG is then transported into egg yolk, resulting in antibody titers in egg yolk which are similar to those seen in serum (Shimizu *et al.*, 1989; Horikoshi *et al.*, 1993). It is interesting to note that both IgM and IgA antibodies are found in egg white, but not in egg yolk. Thus, the latter is an excellent source of IgG (IgY) antibody for passive immunity (Rose *et al.*, 1974).

For purification of egg yolk antibodies (yAb), egg yolks separated from whites must first be delipidated by addition of saline and chloroform (Peralta *et al.*, 1994; Hamada *et al.*, 1991), propane-2-ol, and acetone (Bade and Stegemann, 1984), or by hydration and sedimentation (O'Farrelly *et al.*, 1992; Horikoshi *et al.*, 1993). After removing lipids, yAb present in the water-soluble fraction (WSF) were separated by differential precipitation with ethanol (Hamada *et al.*, 1991; Horikoshi *et al.*, 1993), ammonium sulfate precipitations (O'Farrelly *et al.*, 1992; Kuroki *et al.*, 1993), and other procedures. Highly purified antibodies can be obtained by DEAE-Sephacel and Sephacryl S-300 chromatography to give a single protein band with a molecular mass of 220 kDa (Fig. 1). This protein is dissociated into 76 kDa heavy (H) and 28 kDa light (L) chains after reduction with of 2-mercaptoethanol (2ME). On the other hand, serum antibodies give a 165-kDa protein band in SDS–polyacrylamide gel electrophoresis (PAGE). Since the 220-kDa yAb and 165-kDa serum antibodies were reactive with anti-hen IgG, it was established that both are of the IgG class. Although yAb have been described as IgY in the literature, these antibodies should be more correctly defined as the IgG class of antibodies (Hamada *et al.*, 1991; Horikoshi *et al.*, 1993).

Oral administration or feeding of egg yolk IgG (yIgG) with anti-pathogen specificity may provide a means for the prevention of oral and GI tract infectious diseases. Since ca. 100 mg yIgG can be obtained from hen eggs, yIgG offers strong advantages as a source of exogenous antibodies that can be used for passive immunization (Yolken *et al.*, 1988).

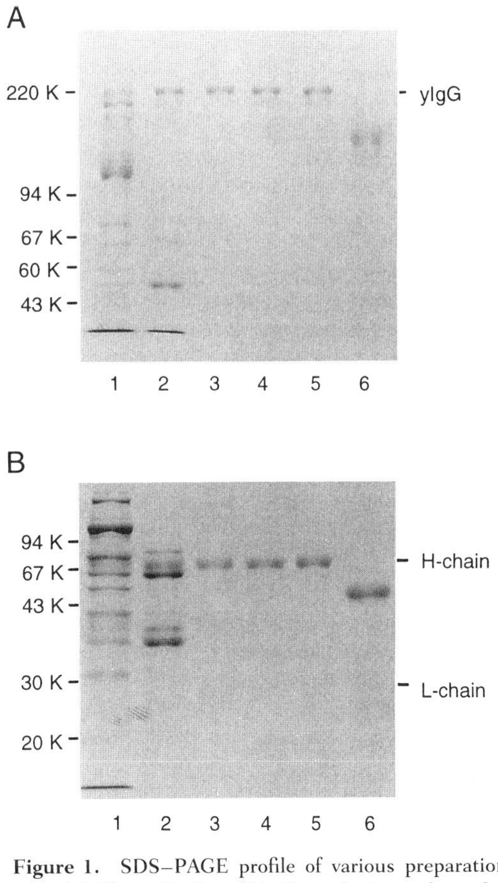

Figure 1. SDS–PAGE profile of various preparations of hen egg yolk (yIgG) antibodies. (A) Nonreducing gels without 2-mercaptoethanol (ME). Yolk proteins (1), WSF (2), chromatographically purified yIgG (3), ethanol-purified yIgG (4), purified hen serum IgG (5), purified rabbit serum IgG (6). (B) Reducing gel in the presence of 2ME. The same samples were applied to the gel as listed in (A). The location of heavy (H) and light (L) chains are indicated. Molecular sizes are shown in kDa. Adapted from Hamada *et al.* (1991) with permission.

4. *Monoclonal Antibodies*

The advantage of using mAb lies in the inherent homogeneity with respect to their immunological specificity, the class of immunoglobulins, and the theoretically limitless supply of antibodies. For production of mAb, hybridoma cells producing mAb are injected intraperitoneally into BALB/c mice that have been primed with pristane. Ascites fluid containing mAb can be taken from mice which exhibit tumor growth following inoculation of the hybridoma. The mAb can be purified by conventional methods (Renegar and Small, 1991a; Ma *et al.*, 1987; Mazenec *et al.*, 1992).

B. Passive Immunization for Protection against Mucosal Infections

1. *Passive Mucosal Protection from Bacterial Infections*

An earlier study reported that bovine milk antibodies obtained from lactating cows immunized with enteropathogenic *Escherichia coli* rapidly eradicated enteropathogenic *E. coli* from the intestine of infants suffering from diarrhea caused by this pathogen (Mietens *et al.*, 1979). The milk immunoglobulin concentrate used in this study was found to neutralize the action of *E. coli* enterotoxin by the rabbit ileal loop test and withstand proteolysis in the digestive tract to a considerable extent. Similar results were found in hamsters given bovine colostral IgG concentrate; bovine IgG specific for *Clostridium difficile* toxins A and B and other antigens protects against disease induced by *C. difficile* in a suckling hamster model of infection (Lyerly *et al.*, 1991).

Mouse IgG1 mAb to *E. coli* K99 pilus was also found to protect calves from experimental infections caused by *E. coli* K99. The mAb was given as ascites fluid at 10 hr of age and this treatment resulted in reduced weight loss, a shorter bout of diarrhea, and a lower mortality rate (Sherman *et al.*, 1983).

The offspring of mammals receive antibodies postnatally through colostrum and mother's milk, and these empirical observations have been experimentally confirmed. For example, foster mouse pups kept with mothers immunized orally by a virulent *Salmonella typhimurium* survived longer than control pups raised with naive mothers, suggesting that mucosal S-IgA antibodies prevent colonization by this pathogen. Since S-IgA is present predominantly in secretions, pooled human saliva is a good source for its isolation. Affinity-purified salivary S-IgA antibodies specific for type 6 M protein of group A *Streptococcus pyogenes* were given to mice intranasally, and it was found that passively administered S-IgA, but not serum IgG, protected mice from streptococcal infection at the mucosal surface. Of interest was the finding that S-IgA alone protected by preventing the initiation of the *S. pyogenes* infection (Bessen and Fischetti, 1988). In other studies, it was clearly demonstrated that mice given ascites containing IgA mAb specific for *Helicobacter felis* intragastrically were protected from *H. felis* infection of the gastric mucosa, although the IgA mAb did not contain secretory component-like serum IgA (Czinn *et al.*, 1993).

A unique model has been devised to provide continuous *in vivo* delivery of antigen-specific monoclonal S-IgA antibody passively into the small intestine of mice by using syngeneic "backpack" hybridoma tumors (Winner *et al.*, 1991). If hybridoma cells secreting IgA mAb specific for *Vibrio cholerae* LPS were injected subcutaneously into mice, the backpack tumors released specific mAb that resulted in increased appearance of this mAb in serum and in the lumen of the GI tract. On the other hand, IgG mAb to *V. cholerae* was not transported into the intestine, even though serum IgG mAb levels were increased. Neonatal mice are known to be highly susceptible to infection by *V. cholerae;* however, neonates injected with the IgA hybridoma cells were resistant to the challenge of *V. cholerae,* while control neonates became ill or died from a severe diarrhea during the same time interval. From these experimental results, it was concluded that the IgA hybridoma tumors backpacked in mice produce a single mAb that identifies a protective epitope and the IgA mAb could protect from mucosal infections by the same or related organisms (Winner *et al.*, 1991).

In this regard, it is essential to identify virulence factors of the pathogenic microorganisms in order to prepare protective antibodies in other animals. Recent progress in gene technology has made it possible to use cloned genes coding for a target virulence factor for production of molecular vaccines. Rabbit polyclonal IgG directed against a virulence factor protein (V antigen) of *Yersinia* species was prepared by using a fusion peptide, PAV. The IgG was found to provide excellent passive immunity in mice against *Yersinia pestis* and *Yersinia pseudotuberculosis,* but not *Y. enterocolitica* (Motin et al., 1994). Recombinant outer membrane proteins, OMPs, of *Pseudomonas aeruginosa* were also used to immunize rabbits to prepare protective serum antibodies. The antisera were found to protect severe combined immunodeficient mice, which do not have mature lymphocytes, against challenge with 1000 LD_{50} doses of *P. aeruginosa* (von Specht *et al.*, 1995).

Another important approach is to develop more simplified and reliable ways for production of mAb or yAb. For this purpose, the technique of development of yAb has been studied extensively for prevention of bacterial infectious diseases during the past 4 years. For example, it was shown that powdered WSF containing yAb to pilus antigens (K88, K99, and 987P) of enterotoxigenic *E. coli* (ETEC) protected neonatal piglets against infection with each of the three strains of ETEC when administered orally (Yokoyama *et al.*, 1992). The protection was found to be dose-dependent, and adsorption of yAb with the pilus antigen removed antibody reactivity and resulted in a significant reduction in the protective nature of the yAb preparation. The yAb were shown to inhibit the adherence of *E. coli* 987 to the intestinal mucosa of antibody-treated but not control piglets (Fig. 2). Similar results have been obtained in rabbits passively administered with yAb directed against heat-treated whole cells of *E. coli*. The rabbits given this yAb were protected from a diarrhea syndrome induced by ETEC, and remained well (O'Farrelly *et al.*, 1992; Ikemori *et al.*, 1992). Furthermore, when yAb specific for *Salmonella enteritidis* 14-kDa fimbriae were given orally to mice, the antibodies protected the host from a challenge with live *S. enteritidis* (2×10^{10} CFU/mouse). In contrast, control mice fed normal yAb manifested various clinical signs with high mortality rates. Thus, oral administration of yAb with specificity for *Salmonella* virulence determinants could serve as an effective tool for the control of intestinal colonization and disease manifestation caused by *Salmonella* infections (Peralta *et al.*, 1994).

2. *Passive Mucosal Protection from Viral Infections*

A large array of viruses infect the mucosal surfaces of the host, including those of the gastrointestinal and respiratory tracts, and are major causes of active infectious diseases on these surfaces, including rotaviruses and influenza viruses, respectively. The host's mucosal immune responses to these viral infections are transient in many cases, and therefore reinfection occurs frequently. Secretory IgA antibodies have been shown to protect mucosal surfaces from various viral infections. In addition to S-IgA, some evidence indicates that the transudation of antiviral IgG into mucosa secretions or passively transferred IgG antibodies can contribute to local mucosal immunity (Childers *et al.*, 1989).

Rotaviruses are ubiquitous in humans and infect animals worldwide. Thus, these viruses are the principal cause of acute infectious diarrhea in young infants both in developed and in third-world countries. Rotavirus infection may result in death from dehydration from the severe diarrhea and vomiting. Only *V. cholerae* infection can cause dehydration with a frequency equal to or greater than rotavirus gastroenteritis. No acceptable vaccine has been produced to date. Passive administration of exogenously produced antibodies elaborated against rotaviruses has been considered as an alternative to active vaccination for prevention of rotavirus infections and subsequent symptoms. It appears that passive immunity to rotavirus is acquired by the newborn from its mother through colostrum (DuPont, 1984; Hilpert *et al.*, 1987; Turner and Kelsey, 1993).

This problem has also been approached by use of passive yAb and it was shown that feeding of WSF containing yAb obtained from hens immunized with simian rotavirus protected 3-day-old mice from infection with murine rotavirus (Bartz *et al.*, 1980). This cross-protection could be achieved due to the antigenic relatedness of rotaviruses from various animal species. Further, passive anti-rotavirus colostral antibody to the human pathogen has been produced in immune cows (Ebina *et al.*, 1985; Tsunemitsu *et al.*, 1989) and from hen egg yolks (Yolken *et al.*, 1988; Ebina *et al.*, 1990). Oral administration of these colostral IgG antibodies prevented the development of diarrhea in infants (Ebina *et al.*, 1985; Turner and Kelsey, 1993). Infants given immune cow's milk concentrate with high rotavirus neutralizing activities in stools showed significantly shorter intervals of virus secretion (Hilpert *et al.*, 1987). yIgG to either homotypic or heterotypic strains of rotavirus prevented the development of gastroenteritis in a suckling mouse model (Yolken *et al.*, 1988; Ebina *et al.*, 1990; Kuroki *et al.*, 1993) as well as in calves challenged with virulent rotavirus (Kuroki *et al.*, 1994).

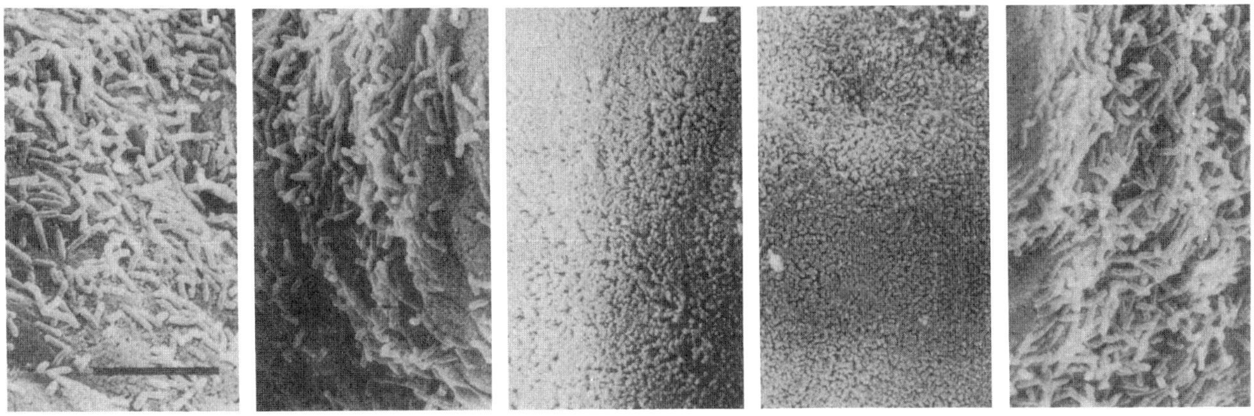

Figure 2. Scanning electron microscopic examination of cellular adherence of an ETEC strain in the ileum of piglets. Villi from the ileum of a nontreated piglet showing adherent enteric bacilli (C), villi of a piglet treated with yIgG to ETEC fimbriae at titers of 156 (1), 623 (2), and 2500(3). The ETEC-laden villus surface of the ileum from a piglet treated with yIgG absorbed with fimbriae. Bar, 10 μm. Adapted from Yokoyama *et al.* (1992) with permission.

Influenza A virus infection is restricted to the upper respiratory tract. Influenza A virus possesses surface glycoproteins, i.e. hemagglutinin (HA) and neuraminidase (NA), that may contribute to attachment and virus penetration during the initial phase of infection. Several major types of HA have been delineated; however, frequent antigenic drift and/or shift of HA occurs. Attachment of viruses to the host cell receptors involves interaction between the HA spike and a sialic acid moiety on epithelial cells lining the mucosal surface of the respiratory tract. Passive antibodies specific for the HA would be expected to prevent adsorption of the viruses. It appears logical to hypothesize that increased levels of anti-HA S-IgA secreted onto the respiratory tract mucosa would be responsible for protective immunity against influenza. Renegar and Small (1991a) demonstrated that intravenously injected polymeric IgA (pIgA) antibody to influenza virus HA was transported physiologically into nasal secretions. The IgA transported into the secretions was functional, as evidenced by antibody to the virus in an ELISA assay which protected mice from actual influenza infection. The protection was abrogated by the intranasal instillation of goat anti-mouse α-chain but not anti-mouse γ-chain, again providing evidence that the monoclonal IgA antibody was protective (Renegar and Small, 1991b).

Mice immunized intranasally with influenza virus A and cholera toxin B subunit (CT-B) induced mucosal S-IgA responses; HA-reactive S-IgA was recovered from the respiratory tract washings. Purified S-IgA from these samples clearly protected mice from the viral challenge when applied to the respiratory tract of naive mice subsequently challenged with virus (Tamura *et al.*, 1991). Purified goat IgG specific for influenza A virus was encapsulated within liposomes and was given to mice intranasally 24 hr before challenge with influenza viruses. These passively immunized mice were found to be fully protected. It was shown that the duration of protection offered by the liposome–antibody complex was relatively longer than of goat antibody not protected by liposomes. The liposome–antibody complex may be protected from *in vivo* dilution and degradation in the upper respiratory tract and lungs (Wong *et al.*, 1994).

Protection against other respiratory viruses with passively derived antibodies has also been reported. For example, it was found that IgA mAb against Sendai virus neutralized the viral activity *in vitro,* and prevented infection of mice challenged with this virus (Mazanec *et al.*, 1987). In a later study, IgG mAb to this virus was reported to be as protective as the IgA mAb in mice challenged intranasally with Sendai virus (Mazanec *et al.*, 1992). Infection of respiratory syncytial virus (RSV) in cotton rats was clearly suppressed by topical administration of human IgG; parenteral application of the IgG was much less effective (Prince *et al.*, 1987).

Several approaches using passive immune therapy for immunodeficiency virus infections have been reported (Zolla-Pazner and Gorny, 1992; Stein *et al.*, 1993). For example, investigators were able to prevent the infection of simian immunodeficiency virus (SIV) and human immunodeficiency virus (HIV) in monkeys as well as feline immunodeficiency virus (FIV) in cats with passive antibody administration (Putkonen *et al.*, 1991; Emini *et al.*, 1992; Hohdatsu *et al.*, 1993). It has been shown that immunization of chimpanzees with human recombinant soluble CD4 molecule elicits an anti-CD4 antibody response that inhibits HIV replication in chimpanzee and human lymphocytes (Watanabe *et al.*, 1992). The administration of serum IgG from AIDS patients which contained antibodies to HIV has been suggested to inhibit HIV replication and spread (Stein *et al.*, 1993). Interruption of the maternal–fetal transmission of HIV could be achieved by passive immunotherapies with human IgG exhibiting high titered antibodies to HIV structural proteins (Prince *et al.*, 1991; Lambert and Stiehm, 1993). These approaches may provide us with valuable insight into the pathogenetic nature of HIV infection (Karpas *et al.*, 1990; Marasco *et al.*, 1993). It should be noted, however, that results obtained by other investigators did not necessarily confer protection by passive antibody immunotherapy (Jacobson *et al.*, 1993; Kent *et al.*, 1994).

3. *Passive Mucosal Antibody Protection from Protozoan Infections*

Cryptosporidium is a protozoan parasite that infects the intestinal epithelium of a wide range of mammals including humans, and is a cause of gastroenteritis and diarrhea. This disease is basically self-limiting in normal hosts; however, it becomes persistent and life-threatening in immunocompromised hosts such as the AIDS patient. No efficacious vaccines or therapeutic agents are available for prevention or treatment of cryptosporidiosis (Fayer and Ungar, 1986). Attempts have been made to determine the efficacy of transfer of passive immunity to cryptosporidiosis through use of mAb, colostral antibodies, or yAb. All of these antibodies were found to neutralize infectivity of *Cryptosporidium parvum* sporozoites for mice. Immune bovine colostral whey was the most effective for neutralization of sporozoites and reduced infectivity in mice challenged with oocysts (Perryman *et al.*, 1990). Antibodies to *C. parvum* were prepared from egg yolks obtained from hyperimmunized hens. The yAb given by gastric gavage were found to reduce the number of parasites on villi of the neonatal mice orally infected with *C. parvum* oocytes (Cama and Sterling, 1991).

Hyperimmune bovine colostrum from pregnant cows immunized with oocytes of *C. parvum* provided protection of neonatal cows and mice against challenge with *C. parvum* oocytes (Fayer *et al.*, 1989a,b). It was also shown that hyperimmune bovine colostrum suppressed infection of *Cryptosporidium* to monolayers of human intestinal epithelial cells (Flanigan *et al.*, 1991). Furthermore, remission of diarrhea in a child with hypogammaglobulinemia was obtained by treatment with hyperimmune bovine colostrum (Tzipori *et al.*, 1986). Similarly, administration of hyperimmune bovine colostrum to *Cryptosporidium* oocysts by direct duodenal infusion of an adult patient with AIDS and with severe symptoms of diarrhea resulted in both remission of symptoms and elimination of oocysts in stool of the patient (Ungar *et al.*, 1990). More studies, however, are required before this approach can be adapted to the general population (Nord *et al.*, 1990).

IV. Vaccination and Passive Immunization against Dental Caries

Dental caries is an infectious disease in which the principal causative agents are mutans streptococci including *Streptococcus mutans* and *Streptococcus sobrinus*. Based on the antigenic specificity of cell wall carbohydrate antigen expressed by these organisms, one can distinguish *S. mutans* by expression of serotypes *c, e,* or *f,* while *S. sobrinus* only expresses either serotype *d* or *g*. Mutans streptococci of serotypes *a, b,* or *h* have been isolated almost exclusively from animals and are not considered as human pathogens. Epidemiological surveys have revealed that serotype *c* organisms are most frequently isolated from human dental caries (Hamada and Slade, 1980). The abilities of mutans streptococci to adhere to the tooth surface in the presence of sucrose and to release acids (mainly lactic acid) from various dietary sugars are etiologically important. Therefore, these two properties, i.e., adherence and acid production, can be considered virulence factors for mutans stretptococci. Adherence of the organisms to the tooth surface is promoted by cell-surface protein antigen (PA) and glucosyltransferases (GTases) catalyzing insoluble, adherent glucan systhesis. Inhibition of cellular adherence by vaccination or passive introduction of preformed antibodies may confer protection against dental caries (Russell and Johnson, 1987; Michalek and Childers, 1990).

A. Vaccination against Dental Caries

Immunization of susceptible hosts with *S. mutans* or virulence-related substance(s) (i.e., a caries vaccine) should induce immune responses that might prevent the organisms from colonizing the tooth surface and/or inhibit biochemical processes/virulence factors of the bacterium. This rationale has been verified, at least experimentally, in rodents and monkeys, but a divergence of opinion exists regarding the determinants for induction of protection among research groups (Hamada and Slade, 1980; Russell and Johnson, 1987). In brief, local or oral immunization with whole cells or isolated antigens of *S. mutans* or *S. sobrinus* induced enhanced levels of salivary S-IgA antibodies specific for immunogen used, which eventually lead to reduced development of dental caries. A variety of antigens including GTase, cell wall lysates, serotype carbohydrate, surface protein antigens (e.g., antigen I/II or PAc, Spa A and 74K protein) and other components have been used (McGhee and Michalek, 1981; Krasse *et al.*, 1987). Oral and/or systemic administration of immunogen has been studied largely in the rat model. Oral administration of purified antigens with liposome–adjuvant complex to rats resulted in higher levels of IgA in saliva and greater protection against caries induction in rats infected with *S. mutans* or *S. sobrinus* (Michalek and Childers, 1990). Enhanced salivary IgA responses were noted in humans following oral administration of GTase derived from *S. sobrinus* (Smith and Taubman, 1987).

In a series of studies by Lehner's group, it was shown that systemic immunization of monkeys with *S. mutans* whole cells or purified protein antigen I/II plus adjuvant induced significant serum IgG responses which correlated with reductions in caries development (Lehner, 1992). It is thought that the serum IgG gains access to the tooth surface through the gingival crevice to exhibit anti-caries activity. However, the mechanism for this transport remains to be elucidated.

B. Passive Immunization against Dental Caries

Passive immunization has been carried out by several research groups in an effort to avoid possible systemic side effects which could result from active immunization. Systemic and local passive immunizations using IgG from immune monkeys or mAb to protein antigen I/II protected monkeys against infection of *S. mutans* and the subsequent development of dental caries in monkeys (Lehner *et al.*, 1992). In rats, passive transfer from dams to their offsprings via colostral IgA/IgG antibodies specific for *S. mutans* antigens resulted in caries reduction (Michalek and Childers, 1990). Good sources of antibodies other than those from the mother must be found for passive immunization. Milk obtained from cows hyperimmunized with *S. mutans* was shown to contain high levels of anti-*S. mutans* IgG1 antibodies. Rats monoinfected with *S. mutans* and given a diet containing the IgG1 exhibited lower plaque scores, numbers of *S. mutans* in plaque, and development of dental caries (Michalek *et al.*, 1987).

Successful trials of passive immunity in enteric infectious diseases using yIgG (*vide supra*) raised the possibility of conferring protection against *S. mutans*-induced dental caries. Therefore, hens were immunized with various *S. mutans* antigens. Special attention was given to purified cell-associated GTase (CA-GTase) as immunogen, since the enzyme was critically important in synthesizing water-insoluble glucan from sucrose. Hyperimmune yIgG specific for CA-GTase and whole cells but not cell free GTase inhibited cell adherence to the glass surface. Only yIgG to CA-GTase reduced plaque accumulation and dental caries development, indicating that CA-GTase is a major virulence attribute of *S. mutans* (Hamada *et al.*, 1991). On the other hand, other investigators claimed that immune yolk powder from hens immunized with whole cells of *S. mutans* resulted in fewer caries lesions (Otake *et al.*, 1991). The immunological specificities of the yolk powder were not determined. In addition, our preliminary studies have indicated that yIgG specific for PAc showed less caries development; however, yIgG to CA-GTase was more efficacious than anti-PAc yIgG. Thus, egg yolks from hyperimmunized hens should provide a convenient and economical source of antibodies for passive immunization. For production of yIgG, it is not necessary to process antibodies from peripheral blood or ascites; thus the production is suited to current regulations for experimental animal protection.

It should be noted here that transgenic plants capable of generating functional S-IgA specific for antigen I/II of *S. mutans* have been developed. Transgenic plants may be suitable for a large-scale production of recombinant S-IgA for passive immunotherapy to infectious diseases (Ma *et al.*, 1995).

IV. Summary and Prospects

In this chapter, we have summarized recent progress for passive immunity against various infectious diseases which affect the mucosal surfaces in humans and in experimental animal models. Passive immunization may be meaningful under the current situation that many oral vaccines exhibit limited efficacy, although oral vaccines are more desirable than other administration routes in many respects. Large quantities of antibodies should be prepared in other animals or *ex vivo*. We have emphasized in this chapter here that hen egg yolk antibodies can be isolated and purified for use in passive immunization. yIgG antibodies have been demonstrated to be efficacious by providing passive immune protection against a variety of microbial diseases. yIgG are superior in various aspects to other antibodies including those from bovine colostrum and milk as well as monoclonal antibodies. The advances in biotechnology and genetic engineering should lead to the development of molecular vaccines that can be used for preparation of antibodies in other animals for passive immunization. In conclusion, existing experimental results suggest that passive immune vaccines may be a promising research area in the health sciences.

References

Bade, H., and Stegemann, H. (1984). Rapid method of extraction of antibodies from hen egg yolk. *J. Immunol.* **74,** 421–426.

Bartz, C. R., Conklin, R. H., Tunstall, C. B., and Steele, J. H. (1980). Prevention of murine rotavirus infection with chicken egg yolk immunoglobulins. *J. Infect. Dis.* **142,** 439–441.

Bessen, D., and Fischetti, V. A. (1988). Passive acquired mucosal immunity to group A streptococci by secretory immunoglobulin A. *J. Exp. Med.* **167,** 1945–1950.

Besser, T. E., and Gay, C. C. (1994). The importance of colostrum to the health of the neonatal calf. *Vet. Clin. North Am. Food Anim. Pract.* **10,** 107–117.

Cama, V. A., and Sterling, C. (1991). Hyperimmune hens as a novel source of anti-*Cryptosporidium* antibodies suitable for passive immune transfer. *J. Protozool.* **38,** 42S–43S.

Childers, N. K., Bruce, M. G., and McGhee, J. R. (1989). Molecular mechanisms of immunoglobulin A defense. *Annu. Rev. Microbiol.* **43,** 503–536.

Czinn, S. J., Cai, A., and Nedrud, J. G. (1993). Protection of germ-free mice from infection by *Helicobacter felis* after active oral or passive IgA immunization. *Vaccine* **11,** 637–642.

DuPont, H. L. (1984). Rotaviral gastoenteritis—some recent developments. *J. Infect. Dis.* **149,** 663–666.

Ebina, T., Sato, A., Umezu, K., Ishida, N., Ohyama, S., Oizumi, A., Aikawa, K., Katagiri, S., Katsushima, N., Imai, A., Kitaoka, S., Suzuki, H., and Konno, T. (1985). Prevention of rotavirus infection by oral administration of cow colostrum containing antihumanrotavirus antibody. *Med. Microbiol. Immunol.* **174,** 177–185.

Ebina, T., Tsukada, K., Umezu, K., Nose, M., Tsuda, K., Hatta, H., Kim, M., and Yamamoto, T. (1990). Gastroenteritis in suckling mice caused by human rotavirus can be prevented with egg yolk immunoglobulin (IgY) and treated with a protein-bound polysaccharide preparation (PSK). *Microbiol. Immunol.* **34,** 617–629.

Emini, E. A., Schleif, W. A., Nunberg, J. H., Conley, A. J., Eda, Y., Tokiyoshi, S., Putney, S. D., Matsushita, S., Cobb, K. E., Jett, C. M., Eichberg, J. W., and Murthy, K. K. (1992). Prevention of HIV-1 infection in chimpanzees by gp120 V3 domain-specific monoclonal antibody. *Nature (London)* **335,** 728–730.

Fayer, R., and Ungar, B. L. P. (1986). *Cryptosporidium* spp. and cryptosporidiosis. *Microbiol. Rev.* **50,** 458–483.

Fayer, R., Andrews, C., Ungar, B. L. P., and Blagburn, B. (1989a). Efficacy of hyperimmune bovine colostrum for prophylaxis of cryptosporidiosis in neonatal calves. *J. Parasitol.* **75,** 393–397.

Fayer, R., Perryman, L. E., and Riggs, M. W. (1989b). Hyperimmune bovine colostrum neutralizes *Cryptosporidium* sporozoites and protects mice against oocyst challenge. *J. Parasitol.* **75,** 151–153.

Flanigan, T., Marshall, R., Redman, D., Kaetzel, C., and Ungar, B. (1991). *In vitro* screening of therapeutic agents against *Cryptosporidium*: Hyperimmune cow colostrum is highly inhibitory. *J. Protozool.* **38,** 225S–227S.

Glass, R. I., Svennerholm, A.-M., Stoll, B. J., Khan, M. R., Hossain, K. M. B., Huq, M. I., and Holmgren, J. (1983). Protection against cholera in breast-fed children by antibodies in breast milk. *N. Engl. J. Med.* **308,** 1389–1392.

Goldman, A. S., Pong, A. J. H., and Goldblum, R. M. (1985). Host defenses: Development and maternal contributions. *Adv. Pediatr.* **32,** 71–100.

Hamada, S., and Slade, H. D. (1980). Biology, immunology, and cariogenicity of *Streptococcus mutans. Microbiol. Rev.* **44,** 331–384.

Hamada, S., Horikoshi, T., Minami, T., Kawabata, S., Hiraoka, J., Fujiwara, T., and Ooshima, T. (1991). Oral passive immunization against dental caries in rats by use of hen egg yolk antibodies specific for cell-associated glucosyltransferase of *Streptococcus mutans. Infect. Immun.* **59,** 4161–4167.

Haneberg, B. (1974). Immunoglobulins in feces from infants fed human or bovine milk. *Scand. J. Immunol.* **3,** 191–197.

Hilpert, H., Brüssow, H., Mietens, C., Sidoti, J., Lerner, L., and Werchau, H. (1987). Use of bovine milk concentrate containing antibody to rotavirus to treat rotavirus gastroenteritis in infants. *J. Infect. Dis.*, **156,** 158–166.

Hohdatsu, T., Pu, R., Torres, B. A., Trujillo, S., Gardner, M. B., and Yamamoto, J. K. (1993). Passive antibody protection of cats against feline immunodeficiency virus infection. *J. Virol.* **67,** 2344–2348.

Horikoshi, T., Hiraoka, J., Saito, M., and Hamada, S. (1993). IgG antibody from hen egg yolks: Purification by ethanol fractionation. *J. Food Sci.* **58,** 739–742.

Ikemori, Y., Kuroki, M., Peralta, R. C., Yokoyama, H., and Kodama, Y. (1992). Protection of neonatal calves against fatal enteric cilibacillosis by administration of egg yolk powder from hens immunized with K99-piliated enterotoxigenic *Escherichia coli. Am. J. Vet. Res.* **53,** 2005–2008.

Jacobson, J. M., Colman, N., Ostrow, N. A., Simson, R. W., Tomesch, D., Marlin, L., Rao, M., Mills, J. L., Clemens, J., and Prince, A. M. (1993). Passive immunotherapy in the treatment of advanced human immnodeficiency virus infection. *J. Infect. Dis.* **168,** 298–305.

Karpas, A., Hewlett, I. K., Hill, F., Gray, J., Byron, N., Gilgen, D., Bally, V., Oates, J. K., Gazzard, B., and Epstein, J. E. (1990). Polymerase chain reaction evidence for human immunodeficiency virus 1 neutralization by passsive immunization in patients with AIDS and AIDS-related complex. *Proc. Natl. Acad. Sci. U.S.A.* **87,** 7613–7617.

Kent, K. A., Kitchin, P., Mills, K. H. G., Page, M., Taffs, F., Corcoran, T., Silvera, P., Flanagan, B., Powell. C., Rose, J., Ling, C., Aubertin, A. M., and Stott, E. J. (1994). Passive immunization of cynomolgue macaques with immune sera or a pool of neutralizing monoclonal antibodies failed to protect against challenge with SIVmac251. *AIDS Res. Hum. Retroviruses* **10,** 189–194.

Krasse, B., Emilson, C.-G., and Gahnberg, L. (1987). An anticaries vaccine: Report on the status of research. *Caries Res.* **21,** 255–276.

Kuroki, M., Ikemori, Y., Yokoyama, H., Peralta, R. C., Icatlo, Jr., F. C., and Kodama, Y. (1993). Passive protection against bovine rotavirus-induced diarrhea in murine model by specific immunoglobulins from chicken egg yolk. *Vet. Microbiol.* **37,** 135–146.

Kuroki, M., Ohta, M., Ikemori, Y., Peralta, R. C., Yokoyama, H., and Kodama, Y. (1994). Passive protection against bovine rotavirus in calves by specific immunoglobulins from chicken egg yolk. *Arch. Virol.* **138,** 143–148.

Lambert, J. S., and Stiehm, E. R. (1993). Passive immunity in the prevention of maternal–fetal transmission of human immunodeficiency virus infection. *Ann. N.Y. Acad. Sci.* **693,** 186–193.

Lehner, T. (1992). "Immunology of Oral Disease," Third Ed., pp. 68–114. Blackwell, Oxford.

Lehner, T., Ma, J. K.-C., and Kelly, C. G. (1992). A mechanism of passive immunization with monoclonal antibodies to a 185,000 Mr streptococcal antigen. *Adv. Exp. Med. Biol.* **327,** 151–163.

Lydyard, P., and Grossi, C. (1989). Development of the immune system. *In* "Immunology" (I. Roitt, J. Brostoff, and D. Male, eds.), 2nd Ed. pp. 14.1–14.10. Gower Medical Publishing, London.

Lyerly, D. M., Bostwick, E. F., Binion, S. B., and Wilkins, T. D. (1991). Passive immunization of hamsters against disease caused by *Clostridium difficile* by use of bovine immunoglobulin G concentrate. *Infect. Immun.* **59,** 2215–2218.

Ma, J. K.-C., Smith, R., and Lehner, T. (1987). Use of monoclonal antibodies in local passive immunization to prevent colonization of human teeth by *Streptococcus mutans. Infect. Immun.* **55,** 1274–1278.

Ma, J. K.-C., Hiatt, A., Hein, M., Vine, N. D., Wang, F., Stabila, P., Van Dolleeweerd, C., Mostov, K., and Lehner, T. (1995). Generation and assembly of secretory antibodies in plants. *Science* **268,** 716–719.

McGhee, J. R., and Michalek, S. M. (1981). Immunobiology of dental caries: Microbial aspects and local immunity. *Annu. Rev. Microbiol.* **35,** 595–638.

Marasco, W. A., Haseltine, W. A., and Chen, S. Y. (1993). Design, intracellular expression, and activity of a human anti-human immunodeficiency virus type 1 gp120 single-chain antibody. *Proc. Natl. Acad. Sci. U.S.A.* **90,** 7889–7893.

Marchalonis, J. J., and Warr, G. W. (1982). "Antibody as a Tool—The Applications of Immunochemistry." Wiley, Chichester.

Mazanec, M. B., Nedrud, J. G., and Lamm, M. E. (1987). Immunoglobulin A monoclonal antibodies protect against Sendai virus. *J. Virol.* **61,** 2624–2626.

Mazanec, M. B., Lamm, M. E., Lyn, D., Portner, A., and Nedrud, J. G. (1992). Comparison of IgA versus IgG monoclonal antibodies for passive immunization of the murine respiratory tract. *Virus Res.* **23,** 1–12.

Mehta, P. D., Mehta, S. P., and Isaacs, C. E. (1989). Distribution of IgG subclasses in human colostrum and milk. *Immunol. Lett.* **22,** 235–238.

Michalek, S. M., and Childers, N. K. (1990). Development and outlook for a caries vaccine. *Crit. Rev. Oral Biol. Med.* **1,** 37–54.

Michalek, S. M., Gregory, R. L., Harmon, C. C., Katz, J.,

Richardson, G. J., Hilton, T., Filler, S. J., and McGhee, J. R. (1987). Protection of gnotobiotic rats against dental caries by passive immunization with bovine milk antibodies to *Streptococcus mutans*. *Infect. Immun.* **55**, 2341–2347.

Mietens, C., Keinhorst, H., Hilpert, H., Gerber, H., Amster, H., and Pahud, J. J. (1979). Treatment of infantile *E. coli* gastroenteritis with specific bovine anti-*E. coli* milk immunoglobulins. *Eur. J. Pediatr.* **132**, 239–252.

Motin, V. L., Nakajima, R., Smirinov, G. B., and Brubaker, R. R. (1994). Passive immunity to yersiniae mediated by anti-recombinant V antigen and protein A-V antigen fusion peptide. *Infect. Immun.* **62**, 4192–4201.

Nord, J., Ma, P., Dijohn, D., Tzipori, S., and Tacket, C. O. (1990). Treatment with bovine hyperimmune colostrum of cryptosporidial diarrhea in AIDS parients. *AIDS* 4, 581–584.

O'Farrelly, C., Branton, D., and Wanke, C. A. (1992). Oral ingestion of egg yolk immunoglobulin from hens immunized with an enterotoxigenic *Escherichia coli* strain prevents diarrhea in rabbits challenged with the same strain. *Infect. Immun.* **60**, 2593–2597.

Otake, S., Nishihara, Y., Makimura, M., Hatta, H., Kim, M., Yamamoto, T., and Hirasawa, M. (1991). Protection of rats against dental caries by passive immunization with hen–egg–yolk antibody (IgY). *J. Dent. Res.* **70**, 162–166.

Peralta, R.C., Yokoyama, H., Ikemori, Y., Kuroki, M., and Kodama, Y. (1994). Passive immunisation against experimental salmonellosis in mice by orally administered hen egg-yolk antibodies specific for 14-kDa fimbriae of *Salmonella* Enteritidis. *J. Med. Microbiol.* **41**, 29–35.

Perryman, L. E., Riggs, M. W., Mason, P. H., and Fayer, R. (1990). Kinetics of *Cryptosporidium parvum* sporozoite neutralization by monoclocal antibodies, immune bovine serum, and immune bovine colostrum. *Infect. Immun.* **58**, 257–259.

Petschow, B. W., and Talbott, R. D. (1994). Reduction in virus-neutralizing activity of a bovine colostrum immunoglobulin concentrate by gastric acid and digestive enzymes. *J. Pediatr. Gastroenterol. Nutr.* **19**, 228–235.

Prentice, A. (1987). Breast feeding increases concentrations of IgA in infants' urine. *Arch. Dis. Childfood* **62**, 792–795.

Prince, A. M., Reesink, H., Pascual, D., Horowitz, B., Hewlett, I., Murthy, K. K., Cobb, K. E., and Eichberg, J. W. (1991). Prevention of HIV infection by passive immunization with HIV immunoglobulin. *AIDS Res. Hum. Retroviruses* 7, 971–973.

Prince, G. A., Hemming, V. G., Horswood, R. L., Baron, P. A., and Chanock, R. M. (1987). Effectiveness of topically administered neutralizing antibodies in experimental immunotherapy of respiratory syncytial virus infection in cotton rats. *J. Virol.* **61**, 1851–1854.

Putkonen, P., Thorstensson, R., Ghavamzadeh, L., Albert, J., Hild, K., Biberfeld, G., and Norrby, E. (1991). Prevention of HIV-2 and SIV_{sm} infection by passive immunization in cynomolgue monkeys. *Nature (London)* **352**, 436–438.

Renegar, K. B., and Small, P. A., Jr. (1991a). Passive transfer of local immunity to influenza virus infection by IgA antibody. *J. Immunol.* **146**, 1972–1978.

Renegar, K. B., and Small, Jr., P. A. (1991b). Immunoglobulin A mediation of murine nasal anti-influenza virus immunity. *J. Virol.* **65**, 2146–2148.

Renegar, K. B., and Small, P. A., Jr. (1994). Passive immunization systemic and mucosal. *In* "Handbook of Mucosal Immunology" (P. L. Ogra, J. Mestecky, M. E. Lamm, W. Strober, J. R. McGhee, and J. Bienenstock, eds.), pp. 347–356. Acadamic Press, Orlando, Florida.

Rolfe, R. D., and Song, W. (1995). Immunoglobulin and non-immunoglobulin components of human milk inhibit *Clostridium difficile* toxin A-receptor binding. *J. Med. Microbiol.* **42**, 10–19.

Rose, M. E., Orlans, E., and Buttress, N. (1974). Immunoglobulin classes in the hen's egg: Their segregation in yolk and white. *Eur. J. Immunol.* **4**, 521–523.

Russell, R. R. B., and Johnson, N. W. (1987). The prospects for vaccination against dental caries. *Br. Dent. J.* **162**, 29–34.

Sherman, D. M., Acres, S. D., Sadowski, P. L., Springer, J. A., Bray, B., Raybould, T. J. G., and Muscoplat, C. C. (1983). Protection of calves against fatal enteric colibacillosis by orally administered *Escherichia coli* K99-specific monoclonal antibody. *Infect. Immun.* **42**, 653–658.

Shimizu, M., Fitzsimmons, R. C., and Nakai, S. (1989). Serum and egg antibody responses in chicken to *Escherichia coli*. *Agric. Biol. Chem.* **53**, 3233–3238.

Shope, S. R., and Schiemann, D. A. (1991). Passive secretory immunity against *Salmonella typhimurium* demonstrated with foster mouse pups. *J. Med. Microbiol.* **35**, 53–59.

Smith, D. J., and Taubman, M. A. (1987). Oral immunization of humans with *Streptococcus sobrinus* glucosyltransferase. *Infect. Immun.* **55**, 2562–2569.

Stein, D. S., Timpone, J. G., Gradon, J. D., Kagan, J. M., and Schnittman, S. M. (1993). Immune-based therapeutics: Scientific rationale and the promising approaches to the treatment of the human immunodehiciency virus—infected individual. *Clin. Infect. Dis.* **17**, 749–771.

Tamura, S., Funato, H., Hirabayashi, Y., Suzuki, Y., Nagamine, T., Aizawa, C., and Kurata, T. (1991). Cross-protection against influenza A virus infection by passively transferred respiratory tract IgA antibodies to different hemagglutinin molecules. *Eur. J. Immunol.* **21**, 1337–1344.

Tsunemitsu, H., Shimizu, M., Hirai, T., Yonemichi, H., Kudo, T., Mori, K., and Onoe, S. (1989). Protection against bovine rotaviruses in newborn calves by continuous feeding of immune colostrum. *Jpn. J. Vet. Sci.* **51**, 300–308.

Turner, R. B., and Kelsey, D. K. (1993). Passive immunization for prevention of rotavirus illness in healthy infants. *Pediatr. Infect. Dis. J.* **12**, 718–722.

Tzipori, S., Roberton, D., and Chapman, C. (1986). Remission of diarrhoea due to cryptosporidiosis in an immunodeficient child treated with hyperimmune bovine colostrum. *Br. Med. J.* **293**, 1276–1277.

Ungar, B. L. P., Ward, D. J., Fayer, R., and Quinn, C. A.

(1990). Cessation of Cryptosporidium-associated diarrhea in an acquired immunodeficiency syndrome patient after treatment with hyperimmune bovine colostrum. *Gastroenterology* **93**, 486–489.

von Behring, E., and Kitasato, S. (1890). Ueber das Zustandekommen der Diphtherie-Immunität und der Tetanus-Immunität bei Thiern. *Dtsch. Med. Wochenschr.* **16**, 1113–1114.

von Specht, B.-U., Knapp, B., Muth, G., Bröker, M., Hungerer, K.-D., Diehl, K. -D., Massarrat, K., Seemann, A., and Domdey, H. (1995). Protection of immunocompromised mice against lethal infection with *Pseudomonas aeruginosa* by active or passive immunization with recombinant *P. aeruginosa* outer membrane protein F and outer membrane protein I fusion proteins. *Infect. Immun.* **63**, 1855–1862.

Watanabe, M., Boyson, J. E., Lord, C. I. and Letvin, N. L. (1992). Chimpanzees immunized with recombinant soluble CD4 develop anti-self CD4 antibody responses with anti-human immunodeficiency virus activity. *Proc. Natl. Acad. Sci. U.S.A.* **89**, 5103–5107.

Winner III, L., Mack, J., Weltzin, R., Mekalanos, J. J., Kraehenbuhl, J.-P., and Neutra, M. R. (1991). New model for analysis of mucosal immunity: Intestinal secretion of specific monoclonal immunoglobulin A from hybridoma tumors protects against *Vibrio cholerae* infection. *Infect. Immun.* **59**, 977–982.

Wong, J. P., Stadnyk, L. L., and Saravolac, E. G. (1994). Enhanced protection against respiratory influenza A infection in mice by liposome-encapsulated antibody. *Immunology* **81**, 280–284.

Yokoyama, H., Peralta, R. C., Diaz R., Sendo, S., Ikemori, Y., and Kodama, Y. (1992). Passive protective effect of chicken egg yolk immunoglobulins against experimental enterotoxigenic *Escherichia coli* infection in neonatal piglets. *Infect. Immun.* **60**, 998–1007.

Yokayama, H., Peralta, R. C., Sendo, S., Ikemori, Y., and Kodama, Y. (1993). Detection of passage and absorption of chicken egg yolk immunoglobulins in the gastrointestinal tract of pigs by use of enzyme-linked immunosorbent assay and fluorescent antibody testing. *Am. J. Vet. Res.* **54**, 867–872.

Yolken, R. H., Leister, F., Wee, S.-B., Miskuff, R., and Vonderfecht, S. (1988). Antibodies to rotaviruses in chickens' eggs: A potential source of antiviral immunoglobulins suitable for human consumption. *Pediatrics* **81**, 291–295.

Zimmerman, D. H., Mundon, F. K., and O'Neill, S. P. (1985). Industrial applications of monoclonal antibodies against bacteria. *In* "Monoclonal Antibodies against Bacteria," volume II. (A. J. L. Macario and E. Conway de Macario, eds.), Vol. 2, pp. 283–320. Academic Press, Orlando, Florida.

Zolla-Pazner, S., and Gorny, M. K. (1992). Passive immunization for the prevention and treatment of HIV infection. *AIDS* **6**, 1235–1247.

V

Mucosal Vaccines for Bacterial Diseases

15

Human Mucosal Vaccines for Salmonella typhi *Infections*

MYRON M. LEVINE
MARCELO B. SZTEIN
Center for Vaccine Development
University of Maryland School of Medicine
Baltimore, Maryland 21201

I. Introduction

Typhoid fever, an acute generalized infection of the reticuloendothelial system, intestinal lymphoid tissue, and gall bladder caused by *Salmonella typhi,* is restricted to human hosts and humans (chronic carriers) serve as the epidemiologic reservoir of infection. A broad spectrum of clinical illness can ensue with more severe forms being characterized by persisting high fever, abdominal discomfort, malaise, and headache. In the preantibiotic era, the disease ran its course over several weeks during which time 10–20% of cases ended in death. In populations in less-developed countries that are not served by treated water supplies and sanitation to remove human waste, typhoid fever is often endemic and typically constitutes the most important enteric disease public health problem of school-age children. The increasing prevalence of *S. typhi* strains exhibiting resistance to multiple, previously effective, antibiotics (Gupta, 1994; Rowe *et al.*, 1990) has complicated the therapy of typhoid fever and has rekindled interest in the programmatic use of new or improved vaccines to prevent typhoid fever (Levine *et al.*, 1989b).

II. Pathogenesis

Understanding the pathogenesis of wild-type *S. typhi* infection is fundamental for designing strategies to attenuate typhoid bacilli in a rational manner so that they can be used as live oral vaccines (Levine *et al.*, 1990b). *S. typhi* are highly invasive, human host-adapted bacteria that rapidly and efficiently pass through the intestinal mucosa of man to eventually reach the reticuloendothelial system where, after an 8- to 14-day incubation period, they precipitate a systemic illness. Susceptible human hosts ingest the causative organisms in contaminated food and water. The inoculum size and the type of vehicle in which it is ingested greatly influence the attack rate for typhoid fever and also affect the incubation period, a relationship that was documented in volunteer studies in the 1960s (Hornick *et al.*, 1970).

After passing through the pylorus and reaching the small intestine, the bacilli rapidly penetrate the mucosa by one of two mechanisms to arrive in the lamina propria. One mechanism involves uptake of the bacilli into endocytic vacuoles and their passage through the enterocytes to be ultimately released into the lamina propria without destroying the enterocyte (Takeuchi, 1967). In the second, quite distinct, invasive mechanism, typhoid bacilli are actively taken up by M cells, the specialized epithelial cells that cover the dome of Peyer's patches and other organized lymphoid tissue of the gut. From here they enter the underlying lymphoid cells (Kohbata *et al.*, 1986).

On reaching the lamina propria in the nonimmune host, typhoid bacilli elicit an influx of macrophages which ingest the organisms but are generally unable to kill them (Sprinz *et al.*, 1966). Some bacilli apparently remain within macrophages of the small intestinal lymphoid tissue. Other typhoid bacilli are drained into mesenteric lymph nodes where further multiplication and ingestion by macrophages takes place. It has recently been reported that upon invasion by gram negative bacteria, including *Salmonella,* there is a release of proinflammatory cytokines, including interleukin-8, monocyte chemotactic protein-1, granulocyte-monocyte colony-stimulating factor, and tumor necrosis factor-α by human colon epithelial cell lines (Jung *et al.*, 1995). Postmortem studies have documented the marked inflammatory responses that occur in the distal ileum in the Peyer's patches and other organized lymphoid aggregations.

MUCOSAL VACCINES

Presumably, cytokine release elicited by intracellular *S. typhi* is responsible, at least in part, for these cellular changes.

Shortly after invasion of the intestinal mucosa, a primary bacteremia takes place during which *S. typhi* are filtered from the circulation by fixed phagocytic cells of the reticuloendothelial system (Hornick *et al.*, 1970). It is believed that the main route by which typhoid bacilli reach the bloodstream in this early stage is by lymph drainage from mesenteric nodes, thereupon entering the thoracic duct and then the general circulation. Conceivably, ingestion of a massive inoculum followed by widespread invasion of the intestinal mucosa could result in rapid and direct invasion of the bloodstream. As a result of this primary bacteremia, the pathogen rapidly attains an intracellular haven throughout the organs of the reticuloendothelial system where it resides during the incubation period (usually 8–14 days) until the onset of clinical typhoid fever (Hornick *et al.*, 1970). Clinical illness is accompanied by a fairly sustained "secondary" bacteremia.

The Vi antigen is a virulence property and virtually all strains freshly isolated from patients possess this polysaccharide capsule (Robbins and Robbins, 1984). Both epidemiological observations and studies in volunteers support the contention that *S. typhi* strains that possess Vi are more virulent than strains lacking this polysaccharide (Hornick *et al.*, 1970).

III. Vaccines

Because of the complex nature of the pathogenesis of *S. typhi* clinical infection, a protective role is probably played by secretory intestinal antibody (in preventing mucosal invasion), circulating antibody (against bacteremic organisms), and cell-mediated immunity (to eliminate intracellular bacilli). With parenteral vaccines, the circulating antibody response is substantial and presumably provides the predominant protective effect. In contrast, with live-attenuated oral vaccines the circulating antibody response may be modest, whereas vigorous intestinal secretory IgA (S-IgA) and cell-mediated immune responses occur which are believed to be responsible for the protection conferred by that type of vaccine.

A. Parenteral Whole-Cell Vaccine

Inactivated (heat-killed, phenol-preserved) *S. typhi* were utilized as parenteral vaccines as far back as 1896 by Pfeiffer and Kolle in Germany and by Wright in England. Randomized, placebo-controlled field trials in the 1960s established the efficacy of the heat-phenolized and acetone inactivated parenteral whole cell vaccines (reviewed by Levine, 1994). Although these vaccines were shown to confer moderate protection that persisted for up to 7 years, they never became well-accepted public health tools because they caused adverse systemic reactions with high frequency (about 25% of recipients develop fever and malaise). The parenteral-killed whole cell vaccines have been supplanted by two newer vaccines, attenuated *S. typhi* strain Ty21a used as a live oral vaccine and purified Vi capsular polysaccharide utilized as a parenteral vaccine (Levine *et al.*, 1989b; Levine, 1994). These newer vaccines, which are at least as effective as the parenteral whole-cell vaccines but are well-tolerated, are licensed and available in many countries and constitute credible public health tools (Levine *et al.*, 1989b; Levine, 1994).

B. Ty21a Live Oral Typhoid Vaccine

In the 1970s, Phase 1 and 2 trials in North American volunteers with streptomycin-dependent *S. typhi* (Levine *et al.*, 1976) and with Vi-negative, *galE* mutant strain Ty21a (Gilman *et al.*, 1977) demonstrated that attenuated *S. typhi* strains could function as well-tolerated, protective live oral vaccines. Although these early attenuated vaccines had to be administered in multiple spaced doses, they nevertheless were protective. In contrast, it must be emphasized that multiple doses of inactivated *S. typhi* were not protective in experimental challenge studies in volunteers (DuPont *et al.*, 1971), nor were such oral killed typhoid bacilli vaccines efficacious in field trials in endemic areas (Chuttani *et al.*, 1973, 1977).

Six large-scale controlled field trials of efficacy were carried out in the 1980s that clearly established the protective activity of Ty21a (Wahdan *et al.*, 1982; Levine *et al.*, 1987a, 1990a; Black *et al.*, 1990; Ferreccio *et al.*, 1989; Simanjuntak *et al.*, 1991). However, these trials also demonstrated that the extent and duration of immunity are greatly influenced by the formulation of the vaccine and the immunization regimen. In the first field trial of Ty21a in Alexandria, Egypt, 32,000 6- to 7-year-old school children received three doses of a liquid suspension of vaccine or placebo on the Monday, Wednesday, and Friday of 1 week (Wahdan *et al.*, 1982); to neutralize gastric acid, the children chewed a 1.0-g tablet of $NaHCO_3$ several minutes before ingesting the vaccine or placebo. During 3 years of surveillance, 96% protective efficacy against confirmed typhoid fever was observed (Wahdan *et al.*, 1982).

A more recent formulation (that is the current commercial product) consists of lyophilized vaccine in enteric-coated, acid-resistant capsules. In a randomized, placebo-controlled field trial in Santiago, Chile, three doses of this enteric-coated formulation given within 1 week provided 67% efficacy during the first 3 years of follow-up (Levine et al., 1987a) and 63% protection over 7 years of follow-up (Levine, 1994). Four doses of Ty21a in enteric-coated capsules given within 8 days are significantly more protective than two or three doses (Ferreccio *et al.*, 1989). When Ty21a was licensed in the United States by the Food and Drug Administration in late 1989, it was with a recommended schedule of four doses to be given at an every other day interval; other countries use a three-dose immunization schedule.

In the mid 1980s the Swiss Serum and Vaccine Institute succeeded in preparing for large-scale field trials a "liquid suspension" formulation of Ty21a that was amenable to large-scale manufacture. The new formulation consists of two packets, one containing a dose of lyophilized vaccine and the other containing buffer. Contents of the two packets are mixed in a cup containing 100 ml of water and the suspension is then ingested by the subject to be vaccinated. A fourth field trial was initiated in Santiago, Chile (Levine *et al.*, 1990a) and a parallel trial was carried out in Plaju, Indonesia (Simanjuntak *et al.*, 1991) to compare directly this new liquid formulation of Ty21a (that somewhat resembles what was used in the Alexandria, Egypt field trial) with the enteric-coated capsule formulation. Vaccine administered as a liquid suspension was superior to vaccine in enteric-coated capsules. In the Santiago trial the difference was highly significant. Ty21a given as a liquid suspension protected young children as well as older children. In previous trials with enteric-coated vaccine, young children were not as well-protected as older children (Levine *et al.*, 1990a).

1. Immune Response to Ty21a

Although Ty21a is only modestly immunogenic and requires three or four spaced doses (administered every other day) to elicit protection, the efficacy is surprisingly long-lasting, enduring for 5–7 years (Levine, 1994). As is summarized below, measurements made with two immunologic assays were found to correlate with the protection conferred by different formulations and immunization schedules of Ty21a in field trials. These include serum IgG O antibody-seroconversions (Levine *et al.*, 1989a) and enumeration of gut-derived IgA O antibody secreting cells (ASCs) detected among peripheral blood mononuclear cells (Kantele, 1990).

2. Serum Antibody Response

The serum antibody response has been extensively studied with Ty21a, beginning with Gilman *et al.* (Jung *et al.*, 1995) who noted that Ty21a vaccine grown in the presence of galactose (which leads to organisms bearing smooth LPS O antigen) was highly protective, whereas vaccine grown in the absence of galactose (resulting in rough organisms) was not. These investigators reported that there was a significantly greater seroconversion of O antibody in recipients of vaccine grown in the presence of galactose.

Using serum IgG O antibody measured by ELISA in Chilean 15- to 19-year-olds, Levine *et al.* (1989a) showed a correlation between seroconversion to various dosage schedules and formulations and protective efficacy in field trials. With the currently licensed enteric-coated capsule formulation, there is a stepwise increase in the proportion of vaccinees who manifest significant rises in serum IgG O antibody depending on whether one administers one, two, or three doses of vaccine within 1 week. Thus, although serum O antibody is not believed to be the main operative mechanism of immunity elicited by attenuated strains, it clearly correlates with protection. Since measurement of serum IgG antibody to *S. typhi* O antigen by ELISA (Levine *et al.*, 1987b) is a simple technique, this provides a practical tool for comparing immunization schedules, formulations and for evaluating new candidate live oral vaccines.

3. Mucosal Immune Response

Most recipients of the usual three-dose oral regimen of Ty21a develop local antibody responses to O antigen (Kantele, 1990, 1991; Bartholomeusz *et al.*, 1986; Sarasombath *et al.*, 1987b; Panero *et al.*, 1972; Cancellieri and Fara, 1985; Kantele and Makela, 1991; Kantele *et al.*, 1986, 1991a,b). The propensity to develop a significant rise in intestinal S-IgA O antibody following immunization with Ty21a is inversely correlated with the preimmunization baseline level of intestinal antibody (Forrest, 1992). Subjects who have elevated baseline titers of S-IgA O antibody mount significantly lower-level increases than vaccinees with absent or low titers. An inverse correlation between baseline titer and propensity to seroconvert has also been reported for the serum vibriocidal antibody response following immunization with live oral cholera vaccines (Su-Arehawaratana *et al.*, 1992).

Kantele and coworkers (Kantele, 1990, 1991; Kantele and Makela, 1991; Kantele *et al.*, 1986, 1991a,b) and Forrest (1988) have shown that gut-derived migrating antibody secreting cells can be detected in peripheral blood following oral immunization with Ty21a and that the ability of these cells to secrete specific IgA antibody in the presence of specific antigen can be quantitated by means of the ELISPOT (Czerkinsky *et al.*, 1987) or similar techniques (Forrest, 1988). These IgA-producing migrating cells are only detectable a few days after immunization. The peak detection of gut-derived IgA antibody-secreting cells (ASCs) in peripheral blood following oral immunization occurs approximately 7 days after vaccination.

Kantele (1990) immunized adult Finnish volunteers with different formulations and immunization schedules of Ty21a, attempting to parallel the different regimens that were used in field trials of the efficacy of Ty21a in Chile (Levine *et al.*, 1987a, 1990a; Black *et al.*, 1990; Ferreccio *et al.*, 1989) and Indonesia (Simanjuntak *et al.*, 1991). Kantele demonstrated that the gut-derived IgA ASC response closely correlates with the efficacy results recorded in field trials. Three doses (every-other-day interval) of Ty21a in enteric-coated capsules were markedly more immunogenic than one dose and Ty21a in a liquid suspension was more immunogenic than vaccine in enteric-coated capsules. Overall, even following three doses of Ty21a the ASC responses were modest.

Forrest *et al.* (1990) studied the mucosal immune response when three doses of Ty21a were administered per rectum on Days 0, 2, and 5. Each dose of vaccine contained 2×10^{11} CFU, a 100-fold larger dose than is contained in the commercial Ty21a preparation. These vaccinees showed a significant increase in S-IgA anti-*S. typhi* O antibody in jejunal fluid, serum, and saliva and in gut-derived IgA ASCs (Forrest *et al.*, 1990).

4. *Cell-Mediated Immune Responses (CMI)*

Although only limited information is currently available, it has long been assumed that cell-mediated immune mechanisms elicited by attenuated *S. typhi* play an important role in protection against this intracellular pathogen. Cell-mediated immune responses, including lymphocyte replication and leukocyte migration inhibition (LMI) in the presence of soluble or particulate antigens and inhibition of *S. typhi* growth by mononuclear cells in the presence of antibody have been measured in typhoid fever patients and following vaccination with live oral vaccines.

Several groups (Rajagopalan *et al.*, 1982; Sarasombath *et al.*, 1987a; Sarma *et al.*, 1977; Dham and Thompson, 1982a) reported that typhoid fever patients and volunteers immunized with killed particulate *S. typhi* vaccines develop specific proliferative and LMI responses to *S. typhi* antigens. LMI responses are measured by the ability of supernatants from activated lymphocytes to inhibit macrophage migration. When these studies were conducted, the specific cytokines responsible for this effect were unknown. We now know that cytokines that mediate LMI responses include the recently cloned migration inhibitory factor (MIF) (Weiser *et al.*, 1989), and IFNγ (Thurman *et al.*, 1985). Therefore, those early LMI tests, which probably measured the combined effects of several cytokines, represent a good indicator of the production of cytokines resulting in macrophage activation. Significant LMI responses were measured as early as the first week of the illness and persisted in some patients for over a year (Sarasombath *et al.*, 1987a; Dham and Thompson, 1982a; Sarma *et al.*, 1977). Interestingly, although antibodies to O and H antigens and positive LMI responses develop almost simultaneously during the *S. typhi* infection, no correlation was found between antibody titers and degree of LMI positivity (Dham and Thompson, 1982a). Espersen *et al.* reported that proliferative responses to heat-phenolized *S. typhi* in patients with typhoid fever were higher, albeit not significantly different, in noncarriers than in chronic carriers, a finding consistent with the notion that more pronounced CMI responses may favor the elimination of *S. typhi* infection (Espersen *et al.*, 1982). Of interest, impairment of cellular reactivity to a heat-killed *S. typhi* suspension by peripheral blood mononuclear cells (PBMC) isolated from chronic typhoid carriers was observed in the presence of high antibody titers to O, Vi, and H antigens (Dham and Thompson, 1982b) and CMI responses were absent or depressed in complicated cases (Rajagopalan *et al.*, 1982).

Proliferative responses to heat-phenol-killed *S. typhi* Ty2 strain are seen in the vast majority of volunteers orally vaccinated with Ty21a and in typhoid fever patients (Murphy *et al.*, 1987, 1989). Low but significant proliferative responses to purified O polysaccharides free of intact LPS were also observed (Murphy *et al.*, 1987, 1989). Proliferative responses to *S. typhi* particulate and purified O polysaccharide antigens, were also found in the majority of volunteers vaccinated with *aroA* mutant strains 541Ty and 543Ty (Levine *et al.*, 1987b). Interestingly, only 10% of these vaccinees mounted a serum antibody response.

No data are available on the production of well-characterized cytokines or proliferative responses to purified *S. typhi* antigens other than O-polysaccharides in typhoid fever patients or volunteers vaccinated with killed *S. typhi* or Ty21a, 541Ty, or 543Ty attenuated strains of *S. typhi.*

Studies in typhoid patients and volunteers orally immunized with attenuated *S. typhi* strains have uncovered a novel mechanism of immune response against enteric pathogens that appears to be a form of antibody-dependent cellular cytotoxicity (ADCC) involving PBMC cells and immune serum. Coculture of PBMC from naive donors with postimmunization sera from volunteers immunized with Ty21a results in a marked inhibition of *S. typhi* growth (Tagliabue *et al.*, 1985, 1986). Neither mononuclear cells by themselves nor postvaccination serum alone had this effect. These investigators reported that the effector cells in this system are $CD4^+$ T cells and the specificity is determined by IgA against *S. typhi* bound to $CD4^+$ cells (Tagliabue *et al.*, 1985, 1986). This group also showed that intestinal S-IgA could substitute for serum IgA. Levine *et al.* (1987b) described a plasma-dependent mononuclear cell inhibition of the growth of *S. typhi* following immunization of North Americans with *aroA* mutant strains 541Ty and 543Ty that appeared to be analogous to the inhibition reported by Tagliabue and co-workers with Ty21a. However, Levine *et al.* (1987b) did not identify the effector cell or the immunoglobulin class of the postvaccination antibody that was involved. Recent studies (Sztein *et al.*,

1996) confirmed the appearance of this ADCC-type reactivity in the majority of volunteers orally immunized with attenuated *S. typhi* vaccine strains CVD 906 and CVD 908. However, cell sorting experiments demonstrated that the ADCC activity is associated with $CD14^+$ monocyte/macrophage populations. The appearance during typhoid fever or following vaccination of effector cells capable of suppressing the *in vitro* growth of *S. typhi* supports the notion that this mechanism might play an *in vivo* role in protection against infection.

C. New Generation of Engineered Attenuated *S. typhi* Strains

Various investigators have attempted to engineer new candidate vaccine strains that are well-tolerated yet considerably more immunogenic than Ty21a; it is expected that a single oral dose of such strains will elicit protective immunity. As a result, candidate vaccine strains have been prepared by inactivating genes encoding various biochemical pathways (Hone *et al.*, 1988), global regulatory systems (Curtiss and Kelly, 1987), other regulatory genes (Pikard *et al.*, 1994), and putative virulence properties (Miller *et al.*, 1993). The relative attenuating potential of these mutations has typically been assessed by measuring changes in LD_{50} after feeding *S. typhimurium* strains harboring these mutations to mice, in comparison with isogenic wild-type strains. Regrettably, the behavior of attenuated *S. typhimurium* strains in mice has not proven to be reliable for predicting the behavior of analogous *S. typhi* mutants in humans. There are several examples in which specific mutations that successfully attenuated *S. typhimurium* for mice failed to adequately attenuate *S. typhi* for humans (Hone *et al.*, 1988; Tacket *et al.*, 1992a). These observations underscore the critical importance of careful clinical trials.

D. *S. typhi* Strain CVD 908

One vaccine strain that has proven to be well-tolerated and impressively immunogenic following administration of a single oral dose in Phase 1 clinical trials in humans is strain CVD 908 (Tacket *et al.*, 1992a,b). This strain harbors precise deletion mutations in *aroC* and *aroD* (Hone *et al.*, 1991), rendering the strain nutritionally dependent on substrates (*para*-aminobenzoic acid and 2,3-dihydroxybenzoate) that are not available in sufficient quantity in human tissues. A summary of results of clinical trials with CVD 908 is shown in Table I. CVD 908 is the first engineered *S. typhi* vaccine candidate to be highly immunogenic yet well-tolerated.

1. *Serum Antibody Responses*

At a well-tolerated dose of 5×10^7 colony forming units (cfu) (which is the dosage level selected for Phase 2 trials), 92% of subjects manifested IgG O antibody seroconversions (Table I). Since IgG O antibody seroconversion was a correlate of protection induced by Ty21a (Levine *et al.*, 1989a), this is considered highly encouraging. In contrast, only 14% of healthy, young-adult Marylanders seroconverted following ingestion of a single oral dose of Ty21a containing 10^9 CFU. A single 5×10^7 CFU dose of CVD 908 also elicited serum anti-flagella antibodies measured by ELISA against purified *S. typhi* flagella (H antigen) in 75% of the volunteers (Table I).

2. *Mucosal Priming*

It appears that single oral doses of CVD 908 induce potent priming of the intestinal immune system, as

TABLE I
Response to Single-Dose *CVD* 908 Live Oral Typhoid Vaccine

Dose (cfu)[a]	N	% Fever		% Stool excretion on Days:		% Rise in: Serum IgG AB		% Rise in: Gut IgA ASCs	% Vaccinemia
		>38	>39	1–2	>3	O	H	O	
5×10^8	6	1	0	100	0	100	100	100 (1062)[b]	100
5×10^7	12	0	0	58	0	92	75	92 (221)	50
5×10^5	7	0	0	40	0	40	40	60 (54)	0
5×10^4	5	0	0	0	0	83	14	83 (17)	0

[a]cfu, colony forming units.
[b]Mean number of IgA ASCs is given in parentheses.

measured by quantitating the number of IgA ASCs against purified S. *typhi* LPS and flagella. For example, following a single 5×10^7 CFU dose of CVD 908, IgA ASCs that react with purified S. *typhi* LPS were observed in 92% of subjects, most having large numbers of such ASCs per 10^6 PBMC (Table I).

3. *Cell-Mediated Immune Responses*

It is well accepted that individual T-cell clones in long-term culture differentiate with a tendency to have specialized patterns of cytokine production, and are termed Th1 (IL-2, lymphotoxin, and IFNγ) or Th2 (IL-4, IL-5, IL-6, and IL-10) (Cherwinski *et al.*, 1987; Mosmann *et al.*, 1986; Street and Mosmann, 1991). In general, Th1 cells have helper activity for DTH responses and Th2 for antibody synthesis. IFNγ and IL-2 produced by Th1 cells may also have important roles in B cell differentiation. Studies in both murine and human clonal populations have also revealed individual cells that secrete different patterns of cytokines that do not fall into the Th1 and Th2 patterns; these cells have been named Th0. Studies in mice have shown that Th2-type cells favor the generation of IgA, IgE, IgM, and IgG1 specific antibodies, while Th1-type cells favor the generation of IgG2a specific antibodies (Street and Mosmann, 1991; Mosmann and Coffman, 1989). The differentiation of T cells into Th1- or Th2-like cells is a process dependent on cytokines present in the microenvironment (Chang *et al.*, 1990). It is generally accepted that IL-4 is important in driving Th2 differentiation and that IL-10 inhibits Th1 differentiation. The Th1–Th2 model has served as an important foundation for understanding the pathophysiology of certain infectious diseases. Convincing evidence for the importance of differences in the patterns of cytokine production in the *in vivo* regulation of immune responses to pathogens was provided by studies of murine leishmaniasis, an intracellular infection in which the cellular immune response is thought to be critical for recovery. Mouse strains that respond with a high Th1-like response have much lower morbidity than animals having a Th2-like cytokine response (Scott *et al.*, 1989). In humans, predominance of Th1- or Th2-like cytokine production patterns in response to various antigens has been reported in PBMC isolated from patients with helminth infections and tuberculoid and lepromatous leprosy (King and Nutman, 1993; Sieling *et al.*, 1993; Mutis *et al.*, 1993; Romagnani, 1994). Human $CD8^+$ T lymphocytes can also be divided into two subsets (types 1 and 2) based on their patterns of cytokine production (Bloom *et al.*, 1992a,b). Type-1 $CD8^+$ T lymphocytes secrete IFNγ but not IL-4, while type-2 $CD8^+$ T lymphocytes produce IL-4 with little or no IFNγ (Bloom *et al.*, 1992a,b).

We have recently observed that when administered to healthy adults, live oral S. *typhi* vaccine strain CVD 908 triggers CMI to S. *typhi* antigens, including cytokine production and proliferative responses (Sztein *et al.*, 1994). Oral immunization with CVD 908 and CVD 906 (a double *aro* mutant derived from a different wild-type parent than CVD 908) resulted in the appearance in peripheral blood of sensitized lymphocytes that exhibit significantly increased proliferative responses to purified S. *typhi* flagella and to whole-cell heat-phenolized S. *typhi* particles, compared to preimmunization levels (Sztein *et al.*, 1994). Significant increases in the proliferative responses to S. *typhi* flagella were also observed in all volunteers in a recent vaccine trial involving immunization with CVD 908 expressing the circumsporozoite protein of *Plasmodium falciparum* (CSP) (Sztein *et al.*, 1994; Gonzalez *et al.*, 1994). Thus, the immune response to at least some components of the vector is unaffected by the expression of a foreign antigen, in this case CSP. Supernatants from PBMC cultures from CVD 908-immunized volunteers showed significant increases in IFNγ production against S. *typhi* flagella in four out of six vaccinees, and significant negative correlations were observed between IL-4 production and both IFNγ production and proliferative responses to S. *typhi* flagella (Fig. 1). These results suggest a predominance of type-1 T lymphocyte responses at the systemic level in CVD 908 vaccinees (Fig. 1).

Because cytokines play a critical role in determining resistance or susceptibility to infection by influencing the outcome of immunological responses, this first demonstration of significant proliferative responses and distinct cytokine secretion patterns (e.g., IFNγ) by PBMC obtained from volunteers vaccinated with attenuated strains of S. *typhi* in response to purified S. *typhi* antigens may represent important immunological mechanisms underlying resistance to S. *typhi* infection. Indeed, this is the type of T lymphocyte response(s) that would be expected to play a critical role in the resistance to S. *typhi* infection at the systemic level, by contributing to the elimination of S. *typhi* in fixed macrophages of the reticuloendothelial system and other cells.

Although cytotoxic T lymphocytes (CTL) play a role in resistance against viral infections, only recently have studies demonstrated that CTL can also play an important role in the defense against intracellular bacteria (Kaufmann, 1988, 1993). Since S. *typhi* are intracellular pathogens, we speculated that CTL responses might play a crucial role in limiting progression of typhoid infection by destroying host cells harboring bacilli. We developed a CTL assay to evaluate whether immunization of volunteers with attenuated strains of S. *typhi* elicits the appearance in peripheral blood of CTL effectors capable of killing Epstein-Barr virus (EBV)-transformed autologous B lymphocytes infected with wild-type S. *typhi* (Sztein *et al.*, 1995). For these studies we used PBMC obtained from individuals immunized with the attenuated S. *typhi* CVD 908 strain carrying a

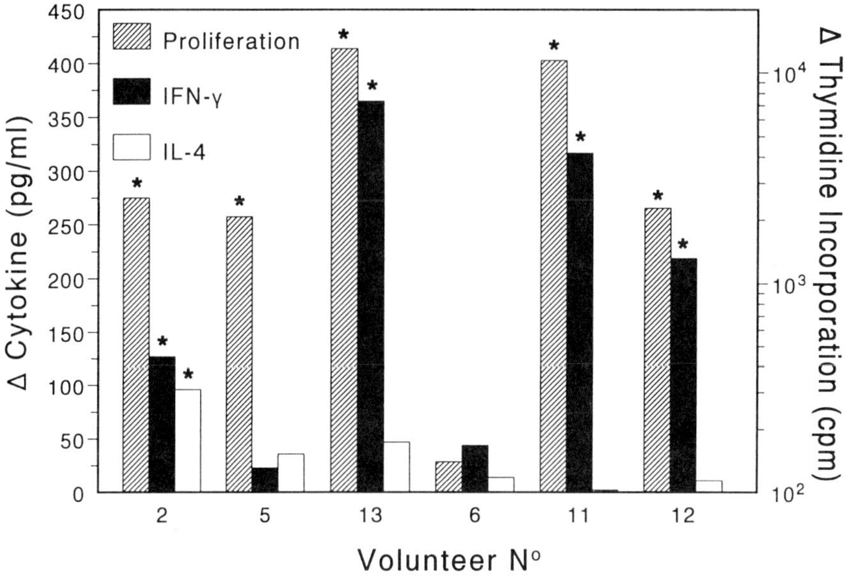

Figure 1. Proliferative responses and cytokine production of volunteers orally immunized with *S. typhi* candidate vaccine strain CVD 908. PBMC obtained prior to and 22 days after oral immunization were isolated by density gradient fractionation and frozen in liquid N_2. PBMC from both time points were thawed and tested simultaneously for proliferative responses and IFNγ and Il-4 production to purified *S. typhi* flagella. Data are presented as Δcpm or Δcytokine at Day 22 minus Δcpm or Δcytokine at Day 0, for each individual volunteer. Δcpm was calculated as ^{3}H-TdR incorporation in the presence of antigen minus ^{3}H-TdR incorporation in the absence of antigen at each time point. Δcytokine production was calculated as cytokine produced in the presence of antigen minus cytokine produced in the absence of antigen at each time point. Values designated with * were significantly increased after immunization as compared to the preimmunization responses in each individual ($P < 0.05$).

gene encoding the CSP of *P. falciparum.* Volunteers received two doses of 5×10^7 organisms at Days 0 and 8. CTL activity was evaluated by using PBMC isolated before and at 14 and 29 days after the first immunization (Fig. 2). PBMC were either used immediately in CTL assays or expanded *in vitro* for 6–8 days in the presence of *S. typhi*-infected autologous EBV-transformed cells prior to the measurement of CTL responses. Using this system we have observed the presence of CTL effectors able to lyse *S. typhi*-infected autologous EBV-transformed cells in all five volunteers examined (Fig. 2). The specific CTL activity was observed in PBMC preparations obtained 14 days after immunization and following 7 to 8 days of *in vitro* expansion in the presence of *S. typhi*-infected autologous EBV-transformed cells. PBMC isolated before immunization with CVD 908-CSP and expanded in the presence of *S. typhi*-infected autologous EBV-transformed cells failed to show CTL activity, and no CTL activity was observed in the absence of expansion. Furthermore, the development of CTL activity requires live organisms, since it was not observed when heat-phenol-killed whole-cell bacteria, purified *S. typhi* flagella, or gentamicin-killed *S. typhi* were used instead of *S. typhi*-infected EBV-transformed cells during expansion. PBMC obtained 29 days after immunization exhibited CTL activity levels comparable or greater than those observed in cells isolated 14 days after immunization (Fig. 2). Finally, we observed that the CTL effector cell

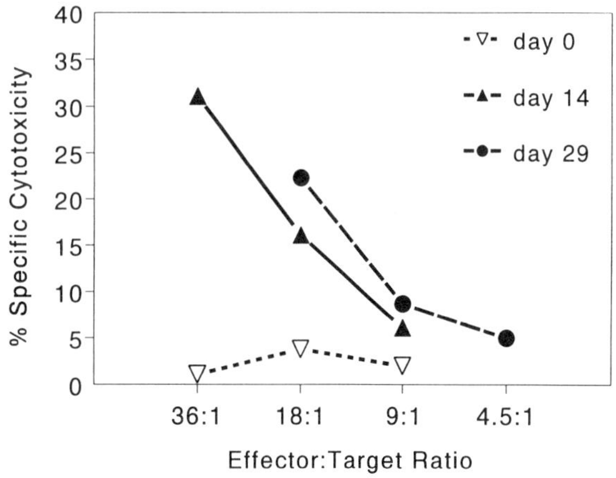

Figure 2. Induction of CTL activity in volunteers orally immunized with the CVD 908-CSP construct. PBMC obtained prior to (Day 0) and 14 and 29 days after oral immunization were isolated by density gradient fractionation and frozen in liquid N_2. PBMC from all time points were thawed and tested simultaneously for CTL activity after an *in vitro* expansion for 6 days in the presence of *S. typhi*-infected autologous Epstein Barr virus (EBV)-transformed cells. Results are expressed as % specific cytotoxicity at the indicated effector:target ratios. Percentage specific lysis was calculated as: (experimental release − spontaneous release) / (maximal release − spontaneous release) × 100, where spontaneous release = cpm released in the absence of effectors and maximal release = cpm released in the presence of 5% Triton X-100. For clarity, data are presented as % specific cytotoxicity = (% specific lysis by PBMC effectors incubated with *S. typhi*-infected autologous EBV-transformed targets) − (% specific lysis by PBMC effectors incubated with mock-infected autologous EBV-transformed targets).

population in these PBMC cultures was a classic $CD8^+$, MHC class I-restricted, cytotoxic T lymphocyte population (Sztein *et al.*, 1995). We also evaluated whether a single dose of CVD 908 was sufficient to elicit CTL activity by investigating the presence of CTL activity in PBMC from volunteers immunized orally with a single dose of 5×10^7 attenuated *S. typhi* strain CVD 908 organisms. In contrast to the results obtained in the CVD 908-CSP vaccine trial in which CTL activity was observed in all five volunteers tested, significant CTL activity was seen in PBMC obtained 22 days after immunization in only one of the four CVD 908 vaccinees evaluated. These results suggest that higher levels of CTL precursors in circulation are elicited by two immunizations.

In summary, the observation that immunization elicits the appearance in the circulation of $CD8^+$, MHC class I-restricted, CTL effector cells capable of killing autologous *S. typhi*-infected targets suggests that CTL responses may play a crucial role in limiting the progression of typhoid infection. Future clinical studies attempting to correlate the induction of CTL activity and/or a predominance of type-1 or type-2 T-cell responses with protection to challenge with virulent *S. typhi* will be critical in establishing the significance of the findings discussed above.

E. *S. typhi* Strain CVD 908-*htrA*

The one possible drawback observed in the Phase 1 and 2 clinical trials with CVD 908 is that 50% of subjects who ingested this vaccine strain at a dose of 5×10^7 CFU and 100% of subjects who received a 5×10^8 CFU dose manifested silent vaccinemias wherein vaccine organisms were recovered from blood cultures collected at one or more time points between Days 4 and 8 after vaccination (Table I). The blood cultures were collected systematically in these individuals at 2 and 12 hr after they ingested vaccine and then on Days 2, 4, 5, 7, 8, 10, 14, 20, 27, and 60. No blood cultures from any vaccinee were positive prior to Day 4 or after Day 8. The vaccinemias appeared to have no clinical consequence (for example, they were not associated with fever) and they were short-lived, spontaneously disappearing without the use of antibiotics.

Chatfield *et al.* (1992) found that inactivation of *htrA*, a gene encoding a heat-shock protein that also functions as a serine protease, attenuates wild-type *S. typhimurium* in the mouse model. Nevertheless, mice immunized orally with Δ*htrA S. typhimurium* are protected against subsequent challenge with a lethal dose of wild-type *S. typhimurium*. Chatfield and coinvestigators introduced a deletion mutation in *htrA* of CVD 908, resulting in strain CVD 908–*htrA*. This strain was fed as a single dose to three groups of subjects at a dose of 5×10^7 ($N = 7$), 5×10^8 ($N = 8$), or 5×10^9 ($N = 7$) cfu (Levine *et al.*, 1995). The CVD 908–*htrA* strain was as well tolerated as the CVD 908 parent. Only one of these 22 subjects developed a low-grade fever which was detected by routine surveillance and was not associated with any complaints of malaise. Similarly, the immune response was excellent: 20/22 individuals manifested significant rises in serum IgG O antibody and in 100% of the subjects gut-derived IgA antibody-secreting cells were detected that made antibody to O antigen. These responses are virtually identical to what was observed in Phase 1 clinical trials in subjects immunized with comparable doses of CVD 908. The one striking difference concerned vaccinemias. Whereas vaccinemias were detected in 12 of 18 subjects who received a 5×10^7 or 5×10^8 cfu dose of CVD 908, no vaccinemias were detected in any of the 22 individuals who ingested well-tolerated, highly immunogenic $5 \times 10^{7-9}$ cfu doses of CVD 908–*htrA* ($P < 0.001$).

IV. Summary Comment

The application of recombinant DNA technology has allowed the rational attenuation of *S. typhi* to yield strains to serve as candidate live oral vaccines to prevent typhoid fever. Results of Phase 1 clinical trials have identified at least two vaccine strains, CVD 908 and CVD 908–*htrA*, that are well-tolerated and elicit potent mucosal IgA, serum IgG, and various cell-mediated immune responses following oral immunization. Preliminary evidence also shows that these strains hold great promise as live vector vaccines to express foreign antigens and to deliver those antigens to the immune system following mucosal immunization.

Acknowledgments

This work was supported in part by Research Contract NO1 AI45251, Grant RO1 AI29471, and Cooperative Research Agreements UO1 AI37546 and UO1 AI35948 to M.M.L. and Grant RO1 AI36525 to M.B.S., all from the National Institute of Allergy and Infectious Diseases.

References

Bartholomeusz, R. C. A., LaBrooy, J. T., Johnson, M., Shearman, D. J. C., and Rowley, D. (1986). Gut immunity to typhoid—The immune response to a live oral typhoid vaccine, Ty21a. *J. Gastroenterol. Hepatol.* **1**, 61.

Black, R. E., Levine, M. M., Ferreccio, C., Clements, M. L., Lanata, C., Rooney, J., and Germanier, R. (1990). Efficacy of one or two doses of Ty21a *Salmonella typhi* vaccine in enteric-coated capsules in a controlled field trial. Chilean Typhoid Committee. *Vaccine* **8**, 81–84.

Bloom, B. R., Modlin, R. L., and Salgame, P. (1992a). Stigma variations: Observations on suppressor T cells and leprosy. *Annu. Rev. Immunol.* **10,** 453–488.

Bloom, B. R., Salgame, P., and Diamond, B. (1992b). Revisiting and revising suppressor T cells. *Immunol. Today* **13,** 131–136.

Cancellieri, V., and Fara, G. M. (1985). Demonstration of specific IgA in human feces after immunization with line T21a *Salmonella typhi* vaccine. *J. Infect. Dis.* **151,** 482–484.

Chang, T. L., Shea, C. M., Urioste, S., Thompson, R. C., Boom, W. H., and Abbas, A. K. (1990). Heterogeneity of helper/inducer T lymphocytes. III. Responses of IL-2- and IL-4-producing (Th1 and Th2) clones to antigens presented by different accessory cells. *J. Immunol.* **145,** 2803–2808.

Chatfield, S. N., Strahan, K., Pickard, D., Charles, I. G., Hormaeche, C. E., and Dougan, G. (1992). Evaluation of *Salmonella typhimurium* strains harbouring defined mutations in *htr*A and *aro*A in the murine salmonellosis model. *Microbial. Pathogen.* **12,** 145–151.

Cherwinski, H. M., Schumacher, J. H., Brown, K. D., and Mosmann, T. R. (1987). Two types of mouse helper T cell clone. III. Further differences in lymphokine synthesis between Th1 and Th2 clones revealed by RNA hybridization, functionally monospecific bioassays, and monoclonal antibodies. *J. Exp. Med.* **166,** 1229–1244.

Chuttani, C. S., Prakash, K., Vergese, A., Gupta, P., Chawla, R. K., Grover, V., and Agarwal, D. S. (1973). Ineffectiveness of an oral killed typhoid vaccine in a field trial. *Bull. WHO* **48,** 754–755.

Chuttani, D. S., Prakash, K., Gupta, P., Groven, V., and Kumar, A. (1977). Controlled field trial of a high dose oral killed typhoid vaccine in India. *Bull. WHO* **55,** 643–644.

Curtiss, III, R., and Kelly, S. M. (1987). *Salmonella typhimurium* deletion mutants lacking adenylate cyclase and cyclic AMP receptor protein are avirulent and immunogenic. *Infect. Immun.* **55,** 3035–3043.

Czerkinsky, C. C., Prince, S. J., Michalek, S. M., Jackson, S., Russell, M. W., Moldoveanu, Z., McGhee, J. R., and Mestecky, J. (1987). IgA antibody-producing cells in peripheral blood after ingestion of antigen: Evidence for a common mucosal immune system in humans. *Proc. Natl. Acad. Sci. U.S.A.* **84,** 2449–2553.

Dham, S. K., and Thompson, R. A. (1982a). Studies of cellular and humoral immunity in typhoid fever and TAB vaccinated subjects. *Clin. Exp. Immunol.* **48,** 389–395.

Dham, S. K., and Thompson, R. A. (1982b). Humoral and cell mediated immune responses in chronic typhoid carriers. *Clin. Exp. Immunol.* **50,** 34–40.

DuPont, L. H., Hornick, R. B., Snyder, M. J., Dawkins, A. T., Heiner, G. G., and Woodward, T. E. (1971). Studies of immunity in typhoid fever. Protection induced by killed oral antigens or by primary infection. *Bull. WHO* **44,** 667–672.

Espersen, F., Mogensen, H. H., Hoiby, N., Hoj, L., Greibe, J., Rasmussen, S. N., and Gaarslev, K. (1982). Humoral and cellular immunity in typhoid and paratyphoid carrier state, investigated by means of quantitative immunoelectrophoresis and *in vitro* stimulation of blood lymphocytes. *Acta Pathol. Microbiol. Immunol. Scand. (C)* **90,** 293–299.

Ferreccio, C., Levine, M. M., Rodriguez, H., and Contreras, R. (1989). Comparative efficacy of two, three, or four doses of TY21a live oral typhoid vaccine in enteric-coated capsules: A field trial in an endemic area. *J. Infect. Dis.* **159,** 766–769.

Forrest, B. D. (1988). Identification of an intestinal immune response using peripheral blood lymphocytes. *Lancet* **1,** 81–83.

Forrest, B. D. (1992). Impairment of immunogenicity of *Salmonella typhi* T21A due to preexisting cross-reacting intestinal antibodies. *J. Infect. Dis.* **166,** 210–212.

Forrest, B. D., Shearman, D. J. C., and LaBrooy, J. T. (1990). Specific immune response in humans following rectal delivery of live typhoid vaccine. *Vaccine* **8,** 209–211.

Gilman, R. H., Hornick, R. B., Woodward, W., DuPont, H. L., Snyder, M. J., Levine, M. M., and Libonati, J. P. (1977). Immunity in typhoid fever: Evaluation of Ty21a—an epimeraseless mutant of *S. typhi*—as a live oral vaccine. *J. Infect. Dis.* **136,** 717–723.

Gonzalez, C., Hone, D., Noriega, F. R., Tacket, C. O., Davis, J. R., Losonsky, G. A., Nataro, J. P., Hoffman, S., Malik, A., Nardin, E., Sztein, M. B., Heppner, D. G., Fouts, T. R., Isibasi, A., and Levine, M. M. (1994). *Salmonella typhi* vaccine strain CVD 908 expressing the circumsporozoite protein of *Plasmodium falciparum*: Strain construction and safety and immunogenicity in humans. *J. Infect. Dis.* **169,** 927–931.

Gupta, A. (1994). Multidrug-resistant typhoid fever in children: Epidemiology and therapeutic approach. *Pediatr. Infect. Dis.* **13,** 124–140.

Hone, D. M., Attridge, S. R., Forrest, B., Morona, R., Daniels, D., LaBrooy, J. T., Bartholomeusz, R. C., Shearman, D. J., and Hackett, J. (1988). A galE via (Vi antigen-negative) mutant of *Salmonella typhi* Ty2 retains virulence in humans. *Infect. Immun.* **56,** 1326–1333.

Hone, D. M., Harris, A. M., Chatfield, S., Dougan, G., and Levine, M. M. (1991). Construction of genetically defined double *aro* mutants of *Salmonella typhi. Vaccine* **9,** 810–816.

Hornick, R., Griesman, S., Woodward, T., DuPont, H., Dawkins, A., and Snyder, M. (1970). Typhoid fever; pathogenesis and immunologic control. *N. Engl. J. Med.* **283,** 686–691 and 739–746.

Jung, H. C., Eckmann, L., Yang, S. K., Panja, A., Fierer, J., Morzycka-Wroblewska, E., and Kagnoff, M. F. (1995). A distinct array of proinflammatory cytokines is expressed in human colon epithelial cells in response to bacterial invasion. *J. Clin. Invest.* **95,** 55–65.

Kantele, A. (1990). Antibody-secreting cells in the evaluation of the immunogenicity of an oral vaccine. *Vaccine* **8,** 321–326.

Kantele, A. (1991a). Immune response to prolonged intestinal exposure to antigen. *Scand. J. Immunol.* **33,** 225–229.

Kantele, A., and Makela, P. H. (1991). Different profiles of the human immune response to primary and secondary immunization with an oral *Salmonella typhi* Ty21a vaccine. *Vaccine* **9,** 423–427.

Kantele, A., Arvilommi, H., and Jokinen, I. (1986). Specific immunoglobulin-secreting human blood cells after peroral vaccination against *Salmonella typhi*. *J. Infect. Dis.* **153**, 1126–1131.

Kantele, A., Arvilommi, H., Kantele, J. M., Rintala, L., and Makela, P. H. (1991a). Comparison of the human immune response to live oral, killed oral or killed parenteral *Salmonella typhi* Ty21a vaccines. *Microbial Pathogen.* **10**, 117–126.

Kantele, A., Kantele, J. M., Arvilommi, H., and Makela, P. H. (1991b). Active immunity is seen as a reduction in the cell response to oral live vaccine. *Vaccine* **9**, 428–431.

Kaufmann, S. H. (1988). $CD8^+$ T lymphocytes in intracellular microbial infections. *Immunol. Today* **9**, 168–174.

Kaufmann, S. H. (1993). Immunity to intracellular bacteria. *Annu. Rev. Immunol.* **11**, 129–163.

King, C. L., and Nutman, T. B. (1993). IgE and IgG subclass regulation by IL-4 and IFN-gamma in human helminth infections. Assessment by B cell precursor frequencies. *J. Immunol.* **151**, 458–465.

Kohbata, S., Yokoyama, H., and Yabuchi, E. (1986). Cytopathogenic effect of *Salmonella typhi* GIFU 10007 on M cells of murine ileal Peyer's patches in ligated ileal loops: An ultrastructural study. *Microbiol. Immunol.* **30**, 1225–1237.

Levine, M. M. (1994). Typhoid fever vaccines. *In* "Vaccines" (S. A. Plotkin and E. A. Mortimer, eds.), pp. 597–633. Saunders, Philadelphia, Pennsylvania.

Levine, M. M., DuPont, L. H., Hornick, R. E., Snyder, M. J., Woodward, W., Gilman, R. H., and Libonati, J. P. (1976). Attenuated streptomycin-dependent *Salmonella typhi* oral vaccine: Potential deleterious effects of lyophilization. *J. Infect. Dis.* **133**, 424–429.

Levine, M. M., Ferreccio, C., Black, R. E., and Germanier, R. (1987a). Large-scale field trial of Ty21a live oral typhoid vaccine in enteric-coated capsule formulation. *Lancet* **1**, 1049–1052.

Levine, M. M., Herrington, D., Murphy, J. R., Morris, J. G., Losonsky, G., Tall, B., Lindberg, A. A., Svenson, S., Baqar, S., Edwards, M. F., and Stocker, B. (1987b). Safety, infectivity, immunogenicity, and *in vivo* stability of two attenuated auxotrophic mutant strains of *Salmonella typhi,* 541Ty and 543Ty, as live oral vaccines in humans. *J. Clin. Invest.* **79**, 888–902.

Levine, M. M., Ferreccio, C., Black, R. E., Tacket, C. O., Germanier, R., and Chilean Typhoid Committee (1989a). Progress in vaccines to prevent typhoid fever. *Rev. Infect. Dis.* **11**, S552–S567.

Levine, M. M., Taylor, D. N., and Ferreccio, C. (1989b). Typhoid vaccines come of age. *Pediatr. Infect. Dis. J.* **8**, 374–381.

Levine, M. M., Ferreccio, C., Cryz, S., and Ortiz, E. (1990a). Comparison of enteric-coated capsules and liquid formulation of Ty21a typhoid vaccine in randomised controlled field trial. *Lancet* **336**, 891–894.

Levine, M. M., Hone, D., Heppner, D. G., Noriega, F., and Sriwathana, B. (1990b). Attenuated *Salmonella* as carriers for the expression of foreign antigens. *Microecol. Ther.* **19**, 23–32.

Levine, M. M., Galen, J., Barry, E., Noriega, F., Chatfield, S., Sztein, M., Dougan, G., and Tacket, C. (1996). Attenuated *Salmonella* as live oral vaccines against typhoid fever and as live vectors. *J. Biotechnol.* **44**, 193–196.

Miller, S. I., Loomis, W. P., Alpuche-Aranda, C., Behlau, I., and Hohmann, E. (1993). The PhoP virulence regulon and live oral *Salmonella* vaccines. *Vaccine* **11**, 122–125.

Mosmann, T. R., Cherwinski, H., Bond, M. W., Giedlin, M. A., and Coffman, R. L. (1986). Two types of murine helper T cell clone. I. Definition according to profiles of lymphokine activities and secreted proteins. *J. Immunol.* **136**, 2348–2357.

Mosmann, T. R., and Coffman, R. L. (1989). Th1 and Th2 cells: Different patterns of lymphokine secretion lead to different functional properties. *Annu. Rev. Immunol.* **7**, 145–173.

Murphy, J. R., Baqar, S., Munoz, C., Schlesinger, L., Ferreccio, C., Lindberg, A. A., Svenson, S., Losonsky, G., Koster, F., and Levine, M. M. (1987). Characteristics of humoral and cellular immunity to *Salmonella typhi* in residents of typhoid-endemic and typhoid-free regions. *J. Infect. Dis.* **156**, 1005–1009.

Murphy, J. R., Wasserman, S. S., Baqar, S., Schlesinger, L., Ferreccio, C., Lindberg, A. A., and Levine, M. M. (1989). Immunity to *Salmonella typhi:* Considerations relevant to measurement of cellular immunity in typhoid-endemic regions. *Clin. Exp. Immunol.* **75**, 228–233.

Mutis, T., Kraakman, E. M., Cornelisse, Y. E., Haanen, J. B., Spits, H., De Vries, R. R., and Ottenhoff, T. H. (1993). Analysis of cytokine production by *Mycobacterium*-reactive T cells. Failure to explain *Mycobacterium leprae*-specific nonresponsiveness of peripheral blood T cells from lepromatous leprosy patients. *J. Immunol.* **150**, 4641–4651.

Panero, C., Saletti, M., and DiTommaso, I. (1972). The detection of intestinal IgA in children following oral typhoid vaccine. *Prog. Immunobiol. Stand.* **5**, 369–372.

Pikard, D., Li, J., Roberts, M., Maskell, D., Hone, D., Levine, M., Dougan, G., and Chatfield, S. (1994). Characterization of defined *ompR* mutants of *Salmonella typhi: ompR* is involved in the regulation of Vi polysaccharide expression. *Infect. Immun.* **62**, 3984–3993.

Rajagopalan, P., Kumar, R., and Malaviya, A. N. (1982). Immunological studies in typhoid fever. II. Cell mediated immune responses and lymphocyte subpopulations in patients with typhoid fever. *Clin. Exp. Immunol.* **47**, 269–274.

Robbins, J., and Robbins, J. (1984). Reexamination of the protective role of the capsular polysaccharide Vi antigen of *Salmonella typhi. J. Infect. Dis.* **150**, 436–449.

Romagnani, S. (1994). Lymphokine production by human T cells in disease states. *Annu. Rev. Immunol.* **12**, 227–257.

Rowe, B., Ward, L. R., and Threlfall, E. J. (1990). Spread of multiresistant *Salmonella typhi. Lancet* **336**, 1065–1066.

Sarasombath, S., Banchuin, N., Sukosol, T., Rungpitarangsi, B., and Manasatit, S. (1987a). Systemic and intestinal immunities after natural typhoid infection. *J. Clin. Microbiol.* **25**, 1088–1093.

Sarasombath, S., Banchuin, N., Sukosol, T., Vanadurongwan, S., Rungpitarasangsi, B., and Dumavibhat, B. (1987b). Systemic and intestinal immunities after different typhoid vacccinations. *Asian Pacific J. Allergy Immunol.* **5**, 53–61.

Sarma, V. N., Malaviya, A. N., Kumar, R., Ghai, O. P., and Bakhtary, M. M. (1977). Development of immune response during typhoid fever in man. *Clin. Exp. Immunol.* **28**, 35–39.

Scott, P., Pearce, E., Cheever, A. W., Coffman, R. L., and Sher, A. (1989). Role of cytokines and CD4 T-cell subsets in the regulation of parasite immunity and disease. *Immunol. Rev.* **112**, 161–182.

Sieling, P. A., Abrams, J. S., Yamamura, M., Salgame, P., Bloom, B. R., Rea, T. H., and Modlin, R. L. (1993). Immunosuppressive roles for IL-10 and IL-4 in human infection. *In vitro* modulation of T cell responses in leprosy. *J. Immunol.* **150**, 5501–5510.

Simanjuntak, C., Paleologo, F., Punjabi, N., Darmowitogo, R., Soeprawato, P., Totosudirjo, H., Haryanto, P., Suprijanto, E., Witham, N., and Hoffman, S. L. (1991). Oral immunisation against typhoid fever in Indonesia with Ty21a vaccine. *Lancet* **338**, 1055–1059.

Sprinz, H., Gangarosa, E. J., Williams, M., Hornick, R. B., and Woodward, T. E. (1966). Histopathology of the upper small intestines in typhoid fever. *Am. J. Dig. Dis.* **11**, 615–624.

Street, N. E., and Mosmann, T. R. (1991). Functional diversity of T lymphocytes due to secretion of different cytokine patterns. *FASEB J.* **5**, 171–177.

Su-Arehawaratana, P., Singharaj, P., Taylor, D. N., Hoge, C., Trofa, A., Kuvanont, K., Migasena, S., Pitisuttitham, P., Lim, Y. L., Losonsky, G., Kaper, J. B., Wasserman, S. S., Cryz, S., Echeverria, P., and Levine, M. M. (1992). Safety and immunogenicity of different immunization regimens of CVD 103-HgR live oral cholera vaccine in soldiers and civilians in Thailand. *J. Infect. Dis.* **165**, 1042–1048.

Sztein, M. B., Wasserman, S. S., Tacket, C. O., Edelman, R., Hone, D., Lindberg, A. A., and Levine, M. M. (1994). Cytokine production patterns and lymphoproliferative responses in volunteers orally immunized with attenuated vaccine strains of *Salmonella typhi*. *J. Infect. Dis.* **170**, 1508–1517.

Sztein, M. B., Tanner, M., Polotsky, Y., Orenstein, J. M., and Levine, M. M. (1995). Cytotoxic T lymphocytes after oral immunization with attenuated vaccine strains of *Salmonella typhi* in humans. *J. Immunol.* **155**, 3987–3993.

Sztein, M. B., *et al.* (1996). AOCC in volunteers immunized with attenuated strains of *Salmonella typhi*. Submitted for publication.

Tacket, C. O., Hone, D. M., Curtiss, R. I., Kelly, S. M., Losonsky, G., Guers, L., Harris, A. M., Edelman, R., and Levine, M. M. (1992a). Comparison of the safety and immunogenicity of *aroC, aroD* and *cya,crp Salmonella typhi* strains in adult volunteers. *Infect. Immun.* **60**, 536–541.

Tacket, C. O., Hone, D. M., Losonsky, G. A., Guers, L., Edelman, R., and Levine, M. M. (1992b). Clinical acceptability and immunogenicity of CVD 908 *Salmonella typhi* vaccine strain. *Vaccine* **10**, 443–446.

Tagliabue, A., Villa, L., Boraschi, D., Peri, G., de Gori, V., and Nencioni, L. (1985). Natural anti-bacterial activity against *Salmonella typhi* by human $T4^+$ lymphocytes armed with IgA antibodies. *J. Immunol.* **135**, 4178–4182.

Tagliabue, A., Villa, L., De Magistris, M. T., Romano, M., Silvestri, S., Boraschi, D., and Nencioni, L. (1986). IgA-driven T cell-mediated anti-bacterial immunity in man after live oral Ty 21a vaccine. *J. Immunol.* **137**, 1504–1510.

Takeuchi, A. (1967). Electron microscope studies of experimental *Salmonella* infection. I. Penetrations into the intestinal epithelium by *Salmonella typhimurium*. *Am. J. Pathol.* **50**, 109–136.

Thurman, G. B., Braude, I. A., Gray, P. W., Oldham, R. K., and Stevenson, H. C. (1985). MIF-like activity of natural and recombinant human interferon-gamma and their neutralization by monoclonal antibody. *J. Immunol.* **134**, 305–309.

Wahdan, M. H., Serie, C., Cerisier, Y., Sallam, S., and Germanier, R. (1982). A controlled field trial of live *Salmonella typhi* strain Ty21a oral vaccine against typhoid: Three year results. *J. Infect. Dis.* **145**, 292–296.

Weiser, W. Y., Temple, P. A., Witek Giannotti, J. S., Remold, H. G., Clark, S. C., and David, J. R. (1989). Molecular cloning of a cDNA encoding a human macrophage migration inhibitory factor. *Proc. Natl. Acad. Sci. U.S.A.* **86**, 7522–7526.

16

Oral Vaccines for Shigella

TIBOR PÁL
Kuwait University
Faculty of Medicine
Safat 13110, Kuwait

ALF A. LINDBERG
Wyeth-Lederle Vaccines and Pediatrics
Pearl River, New York; and
Karolinska Institute
Department of Clinical Bacteriology
Huddinge Hospital
Huddinge, Sweden

I. Bacillary Dysentery: Clinical Picture and Epidemiology

Bacillary dysentery and its association with poor hygienic standards have been known for centuries. Today it still remains one of the main enteric infections of the world. The number of cases has been estimated to be some 200 million per year, mostly among infants and children up to 5 years of age. The mortality data are equally discouraging; annually, ca. 650,000 deaths are attributed to bacillary dysentery (Institute of Medicine, 1986).

The majority of the cases are caused by members of the *Shigella* genus containing four species (*S. dysenteriae, S. flexneri, S. boydii,* and *S. sonnei*), each divided into 12, 13, 18, and 1 serotypes, respectively (Ewing and Lindberg, 1984). Not all of these serotypes occur with equal frequency, however. In the third world, *S. flexneri* 1b, 2a, and 3b and *S. dysenteriae* 1 strains are the most frequent (Lindberg *et al.*, 1991), with *S. dysenteriae* 1 carrying a special importance due to the clinical seriousness of the dysentery.

Cases of similar or somewhat milder symptoms can also be caused by a group of *Escherichia coli* strains called enteroinvasive *E. coli* (EIEC), represented by some 15 O antigenic groups. The pathogenesis of these infections, and the genetic determinants of virulence in EIEC strains, is thought to be identical to that of *Shigellae* (DuPont, 1990). The prevalence of EIEC infections is still poorly known.

Bacillary dysentery is an acute enterocolitis. The patients usually have fever and diarrhea which may progress to dysentery, i.e., intestinal cramps and tenesmus, with frequent passage of small volume, mucoid, often bloody stool samples containing polymorphonuclear leukocytes (DuPont, 1990). While in otherwise healthy individuals the majority of the cases are self-limiting, in young, malnourished children septicemia is relatively frequent, and is often lethal, complication (DuPont, 1990). Infections caused by *S. dysenteriae* 1 strains producing Shiga toxin (see later) have a tendency to present in more serious clinical forms as compared to those caused by nontoxin producers. A particularly serious sequel is the hemolytic uremic syndrome, which has a high mortality rate (DuPont, 1990).

Most of the epidemiological features of bacillary dysentery can be derived from the uniquely low infective dose (ID_{50} 100–1000 cells) of *Shigellae,* which makes the fecal–oral route the primary mode of transmission (DuPont *et al.*, 1989). Bacillary dysentery emerges as an alarming problem every time hygienic standards are inadequate, or can not be maintained, as in asylums, prisons, and military or refugee camps. The relative ease of infection in a poor hygienic environment also explains why *Shigellae* are one of the major causes of diarrhea among travelers visiting endemic areas. Since attempts to improve the hygienic standards in deprived regions of the world meet formidable financial, technical, and cultural barriers, the need for effective immune intervention to prevent shigellosis has long been recognized for those in need, e.g., children in developing countries,

MUCOSAL VACCINES

participants of military field operations, refugee camp habitants, and travelers to endemic areas.

II. Pathogenesis and Molecular Biology of *Shigella* Infections

It has been known for a long time that the characteristic features of the pathology of bacillary dysentery are the extensive inflammation and ulcerative destruction of the colonic mucosa (Takeuchi *et al.*, 1965). LaBrec *et al.* (1964) proposed that the key step of the pathogenesis of bacillary dysentery is the apical infection of the colonic epithelial cells by virulent *Shigellae. In vitro,* undifferentiated epithelial cells were found to be susceptible to *Shigella* infection, thus providing a relatively simple system to study the details of *Shigella*–host cell interactions (Hale and Bonventre, 1979). In this model bacteria enter the target cell by a mechanism called bacterium-directed phagocytosis, resembling classical phagocytosis. The association of the bacteria with the host cell membrane triggers an accumulation of actin beneath the attachment site followed by the engulfment of the bacterium (Clerc and Sansonetti, 1987).

The genetic information of the invasive phenotype is located on a ca. 30-kb segment of a large (140 mDal) extrachromosomal element called the invasion plasmid (IP), which contains more than 30 genes (Sansonetti *et al.* 1981, 1982). A set of these genes codes for proteins (*ipa*—Invasion Protein Antigens), some of which (i.e., proteins Ipa B, Ipa C, and Ipa D) seem to be directly (but in an as yet undetermined way) involved in triggering the host cell to engulf invading bacteria. Another array of proteins (products of the *mxi* and *spa* genes) secure the proper membrane insertion and secretion of the former ones. For details on the arrangements of these plasmid genes see a recent review (Parsot, 1994).

Inside the cell, *Shigellae*—unlike *Salmonellae* or *Yersinia*—rapidly lyse the phagocytic vacuole. This capacity is closely linked to the invasive phenotype, so far no invasive mutants unable to escape from the phagosome have been described (Sansonetti *et al.*, 1986). Once free in the cytoplasm, *Shigellae* start multiplying vehemently (Sansonetti *et al.*, 1986). This extensive intracellular multiplication is now recognized as a characteristic feature of virulent isolates and is an important target in attenuating vaccine candidates (see below). The secreted IcsA product of the plasmid gene *icsA* (or *virG*) has ATPase activity and a unipolar localization, and is associated with the formation of a trail of polymerized host cell actin at one end of the cell (Goldberg *et al.*, 1993). The capability of virulent *Shigella* strains to form this polar, polymerized actin bundle is essential for the intracellular movement of this otherwise nonmotile organism (Bernardini *et al.*, 1989). Nonmotile mutants invariably have a significantly reduced virulence (Pál *et al.*, 1989, Bernardini *et al.*, 1989), thus constituting another promising group of vaccines (see below). By moving in the cytoplasm, *Shigellae* reach the boundaries of the cell, then extrude into an adjacent cell. This double-membrane-bound protrusion eventually gets engulfed by the neighboring cell. The capability to escape from this double-membrane-bound vacuole is associated with the *icsB* gene on the IP (Allaoui *et al.*, 1992). The fast multiplication of *Shigellae* within the cytoplasm disrupts the host cell's metabolism and causes the death of the cell (Sansonetti and Mounier, 1987). This sequence of events eventually leads—in a HeLa cell monolayer—to the formation of plaques, an *in vitro* equivalent of epithelial ulcers (Oaks *et al.*, 1985).

Recently, the *in vivo* relevance of the above scenario, i.e., the apical infection of intestinal epithelial cells, has been challenged. By using more sophisticated tissue culture techniques it was shown that *Shigellae* are actually unable to infect polarized, differentiated epithelial cells from the apical side, but still can invade them from the basolateral side (Pál and Lindberg, 1991; Mounier *et al.*, 1992).

Different mechanisms, probably acting at the same time and in concert, have been proposed to explain how *Shigellae* gain access to the basolateral side of the epithelial cells. In a rabbit model it was shown that *Shigellae* can be taken-up by M cells overlying the intestinal follicular tissues (Wassef, *et al.*, 1989). From the cytoplasm of M cells *Shigellae* could infect the neighboring epithelial cells or, simultaneously, the M cells could transfer the bacteria to the underlying macrophages and leukocytes (Sansonetti *et al.*, 1991). These cells—upon infection—would soon be killed. Infected, apoptotic macrophages secrete proinflammatory cytokines (Zychlinsky *et al.*, 1994). Bacteria released from the lysing macrophages would have access to the basal side of the epithelial layer. At the same time, in response to attracting signals from the luminal microbes, polymorphonuclear leukocytes transmigrating the epithelial layer either would transfer and release the bacteria into the intercellular or subepithelial region, allowing them to infect epithelial cells, or would provide access to the basolateral side by loosening and expanding the paracellular space (Perdomo *et al.*, 1994a,b).

Acute shigellosis induces a significant increase of the numbers of cells producing a broad array of proinflammatory cytokines, of which IL-1β, IL-6, TNFα and INFγ appeared to be associated with the severity of infection (Raqib *et al.*, 1995a). A concomitant significant increase of the levels of most of the cytokines was also seen in feces, correlating well with the disease severity, and exceeding, some 100-times, the corresponding concentrations found in serum (Raqib *et al.*, 1995b). Unlike other cytokines, IFNγ levels were low in the acute phase, and increased gradually thereafter. At the same time, in the acute stage of infection, receptors for IFNγ, TNF, IL-1, IL-3, IL-4, and TGFβ were significantly down-regulated in the rectal mucosa, and the level of receptor density inversely correlated with the severity of the disease (Raqib *et al.*, 1995c). Based on these studies, it is assumed that the initial focal infection might initiate an inflammatory response mediated by a broad range of cytokines released from PMNs, apoptotic macrophages, and other local cytokine-producing cells. These cytokines, beyond regulating the local immune response, induce an extensive inflammatory tissue destruction. The epithelial destruction, in turn, would expose more basolateral (i.e., "infectable") epithelial surfaces to the bacteria, and so the infection and tissue destruction would accelerate as a consequence of the epithelial invasion by *Shigellae* (Perdomo *et al.*, 1994a; Raqib *et al.*, 1995a,b). It is notable that sustained production of cytokines was seen up to 1 month after onset of disease, and at a stage when the patients were asymptomatic since 2 to 3 weeks (Raqib *et al.*, 1995a).

While the genes necessary for the invasive phenotype are located on the IP, their expression is strictly controlled by chromosomal regulators. The *vir*R gene ensures that the invasion-related genes express at 37°C (e.g., body temperature) but not at 30°C (Maurelli and Sansonetti, 1988), while the *omp*R–*env*Z two component regulatory system connects their expression to environmental osmotic signals (Bernardini *et al.*, 1990). The expression of the *vir*G (*ics*A) gene product, and consequently the capability to move intracellularly, is associated with the *pur*E-linked *kcp*A locus of the *Shigella* chromosome (Pál *et al.*, 1989). Earlier it was assumed that this region somehow acts as a positive regulator for the expression of the *vir*G (*ics*A) gene (Pál *et al.*, 1989). Recently, however, it was proposed that the kcpA-positive phenotype in *Shigella* is actually the result of the lack of a functional *omp*T gene present in *E. coli* and coding for a protease. If expressed, i.e., a kcpA-negative phenotype, this protease may degrade the *ics*A (*vir*G) product, rendering the strain intracellularly nonmotile and thus avirulent (Nakata *et al.*, 1993).

The synthesis of the siderophor aerobactin and its receptor is coded for by the *iuc*ABCD and *iut*A genes. Aerobactin mutants obtained through transposon mutagenesis, although not avirulent, were less pathogenic than the wild-type strain, emphasizing the importance of the iron-sequestering system for the bacterial growth within the tissues (Nassif *et al.*, 1987).

The LPS molecule (O antigen) is a major antigenic constituent of the *Shigella* cell surface. Its synthesis and assembly in *S. flexneri* are coded by the chromosomal *rfa* and *rfb* gene clusters (Schnaitman and Klena, 1993). However, in *S. sonnei*, genes coding for the Phase I O antigen are located on an IP which is slightly smaller (120 mDal) in this species than in the other *Shigella* or EIEC strains (Sansonetti *et al.*, 1981). In *S. dysenteriae* 1 some of the genes necessary for the formation of the complete O antigen were found on a type-specific, 6 mDal plasmid (Watanabe and Timmis, 1984). Rough mutants, while still invasive for HeLa cells, are invariably avirulent (Okamura *et al.*, 1983). This may partly be due to the increased sensitivity of hydrophobic R mutants to phagocytosis and intracellular killing by phagocytes. Moreover, it was shown that mutants lacking the O-specific polysaccharide chain are unable to spread to and infect adjacent cells (Okada *et al.*, 1991, Rajakumar *et al.*, 1994).

Strains of *S. dysenteriae* 1 and some *S. flexneri* isolates also produce a potent cytotoxin, called Shiga toxin. The toxin is coded for by genes *stx*A and *stx*B (Stockbine *et al.*, 1988). The main target cell of the toxin seems to be the capillary endothelium (Obrig *et al.*, 1988). The Shiga toxin is not required for induction of the classical symptoms of dysentery. However, infections caused by toxin producer strains are usually present in a clinically more serious form; therefore, the Shiga toxin is considered one of the important virulence factors (Fontaine *et al.*, 1988).

III. Immune Response in Shigellosis

During the course of bacillary dysentery there is a strong antibody response against both major surface antigenic complexes of *Shigellae,* i.e., the LPS molecule (Lindberg *et al.*, 1991), and the IP-coded, invasion related proteins (Ipa-s) (Oaks *et al.*, 1986, Pál and Brasch, 1987). Of this latter group, responses against IpaA, -B, -C, -D, and the virG (icsA) proteins are the most pronounced (Oaks *et al.*, 1986). In endemic areas, by the age of 5, there are high titers against both types of antigens, suggesting that the first encounters with *Shigellae* occurs during the early childhood (Lindberg *et al.*, 1991; Van de Verg *et al.*, 1992). The courses of the peripheral humoral immune responses (Cam *et al.*, 1993) and the immunoglobulin subclasses of serum and secretory antibodies against Ipa-s and LPS (Islam *et al.*, 1995a) differ. Based on our experience with dysenteric patients (Cam *et al.*, 1993) and with vaccinees (Li *et al.*, 1992), the response against LPS seems to be more uniform and easier to stimulate. On the other hand, anti-Ipa responses apparently last longer, especially in endemic areas where the booster effect of repeated infections with other serogroups expressing the same Ipa-s cannot be ruled out.

Most of the epidemiological and experimental data show that the immunity after natural or experimental infections, as well as after vaccines, is serotype specific (Mel *et al.*, 1968; DuPont *et al.*, 1972b; Formal *et al.*, 1990). This points to the cell envelope lipopolysaccharide (LPS) antigen as the main protective antigen. A positive correlation between the LPS-specific peripheral antibody titers and the level of protection was reported (Cohen *et al.*, 1991), and their protective effect proposed (Robbins *et al.*, 1992). Most of the epidemiological and experimental data, however, suggest that although increased levels of peripheral antibodies are good indicators of a previous natural, or artificial antigenic stimulus, which in turn could induce an effective immunity, they are not protective on their own (Shaughnessy *et al.*, 1946; Higgins *et al.*, 1955; Formal *et al.*, 1967; Cohen *et al.*, 1992). Infection (Dinari *et al.*, 1987; Oberhelman *et al.*, 1991) or vaccination (Kärnell *et al.*, 1992a) are usually followed by an antibody response against both the LPS and the Ipa-s at various mucosal sites (Cleary *et al.*, 1989; Cam *et al.*, 1992). Recently, the intensity of the humoral responses at the periphery as well as at mucosal surfaces was shown to correlate with the severity of infection (Islam *et al.*, 1995a). While the protective effect of secretory antibodies for patients (Oberhelman *et al.*, 1991), as well as for breast-fed babies in endemic areas (Clemens *et al.*, 1986; Cam *et al.*, 1992), has been suggested, the immunological mechanism(s) by which these secretory antibodies would interfere with the infective organism still remains a matter of speculation (Lowell *et al.*, 1980, Tagliabue *et al.*, 1983).

The severity of shigellosis in immunodeficient patients (Baskin *et al.*, 1987) indicates the active involvement of cell-mediated effector mechanisms in fighting *Shigellae.* Growing numbers of observations substantiate this assumption. Recently we showed a significant peripheral lymphocyte proliferation response in vaccinees after stimulating their cells with the homologous lipid-free polysaccharide of the LPS antigen (Li *et al.*, 1992). With immunohistological methods, a high level of activation of T cells, as well as other cytokine-producing cells, was detected in rectal biopsies of acute dysenteric patients (Raqib *et al.*, 1995a). Recently, using triple-color flow cytometry, an increased state of activation in peripheral blood T cells was observed in *S. flexneri* and *S. dysenteriae* type 1-infected persons (Islam *et al.*, 1995b). There appeared to be an early T-cell response phase (characterized by CD25, CD54, and CD49c expression), followed by a second phase with increased HLA-DR expression, continued increased CD54 expression, and an increase in CD54RO expressing T memory cells. This may indicate that in shigellosis T cells are specifically activated in the gut early on and are then recirculating, possibly homing to the gut mucosa. The findings in the study were compatible with a multiple-phase model of the inflammatory and immune responses in shigellosis. High NK cell levels, suggested to be effective against *Shigella*-infected cells (Klimpel *et al.*, 1986), were also found, especially in patients suffering from *S. flexneri* dysentery (Islam *et al.*, 1995b).

It has long been a paradigm that LPSs are T-independent antigens. However, our data have strongly suggested that specific cell-mediated immune reactivities can be elicited against the polysaccharide part of the LPS in both *Shigella* (above) and *Salmonella* infections (Robertsson *et al.*, 1982; Lindberg and Robertsson, 1983). Recent studies using mycobacterial glycolipids for the first time provide experimental evidence that glycolipid antigens indeed can be presented to human T cells via CD1 molecules (Sieling *et al.*, 1995). The lipoarabinomannan (LAM) of *M. leprae,* like the LPS of *Shigellae,* is a heterogenous, amphiphilic lipoglycan. The T cells recognized a specific α 1,2-linked mannose polymer and a phosphatidylinositol unit of the LAM. A hypothetical mechanism is that the CD1 molecules transport endosomally targeted glycolipid antigens of the intracellular pathogen (like *M. leprae* and *Shigellae*) to the cell surface, allowing T-cell recognition and killing of infected cells. Should this hypothesis be proven valid this strongly points to the need of a T-cell-dependent anti-LPS immunity for protection against bacillary dysentery, particularly in clearing the tissues from intracellular *Shigellae.*

IV. Vaccine Development

The fact that the majority of bacillary dysentery cases in endemic areas are seen in children up to 5 years of age suggests that the infection(s) experienced in early childhood induce a certain level of protection, i.e., that protective immunity is attainable. This assumption has gained support from challenge studies following artificial infections in humans and monkeys, and lately by vaccine studies as well.

The limits of our understanding of the pathogenesis and the immune defense mechanisms against shigellosis have had important consequences on the efforts to develop anti-dysentery vaccines. Although the steps of the pathogenesis are becoming better understood, the molecular details of the role(s) of the individual bacterial components—maybe with the exception of Shiga toxin—are still incompletely known. This prevents us from attempting specific immune intervention with any particular steps of the pathogenesis. Another important point is that the actual mechanism(s) (even the branch of the immune system, i.e., humoral or cellular) by which *Shigellae* are cleared from the intestinal tract of a protected host is (are) still largely unknown. Therefore the main goal of almost all current *Shigella* vaccine candidates is to deliver as much "protective" antigenic stimulus as possible to trigger the strongest mucosal immune response, in a way still tolerable for the host.

A technical but important difficulty often faced when testing *Shigella* vaccine candidates is the lack of appropriate animal models to judge the safety, immunogenicity, and efficacy of the candidates. Monkeys, in captivity, are frequently colonized, or infected, with *Shigellae* which may interfere with the outcome, and interpretation, of safety/immunogenicity as well as challenge studies (Voino-Yasenetsky, 1977). The disease which develops in monkeys resembles human dysentery; however, the infective dose is several magnitudes higher than for humans. Cheaper, rodent models, e.g., the guinea pig keratoconjunctivitis test (Serény, 1955) or the mouse lung model (Voino-Yasenetskaya and Voino-Yasenetsky, 1977), have long been proposed as virulence assays for *Shigellae*. Both models have recently been shown to be suitable for preliminary testing of safety, immunogenicity, and the protective efficacy of vaccine candidates (Hartman *et al.*, 1991; Mallett *et al.*, 1993). However, the lack of complete adaptability of the results of the various animal models as far as safety and efficacy in humans is concerned calls for Phase I trials early in the course of developing a particular vaccine candidate.

A. Killed Whole-Cell and Acellular Vaccines

1. *Whole Cell Vaccines*

Parenteral whole-cell vaccines made of killed *Shigellae* stimulated a high level of peripheral antibody response. However, no protection was recorded in these studies either in challenged volunteers or in field studies, probably due to the lack of sufficient stimulation of the mucosal immune system by these highly reactogenic vaccines (Shaughnessy *et al.*, 1946; Higgins *et al.*, 1955; Formal *et al.*, 1967).

2. *Ribosomal Vaccines*

It was recently shown that a sufficient level of protection could be induced at mucosal surfaces with subcellular vaccines given subcutaneously (Levenson *et al.*, 1991; Hale, 1995). *S. sonnei* ribosomal extracts were highly protective against the homologous challenge in guinea pigs and monkeys. The serotype-specific nature of protection suggests the involvement of the O-specific polysaccharide chain in inducing the immune response. In fact, it was speculated that the O-repeating unit is covalently bound to the ribosome particles without the presence of KDO and the lipid A moiety, i.e., the other components of the LPS molecule. This latter feature makes this approach particularly attractive, since the toxicity of the LPS complex is clearly associated with the lipid A component. The assumed adjuvant effect of the ribosomes linked to the polysaccharide may contribute to the development of the secretory IgA response and local immune memory (Levenson and Egorova, 1990).

3. *Polysaccharide-Protein/Proteosome Conjugates*

Based on the observation that there was a positive correlation between anti-LPS antibody titers and the level of protection (Cohen *et al.*, 1991) detoxified (i.e., lipid A-free) O-polysaccharide haptens of *S. flexneri* 2a, *S. sonnei*, or *S. dysenteriae* type 1 conjugated to various protein carriers are under investigation as parenteral, single-shot, low-toxicity vaccine candidates (Robbins and Schneerson, 1990; Robbins *et al.*, 1992; Chu *et al.*, 1992). These vaccine candidates were shown to be safe in humans, inducing a high level of peripheral antibody responses against the homologous LPS antigen (Taylor *et al.*, 1993). However, in the guinea pig keratoconjunctivitis model, when administered parenterally, the O-polysaccharide–protein conjugate vaccine did not protect against the homologous challenge, while they induced enhanced protection in a combined, parenteral–mucosal regimen (Hartman *et al.*, 1994). To be protective, sufficiently high antibody titers should be obtained in the gut, transudation of IgG from serum is a likely mechanism to prevent invasion, or antibody-dependent cellular cytotoxicity mechanisms should limit tissue multiplication of the *Shigellae*. The real protective potential can only be judged in humans. A new approach with a nonliving anti-dysentery vaccine candidate attempts to stimulate a mucosal rather than a circulatory antibody response. Complexed by hydrophobic forces to proteosomes made of outer membrane proteins of *Neisseria meningitidis*, the LPS of *S. flexneri* or *S. sonnei* were safe and protective when given orally or intranasally to guinea pigs and mice (Orr *et al.*, 1993). Apparently, the protein carrier part of the complex secured the mucosal immunogenicity of the LPS antigen, inducing significant levels of peripheral LPS-specific IgG, as well as mucosal IgA responses. Guinea pigs immunized by oral or intranasal inoculation were protected from severe infections up to 69 and 74%, respectively, when challenged with the homologous strain in the conjunctival sac. Beyond the promising efficacy data, these experiments demonstrated that an effective protection can be induced at a distant mucosal site with an anti-dysentery vaccine in experimental animals. Similar vaccines with meningococcal polysaccharides were shown to be safe in humans. This, together with the above-described efficacy results, makes the proteosome–LPS conjugate vaccine an interesting vaccine candidate for further investigations.

B. Live Vaccines

1. *Early Attempts*

a. Virulent Cells and Colonial Variants. Similarly to parenteral-killed whole-cell vaccines, live *Shigella* cells administered parenterally were nonprotective (Formal *et al.*, 1967). The fact that naturally acquired, or artificially induced, bacillary dysentery elicits certain level of protection, the majority of subsequent efforts for vaccine development were oriented toward mimicking the course of the natural infections, i.e., using orally administered, live, attenuated vaccines.

A spontaneous avirulent derivative of *S. flexneri* 2a 2457T with an opaque colonial morphology (2457O) was isolated. The molecular basis of attenuation is not known in 2457O, but, although noninvasive, it still harbours the IP. While safe and effective in studies carried out in monkeys, this strain reverted back to the virulent phenotype in human studies. The unknown basis for its attenuation and its instability made 2457O unsuitable for further consideration as a vaccine candidate (Formal *et al.*, 1965; DuPont *et al.*, 1972a,b).

b. Shigella × E. coli, *and* E. coli × Shigella *Hybrids.* The gradual discovery of various loci on the *Shigella* chromosome associated with the virulent phenotype, as well as the relative ease of intergeneric exchange of the genetic material between *Shigella* and *E. coli*, prompted Formal and co-workers to take a new approach during the 1960s. The *xyl–rha* region of an *E. coli* strain was conjugally transferred into a virulent *S. flexneri* strain. The hybrid, while still invasive, was reduced in its capacity to grow within the mucosa (Falkow *et al.*, 1963). It was safe in monkeys and protected them from subsequent challenge (Formal *et al.*, 1966). However, human volunteers developed diarrhea (DuPont *et al.*, 1972a). The reactogenicity of this vaccine was not attributed to reversion, but to the inherent virulence of the clone. Today it is understood that the basis of the relative attenuation was the replacement of the *xyl–rha*-linked *iuc*ABCD–*iut*A cluster responsible for the production of the iron-acquiring aerobactin and its receptor, with the homologous region of the *E. coli* chromosome. Aerobactin negative mutants alone are still virulent, although reduced in capacity to multiply within the mucosa (Nassif *et al.*, 1987).

An effort "in the opposite direction" was the transfer of the *rfb* gene cluster of *S. flexneri* coding for the main protective antigen, i.e., LPS, into a nonpathogenic *E. coli* O8 strain. The hybrid (PGAI42–1-15) was safe in volunteers. However, probably due to its noninvasive character and the likely improper binding of the *Shigella* LPS to the *E. coli* core, it was not immunogenic enough to be protective (Levine *et al.*, 1977).

c. Streptomycin-Dependent Vaccines. During the 1960s Mel and co-workers developed a group of streptomycin-dependent vaccines (Mel *et al.*, 1965a,b, 1968). Clones of *S. sonnei* and several *S. flexneri* serotypes grew only in the presence of streptomycin; therefore, in the absence of this drug (presumably in the intestinal tract, and within the epithelial cells of the intestine) their replicative ability was limited. In field studies they were safe and highly protective (90%) against homologous infection (Mel *et al.*, 1965a,b, 1968). When given to volunteers 25% of them experienced mild diarrhea. In homologous challenge studies the efficacy was between 49 and 60%, depending on the infecting dose (DuPont *et al.*, 1972b). A streptomycin-dependent *S. sonnei* vaccine was successfully used in a custodial institution, virtually eradicating *S. sonnei* cases. A high level of person-to-person transmission of the vaccine strain was observed among the inmates, obviously facilitating the immune-stimulatory effect of the vaccine (Levine *et al.*, 1975). However, when a *S. flexneri* 2a vaccine strain was tested in an institution with a high attack rate of *S. flexneri* 2a, the protective efficacy was disappointingly low (Levine *et al.*, 1974). Moreover, revertants to streptomycin independence, and in some cases to virulence were also observed (Mikhailov *et al.*, 1968; DuPont *et al.*, 1972a). Recently, studying a set of currently developed live anti-dysentery vaccines, the streptomycin-dependent vaccine was less reactogenic in the intranasal mouse model, while still providing significant protection against the homologous challenge (Mallett *et al.*, 1993).

Although the lack of efficacy in the *S. flexneri* 2a trial is not completely understood, we should bear in mind that these streptomycin-dependent mutants were selected well before our present, more advanced understanding of the genetic basis of virulence in *Shigellae.* Lots of the streptomycin-dependent vaccines varied in harbouring the invasion plasmid (S. B. Formal, personal communication, 1988) which might provide an explanation for the variable results. However, the success of these candidates in most of the studies would justify a reevaluation of this approach securing a more stable expression of the streptomycin-dependent (avirulent) phenotype using current molecular biological methods.

2. Vaccines Currently Being Used or Developed

a. Live, Noninvasive Vaccines. The only anti-dysentery vaccine currently in use is the Istrati T32 *S. flexneri* 2a strain (VADIZEN, Cantacuzino Institute, Bucharest, Romania). The strain was selected after 32 successive passage of a wild isolate on artificial media (Meitert *et al.*, 1984). It was repeatedly shown to be safe and avirulent in animals and in man. Originally it was claimed to be invasive, but reduced in its capacity to grow intracellularly. However, recent, independent studies on an aliquot of the vaccine could not confirm its invasive character. Instead, an extensive deletion in the IP was found which prevented it from expressing the invasion-related Ipa-s (Venkatesan *et al.*, 1991).

The safety and efficacy of this *S. flexneri* vaccine was investigated already in the 1970s in large-scale human field studies involving over 30,000 children. Although it took repeated high doses (5×10^{10}–10^{11} cells within 2 weeks, depending on the age of the vaccinee, and booster doses twice a year, thereafter) the vaccine was well tolerated, and the reported side effects were surprisingly mild, even among children as young as 1 year. The protection rate was reported to be as high as 80.9% against the homologous infection. A surprising observation was the even higher (89.2%) rate of heterologous protection against *S. sonnei* infections for which currently we are lacking any sufficient explanation. Previous infection of monkeys even with virulent *S. flexneri* 2a failed to protect animals against *S. sonnei,* while protective against the subsequent homologous challenge (Formal *et al.*, 1990). The T32 Istrati vaccine was safe and highly immunogenic in the intranasal mouse model, but of the vaccines tested, it exhibited the lowest level of protection against the homologous challenge. It should be noted, however, that it was administered to the animals in the same dose as the other vaccines, although its recommended dose for humans is much higher than those of other live vaccine candidates (Mallett *et al.*, 1993). We believe that the reported data with the T32 Istrati (VADIZEN) vaccine certainly justifies more, extensive, and well-documented studies regarding safety and homologous and heterologous protection.

During the 1970s an avirulent strain (Ty21a) of *Salmonella typhi,* with a *gal*E plus other unidentified attenuating mutations, showed promise in volunteers, as well as in some of the field studies in protecting against typhoid fever (Hackett, 1990). Since typhoid fever results in systemic, mucosal, and cell-mediated immune responses it was assumed that Ty21a could be used as vector expressing *Shigella* cell envelope antigens potentially with a resulting protection against bacillary dysentery. The *S. sonnei* IP, which also codes for the O-polysaccharide antigen of this species, was introduced into Ty21a resulting in strain 5076–1C (Formal *et al.*, 1981). The clone expressed both the *Salmonella* and *Shigella* O antigen, but not the Ipa-s. When given orally to volunteers, it was immunogenic eliciting a peripheral, as well as a local humoral response (Black *et al.*, 1987). Its capacity to stimulate LPS-specific, homing antibody secreting cells has also been shown lately (Van de Verg *et al.*, 1990). However, results of protection studies showed an intolerable level of variation with the different vaccine lots (Black *et al.*, 1987; Herrington *et al.*, 1990). Later this lot to lot variation in efficacy was associated with the presence of pili and the flagellar antigen (Schultz *et al.*, 1990). However, when the culture conditions were adjusted to obtain consistent lots similar to the protective ones, the resulting vaccine, for unknown reasons, was still poorly protective (Herrington *et al.*, 1990). We speculate that, although expressed in Ty21a, the lack of the proper linkage of the *Shigella* O chain to its core resulted in insufficient immunogenicity (Seid *et al.*, 1984). Another argument against this approach could be that strain 5076–1C is too attenuated (Hackett, 1990). Several new *S. typhi* candidates attenuated by known deletions are available (Hackett, 1990), and might prove to be suitable alternatives for Ty21a in continuing the improvement of *S. typhi* X *Shigella* hybrid vaccines.

b. Live, Invasive Vaccines. This group of live vaccines, while attenuated, has been designed with the goal of maintaining the invasive nature of the *Shigellae* in order to mimic the natural infection and guarantee antigenic delivery to the immune system. A better understanding of the steps in pathogenesis allowed the disarmament of virulence-related traits other than invasion in order to achieve sufficient attenuation. Two phenotypes have been targeted during these experiments, sometimes combined with each other or with other mutations. One is the capacity of virulent strains to spread intracellularly, which is dependent on the presence of the *vir*G (*ics*A) gene on the plasmid, and the *kcp*A locus of the *Shigella* chromosome (Pál *et al.*, 1989, Bernardini *et al.*, 1989). The other one is the potential for the rapid intracytoplasmic growth after escaping from the phagosome (Sansonetti *et al.*, 1986). Various strategies have been used to develop these candidates (Table I).

An *E. coli* K-12 strain was crossed with a *S. flexneri* 2a Hfr donor in order to transfer the *his*- and *pro*-linked genes coding for the type- and group-specific cell envelope antigens. This was followed by the mobilization of the IP into this hybrid making it invasive for epithelial cells. With the exception of loci responsible for the *S. flexneri* 2a O antigen synthesis, this clone (EC104) lacked all the virulence-related chromosomal genes, in particular the *pur*E-linked *kcp*A locus and the *xyl–rha*-linked cluster coding for aerobactin production. The vaccine was safe and immunogenic in monkeys and protected to a significant level against challenge with the homologous strain (Formal *et al.*, 1984). However, when given to nine volunteers, EC 104 induced diarrhea in four of them (S. B. Formal, personal communication, 1988). Since for the transfer of the IP into the hybrid strain it was tagged by a kanamycin transposon considered unsuitable in vaccines for human use, a similar hybrid (EcSf2a-1) was generated with a mercury resistance transposon-labeled IP (Newland *et al.*, 1992). EcSf2a-1, however, was also too reactogenic in humans (Kotloff *et al.*, 1992). The reasons for the reactogenicity are not entirely clear. Theoretically, the kcpA-negative character preventing intracellular spread of the vaccines should have secured an avirulent phenotype. It was shown, however, that *E. coli* X *Shigella* hybrids harboring the IP could revert to intracellularly motile clones, i.e., to the kcpA-positive phenotype (Pál *et al.*, 1989). This was later shown also for EcSf2a-1 (Newland *et al.*, 1992); kcpA-positive, intracellularly motile revertants of EcSf2a-1, however, were virulent only after a subsequent conjugal transfer of the *rfa* gene of the *Shigella* chromosome, providing the expression of the *Shigellae* core in the hybrid strain (Newland *et al.*, 1992). Apparently, once able to move intracellularly, the remaining

TABLE I
Live, Invasive Anti-dysentery Vaccine Candidates

Vaccine	Species	Altered phenotype (gene)			Safety	Efficacy
		IC[a] spread	IC growth	Others		
EC 104	*E. coli* × *S. flexneri* 2a	(*kcp*A)		(*iuc*A)	Safe in monkeys, diarrhea in humans	Protective in monkeys
EcSf2a-1	*E. coli* × *S. flexneri* 2a	(*kcp*A)		(*iuc*A)	Diarrhea in humans	No protection in humans
SC560	*S. flexneri* 5	(Δ*ics*A)			Mild symptoms in monkeys	Protective in monkeys
SC 445	*S. flexneri* 5	(*ics*A::Tn*pho*A)		(Δ*envZ*, *omp*R)	Safe in monkeys	Dysentery in 1 out of 5 challenged monkeys
SC5700	*S. flexneri* 5	(*ics*A::Tn*pho*A)		(*iuc*::Tn*10*)	Safe in monkeys	Protective in monkeys
vc 77	*S. flexneri* 2a		(*pur*)	(Rif)	Safe in humans	No protection in humans
vc 3359	*S. sonnei*		(*pur*)	(Rif)	Safe in humans	No protection in humans
TSF-21	*S. flexneri* Y		(*thy*A)	(Ts)	Safe in monkeys	Protective in monkeys
SFL124	*S. flexneri* Y		(Δ*aro*D)		Well tolerated in humans up to 2 × 10^9 cfu[b]	Protective in monkeys
SFL1070	*S. flexneri* 2a		(Δ*aro*D)		Well tolerated in humans up to 10^8 CFU	Protective in monkeys
EcSf2a-2	*E. coli* × *S. flexneri* 2a	(kcpA)	(Δ*aro*D)		Well tolerated in humans up to 2 × 10^9 CFU	No protection in humans
CVD1203	*S. flexneri* 2a	(Δ*vir*G)	(Δ*aro*A)		Safe in guinea pig	Protective in guinea pigs

[a]Intracellular.
[b]Colony forming unit.

attenuating trait of this vaccine strain, e.g., the lack of aerobactin production, was not enough to secure the avirulent character. This is not surprising, since mutants in the aerobactin gene, although quantitatively less virulent, still were able to cause the characteristic pathology of virulent *Shigellae* (Nassif *et al.*, 1987). In light of recent findings, i.e., that the kcpA-negative phenotype is actually due to the expression of a protease (Nakata *et al.*, 1993), we should consider the potential difficulties when trying to secure the stable and permanent expression of a functional protein instead of preventing its production. This points to the necessity of either introducing supplementary attenuations into these strains (see below) or looking for different approaches in order to maintain the lack of intracellular motility.

The introduction of a mutation/deletion into the *vir*G(*ics*A) gene harboured by the IP and necessary for the intracellular mobility could provide a solution to the above problem. SC560, a Δ*ics*A derivative of a wild-type *S. flexneri* 5 strain, caused focal lesions only in the intestinal mucosa, in accordance with its inability to spread from cell-to-cell (Sansonetti *et al.*, 1991). Although protective against subsequent challenge, clinically this strain still caused mild dysentery in monkeys. In order to achieve a more complete attenuation, an *ics*A::Tn*pho*A mutation was combined with a Δ*env*Y, *omp*R deletion disconnecting the strain from one of its main regulatory signals, *i.e.*, the osmotic pressure of its milieu. While a strain with the Δ*env*Y, *omp*R deletion only (SC433) still caused dysentery in monkeys, the double mutant (SC445) was well tolerated by the vaccinated animals. However, when challenged, one out of five animals developed dysentery, suggesting that with this combination of mutations SC445 might be too attenuated (Sansonetti *et al.*, 1991). In another set of experiments Sansonetti and Arondel combined the *ics*A::Tn*pho*A mutation with an *iuc*::Tn10 mutation limiting the capacity of the strain (SC5700) not only to spread, but also, due to the lack of aerobactin, to multiply within tissues. This vaccine was well tolerated by the animals, induced a significant immune response, and was fully protective in challenge studies in monkeys, giving an excellent example for rational, experimental vaccine design (Sansonetti and Arondel, 1989). The final evaluation of this vaccine candidate's safety and immunogenicity requires human trials.

After recognizing the importance of the capability of *Shigellae* to multiply intracellularly, attempts were made to generate vaccines unable to grow in the cytoplasm. Mutagen-induced purine auxotroph mutants were selected from *S. flexneri* 2a (vc 77) and from *S. sonnei* (vc 3359) combined with spontaneous *rif* (Rifampicin resistant, RNA polymerase) mutations (Linde *et al.*, 1990). The strains were invasive and unable to grow intracellularly. As expected, they were safe and immunogenic in human volunteers; however, they failed to protect two out of the four vaccinees upon challenge (Dentchev *et al.*, 1990).

Ahmed and co-workers reported on the development of a thymine auxotroph, temperature-sensitive double mutant (TSF21) of *S. flexneri* Y. It was speculated that the main attenuating factor in TSF21 is the lack of intracellular growth due the requirement for thymine (Ahmed *et al.*, 1990). The attenuating mutation was shown to be due to a single base substitution in the *thy*A gene, resulting in the change of glutamine at position 44 in the wild type thymidilate synthase to leucine in the mutant (Nur-E-Kamal *et al.*, 1994). The vaccine was safe in monkeys and protective against the homologous challenge (Ashraf *et al.*, 1991). No data on human trials are available at the moment. Remarkably, in monkeys, the *S. flexneri* Y strain was fully protective against the quasi-heterologous challenge with serotype 3a, and partially protective (short-term diarrhea in two of four animals) against a *S. dysenteriae* type 1 strain (Giri *et al.*, 1993). The vaccine induced antibody response against both the homologous, as well as the heterologous LPS antigens. The cross-protection data between the serotype Y vaccine and the 3a type challenge strain can be attributed to the group-specific backbone structure shared by all but type 6 *S. flexneri* serotypes (Ewing and Lindberg, 1984). We speculate that one explanation for the efficacy against the *S. dysenteriae* 1 challenge could be the LPS epitope we recently described with monoclonal antibody MASF B. This antibody, beyond recognizing all *S. flexneri* serotypes, reacts with *S. dysenteriae* strains, indicating the presence of a shared epitope by all of these strains (Carlin and Lindberg, 1987). Whether immune responses elicited against this epitope bear any protective value, indeed, needs further investigations.

The recent success of aromatic-dependent *Salmonella* vaccines (Stocker, 1988) encouraged several groups to take a similar approach to attenuate *Shigella* vaccines. The precursor of folic acid, *p*-aminobenzoic acid and 2,3-dihydropholic acid, are not vertebrate metabolites, and therefore the cytoplasm of eukaryotic cells do not contain these compounds. *E. coli* and *Shigellae* cannot assimilate folic acid if mutations in the *aro* genes prevent them from synthesizing it from the above metabolites; further, if they are not available from the environment, they stop multiplying. This prompted us to first construct an *aro*D::Tn10 mutated derivative (SFL114) of a virulent *S. flexneri* Y strain, SFL1 (Lindberg *et al.*, 1988). The strain had significantly reduced intracellular growth capacity (Lindberg *et al.*, 1990), was well tolerated and highly protective in monkeys (Lindberg *et al.*, 1988, 1990). Later, SFL114 was further improved by deleting the *aro*D gene, resulting in strain SFL124 (Kärnell *et al.*, 1992a). SFL124 proved to be as safe and as effective in monkeys as the mutant version, SFL114 (Kärnell *et al.*, 1992b). Recently, the protective efficacy of SFL124 was also shown in the guinea pig keratoconjunctivitis assay (Hartman *et al.*, 1991) and in the intranasal mouse model (Mallett *et al.*, 1993). When administered to volunteers living in Sweden, SFL124 was safe, inducing a short-lasting mild diarrhea in only 2 of the 21 vaccinees (Li *et al.*, 1992). It was also highly effective to stimulate peripheral as well as local LPS-specific responses, especially after a three-dose regimen. Interestingly, peripheral anti-Ipa responses were noted only in volunteers who had experienced bacillary dysentery infections earlier in their life. When tested in 30 Vietnamese volunteers, the vaccine was completely safe and induced a significant increase of LPS-specific antibody-secreting cells in 90% and Ipa-specific antibody-secreting cells in 87% of the vaccinees. The nature of responses observed after booster doses given 6 and 12 months later indicated that the primary vaccination also stimulated a mucosal memory lasting for at least a year (Li *et al.*, 1993). Recently, the vaccine was also tested, in a single dose regimen, in Vietnamese children between 9 and 14 years of age. SFL124 was remarkably well tolerated by the children even when receiving 10^9 cells. In a dose–response manner, the vaccine was immunogenic in the children, and the characteristics of the immune response resembled that of a secondary response. This was an important observation of the study, suggesting that when using the vaccine in an endemic environment, priming is likely because of natural infections, and the vaccine would serve as a booster stimulus (Li *et al.*, 1994).

It should be noted that an advantage of *S. flexneri* serotype Y vaccines is that this serotype represents the backbone structure of the O antigen of all but type six serotypes. For the individual types this is then modified by glucosylating or acetylating phages (Ewing and Lindberg, 1984). The corresponding genes from some of these phages have been cloned, allowing the easy conversion of the tested vaccine strains into other serotypes (Verma *et al.*, 1991).

A similar attenuating marker was introduced into a virulent *S. flexneri* 2a strain (2457T) resulting in a Δ*aro*D derivative (SFL1070) (Kärnell *et al.*, 1993). The strain was impaired in growing within the cytoplasm of the host cell. It was safe in monkeys, and elicited a significant sIgA response against the homologous LPS antigen. Seven of the eight monkeys challenged were completely protected after vaccination. SFL1070 was given in graded doses between 10^5 and 10^9 cells to Swedish volunteers. It was found that the optimal balance between reactogenicity and immunogenicity was 10^8 cells, some 20 times lower than was found in case of the Y serotype SFL114 or SFL124 (Kärnell *et al.*, 1995). SFL1070 stimulated a significant response in a dose-dependent way, a dose of 10^8 cells being immunogenic in all the vaccinees. The promising safety and immunogenicity data obtained so far with the aromatic-dependent *S. flexneri* vaccines encourages us to further evaluate its potential.

In order to secure complete attenuation, two recent vaccine candidates combine the lack of motility with the inability for intracellular multiplication achieved by auxotrophy for aromatic compounds. To overcome the problem posed by the reversion to the kcpA-positive phenotype seen in EcSf2a-1, an *aro*D deletion was also introduced into this strain, resulting in vaccine candidate EcSf2a-2 (Newland *et al.*, 1992). The strain was safe and protective (60%) in monkeys. When given to volunteers, it was well tolerated up to a dose of 2.1×10^9 cfu. However, from a dose of 2.5×10^9, 17% of the patients reacted with fever and diarrhea, and two of the four volunteers developed dysentery when given a dose of 1.8×10^{10} cfu (Kotloff *et al.*, 1992). Although immunogenic, EcSf2a-2 exhibited only a 36% protection against a subsequent challenge (Kotloff *et al.*, 1992). With regard to the reactogenicity of this strain it should be noted that our *S. flexneri* Y strain attenuated only by a similar *aro*D deletion also induced mild enteric symptoms when given in the same dose in some of the volunteers. However, according to our experience, the severity of these symptoms was well within the acceptable level for an enteric vaccine containing invasive organisms, and the vaccine was nonreactogenic in people living in endemic areas. When lowering the dose of EcSf-2a to 5×10^8 cfu administered on Days 0, 3, 14, and 17, the vaccine was safe and immunogenic in a phase II study involving 244 adult volunteers (Taylor *et al.*, 1994).

Recently, a candidate with similar phenotypic character, but a different genetic background has been developed. Introducing an *aro*A deletion into the chromosome, and subsequently a *vir*G (*ics*A) deletion into the IP of the wild-type *S. flexneri* 2a (2457T), strain CVD 1203 was constructed. A clone (CVD 1201.1) with only the Δ*aro*A deletion still caused transient, mild symptoms in some of the guinea pigs infected. This is in agreement with our observation that the Δ*aro*D deletion provided less effective attenuation in this background (i.e., 2457T) than using a *S. flexneri* Y parent strain (Kärnell *et al.*, 1995). When the Δ*aro*A mutation was combined with the Δ*vir*G genotype, the resulting CVD 1203 vaccine candidate was safe but still immunogenic and protective against the homologous challenge in the guinea pig keratoconjunctivitis model (Noriega *et al.*, 1994). A phase I human trial was started in 1995.

These results certainly point to the importance of the inherent virulence of the parent strains. Recently, B. A. Hartman and M. Venkatesan showed that *S. flexneri* strains express different levels of virulence (personal communication, 1995). The level of pathogenicity correlated with the restriction fragment length pattern of the IP as tested with a probe specific to the conserved part of the multicopy *ipa*H gene (B. A. Hartman and M. Venkatesan, personal communication, 1995; Hartman *et al.*, 1990). The parent strain of SFL124, SFL1, was less virulent than the highly pathogenic strain 2457T used to construct SFL1070. One may assume that the donor strain (M90T) for the IP (pWR100) carried by EcSf2a-2 also would fall to the highly virulent category. This may explain why vaccine candidates with identical or similar attenuating markers (deletions in the *aro* genes) are not equally reactogenic.

V. Conclusions

Over the past 50 years a great deal of effort has been dedicated to develop a safe and effective vaccine formulation against bacillary dysentery. Still, we do not have a vaccine with proven efficacy and safety record sufficient for broad-scale introduction. We do not even know which type of vaccine will finally comply with the need for the delicate balance between safety and efficacy, or whether it will be a parenteral subunit, or a live, attenuated, oral vaccine.

Why have all efforts so far been in vain? There are several reasons for this. We still do not know what immune defense mechanisms to stimulate, nor do we know how the memory mechanisms are regulated. The fact that children in developing countries acquire immunity, which appears to be long-lasting, may be more an effect of repeated encounters with *Shigellae, i.e.*, boosters, in a *Shigellae*-endemic environment than an indication of a lasting memory. The notion that anti-O antigen immunity correlates with protection may be a surrogate marker, but in light of the recent observation that human CD1 molecules present microbial glycolipids so they are recognized by T cells it is conceivable that a mechanism and an explanation for the observed species and serotype-specific immunity against the intracellular *Shigellae* have been found.

Recent studies by our own group confirm earlier observations that the inflammatory response is a significant part of the pathogenesis of shigellosis. A production of proinflammatory cytokines occurs in the colonic tissues in acute shigellosis with a sustained mucosal production up to 1 month after the onset of dysentery. A simultaneous downregulation of cytokine surface receptors in the acute stage and a gradual reappearance in the convalescent stage suggests a tight regulation of cytokine activities at the mucosal level. The net effect is an increased and prolonged infiltration of granulocytes, monocytes, and lymphocytes into the colonic mucosa. The cytokine profile did not show a selective activation of Th1 (IFNδ, TGFβ) or Th2 (IL-4, IL-10) subsets in either the acute or convalescent stages of shigellosis. Thus cellular as well as humoral immune responses are elicited. The Th2 responses may balance, in part, the immunopathologic potentials of the Th1 response. A less desired consequence, however, is that the down-regulation of the Th1 response impairs eradication of the intracellular *Shigellae,* thereby favoring persistence of the infection.

The best prophylactic measure would be to prevent the *Shigellae* from invading the mucosal lining of the intestine, and if a high infective bolus overcomes that defense line, to limit the intracellular multiplication and spread of the bacteria in the tissues. This would prevent, or limit, the release of the proinflammatory cytokines. This strongly suggests that a mucosal delivery of a *Shigella* vaccine formulation should be preferred. The elicited immune response should aid both in preventing invasion and in eradication of *Shigellae* that are intracellular and multiplying.

Among vaccine candidates presently under development, at a preclinical or Phase I stage, several have the desired characteristics:

1. Live-attenuated *Shigellae,* which will provide an array of surface antigens. The balance between safety and immunogenicity, and consequently efficacy, will have to be established in trials. This approach comes closest to mimicking a natural infection without the characteristics of bacillary dysentery, and the antigens will be targeted to the same tissues as wild-type *Shigellae.*
2. Live-attenuated vector strain expressing one or more of presently known critical surface components such as LPS (or its O-antigenic epitopes), a few selected Ipa antigens (or immunodominant peptides thereof), and perhaps the B subunit of the Shiga toxin. The nature of the immune response will be dependent on the characteristics of the vector strain.
3. Subunit vaccine, composed of LPS (or O-antigenic epitopes in a glycoconjugate), Ipa proteins (peptides), and perhaps the Shiga toxin B subunit and delivered at a mucosal surface. The formulation can be as a liposome, proteosome, or lactide–glycolide particle which may have to be targeted to M cells for an optimal uptake. The formulation most likely will be given together with an adjuvant. Currently subunit vaccines are expensive compared to live vaccine strains (as *Shigellae* or in vectors) which may delay their development.

All of the three categories of vaccine formulations can be made and tested. The need for conducting field trials is obvious since none of the available animal models can predict safety and efficacy in humans. Unfortunately, shigellosis is a disease of developing countries, and the market in industrialized countries (which will pay for the development costs) is restricted to travelers and potentially the military. Therefore, development of efficacious *Shigella* vaccines is a low priority among major vaccine manufacturers.

References

Ahmed, Z. U., Sarker, M. R., and Sack, D. A. (1990). Protection of adult rabbits and monkeys from lethal shigellosis by oral immunization with a thymine-requiring and temperature-sensitive mutant of *Shigella flexneri* Y. *Vaccine* **8,** 153–158.

Allaoui, A., Mounier, J., Prevost, M. C., Sansonetti, P. J., and Parsot, C. (1992). *icsB*: A *Shigella flexneri* virulence gene necessary for the lysis of protrusions during intercellular spread. *Mol. Microbiol.* **6,** 1605–1616.

Ashraf, M. M., Giri, D. K., Batra, H. V., Khandekar, P., Ahmed, Z. U., and Talwar, G. P. (1991). Potentials of *Shigella flexneri* Y strain TSF21 as a candidate vaccine against shigellosis: Safety, immunogenicity and protective efficacy in Bonnet monkeys. *FEMS Microbiol. Immunol.* **76,** 165–170.

Baskin, D. H., Lax, J. D., and Barenberg, D. (1987). *Shigella* bacteremia in patients with the Acquired Immune Deficiency Syndrome. *Am. J. Gastroenterol.* **82,** 338–341.

Bernardini, M. L., Mounier, J., d'Hauteville, H., Coquis-Rondon, M., and Sansonetti, P. J. (1989). Identification of *icsA*, a plasmid locus of *Shigella flexneri* that governs intra- and intercellular spread through interaction with F-actin. *Proc. Natl. Acad. Sci. U.S.A.* **86,** 3867–3871.

Bernardini, M. L., Fontaine, A., and Sansonetti, P. J. (1990). The two-component regulatory system *OmpR-EnvZ* controls the virulence of *Shigella. J. Bacteriol.* **172,** 6274–6281.

Black, R. E., Levine, M. M., Clements, M. L., Losonsky, G., Herrington, D., Berman, S., and Formal, S. B. (1987). Prevention of shigellosis by a *Salmonella typhi–Shigella sonnei* bivalent vaccine. *J. Infect. Dis.* **155,** 1260–1265.

Cam, P. D., Achi, R., Lindberg, A. A., and Pál, T. (1992). Antibodies against plasmid coded antigens of *Shigellae* in human colostrum and milk. *Acta Microbiol. Hung.* **39,** 263–270.

Cam, P. D., Pál, T., and Lindberg, A. A. (1993). Immune response against lipopolysaccharide and invasion plasmid coded antigens of *Shigellae* in Vietnamese and Swedish dysenteric patients. *J. Clin. Microbiol.* **31,** 454–457.

Carlin, N. I. A., and Lindberg, A. A. (1987). Monoclonal antibodies specific for *Shigella flexneri* lipopolysaccharides: Clones binding to type IV, V and VI antigens, group 3,4 antigen and an epitope common to all *S. flexneri* and *S. dysenteriae* type 1. *Infect. Immun.* **55,** 1412–1420.

Chu, C.-Y., Liu, B., Watson, D., Szu, S. C., Bryla, K., Shiloach, J., Schneerson, R., and Robbins, J. B. (1992). Preparation, characterization, and immunogenicity of conjugates composed of the O-specific polysaccharide of *Shigella dysenteriae* type 1 (Shiga's bacillus) bound to tetanus toxoid. *Infect. Immun.* **40,** 245–256.

Cleary, T. G., Winsor, D. K., Reich, D., Ruiz-Palacios, G., and Calva, J. J. (1989). Human milk immunoglobulin A antibodies to *Shigella* virulence determinants. *Infect. Immun.* **57,** 1675–1679.

Clemens, J. D., Stanton, B., Stoll, B., Shahid, N. S., Banu, H. and Alauddin Chowdhury, A. K. M. (1986). Breast feeding as a determinant of severity in shigellosis. *Am. J. Epidemiol.* **123,** 710–720.

Clerc, P., and Sansonetti, P. J. (1987). Entry of *Shigella flexneri* into HeLa cells; evidence for directed phagocytosis involving actin polymerization and myosin accumulation. *Infect. Immun.* **55**, 2681–2688.

Cohen, D., Green, M. S., Block, C., Slepon, R., and Ofek, I. (1991). Prospective study of the association between serum antibodies to lipopolysaccharide O antigen and the attack rate of shigellosis. *J. Clin. Microbiol.* **29**, 386–389.

Cohen, D., Green, M. S., Block, C., Slephon, R., and Lerman, Y. (1992). Natural immunity to shigellosis in two groups with different previous risks of exposure to *Shigella* is only partly expressed by serum antibodies to lipopolysaccharide. *J. Infect. Dis.* **165**, 785–787.

Dentchev, V., Marinova, S., Vassilev, T., Bratoyeva, M., and Linde, K. (1990). Live *Shigella flexneri* 2a and *Shigella sonnei* I vaccine candidate strains with two attenuating markers. II. Preliminary results of vaccination of adult volunteers and children aged 2–17 years. *Vaccine* **8**, 30–34.

Dinari, G., Hale, T. L., Austin, S. W., and Formal, S. B. (1987). Local and systemic antibody response to *Shigella* infection in *Rhesus* monkeys. *J. Infect. Dis.* **155**, 1065–1069.

DuPont, H. L. (1990). *Shigella* species (Bacillary Dysentery). *In* "Principles and Practice of Infectious Disease" (G. L. Mandell, R. G. Douglas, Jr., and J. E. Bennett, eds.), pp. 1716–1722. Churchill Livingstone, London.

DuPont, H. L., Hornick, R. B., Snyder, M. J., Libonati, J. P., Formal, S. B., and Gangarosa, E. J. (1972a). Immunity in shigellosis: I. Response of man to attenuated strains of *Shigella*. *J. Infect. Dis.* **125**, 5–11.

DuPont, H. L., Hornick, R. B., Snyder, M. J., Libonati, J. P., Formal, S. B., and Gangarosa, E. J. (1972b). Immunity to shigellosis. II. Protection induced by oral live vaccine or primary infection. *J. Infect. Dis.* **125**, 12–16.

DuPont, H. L., Levine, M. M., Hornick, R. B., and Formal, S. B. (1989). Inoculum size in shigellosis and implications for expected mode of transmission. *J. Infect. Dis.* **159**, 1126–1128.

Ewing, W. H., and Lindberg, A. A. (1984). Serology of *Shigella*. *In* "Methods in Microbiology" (T. Bergan, ed.), Vol. 1, pp. 113–142, Academic Press, New York.

Falkow, S., Schneider, H., Baron, L. S., and Formal, S. B. (1963). Virulence of *Escherichia–Shigella* genetic hybrids for the guinea pig. *J. Bacteriol.* **86**, 1251–1258.

Fontaine, A., Arondel, J., and Sansonetti, P. J. (1988). Role of Shiga toxin in the pathogenesis of bacillary dysentery, studied by using a Tox^- mutant of *Shigella dysenteriae* 1. *Infect. Immun.* **56**, 3099–3109.

Formal, S. B., LaBrec, E., Palmer, A., and Falkow, S. (1965). Protection of monkeys against experimental shigellosis with attenuated vaccines. *J. Bacteriol.* **90**, 63–68.

Formal, S. B., Kent, T. H., May, H. C., Palmer, A., Falkow, S., and LaBrec, E. H. (1966). Protection of monkeys against experimental shigellosis with a living attenuated oral polyvalent dysentery vaccine. *J. Bacteriol.* **92**, 17–22.

Formal, S. B., Maenza, R. M., Austin, S., and LaBrec, E. H. (1967). Failure of parenteral vaccines to protect monkeys against experimental shigellosis. *Proc. Soc. Exp. Biol. Med.* **125**, 347–349.

Formal, S. B., Baron, L. S., Kopecko, D. J., Washington, O., Powell, C., and Life, C. A. (1981). Construction of a potential bivalent vaccine strain: Introduction of *Shigella sonnei* form I antigen genes into the galE *Salmonella typhi* Ty21a typhoid vaccine strain. *Infect. Immun.* **34**, 746–750.

Formal, S. B., Hale, T. L., Kapfer, C., Cogan, J. P., Snoy, P. J., Chung, R., Wingfield, M. E., Elisberg, B. L., and Baron, L. S. (1984). Oral vaccination of monkeys with an invasive *Escherichia coli* K12 hybrid expressing *Shigella flexneri* 2a somatic antigen. *Infec. Immun.* **46**, 465–469.

Formal, S. B., Oaks, E. V., Olsen, R. E., Wingfield-Eggleston, M., Snoy, P. J., and Cogan J. P. (1990). Effect of prior infection with virulent *Shigella flexneri* 2a on the resistance of monkeys to subsequent infection with *Shigella sonnei*. *J. Infect. Dis.* **164**, 533–537.

Giri, D. K., Ashraf, M. M., and Ahmed Z. U. (1993). Heterologous protection of Bonnet monkeys from experimental shigellosis after oral immunization with *Shigella flexneri* serotype Y thymine-dependent temperature-sensitive mutant TSF21. *Immunol. Infect. Dis.* **3**, 23–26.

Goldberg, M. B., Barzu, O., Parsot, C., and Sansonetti, P. J. (1993). Unipolar localization and ATPase activity of *IcsA*, a *Shigella flexneri* protein involved in intracellular movement. *J. Bacteriol.* **175**, 2189–2196.

Hackett, J. (1990). *Salmonella*-based vaccines. *Vaccine* **8**, 5–11.

Hale, T. L. (1995). *Shigella* vaccines. *In* "Molecular and Clinical Aspects of Bacterial Vaccine Development" (D. A. A. Ala'Aldeen and C. E. Hormaeche, eds.), pp. 179–204. Wiley, New York.

Hale, T. L., and Bonventre, P. F. (1979). *Shigella* infection of Henle intestinal epithelial cells: Role of the bacterium. *Infect. Immun.* **24**, 879–886.

Hartman, A. B., Venkatesan, M., Oaks, E. V., and Buysse, J. M. (1990). Sequence and molecular characterization of a multicopy invasion plasmid antigen gene, *ipa*H, of *Shigella flexneri*. J. Bacteriol. **172**, 1905–1915.

Hartman, A. B., Powell, C. J., Schultz, C. L., Oaks, E. V., and Eckels, K. H. (1991). Small-animal model to measure efficacy and immunogenicity of *Shigella* vaccine strains. *Infect. Immun.* **59**, 4075–4083.

Hartman, B. A., Van de Verg, L. L., Collins, H. H., Jr., Tang, D. B., Bendiuk, N. O., Taylor, D. N., and Powell, C. J. (1994). Local immune response and protection in the guinea pig keratoconjunctivitis model following immunization with *Shigella* vaccines. *Infect. Immun.* **62**, 412–420.

Herrington, D. A., Van der Berg, L., Formal, S. B., Hale, T. L., Tall, B. D., Cryz, S. J., Tramont, E. C., and Levine, M. M. (1990). Studies in volunteers to evaluate candidate *Shigella* vaccines: Further experience with a bivalent *Salmonella typhi–Shigella sonnei* vaccine and protection conferred by previous *Shigella sonnei* disease. *Vaccine* **8**, 353–357.

Higgins, A. R., Floyd, T. M., and Kader, M. A. (1955). Studies in shigellosis. III. A controlled evaluation of monovalent *Shigella* vaccine in a highly endemic environment. *Am. J. Trop. Med. Hyg.* **4**, 281–288.

Institute of Medicine (1986). The prospect for immunizing against *Shigella* spp. *In* "New Vaccine Development: Establishing Priorities. Volume 2. Diseases of importance in developing countries," pp. 329–337. National Academy Press, Washington, D.C.

Islam, D., Wretlind, B., Ryd, M., Lindberg, A. A., and Christenson, B. (1995a). Immunoglobulin subclass distribution and dynamics of *Shigella*-specific antibody responses in serum and stool samples in shigellosis. *Infect. Immun.* **63,** 2054–2061.

Islam, D., Bardhan, P. K., Lindberg, A. A., and Christensson, B. (1995b). *Shigella* infection induces cellular activation of T and B cells and distinct species-related changes in peripheral blood lymphocyte subsets during the course of disease. *Infect. Immun.* **63,** 2941–2949.

Kärnell, A., Stocker, B. A. D., Katakura, S., Reinholt, F. P., and Lindberg, A. A. (1992a). Live oral auxotrophic *Shigella flexneri* SFL124 vaccine with a deleted *aro*D gene: Characterization and monkey protection studies *Vaccine* **10,** 389–394.

Kärnell, A., Sweiha, H., and Lindberg, A. A. (1992b). Auxotrophic live oral *Shigella flexneri* vaccine protects monkeys against challenge with *Shigella flexneri* of different serotypes. *Vaccine* **10,** 167–174.

Kärnell, A., Cam, P. D., Verma, N., and Lindberg, A. A. (1993). *Aro*D deletion attenuates *Shigella flexneri* strain 2457T an makes it a safe and efficacious oral vaccine in monkeys. *Vaccine* **11,** 830–836.

Kärnell, A., Li, A., Zhao, C. R., Karlsson, K., Minh, N. B., and Lindberg, A. A. (1995). Safety and immunogenicity study of the auxotrophic *Shigella flexneri* 2a vaccine SFL1070 with a deleted *aro*D gene in adult Swedish volunteers. *Vaccine* **13,** 88–99.

Klimpel, G. R., Niesel, D. W., and Klimpel, K. D. (1986). Natural cytotoxic effector cell activity against *Shigella flexneri*-infected HeLa cells. *J. Immunol.* **136,** 1081–1086.

Kotloff, K. L., Herrington, D. A., Hale, T. L., Newland, J. W., Van de Berg, L., Cogan, J. P., Snoy, P. J., Sadoff, J. C., Formal, S. B., and Levine, M. M. (1992). Safety, Immunogenicity, and efficacy in monkeys and humans of invasive *Escherichia coli* K-12 hybrid vaccine candidates expressing *Shigella flexneri* 2a somatic antigen. *Infect. Immun.* **60,** 2218–2224.

LaBrec, E. H., Schneider, H., Magnani, T. J., and Formal, S. B. (1964). Epithelial cell penetration as an essential step in the pathogenesis of bacillary dysentery. *J. Bacteriol.* **88,** 1503–1518.

Levenson, V. I., and Egorova, T. P. (1990). Polysaccharide nature of O-antigen in protective ribosomal preparations from *Shigella*: Experimental evidence and implications for the ribosomal vaccine concept. *Res. Microbiol.* **141,** 707–720.

Levenson, V. I., Egorova, T. P., Belkin, Z. P., Fedosova, V. G., Subbotina, J. L., Rulhadze, E. Z., Dzhikidze, E. K., and Stassilevich, Z. K. (1991). Protective ribosomal preparation from *Shigella sonnei* as a parenteral candidate vaccine. *Infect. Immun.* **59,** 3610–3618.

Levine, M. M., Gangarosa, E. J., Werener, M., and Morris, G. K. (1974). Shigellosis in costudial institutions III. Prospective clinical and bacteriologic surveillance of children vaccinated with oral attenuated *Shigella* vaccines. *J. Pediatr.* **84,** 803–806.

Levine, M. M., Gangarosa, E. J., Barrow, W. B., Morris, G. K., Wells, J. G., and Weiss, C. F. (1975). Shigellosis in costudial institutions: IV. *In vivo* stability and transmissibility of oral attenuated streptomycin-dependent *Shigella* vaccines. *J. Infect. Dis.* **131,** 704–705.

Levine, M. M., Woodward, W. E., Formal, S. B., Gemski, P., Jr, DuPont, H. L., Hornick, R. L., and Snyder, M. J. (1977). Studies with a new generation of oral attenuated *Shigella* vaccine: *Escherichia coli* bearing surface antigens of *Shigella flexneri*. *J. Infect. Dis.* **136,** 577–581.

Li, A., Pál, T., Forsum, U., and Lindberg, A. A. (1992). Safety and immunogenicity of the live oral auxotrophic *Shigella flexneri* SFL124 in volunteers. *Vaccine* **10,** 395–404.

Li, A., Kärnell, A., Huan, P. T., Cam, P. D., Minh, N. B., Tram, L. N., Quy, N. P., Trach, D. D., Karlsson, K., Lindberg, G., and Lindberg, A. A. (1993). Safety and immunogenicity of the live oral auxotrophic *Shigella flexneri* SFL124 in adult Vietnamese volunteers. *Vaccine* **11,** 180–190.

Li, A., Cam, P. D., Islam, D., Minh, N. B., Huan, P. T., Rong, Z. C., Karlsson, K., Lindberg, G., and Lindberg, A. A. (1994). Immune response in Vietnamese children after a single dose of the auxotrophic, live *Shigella flexneri* Y vaccine strain SFL124. *J. Infect.* **28,** 11–23.

Lindberg, A. A., and Robertsson, J. A. (1983). *Samonella typhimurium* infection in calves: Cell-mediated and humoral immune reactions before and after challenge with live virulent bacteria in calves given live or inactivated vaccines. *Infect. Immun.* **41,** 751–757.

Lindberg, A. A., Kärnell, A., Stocker, B. A. D., Katakura, S., Sweiha, H., and Reinholt, F. P. (1988). Development of an auxotrophic oral live *Shigella flexneri* vaccine. *Vaccine* **6,** 146–150.

Lindberg, A. A., Kärnell, A., Pál, T., Sweiha, H., Hultenby, K., and Stocker, B. A. D. (1990). Construction of an auxotrophic *Shigella flexneri* strain for use as a live vaccine. *Microbial Pathogen.* **8,** 433–440.

Lindberg, A. A., Cam, P. D., Chan, N., Phu, L. K., Trach, D. D., Lindberg, G., Karlsson, K., Kärnell, A., and Ekwall, E. (1991). Shigellosis in Vietnam: Seroepidemiologic studies with use of lipopolysaccharide antigens in enzyme immunoassays. *Rev. Infect. Dis.* **13**(Suppl. 4), S231–S237.

Linde, K., Dentchev, V., Bondarenko, V., Marinova, S., Randhagen, B., Bratoyeva, M., Tsvetanov, Y., and Romanova, Y. (1990). Live *Shigella flexneri* 2a and *Shigella sonnei* I vaccine candidate strains with two attenuating markers. I. Construction of vaccine candidate strains with retained invasiveness but reduced intracellular multiplication. *Vaccine* **8,** 25–29.

Lowell, G. H., MacDermott, R. P., Summers, P. L., Reeder, A. A., Bertovich, M. J., and Formal, S. B. (1980). Antibody-dependent cell-mediated antibacterial activity: K lymphocytes, monocytes, and granulocytes are effective against *Shigella*. *J. Immunol.* **125,** 2778–2784.

Mallett, C. P., Van DeVerg, L., Collins, H. H., and Hale, T. L. (1993). Evaluation of *Shigella* vaccine safety and efficacy in an intranasal challenged mouse model. *Vaccine* **11,** 190–196.

Maurelli, A. T., and Sansonetti, P. J. (1988). Identification of a chromosomal gene controlling temperature regulated expression of *Shigella* virulence. *Proc. Natl. Acad. Sci. U.S.A.* **85**, 2820–2824.

Meitert, T., Pencu, E., Ciudin, L., and Tonciu, M. (1984). Vaccine strain *Sh. flexneri* T32-Istrati. Studies in animals and in volunteers. Antidysentery immunoprophylaxis and immunotherapy by live vaccine Vadizen (*Sh. flexneri* T32-Istrati). *Arch. Roum. Pathol. Exp. Microbiol.* **43**, 251–278.

Mel, D. M., Rapo, R. G., Terzin, A. L., and Vuksic, L. (1965a). Studies on vaccination against bacillary dysentery: II. Safety tests and reactogenicity studies on a live dysentery vaccine intended for use in field trials. *Bull. WHO* **32**, 637–645.

Mel, D. M., Terzin, A. L., and Vuksic, L. (1965b). Studies on vaccination against bacillary dysentery: III. Effective oral immunization against *Shigella flexneri* 2a in a field trial. *Bull. WHO* **32**, 647–677.

Mel, D. M., Arsic, B. L., Nikoloc, B. D., and Radovanic. M. L. (1968). Studies on vaccination against bacillary dysentery. 4. Oral Immunization with live monotypic and combined vaccines. *Bull. WHO* **39**, 375–380.

Mikhailov, F. F., Sergeev, V. V., and Elkina, S. I. (1968). Pathogenic revertants of streptomycin dependent mutants of *Shigella flexneri* and their revertants. (in Russian) *J. Microbiol. Epidemiol. Immunol.* **39**, 375–380.

Mounier, J., Vasselon, T., Hellio, R., Lesourd, M., and Sansonetti, P. (1992). *Shigella flexneri* enters human colonic Caco-2 epithelial cells through the basolateral pole. *Infect. Immun.* **60**, 237–248.

Nakata, N., Tobe, T., Fukuda, I., Suzuki, T., Komatsu, K., Yoshikawa, M., and Sasakawa, C. (1993). The absence of a surface protease, *Omp*T, determines the intercellular spreading ability of *Shigella*: the relationship between *omp*T and *kcp*A loci. *Mol. Microbiol.* **9**, 459–468.

Nassif, X., Mazert, M. C., Mounier, J., and Sansonetti, P. J. (1987). Evaluation with an *iuc*::Tn*10* mutant of the role of aerobactin production in the virulence of *Shigella flexneri*. *Infect. Immun.* **55**, 1963–1969.

Newland, J. W., Hale, T. L., and Formal, S. B. (1992). Genotypic and phenotypic characterization of an *aro*D deletion-attenuated *Escherichia coli* K12-*Shigella flexneri* hybrid vaccine expressing *S. flexneri* somatic antigen. *Vaccine* **10**, 766–776.

Noriega, F. R., Wang, J. Y., Losonsky, G., Maneval, D. R., Hone, D. M., and Levine, M. M. (1994). Construction and characterization of attenuated Δ*aroA* Δ*virG Shigella flexneri* 2a strain CVD 1203, a prototype live oral vaccine. *Infect. Immun.* **62**, 5168–5172.

Nur-E-Kamal, M. S. A., Mamun, A. A. M. A., and Ahmed, Z. U. (1994). Molecular cloning of the wild-type and mutant *thy*A gene from *Shigella flexneri* Y. *Microbiol. Immunol.* **38**, 309–312.

Oaks, E. V., Wingfield, M. E., and Formal, S. B. (1985). Plaque formation by virulent *Shigella flexneri*. *Infect. Immun.* **48**, 124–129.

Oaks, E. V., Hale, T. L., and Formal, S. B. (1986). Serum immune response to *Shigella* protein antigens in *Rhesus* monkeys and humans infected with *Shigella* spp. *Infect. Immun.* **53**, 57–63.

Oberhelman, R. A., Kopecko, D. J., Salazar-Lindo, E., Gotuzzo, E., Buysse, J. M., Venkatesan, M. M., Yi, A., Fernandez-Prada, C., Guzman, M., León-Barúa, R., and Sack, R.B. (1991). Prospective study of systemic and mucosal immune responses in dysenteric patients to specific *Shigella* invasion plasmid antigens and lipopolysaccharides. *Infect. Immun.* **59**, 2341–2350.

Obrig, T. G., DelVecchi, P. J., Brown, J. E., Morgan, T. P., Rowland, B. M., Judge, T. K., and Rothman, S. W. (1988). Direct cytotoxic action of Shiga toxin on human vascular endothelial cells. *Infect. Immun.* **56**, 2373–2378.

Okada, N., Sasakawa C., Tobe, T., Yamada, M., Nagai, S., Talukder, K. A., Komatsu, K., Kanegasaki, S., and Yoshikawa, M. (1991). Virulence-associated chromosomal loci of *Shigella flexneri* identified by random Tn5 insertion mutagenesis. *Mol. Microbiol.* **5**, 187–195.

Okamura, N., Nagai, T., Nakaya, R., Kondo, S., Murakami, M., and Hisatsune, K. (1983). HeLa cell invasiveness and O antigen of *Shigella flexneri* as separate and prerequisite attributes of virulence to evoke keratoconjunctivitis in guinea pigs. *Infect. Immun.* **39**, 505–513.

Orr, N., Robin, G., Cohen, D., Arnon, R., and Lowell, G. H. (1993). Immunogenicity and efficacy of oral or intranasal *Shigella flexneri* 2a and *Shigella sonnei* proteosome–lipopolysaccharide vaccines in animal models. *Infect. Immun.* **61**, 2390–2395.

Pál, T., and Brasch, G. (1987). IgG response of dysenteric patients to antigens coded by the virulence plasmid of enteroinvasive pathogens. *Acta Microbiol. Hung.* **34**, 159–163.

Pál, T., and Lindberg, A. A. (1991). Association of invasive *Shigella* strains with epithelial cells. *In* "Molecular Pathogenesis of Gastrointestinal Infections" (T. Wadström, P. H. Mäkelä, A.-M. Svennerholm, and H. Wolf-Watz, eds.), pp. 223–229, Plenum Press, New York.

Pál, T., Newland, J. W., Tall, B. D., Formal, S. B., and Hale, T. L. (1989). Intracellular spread of *Shigella flexneri* associated with the *kcp*A locus and a 140-kilodalton protein. *Infect. Immun.* **57**, 477–486.

Parsot, C. (1994). *Shigella flexneri*: Genetics of entry and intracellular dissemination in epithelial cells. Bacterial pathogenesis of plants and animals. *Curr. Top. Microbiol. Immunol.* **192**, 217–241.

Perdomo, O. J. J., Cavaillon, J. M., Huerre, M., Ohayon, H., Gounon, P., and Sansonetti, P. J. (1994a). Acute inflammation causes epithelial invasion and mucosal destruction in experimental shigellosis. *J. Exp. Med.* **180**, 1307–1319.

Perdomo, J. J., Gounon, P., and Sansonetti, P. J. (1994b). Polymorphonuclear leukocyte transmigration promotes invasion of colonic epithelial monolayer by *Shigella flexneri*. *J. Clin. Invest.* **93**, 633–643.

Rajakumar, K., Jost, B. H., Sasakawa, C., Okada, N., Yoshikawa, M., and Adler, B. (1994). Nucleotide sequence of the rhamnose biosynthetic operon of *Shigella flexneri* 2a and role of lipopolysaccharide in virulence. *J. Bacteriol.* **176**, 2362–2373.

Raqib, R., Lindberg, A. A., Wretlind, B., Bardhan, P. K., Andersson, U., and Andersson, J. (1995a). Persistence of local cytokine production in shigellosis in acute and convalescent stages. *Infect. Immun.* **63**, 289–296.

Raqib, R., Wretlind, B., Andersson, J., and Lindberg, A. A.

(1995b). Cytokine secretion in acute shigellosis is correlated to disease activity and directed more to stool than to plasma. *J. Infect. Dis.* **171**, 376–384.

Raqib, R., Lindberg, A. A., Bjork, L., Bardhan, P. K., Wretlind, B., Andersson, U., and Andersson, J. (1995c). Down-regulation of gamma interferon, tumor necrosis factor type 1, interleukin 1 (IL-1) type 1, IL-3, IL-4, and transforming growth factor β type 1 receptors at the local site during the acute phase of *Shigella* infection. *Infect. Immun.* **63**, 3079–3087.

Robbins, J. B., and Schneerson, R. (1990). Polysaccharide–protein conjugates: A new generation of vaccines. *J. Infect. Dis.* **161**, 821–832.

Robbins, J. B., Chu, C.-Y., and Schneerson, R. (1992). Hypothesis for vaccine development: serum IgG LPS antibodies confer protective immunity to non-typhoidal *Salmonellae* and *Shigellae*. *Clin. Infect. Dis.* **15**, 346–361.

Robertsson, J. A., Svensson, S. B., and Lindberg, A. A. (1982). *Salmonella typhimurium* infection in calves: Delayed skin reactions directed against the O-antigenic polysaccharide chain. *Infect. Immun.* **37**, 737–748.

Sansonetti, P. J., and Arondel, J. (1989). Construction and evaluation of a double mutant of *Shigella flexneri* as a candidate for oral vaccination against shigellosis. *Vaccine* **7**, 443–450.

Sansonetti, P. J., and Mounier, J. (1987). Metabolic events mediating early killing of host cells infected by *Shigella flexneri*. *Microbial Pathogen.* **3**, 53–61.

Sansonetti, P. J., Kopecko, D. J., and Formal, S. B. (1981). *Shigella sonnei* plasmids: Evidence that a large plasmid is necessary for virulence. *Infect. Immun.* **34**, 75–83.

Sansonetti, P. J., Kopecko, D. J., and Formal, S. B. (1982). Involvement of a plasmid in the invasive ability of *Shigella flexneri*. *Infect. Immun.* **35**, 852–860.

Sansonetti, P. J., Ryter, A., Clerc, P., Maurelli, A. T., and Mounier, J. (1986). Multiplication of *Shigella flexneri* within HeLa cells: Lysis of the phagocytic vacuole and plasmid-mediated contact hemolysis. *Infect. Immun.* **51**, 461–469.

Sansonetti, P. J., Arondel, J., Fontaine, A., d'Hauteville, H., and Bernardini, M. L. (1991). *OmpB* (osmo regulation) and *icsA* (cell-to-cell spread) mutants of *flexneri*: Vaccine candidates and probes to study the pathogenesis of shigellosis. *Vaccine* **9**, 416–422.

Schnaitman, C., and Klena, J. D. (1993). Genetics of lipopolysaccharide biosynthesis in enteric bacteria. *Microbiol. Rev.* **57**, 655–682.

Schultz, C. L., Kaufman, B., Hamilton, D., Hartman, A., Ruiz, M., Powell, C., and Berman, S. (1990). Cell wall structures which may be important for successful immunization with *Salmonella–Shigella* hybrid vaccines. *Vaccine* **8**, 115–120.

Seid, R. C., Jr., Kopecko, D. J., Sadoff, J. C., Schneider, H., Baron, L. S., and Formal, S. B. (1984). Unusual lipopolysaccharide antigen of a *Salmonella typhi* oral vaccine strain expressing the *Shigella sonnei* form I antigen. *J. Biol. Chem.* **259**, 9028–9034.

Serény, B. (1955). Experimental *Shigella* keratoconjunctivitis. *Acta Microbiol. Acad. Sci. Hung.* **2**, 293–296.

Shaughnessy, H. J., Olsson, R. C., Bass, K., Friewer, F., and Levison, S. O. (1946). Experimental human bacillary dysentery: Polyvalent dysentery vaccine in its prevention. *J. Am. Med. Assoc.* **132**, 362–368.

Sieling, P. A., Chatterjee, D., Porcelli, S. A., Prigozi, T. I., Mazzaccaro, R. J., Soriano, T., Bloom, B. R., Brenner, M. B., Kronenberg, M., Brennan, P. J., and Modlin, R. L. (1995). CDI restricted T cell recognition of microbial lipoglycan antigens. *Science* **269**, 227–230.

Stockbine, N. A., Jackson, M. P., Sung, L. M., Holmes, R. K., and O'Brien, A. D. (1988). Cloning and sequencing of the genes for Shiga toxin from *Shigella dysenteriae* type 1. *J. Bacteriol.* **170**, 1116–1122.

Stocker, B. A. D. (1988). Auxotrophic *Salmonella typhi* as a live vaccine. *Vaccine* **6**, 141–145.

Tagliabue, A., Nencioni, L., Villa, L., Keren, D. F., Lowell, G. H., and Boraschi, D. (1983). Antibody-dependent cell mediated antibacterial activity of intestinal lymphocytes with secretory IgA. *Nature (London)* **306**, 184–185.

Takeuchi, A., Sprinz, H., LaBrec, E. H., and Formal, S. B. (1965). Experimental bacillary dysentery. An electron-microscopic study of the response of the intestinal mucosa to bacterial invasion. *Am. J. Pathol.* **47**, 1011–1044.

Taylor, D. N., Trofa, A. C., Sadoff, J., Chu, C., Bryla, D., and Shiloach, J. (1993). Synthesis, characterization, and clinical evaluation of conjugate vaccines composed of the O-specific polysaccharide of *Shigella flexneri* 2a, and *Shigella sonnei* (*Plesiomonas shigelloides*) bound to bacterial toxoids. *Infect. Immun.* **61**, 3678–3687.

Taylor, D. N., Phillip, D. F., Yapor, M., Trofa, A., Van de Verg, L., Hartman, A., Bendiuk, N., Newland, J. W., Formal, S. B., Sadoff, J. C., and Hale, T. L. (1994). Outpatient studies of the safety and immunogenicity of an auxotrophic *Escherichia coli* K-12–*Shigella flexneri* 2a hybrid vaccine candidate, EcSf2a-2. *Vaccine* **12**, 565–568.

Van de Verg, L., Herrington, D. A., Murphy, J. R., Wasserman, S. S., Formal, S. B., and Levine, M. M. (1990). Specific immunoglobulin A-secreting cells in peripheral blood of humans following oral immunization with a bivalent *Salmonella typhi–Shigella sonnei* vaccine or infection by pathogenic *S. sonnei*. *Infect. Immun.* **58**, 2002–2004.

Van de Verg, L. L., Herrington, D. A., Boslego, J., Lindberg, A. A., and Levine, M. M. (1992). Age-specific prevalence of serum antibodies to the invasion plasmid and lipopolysaccharide antigens of *Shigella* species in Chilean and North American populations. *J. Infect. Dis.* **166**, 158–161.

Venkatesan, M., Fernandez-Prada, C., Buysee, J. M., Formal, S. B., and Hale, T. L. (1991). Virulence phenotype and genetic characteristics of the T32-Istrati *Shigella flexneri* 2a vaccine strain. *Vaccine* **9**, 358–363.

Verma, N. K., Brandt, J. M., Verma D. J., and Lindberg, A. A. (1991). Molecular characterization of the O-acetyl transferase gene of converting bacteriophage SF6 that adds group antigen 6 to *Shigella flexneri*. *Mol. Microbiol.* **5**, 71–75.

Voino-Yasenetskaya, M. K., and Voino-Yasenetsky M. V. (1977). Intranasal challenge of laboratory animals with *Shigellae* (The *Shigella* lung model). *In* "Pathogenesis of

Intestinal Infections" (M. V. Voino-Yasenetsky and T. Bakács, eds.), pp. 114–125. Akadémai Kiadó, Budapest.

Voino-Yasenetsky, M. V. (1977). Dysentery in monkeys. *In* "Pathogenesis of Intestinal Infections" (M. V. Voino-Yasenetsky and T. Bakács, eds.), pp. 141–155. Akadémai Kiadó, Budapest.

Wassef, J. W., Keren, D. F., and Mailloux, J. L. (1989). Role of M cells in initial antigen uptake and in ulcer formation in the rabbit intestinal loop model of shigellosis. *Infect. Immun.* **57**, 858–863.

Watanabe, H., and Timmis, K. N. (1984). A small plasmid in *Shigella dysenteriae* 1 specifies one or more functions essential for O antigen production and bacterial virulence. *Infect. Immun.* **43**, 391–396.

Zychlinsky, A., Fitting, C., Cavaillon, J.-M., and Sansonetti, P. J. (1994). Interleukin 1 is released by murine macrophages during apoptosis induced by *Shigella flexneri*. *J. Clin. Invest.* **94**, 1328–1332.

17

Progress toward Live-Attenuated Cholera Vaccines

Matthew K. Waldor
John J. Mekalanos
Department of Microbiology and Molecular Genetics and
Shipley Institute of Medicine
Harvard Medical School
Boston, Massachusetts 02115

I. Introduction

Cholera is an acute secretory diarrheal disease. The watery diarrhea and vomiting which are characteristic of cholera can be so severe, and the ensuing dehydration so rapid, that death of the human host can occur within hours of the onset of symptoms. Clinical descriptions of cholera exist in Sanskrit texts that date back more than two millennia (Barua, 1992). Despite its ancient history, cholera remains a significant public health problem in the world today. In fact, there has been a resurgence of worldwide cholera in the first few years of the 1990s (World Health Organization, 1994). In 1993 more countries reported cholera to the WHO than ever before (World Health Organization, 1994).

Vibrio cholerae, the etiologic agent of cholera, are mucosal bacterial pathogens. Humans become infected with *V. cholerae* after ingestion of contaminated food or water. Then, these highly motile gram$^-$ organisms colonize the surface of the small intestine and elaborate a protein enterotoxin, cholera toxin, which is largely responsible for the symptoms of cholera. The profuse rice water stool which is the hallmark of cholera contains up to 10^8 *V. cholerae* per milliliter and thus allows the bacterium to be rapidly disseminated in the environment and spread to other people. Microbiologically, *V. cholerae* strains have been divided into serogroups. The O1 serogroup has been further subdivided into two biotypes, classical and El Tor, and two principal serotypes, Ogawa and Inaba (Kaper *et al.*, 1995).

History has recorded seven cholera pandemics. The classical biotype of *V. cholerae* serogroup O1 is believed to have given rise to the first six cholera pandemics (Barua, 1992). The seventh pandemic of cholera began in 1961 on the Indonesian island of Sulawesi. This pandemic, which continues today, is caused by the El Tor biotype of *V. cholerae* O1. The El Tor biotype of *V. cholerae* has now almost entirely replaced the classical biotype of *V. cholerae* as a cause of cholera. The Americas had been free of cholera for nearly a century until 1991 when El Tor *V. cholerae* arrived in Peru. Since then, this strain has spread throughout Latin America and has given rise to more than a million cases of cholera in the western hemisphere (World Health Organization, 1994).

Though there are more than 100 known serogroups of *V. cholerae,* only *V. cholerae* serogroup O1 had been associated with cholera. This changed in late 1992 when a novel serogroup of *V. cholerae, Vibrio cholerae* O139 (synonym Bengal), arose on the Indian subcontinent and subsequently gave rise to a major cholera epidemic in India and Bangladesh (Cholera Working Group, 1993). Molecular characterization of *V. cholerae* O139 has demonstrated that this novel serogroup arose from an El Tor O1 strain which acquired the DNA encoding the O139 serogroup antigen from an unknown donor strain via horizontal gene transfer (Waldor and Mekalanos, 1994c; Bik *et al.*, 1995). Worldwide there are currently two principal causes of epidemic cholera: *V. cholerae* biotype El Tor serogroup O1 and *V. cholerae* O139. The O139 strains are largely confined to Southern Asia (India, Bangladesh, Thailand, Pakistan, Nepal and Myanmar) whereas the El Tor O1 strains are spread worldwide.

The chemical basis for the serogroup antigens resides in the O antigen of lipopolysaccharide (LPS). Compared to O1 strains, O139 strains have a distinct O antigen as well as a polysaccharide capsule which is a polymer of the O antigen (Hisatsune *et al.*, 1993; Waldor *et al.*, 1994). Epidemiological data from the 1993 O139 epidemic in India and Bangladesh have lent credence to the notion that the O antigen is a principal target of protective immunity to cholera since prior immunity to *V. cholerae* O1 appeared to offer no protec-

MUCOSAL VACCINES

tion against *V. cholerae* O139 (Cholera Working Group, 1993).

Given the substantial morbidity and mortality of cholera, efforts to develop cholera vaccines began shortly after the identification of *V. cholerae* as the cause of cholera more than a century ago. These efforts, until fairly recently (see below), have been largely unsuccessful. Contemporary efforts for the development of safe and effective cholera vaccines have been guided by the notion that such vaccines would be most useful if they were cost-effective and widely available. Many factors, reviewed by Clemens *et al.* (1994), must be considered when analyzing the potential cost-effectiveness and usefulness of a cholera vaccine. Foremost, an effective vaccine could prevent the morbidity and mortality of cholera both in residents of cholera-endemic areas and in travelers to endemic areas. This alone is highly significant since there are approximately 500,000 to 1,000,000 clinical cases of cholera worldwide annually. In endemic areas where experienced medical personnel are available for cholera treatment, mortality from cholera is usually 1–3%, but in epidemic situations mortality can exceed 50% (World Health Organization, 1994). For example, in the recent 1994 cholera epidemic in the Rwandian refugee camps of Goma Zaire, an estimated 50,000 cholera fatalities occurred. Furthermore, it has been noted by the World Health Organisation that approximately 80% of all refugee camps worldwide suffer a cholera epidemic during some stage of their existence.

In addition to preventing the direct morbidity and mortality of cholera, an effective vaccine could also have a variety of other secondary beneficial effects including preventing lost work days of cholera patients and their families, preventing the loss of food export income from cholera endemic areas, and increasing tourism. While it can be argued that the provision of safe water supplies globally will lead to the ultimate eradication of cholera, this task will require decades and tens to hundreds of billions of dollars. Thus a safe, easily administered and effective cholera vaccine would certainly be useful in the world right now.

Properties of an ideal cholera vaccine include efficacy, safety, and convenience (Table I). An effective vaccine should confer long-lasting, perhaps life-long, protective immunity against the strains of *V. cholerae* that give rise to cholera in the world today (*V. cholerae* O139 and El Tor O1). The protective immune response should be achievable in a wide range of ages and populations after a single oral dose. The immune response should be rapid to facilitate the possibility of employing the vaccine in epidemic situations. To reduce the spread of *V. cholerae,* the immune response to a cholera vaccine should eliminate shedding of wild-type strains in vaccinees who ingest wild-type *V. cholerae*. Obviously, a safe vaccine would be free of side effects. In live vaccines, another aspect of safety concerns the genetic stability of the vaccine construct. Live vaccines should be engineered so as to be unable to regain toxigenicity by reversion or recombination and, further, should be unable to transfer to other bacteria potentially deleterious genes such as those encoding virulence factors and antibiotic resistance. Since a cholera vaccine would be most useful for the developing world where there are very limited health care resources, the vaccine should be inexpensive and easy to formulate and administer—ideally by a single oral dose.

TABLE I
Properties of an Ideal *V. cholerae* Vaccine

Safety
No adverse side effects
Genetic stability
Inability to reacquire toxigenicity
Inability to transfer potentially deleterious genes to other bacteria
Efficacy
Long-lasting protective immunity to existing strains for all ages and populations after a single dose
Rapid development of immunity following a single dose
Lack of shedding of wild-type strains after challenge
Convenience
Inexpensive
Simple to formulate and administer
Single oral dose

II. Parenteral Cholera Vaccines

Soon after the discovery of *V. cholerae* as the etiologic agent of cholera, there were attempts to make cholera vaccines. Though there were early attempts at oral-killed vaccines, most research until recently focused on the development of parenteral cholera vaccines. In the 1960s and 1970s, large controlled trials of the efficacy of killed whole-cell vaccines were undertaken in Bangladesh, Indonesia, and the Philippines (reviewed in Levine and Pierce, 1992). These trials revealed that parenteral-killed cholera vaccines confer only short-lived immunity to cholera with protective efficacies usually in the 30–80% range in the first 6 months after vaccination, falling to approximately 30% shortly thereafter (Levine and Pierce, 1992).

Parenterally administered purified *V. cholerae* LPS vaccines have also been tested in field trials and have demonstrated efficacy similar to or less than that of the parenteral whole-cell vaccines. Recently Robbins and colleagues have described conjugates of detoxified Ogawa and Inaba LPS to cholera toxin as candidate parenteral vaccines (Szu *et al.*, 1994) but these vaccines have not been clinically evaluated yet. Parenteral vaccines against different formulations of cholera toxin have also been studied. A field trial of a parenterally administered, alum-absorbed, glutaraldehyde-inactivated cholera toxoid in Bangladesh showed almost no protective effect (Levine and Pierce, 1992). Thus, parenteral vaccines to date have been disappointing overall.

III. Oral Cholera Vaccines

Pathogenesis studies have revealed that *V. cholerae* are strictly mucosal pathogens. That is, *V. cholerae* survive and multiply on the surface of the epithelium of the small intestine but the bacteria do not cross this epithelial barrier. Recovery from cholera is known to engender long-lived immunity that is presumably mucosal in nature. Thus, over the past decade there has been considerable effort toward the development of an oral cholera vaccine. Compared with a parenteral vaccine, an oral vaccine would more closely resemble natural infection and therefore be more likely to engender a mucosal immune response.

IV. Infection-Derived Immunity

There is considerable evidence from volunteer studies that infection with wild-type toxigenic *V. cholerae* O1 (Levine and Pierce, 1992) and *V. cholerae* O139 (Tacket *et al.*, 1994) leads to protective immunity against challenge with wild-type strains of the same serogroup. Volunteer studies conducted by Levine and colleagues have demonstrated that protective immunity to classical *V. cholerae* O1 persisted as long as 3 years after experimental infection with classical *V. cholerae* O1 (Levine and Tacket, 1994). Experimental studies with the El Tor biotype of *V. cholerae* O1 have also indicated that an initial infection with an El Tor strain leads to subsequent protection in challenge studies with an El Tor strain (Levine and Tacket, 1994). However, challenge studies years after the experimental infection have not been carried out for the El Tor biotype, so the duration of protective immunity following El Tor infection is not as clearly known as it is for infection with classical *V. cholerae.* The experimental challenge studies have suggested that the potency of the immune response to the El Tor biotype may not be as potent as that to the classical biotype. Thus, no recipients of classical *V. cholerae* had positive *V. cholerae* coprocultures following challenge with classical *V. cholerae*, but this was not the case for recipients of El Tor strains challenged with an El Tor strain (Levine and Tacket, 1994). Unfortunately, volunteer studies to evaluate whether an initial wild-type classical or El Tor infection leads to protection with challenge by the opposite biotype have not been undertaken.

Epidemiologic studies of infection derived immunity to *V. cholerae* from endemic regions have not been as clear as volunteer studies. Some investigators have concluded that there is little protective immunity engendered by natural infection (Woodward, 1971), whereas others have reported up to 90% reduction in the risk of cholera following a clinically apparent case of *V. cholerae* infection (Glass *et al.*, 1982). The significance of the discrepancies between the volunteer studies and the epidemiologic studies with regard to the existence of infection-derived immunity is not understood. Clearly, a live-attenuated vaccine candidate tested in volunteer studies must be further tested in endemic areas to establish its validity in endemic populations. However, the evidence of long-lasting immunity to cholera following experimental infection with *V. cholerae* from volunteer studies has lent substantial impetus to the development of oral live-attenuated *V. cholerae* candidates.

V. Killed Whole-Cell Oral Vaccines

Considerable work has also been devoted to the development of killed whole-cell oral cholera vaccines. In the early 1960s Freter and Gangarosa administered large oral doses of killed *V. cholerae* O1 to volunteers and showed that a large majority of these subjects developed coproantibodies against the immunizing strain (Freter and Gangarosa, 1963). Since these early studies, several studies have evaluated the efficacy of killed whole-cell vaccines in both volunteer and endemic settings. The volunteer studies with wild-type challenges following oral killed whole-cell vaccines have shown 50–60% protective efficacy but the frequency of positive coprocultures following these challenges was not significantly lower in the vaccinee group compared with the control group (Black *et al.*, 1987).

The most widely tested oral killed vaccine candidates have been developed by Svennerholm, Holmgren, and colleagues. This vaccine consists of a combination of heat-killed and formalin-killed classical and El Tor strains of *V. cholerae* of both serotypes (Inaba and Ogawa) in addition to the nontoxic B subunit of cholera toxin. A placebo-controlled field trial of this B-subunit-killed whole-bacterial cell (BS-WC) vaccine involving nearly 90,000 people was conducted in children and adults in Bangladesh. Three oral doses of the BS-WC vaccine, whole-cell vaccine (WC) alone, or placebo were administered at 6-week intervals. Six months after vaccination, the BS-WC vaccine had a protective efficacy of 85% whereas the WC vaccine had a protective efficacy of 58% (Clemens *et al.*, 1986). This difference in the protective efficacy between the BS-WC and WC vaccinee groups was no longer apparent after 6 months of follow-up. Both the WC and BS-WC vaccines led to a protective efficacy of around 50% after 3 years, though the efficacy in children less than 5 years old at this point was only about 25% (Clemens *et al.*, 1990). The protective efficacy was apparently longer lived against classical than El Tor cholera (Clemens *et al.*, 1990). The BS-WC vaccine also gave rise to significant protection against diarrhea caused by enterotoxigenic *E. coli* (which produce an enterotoxin which is immunologically cross reactive with the B subunit of cholera toxin) during the first few months of the trial (Clemens *et al.*, 1988).

Though the results of this large field trial certainly demonstrate that the BS-WC vaccine has value, there are a variety of limitations to the oral killed vaccine approach. These include: (1) the relatively short-lived protective efficacy greater than 50% especially in children, (2) the necessity for more than one vaccine dose, (3) the existence of positive *Vibrio* coprocultures in vaccinees after challenge with wild-type *V. cholerae,* (4) the potentially expensive manufacturing process for this vaccine, and (5) the inability of killed *V. cholerae* cells to present antigens that are only expressed *in vivo* to the mucosal immune system.

VI. Live-Attenuated Oral Vaccines

Live-attenuated oral vaccines offer several potential advantages over nonliving oral vaccines. After a single oral inoculation of a relatively small dose of a live *V. cholerae* vaccine strain, the strain can replicate in the small bowel to a much larger and therefore more immunogenic dose within the vaccinee. This opens the possibility for a single-dose vaccine. During the course of *in vivo* replication, the live vaccine will express antigens that are normally expressed *in vivo* in response to the growth conditions present in the small intestine. The bacterial cell surface antigens present on killed whole-cell vaccines will only be a reflection of the *in vitro* growth conditions that were used to manufacture the vaccine. There is some experimental evidence that antigens that are only expressed *in vivo* are immunogenic (Jonson *et al.*, 1989). The presentation of antigens from the in vivo replicating live vaccine should closely resemble the highly immunizing antigen presentation processes that occur during natural infection—a process which we know leads to long-lived immunity. It is believed that specialized intestinal epithelial cells that overlay intestinal lymphoid tissue known as M cells are crucial for antigen sampling in the intestine (Kraehenbuhl and Neutra, 1992). It has been shown in a rabbit model of cholera that M cells take up live *V. cholerae* significantly better than killed bacteria (Owen *et al.*, 1986). Also, the presentation of antigen to the intestinal mucosal immune system by killed whole-cell vaccines most likely does not lead to the same cytokine cascades that amplify the immune response to replicating *V. cholerae.*

VII. Nonrecombinant Live Oral Vaccines

Once pathogenesis studies made clear that cholera toxin was the principal cause of the diarrhea that is the hallmark of cholera, attempts were made to isolate *V. cholerae* mutants that no longer produced cholera toxin. Following nitrosoguanidine mutagenesis, Honda and Finkelstein (1979) were able to isolate a mutant El Tor strain, designated Texas Star-SR, which did not produce the toxic A subunit of cholera toxin but did produce the nontoxic B subunit of cholera toxin. Volunteer studies with Texas Star-SR showed that this oral live-attenuated vaccine candidate induced significant protection against challenge with wild-type El Tor strains (Levine *et al.*, 1984). However, approximately 25% of the vaccinees experienced mild diarrhea after ingestion of the vaccine indicating that this strain was insufficiently attenuated (Levine *et al.*, 1984). This residual "reactogenicity" following deletion of cholera toxin has been a problem for many oral live attenuated vaccine candidates (see below).

VIII. Recombinant Live-Attenuated Vaccines

The advent of recombinant DNA technology opened new possibilities for the creation of live-attenuated oral *V. cholerae* vaccine strains. The possibility to construct precise deletions of genes encoding virulence factors and to insert genes encoding important antigens became attainable. The merits and drawbacks of some of the live-attenuated oral vaccine constructs that have been engineered to date are discussed below.

Shortly after the cloning of the genes encoding cholera toxin, the *ctxAB* operon (Pearson and Mekalanos, 1982) live vaccine strains derived from a classical strain containing deletions of the A subunit or both the A and B subunits of cholera toxin were constructed by Mekalanos and colleagues (1983). However, an El Tor strain with a deletion of *ctxAB,* JBK70, constructed by Kaper and colleagues (Kaper *et al.*, 1984) was the first genetically engineered *V. cholerae* vaccine strain to be tested in volunteers. One month after ingestion of JBK70, volunteers were challenged with the wild-type toxigenic parental strain of JBK70, N16961. The vaccine had a protective efficacy of 90% (Levine *et al.*, 1988b); however, at all doses of JBK70 tested, a significant fraction of volunteers experienced adverse side effects (Table II) (Levine *et al.*, 1988b). These side effects included diarrhea, though not of the magnitude seen with wild-type strains, abdominal cramps, malaise, nausea, vomitting, or fever. These adverse effects experi-

TABLE II
Properties of Some Recombinant Oral Cholera Vaccines

Vaccine	Parental strain (biotype, serotype)	Properties of vaccine strain	Adverse effects[a]	Colonization of vaccine strain (%)[b]	Protective efficacy (%)[c]	Shedding of challenge strain (%)[d]	Reference
JBK 70	N16961 (El Tor, Inaba)	Δ*ctxAB* mercury resistant	Moderate	100	90	20	Kaper *et al.* (1984)
O395N1	O395 (classical, Ogawa)	Δ*ctxA* streptomycin resistant	Mild	100	75	N.A.[e]	Mekalanos *et al.* (1983)
TCP2	O395 (classical, Ogawa)	Δ*ctxA*, Δ*tcpA* streptomycin resistant	None	0	33	N.A.	Herrington *et al.* (1988)
CVD 102	O395 (classical, Ogawa)	Δ*ctxA* thymine auxotroph	None	40	N.D.[f]	N.D.	Levine *et al.* (1988b)
CVD 104	N16961 (El Tor, Inaba)	Δ*ctxAB*, Δ*hlyA* mercury resistant	Moderate	100	N.D.	N.D.	Levine *et al.* (1988b)
CVD 105	O395 (classical, Ogawa)	Δ*ctxA*, Δ*hlyA*	Moderate	100	N.D.	N.D.	Levine *et al.* (1988b)
CVD 103-HgR	569B (classical, Inaba)	Δ*ctxA* *hlyA::mer*	None	28	100 (classical) 63 (El Tor)	29 (classical) 83 (El Tor)	Levine *et al.* (1988a); Levine and Tacket (1994)
PERU-3	C6709 (El Tor, Inaba)	Δ*attRS1* *recA::htpG-ctxB* streptomycin resistant	Mild	83	87	N.A.	Taylor *et al.* (1994)
BANG-3	P27459 (El Tor, Inaba)	Δ*attRS1* *recA::htpG-ctxB* streptomycin resistant	Moderate	100	N.D.	N.D.	Taylor *et al.* (1994)
BAH-3	E7946 (El Tor, Ogawa)	Δ*attRS1* *recA::htpG-ctxB* streptomycin resistant	Moderate	100	N.D.	N.D.	Taylor *et al.* (1994)
CVD 110	E7946 (El Tor, Ogawa)	Δ*ctxAB zot ace* *hlyA::ctxB mer*	Moderate	100	N.D.	N.D.	Tacket *et al.* (1993)
BENGAL-3	MO10 (O139)	Δ*attRS1* *recA::htpG-ctxB* streptomycin resistant	Mild		N.D.	N.D.	Coster *et al.* (1995)
PERU-14	C6709 (El Tor, Inaba)	Δ*attRS1* *recA::htpG-ctxB* streptomycin resistant, filamentous, motility deficient	None	100	80	N.A.	Taylor *et al.* (1994)
PERU-15	C6709 (El Tor, Inaba)	Δ*attRS1* *recA::htpG-ctxB* streptomycin resistant nonmotile	None	82	60	80	Kenner *et al.* (1995)
BENGAL-15	MO10 (O139)	Δ*attRS1* *recA::htpG-ctxB* streptomycin resistant nonmotile	None	90	83	42	Coster *et al.* (1995)

[a]Adverse effects include diarrhea, abdominal cramps, maliase, anorexia, or fever elicited by the vaccine strain.
[b]Percentage of vaccinees who shed the vaccine strain in their stool.
[c]Percentage of vaccinees challenged with a wild-type strain who do not develop diarrhea.
[d]The percentage of vaccinees in whom wild-type *V. cholerae* could be detected in coprocultures after challenge.
[e]Not available.
[f]Not done.

enced by volunteers who have been the recipients of vaccine strains that contain a deletion of at least the gene encoding the toxic A subunit of cholera toxin have been termed "reactogenicity." Reactogenicity has been a significant problem in almost all live vaccine constructs engineered to date. This occurrence of symptoms in volunteers who have ingested *V. cholerae* strains which do not produce active cholera toxin has stimulated new thinking and research into the pathogenesis of cholera.

Two principal hypotheses have been put forward

to explain the cause of reactogenicity. The first hypothesis proposes the existence of additional toxins in *V. cholerae* strains besides cholera toxin (Levine and Pierce, 1992). The principal alternative explanation is the "colonization = reactogenicity" hypothesis. This proposes that the persistence and mulitplication of *V. cholerae* within the small intestine (bacterial colonization) induces symptoms of gastrointestinal distress by a mechanism that does not involve the action of an enterotoxin per se. Further vaccine candidates have been developed to begin to test these hypotheses.

Toxins that have been considered as the potential source of reactogenicity include a hemolysin, encoded by *hlyA* (Manning *et al.*, 1984), zonula-occludens toxin, encoded by *zot* (Baudry *et al.*, 1992), accessory cholera enterotoxin, encoded by *ace* (Trucksis *et al.*, 1993) and Shiga-like toxin (Levine and Pierce, 1992), whose existence has not been established by molecular cloning. Deletion of *hlyA* from either El Tor or classical cholera toxin deletion strains, CVD104 and CVD105, respectively, did not abrogate the vaccine strains' reactogenicity (Levine and Pierce, 1992) (Table II).

Zot and *ace* are part of the core region of the cholera toxin (CTX) genetic element (Fig. 1) (Pearson *et al.*,

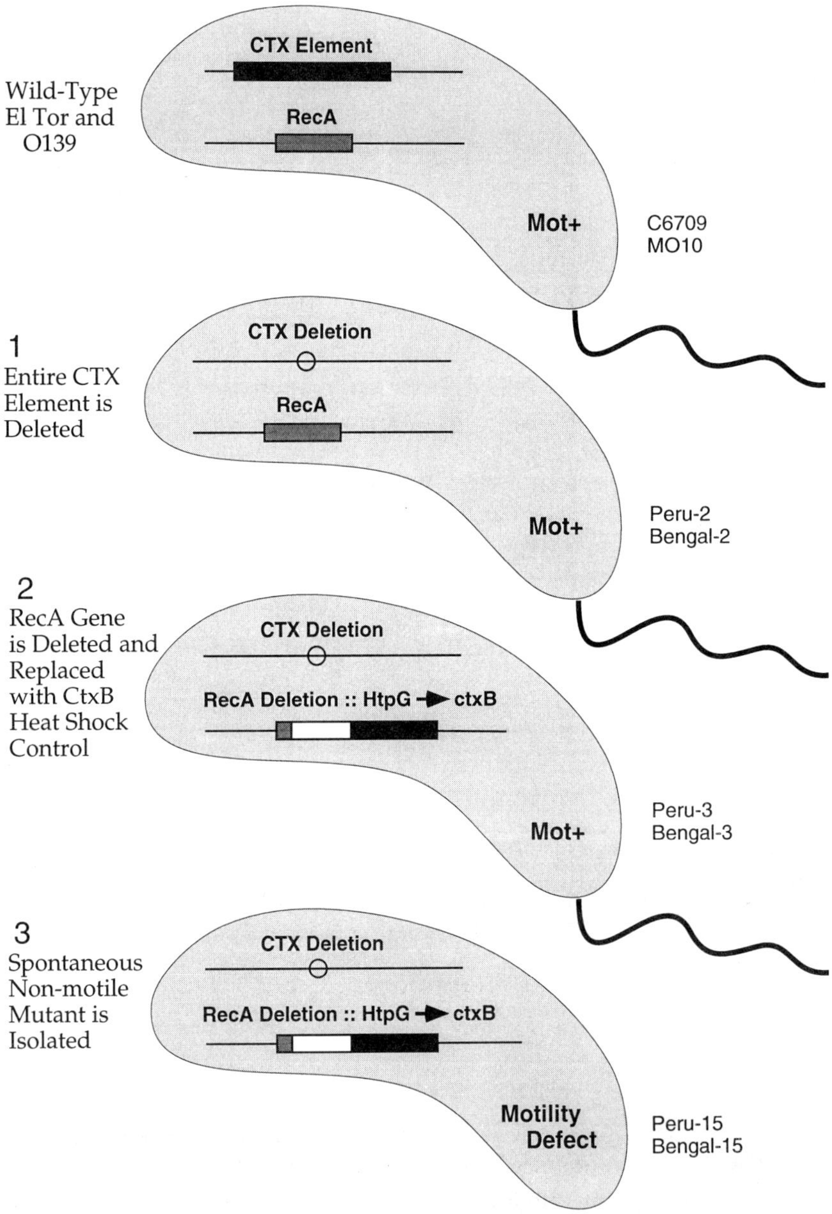

Figure 1. Steps in the construction of oral live-attenuated *V. cholerae* vaccine strains. Step 1: deletions of the entire CTX genetic element from C6709 (El Tor O1) or MO10 (O139) were accomplished by allele exchange. Step 2: The *recA* gene is deleted and replaced with *ctxB* under the control of the heat shock promoter by allele exchange. Step 3: spontaneous nonmotile mutants of these strains were then isolated.

1993). The core region of the CTX genetic element carries the *ctxAB* operon, *zot, ace,* and *cep.* The latter encodes a putative pilin-like colonization factor (Pearson *et al.*, 1993). This core region is flanked by repetitive sequences called RS1 which encode a site-specific recombination system (see below) (Pearson *et al.*, 1993). El Tor and O139 strains which contain deletions of the entire CTX genetic element including the loci *ctxA, ace,* and *zot* (vaccine strains Peru-3, Bah-3, Bang-3, CVD 110, and Bengal-3) still led to some adverse side effects in vaccine recipients (Tacket *et al.*, 1993; Taylor *et al.*, 1994; Coster *et al.*, 1995) (Table II) indicating that *ace* and *zot* are not the cause or at least the sole cause of reactogencity. Thus, to date no gene encoding a toxic moiety has been discovered that can account for reactogenicity.

There is some experimental evidence to support the colonization = reactogenicity hypothesis. In volunteer studies, vaccine strains that have given rise to the least reactogenicity have been those strains that have been the least detectable by coproculture of vaccinees following vaccine ingestion. Detection of the vaccine strain in stool cultures of vaccinees is believed to reflect intestinal colonization (see below). There also appears to be a rough correlation between a vaccine strains' colonization and its immunogenicity. Certainly some degree of colonization is essential for a live vaccine's immunogenicity. This has been seen clearly in volunteers who ingested the vaccine strain TCP2. This strain has an interruption of *tcpA,* a gene which encodes the toxin coregulated pilus TCP, the most important colonization factor for *V. cholerae* that has been identified (Taylor *et al.*, 1987). TCP2 produces no TCP and this vaccine strain was not recoverable in stool cultures from volunteers who ingested this strain (Herrington *et al.*, 1988) suggesting that this strain did not colonize. There was no detectable immune response to *V. cholerae* in the recipients of TCP2 (Herrington *et al.*, 1988). Similarly, CVD102, a thymine auxotrophic derivative of vaccine strain CVD101, is unable to replicate *in vivo* (Levine *et al.*, 1988b) and is only minimally immunogenic. If some colonization is essential for immunogenicity yet too much colonization leads to reactogenicity, then the solution to reactogenicity may be to identify a vaccine strain that colonizes just enough to engender immunity without leading to adverse side effects. However, this formulation reflects an overly simplistic view of bacterial colonization of the small intestine. So far our only measure of *V. cholerae* small intestinal colonization in volunteers is to quantify the amount of bacteria in coprocultures of vaccinees—clearly only a surrogate measurement of small intestinal colonization. More importantly, the precise location of the bacteria which are persisting and multiplying in the small intestine may be a critical determinant of adverse reactions as well as immunogencity (see below).

IX. CVD103-HgR

The most extensively tested oral live attenuated cholera vaccine has been developed at the Center for Vaccine Development by Levine, Kaper, and colleagues. CVD103-HgR is $ctxA^{-}B^{+}$ derivative of the classical Inaba *V. cholerae* O1 strain 569B (Levine *et al.*, 1988a). This vaccine strain also contains *mer,* a gene encoding resistance to mercury, to mark the vaccine strain as distinct from wild-type strains, introduced into the *hlyA* locus. The vaccine has been tested in a wide range of age groups and populations. Currently there is a large field trial of CVD103-HgR underway in Indonesia. A remarkable feature of CVD103-HgR has been its almost complete lack of reactogenicity (Levine *et al.*, 1988a). Although CVD103-HgR contains the same deletions (Δ*ctxA*, Δ*hlyA*) as in vaccine strains that have proved too reactogenic, CVD103HgR has led to almost no adverse effects in vaccinees (Levine *et al.*, 1988a). Thus the molecular basis for the lack of reactogenicity of CVD103-HgR is not entirely clear. This emphasizes the critical role that the wild-type strain background exerts in determining a vaccine candidate's properties. In volunteer studies, after a single dose of CVD103-HgR, volunteers challenged with wild-type strains of *V. cholerae* from 1 to 24 weeks after oral vaccination were significantly protected against cholera (Levine and Tacket, 1994). The protective efficacy was 100% for challenge with a homologous (classical) biotype strain (Levine and Tacket, 1994). However, the protective efficacy for challenge with the heterologous (El Tor) biotype was approximately 63% (Levine and Tacket, 1994). Also, after challenge with an El Tor wild-type strain there was no reduction in the frequency of isolation of the challenge strain in coprocultures from the volunteers. The results of the extensive on-going controlled field trial of CVD103-HgR in Indonesia are eagerly awaited.

X. A New Generation of Cholera Vaccines

Over the past 5 years, our laboratory has undertaken the construction of a new series of live attenuated oral cholera vaccines. These vaccine constructs have been generated in *V. cholerae* strains that are currently giving rise to cholera in the world right now, i.e., in either El Tor O1 or O139 strain backgrounds. A fundamental guiding principal in these strain constructions has been attempts to ensure the genetic stability of the vaccine strains. This is an essential consideration for all live vaccines because reversion to virulence is always a critical concern.

As mentioned above, the operon encoding cholera toxin is part of a larger genetic element termed the CTX genetic element. The core encoded virulence genes in the CTX genetic element, *ctxAB, ace, zot,* and *cep,* are flanked by 1 or more copies of RS1 sequences (Mekalanos 1983; Pearson *et al.*, 1993; Waldor and Mekalanos, 1994a). The RS1 sequences encode a site-specific recombination system that mediates recombination between the CTX genetic element and attRS1, an 18-base pair target sequence on the *V. cholerae* chromosome (Pearson *et al.*, 1993). Taken as a whole, then, the CTX element can be thought of as a site-specific transposon.

The first step in our vaccine constructions has been deletion of the entire CTX element (Fig. 1). This "attRS1" deletion removes the core, RS1, and attRS1 sequences from the starting strain. These deletions have been generated in a variety of El Tor O1 strains including strain C6709, an El Tor Inaba strain isolated in 1991 in Peru soon after the outbreak of cholera in South America, and in MO10, an O139 isolate from the outbreak that began in late 1992 in Madras, India. The deletions have been generated by marker exchange with plasmid pAR62 (Pearson *et al.*, 1993). This plasmid contains an attRS1 deletion flanked by the chromosomal DNA that is adjacent to the CTX genetic element. Since O139 strains arose from an El Tor strain (Waldor and Mekalanos, 1994a,b), we were able to use pAR62 to generate attRS1 deletions in both wild-type O139 strains and El Tor O1 strains. The attRS1 deletion derivative in C6709 was designated Peru-2 while the attRS1 deletion derivative of MO10 was designated Bengal-2 (Fig. 1). Note also that Tacket and colleagues constructed a derivative of *V. cholerae* El Tor (CVD110) which was also deleted in the "core" of the CTX element, but which retains a copy of RS1 on its chromosome (Tacket *et al.*, 1993). Thus, strain CVD110 is still capable in theory of reaquiring the CTX element by site-specific recombination, in contrast to our El Tor attRS1 deletion derivatives which lack this property.

Besides site-specific reacquisition of the CTX element by an RS1-mediated or site-specific recombinational mechanism, vaccine strains could also in theory regain cholera toxin genes by other mechanisms that might involve transformation, transduction, or conjugation followed by homologous recombination. Therefore, after generating attRS1 deletions in our constructs, in a second step, we have also deleted *recA,* a gene which encodes a protein essential for homologous recombination (Fig. 1). Like the attRS1 deletions, these deletions were accomplished by marker exchange. The plasmid used for this marker exchange with Peru-2 and Bengal-2 contains the chromosomal DNA which flanks the *recA* locus and in the place of *recA* has inserted *ctxB* under the control of the powerful heat shock promoter, htpG (Roberts *et al.*, 1992). The resultant derivatives were designated Peru-3 and Bengal-3. These strains produce levels of the B subunit of cholera toxin that far exceed those produced by the respective parental strains. Recall that the B subunit of cholera toxin is nontoxic but the studies of the BS-WC vaccine showed that the addition of the B subunit to this oral killed whole-cell vaccine engendered short-term immunity to enterotoxigenic *E. coli* as well as more solid immunity to *V. cholerae.*

The combination of the deletion of *recA* with the *attRS1* deletion provides an unprecedented level of safety from possible reversion to enterotoxicity. This concern about possible reversion of *ctxA* deletion strains is not strictly theoretical. There is experimental evidence that CVD103-HgR can reacquire *ctxA* from a *V. cholerae* strain possessing a conjugative sex factor (Kaper *et al.*, 1994). While gene transfer and recombination events are undoubtedly rare, they certainly do occur. In fact, *V. cholerae* O139 arose from horizontal gene transfer and recombination (Waldor and Mekalanos, 1994c; Bik *et al.*, 1995).

In initial safety studies in volunteers with Peru-3 and Bengal-3 conducted as collaborative studies by investigators from Walter Reed Army Institute of Research, U.S. Army Medical Research of Infectious Diseases, and Virus Research Institute (Cambridge, MA), these vaccines were found to be generally well tolerated. However, they were mildly reactogenic, with two of six Peru-3 recipients and one of five Bengal-3 recipients experiencing mild diarrhea (Taylor *et al.*, 1994; Coster *et al.*, 1995). Similar constructs generated in the wild-type El Tor O1 strains E7946 and P27459 (vaccine strains Bah-3 and Bang-3, respectively) led to significantly more reactogenicity in volunteers. This reemphasizes the importance of the properties of the starting strain in live vaccine construction.

One hint for a solution to the problem of reactogenicity came from volunteer studies of vaccine strain Peru-14. Peru-14 is a spontaneous filamentous mutant of Peru-3. In soft agar plates these filamentous cells exhibit a markedly reduced motility. In volunteer studies, recipients of a range of doses of Peru-14 experienced almost no adverse side effects. In nine volunteer recipients of 10^9 Peru-14 cells, only two volunteers developed mild abdominal cramps, and none of the volunteers developed diarrhea (Taylor *et al.*, 1994) (Table II). Despite this remarkable lack of reactogenicity, Peru-14 colonized the volunteers and protected vaccinees from subsequent wild-type challenge with a protective efficacy of 80% (Taylor *et al.*, 1994) (Table II). We hypothesized that the impaired motility of Peru-14 might account for its lack of reactogenicity.

Thus, in an attempt to entirely abrogate the reactogenicity of Peru-3 and Bengal-3, spontaneous nonmotile mutants of both strains were isolated (Fig. 1). These nonmotile mutants—Peru-15 and Bengal-15—have been tested in volunteers and have led to virtually no reactogenicity (Kenner *et al.*, 1995) (Coster *et al.*, 1995) (Table II). However, both vaccine strains colonized the volunteers as evidenced by positive stool cultures for the vaccine strain in the vaccinees. Most importantly, in challenge studies with the wild-type El Tor strain N16961, three of five recipients of Peru-15 were completely protected from diarrhea, although four of five vaccine recipients excreted the challenge strain (Kenner *et al.*, 1995). Similarly, when recipients of Bengal-15 were challenged with the O139 wild-type strain MO10, only one of seven volunteers developed mild diarrhea and three of seven excreted the challenge strain (Coster *et al.*, 1995). Thus Peru-15 and Bengal-15 appear to be safe and reasonably effective candidate vaccines for cholera caused by El Tor O1 and O139 strains, respectively. Additional volunteer studies with these vaccine strains are in progress and hopefully field trials in cholera-endemic areas will begin soon.

Why were the nonmotile strains Peru-15 and Bengal-15 nonreactogenic and their isogenic motile parental strains Peru-3 and Bengal-3 reactogenic? Motility and chemotaxis are thought to allow *V. cholerae* to swim toward and penetrate the mucus gel overlying much of the intestinal epithelium and crypts (Freter *et al.*, 1981). Nonmotile mutants are also decreased in adherence to brush border membranes of intestinal epithelial cells (Freter *et al.*, 1981). Thus motility deficient vaccine strains may fail to efficiently penetrate the mucus gel and may fail to adhere intimately to the underlying epithelial cells.

Why might contact of *V. cholerae* with absorptive epithelial cells induce adverse reactions in volunteers? In a variety of *in vitro* systems, investigators have shown that epithelial cells respond to the presence of adherent bacteria with the production of proinflammatory cytokines. For example, Svanborg and colleagues have shown that epithelial cells respond to the presence of adherent *E. coli* with the production of interleukin-6 (Hedges *et al.*, 1992). This potent cytokine has inflammatory properties and also plays an important local role in stimulating IgA-specific immune responses. Similarly, it has been shown that cultured polarized epithelial cells release the neutrophil chemotactic chemokine IL-8 in the presence of *Salmonella typhimurium* (McCormick *et al.*, 1993). The proinflammatory cytokines

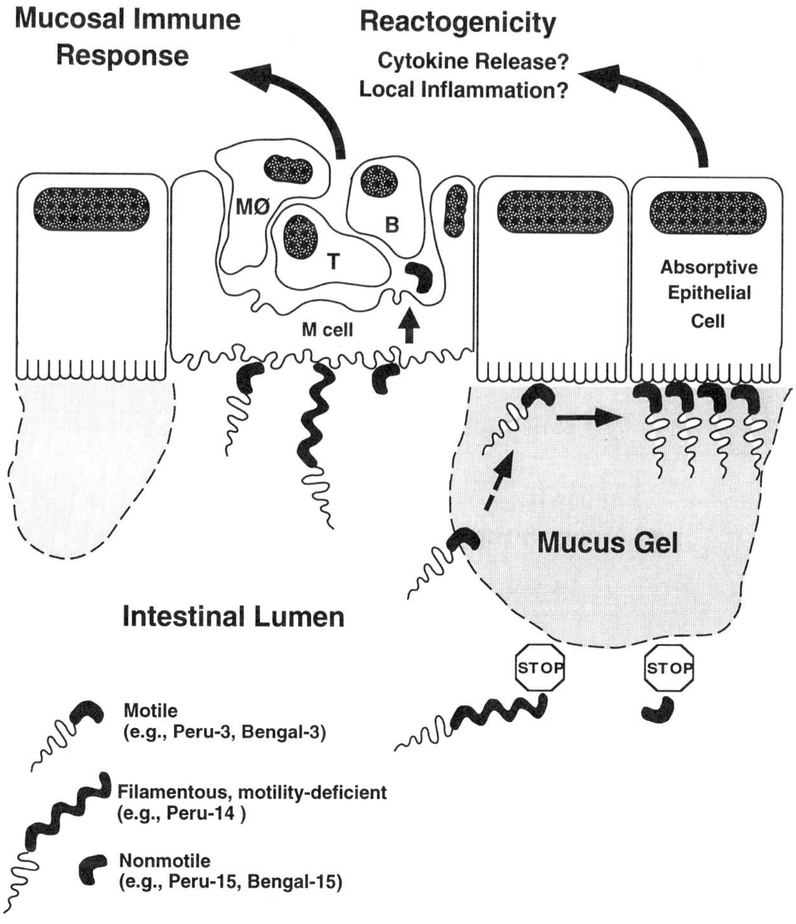

Figure 2. The role of motility in the origin of reactogenicity. The nonmotile vaccine strains Peru-15 and Bengal-15, represented by the nonflagellated vibrios, are unable to penetrate the mucus gel and adhere to underlying epithelial cells. Therefore, we speculate that these vaccine strains do not elicit the release of cytokines and a local inflammatory response which may be the basis for reactogenicity. However, these nonmotile vaccines are taken up by M cells as efficiently as motile strains and therefore lead to the generation of a potent mucosal immune response.

produced by intestinal epithelial cells in response to close contact by live, motile *V. cholerae* strains may be the cause of the adverse symptoms in recipients of motile vaccine strains. This cytokine response may not be induced as efficiently by motility-deficient vaccine strains because these strains do not interact as extensively with the mucus-coated epithelial cells Fig. 2).

Thus the colonization = reactogenicity hypothesis can be refined and restated as the "mucus penetration = reactogencity" hypothesis. This latter proposal begins to take into account the location within the small intestine where vaccine strains are replicating and certain aspects of the *in vivo* physiology of the vaccine strains. The mucus penetration = reactogenicity hypothesis is now being formally tested by evaluating in the same volunteer study the highly reactogenic El Tor vaccine strain Bah-3 with its nonmotile isogenic derivative Bah-15.

The proinflammatory cytokine response which may be elicited in response to *V. cholerae* adhering to epithelial cells not only may lead to reactogenicity but also may contribute to the immunogenicity of a vaccine strain. However, the nonmotile vaccine strains remain highly immunogenic. This is probably because the principal antigen-sampling process operative in the intestinal mucosa involves endocytosis by specialized non-mucus covered epithelial cells known as M cells (Kraehenbuhl and Neutra, 1992). M cells have very little mucus coat or even glycocaylx covering their apical membrane (Kraehenbuhl and Neutra, 1992). Thus, we can postulate that motility-deficient vaccine strains interact with M cells at least as well as motile vaccine strains given the lack of the mechanical barrier imposed by mucus and glycocaylx. Presumably, colonization of motility-deficient vaccine strains occurs within the intestinal lumen and outer mucus layers and the resultant bacterial progeny eventually contact M cells. That motility-deficent strains do indeed colonize well is evidenced by their prominant shedding by volunteers and the immune response they elicit (Taylor *et al.*, 1994; Coster *et al.*, 1995; Kenner *et al.*, 1995) (Table II).

The results of volunteer studies suggest that reasonably safe and effective vaccines for El Tor O1 and O139 *V. cholerae* strains are now in hand. Further volunteer studies and field studies with this new generation of cholera vaccines should be done to begin to answer a variety of questions including: (1) What is the duration of protective immunity engendered by these vaccine strains? (2) How soon after vaccination are individuals protected against cholera? (3) Are these vaccines safe and effective for young children, immunocompromised hosts, and a wide range of human populations? (4) In areas where both El Tor O1 and O139 strains coexist, can a bivalent vaccine be simply achieved by making a "cocktail" consisting of a mixture of oral live-attenuated El Tor and O139 vaccine strains?

Other public health issues such as exploring the usefulness of cholera vaccines in refugee camps and other epidemic situations also need to be addressed. Now that the era of safe and effective cholera vaccines is upon us we can also begin to explore the use of these oral vaccine strains as vectors for delivery of a variety of heterologous antigens to the intestinal mucosal immune system (Butterton *et al.*, 1995). If there is a unity of the mucosal immune system, it may be possible to protect all or some mucosal surfaces from a wide variety of pathogens by simple oral administration of a *V. cholerae* vaccine strain expressing an array of foreign antigens.

Acknowledgments

We thank our many colleagues who were essential participants in the development and testing of the new oral live-attenuated cholera vaccines described here. These include our colleagues at Harvard Medical School, Virus Research Institute, U. S. Army Medical Research Institute of Infectious Diseases, and Walter Reed Army Institute of Research. We give special thanks to the volunteers who participated in the clinical evaluation of our vaccine constructs. We thank Dr. A. Camilli for critically reviewing the manuscript. Matthew K. Waldor is a physician postdoctoral fellow of the Howard Hughes Medical Institute. This work was supported by Grant AI-18045 to J.J.M. from the National Institues of Allergy and Infectious Diseases. J.J.M. is a stockholder in Virus Research Institute, Inc. (Cambridge, MA), and was not involved in the clinical assessment of the vaccine constructs discussed here.

Note added in proof. We have recently discovered that the CTX genetic element encodes a filamentous phage—the CTX phage (Waldor and Mekalanos. Lysogenic conversion by a filamentous phage encoding cholera toxin (1996). *Science,* in press.) The CTX phage uses TCP as its receptor and is capable of infecting live-attenuated *V. cholerae* vaccine constructs. Thus, we are now challenged to engineer another generation of live-attenuated *V. cholerae* vaccine constructs that cannot be infected by the CTX phage.

References

Barua, B. (1992). History of cholera. *In* "Cholera" (D. Barua, and W. B. Greenough III, eds.), pp. 1–36. Plenum, New York.

Baudry, B., Fasano, A., Ketley, J., and Kaper, J. B. (1992). Cloning of a gene (*zot*) encoding a new toxin produced by *Vibrio cholerae. Infect. Immun.* **60,** 428–434.

Bik, E. M., Bunschoten, A. E., Gouw, R. D., and Mooi, F. (1995). Genesis of the novel epidemic *Vibrio cholerae* O139 strain: Evidence for horizontal transfer of genes involved in polysaccharide synthesis. *EMBO J.* **14,** 209–216.

Black, R. E., Levine, M. M., Clements, M. L., Young, C. R., Svennerholm, A. M., and Holmgren, J. (1987). Protective efficacy in humans of killed whole-vibrio oral cholera vaccine with and without the B subunit of cholera toxin. *Infect. Immun.* **55,** 1116–1120.

Butterton, J. R., Beattie, D. T., Gardel, C. L., Carroll, P. A., Hyman, T., Killeen, K. P., Meakalnos, J. J., and Calderwood, S. B. (1995). Heterologous antigen expression in *Vibrio cholerae* vector strains. *Infect. Immun.* **63,** 2689–2696.

Cholera Working Group (1993). Large epidemic of cholera-like disease in Bangladesh caused by *Vibrio cholerae* O139 synonym Bengal. *Lancet* **342,** 387–390.

Clemens, J., Sack, D., Harris, J. R., Chakraborty, J., Khan, M. R., Stanton, B. F., Kay, B., Khan, M. U., Yunus, M., Svennerholm, A.-M., and Holmgren, J. (1986). Field trial of oral cholera vaccines in Bangladesh. *Lancet* **1,** 124–127.

Clemens, J. D., Sack, D. A., Harris, J. R., Chakraborty, J., Neogy, P. K., Stanton, B., Huda, N., Khan, M. U., Kay, B. A., and Khan, M. R. (1988). Cross-protection by B subunit-whole cell cholera vaccine against diarrhea associated with heat-labile toxin-producing enterotoxigenic *Escherichia coli*: Results of a large-scale field trial. *J. Infect. Dis.* **158,** 372–377.

Clemens, J. D., Sack, D. A., Harris, J. R., Loon, F. V., Chakraborty, J., Ahmed, F., Rao, M. R., Khan, M. R., Yunus, M., and Huda, N. (1990). Field trial of oral cholera vaccines in Bangladesh: Results from three-year follow-up. *Lancet* **335,** 270–273.

Clemens, J., Spriggs, D., and Sack, D. (1994). Public health considerations for the use of cholera vaccines in cholera control programs. *In* "*Vibrio cholerae* and Cholera: Molecular to Global Perspectives" (I. Wachsmuth, P. Blake, and O. Olsvik, eds.), pp. 425–440. ASM Press, Washington, D.C.

Coster, T. S., Killeen, K. P., Waldor, M. K., Beattie, D., Spriggs, D., Kenner, J. R., Trofa, A., Sadoff, J., Mekalanos, J. J., and Taylor, D. N. (1995). Safety, immunogenicity and efficacy of a live attenuated *Vibrio cholerae* O139 vaccine protype, Bengal-15. *Lancet* **345,** 949–952.

Freter, R., and Gangarosa, E. J. (1963). Oral immunization and production of coproantibody in human volunteers. *J. Immunol.* **91,** 724–729.

Freter, R., O'Brien, P. C. M., and Macsai, M. M. S. (1981). Role of chemotaxis in the association of motile bacteria with intestinal mucosa: *In vivo* studies. *Infect. Immun.* **34,** 234–240.

Glass, R. I., Becker, S., Huq, I., Stoll, B. J., Khan, M. U., Merson, M. H., Lee, J. V., and Black, R. E. (1982). Endemic cholera in rural Bangladesh, 1966–1980. *Am. J. Epidemiol.* **116,** 959–970.

Hedges, S., Svensson, M., and Svanborg, C. (1992). Interleukin-6 response of epithelial cell lines to bacterial stimulation *in vitro*. *Infect. Immun.* **60,** 1295–1301.

Herrington, D. A., Hall, R. H., Losonsky, G., Mekalanos, J. J., Taylor, R. K., and Levine, M. M. (1988). Toxin, toxin-coregulated pili, and the *toxR* regulon are essential for *Vibrio cholerae* pathogenesis in humans. *J. Exp. Med.* **168,** 1487–1492.

Hisatsune, K., Kondo, S., Isshiki, Y., Iguchi, T., Kawamata, Y., and Shimada, T. (1993). O-antigenic lipopolysaccharide of *Vibrio cholerae* O139 Bengal, a new epidemic strain for recent cholera in the Indian subcontinet. *Biochem. Biophys. Res. Commun.* **196,** 1309–1315.

Honda, T., and Finkelstein, R. A. (1979). Selection and characteristics of a novel *Vibrio cholerae* mutant lacking the A (ADP-ribosylating) portion of the cholera enterotoxin. *Proc. Natl. Acad. Sci. U.S.A.* **76,** 2052–2056.

Jonson, G., Svennerholm, A. M., and Holmgren, J. (1989). *Vibrio cholerae* expresses cell surface antigens during intestinal infection which are not expressed during *in vitro* culture. *Infect. Immun.* **57,** 1809–1815.

Kaper, J. B., Lockman, H., Baldini, M. M., and Levine, M. M. (1984). Recombinant nontoxinogenic *Vibrio cholerae* strains as attenuated cholera vaccine candidates. *Nature (London)* **308,** 655–658.

Kaper, J. B., Michalski, J., Ketley, J. M., and Levine, M. M. (1994). Potential for reacquisition of cholera enterotoxin genes by attenuated *Vibrio cholerae* vaccine strain CVD 103-HgR. *Infect. Immun.* **62,** 1480–1483.

Kaper, J. B., Morris, J. G., and Levine, M. M. (1995). Cholera. *Clin. Microbiol. Rev.* **8,** 48–86.

Kenner, J., Coster, T., Trofa, A., Taylor, D., Barrera-Oro, M., Hyman, T., Adams, J., Beattie, D., Killeen, K., Mekalanos, J. J., and Sadoff, J. C. (1995). Peru-15, a live, attenuated oral vaccine candidate for *Vibrio cholerae* O1 El Tor. *J. Infect. Dis.* **172,** 1126–1129.

Kraehenbuhl, J. P., and Neutra, M. R. (1992). Molecular and cellular basis of immune protection of mucosal surfaces. *Physiol. Rev.* **72,** 853–879.

Levine, M. M., and Pierce, N. F. (1992). Immunity and vaccine development. *In* "Cholera" (D. Barua, and W. B. Greenough, eds.), pp. 285–328. Plenum, New York.

Levine, M. M., and Tacket, C. O. (1994). Recombinant live cholera vaccines. *In* "*Vibrio cholerae* and Cholerae" (I. K. Wachsmuth, P. A. Blake, and O. Olsvik, eds.), pp. 395–413. ASM Press. Washington, D.C.

Levine, M. M., Black, R. E., Clements, M. L., Lanata, C., Sears, S., Honda, T., Young, C. R., and Finkelstein, R. A. (1984). Evaluation in humans of attenuated *Vibrio cholerae* El Tor Ogawa strain Texas Star-SR as a live oral vaccine. *Infect. Immun.* **43,** 515–522.

Levine, M. M., Kaper, J. B., Herrington, D., Ketley, J., Losonsky, G., Tacket, C. O., Tall, B., and Cryz, R. (1988a). Safety, immunogenicity, and efficacy of recombinant live oral cholera vaccines, CVD 103 and CVD 103-HgR. *Lancet* **2,** 467–470.

Levine, M. M., Kaper, J. B., Herrington, D., Losonsky, G., Morris, J. G., Clements, M., Black, R. E., Tall, B., and Hall, R. (1988b). Volunteer studies of deletion mutants of *Vibrio cholerae* 01 prepared by recombinant techniques. *Infect. Immun.* **56,** 161–167.

McCormick, B. A., Colgan, S. P., Archer, C. D., Miller, S. I., and Madara, J. L. (1993). *Salmonella typhimurium* attachment to human intestinal epithelial monolayers: Transcellular signalling to subepithelial neutrophils. *J. Cell Biol.* **123,** 895–907.

Manning, P. A., Brown, M. H., and Heuzenroeder, M. W. (1984). Cloning of the structural gene (*hly*) for the haemolysin of *Vibrio cholerae* El Tor strain 017. *Gene* **31**, 225–231.

Mekalanos, J. J. (1983). Duplication and amplification of toxin genes in *Vibrio cholerae*. *Cell(Cambridge, Mass.)* **35**, 253–263.

Mekalanos, J. J., Swartz, D. J., Pearson, G. D., Harford, N., Groyne, F., and deWilde, M. (1983). Cholera toxin genes: Nucleotide sequence, deletion analysis and vaccine development. *Nature (London)* **306**, 551–557.

Owen, R. L., Pierce, M. F., Apple, R. T., and Cray, W. C. (1986). M cell transport of *Vibrio cholerae* from the intestinal lumen into Peyer's patches: A mechanism for antigen sampling and for microbial transepithelial migration. *J. Infect. Dis.* **153**, 1108–1118.

Pearson, G. D., and Mekalanos, J. J. (1982). Molecular cloning of *Vibrio cholerae* enterotoxin genes in *Escherichia coli* K-12. *Proc. Natl. Acad. Sci. U.S.A.* **79**, 2976–80.

Pearson, G. D. N., Woods, A., Chiang, S. L., and Mekalanos, J. J. (1993). CTX genetic element encodes a site-specific recombination system and an intestinal colonization factor. *Proc. Natl. Acad. Sci. U.S.A.* **90**, 3750–3754.

Roberts, A., Pearson, G. D., and Mekalanos, J. J. (1992). Cholera vaccine strains derived from a 1991 Peruvian isolate of *Vibrio cholerae* and other El Tor strains. *In* "Proceedings of the 28th Joint Conference on Cholera and Related Diarrheal Diseases." pp. 43–47. U.S.—Japan Cooperative Medical Science Program, Tokyo, Japan).

Szu, S., Gupta, R., and Robbins, J. (1994). Induction of serum vibriocidal antibodies by O-specifc polysaccharide–protein conjugate vaccines for prevention of cholera. *In* "*Vibrio cholerae* and Cholera: Molecular to Global Perspectives" (Wachsmuth, I. K., Blake, P. A., and Olsvik, O., eds.), pp. 381–394. ASM Press. Washington, D.C.

Tacket, C. O., Losonsky, G., Nataro, J. P., Cryz, S. J., Edelman, R., Fasano, A., Michalski, J., Kaper, J. B., and Levine, M. M. (1993). Safety and immunogenicity of live oral cholera vaccine candidate CVD 110, a Δ*ctxA* Δ*zot* Δ*ace* derivative of El Tor Ogawa *Vibrio cholerae*. *J. Infect. Dis.* **168**, 1536–1540.

Tacket, C., Morris, G., Losonsky, G., Nataro, J., Michalski, J., Comsock, L., Kaper, J., and Levine, M. (1994). Volunteer studies investigating the pathogenicity of *Vibrio cholerae* O139 and the protective efficacy conferred by both primary infection and by vaccine strain CVD112. *In* "Proceedings of the 30th Joint Conference on Cholera and Related Diarrheal Diseases," pp. 142–147. U.S.–Japan Cooperative Medical Science Program, Fukuoka).

Taylor, D. N., Killeen, K. P., Hack, D. C., Kenner, J. R., Coster, T. S., Beattie, D. T., Ezzell, J., Hyman, T., Trofa, A., Sjogren, M. H., Friedlander, A., Mekalanos, J. J., and Sadoff, J. C. (1994). Development of a live, oral, attenuated vaccine against El Tor cholera. *J. Infect. Dis.* **170**, 1518–1523.

Taylor, R. K., Miller, V. L., Furlong, D. B., and Mekalanos, J. J. (1987). Use of *phoA* gene fusions to identify a pilus colonization factor coordinately regulated with cholera toxin. *Proc. Natl. Acad. Sci. U.S.A.* **84**, 2833–2837.

Trucksis, M., Galen, J., Michalski, J., Fasano, A., and Kaper, J. B. (1993). Accessory cholera enterotoxin (Ace), the third toxin of a *Vibrio cholerae* virulence cassette. *Proc. Natl. Acad. Sci. U.S.A.* **90**, 5267–5271.

Waldor, M. K., and Mekalanos, J. J. (1994a). Emergence of a new cholera pandemic: Molecular analysis of virulence determinants in *Vibrio cholerae* 0139 and development of a live vaccine prototype. *J. Infect. Dis.* **170**, 278–283.

Waldor, M. K., and Mekalanos, J. J. (1994b). ToxR regulates virulence gene expression in non-O1 strains of *Vibrio cholerae* that cause epidemic cholera. *Infect. Immun.* **62**, 72–78.

Waldor, M. K., and Mekalanos, J. J. (1994c). *Vibrio cholerae* O139 specific gene sequences. *Lancet* **343**, 1366.

Waldor, M. K., Colwell, R., and Mekalanos, J. J. (1994). The *Vibrio cholerae* 0139 serogroup antigen includes O-antigen capsule and lipopolysaccharide virulence determinants. *Proc. Natl. Acad. Sci. U.S.A.* **91**, 11388–11392.

Woodward, W. E. (1971). Cholera reinfection in man. *J. Infect. Dis.* **123**, 61–66.

World Health Organization (1994). Cholera in 1993. *Weekly Epidemiological Record* **69**, 205–212.

18

Oral Vaccines against Cholera and Enterotoxigenic Escherichia coli *Diarrhea*

Jan Holmgren
Ann-Mari Svennerholm
Department of Medical Microbiology and Immunology
University of Göteborg
S-413 46 Göteborg, Sweden

I. Introduction

Diarrheal disease remains one of the leading global health problems. It has been estimated that 3–5 billion episodes of diarrhea, resulting in 5–10 million deaths, occur annually in developing countries, with the highest incidence and severity in children below the age of 5 years (Black, 1986; Farthing and Keusch, 1989). About half of these cases are caused by bacteria that produce one or more enterotoxins. Cholera, resulting from infection with *Vibrio cholerae* bacteria, is the most severe of these "enterotoxic" enteropathies, whereas infection with enterotoxigenic *Escherichia coli* (ETEC) causes the largest number of cases.

Vibrio cholerae of serogroup O1 is the prototype for the enterotoxin-producing bacteria and was first isolated by Robert Koch in 1884. Until the beginning of this century all *V. cholerae* O1 isolates were of the same, so-called classical, biotype. In 1906, however, vibrios of a new biotype, El Tor, were isolated and for many years vibrios of either the classical or El Tor biotype were isolated from cholera cases. *V. cholerae* O1 can appear in the form of two different serotypes, Inaba and Ogawa. During the early part of the 19th century cholera started to spread from its likely ancient home in Bengal, and since then seven large pandemics have been described which have affected large parts of the world. The latest pandemic took its departure from Celebes in 1961 and has spread to many countries in Asia and Africa, and from 1991 cholera has also appeared in large numbers in South and Central America for the first time in more than 100 years (Blake, 1994). The causative agent in Latin America appears to be identical to the seventh pandemic O1 El Tor organisms isolated from Asia and Africa.

Very recently *V. cholerae* of a "new" serogroup, O139, has emerged as an additional cause of cholera in India and Bangladesh (Morris, 1994); cholera caused by these bacteria has also been reported from a number of neighbouring countries (Thailand and Nepal). Although it is currently restricted to Southeast Asia, there is obviously a risk that *V. cholerae* O139 may follow the tracks of *V. cholerae* O1, reaching Africa and Latin America.

Although in endemic areas the highest incidence of cholera is seen in children of less than 5 years of age (Mosley *et al.*, 1968), approximately two-thirds of all *V. cholerae* O1 cases still occur in older children and adults. In contrast, when cholera has spread to new countries, all age groups have been equally affected. This is probably due to a lack of natural immunity that normally develops with age in endemic countries (Tauxe *et al.*, 1994). Similarly, cholera caused by the new serogroup O139 has been recorded at least as frequently in adults as in children (Morris, 1994). The total number of cholera cases annually is uncertain since several affected countries and/or areas do not monitor and/or report the disease. The recent outbreaks of *V. cholerae* O1 in Latin America as well as of *V. cholerae* O139 in Asia have probably resulted in a substantially increased number of cholera cases in the last 5 years. Therefore, the often-cited figures of approximately 5 million cases and 200,000 deaths from cholera annually are probably underestimates of the present situation.

ETEC together with rotavirus, is the most common cause of diarrhea in children in developing countries in Asia, Africa, and Latin America, and ETEC continues to be a common cause of diarrhea also in adults. Although it has been estimated that only about one-third of all ETEC infections are symptomatic in children in endemic areas, this is enough to result in at least 650 million episodes of diarrhea and about 800,000 deaths annually in children below the age of 5 years (Black, 1986). ETEC is also without comparison the most common cause of traveller's diarrhea (Black, 1990). Indeed,

MUCOSAL VACCINES

it has been estimated that 50% of persons travelling to developing countries experience diarrheal disease, and ETEC is isolated in one-third to one-half of these episodes.

The disease caused by the enterotoxin-producing bacteria is characterized by watery stools without blood and mucus (Farthing and Keusch, 1989). Although most cases are relatively mild, in other cases the diarrhea may result in moderate to severe dehydration that is sometimes fatal. In cholera, which is the most frequent dehydrating disease, the most severe cases can purge as much as 15–25 liters of water and electrolytes per day; the mortality rate in severe, nontreated cholera is 30–50%. ETEC disease may vary from mild diarrhea to a severe cholera-like disease and is often accompanied by nausea, vomiting, abdominal cramps, anorexia, and fever.

No effective vaccines for use in humans against either cholera or ETEC diarrhea have been available until recently. Thus, previous parenteral cholera vaccines have induced up to 50% protection for only 3–6 months (Feeley and Gangarosa, 1980) and vaccines against ETEC and other enterotoxin-producing organisms have been lacking. The limitations in protection induced by the previous cholera vaccines could be explained primarily by the parenteral administration route used. Thus, injectable cholera vaccines give rise to no or very low immune responses locally in the gut, where both the bacteria and the toxin they produce exert their action during infection and where local immunity is of critical importance.

In recent years, however, an inactivated oral cholera vaccine that has been shown in large field trials to afford 85% protection for the first 6 months and 60–70% protection for 2–3 years has been developed and licensed (Clemens *et al.*, 1990; Holmgren and Svennerholm, 1992). A live oral cholera vaccine, CVD 103-HgR, has also been developed and found to be safe and immunogenic and to give rise to significant protection against challenge with *V. cholerae* O1 in human volunteers (Kaper, 1990; Levine and Tacket, 1995). Different from the inactivated cholera vaccine, the protective efficacy of the live vaccine against natural disease and the duration of protection have not yet been determined but are presently under study in a field trial in Indonesia. Vaccine candidates against ETEC diarrhea in humans have also been developed, and an oral killed ETEC vaccine has been tested with promising results in Phase 1 and Phase 2 trials in both endemic and nonendemic areas (Svennerholm *et al.*, 1989; Holmgren and Svennerholm, 1992; Svennerholm and Holmgren, 1995). In this chapter, we describe the development and testing of oral-inactivated vaccines against cholera and ETEC diarrhea, respectively. The development of these vaccines has to a large extent been based on new insights into the mechanisms of disease and immunity in enterotoxin-induced diarrheas achieved during the last decades (Holmgren and Svennerholm, 1992).

II. Mechanisms of Disease and Immunity

A. Antitoxic Immunity

The major pathogenic mechanisms of enterotoxigenic bacteria include initial bacterial colonization of the small intestine followed by the elaboration of one or more enterotoxins that through various mechanisms can induce electrolyte and water secretion, resulting in diarrhea (Guerrant, 1985; Holmgren and Svennerholm, 1992). These enterotoxins, which have a cytotonic rather than cytotoxic effect on the intestinal epithelium, are believed to stimulate secretion, primarily from the small intestinal crypt cells, by inducing increased formation of cyclic AMP and/or cyclic GMP in the epithelial cells. The prototype enterotoxin is cholera toxin (CT) being produced by *V. cholerae* O1 bacteria, as well as by the novel serogroup O139 (Guerrant, 1985; Waldor and Mekalanos, 1994). Cholera toxin consists of five identical binding (B) subunits associated in a ring into which a single toxic-active (A) subunit is noncovalently inserted; the binding receptor for the cholera toxin on cells is a specific glycolipid, the ganglioside G_{M1} (Holmgren, 1981).

ETEC bacteria may produce either or both a heat-labile enterotoxin (LT) and a heat-stable enterotoxin (ST) (Guerrant, 1985, Holmgren and Svennerholm, 1992). While both geographic and age-related variations may occur, on an average approximately one-third of all clinical ETEC isolates produce LT alone, one-third ST alone, and one-third LT in combination with ST (Svennerholm and Holmgren, 1995). LT is structurally, functionally, and immunologically closely related, although not identical, to CT. Thus, similar to CT, LT consists of five B subunits and one A subunit, and both of these proteins cross-react immunologically with the corresponding CT subunit proteins, although there are also specific A- and B-subunit epitopes on both toxins (Guerrant, 1985; Holmgren and Svennerholm, 1992). Similar to the situation for antitoxic cholera immunity, the anti-LT immune response is mainly directed against the B-subunit portion of the molecule, although some contribution of antibodies to the A subunit may also exist (Svennerholm *et al.*, 1986a).

The identification of the subunit structure of CT and LT and the roles of the different subunits have indicated that the purified cholera or LT B subunits (CT-B or LT-B) are suitable toxoid candidates. Furthermore, B subunits are particularly well suited as oral immunogens, because they are stable in the intestinal milieu and are capable of binding to the intestinal epithelium, including the M cells of the Peyer's patches, which are important properties for stimulating mucosal immunity including local immunological memory (Neutra and Kraehenbühl, 1992). This is probably an important protection factor, since studies in experimental animals have shown a direct correlation between protection against CT-induced fluid secretion and intestinal synthesis of secretory IgA (S-IgA) antibodies, and also between protection and the number of antitoxin-producing cells in the intestine (Holmgren and Svennerholm, 1992). These results, together with the strictly mucosal, noninvasive nature of cholera, suggest that locally formed S-IgA antibodies are of major importance for providing antitoxic immunity in the gut.

Antibodies against CT-B may also cross-protect against *E. coli* LT disease and vice versa, although protection against the homologous toxin may be somewhat stronger (Svennerholm *et al.*, 1986a). Therefore, studies have been undertaken to genetically modify the structural gene for CT-B to encode B subunits that also contain LT-B-specific epitopes (Lebens *et al.*, 1996). However, studies both in endemic areas and in travellers have shown that peroral administration of CT-B may induce highly significant cross-protection against diarrhea caused by LT-producing *E. coli* (Clemens *et al.*, 1988a; Peltola *et al.*, 1991).

E. coli ST, on the other hand, has very distinct properties from the heat-labile toxins. While animal strains of ETEC may produce two different forms of ST (STa and STb), STa is the only form produced by human ETEC isolates (Guerrant, 1985). STa is a small molecule consisting of 18 or 19 amino acids and stimulates guanylate cyclase activity in intestinal cells. Different from LT, which is a strong immunogen, STa is not immunogenic unless coupled to a carrier protein, chemically or by recombinant technology (Frantz and Robertson, 1981; Sanchez *et al.*, 1988; Svennerholm *et al.*, 1986b). Accordingly, STa that is released during infection does not induce any antibody response and it is still unclear whether sufficiently strong anti-ST immunity may be induced by vaccination with artificial STa–carrier protein conjugates to provide significant protection against disease caused by ST-producing *E. coli* in humans.

B. Colonization Factors and Antibacterial Immunity

In previous studies we have shown that *V. cholerae* O1 LPS is the predominant antigen affording antibacterial immunity against experimental cholera (Svennerholm, 1980). Recent studies have suggested that antibacterial immunity against *V. cholerae* O139 to a large extent is also provided by antibodies against LPS. An important observation guiding the design of new cholera vaccines concerns the cooperation between antitoxic and antibacterial immune mechanisms in cholera. The main protective antibodies against cholera have been identified as being directed against the cell-wall LPS and CT-B (Holmgren *et al.*, 1977). Either of these two types of antibodies can confer strong protection against disease by inhibiting bacterial colonization and toxin binding, respectively, and when present together in the gut they can have a strongly synergistic protective effect (Svennerholm and Holmgren, 1976).

Enterotoxin-producing bacteria must colonize the small intestine to cause diarrhea. This colonization is dependent on receptor–ligand interactions between the bacteria and the host cells, which usually are specific for the species. Colonization is promoted by distinct attachment factors on the bacteria, so-called adhesins or colonization factors, that may be fimbrial or fibrillar in nature (Evans and Evans, 1989).

In *V. cholerae* O1 bacteria of the classical biotype, a toxin-coregulated pilus (TCP) has been shown to be of importance for colonization of the small intestine (Taylor *et al.*, 1987), and recent evidence indicates that for *V. cholerae* O1 El Tor and O139 an antigenically distinct form of TCP is also important for colonization and disease (Voss *et al.*, 1996). In addition, *V. cholerae* bacteria have been found to express a number of other fimbrial structures, e.g., the mannose-sensitive hemagglutinin (MSHA), which can mediate bacterial attachment to epithelial cells; the role of these other attachment factors for colonization and infection in humans remains to be defined (Jonson *et al.*, 1991). The identification of TCP as an important colonization factor on *V. cholerae* suggests that it should be possible to raise protective antibacterial immunity against these fimbrial antigens. Indeed, in experimental systems it has been found that monoclonal antibodies or polyclonal antisera against TCP can protect against infection and disease (Osek *et al.*, 1992). However, following natural infection, little if any anti-TCP immunity develops, and as an overall conclusion it remains to be defined whether mucosal immune responses against TCP and other surface antigens on *V. cholerae* can add significantly to the strong protective action mediated by antibodies to the O1 (or O139) LPS antigen.

In ETEC, various species-associated colonization factor fimbriae have been identified. A majority (50–80%) of human clinical ETEC isolates express one of three distinct colonization factor antigens (CFAs), referred to as CFA/I, CFA/II, or CFA/IV (Evans and Evans, 1989; Svennerholm *et al.*, 1989). CFA/I is a homogenous protein consisting of ~100 identical 15-kDa subunits. CFA/II, on the other hand, consists of three different subcomponents, the so-called coli surface antigens CS1, CS2, and CS3. Similar to CFA/II, CFA/IV consists of subcomponents, i.e., CS4, CS5, and CS6. Usually, the fibrillar CS3 is expressed alone or together with the fimbrial CS1 and CS2. In an analogous way

CS6, which has neither a fimbrial or fibrillar structure, is found together with the fimbrial CS4 or CS5. In addition, a number of other putative colonization factors, e.g., PCFO159, PCFO166, CS7, CS17, and CFA/III, have been described but with lower frequencies (McConnell, 1991). The three predominant CFAs (CFA/I, CFA/II, and CFA/IV), like the less frequent ones, are expressed mainly on ST and LT + ST ETEC strains. There is still a high proportion of *E. coli* strains, particularly those producing LT only, in which a specific colonization factor has not yet been identified. All of the different CFAs and their subcomponents, as well as most of the PCFs, have been shown to promote colonization of ETEC in animal models and to induce specific antibody formation following experimental infection (Åhrén and Svennerholm, 1985; Svennerholm *et al.*, 1990; Svennerholm *et al.*, 1992).

The great diversity of O groups associated with human ETEC (Black, 1986) limits the utility of LPS as a protective vaccine antigen against ETEC. Antibodies against the different CFAs, on the other hand, have been highly effective in protecting against diarrhea caused by ETEC expressing the homologous CFA. Furthermore, much in the same way as for the synergistic cooperation between anti-LPS and anti-CT-B antibodies for protection against cholera (Holmgren *et al.*, 1977), anti-CFA antibodies have been found to cooperate synergistically with anti-LT antibodies in protecting against infection with LT-producing CFA-carrying *E. coli* (Åhrén and Svennerholm, 1985). These results suggest that an effective ETEC vaccine should ideally provide anti-CFA as well as anti-toxic immunity and should thus contain the most prevalent CFAs/CS-factors in combination with a suitable LT or LT/ST toxoid.

III. Oral Cholera Vaccines

A. B Subunit Whole-Cell Vaccine

An oral cholera vaccine consisting of the nontoxic, highly immunogenic CT-B protein in combination with heat- and formalin-killed *V. cholerae* O1 classical and El Tor vibrios (Table I) has been developed and is now a licensed vaccine (Holmgren and Svennerholm, 1992). This CT-B whole-cell (B-WC) vaccine, which is given together with a bicarbonate buffer to preserve the CT-B pentameric structure, has proved in extensive clinical trials, including large field trials, to be completely safe and to provide good protection against cholera and also partial protection against diarrhea caused by LT-producing ETEC.

The B-WC vaccine was designed to evoke antitoxic as well as antibacterial intestinal immunity, since in animal studies these types of immunity have been shown to provide synergistic cooperative protection (Svennerholm and Holmgren, 1976; Holmgren and Svennerholm, 1983). Phase I and Phase II clinical studies established that the vaccine does not cause any detectable side effects and that, after either two or three doses, it stimulates a gut mucosal IgA antitoxic and antibacterial immune response (including memory) comparable to that induced by cholera disease itself (Svennerholm *et al.*, 1984; Jertborn *et al.*, 1988; Quiding *et al.*, 1991). Furthermore, immunization with either the complete B-WC vaccine or the WC component alone was found to protect American volunteers against challenge with a dose of live cholera vibrios (biotype El Tor) that caused disease in 100% of concurrently tested unvaccinated controls (Black *et al.*, 1987).

On this basis, a large, double-blind, placebo-controlled field trial with more than 90,000 participants was undertaken in rural Bangladesh. The results established that both the B-WC vaccine and the WC component alone confer long-lasting protection against cholera. The B-WC vaccine had a higher initial efficacy level than the WC vaccine (85% *versus* 58% for the initial 4- to 6-month period); indeed, if for calculation of the protective efficacy of the CT-B component one estimates the protective efficacy of B-WC in comparison with WC by looking at the WC group as "placebo" the protective

TABLE I
Oral B Subunit (B) Whole-Cell (WC) Cholera Vaccines

Per dose composition	Clinical evaluation
A. B-O1 WC (Bangladesh field trial formulation)	
1 mg CT-B (purified from CT) + 1 × 10^{11} killed bacteria 2.5 × 10^{10} heat-killed Inaba vibrios (strain Cairo 48) 2.5 × 10^{10} heat-killed Ogawa vibrios (strain Cairo 50) 2.5 × 10^{10} formalin-killed classical vibrio (strain Cairo 50) 2.5 × 10^{10} formalin-killed El Tor vibrios (strain Phil 6973)	Safe, immunogenic and protective both in volunteers and in large field trials in Bangladesh: 85% efficacy first 6 months; ca 60% first 3 years. Cross-protection against ETEC: ca 70% short-term efficacy. Licensed 1991. Replaced by B (below) in 1993.
B. rB-O1 WC (Currently licensed formulation)	
1 mg recombinant CT-B + same WC composition as in A (above)	Same safety, immunogenicity, and protective efficacy as for A (above). Field trial in Peru showed 86% protection against O1 El Tor cholera. Licensed in 1993.
C. Bivalent rB-O1/O139 WC	
1 mg rCT-B + O1 WC same as in B + 5 × 10^{10} formulin-killed O139 vibrios (bacteria grown and formalin-inactivated to express fimbrial antigens such as MSHA)	Safe and immunogenic in Phase I and Phase II clinical trials. Protective efficacy against O139 cholera not yet determined.

efficacy was 73%, in support of the significant protective immunogenicity of the CT-B component (Clemens *et al.*, 1986). The B-WC continued to be significantly more protective than the WC alone vaccine for the first 8 months after vaccination. Thereafter, however, the efficacy was similar, approximately 60% for both vaccines, if calculated for the whole population above age 2 years, for a 3-year follow-up period (Clemens *et al.*, 1990). Protection was of similar magnitude after two or three doses of vaccine (Clemens *et al.*, 1990). Still higher (ca 70%) long-term protective efficacy was seen in those over age 5 when vaccinated. It is likely that also the age group below 5 years, in which immunity rapidly waned after the initial high-level protection for the first 6–9 months, could also be provided with long-lasting high-level protection by a booster immunization after 1 year.

In the initial vaccine formulation tested in Bangladesh, the CT-B component was prepared by chemical isolation from cholera toxin produced by the high-expression wild-type strain 569B (Tayot *et al.*, 1981) which made the preparation of this component relatively laborious and expensive. It was therefore a significant improvement when Sanchez and Holmgren (1989) were able to construct an efficient recombinant overexpression system for the large-scale production of CT-B. Based on this, it has since been possible to further increase and simplify the production and downstream purification of recombinant CT-B for industrial vaccine production purposes (J. Holmgren and SBL. Vaccin, unpublished data). Extensive clinical testing of a second-generation vaccine formulation based on such recombinantly produced CT-B (rCT-B), designated rB-WC in Table I, has in different settings shown the same degree of safety and immunogenicity as the Bangladesh trial formulation, and therefore this has become the currently produced and licensed vaccine formulation. A recent field trial in Peru has also confirmed the strong protective efficacy of the rB-WC formulation. Thus, Sanchez *et al.* (1994) found that this vaccine given in two doses together with a bicarbonate buffer conferred no less than 86% protection against cholera in Peruvian military recruits. It is especially noteworthy that this high level of protection, being very similar to the 85% protection seen for the first 6-month postvaccination period in Bangladesh, in the Peruvian setting (i) was obtained with two doses of vaccine given only 1–2 weeks apart, (ii) was directed against severe cholera of exclusively the O1 El Tor biotype which is usually more difficult to protect against than classical biotype cholera, and (iii) was achieved in a population almost exclusively of blood group O; these were factors that earlier had been thought by some to possibly reduce the efficacy of the vaccine as compared with the findings in the Bangladesh trial.

In Vietnam, a locally produced vaccine similar to the Swedish version except lacking the CT-B component has also been found to give ca 80% protection against O1 El Tor cholera (Trach *et al.*, 1996).

Through its B subunit component, the B-WC vaccine also has been shown to provide substantial short-term protection against diarrhea caused by ETEC (Clemens *et al.*, 1988a; Peltola *et al.*, 1991). This is discussed in greater depth below.

Both the B-WC and the WC vaccines substantially reduced the overall diarrhea morbidity among those vaccinated, such that there was a 50% reduction in admissions for life-threatening diarrhea in the vaccinated group compared with the placebo group over 3 years of follow-up (Clemens *et al.*, 1988b; J. Clemens, unpublished data). The latter finding provides ample evidence of the public health application potential of the B-WC cholera vaccine in settings such as those found not only in Bangladesh but also in many other countries, where cholera, ETEC, and additional enterotoxic diarrheal diseases account for a large number of life-threatening watery diarrheas, especially in those over the age of 2, and where adequate treatment facilities in rural areas are still scarce (Sack and Freij, 1990; Sack *et al.*, 1991). Interestingly, in the first year of follow-up after vaccination in Bangladesh there was also a dramatic effect of either of the B-WC and WC vaccines as compared with placebo on total mortality. Several additional findings suggested that this reduction in overall mortality was a specific effect rather than a statistical coincidence: (i) the effect was restricted to the high-cholera season, (ii) it was correlated with deaths associated with or preceded by diarrheal disease according to "verbal autopsy" reports by household members, and (iii) it was limited to the underprivileged group of women rather than children participating in the study (Clemens *et al.*, 1988b). However, in contrast to the observation mentioned above that vaccination significantly reduced the incidence of life-threatening watery diarrheas in both adult women and children, during each of the three follow-up study years, the effect on total mortality was restricted to the first year; it remains to be determined whether indeed even in a "well-treated" area such as the field site in Matlab there is a significant number of hidden cholera and severe ETEC diarrhea deaths that might be averted by effective cholera and/or ETEC vaccination programs.

B. CVD103-HgR Vaccine and Other Live Vaccine Candidates

During the past decade, recombinant DNA techniques have been applied to construct various attenuated *V. cholerae* O1 strains to be tested for their utility as live oral vaccines. A series of early vaccine candidates were constructed from wild-type *V. cholerae* O1 strains by introducing deletions in the chromosomal gene(s) encoding the A subunit or both the A and B subunits of CT

(Kaper *et al.*, 1984a,b). Although these first-generation recombinant live vaccine strains, such as JBK 70 and CVD101, were markedly attenuated compared with their wild-type parents, they still caused unacceptable adverse reactions in up to 50% of immunized volunteers resulting in mild-to-moderate diarrhea often associated with additional reactions such as malaise, headache, and vomiting. Thus, it was clear that the removal of even the whole CT gene from at least highly pathogenic *V. cholerae* O1 wild-type strains represented an insufficient attenuation for providing a safe nonreactogenic vaccine strain. At the same time it was evident that even a single-dose immunization with such strains could elicit good-titer serum vibriocidal antibody responses as well as significant protection against later challenge with the wild-type parent strain in volunteers. To overcome safety problems, attempts were then made to use a less pathogenic and relatively poorly colonizing strain, 569B (classical biotype, Inaba serotype), as the parental strain for vaccine construction. This resulted in the first well-tolerated, immunogenic, and protective engineered vaccine strain, CVD103-HgR, obtained by deletion of >90% of the gene encoding the A subunit of cholera toxin leaving intact the expression of CT-B, and as an extra marker to readily differentiate the vaccine strain from wild-type vibrios also containing an introduced gene encoding resistance to Hg^{2+}. CVD103-HgR has now been tested extensively in human subjects for its safety and immunogenicity, both in industrialized countries and in developing countries with and without endemic cholera (Levine and Tacket, 1995). The results have shown that in adult volunteers living in industrialized countries, a single dose of CVD103-HgR containing 5×10^8 colony-forming units (cfu), and given in a bicarbonate buffer to protect the vaccine strain from gastric acid, is safe and gives vibriocidal seroconversion in ≥90% of vaccinees. Furthermore, and of greater significance since serum vibriocidal antibodies do not mediate or necessarily reflect vaccine-induced protective immunity against cholera, vaccination also conferred significant protection against challenge with wild-type *V. cholerae* O1 strains as tested in volunteers in the United States. The overall protection was high (80–100%) against challenge with classical biotype and moderate (49–67%) against challenge with El Tor biotype (Levine and Tacket, 1995). Similar to previous findings with the inactivated B-WC cholera vaccine, which gave 64% protection against any type of cholera after challenge with the El Tor biotype but 100% protection against clinically significant cholera (defined as ≥2 liters total purge) (Black *et al.*, 1987), vaccination with CVD103-HgR provided complete protection against severe (>5 liters total purge) and almost complete protection against clinically significant cholera even after El Tor challenge. Based on these results CVD103-HgR was recently licensed in Switzerland for prevention of cholera in travellers.

However, when studies of CVD103-HgR in adults and children began in less-developed countries where cholera was endemic, it was found that the 5×10^8 cfu dosage elicited vibriocidal antibody seroconversions in <25% of the vaccinees. Apparently the "take" of the vaccine at this dosage was relatively poor in populations already having partial immunity based on previous natural exposure to *V. cholerae* organisms. To overcome this problem, higher doses of vaccine were tested, and the results have shown that administering a single dose of vaccine containing one log higher number of vaccine organisms, i.e., 5×10^9 cfu, markedly increased the vibriocidal conversion rate, usually to >75% (Levine and Tacket, 1995). A large-scale field trial is currently underway in Indonesia to determine the efficacy of a single dose with 5×10^9 cfu of CVD103-HgR in preventing cholera in an endemic area.

Mekalanos and co-workers prepared a series of interesting live vaccine candidates generated from wild-type El Tor strains, which have been tested for safety and immunogenicity in volunteers (Taylor *et al.*, 1994; Coster *et al.*, 1995). The various vaccine constructs have in common a deletion of the whole "virulence cassette" that contains the genes encoding for CT, and the associated virulence factors Zot (zonula occludence toxin), Ace (auxiliary cholera enterotoxin), and Cep (chore-encoded pilus, an accessory colonization factor) as well as of factors RS1 and attRS1 which are involved in site-specific and homologous recombination. Similar to the previous observations with attenuation of strains of the classical biotype, these first-generation El Tor vaccine candidate strains gave rise to unacceptable side reactions with diarrhea and usually additional gastrointestinal adverse reactions. More recently, however, Mekalanos and co-workers have selected a motility-deficient mutant strain, designated Peru-14, from one of the previous vaccine constructs and this strain has to date given much more promising results in clinical studies with little reactogenicity yet good protective immunogenicity (Taylor *et al.*, 1994; Coster *et al.*, 1995). Further clinical evaluation of the Peru-14 vaccine strain is clearly warranted.

C. Combined Vaccines against O1 and O139 Cholera

Based on the emerging significance since late 1992 of *V. cholerae* O139 as an additional cause of epidemic cholera in Southeast Asia, much recent attention has been focused on the possibility of developing a cholera vaccine that also affords protection against this "new" type of cholera.

1. Bivalent B Subunit-O1/O139-Inactivated WC Vaccine

We studied the immune mechanisms and protective antigens of *V. cholerae* O139 in animal models as a basis for vaccine development; then, in collaboration with SBL Vaccin, Sweden (P. Askelöf, U. Bjare, and H. Wigzell), we developed an oral bivalent B subunit-O1/O139 whole cell cholera vaccine, which is now in clinical testing.

Based on a broad characterization of different clinical isolates of *V. cholerae* O139 Bengal with regard to properties deemed to be relevant for vaccine development, we selected one typical strain, 4260B, as a candidate inactivated vaccine strain. This strain, having a well-exposed O antigen and capsule and the capacity to produce large amounts of TcpA, CT, and mannose-sensitive hemagglutinin (MSHA) pili, but minimal production of the proteolytic soluble hemagglutinin, was used as immunogen for production of antibacterial antisera. Antisera against live or killed O139 vibrios (4260B) conferred passive protection against fluid accumulation induced by challenge with the homologous and heterologous O139 strains. The protective effect of antisera was correlated to the anti-LPS antibody titers rather than to titers against whole bacteria that had been grown for TCP expression and was substantially higher than the protection conferred by antisera to CT or CT-B. However, monoclonal antibodies to O139 LPS and CT-B/CT exhibited a strong synergistic protection against O139 challenge irrespective of the level of sensitivity of challenge strains to monoclonal antibodies against O139 LPS in vibriocidal assays *in vitro* (Jonson *et al.*, 1996).

Based on these findings, we (together with SBL Vaccin) have developed an oral bivalent B subunit O1/O139 whole cell (B-O1/O139 WC) cholera vaccine by adding formalin-killed O139 vibrios of strain 4260B to the recently licensed oral rB-O1 WC vaccine (Table I). When tested in Swedish volunteers, this rB-O1/O139 WC vaccine was found to be safe and immunogenic (Jertborn *et al.*, 1996a). Two vaccine doses given 2 weeks apart induced strong intestinal–mucosal IgA antibody responses to CT (100%), O1 vibrios (78%), and O139 vibrios (78%) as tested by ELISAs using pre- and postvaccination intestinal lavage or fecal extract specimens. These gut IgA antibody responses were associated with intestine-derived antibody-secreting cell responses in peripheral blood. A third dose of vaccine given after 5–6 weeks did not result in any further increased immune response. Most volunteers also developed IgA and IgG antitoxin as well as vibriocidal antibody responses in serum that were comparable to those induced by the B-O1 WC vaccine. Thus, the O139 component of the vaccine seemed to have similar capacity as the O1 component to induce intestinal and systemic antibacterial immune responses, and its addition to the vaccine did not interfere with the immunogenicity of the B subunit or O1 WC components.

2. Live O139 Vaccine Candidates

Following similar strategies as used for developing live O1 cholera vaccine candidates, the Kaper–Levine and the Mekalanos–Sadoff–Taylor teams have recently constructed live oral vaccine candidates based on *V. cholerae* O139 strains. Thus, Tacket *et al.* (1995) engineered an attenuated *V. cholerae* O139 vaccine candidate (CVD112-RM) by deleting the entire "virulence cassette" chromosomal region and introducing a deletion mutation in *recA* in order to diminish the ability of the vaccine strain to recombine foreign DNA into its chromosome. Waldor and Mekalanos (1994) constructed an attenuated vaccine candidate (Bengal-3) from another wild-type strain of *V. cholerae* O139 by deleting the whole virulence cassette plus the RS1 and attRS1 factors involved in virulence cassette recombination; in addition, they inserted a recombinant gene encoding CT-B into *recA* to both inactivate the latter gene and provide overexpression of CT-B. Both CVD112-RM and Bengal-3 have been found in initial volunteer studies to have low reactogenicity and to induce protective immunity against challenge with wild-type homologous *V. cholerae* O139 organisms (Tacket *et al.*, 1995; Coster *et al.*, 1995). However, as opposed to the situation with the bivalent B-O1/O139 vaccine in which there was no indication of any competition between different vaccine components with regard to immunogenicity, there is evidence that it may be difficult to combine live vaccines against O1 and O139 cholera without the risk of reducing the immunogenicity of either or both vaccine strains (J. Mekalanos, personal communication). This problem clearly deserves further study in different settings.

IV. Oral B Subunit Whole-Cell ETEC Vaccine

The findings of drastically decreased rates of ETEC diarrhea in children in developing countries with age (Black, 1986) and a decreased disease to infection rate in highly endemic areas (Cravioto *et al.*, 1988; López-Vidal *et al.*, 1990) suggest that protective immunity may develop against ETEC. Studies in human volunteers have also shown significant protection against reinfection with the homologous ETEC strain, whereas protection was not effective against rechallenge with ETEC strains expressing heterologous surface antigens (Levine, 1990).

Another strong indication of the potential of inducing effective protective immunity against ETEC disease in humans is the finding in the Bangladeshi cholera vaccine trial that the oral B-WC cholera vaccine through its CT-B component, which cross-reacts immunologically with *E. coli* LT-B, afforded significant protection against diarrhea caused by LT-producing ETEC (Clemens *et al.*, 1988a). Interestingly, the protection observed (about 67% for 3 months) was equally strong against bacteria producing LT alone as against bacteria producing LT in combination with ST. The protection was also more pronounced against ETEC diarrhea associated with severe life-threatening dehydration, which was reduced by 86% during the first few months after immunization, than against milder disease (56% efficacy). The oral B-WC cholera vaccine also afforded highly significant protection, ca. 60% protective efficacy, against LT producing *E. coli* (LT or LT + ST strains) in Finnish travellers going to Morocco for a limited vacation period (Peltola *et al.*, 1991).

Thus, there is strong support for the potential of developing an effective ETEC vaccine for use in humans. As for cholera, however, a broader and stronger protective efficacy is to be expected if the mucosal immunity against LT achieved by immunization either with LT-B or, as in the examples mentioned above, with CT-B can be combined with antibacterial immunity directed mainly, if not exclusively, against the predominant CFAs on human ETEC strains (i.e., CFA/I, CFA/II and CFA/IV). Different ETEC vaccine candidates have recently been considered based on these premises, e.g., live or inactivated vaccines that may provide both anticolonization and antitoxic immunities.

Attempts to use purified CFA antigens for immunization have yielded disappointing results. Not only are such antigens relatively expensive to prepare, but they have also proven to be very sensitive to proteolytic degradation in the human gastrointestinal tract, which probably explains their poor immunogenicity in human volunteer studies (Levine, 1990). Live bacteria expressing the major CFAs and producing LT-B may also be considered as ETEC vaccine candidates. If such strains could effectively colonize and multiply in the gut, they might provide a sustained antigen stimulation for the local intestinal immune system (Levine, 1990). However, since the different colonization factors are normally not expressed on the same strains and it has not yet been possible to successfully clone the genes for different CFAs in the same host organisms to allow stable surface expression of the different fimbriae, such vaccines must, at least for the time being, be based on a cocktail of several different strains. Thus, with any mixed vaccines there is a risk of overgrowth of one of the included vaccine strains with suppression of the others. Furthermore, live vaccines may have the risk of reverting to toxicity by uptake of toxin-encoding plasmids, low production of LT-B during growth *in vivo,* and poor survival of the vaccine strains during storage. Based on such considerations we have concluded that a more practical way to construct a vaccine is probably to prepare killed ETEC bacteria that express the most important CFAs on their surface and combine these organisms with an appropriate B-subunit component. Based on the cross-protection against LT-producing ETEC diarrhea noticed after immunization with CT-B-containing oral cholera vaccine and the availability of a very high-yield production system of recombinant CT-B, we regard CT-B to be an acceptable replacement of LT-B in such an ETEC vaccine. Therefore, in collaboration with SBL Vaccin we have developed a CT-B–CFA whole-cell ETEC (B-CFA ETEC) vaccine with the potential of providing broad protection against ETEC diseases in different countries.

A. Testing of a Prototype ETEC Vaccine

The first prototype vaccine consisting of a mixture of killed *E. coli* expressing CFA/I and the different CS-components of CFA/II and CT-B (Table II) has been produced. The B-subunit component was provided as conventionally purified subunits in the oral B-WC cholera vaccine. Strains that belong to common ETEC-γ sero-groups, i.e., O6, O78, and O139, and that express the different fimbriae in high concentrations were selected for preparation of the whole-cell component. The bacteria were inactivated by mild formalin-treatment, which resulted in complete killing of the bacteria without significant losses in antigenicity of the different CFAs and O-antigens (Svennerholm *et al.*, 1989). At variance with purified CFA, the CFA-antigens of the inactivated bacteria were stable after incubation in human gastrointestinal secretions containing acid and proteolytic enzymes (Svennerholm *et al.*, 1989).

The safety and immunogenicity of the prototype B-CFA ETEC vaccine have been studied in approximately 100 adult Swedish volunteers given two or three oral doses at 2-week intervals. Surveillance for side-effects revealed that the vaccine was safe, i.e., it did not give rise to any significant side effects (Wennerås *et al.*,

TABLE II
Oral B Subunit Whole-Cell ETEC Vaccines

Per dose composition
A. B-ETEC WC (prototype vaccine) 1 mg CT-B + 1 × 10^{11} formalin-killed ETEC expressing CFA/I and CFA/II (CS1 and CS2 + CS3) (the CT-B component is prepared by mixing the CFA ETEC WC with B-WC cholera vaccine, prep. A in Table I)
B. Recombinant B-CFA ETEC vaccine ("definitive" vaccine formulation) 1 mg rCT-B + 1 × 10^{11} formalin-killed ETEC expressing CFA/I, CFA/II (CS1 and CS2 + CS3) and CFA/IV [CS4 + (CS6) and CS5 + (CS6)]

1992; Åhrén *et al.*, 1993). Determination of specific immune responses in intestinal lavages was performed by determining specific ELISA IgA titers in relation to the total IgA content of each specimen. As shown in Table III, significant IgA antibody responses were observed against CFA/I, CFA/II, and CT-B in a majority of the vaccinees. In most cases maximal intestinal antibody responses were already achieved after two doses of vaccine (Åhrén *et al.*, 1993). The prototype ETEC vaccine also gave rise to significant increases in peripheral blood ASCs with specificities for CFA/I, CFA/II, and CT-B in 85–100% of the volunteers (Wennerås *et al.*, 1992). Responses were predominantly in IgA-producing cells, but high frequencies of IgM ASC responses against CFAs and of IgG ASCs against CT-B were also seen (Table III). Two oral immunizations seemed to be optimal in inducing specific immune reponses since neither specific IgA levels in intestinal lavages nor the number of CFA-specific ASCs increased after administration of a third dose of vaccine (Wennerås *et al.*, 1992; Åhrén *et al.*, 1993).

In spite of inducing significant immune responses locally in the intestine, the CFA component of the prototype ETEC vaccine was relatively inefficient in eliciting specific antibody responses against the different CFAs in serum. This was particularly evident when determining serum IgG responses against CFA/II, whereas IgA responses against CFA/I were more frequent. Particularly, the magnitude of the serum antibody responses against CFAs was considerably lower than that of the responses against either CFA/I or CFA/II in intestinal lavage fluid or that of corresponding ASC responses in peripheral blood (Wennerås *et al.*, 1992; Åhrén *et al.*, 1993). However, both the frequency and the magnitude of the immune responses against the CT-B component in serum were comparable to those in intestinal lavage fluid. Furthermore, whereas ASC responses against CFAs were predominant in IgA and IgM producing cells, significant ASC responses against the CT-B component were found only in IgA and IgG cells (Wennerås *et al.*, 1992). We also showed that a majority of volunteers given one or two oral immunizations with the prototype vaccine had responded with increased levels of circulating T cells capable of producing large quantities of interferon gamma (IFNγ) following *in vitro* exposure to either CFA/I or CFA/II (Wennerås *et al.*, 1994). The capacity of the CFA component of the vaccine to selectively induce a mucosal immune response has complicated evaluation of the immunogenicity of the vaccine in extended phase I/II trials. This is particularly true for children in endemic areas, in whom neither the intestinal lavage method nor determination of mucosal derived T or B cells in peripheral blood (which requires 20–30 ml whole blood for each specimen) could readily be used. Therefore, alternative methods to assess intestinal immune responses to peroral ETEC vaccines in large population groups, particularly in children, are required.

2. An Oral rB-CFA ETEC Vaccine

Based on the promising results from studies of the prototype ETEC vaccine in adult Swedish volunteers, a

TABLE III

Immune Responses against Oral CT-B-WC ETEC Vaccines in Swedish Volunteers

	Frequency (%) with significant responses						
	Prototype vaccine				rCT-B-CFA vaccine		
	Intestinal lavage	Blood ASC	Serum[a]		Blood ASC	Serum[c]	
Response to	IgA[a]	IgA[b]	IgA	IgG	IgA[c]	IgA	IgG
CFA/I	9/11 (82)	18/21 (86)	13/20 (65)	6/20 (30)	22/28 (79)	19/32 (59)	14/32 (44)
CS1 + CS3	9/11 (82)	19/21 (90)	3/20 (15)	2/20 (10)	25/32 (78)	N.T.	N.T.
CS2	8/11 (73)	N.T.	8/20 (40)	3/20 (15)	8/11 (73)	9/32 (28)	7/32 (22)
CS4	N.T.	N.T.	N.T.	N.T.	20/32 (63)	3/32 (9)	1/32 (3)
CS5	N.T.	N.T. (92)	N.T.	N.T.	26/32 (81)	5/32 (16)	3/32 (9)
CT-B	10/11 (91)	21/21 (100)	19/20 (95)	20/20 (100)	32/32 (100)	29/32 (91)	27/32 (84)

[a]Data from Åhrén *et al.* (1993).
[b]Data from Wennerås *et al.* (1992).
[c]Data from Jertborn *et al.* (1996b).

modified, more definitive formulation of the ETEC vaccine was produced by SBL Vaccin. This vaccine (Table II) contains recombinantly produced CT-B (the same as in the rB-WC cholera vaccine) in combination with five different *E. coli* strains expressing CFA/I and the different fimbrial subcomponents of CFA/II and CFA/IV. Based on numerous epidemiological studies of ETEC CFAs in different geographic areas, this modified ETEC vaccine has a potential protective coverage of at least 70–80%.

The rB-CFA ETEC vaccine has been evaluated for safety and immunogenicity in various Phase I/Phase II trials in different countries. Peroral administration of one, or in most instances, two doses of the vaccine 2 weeks apart to more than 300 Swedish, Bangladeshi, Egyptian, or American volunteers has shown that the vaccine is safe. The capacity of the rB-CFA vaccine to induce a mucosal immune response has been assessed predominately by determining ASC responses in peripheral blood against CT-B as well as the different CFAs in the vaccine, since our studies have suggested that peripheral blood ASC responses may be good proxy measures of intestinal immune responses. As shown in Table III the rB-CFA vaccine induced comparable frequencies of ASC responses against CFA/I, CFA/II, and CT-B as the prototype vaccine in Swedish adult volunteers. Furthermore, the rB-CFA ETEC vaccine, which also contains bacteria expressing CS4 and CS5, has induced ASC responses against these latter colonization factors in most instances (Jertborn *et al.*, 1996b).

In recent studies in Sweden, immune responses against CFAs and CT-B in intestinal lavage fluids have been compared with corresponding responses in serum and stool extracts, as well as with ASC-responses in peripheral blood. These analyses have shown a strong relationship between specific IgA responses in intestinal lavage fluid and peripheral blood IgA ASC responses (Åhrén *et al.*, 1996). The studies have also suggested that determination of anti-CFA antibodies in fecal extracts may be used as a proxy measure of immune responses in intestinal lavage fluid, although the sensitivity of determining immune responses in stool has been somewhat lower. Similar to the prototype vaccine, the rB-CFA ETEC vaccine has been considerably less efficient in inducing a serum antibody response against the different CFAs. In keeping with results from studies of the prototype vaccine, the CFA/I component has been more efficient than the other CFAs to elicit a specific IgA or IgG response in serum. A reason for this discrepancy between different CFA components of the vaccine to elicit systemic immune responses is unclear.

Phase I or Phase II trials of the rB-WC ETEC vaccine in different countries, e.g., Egypt and Bangladesh, have shown that the vaccine gives rise to frequencies of ASC responses in volunteers in all these ETEC endemic countries comparable to those in Sweden. Studies are also in progress in Bangladesh to compare immune responses induced by the ETEC vaccine and clinical disease in patients convalescing from ETEC diarrhea.

The promising results obtained from the studies of the rB-CFA ETEC vaccine in different countries have encouraged the planning of several phase III trials of the vaccine, both in children in endemic areas and in travellers to these areas. Due to the very high incidence of ETEC disease, e.g., in travellers to certain ETEC endemic areas, >50% incidence during a 3-week period (Sack, 1985), phase III studies could be undertaken in relatively small groups of volunteers. In a study that was initiated during Spring 1996, European travellers going for cruises on the Nile are given two doses of the vaccine or an *E. coli* K12 placebo in a double-blind fashion and the incidence of ETEC disease in the two study groups is evaluated during follow-up. In another trial, the ETEC vaccine will be tested for protective efficacy in Austrian travellers going to different countries in Asia, Africa, and Latin America. Studies are also planned, initially in Egypt and then in other ETEC-endemic countries (e.g., Bangladesh and Nicaragua) to test the vaccine for capacity to protect against ETEC diarrhea in children less than 5 years. The Phase III trials are preceded by extensive Phase II trials to confirm that the vaccine is safe and immunogenic also in young children. The results from these different studies may reveal the possibility of using an inactivated ETEC vaccine for immunoprophylaxis against traveller's diarrhea caused by ETEC as well as for use as a public health tool to control the most prevalent form of diarrhea in children in developing countries.

V. Summary

During the last decade there has been rapid progress in the development of new, much improved vaccines against cholera. These vaccines, which are given orally to stimulate specifically secretory IgA formation and immunologic memory in the gut mucosal immune system, are based either on a combination of purified cholera B subunit (CT-B) and killed *V. cholerae* O1 vibrios of the different serotypes and biotypes (B-WC vaccine) or on live attenuated mutant strains of *V. cholerae* producing CT-B (e.g., CVD103-HgR). The most extensively tested of these new vaccines, the oral B-WC cholera vaccine, has proved to be completely safe. Its excellent immunogenicity associated with high-level short-term protective efficacy (85% for the first 6 months in both children and adults) as well as good long-term protection (ca 70% over 3 years in vaccinees more than 5 years of age) against cholera has been documented, e.g., in a large, randomized, placebo-controlled field trial in 90,000 persons living in a cholera-endemic area. The newly emerging cholera endemic caused by a new serogroup of *V. cholerae,* O139, has also led us to develop a second-generation CT-B-WC cholera vaccine containing the new serotype as an additional WC vaccine component. Because of the cross-reacting enterotoxins, the B-WC cholera vaccine also confers significant (60–70%) short-term protection against diarrhea caused by LT-producing enterotoxigenic *E. coli.* Based on the latter finding, a specific oral vaccine against ETEC diarrhea based on a combination of CT-B and different colonization antigens (CFA/I, CFA/II, and CFA/IV) expressed on killed *E. coli* has now been developed and proved to be safe and immunogenic in Phase I/II trials in humans. The introduction of recombinant DNA technology for production of the B-subunit component has facilitated inexpensive large-scale manufacturing of both the cholera and ETEC vaccines. In addition to being useful prophylactic agents in travellers, these vaccines will hopefully become cost-effective public health tools in future strategies to control cholera and *E. coli* diarrhea in developing countries.

Acknowledgments

The authors thank Drs. M. Jertborn, C. Åhrén and C. Wennerås for their important contributions to the Phase I and Phase II trials of cholera and ETEC vaccines in Sweden, F. Qadri, P. K. Bardhan, C. Wennerås, and R. B. Sack for conducting the ETEC vaccine trial in Bangladesh, and Dr. S. Savarino, M. Brown, E. Hall, J. Clemens *et al.* for performing Phase I and Phase II studies of ETEC vaccines in Egypt. We remain indebted to Dr. J. Clemens, D. A. Sack, and ICDDR,B for invaluable collaboration over many years, especially with the field testing of oral cholera vaccines. We also thank SBL Vaccin AB, Stockholm, Sweden, for their active participation over many years in the development and production of the different vaccines described in this chapter. Financial support for our studies has been obtained from the Swedish Medial Research Council, The Swedish Agency for Research Cooperation with Developing Countries, and the World Health Organization.

References

Åhrén, C. M., and Svennerholm, A.-M. (1985). Experimental enterotoxin-induced *Escherichia coli* diarrhea and protection induced by previous infection with bacteria of the same adhesin or enterotoxin type. *Infect. Immun.* **50,** 255–261.

Åhrén, C., Wennerås, C., Holmgren, J., and Svennerholm, A.-M. (1993). Intestinal antibody response after oral immunization with a prototype enterotoxigenic *Escherichia coli* vaccine. *Vaccine* **11,** 929–934.

Åhrén, C., Jertborn, M., and Svennerholm, A.-M. (1996). Intestinal immune response and its reflection in blood after immunization with an oral ETEC vaccine. In preparation.

Black, R. E. (1986). The epidemiology of cholera and enterotoxigenic *E. coli* diarrheal disease. *In* "Development of Vaccines and Drugs against Diarrhea" (J. Holmgren, A. Lindberg, and R. Möllby, eds.), pp. 23–32. 11th Nobel Conference, Stockholm, Lund, Studentlitteratur.

Black, R. E. (1990). Epidemiology of traveller's diarrhea and relative importance of various pathogens. *Rev. Infect. Dis.* **12,** S73-S79.

Black, R. E., Levine, M. M., Clemens, M. L., Young, C. R., Svennerholm, A.-M., and Holmgren, J. (1987). Protective efficacy in man of killed whole vibrio oral cholera vaccine with and without the B subunit of cholera toxin. *Infect. Immun.* **77,** 1116–1129.

Blake, P. A. (1994). Historical perspectives on pandemic cholera. *In* "*Vibrio cholerae* and Cholera: Molecular to Global Perspectives" (I. K. Wachsmuth, P. A. Blake, and Ø. Olsvik, eds.), pp. 293–295. American Society for Microbiology, Washington, D.C.

Clemens, J., Sack, D. A., Harris, J. R., Chakraborty, J., Khan, M. R., Stanton, B. F., (1986). Field trial of oral cholera vaccines in Bangladesh. *Lancet* **1,** 124–127.

Clemens, J., Sack, D. A., Harris, J. R., Chakraborty, J., Neogy, P. K., Stanton, B. F., Kay, B. A., Khan, M. U., Yunus, M. D., Atkinson, W., Svennerholm, A.-M., and Holmgren, J. (1988a). Cross-protection by B subunit–whole cell cholera vaccine against diarrhea associated with heat-labile toxin-producing enterotoxigenic *Escherichia coli*: Results of a large-scale field trial. *J. Infect. Dis.* **158,** 372–377.

Clemens, J. D., Sack, D. A., Harris, J. R., Chakraborty, J., Khan, M. R., Stanton, B. F., Ali, M., Ahmed, F., Yunus, M., Kay, B. A., Khan, M. U., Rao, M. R., Svennerholm, A.-M., and Holmgren, J. (1988b). Impact of B subunit killed whole-cell and killed whole-cell-only oral vaccines against cholera upon treated diarrhoeal illness and mortality in an area endemic for cholera. *Lancet* **1,** 1375–1379.

Clemens, J. D., Sack, D. A., Harris, J. R., van Loon, F., Chakraborty, J., Ahmed, F., Rao, M. R., Khan, M. R., Yunus, M. D., Huda, N., Stanton, B. F., Kay, B. A., Walter, S., Ecckels, R., Svennerholm, A.-M., and Holmgren, J. (1990). Field trial of oral cholera vaccines in Bangladesh: Results from three-year follow-up. *Lancet* **355,** 270–273.

Coster, T. S., Killeen, K. P., Waldor, M. K., Beattie, D. T., Spriggs, D. R., Kenner, J. R., Trofa, A., Sadoff, J. C., Mekalanos, J. J., and Taylor, D. N. (1995). Safety, immunogenicity, and efficacy of live attenuated *Vibrio cholerae* O139 vaccine prototype. *Lancet* **345,** 949–952.

Cravioto, A., Reyes, R. E., Ortega, R., Fernandéz, G., Hernandez, R., and López, D. (1988). Prospective study of diarrhoeal diseases in a cohort of rural Mexican children: Incidence and isolated pathogens during the first two years of life. *Epidemiol. Infect.* **101,** 123–134.

Evans, D. J., and Evans, D. G. (1989). Determinants of microbial attachment and their genetic control. *In* "Enteric

Infection. Mechanisms, Manifestations and Management" (M. J. G. Farthing and G. T. Keusch, eds.), pp. 31–40. Chapman & Hall, London.

Farthing, M. J. G., and Keusch, G. T. (eds.) (1989). "Enteric Infection. Mechanisms, Manifestations and Management." Chapman & Hall, London.

Feeley, J. C., and Gangarosa, E. J. (1980). Field trials of cholera vaccine. *In* "Cholera and Related Diarrheas" (Ö. Ouchterlony and J. Holmgren, eds.), pp. 204–210. 43rd Nobel Symp., Stockholm, 1978. Karger, Basel.

Frantz, J. C., and Robertson, D. C. (1981). Immunological properties of *Escherichia coli* heat-stable enterotoxins: Development of a radioimmunoassay specific for heat-stable enterotoxins with suckling mouse activity. *Infect. Immun.* **33,** 193–198.

Guerrant, R. L. (1985). Microbial toxins and diarrhoeal disease: Introduction and overview. *In* "Microbial Toxins and Diarrhoeal Disease" (D. Evered and J. Whelan, eds.), pp. 1–13. Ciba Foundation Symposium 112, Pitman, London.

Holmgren, J. (1981). Actions of cholera toxin and the prevention and treatment of cholera. *Nature (London)* **292,** 413–417.

Holmgren, J., and Svennerholm, A.-M. (1983). Cholera and the immune response. *Prog. Allergy* **33,** 106–119.

Holmgren, J., and Svennerholm, A.-M. (1992). Bacterial enteric infections and vaccine development. *In* "Mucosal Immunology, Gastroenterology Clinics of North America" (R. P. McDermott and C. O. Elson, eds.), pp. 283–302. Saunders, Philadelphia, Pennsylvania.

Holmgren, J., Svennerholm, A.-M., Lönnroth, I., Fall-Persson, M., Markman, B., and Lundbäck, H. (1977). Development of improved cholera vaccine based on subunit toxoid. *Nature (London)* **269,** 602–604.

Jertborn, M., Svennerholm, A.-M., and Holmgren, J. (1988). Five-year immunologic memory in Swedish volunteers after oral cholera vaccination. *J. Infect. Dis.* **157,** 374–377.

Jertborn, M., Svennerholm, A.-M., and Holmgren, J. (1996a). Intestinal and systemic immune responses in humans after oral immunization with a bivalent B subunit–O1/O139 whole cell cholera vaccine. *Vaccine.* In press.

Jertborn, M., Åhrén, C., Holmgren, J., and Svennerholm, A.-M. (1996b). Clinical trials of an oral inactivated enterotoxigenic *Escherichia coli* vaccine. Submitted for publication.

Jonson, G., Holmgren, J., and Svennerholm, A.-M. (1991). Identification of a mannose-binding pilus on *Vibrio cholerae* El Tor. *Microbial Pathogen.* **11,** 433–441.

Jonson, G., Osek, J., Svennerholm, A.-M., and Holmgren, J. (1996). Immune mechanisms and protective antigens of *Vibrio cholerae* serogroup O139 as a basis for vaccine development. *Infect. Immun.* In press.

Kaper, J. B. (1990). Attenuated *Vibrio cholerae* strains prepared by recombinant DNA techniques used as live oral vaccines. *In* "New Generation Vaccines" (G. C. Woodrow and M. M. Levine, eds.), pp. 304–310. Dekker, Basel.

Kaper, J. B., Lockman, H., Baldini, M. M., and Levine, M. M. (1984a). A recombinant live oral cholera vaccine. *Bio/Technology* **2,** 345–349.

Kaper, J. B., Lockman, H., Baldini, M. M., and Levine, M. M. (1984b). Recombinant nontoxigenic *Vibrio cholerae* strains as attenuated cholera vaccine candidates. *Nature (London)* **308,** 655–658.

Lebens, M., Shahabi, V., Bäckström, M., Houze, T., Lindblad, M., and Holmgren, J. (1996). Synthesis of hybrid molecules between heat-labile entertoxin and cholera toxin B subunits: Potential for use in broad spectrum vaccine. *Infect. Immun.* **64,** 2144–2150.

Levine, M. M. (1990). Vaccines against enterotoxigenic *Escherichia coli* infections. *In* "New Generation Vaccines" (G. C. Woodrow and M. M. Levine, eds.), pp. 649–660. Dekker, New York.

Levine, M. M., and Tacket, C. O. (1995). Live oral vaccines against cholera. *In* "Molecular and Clinical Aspects of Bacterial Vaccine Development" (D. A. A. Ala'Aldeen and C. E. Hormaeche, eds.), pp. 233–258. Wiley, Chichester, England.

López-Vidal, Y., Calva, J. J., Trujillo, A., de León, A. P., Ramos, A., Svennerholm, A.-M., and Ruiz-Palacios, G. M. (1990). Enterotoxins and adhesins of enterotoxigenic *Escherichia coli*: Are they risk factors for acute diarrhea in the community? *J. Infect. Dis.* **162,** 442–447.

McConnell, M. M. (1991). Newly characterized putative colonization factors of human enterotoxigenic *Escherichia coli. In* "Molecular Pathogenesis of Gastrointestinal Infections" (T. Wadström, P. H. Mäkelä, A.-M. Svennerholm, and H. Wolf-Watz, eds.), pp. 79–85. FEMS Symposium Number 58, Helsingør. Plenum, New York and London.

Morris, J. G. (1994). *Vibrio cholerae* O139 Bengal. *In* "*Vibrio cholerae* and Cholera: Molecular to Global Perspectives" (I. K. Wachsmuth, P. A. Blake, and Ø. Olsvik, eds.), pp. 95–102. American Society for Microbiology, Washington, D.C.

Mosley, W. H., Ahmed, S., Benenson, A. S., and Ahmed, A. (1968). The relationship of vibriocidal antibody titre to susceptibility to cholera in family contacts of cholera patients. *Bull. WHO* **38,** 777–785.

Neutra, M. R., and Kraehenbühl, J.-P. (1992). Transepithelial transport and mucosal defence I: The role of M cells. *Trends Cell. Biol.* **2,** 134–138. Elsevier Science Publishers Ltd.

Osek, J., Svennerholm, A.-M., and Holmgren, J. (1992). Protection against *Vibrio cholerae* El Tor infection by specific antibodies against mannose-binding hemagglutinin pili. *Infect. Immun.* **60,** 4961–4964.

Peltola, H., Siitonen, A., Kyrönseppä, H., Simula, I., Mattila, L., Oksanen, P., Kataja, M. J., and Cadoz, M. (1991). Prevention of travellers' diarrhoea by oral B-subunit/whole cell cholera vaccine. *Lancet* **338,** 1285–1289.

Quiding, M., Nordström, I., Kilander, A., Andersson, G., Hanson, L.-Å., Holmgren, J., and Czerkinsky, C. (1991). Intestinal immune responses in humans. Oral cholera vaccination induces strong intestinal antibody responses, gamma-interferon production, and evokes local immunological memory. *J. Clin. Invest.* **88,** 143–148.

Sack, R. B. (1985). Treatment and prevention of travellers diarrhea. *In* "Development and Drugs against Diarrhea" (J. Holmgren, A. Lindberg, and R. Möllby, eds.), pp. 298–301. 11th Nobel Conference Stockholm. Studentlitteratur, Lund, Sweden.

Sack, D. A., and Freij, L. (1990). Prospects for public health benefits in developing countries from new vaccines against enteric infections. SAREC documentation, conference report 1990:2, SAREC symposium, Gothenburg, Sweden, 28–29 May.

Sack, D. A., Freij, L., and Holmgren, J. (1991). Prospects for public health benefits in developing countries from new vaccines against enteric infections. *J. Infect. Dis.* **163**, 503–506.

Sanchez, J., and Holmgren, J. (1989). Recombinant system for overexpression of cholera toxin B subunit in *Vibrio cholerae* as a basis for vaccine development. *Proc. Natl. Acad. Sci. U.S.A.* **86**, 481–485.

Sanchez, J., Svennerholm, A.-M., and Holmgren, J. (1988). Genetic fusion of a non-toxic heat-stable enterotoxin-related decapeptide antigen to cholera toxin B-subunit. *FEBS Lett.* **241**, 110–114.

Sanchez, J. L., Vasques, B., Begue, R. E., Meza, R., Castellares, G., Cabezas, C., Watts, D. M., Svennerholm, A.-M., Sadoff, J. C., and Taylor, D. N. (1994). Protective efficacy of the oral, whole cell/recombinant B subunit cholera vaccine in Peruvian military recruits, *Lancet* **344**, 1273–1276.

Svennerholm, A.-M. (1980). The nature of protective immunity in cholera. *In* "Cholera and Related Diarrheal Disease" (Ö. Ouchterlony and J. Holmgren, eds.), pp. 171–184. 43rd Nobel Symposium, Stockholm, 1978. Karger, Basel.

Svennerholm, A.-M., and Holmgren, J. (1976). Synergistic protective effect in rabbits of immunization with *Vibrio cholerae* lipopolysaccharide and toxin/toxoid. *Infect. Immun.* **13**, 735–740.

Svennerholm, A.-M., and Holmgren, J. (1995). Oral B-subunit whole-cell vaccines against cholera and enterotoxigenic *Escherichia coli* diarrhoea. *In* "Molecular and Clinical Aspects of Bacterial Vaccine Development" (D. A. A. Ala'Aldeen and C. E. Hormaeche, eds.), pp. 205–232. Wiley, Chichester, England.

Svennerholm, A.-M., Jertborn, M., Gothefors, L., Karim, M., Sack, D. A., and Holmgren, J. (1984). Mucosal antitoxic and antibacterial immunity after cholera disease and after immunization with a combined B subunit–whole cell vaccine. *J. Infect. Dis.* **149**, 884–893.

Svennerholm, A.-M., Wikström, M., Lindblad, M., and Holmgren, J. (1986a). Monoclonal antibodies to *Escherichia coli* heat-labile enterotoxins: Neutralizing activity and differentiation of human and porcine LTs and cholera toxin. *Med. Biol.* **64**, 23–30.

Svennerholm, A.-M, Wikström, M., Lindblad, M., and Holmgren, J. (1986b). Monoclonal antibodies against *E. coli* heat-stable toxin (STa) and their use in diagnostic ST ganglioside G_{M1}-enzyme-linked immunosorbent assay. *J. Clin. Microbiol.* **24**, 585–590.

Svennerholm, A.-M., Holmgren, J., and Sack, D. A. (1989). Development of oral vaccines against enterotoxigenic *Escherichia coli* diarrhoea. *Vaccine* **7**, 196–198.

Svennerholm, A.-M., Wennerås, C., Holmgren, J., McConnell, M. M., and Rowe, B. (1990). Roles of different coli surface antigens of colonization factor antigen II in colonization by and protective immunogenicity of enterotoxigenic *Escherichia coli* in rabbits. *Infect. Immun.* **58**, 341–346.

Svennerholm, A.-M., McConnell, M. M., and Wiklund, G. (1992). Roles of different putative colonization factor antigens in colonization of human enterotoxigenic *Escherichia coli* in rabbits. *Microbial Pathogen.* **13**, 381–389.

Tacket, C. O., Losonsky, G., Nataro, J. P., Comstock, L., Michalski, J., Edelman, R., Kaper, J. B., and Levine, M. M. (1995). Initial clinical studies of CVD 112 *Vibrio cholerae* O139 live oral vaccine: Safety and efficacy against experimental challenge. *J. Infect. Dis.* **172**, 883–886.

Tauxe, R., Seminario, L., Tapia, R., and Libel, M. (1994). The Latin American epidemic. *In* "*Vibrio cholerae* and Cholera: Molecular to Global Perspectives" (I. K. Wachsmuth, P. A. Blake, and Ø. Olsvik, eds.), pp. 321–344. American Society for Microbiology, Washington, D.C.

Taylor, D. N., Killeen, K. P., Hack, D. C., Kenner, J. K., Coster, T. S., Beattie, D. T., Ezzell, J., Hyman, T., Trofa, A., Sjogren, M. H., Friedlander, A., Mekalanos, J. J., and Sadoff, J. C. (1994). Development of a live, oral and attenuated vaccine against El Tor cholera. *J. Infect. Dis.* **170**, 1518–1523.

Taylor, R. K., Miller, V. L., Furlong, D. B., and Mekalanos, J. J. (1987). Use of *phoA* gene fusions to identify a pilus colonization factor coordinately regulated with cholera toxin. *Proc. Natl. Acad. Sci. USA* **84**, 2833–2837.

Tayot, J.-L., Holmgren, J., Svennerholm, L., Lindblad, M., and Tardy, M. (1981). Receptor-specific large scale purification of cholera toxin on silica beads derivatized with lyso-G_{M1} ganglioside. *Eur. J. Biochem.* **113**, 249–258.

Trach, D. D., Clemens, J. D., Ke, N. T., Thuy, H. T., Son, N. D., Canh, D. G., Hang, P. V. D., and Rao, M. R. (1996). Field trial of a locally produced, killed oral cholera vaccine in Vietnam. Submitted for publication.

Waldor, M. K., and Mekalanos, J. J. (1994). Emergence of a new cholera pandemic: Molecular analysis of virulence determinants in *Vibrio cholerae* O139 and development of a live vaccine prototype. *J. Infect. Dis.* **170**, 278–283.

Wennerås, C., Svennerholm, A.-M., Åhrén, C., and Czerkinsky, C. (1992). Antibody-secreting cells in human peripheral blood after oral immunization with an inactivated enterotoxigenic *Escherichia coli* vaccine. *Infect. Immun.* **60**, 2605–2611.

Wennerås, C., Svennerholm, A.-M., and Czerkinsky, C. (1994). Vaccine-specific T cells in human peripheral blood after oral immunization with an inactivated enterotoxigenic *Escherichia coli* vaccine. *Infect. Immun.* **62**, 874–879.

Voss, E., Manning, P., and Attridge, S. (1996). The toxin-coregulated pilus is a colonization factor and protective antigen of Vibrio cholerae El Tor. *Microbial Pathogen.* **20**, 141–153.

19

Mucosal Immunity to H. pylori: *Implications for Vaccine Development*

PETER B. ERNST*,†
VICTOR E. REYES*
*Department of Pediatrics and
†Sealy Center for Molecular Sciences
University of Texas Medical Branch
Galveston, Texas 77555

JOHN G. NEDRUD‡
STEVEN J. CZINN§
‡Institute of Pathology and
§Department of Pediatrics
Case Western Reserve University
Cleveland, Ohio 44106

I. Introduction

Over half the population on Earth is persistently infected with *Helicobacter pylori*. Although this bacteria will cause gastritis in all infected individuals, most will remain asymptomatic even though they are infected for life. However, *H. pylori* is necessary for most recurrent peptic ulcers and is also implicated as an important factor in the pathogenesis of gastric cancer (Blaser, 1990; Rauws and Tytgat, 1990; Loffeld *et al.*, 1991; Graham, 1991a; Fonthan *et al.*, 1995; Correa, 1995). Humans appear to be the major reservoir for *H. pylori* and the infection is virtually endemic in developing countries. Unfortunately, specific preventive measures that would curtail new infections are not currently known. The organism is susceptible to antimicrobial therapy but the regimes are somewhat cumbersome and expensive. Antibiotic resistance is also emerging. It is unlikely that antibiotics and altered practices in prevention will be sufficient to eliminate this infection. Thus, the development of a vaccine offers a tremendous opportunity to treat as well as prevent infection and thereby virtually eliminate many severe gastroduodenal diseases. This chapter will summarize some of the bacteriological properties of *H. pylori* that identify useful antigens for vaccine development. In addition, the interesting immunobiology of this infection will be discussed and contrasted to immunological responses that should allow the host to develop protective immunity after oral immunization.

II. Overview of *H. pylori* Infection

Organisms we now know as *H. pylori* have been recognized in the human gastric mucosa for many years. However, it was only after a more recent series of provocative reports that investigators renewed their interest in the role of *H. pylori* in gastroduodenal disease (Marshall and Warren, 1984; Marshall *et al.*, 1985). It is now clear that *H. pylori* is sufficient to cause gastritis (Blaser, 1992; Fonthan *et al.*, 1995). In addition, cure of *H. pylori* infection with antibiotics can prevent most gastric ulcers and virtually all duodenal ulcers (Rauws and Tytgat, 1990; Graham *et al.*, 1992). Other changes in the gastric mucosa are also associated with *H. pylori* infection, including the accumulation of lymphoid aggregates as well as epithelial cell metaplasia and atrophy (Correa, 1995). Thus, the scope of diseases associated with this bacteria has been expanded to include gastric cancers including B cell lymphomas (maltomas) as well as adenocarcinoma (Talley *et al.*, 1991; Parsonnet *et al.*, 1991; Correa, 1995).

With the recognition of *H. pylori* infection in the pathogenesis of gastric disease, several epidemiological studies have been pursued. These are reviewed in detail elsewhere (Blaser, 1992; Talley *et al.*, 1991) but some of these findings have implications for vaccine development. First of all, it is clear that more people on this planet are infected than are uninfected. The rate of infection has been decreasing in developed countries; however, the incidence approaches 95% in economically developing nations. The linkage of infection with economic factors is illustrated by the observation that the prevalence of infection in the United States is far greater in people with lower incomes than in those with higher incomes (Graham *et al.*, 1991b; Hoda *et al.*, 1992). Although some animals may be infected with *H. pylori,* humans are a major reservoir and may spread the infection through oral–oral or fecal–oral modes of transmission. It is believed that infection occurs primarily in childhood (Fiedorek *et al.*, 1991; Banatvala *et al.*, 1993) and persists for life. These findings point to the inadequacies of natural immunity since it is ineffective at clearing the infection. Moreover, any strategy for preventive vaccines will have to be applied to children since they are the population at highest risk of becoming infected.

The organism has many properties that facilitate its ability to exist in the harsh, acidic environment of the stomach. *H. pylori* produces a urease enzyme that catalyzes the conversion of urea to ammonia that in turn can act as a base and buffer luminal acidity (Mobley *et al.*, 1991). This activity is believed to be necessary in order to permit infection. *H. pylori* is also quite motile and moves through the mucus to the area adjacent to the epithelial surface. Once under the mucus layer, *H. pylori* enjoys the same cytoprotective environment that protects the gastric epithelium from autodigestion by luminal acid. *H. pylori* binds to gastric epithelial cells, although the structure or structures responsible for the binding remain to be completely defined (Dytoc *et al.*, 1992; Clyne and Drumm, 1993). The molecules and structures involved in colonization, motility, and binding have been considered to be of potential use as vaccine antigens.

One of the interesting features of *H. pylori* is the remarkable genetic diversity of the different isolates. Although this has been an extremely useful epidemiological tool, the purpose of this diversified genome is unclear. It does not appear, at least as of yet, that this heterogeneity provides the organism with a phenotypic diversity that would enhance immune avoidance. Since most people who are infected with *H. pylori* will remain asymptomatic, it is believed that some of the heterogeneity among the different isolates will reflect virulence factors that may be associated with a higher risk of gastroduodenal disease (Yoshimura *et al.*, 1994; Xiang *et al.*, 1995). In fact, *H. pylori* have been classified as Type I or Type II based on their expression of *cagA* and *vacA*—two genes that mark strains found in greater frequency in diseased individuals than in asymptomatic controls. Thus, virulence factors may also be useful as antigens for an effective vaccine.

III. Gastric Immune and Inflammatory Responses to *H. pylori* Infection

A. Induction of Gastric Immunity

Perhaps due to the bias that the stomach was rarely infected, relatively few reports have described immunological mechanisms in the human stomach. Most of the current opinion on the induction of gastric immune and inflammatory responses has been based on our knowledge of similar responses in the intestine that are discussed extensively elsewhere in this volume. However, the recognition of *H. pylori* has stimulated additional research into the tissue-specific properties of gastric immunity.

In general, the first step in developing immunity to infection requires the host to recognize that a microbe is in fact a pathogen and not a commensal. In the stomach, this process is triggered by damage and the ability of *H. pylori* to induce a nonspecific, acute inflammatory response. In order to fulfill the requirement that the host responds appropriately, regulatory T cells must be optimally activated. This model suggests that effective gastric immunity will require that *H. pylori* induces sufficient inflammation and damage to trigger a response. The inability to clear infection and the subsequent development of gastroduodenal disease likely results from inappropriate T-cell regulation.

B. The Role of Epithelial Cells in the Induction of Gastric Immune/Inflammatory Responses

The importance of local antigen stimulation in the recruitment and activation of mucosal immunity is supported by two observations. First of all, there is a paucity of lymphocytic infiltration throughout the entire digestive tract in germfree animals. Second, very few T or B cells are observed in the gastric mucosa in the absence of *H. pylori* or some other local stimulus such as nonsteroidal anti-inflammatory drugs. Thus, factors within the effector sites, including antigen, chemokines, and adhesion molecules, may be particularly important for the accumulation of immune and inflammatory cells required for the induction of immunity against a gastric infection with *H. pylori.*

Crabtree and colleagues have conducted several studies documenting the ability of *H. pylori* to activate neutrophils by stimulating IL-8 production in the gastric mucosa and in the epithelium (Crabtree *et al.*, 1993, 1994b). These original observations have been extended in other reports showing that *H. pylori* induces the accumulation of mRNA for IL-8 and stimulates the secretion of immunoreactive as well as biologically active IL-8 from gastric epithelial cell lines (Crowe *et al.*, 1995; Sharma *et al.*, 1995; Huang *et al.*, 1995). This *in vitro* evaluation correlates with the increase in neutrophils and IL-8 in the mucosa (Mai *et al.*, 1992; Moss *et al.*, 1995). Moreover, *H. pylori* induces IL-8 without invasion in gastric cell lines (Crowe *et al.*, 1995) suggesting that the natural tropism between *H. pylori* and gastric epithelium is mimicked in these *in vitro* approaches.

Several reports suggest that killed *H. pylori* do not stimulate IL-8 production from the epithelium (Crowe *et al.*, 1995; Sharma *et al.*, 1995) while another report indicates that secreted products from *H. pylori* do, particularly in nongastric cells (Huang *et al.*, 1995). This apparent discrepancy may result from the use of different strains of *H. pylori* and the length of time used for epithelial stimulation. Strain differences in the IL-8 response became apparent when *H. pylori* bearing the cytotoxin associated gene *CagA* were associated with more severe gastric pathology and IL-8 production. This conclusion was based on the fact that natural mutants lacking *CagA* did not induce IL-8 *in vitro* (Crabtree *et al.*, 1994a). A more recent study shows that isogenic mutants lacking *CagA* and/or *VacA* are still capable of inducing IL-8 (Sharma *et al.*, 1995). Therefore, while these genes may mark virulence, other genes in close physical association with *CagA* and/or *VacA* loci may be necessary for IL-8 induction. Molecules such as the *CagA* and *VacA* products that may be important in inflammatory responses could also be excellent candidates for vaccine antigens. However, since the *CagA*/*VacA* products are expressed by only 50–60% of *H. pylori* strains, it would also be important that any vaccine include other antigens which are common to all strains.

C. Induction of Inflammation within the Gastric Lamina Propria

Although *H. pylori* is rarely invasive, proinflammatory material is shed and reaches the underlying fibroblasts and inflammatory cells, particularly if the epithelial barrier function is compromised. The gene coding for a novel neutrophil-activating protein (HP-NAP) has recently been cloned from *H. pylori* and shown to enhance the binding of neutrophils to endothelium (Evans *et al.*, 1995). Formylated tripeptides, LPS (Nielsen *et al.*, 1994), urease (Mai *et al.*, 1992), or other factors produced by the bacterium may also lead to changes in the migration (Mai *et al.*, 1992), adhesion (Evans *et al.*, 1995; Ender *et al.*, 1995), and activation of neutrophils (Nielsen and Andersen, 1992; Norgaard *et al.*, 1995) or monocytes (Mai *et al.*, 1991; Perez-Perez *et al.*, 1995). Stimulated monocytes/macrophages and fibroblasts produce other cytokines such as IL-1, IL-6, or TNFα (Crabtree *et al.*, 1991; Noach *et al.*, 1994; Fuachere and Andersen, 1995) and RANTES (H. Häberle and P. B. Ernst, unpublished observation, 1995). These cytokines can recruit and activate immune and inflammatory cells as well as increase the expression of adhesion molecules that facilitate the adherence and activation of these cells.

Gastritis can occur in the absence of T and B cells following infection of immunodeficient mice with *H. felis* (Blanchard *et al.*, 1995b). This suggests that a significant portion of the changes in patients infected with *H. pylori* result from nonspecific inflammatory responses. Although *H. pylori* can induce gastritis in T- and B-cell-deficient mice (Blanchard *et al.*, 1995b), it is likely that both lymphoid and myeloid cells collaborate with the organism itself to cause gastritis and possibly gastroduodenal disease, including peptic ulcer (Ernst *et al.*, 1995).

D. Regulatory T Cells in Gastric Tissue during Infection with *H. pylori*

Immunological effector mechanisms may be driven by antigen but the magnitude and type of immune response that develops is largely dictated by cytokines derived from T cells. In the healthy stomach, there are very few lymphocytes in the lamina propria while a few $CD8^+$ T cells are found within the epithelium (Kirchner *et al.*, 1990). However, during gastritis, including that seen with an infection with *H. pylori,* there is an increase in both $CD8^+$ (Fan *et al.*, 1994) and $CD4^+$ T cells (Valnes *et al.*, 1990) within the gastric mucosa. Karttunen and colleagues (1995) have made the observation that the number of interferon-γ (IFNγ)-producing cells is increased during infection with *H. pylori*, suggesting that Th1 cells may predominate. The presence of Th1 cells and IFNγ production are likely to lead to immunophysiological interactions that directly promote tissue damage. For example, IFNγ alters epithelial barrier function in intestinal cell lines (Madara and Stafford, 1989). Other cytokines, including TNFα, can collaborate with IFNγ to alter epithelial cell IL-8 gene expression (Yasumoto *et al.*, 1992).

The evidence that Th1 cells may be increased relative to Th2 cells during *H. pylori* infection suggests that a marked skewing in this response may lead to disease as implicated in the pathogenesis of more classical autoimmune diseases (Liblau *et al.*, 1995).

This notion is supported by a report describing the development of colitis in mice following the ablation of the gene coding for IL-10, a cytokine which selects for Th2 responses (Kuhn *et al.*, 1993). This disease is driven by luminal bacteria as animals maintained in an environment free of flora do not develop colitis. Moreover, recent observations showed that treating *H. felis*-infected mice with neutralizing antibodies recognizing IFNγ markedly attenuated gastric inflammation suggesting that Th1 cells contribute to the magnitude of the inflammatory response following infection with *Heli-*

cobacter (Mohammadi *et al.*, 1996). Thus, the inappropriate regulation of the host response to luminal flora is paramount in determining whether a host will develop protective immunity or chronic inflammation.

E. B-Cell Responses to *H. pylori*

Many B cells and plasma cells are evident in the gastric mucosa during infection with *H. pylori.* In fact, lymphoid aggregates that contain many B cells are an extremely common finding in the gastric mucosa during infection (Isaacson, 1982). Several reports have documented an increase in IgM, IgG, and IgA antibodies in serum or gastric tissue (Wyatt *et al.*, 1986; Witt, 1991; Stacey *et al.*, 1990; Rathbone *et al.*, 1988) following *H. pylori* infection as well as increases in IgG and IgA antibody-producing cells in the mucosa in association with gastritis (Isaacson, 1982; Valnes *et al.*, 1986). The inability of these antibodies to confer adequate protection may reflect the fact that they are of the wrong isotype or specificity. In fact, evidence suggests that the antibodies induced with natural infection may contribute to local inflammation through antigen–antibody complex formation. For example, IgM antibodies produced from immortalized B cells obtained from the gastric mucosa have been shown to recognize the gastric epithelium (Vollmers *et al.*, 1994). Other evidence suggests that B cells within a gastric maltoma express an idiotype that recognizes a determinant shared by both IgA and IgM (Greiner *et al.*, 1994). These autoantibodies may be of importance in the phenomenon of postimmunization gastritis discussed below.

F. Implications for Immunotherapy

Given that individuals remain persistently infected with *H. pylori,* one can assume that the host response is qualitatively or quantitatively inappropriate. While this may have implications for the development of gastroduodenal disease, it also creates a window of opportunity to use immunotherapy for the treatment or prevention of *H. pylori* infection. For example, if in fact it is correct that Th1 cells predominate, then one could predict that increasing the relative numbers of Th2 cells may be sufficient to enhance immunity and eliminate or prevent the infection (Fig. 1). Shifting the Th cell phenotype by artificial immunization may affect the isotype, specificity, and avidity of antibodies that emerge from a B-cell

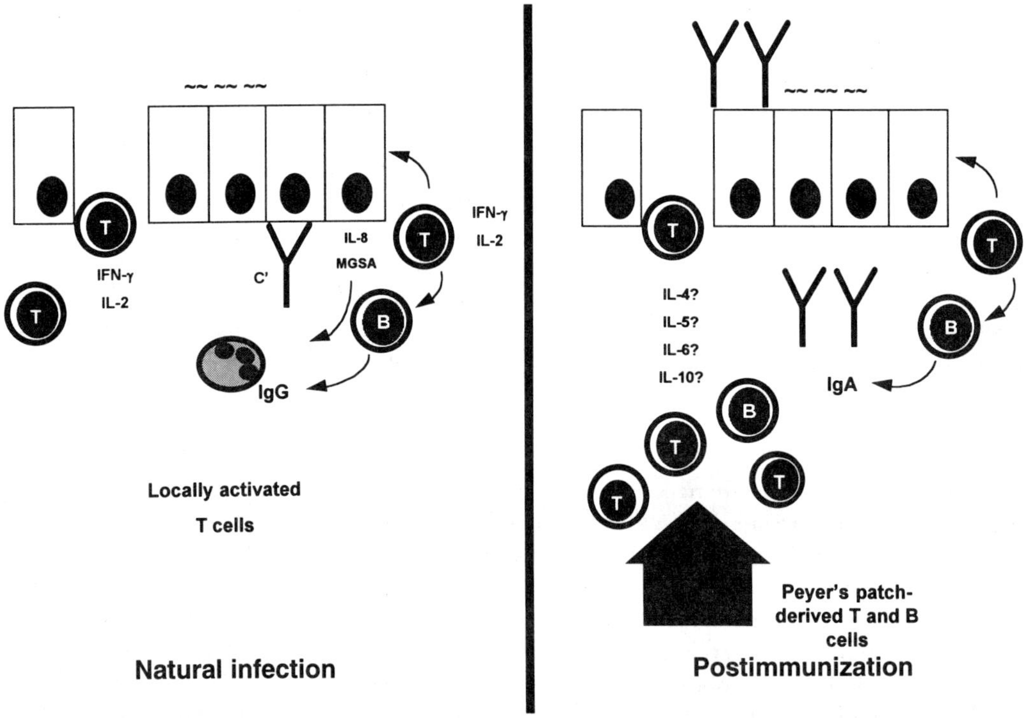

Figure 1. The mucosal inflammation associated with a persistent, natural infection with *H. pylori* leads to a Th1 response and the accumulation of B cells and neutrophils in the gastric mucosa of the inflamed stomach. This response may subvert the preferred strategy of developing protection without inflammation. Effective immunity may be induced by vaccines that increase the relative magnitude of the cytokines associated with a Th2 response since Th2 cells satisfy the criterion of selecting for protective mucosal IgA responses while inhibiting potentially proinflammatory cell-mediated immunity. Oral immunization may induce IgA-enhancing Th2 cells from Peyer's patches which, in turn, will migrate to the stomach in response to gastric inflammation. This process could provide a more complementary, overlapping immune response to *H. pylori* and allow the host to clear an ongoing or future infection.

response. For example, if the predominant regulatory T-cell population induced during natural infection selects for IgG, the use of antigens and adjuvants that enhance IgA responses of the appropriate specificity could be sufficient to induce protection.

IV. Why Develop a Vaccine for *H. pylori*?

Although people become infected in childhood and remain so for the rest of their life, combinations of antimicrobials called "triple therapy" can be used to successfully clear the infection in a majority of patients. Why, then, is a vaccine needed?

The threat of antibiotic resistance is certainly one reason for considering the need for a vaccine. In addition, antimicrobial protocols for treating *H. pylori* infection tend to use antibiotics for a long time and may also include inhibitors of acid secretions. Together, these factors add to the cost and jeopardize the compliance of patients. Perhaps the most compelling reason for a vaccine, however, lies in the nature of the sequelae to the infection. Although all infected patients have chronic active gastritis, only a minority of these patients develop severe gastrointestinal disease, including peptic ulcers which require medical attention. The remaining patients exhibit few, if any, overt signs of infection, but the underlying chronic gastritis is a significant risk factor for gastric cancer (Owen, 1977; Correa, 1995). Thus, while symptomatic patients can be cured of their infection and subsequently resolve their gastritis, a large number of otherwise asymptomatic, but infected, individuals have chronic active gastritis for decades and may eventually go on to develop gastric cancer. Thus an *H. pylori* vaccine might be able to break the infectious cycle and significantly reduce the risk of gastric cancer and peptic ulcers.

The widely accepted cohort theory for *H. pylori* infection suggests that *H. pylori* infection is primarily acquired in childhood and that as the population ages, new infections of adults are relatively rare (Banatvala *et al.*, 1993). In addition, recurrence rates after triple therapy have been reported to be low, which may have more to do with exposure rates and opportunity for reinfection than the existence of effective immunity after antimicrobial cure. Indeed, animal studies have shown that in contrast to vaccination, triple-therapy cure of *Helicobacter* infections does not lead to immunity to reinfection (Chen *et al.*, 1993; Fox *et al.*, 1994; S. J. Czinn, unpublished results, 1994). If this hypothesis is true, then in a situation where adults do have high exposure rates, such as in a developing country, one might expect a relatively high rate of reinfection after triple therapy cure. In fact, one recent study from Brazil showed exactly this result (Coelho *et al.*, 1992). However, as some studies in developing countries do not always definitively document successful eradication, it is possible that the "new" infection is due to recrudescence or even inoculation by subsequent endoscopy. Nonetheless, these situations provide additional rationale for a vaccine: immunization will yield a more effective immune response than infection, which seems to provide no protection at all.

Another rationale for an effective *H. pylori* vaccine lies in the adverse effects of triple therapy (Chiba *et al.*, 1992): First, triple therapy leads to drug resistance in patients who are not cured. Second, triple therapy leads to moderate side effects such as nausea, diarrhea, abdominal pain, and/or pseudomembranous colitis in 30% of patients, which can result in poor patient compliance and failure to cure the infection. Third, with the growing realization that *H. pylori* infection is the causative agent for the majority of peptic ulcers, there will likely be increased indiscriminate use of antibiotics for all patients suffering from dyspepsia. Such large-scale use of antibiotics may lead to increased drug resistance in *H. pylori* and the emergence of other drug-resistant human pathogens.

Thus the development of a safe and effective vaccine for the prevention of *H. pylori* infection should reduce the incidence of both peptic ulcers and gastric cancer. Even though such a vaccine could be of great benefit to future generations, infection with *H. pylori* generally lasts for life. Recent experiments (discussed below) have shown that a therapeutic vaccine can cure *Helicobacter*-infected animals (Doidge *et al.*, 1994; Corthesy-Theulaz *et al.*, 1995). This fact provides another strong rationale for the development of an *H. pylori* vaccine: vaccination alone or as an adjunct to antimicrobial therapy could be of great benefit to individuals who are already infected.

V. Strategies for Successful Vaccination against *H. pylori*

A prerequisite for preclinical vaccine development and testing was the development of suitable animal models for *H. pylori* infection. Several animal models now exist for the study of *Helicobacter*-related disease and immunology. Although both gnotobiotic pigs (Eaton and Krakowa, 1992) and dogs (Radin *et al.*, 1990) can be colonized by *H. pylori,* these models are expensive and impractical, particularly for performing large experiments. Primate models (Fujioka *et al.*, 1993; Hazell *et al.*, 1992) are generally even more expensive, but may find use after vaccine candidates are screened in smaller animal models but before human trials. Natural infection of a colony of cats by *H. pylori* has recently been reported (Handt *et al.*, 1994) and it is possible that these cats may ultimately be a valuable model for vaccine studies.

Infection of mice with *H. pylori* has also been recently reported by several groups (Karita *et al.*, 1991; Marchetti *et al.*, 1995). In these models, recovery of *H. pylori* organisms was low, and whether chronic infections will occur is not yet known. Additionally, although the morphology of the infected epithelium seemed altered in these models the inflammation associated with infection was minimal compared to that in the human and in the *H. felis* mouse model (Lee *et al.*, 1990; Fox *et al.*, 1993; Blanchard *et al.*, 1995b). It is possible that different mouse-adapted strains of *H. pylori* as well as the strain of the mouse will determine the degree of inflammation in these models.

Two models now in general use include *H. felis* (isolated from the domestic cat) infection of conventional mice (Lee *et al.*, 1990) and infection of ferrets with the indigenous *H. mustelae* (Fox *et al.*, 1990). Both models generate an inflammatory response similar to that seen in humans, which includes a persistent neutrophilic infiltrate and the development of lymphoid aggregates (Lee *et al.*, 1990; Fox *et al.*, 1991, 1993). Both models have been demonstrated to require the same detailed antimicrobial therapy for eradication of the respective bacteria (Leunk *et al.*, 1994), and perhaps most significantly, *H. felis* infection of mice results in inflammation that is mouse strain dependent (Sakagami *et al.*, 1994; Mohammadi *et al.*, 1995b), allowing for an investigation that might determine why some humans respond differently to *H. pylori* infection than others. The mouse model allows for experiments with large groups of animals with a well-characterized immune system and an extensive array of reagents. The ferret model has the advantage of allowing long-term monitoring of infection or immunization by gastric endoscopy/biopsy.

Parenteral vaccination against *Helicobacter* infection in animal models has been ineffective in preventing infection even though serum antibodies are induced (Chen *et al.*, 1993; Eaton and Krakowa, 1992; Lee *et al.*, 1995). In contrast, oral immunization with an appropriate mucosal adjuvant has protected animals from *Helicobacter* infection (Chen *et al.*, 1993; Czinn *et al.*, 1993; Ferrero *et al.*, 1994; Lee *et al.*, 1995; Marchetti *et al.*, 1995; Michetti *et al.*, 1994; Pappo *et al.*, 1995). These studies are summarized in more detail below. Thus stimulation of the mucosal immune system appears to be necessary for a vaccine to be effective against *H. pylori*.

Based on what we know of the biology of *H. pylori* and what we know from other pathogenic bacteria, it is a reasonable assumption that a vaccine should induce a mucosal IgA anti-*Helicobacter* response in the stomach. There are, however, no data to actually support this contention. Although it seems unlikely that T cells actually confer immunity directly, T-cell-derived cytokines may be required for the induction of anti-*Helicobacter* immunity. Finally, even assuming that a gastric IgA anti-*H. pylori* immune response is what is required, no one has ever before attempted to induce an antigen-specific response in the stomach of humans. Thus, while the prospect of developing an *H. pylori* vaccine is an exciting one, it is also a daunting one as there are many unanswered yet fundamental questions about what may be required.

VI. Experimental Evidence That Immunization Can Prevent and/or Cure *Helicobacter* Infection

A. Prophylactic Immunization

In the *H. felis* mouse model, mice remain persistently infected and display many histologic findings that are similar to *H. pylori*-infected humans (Fox *et al.*, 1993; Pappo *et al.*, 1995; Sellman *et al.*, 1995). Based on the previously established immunization strategy for generating a significant gastric antibody response (Czinn and Nedrud, 1991) germfree, outbred mice were orally immunized with *H. felis* lysates (Czinn *et al.*, 1993). A significant IgA and IgG anti-*H. felis* response was generated in serum and in gastric and intestinal secretions in immunized mice relative to nonimmunized controls. Additionally, significant protection was observed when the mice were challenged with 10^6 cfu *H. felis* as only 20% of the immunized animals became colonized compared with 80% of the non immunized controls. Simultaneously, Chen *et al.* (1993) made similar observations. We have also performed similar experiments with ferrets using *H. mustelae* and have shown protection in this model.

Since it has been shown that immunized (protected) and infected animals acquire similar magnitudes of antibody responses (Sellman *et al.*, 1995), it appears that the difference between immune and infected mice cannot simply be that immunized animals respond more vigorously. We are thus left with the hypothesis that the **quality** of the immune response might differ after immunization versus infection. In fact, Western blots of *H. felis* antigens using serum from infected and immunized mice demonstrate clear differences in antibody repertoire (T. G. Blanchard, S. J. Czinn, and J. Nedrud, unpublished observations, 1995). In addition, recent studies where purified *H. pylori* urease was used as a vaccine showed that mice immunized by a protective protocol developed a significant mucosal IgA anti-urease immune response, whereas naive, challenged mice or mice immunized by a nonprotective protocol did not (Lee *et al.*, 1995).

Although antibodies and/or T-cell-mediated immune responses could theoretically be involved in protecting animals from infection after immunization, the adoptive transfer of splenic T cells or a T-cell line from immunized mice was unable to protect the recipients from *H. felis* infection (Mohammadi *et al.*, 1995a). Thus, while antibody alone could protect from infection in the *H. felis* model (Blanchard *et al.*, 1995a; Czinn *et al.*, 1993) splenic T cells could not.

The mechanism(s) by which antibodies protect from infection are not known, although a reasonable assumption might be that antibody binds to the bacterial surface and acts as a barrier to infection ("immune exclusion"). We have demonstrated that antibodies are sufficient for protection of the host in a series of passive protection studies employing a panel of *H. felis*-specific monoclonal antibodies (MAbs) (Blanchard *et al.*, 1995a; Czinn *et al.*, 1993). Incubation of the bacteria with several of our MAbs prior to inoculation of the host results in almost complete protection as demonstrated by gastric biopsy examination for urease activity. These antibodies all agglutinated *H. felis* which would facilitate bacterial clearance via the peristaltic movement of the gastrointestinal tract. Further evidence that *Helicobacter*-specific IgA is sufficient for conferring protection to the host was provided when resistance of West African infants to *H. pylori* infection was shown to correlate with *H. pylori*-specific IgA levels in the nursing mother's breast milk (Thomas *et al.*, 1993).

The identification of protective epitopes that might serve as potential vaccine candidates was a rapid development which has been the result of two separate approaches. The possession of several MAbs which could effectively prevent the colonization of *H. felis* in the mouse stomach helped identify antigens recognized by the respective antibodies. The first two protective MAbs identified, IgA 71 and IgG 40, were used to screen an expression library and their respective antigens were subcloned and sequenced (Blanchard *et al.*, 1995a). Both were specific for the large subunit of urease. Immunoprecipitation with *H. felis* outer membrane proteins was consistent with this observation and the ability of IgA 71 but not IgG 40 to immunoprecipitate *H. pylori* urease demonstrated that the two MAbs recognized separate epitopes. This was confirmed by competitive radioimmunoassay.

The second approach used by others has been to purify the dominant *Helicobacter* proteins and test for vaccine efficacy in mice when given in combination with cholera toxin. Several laboratories have successfully used urease as a protective antigen against *H. felis* infection when delivered to mice with cholera toxin (Ferrero *et al.*, 1994; Michetti *et al.*, 1994; Pappo *et al.*, 1995; Lee *et al.*, 1995). Because urease shares a high degree of homology between *Helicobacter* species, these studies have all been performed by oral immunization with the *H. pylori* urease. To date urease seems to be the most likely vaccine candidate and therefore has been examined in greater detail for protective epitopes. Ferrero *et al.* have used recombinant ureA and ureB subunits from both *H. felis* and *H. pylori* and tested their efficacy in the mouse model (Ferrero *et al.*, 1994). The ureB proteins were able to confer protection 17 weeks after immunization, providing evidence for a prolonged protective immune response. The UreA proteins from both species failed to induce protective immunity, thus demonstrating the importance of immunizing with the large subunit (Ferrero *et al.*, 1994).

Other studies have shown that the GroES homolog of *H. pylori* is also an effective antigen for the induction of immunity in mice (Ferrero *et al.*, 1995). However, as human heat shock proteins may have structural homology to microbial GroES molecules it will be important to determine if vaccine antigens with these molecular similarities induce deleterious side effects.

The *H. pylori* cytotoxin has been used to induce protective immunity to cytotoxin positive strains in the *H. pylori* mouse model (Marchetti *et al.*, 1995). This group has suggested that *H. pylori* strains expressing the cytotoxin are more likely to be associated with disease (Xiang *et al.*, 1995) and thus, the cytotoxin may be a useful vaccine antigen. However, as cytotoxin-negative strains do cause chronic inflammation, and since urease is ubiquitously expressed by all gastric *Helicobacter* strains, urease, and other antigens expressed on all strains of *H. pylori*, remain favored candidates for an *H. pylori* vaccine.

Although the results to date have been encouraging, several areas have to be investigated in order to select the best candidate vaccines for use in man. It now seems evident that urease and possibly other well characterized proteins might serve as efficient antigens for the induction of protective antibodies to *H. pylori*. Interestingly, all antigens tested to date appear to be effective. It is possible that **any** antigen, in combination with an effective adjuvant, will induce the appropriate regulatory T cells to induce specific immunity. In addition, immunity to other antigens may be enhanced through a bystander mechanism in which the vaccine antigen drives T cells that expand B cells recognizing both the vaccine and other antigens on *H. pylori*.

B. Therapeutic Immunization

In view of the initial success of oral immunization for the prevention of *Helicobacter* infections in mice, the next logical step was to determine if immunization could **cure** a chronic infection. Mice that were infected with *H. felis* were given the oral vaccine and assessed for evidence of infection. Using this approach, two groups have recently demonstrated that mice were able to clear their infection after oral immunization (Doidge *et al.*, 1994; Corthesy-Theulaz *et al.*, 1995). These findings have been confirmed in ferrets where the animals had a natural, chronic infection with *H. mustelae*. Therapeutic immunization cleared 30% of the animals of their infection, and significantly reduced inflammation in all immunized animals. If these experiments in mice and ferrets continue to yield positive results, it could lead to immunotherapy for *H. pylori* infection of humans. If this is successful in humans, vaccination could be applied to the entire infected population, alone or in combination with antibiotics, and virtually remove *H. pylori*-associated diseases. Combinations of vaccines and antibiotics would be superior to antibiotics alone since they would prevent the treatment failures due to antibiotic resistance or problems with compliance. Moreover, vaccine-induced immunity could prevent future disease in populations with a high risk of reinfection.

VII. Future Challenges in Mucosal Vaccines for *H. pylori*

A. Adjuvants

One of the most challenging aspects of developing a vaccine for *H. pylori* is enhancing the efficacy of immunization using a mucosal adjuvant. All of the animal studies to date which have shown protection versus *Helicobacter* infections after oral immunization have used cholera toxin or the closely related *E. coli* heat-labile toxin as an adjuvant. Mucosal immunization without any adjuvant or with other adjuvants has not been as effective. Since cholera toxin is highly toxic in man, development of a mucosal adjuvant suitable for a human *Helicobacter* vaccine will be of prime importance. One study has reported using the nontoxic B subunit of cholera toxin as an adjuvant to induce protection in mice against subsequent infection with *H. felis* (Lee and Chen, 1994). Similar preparations of cholera toxin B subunit have been safely used as an antigen in tens of thousands of people as part of a whole cell cholera vaccine (Clemens *et al.*, 1988), but whether purified B subunit will act as an adjuvant for heterologous antigens in humans is not known. On this matter, we and others have demonstrated that recombinant cholera toxin B or heat-labile B subunit have no adjuvanticity when used orally and that commercially prepared B subunits typically have contaminating A subunit present, which is most likely responsible for the adjuvant effects (Lycke *et al.*, 1992; Nedrud *et al.*, 1995). Another approach which has been taken recently is the generation of mutant cholera toxin or heat-labile toxin molecules which retain adjuvanticity but have reduced or eliminated toxicity (Dickinson and Clemens, 1995; Douce *et al.*, 1995; Grant *et al.*, 1994); the reported adjuvant effects may be due to small amounts of residual pharmacologic activity. Other approaches including live-attenuated vectors, microspheres, liposomes, and ISCOMs might be used for effective delivery and enhancement of an *H. pylori* vaccine and are discussed extensively elsewhere in this volume.

B. Duration of Gastric Immunity

Another important issue for the future in *Helicobacter* vaccine development is durability of protection. Protein antigens administered orally with cholera toxin adjuvant have been shown to elicit mucosal IgA immune memory responses for up to 2 years after immunization (Vajdy and Lycke, 1992; Lycke and Holmgren, 1987). Protection for up to 2 years has also been demonstrated in an experimental Sendai virus system utilizing cholera toxin adjuvant and oral immunization of mice (Nedrud, 1996). Thus, essentially life-long immunity could be induced in mice after mucosal immunization using a cholera toxin adjuvant. In addition, a preliminary report using the *H. felis* mouse model showed that animals were protected from infection for 15 months after immunization with *H. felis* sonicate plus cholera toxin (Radcliff *et al.*, 1995). These encouraging results suggest that it may be possible to induce long-term immunity toward *H. pylori* with the kinds of first generation vaccines now under development, and live-attenuated vector vaccines have the potential for even greater durability.

C. Postimmunization Gastritis

Finally, it is important that future studies consider the adverse effects of *H. pylori* immunization. Eaton and Krakowka have shown that parental immunization of pigs with killed whole *H. pylori* resulted in elevated levels of inflammation of the gastric mucosa upon oral challenge with live *H. pylori* (Eaton and Krakowa, 1992). Although the medical profession is well aware of many side effects associated with parenterally administered vaccines, the potential risks of oral immunization remain to be determined since there are few precedents for oral immunization that would let us say with complete confidence that these vaccines will always be safe. For example, protective immunity to *H. felis* infection in mice does not preclude an inflammatory response from developing following challenge with *H. felis* (Michetti *et al.*, 1994; Mohammadi *et al.*, 1994; Pappo *et al.*, 1995). This is consistent with the observation that immunization of mice with *H. pylori* leads to the production of antibodies that recognize human and murine gastric epithelium (Negrini *et al.*, 1991). Moreover, these authors have shown that the administration of these antibodies to mice will induce an erosive gastritis. These data are consistent with the reports described above that *H. pylori* induces autoreactive antibodies in the gastric mucosa of infected humans. Obviously this issue must be examined in detail when evaluating candidate vaccines.

Although the mechanism for postimmunization gastritis is not clear, it may be possible to predict some problems when one considers the goal of the mucosal immune response. The immune response is designed to discriminate between "self" and "non-self", however, in the gastrointestinal tract, you are, immunologically speaking, what you eat. Therefore, local immune responses are designed to limit many immune responses to antigens that are persistently found within the lumen as well as tissue antigens. This is critical since the luminal antigen pool is immense and many may cross-react with tissue antigens. In addition, immunologically significant amounts of luminal antigen cross the epithelial barrier and must not induce persistent inflammation. Using adjuvants that are well know to circumvent the normal processes that control oral tolerance, one may induce responses to tissue or luminal antigens (Manganaro *et al.*, 1994). Clearly, antigen selection will be also important. For example, the heat shock protein on *H. pylori* has been used successfully as a vaccine antigen in mice; however, there is some question that a host response to this antigen may cross-react with human heat shock proteins. In addition, structurally homologous urease is expressed on other bacteria and is found in various dietary constituents such as legumes. Thus, the induction of a strong anti-urease response may sensitize the host and predispose to persistent immune activation and inflammation after subsequent encounters with cross-reactive antigens.

In addition to the magnitude of the induced immune response, the isotype of the antibody may also be important. Considering that natural infection with *H. pylori* may induce primarily Th1 cell responses, oral vaccines have been designed to stimulate Th2 cells in the hope of inducing higher titers of IgA (Xu-Amano *et al.*, 1993). However, cytokines from Th2 cells can also induce IgE responses (Stevens *et al.*, 1988) and in fact, Snider and colleagues have shown that cholera toxin also induces IgE responses when used as an oral adjuvant (Snider *et al.*, 1994). Thus, subsequent stimulation with antigens that cross-react with the vaccine may bind IgE which, in turn, can lead to altered electrolyte secretion (Castro *et al.*, 1987; Vermillion *et al.*, 1989; Crowe *et al.*, 1990), muscle contractility (Russell and Castro, 1985; Marzio *et al.*, 1992), and significant discomfort.

Whether postimmunization gastritis represents autoimmunity, a persistent low-level infection, a beneficial inflammatory response responsible for clearing a transient infection, or an altered mucosal immune system remains to be determined. It should be remembered that the presence of some inflammation is probably required for effective immunity, particularly in the stomach which is usually devoid of immune and inflammatory cells. Nonetheless, the risks associated with any postimmunization gastritis must be resolved.

VIII. Summary

In conclusion, many striking and potentially significant observations have been made since the recognition of *H. pylori* as a human pathogen. Excellent animal models are available in which promising vaccine antigens and adjuvants have been shown to induce protection or treat an ongoing infection. The effort to develop an effective *H. pylori* vaccine may yield a successful oral vaccine that could virtually eliminate the major reservoir for *H. pylori.* It is quite possible that the history of *H. pylori* will show a very rapid evolution from understanding its pathogenesis to preventing its colonization and subsequent disease.

References

Banatvala, N., Mayo, K., Megraud, F., Jennings, R., Deeks, J. J., and Feldman, R. A. (1993). The cohort effect and *Helicobacter pylori*. *J. Infect. Dis.* **168,** 219–221.

Blanchard, T. G., Czinn, S. J., Maurer, R., Thomas, W. D., Soman, G., and Nedrud, J. G. (1995a). Urease-specific monoclonal antibodies prevent *Helicobacter felis* infection in mice. *Infect. Immun.* **63,** 1394–1399.

Blanchard, T. G., Czinn, S. J., Nedrud, J. G., and Redline, R. W. (1995b). *Helicobacter*-associated gastritis in SCID mice. *Infect. Immun.* **63,** 1113–1115.

Blaser, M. J. (1990). *Helicobacter pylori* and the pathogenesis of gastroduodenal inflammation. *J. Infect. Dis.* **161,** 626–633.

Blaser, M. J. (1992). Hypotheses on the pathogenesis and natural history of *Helicobacter pylori*-induced inflammation. *Gastroenterology* **102,** 720–727.

Castro, G. A., Harari, Y., and Russell, D. A. (1987). Mediators of anaphylaxis-induced ion transport changes in small intestine. *Am. J. Physiol.* **253,** G540-G548.

Chen, M., Lee, A., Hazell, S., Hu, P., and Li, Y. (1993). Immunisation against gastric infection with *Helicobacter* species: First step in the prophylaxis of gastric cancer. *Zentralbl. Bakteriol.* **280,** 155–165.

Chiba, N., Babu, V. R., Rademaker, J. W., and Hunt, R. H. (1992). Meta-analysis of the efficiency of antibiotic therapy in eradicating *Helicobacter pylori, Am. J. Gastroenterol.* **87,** 1716–1727.

Clemens, J. D., Harris, J. R., Khan, M. R., Ali, M., Yunus, M., Khan, M. U., Svennerholm, A. M., Sack, D. A., Chakraborty, J., Stanton, B. F., Ahmed, F., Kay, B. A., Rao, M. R., and Holmgren, J. (1988). Impact of B subunit killed whole-cell and killed whole-cell only oral vaccines against cholera upon treated diarrhoeal illness and mortality in an area endemic for cholera. *Lancet,* **335,** 1375–1379.

Clyne, M., and Drumm, B. (1993). Adherence of *Helicobacter pylori* to primary human gastrointestinal cells. *Infect. Immun.* **61,** 4051–4057.

Coelho, J. G. V., Passos, M. C. F., Chausson, T., Costa, E. L., Maia, A. F., Brandao, M. J. C. C., Rodrigues, D. C., and Castro, L. P. (1992). Duodenalulcer and eradication of *Helicobacter pylori* in a developing country. An 18 month follow-up study. *Scand. J. Gastroenterol.* **27,** 362–366.

Correa, P. (1995). *Helicobacter pylori* and gastric carcinogenesis. *Am. J. Surg. Pathol.* **19,** S37-S43.

Corthesy-Theulaz, I., Porta, N., Glauser, M., Saraga, E., Vaney, A.-C., Hass, R., Kraehenbuhl, J.-P., Blum, A. L., and Michetti, P. (1995). Oral immunization with *Helicobacter pylori* urease B subunit as a treatment against *Helicobacter* infection in mice. *Gastroenterology* **109,** 115–121.

Crabtree, J. E., Shallcross, T. M., Heatley, R. V., and Wyatt, J. I. (1991). Mucosal tumour necrosis factor α and interleukin-6 in patients with *Helicobacter pylori* associated gastritis. *Gut* **32,** 1473–1477.

Crabtree, J. E., Peichl, P., Wyatt, J. I., Stachl, U., and Lindley, I. J. D. (1993). Gastric interleukin-8 and IgA IL-8 autoantibodies in *Helicobacter pylori* infection. *Scand. J. Immunol.* **37,** 65–70.

Crabtree, J. E., Covacci, A., Farmery, S. M., Xiang, Z., Tompkins, D. S., Perry, S., Lindley, I. J. D., and Rappuoli, R. (1994a). *Helicobacter pylori* induced interleukin-8 expression in gastric epithelial cells is associated with CagA positive phenotype. *J. Clin. Pathol.* **48,** 41–45.

Crabtree, J. E., Wyatt, J. I., Trejdosiewicz, L. K., Peichl, P., Nichols, P. H., Ramsay, N., Primrose, J. N., and Lindley, I.J.D. (1994b). Interleukin-8 expression in *Helicobacter pylori* infected, normal, and neoplastic gastoduodenal mucosa. *J. Clin. Pathol.* **47,** 61–66.

Crowe, S. E., Sestini, P., and Perdue, M. H. (1990). Allergic reactions of rat jejunal mucosa. Ion transport responses to luminal antigen and inflammatory mediators. *Gastroenterology* **99,** 74–82.

Crowe, S. E., Alvarez, L., Sherman, P. M., Jin, Y., Dytoc, M., Hunt, R. H., Patel, J., Muller, M. J., and Ernst, P. B. (1995). Expression of interleukin-8 and CD54 by human gastric epithelium after *H. pylori* infection *in vitro.* *Gastroenterology* **108,** 65–74.

Czinn, S. J., and Nedrud, J. G. (1991). Oral immunization against *Helicobacter pylori, Infect. Immun.* **59,** 2359–2363.

Czinn, S. J., Cai, A., and Nedrud, J. G. (1993). Protection of germfree mice from infection by *Helicobacter felis*-induced inflammation. *Infect. Immun.* **61,** 637–642.

Dickinson, B. L., and Clemens, J. D. (1995). Dissociation of *Escherichia coli* heat-labile enterotoxin adjuvanticity from ADP-ribosyltransferase activity. *Infect. Immun.* **63,** 1617–1623.

Doidge, C., Gust, I., Lee, A., Buck, F., Hazell, S., and Manne, U. (1994). Therapeutic immunization against *Helicobacter pylori* infection. *Lancet* **343,** 913–914.

Douce, G., Trucotte, C., Cropley, I., Roberts, M., Pizza, M., Domenighini, M., Rappuoli, R., and Dougan, G. (1995). Mutants of *Escherichia coli* heat labile toxin lacking ADP-ribosyltransferase activity act as nontoxic, mucosal adjuvants. *Proc. Natl. Acad. Sci. U.S.A.* **92,** 1644–1648.

Dytoc, M., Gold, B., Louie, M., Heusca, M., Fedorko, L., Crowe, S. E., Lingwood, C., Brunton, J., and Sherman, P. M. (1992). Comparison of *Helicobacter pylori* and attaching-effacing *Escherichia coli* adhesion to eukaryotic cells. *Infect. Immun.* **61,** 448–456.

Eaton, K. A., and Krakowa, S. (1992). Chronic active gastritis due to *Helicobacter pylori* in immunized gnotobiotic piglets. *Gastroenterology* **103,** 1580–1586.

Ender, G., Brooks, W., von Jan, N., Lehn, N., Bayerdorffer, E., and Hatz, R. (1995). Expression of adhesion molecules on human granulocytes after stimulation with *Helicobacter pylori* membrane proteins: Comparison with membrane proteins from other bacteria. *Infect. Immun.* **63,** 2473–2477.

Ernst, P. B., Crowe, S. E., and Reyes, V. E. (1995). The immunopathogenesis of gastroduodenal disease associated with *Helicobacter pylori* infection. *Curr. Opin. Gastroenterol.* **11,** 512–518.

Evans, D. J., Evans, D. G., Takemura, T., Nakano, H., Lampert, H. C., Graham, D. Y., Granger, D. N., and Kvietys, P. R. (1995). Characterization of a *Helicobacter pylori* neutrophil-activating protein. *Infect. Immun.* **63,** 2213–2220.

Fan, X. J., Chua, A., Shahi, C. N., McDevitt, J., Keeling, P. W. N., and Kelleher, D. (1994). Gastric T lymphocyte response to *Helicobacter pylori* in patients with *H. pylori* colonisation. *Gut* **35,** 1379–1384.

Ferrero, R. L., Thiberge, J.-M., Huerre, M., and Labigne, A. (1994). Recombinant antigens prepared from the urease subunits of *Helicobacter* spp.: Evidence of protection in a mouse model of gastric infection. *Infect. Immun.* **62,** 4981–4989.

Ferrero, R. L., Thiberge, J.-M., Kansau, I., Wuscher, N., Huerre, M., and Labigne, A. (1995). The GroES homolog of *Helicobacter pylori* confers protective immunity against mucosal infection in mice. *Proc. Natl. Acad. Sci. U.S.A.* **92,** 6499–6503.

Fiedorek, S. C., Malaty, H. M., Evans, D. L., Pumphrey, C. L., Casteel, H. B., Evans, D. J., Jr., and Graham, D. Y. (1991). Factors influencing the epidemiology of *Helicobacter pylori* infection in children. *Pediatrics* **88,** 578–582.

Fonthan, E. T., Ruiz, B., Perez, A., Hunter, F., and Correa, P. (1995). Determinants of *Helicobacter pylori* infection and chronic gastritis. *Am. J. Gastroenterol.* **90,** 1094–1101.

Fox, J. G., Correa, P., Taylor, N. S., Lee, A., Otto, G., Murphy, J. C., and Rose, R. (1990). *Helicobacter mustelae*-associated gastritis in ferrets: An animal model of *Helicobacter pylori* gastritis in humans. *Gastroenterology* **99,** 352–361.

Fox, J. G., Otto, G., Taylor, N. S., Rosenblad, W., and Murphy, J. C. (1991). *Helicobacter mustulae*-induced gastritis and elevated gastric pH in the ferret (*Mustela putorius furo*). *Infect. Immun.* **59,** 1875–1880.

Fox, J. G., Blanco, M., Murphy, J. C., Taylor, N. S., Lee, A., Kabok, Z., and Pappo, J. (1993). Local and systemic immune responses in *Helicobacter felis* active chronic gastritis. *Infect. Immun.* **61,** 2309–2315.

Fox, J. G., Batchelde, M., Hayward, A., Yan, L., Palley, L., Murphy, J. C., and Shames, B. (1994). Prior *Helicobac-*

ter mustelae infection does not confer protective immunity against experimental reinfection in ferrets. *Am. J. Gastroenterol.* **89,** 1318–1322.

Fuachere, J.-L., and Andersen, L. P. (1995). Immunological aspects. *Curr. Opin. Gastroenterol.* **11,** 21–24.

Fujioka, T., Shuto, R., Kodama, R., Fujiyama, K., Kubato, T., Murakami, K., and Nasu, M. (1993). Experimental model for chronic gastritis with *Helicobacter pylori*: Long-term follow-up study in *H. pylori*-infected Japanese macaques. *Eur. J. Gastroenterol. Hepatol.* **5,** S73-S77.

Graham, D. Y. (1991a). *Helicobacter pylori*: Its epidemiology and its role in duodenal ulcer disease. *J. Gastroenterol. Hepatol.* **6,** 105–113.

Graham, D. Y., Malaty, H. M., Evans, D. G., Evans, D. J., Jr., Klein, P. D., and Adam, E. (1991b). Epidemiology of *Helicobacter pylori* in an asymptomatic population in the United States. Effect of age, race, and socioeconomic status. *Gastroenterology* **100,** 1495–1501.

Graham, D. Y., Lew, G. M., Klein, P. D., Evans, D. G., Evans, D. J., Jr., Saeed, Z. A., and Malaty, H. M. (1992). Effect of treatment of *Helicobacter pylori* infection on the long-term recurrence of gastric or duodenal ulcer. A randomized, controlled study. *Ann. Intern. Med.* **116,** 705–708.

Grant, C. C. R., Messer, R. J., and Cieplak, W. J. (1994). Role of trypsin-like cleavage at arginine 192 in the enzymatic and cytotoxic activities of *Escherichia coli* heat-labile enterotoxin. *Infect. Immun.* **62,** 4270–4278.

Greiner, A., Marx, A., Heesemann, J., Leebmann, J., Schmausser, B., and Muller-Hermelink, H. K. (1994). Idiotype identity in a MALT-type lymphoma and B cells in *Helicobacter pylori* associated chronic gastritis. *Lab. Invest.* **70,** 572–578.

Handt, L. K., Fox, J. G., Dewirst, F. E., Fraser, G. J., Paster, B. J., Yan, L. L., Rozmiarek, H., Rufo, R., and Stalis, I. H. (1994). *Helicobacter pylori* isolated from the domestic cat: Public health implications. *Infect. Immun.* **62,** 2367–2374.

Hazell, S., Eichberg, J. W., Lee, D. R., Alpert, L., Evans, D. G., Evans, D. J., Jr., and Graham, D. Y. (1992). Selection of the chimpanzee over the baboon as a model for *Helicobacter pylori* infection. *Gastroenterology* **103,** 848–854.

Hoda, M. M., Evans, D. G., Evans, D. J., Jr., and Graham, D. Y. (1992). *Helicobacter pylori* in Hispanics: Comparison with blacks and whites of similar age and socioeconomic class. *Gastroenterology* **103,** 813–816.

Huang, J., O'Toole, P. W., Doig, P., and Trust, T. J. (1995). Stimulation of interleukin-8 production in epithelial cell lines by *Helicobacter pylori, Infect. Immun.* **63,** 1732–1738.

Isaacson, P. (1982). Immunoperoxidase study of the secretory immunoglobulin system and lysozyme in normal and diseased gastric mucosa. *Gut* **23,** 578–588.

Karita, M., Kouchiyama, T., Okita, K., and Nakazawa, T. (1991). New small animal model for human gastric *Helicobacter pylori* infection: Success in both nude and euthymic mice. *Am. J. Gastroenterol.* **86,** 1596–1603.

Karttunen, R., Karttunen, T., Ekre, H.-P. T., and MacDonald, T. T. (1995). Interferon-γ and interleukin 4 secreting cells in the gastric antrum in *Helicobacter pylori* positive and negative gastritis. *Gut* **36,** 341–345.

Kirchner, T., Melber, A., Fischbach, W., Heilmann, K. L., and Muller-Hermelink, H. K. (1990). Immunohistological patterns of the local immune response in *Helicobacter pylori* gastritis. *In "Helicobacter pylori,* Gastritis and Peptic Ulcer" (P. Malfertheiner and H. Ditschuneit, eds.), pp. 213–222. Springer-Verlag, Berlin.

Kuhn, R., Lohler, J., Rennick, D., Rajewsky, K., and Muller, W. (1993). Interleukin-10-deficient mice develop chronic enterolcolitis. *Cell (Cambridge, Mass.)* **75,** 263–274.

Lee, A., and Chen, M. (1994). Successful immunization against gastric infection with *Helicobacter* species: Use of a cholera toxin B-subunit–whole-cell vaccine. *Infect. Immun.* **62,** 3594–3597.

Lee, A., Fox, J. G., Otto, G., and Murphy, J. (1990). A small animal model of human *Helicobacter pylori* active chronic gastritis. *Gastroenterology* **99,** 1315–1323.

Lee, C. K., Weltzin, R., Thomas, W. D. J., Kleanthous, H., Ermak, T. H., Soman, G., Hill, J., Ackerman, S. K., and Monath, T. P. (1995). Oral immunization with recombinant *Helicobacter pylori* urease induces secretory IgA antibodies and protects mice from challenge with *Helicobacter felis, J. Infect. Dis.* **172,** 161–172.

Leunk, R. D., Czinn, S. J., and Bierman, J. C. (1994). An *in vivo* model to evaluate therapies for gastric infection in humans. *Gastroenterology* **106,** A124.

Liblau, R. S., Singer, S. M., and McDevitt, H. O. (1995). Th1 and Th2 $CD4^+$ T cells in the pathogenesis of organ-specific autoimmune diseases. *Immunol. Today* **16,** 34–38.

Loffeld, R. J. L. F., Willems, I., Flendrig, J. A., and Arends, J. W. (1991). *Helicobacter pylori* and gastric carcinoma. *Histopathology* **17,** 537–541.

Lycke, N., and Holmgren, J. (1987). Long-term cholera antitoxin memory in the gut can be triggered to antibody formation associated with protection within hours of an oral challenge immunization. *Scand. J. Immunol.* **25,** 407–412.

Lycke, N., Tsuji, T., and Holmgren, J. (1992). The adjuvant effect of *Vibrio cholerae* and *E. coli* heat labile interotoxins is linked to their ADP-ribosyltransferase activity. *Eur. J. Immunol.* **22,** 2277–2281.

Madara, J. L., and Stafford, J. (1989). Interferon-γ directly affects barrier function of cultured intestinal epithelial monolayers. *J. Clin. Invest.* **83,** 724–727.

Mai, U. E. H., Perez-Perez, G. I., Wahl, L. M., Wahl, S. M., Blaser, M. J., and Smith, P. D. (1991). Soluble surface proteins from *Helicobacter pylori* activate monocytes/macrophages by lipopolysaccharide-independent mechanism. *J. Clin. Invest.* **87,** 894–900.

Mai, U. E. H., Perez-Perez, G. I., Allen, J. B., Wahl, S. M., Blaser, M. J., and Smith, P. D. (1992). Surface proteins from *Helicobacter pylori* exhibit chemotactic activity for human leukocytes and are present in gastric mucosa. *J. Exp. Med.* **175,** 517–525.

Manganaro, M., Ogra, P. L., and Ernst, P. B. (1994). Oral Immunization: Turning fantasy into reality. *Int. Arch. Allergy Appl. Immunol.* **103,** 223–233.

Marchetti, M., Arico, B., Burroni, D., Figura, N., Rappuoli, R., and Ghiara, P. (1995). Development of a mouse model of *Helicobacter pylori* infection that mimics human disease. *Science* **267,** 1655–1658.

Marshall, B. J., and Warren, J. R. (1984). Unidentified curved bacilli in the stomach of patients with gastritis and peptic ulceration. *Lancet* **8390,** 1311–1315.

Marshall, B. J., Armstrong, J. A., McGechie, D. B., and Glancy, R. J. (1985). Attempt to fulfill Koch's postulates for pyloric *Campylobacter, Med. J. Aust.* **142,** 436–439.

Marzio, L., Blennerhassett, P., Vermillion, D., Chiverton, S., and Collins, S. (1992). Distribution of mast cells in intestinal muscle of nematode-sensitized rats. *Am. J. Physiol.* **262,** G477-G482.

Michetti, P., Corthesy-Theulaz, I., Davin, C., Haas, R., Vaney, A.-C., Heitz, M., Bille, J., Kraehenbuhl, J.-P., Saraga, E., and Blum, A. L. (1994). Immunization of Balb/c mice against *Helicobacter felis* infection with *Helicobacter pylori* urease. *Gastroenterology* **107,** 1002–1011.

Mobley, H. L. T., Hu, L.-T., and Foxall, P. A. (1991). *Helicobacter pylori* urease: Properties and role in pathogenesis. *Scand. J. Gastroenterol.* **26** (Suppl. 187), 39–46.

Mohammadi, M., Czinn, S., and Nedrud, J. (1994). Oral immunization prevents *Helicobacter felis* colonization of conventional mice but does not prevent inflammation. *Am. J. Gastroenterol.* **89,** 1343.

Mohammadi, M., Nedrud, J. G., and Czinn, S. (1995a). Adoptive transfer of *Helicobacter*-specific lymphocytes enhances inflammation in mice. *Clin. Immunol. Immunopathol.* **76,** S8.

Mohammadi, M., Redline, R., Nedrud, J., and Czinn, S. (1995b). Role of the host in pathogenesis of *Helicobacter* associated gastritis: *H. felis* infection of inbred and congenic mouse strains. *Infect. Immun.* **64,** 238–245.

Mohammadi, M., Czinn, S., Redline, R., and Nedrud, J. (1996). Helicobacter-specific cell-mediated immune responses display a predominant Th1 phenotype and promote a DTH response in the stomachs of mice. *J. Immunol.* **156,** 4729–4738.

Moss, S. F., Legon, S., Davies, J., and Calam, J. (1995). Cytokine gene expression in *Helicobacter pylori* associated antral gastritis. *Gut* **35,** 1567–1570.

Nedrud, J., Blanchard, T. G., Czinn, S., and Lycke, N. (1995). Recombinant cholera toxin B subunit is not an adjuvant for oral immunization against *Helicobacter felis* in mice. *J. Cell. Biochem.* **19,** A261.

Nedrud, J. G., Taraszka, K., and Sigmund, N. (1996). Oral immunization of mice using inactivated virus and cholera toxin adjuvant confers complete and life long protection from Sendai virus infection when combined with intranasal boosting. Submitted for publication.

Negrini, R., Lisato, L., Zanella, I., Cavazzini, L., Gullini, S., Villanacci, V., Poiesi, C., Albertini, A., and Ghielmi, S. (1991). *Helicobacter pylori* infection induces antibodies cross-reacting with human gastric mucosa. *Gastroenterology* **101,** 437–445.

Nielsen, H., and Andersen, L. P. (1992). Activation of human phagocyte oxidative metabolism by *Helicobacter pylori, Gastroenterology* **103,** 1747–1753.

Nielsen, H., Birkholz, S., Andersen, L. P., and Moran, A. P. (1994). Neutrophil activation by *Helicobacter pylori* lipopolysaccarides. *J. Infect. Dis.* **170,** 135–139.

Noach, L. A., Bosma, N. B., Jansen, J., Hoek, F. J., van-Deventer, S. J., and Tytgat, G. N. (1994). Mucosal tumor necrosis factor-alpha, interleukin-1 beta and interleukin-8 production in patients with *Helicobacter pylori, Scand. J. Gastroenterol.* **29,** 425–429.

Norgaard, A., Andersen, L. P., and Nielsen, H. (1995). Neutrophil degranulation by *Helicobacter pylori* proteins. *Gut* **36,** 354–357.

Owen, R. L. (1977). Sequential uptake of horseradish peroxidase by lymphoid follicle epithelium of Peyer's patches in the normal unobstructed mouse intestine: An ultrastructural study. *Gastroenterology* **72,** 440–451.

Pappo, J., Thomas, W. D., Kabok, Z., Taylor, N. S., Murphy, J. C., and Fox, J. G. (1995). Effect of oral immunization with recombinant urease on murine *Helicobacter felis* gastritis. *Infect. Immun.* **63,** 1246–1252.

Parsonnet, J., Friedman, G. D., Vandersteen, D. P., Chang, Y., Vogelman, J. H., Orentreich, N., and Sibley, R. K. (1991). *Helicobacter pylori* infection and the risk of gastric carcinoma. *N. Engl. J. Med.* **325,** 1127–1131.

Perez-Perez, G. I., Shepherd, V. L., Morrow, J., and Blaser, M. J. (1995). Activation of human THP-1 cells and rat bone marrow-derived macrophages by *Helicobacter pylori* lipopolysaccharide. *Infect. Immun.* **63,** 1183–1187.

Radcliff, F., Chen, M., and Lee, A. (1995). Protective immunisation against *Helicobacter* stimulates long-term immunity. *Clin. Immunol. Immunopathol.* **76,** S19.

Radin, M. J., Eaton, K. A., Krakowa, S., Morgan, D. R., Lee, A., Otto, G., and Fox, J. (1990). *Helicobacter pylori* gastric infection in gnotobiotic beagle dogs. *Infect. Immun.* **58,** 2606–2612.

Rathbone, B. J., Wyatt, J., Tompkins, D., Heatley, R. V., and Losowsky, M. S. (1988). *In vitro* production of *Campylobacter pyloridis* specific antibodies by gastric mucosal biopsies. *Gut* **29,** A607 (abstract).

Rauws, E., and Tytgat, G. N. J. (1990). Eradication of *Helicobacter pylori* cures duodenal ulcer. *Lancet* **1,** 1233–1235.

Russell, D. A., and Castro, G. A. (1985). Anaphylactic-like reaction of small intestinal epithelium in parasitized guinea pigs. *Immunology* **54,** 573–579.

Sakagami, T., Shimoyama, T., O'Rourke, J., and Lee, A. (1994). Back to the host: Severity of inflammation induced by *Helicobacter felis* in different strains of mice. *Am. J. Gastroenterol.* **89,** 1345.

Sellman, S., Blanchard, T. G., Nedrud, J. G., and Czinn, S. J. (1995). Vaccine strategies for prevention of *Helicobacter pylori* infections. *Eur. J. Gastroenterol. Hepatol.* 7(Suppl. 1), 151–156.

Sharma, S. A., Tummuru, M.K.R., Miller, G. G., and Blaser, M. J. (1995). Interleukin-8 response of gastric epithelial cell lines to *Helicobacter pylori* stimulation *in vitro. Infect. Immun.* **63,** 1681–1687.

Snider, D. P., Marshall, J. S., Perdue, M. H., and Liang, H. (1994). Production of IgE antibody and allergic sensitization of intestinal peripheral tissues after oral immunization with protein Ag and cholera toxin. *J. Immunol.* **153,** 647–657.

Stacey, A. R., Hawtin, P. R., and Newell, D. G. (1990). Local immune responses to *Helicobacter pylori* infections. *In* "*Helicobacter pylori,* Gastritis and Peptic Ulcer" (P. Malfertheiner and H. Ditschuneit, eds.), pp. 162–166. Springer-Verlag, New York.

Stevens, T. L., Bossie, A., Sanders, V. M., Fernandez-Botran, R., Coffman, R. L., Mosmann, T. R., and Vitetta, E. S. (1988). Regulation of antibody isotype secretion by subsets of antigen-specific helper T cells. *Nature (London)* **334,** 255–258.

Talley, N. J., Zinsmeister, A. R., Weaver, A., DiMagno, E. P., Carpenter, H. A., Perez-Perez, G. I., and Blaser, M. J. (1991). Gastric adenocarcinoma and *Helicobacter pylori* infection. *J. Natl. Cancer Inst.* **83,** 1734–1739.

Thomas, J. E., Austin, S., Dale, A., McClean, P., Harding, M., Coward, W. A., and Weaver, L. T. (1993). Proection by human milk IgA against *Helicobacter pylori* infection in infancy. *Lancet* **342,** 121.

Vajdy, M., and Lycke, N. Y. (1992). Cholera toxin adjuvant promotes long-term immunological memory in the gut mucosa to unrelated immunogens after oral immunization. *Immunology* **75,** 488–492.

Valnes, K., Brandtzaeg, P., Elgjo, K., and Stave, R. (1986). Quantitative distribution of immunoglobulin-producing cells in gastric mucosa: Relation to chronic gastritis and glandular atrophy. *Gut* **27,** 505–514.

Valnes, K., Huitfeldt, H. S., and Brandtzaeg, P. (1990). Relation between T cell number and epithelial HLA class II expression quantified by image analysis in normal and inflamed human gastric mucosa. *Gut* **31,** 647–652.

Vermillion, D. L., Ernst, P. B., Scicchitano, R., and Collins, S. M. (1989). Antigen-induced contraction of jejunal smooth muscle in the sensitized rat. *Am. J. Physiol.* **255,** G701-G708.

Vollmers, H. P., Dammrich, J., Ribbert, H., Grassel, S., Debus, S., Heesemannn, J., and Muller-Hermelink, H. K. (1994). Human monoclonal antibodies from stomach carcinoma patients react with *Helicobacter pylori* and stimulate stomach cancer cells *in vitro. Cancer* **74,** 1525–1532.

Witt, C. S. (1991). The mucosal immune response to *Helicobacter pylori. In* "Mucosal Immunology" (A. W. Cripps, ed.), pp. 149–153. Newey and Beath, Newcastle.

Wyatt, J. I., Rathbone, B. J., and Heatley, R. V. (1986). Local immune response to gastric *Campylobacter* in non-ulcer dyspepsia. *J. Clin. Pathol.* **39,** 863–870.

Xiang, Z., Censini, S., Bayeli, P. F., Telford, J. L., Figura, N., Rappuoli, R., and Covacci, A. (1995). Analysis of expression of CagA and VacA virulence factors in 43 strains of *Helicobacter pylori* reveals that clincial isolates can be divided into two major types and that CagA is not necessary for expression of the vacuolating toxin. *Infect. Immun.* **63,** 9463–9498.

Xu-Amano, B. J., Kiyono, H., Jackson, R. J., Staats, H. F., Fujihashi, K., Burrows, P. D., Elson, C. O., Pillai, S., and McGhee, J. R. (1993). Helper T cell subsets for immunoglobulin A responses: Oral immunization with tetanus toxoid and cholera toxin as adjuvant selectively induces Th2 cells in mucosa associated tissues. *J. Exp. Med.* **178,** 1309–1320.

Yasumoto, K., Okamoto, S., Mukaida, N., Murakami, S., Mai, M., and Matsushima, K. (1992). Tumor necrosis factor α and interferon γ synergistically induce interleukin 8 production in a human gastric cancer cell line through acting concurrently on AP-1 and NF-kappaB-like binding sites of the interleukin 8 gene. *J. Biol. Chem.* **267,** 22506–22511.

Yoshimura, H. H., Evans, D. G., and Graham, D. Y. (1994). DNA–DNA hybridization demonstrates apparent genetic differences between *Helicobacter pylori* from patients with duodenal ulcer and asymptomatic gastritis. *Dig. Dis. Sci.* **38,** 1128–1131.

20

Mucosal Immunity Induced by Oral Administration of Bacille Calmette–Guérin

DANIEL F. HOFT
Division of Infectious Diseases and Immunology
Department of Internal Medicine
St. Louis University Health Sciences Center
St. Louis, Missouri 63110

MARINA GHEORGHIU
Laboratoire du BCG
Institut Pasteur
75724 Cedex, Paris, France

I. General Background on Bacille Calmette–Guérin

The *Mycobacterium bovis* Bacille Calmette–Guérin (BCG) vaccine strain was originally developed between 1904 and 1908 in France at the Institut Pasteur de Lille by Albert Calmette and Camille Guérin. They attenuated the virulence of this *M. bovis* strain by successive passages on glycerinated bile–potato medium. Extensive animal studies conducted between 1908 and 1921 failed to identify reversion of this attenuated *M. bovis* strain to virulence. On the contrary, immunization of animals with the *M. bovis* BCG strain conferred resistance to challenges with virulent mycobacteria. Thus, BCG was first used as a vaccine against human tuberculosis (TB) in 1921. The detailed history of BCG has been reviewed (Gheorghiu, 1996).

The BCG vaccine is still the only one currently available for infections related to all species of mycobacteria. The BCG vaccine has been used extensively in areas with high rates of infection with *Mycobacterium tuberculosis* (Mtb). Even now, most countries in the world vaccinate their populations in childhood with BCG. The BCG vaccine is included by the World Health Organization in the expanded program of immunization. It has been estimated that a total of more than 3 billion doses of BCG have been administered since 1921, making BCG one of the most widely used vaccines in the world.

There has been considerable controversy concerning the protective efficacy of BCG vaccination over the last several decades. The prevention of mycobacterial infection and the measurement of BCG vaccine efficacy are challenging goals because of the complex biological interactions between the mycobacterial pathogen and host immunity. It has not been possible to determine accurately the efficacy of BCG in the prevention of Mtb infection. Approximately 90% of immunocompetent individuals infected with Mtb will never develop disease, and the standard method used for detection of asymptomatic Mtb infection is the delayed type hypersensitivity (DTH) response to tuberculin purified protein derivative (PPD). Vaccination with BCG may induce a positive DTH response to PPD, and, therefore, previous vaccination with BCG can make it difficult to detect asymptomatic cases of Mtb infection that occur postvaccination. An increase in the DTH response above the baseline levels postvaccination ("virage tuberculinique") can be used to detect recent infection with Mtb (Mande, 1996), but the interpretation of this response requires close follow-up of the PPD status in a given individual because of the possibility of waning vaccine-induced immunity over time. For these reasons, it has not been feasible to determine the efficacy of BCG in the prevention of asymptomatic Mtb infection in large-scale, long-term clinical trials.

The major end points studied in BCG efficacy trials have been the differences in disease rates that occur in a minority of the Mtb-infected persons. Different BCG trials have detected highly variable efficacy rates ranging from 0 to 80% for the prevention of active tuberculous disease (reviewed in Fine, 1989; Fine & Rodrigues, 1990; Bloom and Fine, 1994). The latency of disease associated with Mtb infection provides a formidable challenge for any preventative vaccine strategy, as well as another obstacle for efforts to measure accurately the protective efficacy induced by BCG. The majority of cases of active tuberculous disease occur through reactivation of remote Mtb infection, when immune defenses are depressed by chronic illness, age, or immunosuppressive therapies. Prolonged vaccine-induced immunity is difficult to achieve and is susceptible to the same conditions that depress general immunity. Thus, partial protection may be the best we can hope for with any vaccination strategy designed to prevent the latent disease associated with TB. The measurement of BCG efficacy in the prevention of reactivation of remote Mtb infection requires long-term follow-up, making clinical trials expensive and logistically difficult. Despite these problems associated with the study of TB vaccines, meta-analyses evaluating all published BCG efficacy trials have concluded that BCG significantly reduces the risk of pulmonary TB by 50% and decreases TB related deaths by 71% (Colditz *et al.*, 1994, 1995).

Vaccination with BCG has not been utilized to any great extent in the United States. The U.S. public health strategy for TB prevention has consisted of case detection by PPD screening, followed by preventive chemotherapy with isoniazid in PPD-positive healthy individuals to inhibit the development of active disease. This strategy has been appropriate in view of the low prevalence of TB in the United States. However, the resurgence of the overall rates of tuberculosis as well as the increasing rates of multiple-drug-resistant TB in the United States have renewed interest in BCG. Studies of BCG are important for other reasons unrelated to protective efficacy against mycobacterial infections. Molecular techniques required to insert foreign genes into BCG have been developed (Jacobs *et al.*, 1989; Husson *et al.*, 1990; Barletta *et al.*, 1990; Collins, 1991; Winter *et al.*, 1991; Connell *et al.*, 1993). Because BCG vaccination is known to induce long-term mycobacterial specific immunity, the use of recombinant BCG expressing foreign proteins may be an excellent method to induce protective immunity against many other pathogens (see Chapter 9 by Langermann in this volume).

II. History of Oral Bacille Calmette–Guérin

Oral vaccination was the original method of BCG administration used to prevent human TB. In July of 1921, B. Weill-Hallé, chief physician at the Hospital de la Charité in Paris, in collaboration with Calmette and Guérin, vaccinated the first human infant born into a home with family members suffering from active TB. Three administrations of 2 mg of BCG each [total dose $\sim 240 \times 10^6$ "bacillary elements," probably equivalent to colony-forming units (cfu)] were given on the third, fifth, and seventh days of life (Calmette *et al.*, 1926; Rosenthal, 1980). During the next 4 years, more than 300 infants were orally vaccinated with BCG in the maternity ward of the Hospital de la Charité using larger doses of up to 10 mg each or 1200×10^6 cfu. There were no significant adverse effects noted among these children, and only one of the vaccinated children died of TB despite chronic exposure to the disease (Weill-Halle, 1924; Calmette *et al.*, 1924). Calmette later reported the results of nonrandomized studies involving more than 50,000 children (Calmette *et al.*, 1926). Mortality from TB was 1.8% among vaccinated compared with 25–32% among unvaccinated infants. These results indicated that oral vaccination with BCG is relatively safe and suggested that oral BCG could induce human immunity protective against TB. The League of Nations compiled the results of all reported animal and human BCG trials in 1928 and submitted the compiled reports to expert commissions of bacteriologists, clinicians, and veterinary surgeons for review. The conclusions of this review process were that BCG was a safe vaccine, and that BCG used orally as a "preimmunition" vaccine against TB could induce a "certain degree of immunity" (Société des Nations, 1928). During the next 30 years oral BCG vaccination in infants was used widely throughout Europe, Asia, Canada, and South America.

Calmette chose the oral route for initial BCG vaccination partially because of its simplicity and its requirement for minimal administration materials and equipment. In addition, it had been shown previously, and was confirmed by Calmette, that the intestinal epithelium of newborn animals was permeable to bacteria (Calmette *et al.*, 1925, 1936; Weigert, 1883). Therefore, Calmette reasoned that BCG could penetrate the intestinal mucosa of newborn infants and stimulate systemic mycobacterial specific immunity. He recommended that babies be vaccinated orally with BCG within the first 10 days of life. This recommendation provided the added advantage that the infants, considered to be the major target population for prevention of TB, would be vaccinated prior to leaving the maternity ward and thus prior to TB infection from family contacts. Definitive proof for the transit of BCG across human intestinal mucosa was obtained by the isolation of BCG from the mesenteric ganglia of children vaccinated in infancy who died within 2–3 months of birth from unrelated causes (Zeyland and Piasecka-Zeyland, 1928). Calmette *et al.* (1933) provided further evidence for the systemic spread of BCG after mucosal invasion by isolating BCG from the blood of infants 3–5 hr after ingestion of the vaccine. More recently, it has been shown that, like other bacteria, BCG is taken up from the intestinal lumen through the M cells of the Peyer's patches lining the small bowel (Fujimura, 1986), as shown in Fig. 1. In addition, the data presented in Table I indicate that BCG can be translocated across rhinopharyngeal mucosa, as discussed in more detail later in this chapter.

Despite the relatively low risk of adverse reactions and the apparent successful induction of protective immunity associated with its use, oral BCG vaccination was perceived to have certain drawbacks. Suppurative cervical lymphadenitis was the most frequent complication of oral BCG vaccination. The first investigations of the incidence of this complication among orally vaccinated children were reported at the First International Congress on BCG, held in Paris in 1948 (Van Deinse, 1948; Domingo, 1948). The incidence was low and variable: in France from 0.05 to 0.008%; in Belgrade from 1 to 4%. Otitis media and retropharyngeal abscesses were reported, but with even lower frequencies than found for lymphadenitis. These complications were thought to occur in infants who did not completely swallow vaccine preparations that were not well standardized, well dispersed, or appropriately diluted (reviewed in Domingo, 1948). The most detailed analyses of BCG complications associated with different routes of vaccine administration were published by Lotte *et al.* (1984). They found that in 11 studies reporting complications associated with oral BCG use, the rates of cervical suppurative lymphadenitis ranged from 0.08 to 26 cases per 1000 vaccinated subjects. After intradermal BCG vaccination, the rates of regional suppurative lymphadenitis ranged from 0.0006 to 38 cases per 1000 vaccinated subjects in the 22 studies reporting complication rates. Therefore, it is unclear whether oral BCG vaccination is associated with higher complication rates in comparison with intradermal administration of BCG. In addition, vaccines that are well dispersed, appropriately diluted, and administered with modern techniques of vaccine microencapsulation could be used to minimize these complications by preventing inadvertent pharyngeal high-dose inoculation.

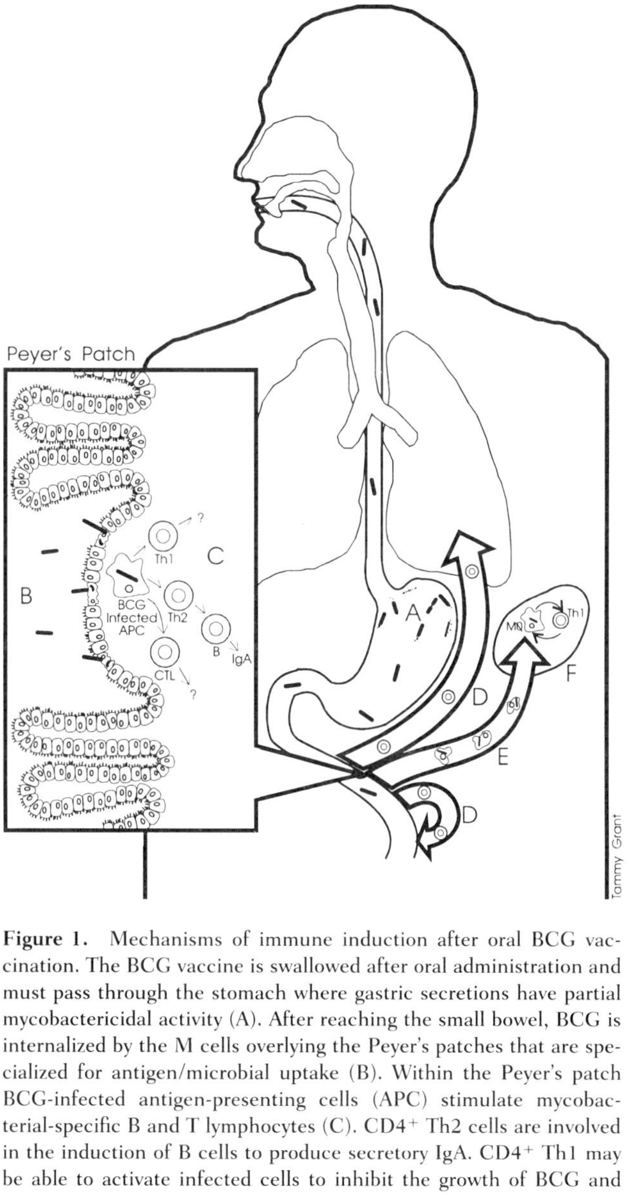

Figure 1. Mechanisms of immune induction after oral BCG vaccination. The BCG vaccine is swallowed after oral administration and must pass through the stomach where gastric secretions have partial mycobactericidal activity (A). After reaching the small bowel, BCG is internalized by the M cells overlying the Peyer's patches that are specialized for antigen/microbial uptake (B). Within the Peyer's patch BCG-infected antigen-presenting cells (APC) stimulate mycobacterial-specific B and T lymphocytes (C). $CD4^+$ Th2 cells are involved in the induction of B cells to produce secretory IgA. $CD4^+$ Th1 may be able to activate infected cells to inhibit the growth of BCG and virulent mycobacteria. $CD8^+$ CTL may be able to lyse cells infected with mycobacteria. After stimulation of mycobacterial-specific B and T lymphocytes in Peyer's patches, these cells disseminate through the blood and lymphatics to mucosal immune effector sites in the lamina propria and epithelia of the lungs, gut, etc. (D). The BCG infected macrophages migrate through the blood and lymphatics to the spleen and other reticuloendothelial organs (E) where they can activate Th1 cells to produce IFN-γ and other macrophage activating products (F). Finally, mycobacterial specific humoral immune responses and $CD8^+$ CTL may be stimulated in the spleen and other reticuloendothelial sites by infected macrophages.

Another problem associated with the early use of oral BCG vaccination was that a large proportion of French children did not develop DTH responses to PPD after oral ingestion of BCG, or the DTH responses were low, variable (30 to 80%), and of short duration (1 year or less). The standard total dose used by Calmette for oral vaccination of infants was 30 mg of BCG (or ~1200 $\times 10^6$ cfu). Studies by de Assis in Brazil published in the late 1940s have clearly shown that total doses up to 10-fold higher than the doses recommended by Calmette are required for the consistent induction of positive DTH responses to PPD after oral vaccination with BCG (de Assis, 1948). Therefore, the weakness of tuberculin reactivity in French children vaccinated orally with BCG in the third and fourth decades of the twentieth century could be explained by the use of suboptimal doses of vaccine. The increased doses required for oral BCG vaccination do increase the cost of TB vaccination. However, the original method of oral BCG vaccination consisted of administering the vaccine in water or fruit juice. Chemical buffering (simply in milk or in a bicarbonate solution), or microencapsulation of the vaccine, may prevent exposure to mycobactericidal effects of gastric secretions and allow low doses of oral BCG vaccina-

TABLE I

Recovery of BCG in Gastrointestinal Lymphoid Tissues and Target Organs after Oral Immunization[a]

Day	Feces (per g)	PP	SMG	PGLN	CLN	MLN	Liver	Spleen	Lungs
1	ND	15 ± 10	25 ± 5	0	0	0	0	0	0
2	$2 \times 10^5 \pm 0.05$	42 ± 10	24 ± 11	0	0	0	0	0	0
3	$1 \times 10^6 \pm 0.2$	93 ± 9	28 ± 16	0	0	0	0	0	0
4	$2 \times 10^6 \pm 0.1$	110 ± 14	83 ± 23	45 ± 18	25 ± 4	0	0	0	0
5	$3 \times 10^6 \pm 0.3$	260 ± 43	128 ± 72	63 ± 12	15 ± 4	0	0	0	0
6	$4 \times 10^6 \pm 0.5$	193 ± 9	73 ± 2	41 ± 1	18 ± 2	0	0	0	0
8	$5 \times 10^4 \pm 0.004$	26 ± 1	73 ± 6	57 ± 5	17 ± 5	0	0	0	0
10	0	15 ± 4	60 ± 14	69 ± 3	22 ± 2	0	50 ± 12	0	0
12	ND	10 ± 0	137 ± 12	78 ± 8	42 ± 2	17 ± 11	170 ± 24	18 ± 2	0
15	ND	0	130 ± 38	220 ± 43	550 ± 41	13 ± 2	167 ± 12	510 ± 53	45 ± 35
30	ND	0	92 ± 13	885 ± 71	820 ± 52	50 ± 15	21 ± 1	858 ± 51	23 ± 20
60	ND	0	23 ± 2	320 ± 20	0	32 ± 2	0	102 ± 2	0

[a]BALB/c mice were immunized with 10^9 cfu of BCG given orally for five consecutive days (total dose: 5×10^9 BCG cfu). Results are given as mean numbers of colony-forming units per mouse organ (PP, Peyer's patches; SMG, submandibular gland; PGLN, periglandular lymphnodes; CLN, cervical lymph nodes; MLN, mesenteric lymph nodes). ND, Not determined.

tion to be effective in the induction of mucosal and systemic immune responses. In addition, tuberculin reactivity has not always correlated with protective immunity against tuberculosis (Hart, 1967; Comstock, 1988), and it is unknown whether mucosal immune responses stimulated by oral BCG vaccination in the absence of systemic delayed type hypersensitivity can be protective against mycobacterial infection. In theory, mucosal immune responses alone could prevent infection through mucosal surfaces. However, despite widespread use of oral BCG prior to 1976, there are no published reports of controlled human trials of the protective efficacy of oral BCG vaccination. The BCG efficacy trials included in the meta-analyses referred to above involved parenteral routes of vaccination only.

The third drawback perceived for oral BCG vaccination was assumed by Calmette even prior to use of BCG in humans. Because the animal studies had shown that the first 10 days of life was the period of optimal intestinal epithelial permeability to microbes, Calmette believed that only infants could be successfully immunized by oral administration of BCG. After this newborn period, the intestinal mucosa was assumed to become impermeable to microbial transit, and increases in gastric acid secretion were thought to provide high levels of mycobacericidal activity. Because of these assumptions, the use of subcutaneous BCG vaccination in adults was evaluated as early as the mid-1920s (Heimbeck and Scheel, 1928). However, the work of de Assis in Brazil has clearly demonstrated that older children and adults can be successfully immunized (assessed by DTH responses to PPD) by oral administration of BCG, albeit with higher doses than used in infants (de Assis, 1948). On the basis of the results of de Assis and colleagues, the Brazilian government maintained a national policy of monthly oral BCG booster vaccinations for the first 6 months of life for more than three decades. This policy was claimed to lower the mortality from TB in Brazil. Unfortunately, careful epidemiological studies were not conducted that could support this assertion. As mentioned above, chemical buffering or microencapsulation of the vaccine may make it possible to successfully administer lower doses of BCG by preventing exposure to the mycobactericidal effects of gastric secretions. In addition, targeting strategies that deliver vaccine directly to the M cells in the small bowel, specialized for antigen uptake into the induction sites of mucosal immunity, could result in increased efficiency of oral BCG vaccination.

A fourth drawback perceived for oral BCG that stimulated the evaluation of parenteral routes of administration was related to the identification of TB deaths in some children vaccinated orally in infancy (Calmette, 1927). Oral BCG vaccination did not provide complete protection against TB. However, as mentioned above, no method of BCG vaccination has been associated with complete protection against TB, and there have been no trials that have compared the protective efficacy of oral and parenteral routes of BCG vaccination. Therefore, we do not know whether parenteral routes of BCG vaccination are any better than oral BCG vaccination in the prevention of TB.

Because of these perceived drawbacks for oral BCG vaccination, intradermal and percutaneous routes of BCG vaccination have become standard in tuberculosis control programs worldwide. However, mucosal BCG vaccination may provide the only method of stimulating immune responses that could prevent initial mucosal infection with Mtb. In addition, the ability to genetically manipulate BCG for its use as a vaccine vector make further studies of oral BCG vaccination important to pursue. The possibility that lower oral doses of BCG can stimulate mucosal immune responses, or systemic immune responses other than DTH responses to PPD, has not been carefully studied. If low doses of recombinant BCG can induce protective mucosal immunity against the foreign antigens expressed, without stimulating DTH responses to PPD, the usefulness of the PPD screening test could be preserved. Therefore, it is important to study mucosal and systemic immunity after low- and high-dose oral BCG vaccination to gain insight into the potential uses of oral BCG for the prevention of mucosal infection with mycobacteria, as well as for the induction of immunity against foreign antigens expressed by recombinant BCG.

III. Protective Mycobacterial Immune Responses

It is generally accepted that cellular immune responses are the most important protective responses that develop naturally after resolution of primary infection with Mtb and after BCG vaccination. Splenic T cells harvested from mice protected against a normally lethal Mtb challenge by a preceding vaccination are capable of transferring protective immunity to naive mice (Orme and Collins, 1983; Orme, 1988a). Adoptive transfer studies have demonstrated that CD4$^+$ T lymphocytes are necessary for the resistance mediated by acquired immunologic memory (Orme, 1988b). In addition, BCG challenges normally sublethal in wild-type mice result in death in MHC class II deficient mice, further demonstrating the importance of CD4$^+$ T cells for mycobacterial protective immunity since class II antigen presentation is required for the stimulation of CD4$^+$ T cells (Kaufmann and Ladel, 1994). However, CD4$^+$ T cells are not the only important immune subset in protective mycobacterial immunity. Animals genetically devoid of β_2-microglobulin that are deficient in class I MHC surface expression, as well as MHC class I genetic knockout mice, are more susceptible to Mtb challenge (Flynn *et al.*, 1992; Bloom *et al.*, 1994). Because MHC class I molecules present antigens to CD8$^+$ T cells, these latter experiments suggest that CD8$^+$ T lymphocytes provide some protective activity against a lethal Mtb challenge. Vaccination with BCG has been shown to stimulate both CD4$^+$ and CD8$^+$ memory T cell responses against mycobacterial antigens, as well as foreign antigens expressed by recombinant BCG (Aldovini and Young, 1991; Lagranderie *et al.*, 1993a, 1996; Yasutomi *et al.*, 1993; Winter *et al.*, 1995; Gheorghiu *et al.*, 1995; Belyakoff *et al.*, 1995).

Evidence has shown that two populations of CD4$^+$ T helper (Th) lymphocytes, which produce distinct profiles of cytokines after antigenic stimulation, can be differentially stimulated and can have opposing effects on resistance and susceptibility (Mosmann *et al.*, 1986, 1991; Salgame *et al.*, 1991; Yamamura *et al.*, 1991; Maggi *et al.*, 1991; Scott *et al.*, 1989). Th1 cells, which produce γ-Interferon (IFN-γ), TNF-β, and interleukin-2 (IL-2) after antigenic stimulation, are increased in animals resistant to infection with several different intracellular parasites. γ-Interferon, one of the cytokines produced by the Th1-type of CD4$^+$ T lymphocytes, can increase the killing activity of murine macrophages for mycobacteria (Rook *et al.*, 1985; Flesch and Kaufmann, 1987). Tumor necrosis factor (TNF), produced by Th1 cells and macrophages, has been shown to be important for macrophage activation and the induction of granulomatous responses (Dannenberg and Rook, 1994). Studies have clearly demonstrated that CD4$^+$ Th1 cell responses are necessary for protection in the mouse model of Mtb infection (Cooper *et al.*, 1995; Flynn *et al.*, 1993, 1995; Kamijo *et al.*, 1994). However, the human macrophage may receive activation signals by mechanisms other than IFN-γ (Douvas *et al.*, 1985), and it has been more difficult to confirm that Th1 cells are important in protective human immunity to mycobacteria. Th2 cells secrete IL-4, IL-5, IL-6, and IL-10 after antigenic stimulation, and they are preferentially expanded in mice with increased susceptibility to systemic infection with intracellular parasites. The cytokines produced by the Th2 cell subset are essential for the regulation of B cell responses, including the induction of mucosal immunoglobulin A (IgA) responses.

As stated above, the role of differential Th lymphocyte stimulation in human resistance and susceptibility to mycobacteria has not been well defined. However, three separate models of protective mycobacterial immunity support a role for Th1 cells in human resistance to mycobacterial disease. First, tuberculous pleuritis has been studied as a model of protective immunity because this clinical manifestation of Mtb infection is usually self-limited in immunocompetent individuals. The mononuclear cells that accumulate in the pleural fluid of persons with tuberculous pleuritis have been shown to produce high levels of IFN-γ in response to mycobacterial antigens (Barnes *et al.*, 1992). A second model of protective immunity focuses on persons that are PPD positive after infection with Mtb, but who remain asymptomatic presumably because they have successfully controlled mycobacterial replication. Sanchez *et al.* (1994) demonstrated that the mycobacterial-specific immune responses detectable in the peripheral blood mononuclear cells from asymptomatic PPD$^+$ individuals are predominately Th1-like, with increases in IFN-γ and IL-2 and decreases in IL-4, compared with controls suffering from active TB disease. We have been studying the Th1 and Th2 responses in a third model of protective human immunity to mycobacteria: the antigen specific immune responses induced by intradermal BCG vaccination. Our results are consistent with the extensive animal data and the other two models of protective human immunity to mycobacteria. Persons vaccinated with BCG develop increases in IFN-γ responses and decreases in IL-4 responses to mycobacterial antigens in their peripheral blood mononuclear cells (Hoft *et al.*, 1996; Kemp *et al.*, 1996).

Studies have emphasized the importance of innate immunity in mycobacterial infections, and have suggested that $\gamma\delta$ T cells and/or CD4, CD8 double-negative $\alpha\beta$ T cells induced by nonpeptidic ligands (prenyl pyrophosphate derivatives and mycobacterial lipids, respectively) may be involved in the early control of mycobacterial infections (Pfeffer *et al.*, 1992; Lang *et al.*, 1995; Tanaka *et al.*, 1995; Morita *et al.*, 1995; Tsukaguchi *et al.*, 1995; Procelli *et al.*, 1992; Beckman *et al.*, 1994). It is unknown whether it is possible to induce antigen-specific memory $\gamma\delta$ T cells and/or CD4,CD8 double-negative $\alpha\beta$ T cells. In addition, it is unknown whether BCG vaccination induces these responses. It will be important in future trials to determine whether $\gamma\delta$ T cells and/or CD4,CD8 double-negative $\alpha\beta$ T cells are important for the protective immunity induced by BCG vaccination.

All of the above studies have focused on systemic immune responses protective against disseminated Mtb infection. Relatively little attention has been given to the potential importance of mucosal immunity to mycobacterial antigens. Infection with Mtb is transmitted through mucosal surfaces, and, in theory, mucosal immune responses could prevent infection with Mtb. This possibility has not been adequately considered during the transition from oral to parenteral methods of BCG for TB vaccination. Investigations of the administration of aerosilized BCG to guinea pigs have demonstrated that mucosal BCG vaccination can induce high levels of bronchoalveolar macrophage activation and protection against virulent Mtb challenge (Lagranderie *et al.*, 1993b).

IV. Immunity Stimulated by Oral Bacille Calmette–Guérin Vaccination

The most well characterized immune response at mucosal surfaces is the local production of antibodies of the secretory IgA isotype (reviewed in McGhee *et al.*, 1992). Orally administered antigens are taken up in the small bowel via the specialized M cells overlying the lymphoid aggregates (Peyer's patches) known as the gut-associated lymphoid tissues (GALT). Stimulation of IgA precursor B cells in GALT leads to the disemination of mature B cells to mucosal effector immune sites including the lamina propria of the intestinal, respiratory, and genitourinary tracts, as well as various secretory glands (e.g., salivary glands) in communication with mucosal surfaces. T lymphocytes stimulated by antigens in mucosal inductive sites are involved in the generation of mucosal IgA responses, and they contribute other mucosal immune effector functions through cytokine production or direct cytolytic activity (reviewed in McGhee *et al.*, 1989). Investigations in gene knockout mice deficient in IL-4 and IL-6 (cytokines produced by $CD4^+$ Th2 lymphocytes) have confirmed important roles for these cytokines in the generation of antigen specific mucosal IgA responses (Vajdy *et al.*, 1995; Ramsay *et al.*, 1994), and increased numbers of Th2 cells have been identified in mucosal immune induction and effector sites. $CD4^+$ T lymphocytes that secrete cytokine patterns consistent with Th1 cells (IFN-γ, IL-2, and TNF-β), as well as $CD8^+$ cytotoxic T lymphocytes (CTL), have been identified in mucosal immune effector sites, but the functions of these cells have not been clearly defined. T lymphocytes activated by antigens in mucosal inductive sites also circulate throughout the blood and lymphatics, and disseminate to the lamina propria and epithelia of multiple mucosal tissues.

The mechanisms of human lymphocyte recirculation and emigration that direct lymphocytes to migrate from the peripheral blood to mucosal immune effector sites are only partially understood (Springer, 1994). These processes involve at least three steps, with multiple molecular events at each step, providing for a high level of diversity. Naive T lymphocytes express high levels of the L-selection adhesion molecule, which binds to ligands found on the high endothelial venules (HEV) or peripheral lymph nodes and mucosal associated lymphoid tissue. After initial binding of lymphocytes to HEV, a signal is transmitted via G protein-coupled receptors on the lymphocyte to activate the expression of specific secondary adhesion molecules known as integrins. The expression of different integrins can determine whether the lymphocyte will emigrate through the HEV in different lymphoid tissue. The $\alpha_4\beta_7$ integrin has been shown to be involved in the directional trafficking of murine lymphocytes to Peyer's patches and other gut-associated lymphoid tissue, and therefore it would seem to be an adhesion molecule specific for mucosal immunity (Holzmann *et al.*, 1989; Bell and Issekutz, 1993).

B and T lymphocytes primed at local mucosal immune induction sites and dispersed to mucosal immune effector sites can respond to further mucosal challenges with antigen-specific secretory antibody responses, T cell cytokine production, and cytolytic activity. Secretory IgA responses are known to be important in protective immunity against extracellular bacteria that cause diarrheal diseases as well as certain viruses susceptible to antibody neutralization (e.g., influenza virus), and may be important in the prevention of mucosal infection with Mtb. It is likely that T cell cytokine responses and cytolytic activity contribute other important functions in protective immunity at mucosal surfaces as well.

It has been shown that after oral administration BCG is taken up from the intestinal lumen through M cells in Peyer's patches similar to other orally ingested antigens and bacteria (Fujimura, 1986). However, the uptake and induction of mucosal immune responses by BCG, may be more complicated than the general outline for mucosal immune responses described above. Gheorghiu *et al.* (1995) found that BCG could translocate through rhinopharyngeal epithelia as well as intestinal mucosa (Table I). The BCG vaccine was administered orally to mice on five consecutive days at a dose of 5×10^9 cfu per day. During the first 5 days of the immunization protocol, in addition to being recovered from intestinal Peyer's patches and mesenteric lymph nodes, BCG was cultivated from submandibular glands, periglandular lymph nodes, and cervical lymph nodes. The recovery of BCG from head and neck internal tissues, prior to recovery from widely disseminated systemic sites (e.g., liver and spleen), strongly suggests that BCG translocates across rhinopharnygeal mucosa after oral ingestion. The development of suppurative cervical lymphadenitis after oral BCG administration, in some infants, further indicates that BCG can cross mucosa in the oropharynx, esophagus, or nasal epithelia. This rhinopharyngeal mucosal translocation of BCG may be important for the mucosal immune responses stimulated by oral BCG vaccination. The epidemiological data indicating that both achlorhydric persons and individuals that have undergone partial gastrectomy are at increased risk of developing TB has led to the general belief that gastric acidity is mycobactericidal. The murine experiments presented in Table I demonstrate that a substantial portion of the recoverable colony-forming units of ingested BCG are eliminated viable in feces. These results document that viable BCG traverses the entire length of the gastrointestinal tract; this suggests that BCG may induce immune responses by invading and replicating in any segment of the gut. It will be important to determine whether rhinopharyngeal or distal intestinal mucosal translocation is critical for the induction of any of the subsets of mucosal immunity induced by oral BCG vaccination.

Oral BCG vaccination in mice has been shown to be capable of stimulating high levels of secretory IgA responses (Lagranderie *et al.*, 1993a, 1996; Gheorghiu *et al.*, 1995). Recombinant strains of BCG expressing the *lacZ* gene were used to orally immunize guinea pigs and mice. Both antibody and cell-mediated immune responses to β-galactosidase were induced in guinea pigs, and mice developed antigen-specific secretory IgA responses directed against the foreign protein expressed by these recombinant BCG (Lagranderie *et al.*, 1993a; Gheorghiu *et al.*, 1995). In addition, mice orally immunized with BCG developed high levels of secretory IgA responses directly against mycobacterial antigens in intestinal secretions, as well as in bronchoalveolar lavages and sera (Lagranderie *et al.*, 1996). The induction of secretory IgA responses by mucosal BCG vaccination strongly suggests that Th2 cells are stimulated by mucosal BCG vaccination. In addition, Belyakoff *et al.* (1995) have demonstrated that oral BCG administration to mice can induce the antigen-specific production of IL-6 in $CD4^+$ T cells isolated from Peyer's patches postvaccination. These results provide direct evidence for the induction of Th2 responses by oral vaccination with BCG. This is in contrast to previous studies demonstrating a strong bias for the induction of Th1 responses in both humans and animal models after parenteral BCG vaccination (Del Prete *et al.*, 1991; Haanen *et al.*, 1991; Pearlman *et al.*, 1993; Hoft *et al.*, 1996; Kemp *et al.*, 1996).

In response to Mtb infection in mucosal tissue, Th1 cells could activate macrophages and lead to increased killing activity against intracellular mycobacteria. Mycobacterial-specific CTL could directly lyse epithelial cells and macrophages infected with Mtb in mucosal tissue. In the murine studies conducted by Belyakoff *et al.* (1995) mentioned above, $CD4^+$ T cells purified from the Peyer's patches of animals immunized orally with BCG were found to produce IFN-γ in response to *in vitro* stimulation with mycobacterial antigens. Gheorghiu *et al.* (1995) demonstrated that T cells harvested from intestinal Peyer's patches, intraepithelial lymphocytes (i-IEL), and splenocytes of mice orally immunized with a recombinant BCG expressing the Nef protein of simian immunodeficiency virus (SIV) produced IFN-γ and TNF-α after *in vitro* stimulation with mycobacterial antigens or Nef-specific peptide (Gheorghiu *et al.*, 1995, and Table II). These results indicate that oral BCG vaccination can stimulate Th1 cells, or Th0 cells that produce both Th1 and Th2 cytokines (IFN-γ and IL-6, respectively) in both local mucosal and systemic tissues. In addition, at the Institut Pasteur, oral vaccination of mice with BCG has been shown to induce $CD8^+$ lymphocytes purified from intestinal intraepithelia and spleen with antigen specific cytotoxicity for both mycobacterial antigens and the SIV Nef protein expressed in a recombinant strain of BCG (Gheorghiu *et al.*, 1995).

Therefore, at least in mice, oral BCG vaccination can be used to stimulate all the major subsets of cellular and humoral immunity that could provide protective mucosal and systemic immunity. Whether oral BCG vaccination can stimulate these same immune responses in humans is unknown at the present time, but we are conducting a dose escalation trial of oral BCG vaccination in human volunteers to address this question. Figure 1 summarizes proposed mechanisms of in-

TABLE II
Enumeration of Cytokine-Producing Cells from Orally Immunized BALB/c Mice[a]

		IFN-γ SFC[b] after stimulation *in vitro* with		TNF-α SFC after stimulation *in vitro* with	
Cells from	Immunization with	SIV-Nef peptide (1 μg/ml)	PPD (10 μg/ml)	SIV-Nef peptide (1 μg/ml)	PPD (10 μg/ml)
PP	rBCG SIV-Nef	70 ± 10	90 ± 12	105 ± 20	100 ± 15
	BCG 1173P2	6 ± 2	100 ± 30	8 ± 2	115 ± 30
IEL	rBCG SIV-Nef	30 ± 5	35 ± 6	30 ± 10	35 ± 5
	BCG 1173P2	3 ± 1	30 ± 5	2 ± 0	30 ± 4
SP	rBCG SIV-Nef	100 ± 18	120 ± 18	350 ± 60	480 ± 35
	BCG 1173P2	10 ± 4	150 ± 25	40 ± 8	350 ± 55

[a]BALB/c mice (five per group) were orally immunized with 5×10^9 cfu of rBCG SIV-Nef or 1173P2 BCG. Four weeks later, cells from Peyer's patches (PP), intraepithelial lymphocytes (IEL), and spleen (SP) were harvested, and cytokine-producing cells were detected after stimulation with 146–160 SIV-Nef peptide or with PPD.

[b]Number of spot-forming cells per 10^6 cells.

duction of cellular and humoral immune responses after oral BCG vaccination.

V. Summary

The oral administration of BCG may be a way to improve the protective efficacy of BCG against TB by providing mucosal immunity that can prevent Mtb infection, as well as a way to improve the ease of BCG administration and lower the cost of mass vaccination. In addition, the use of oral BCG as a vaccine vector may be an ideal means of inducing both mucosal and systemic protective immunity against other human pathogens. The perceived drawbacks of oral BCG have included adverse effects, mycobactericidal activity of gastric secretions, relative impermeability of adult intestinal mucosa to microbes, and previous observations that oral BCG vaccination had provided only incomplete protection against TB. However, it is unclear whether oral BCG vaccination is associated with increased risks compared with intradermal BCG vaccination, which is used safely in millions of infants every year. In addition, new methods of oral delivery may decrease the risks of adverse effects as well as enhance the potency of mucosal and systemic immune responses induced by oral BCG vaccine. Oral administration of BCG to animals has been shown to stimulate both cellular and humoral subsets of mucosal and systemic immunity. Investigations of the mucosal and systemic immune responses stimulated by oral BCG vaccination in humans are now underway.

References

Aldovini, A., and Young, R. A. (1991). Humoral and cell-mediated immune responses to live recombinant BCG-HIV vaccines. *Nature (London)* **351**, 479–482.

Barletta, R. G., Snapper, B., Cirillo, J. D., Connell, N. D., Kim, D. D., Jacobs, W. R., and Bloom, B. R. (1990). Recombinant BCG as a candidate oral vaccine vector. *Res. Microbiol.* **141**, 931–939.

Barnes, P. F., Mehra, V., Rivoire, B., Fong, S. J., Brennan, P. J., Voegtline, M. S., Minden, P., Houghten, R. A., Bloom, B. R., and Modlin, R. L. (1992). Immunoreactivity of a 10-kDa antigen of *Mycobacterium tuberculosis*. *J. Immunol.* **148**, 1835–1840.

Beckman, E. M., Procelli, S. A., Morita, C. T., Behar, S. M., Furlong, S. T., and Brenner, M. B. (1994). Recognition of a lipid antigen by CD1-restricted alpha beta$^+$ T cells. *Nature (London)* **372**, 691–694.

Bell, R. G., and Issekutz, T. (1993). Expression of a protective intestinal immune response can be inhibited at three distinct sites by treatment with anti-alpha 4 integrin. *J. Immunol.* **151**, 4790–4802.

Belyakoff, I. M., VanCott, J. E., Carter, P. B., Hiroi, T., Yamamoto, M., Hoft, D. F., McGhee, J. R., and Kiyono, H. (1995). Antigen-specific B-cell responses in mucosal immunity after oral administration of BCG. *FASEB 9th Int. Cong. Immunol.* 4870.

Bloom, B. R., and Fine, P. E. M. (1994). The BCG experience: Implications for future vaccines against tuberculosis. *In* "Tuberculosis: Pathogenesis, Protection, and Control" (B. R. Bloom, ed.), pp. 531–557. American Society for Microbiology, Washington, D.C.

Bloom, B. R., Flynn, J., McDonough, K., Kress, Y., and Chan, J. (1994). Experimental approaches to mechanisms of protection and pathogenesis in *M. tuberculosis* infection. *Immunobiology* **191**, 526–536.

Calmette, A. (1927). "La Vaccination Preventive Contre la Tuberculose par le BCG." Masson et Cie, Paris.

Calmette, A., Guérin, C., and Weill-Halle, B. (1924). Essais d'immunisation contre l'infection tuberculeuse. *Bull. Acad. Med.* **91**, 787–797.

Calmette, A., Guérin, C., Weill-Halle, B., Nègre, L., Boquet, A., and Turpin, R. (1925). Essais de premunition par le BCG contre l'infection tuberculeuse de l'homme et des animaux. *Bull. Acad. Med.* **93**, 681–696.

Calmette, A., Guérin, C., Nègre, L., and Bocquet, A. (1926). Prémunition des nouveau-nés contre la tuberculose par le vaccin BCG. *Ann. Inst. Pasteur* **2**, 89–120.

Calmette, A., Weill-Halle, B., Saenz, A., and Costil, L. (1933). Demonstration experimentale du passage des bacilles-vaccines BCG a travers la muquesuse del'intestin chez l'enfant et chez le singe. *Bull. Acad. Med.* **110**, 203–212.

Calmette, A., Boquet, A., and Nègre, L. (1936). "L'infection Bacillaire et al Tuberculose." Masson et Cie, Paris.

Colditz, G. A., Brewer, T. F., Berkey, C. S., Wilson, M. E., Burdick, E., Fineberg, H. V., and Mosteller, F. (1994). Efficacy of BCG vaccine in the prevention of tuberculosis: Meta-analysis of the published literature. *JAMA, J. Am. Med. Assoc.* **271**, 698–702.

Colditz, G. A., Berkey, C. S., Mosteller, F., Brewer, T. F., Wilson, M. E., Burdick, E., and Fineberg, H. V. (1995). The efficacy of Bacillus Calmette–Guerin vaccination of newborns and infants in the prevention of tuberculosis: Meta-analyses of the published literature. *Pediatrics* **96**, 29–35.

Collins, F. M. (1991). Antituberculous immunity: New solutions to an old problem. *Rev. Infect. Dis.* **13**, 940–950.

Comstock, G. W. (1988). Identification of an effective vaccine against tuberculosis. *Am. Rev. Respir. Dis.* **138**, 479–480.

Connell, N. D., Medina-Acosta, E., McMaster, W. R., Bloom, B. R., and Russell, D. G. (1993). Effective immunization against cutaneous leishmaniasis with recombinant bacille Calmette–Guerin expressing the *Leshmania* surface proteinase gp63. *Proc. Natl. Acad. Sci. U.S.A.* **90**, 11473–11477.

Cooper, A. M., Dalton, D. K., Stewart, T. A., Griffin, J. P., Russell, D. G., and Orme, I. M. (1993). Disseminated tuberculosis in interferon gamma gene-disrupted mice. *J. Exp. Med.* **178**, 2243–2247.

Cooper, A. M., Roberts, A. D., Rhoades, E. R., Callahan, J. E., Getzy, D. M., and Orme, I. M. (1995). The role of interleukin-12 in acquired immunity to *Mycobacterium tuberculosis* infection. *Immunology* **84**, 423–432.

Dannenberg, A. M., Jr., and Rook, G. A. W. (1994). Pathogenesis of pulmonary tuberculosis: An interplay of tissue damaging and macrophage activating immune responses. *In* "Tuberculosis: Pathogenesis, Protection and Control" (B. R. Bloom, ed.), pp. 459–483. American Society for Microbiology, Washington, D.C.

de Assis, A. (1948). Vaccination concomitante au BCG, 1st International Congress on BCG. *Ann. Inst. Pasteur* **75**, 205–225.

Del Prete, G. F., De Carli, M., Mastromauro, C., Biagiotti, R., Macchia, D., Falagiani, P., Ricci, M., and Romagnani, S. (1991). Purified protein derivative of *Mycobacterium tuberculosis* and excretory–secretory antigen(s) of *Toxocara canis* expand *in vitro* human T cells with stable and opposite (type 1 T helper or type 2 T helper) profile of cytokine production. *J. Clin. Invest.* **88**, 346–350.

Domingo, P. (1948). Valeur de la voie gastrique dans la vaccination antituberculeuse par le BCG. *In* "Premier Congrès International du BCG 1948," pp. 230–240. Institut Pasteur, Paris.

Douvas, G. S., Looker, D. L., Vatter, A. E., and Crowle, A. J. (1985). Gamma interferon activates human macrophages to become tumoricidal and leishmanicidal but enhances replication of macrophage-associated mycobacteria. *Infect. Immun.* **50**, 1–8.

Fine, P. E. M. (1989). The BCG story: Lessons from the past and implications for the future. *Rev. Infect. Dis.* **11**, S353–S359.

Fine, P. E. M., and Rodrigues, L. C. (1990). Modern vaccines: Mycobacterial diseases. *Lancet* **335**, 1016–1020.

Flesch, I., and Kaufmann, S. H. E. (1987). Mycobacterial growth inhibition by interferon-activated bone marrow macrophages and differential susceptibility amongst strains of *Mycobacterium tuberculosis*. *J. Immunol.* **138**, 4408–4413.

Flynn, J. L., Goldstein, M. M., Triebold, K. J., Koller, B., and Bloom, B. R. (1992). Major histocompatibility complex class I-restricted T cells are required for resistance to *Mycobacterium tuberculosis* infection. *Proc. Natl. Acad. Sci. U.S.A.* **89**, 12013–12017.

Flynn, J. L., Chan, J., Triebold, K. J., Dalton, D. K., Stewart, T. A., and Bloom, B. R. (1993). An essential role for interferon gamma in resistance to *Mycobacterium tuberculosis* infection. *J. Exp. Med.* **178**, 2249–2254.

Flynn, J. L., Goldstein, M. M., Triebold, K. J., Sypek, J., Wolf, S., and Bloom, B. R. (1995). IL-12 increases resistance to BALB/c mice to *Mycobacterium tuberculosis* infection. *J. Immunol.* **155**, 2515–2524.

Fujimura, Y. (1986). Financial morphology of microfold cells (M cells) in Peyer's patches phagocytosis and transport of BCG by M cells into rabbit Peyer's patches. *Gastroenterol. Jpn.* **21**, 325–335.

Gheorghiu, M. (1996). Antituberculosis BCG vaccine, lessons from the past. *In* "History of Vaccinology" (S. Plotkin, ed.), in press. Elsevier, Paris.

Gheorghiu, M., Lagranderie, M., Balazuc, A. M., and Gicquel, B. (1995). Mucosal induced immune responses after oral BCG vaccination. *Clin. Immunol. Immunopathol.* **76**, S94 and 547.

Haanen, J. B. A. G., de Waal Malefijt, R., Res, P. C. M., Kraakman, E. M., Ottenhoff, T. H. M., de Vries, R. R. P., and Spits, H. (1991). Selection of a human T helper type 1-like T cell subset by mycobacteria. *J. Exp. Med.* **174**, 583–592.

Hart, P. D. (1967). Efficacy and applicability of mass BCG vaccination in tuberculosis control. *Br. Med. J.* **1**, 293–295.

Heimbeck, J., and Scheel, O. (1928). Le reaction tuberculinique et le vaccin BCG chez les adultes. Experiences faites a l'hopital Ulleval d'Oslo (Norvege). *Bull. Acad. Med.* **99**, 44–51.

Hoft, D. F., Kemp, E. B., Mariano, M., Cruz, O., Kiyono, H., McGhee, J. R., Belisle, J. T., Milligan, T. W., Miller, J. P., and Belshe, R. B. (1996). Mycobacterial specific human immunity induced by intradermal BCG vaccination. Submitted for publication.

Holzmann, B., McIntyre, B. W., and Weissman, I. L. (1989). Identification of a murine Peyer's patch-specific lymphocyte homing receptor as an integrin molecule with an alpha chain homologous to human VLA-4. *Cell (Cambridge, Mass.)* **56**, 37–47.

Husson, R. N., James, B. E., and Young, R. A. (1990). Gene replacement and expression of foreign DNA in mycobacteria. *J. Bacteriol.* **172**, 519–524.

Jacobs, W. R., Snapper, S. B., Tuckman, M., and Bloom, B. R. (1989). Mycobacteriophage vector systems. *Rev. Infect. Dis.* **11**, S404–S410.

Kamijo, R., Shapiro, D., Gerecitano, J., Le, J., Bosland, M., and Vilcek, J. (1994). Biological functions of IFN-gamma and IFN-alpha/beta: Lessons from studies in gene knockout mice. *Hokkaido J. Med. Sci.* **69**, 1332–1338.

Kaufmann, S. H. E., and Ladel, C. H. (1994). Role of T cell subsets in immunity against intracellular bacteria: Experimental infections of knock-out mice with *Listeria monocytogenes* and *Mycobacterium bovis. Immunobiology* **191**, 509–519.

Kemp. E. B., Belshe, R. B., and Hoft, D. F. (1996). Immune response stimulated by percutaneous and intradermal BCG. *J. Infect. Dis.* **174**, 113–119.

Lagranderie, M., Murray, A., Gicquel, B., Leclerc, C., and Gheorghiu, M. (1993a). Oral immunization with recombinant BCG induces cellular and humoral immune responses against the foreign antigen. *Vaccine* **11**, 1283–1290.

Lagranderie, M., Ravisse, P., Marchal, G., Gheorghiu, M., Balasubramanian, V., Wiegeshaus, E. H., and Smith, D. W. (1993b). BCG-induced protection in guinea pigs vaccinated and challanged via the respiratory route. *Tubercle and Lung Disease* **74**, 38–46.

Lagranderie, M. R., Balazuc, A. M., Deriaud, E., Leclerc, C. D., and Gheorghiu, M. (1996). Comparison of immune responses of mice immunized by five different BCG vaccine strains. *Infect. Immun.* **64**, 1–9.

Lang, F., Peyrat, M. A., Constant, P., Davodeau, F., David-Ameline, J., Poquet, Y., Vié, H., Fournié, J. J., and Bonneville, M. (1995). Early activation of human Vgamma9delta2 T cell broad cytotoxicity and TNF production by nonpeptidic mycobacterial ligands. *J. Immunol.* **154**, 5986–5994.

Lotte, A., Wasz-Hockert, O., Poisson, N., Dumitrescu, N., Vernon, M., and Couvet, E. (1984). BCG complications: Estimates of the risks among vaccinated subjects and statistical analysis of their main characteristics. *Adv. Tuberc. Res.* **21**, 107–193.

McGhee, J. R., Mestecky, J., Elson, C. O., and Kiyono, H. (1989). Regulation of IgA synthesis and immune response by T cells and interleukins. *J. Clin. Immunol.* **9**, 175–199.

McGhee, J. R., Mestecky, J., Dertzbaugh, M. T., Eldridge, J. H., Hirasawa, M., and Kiyono, H. (1992). The mucosal immune system: From fundamental concepts to vaccine development. *Vaccine* **10**, 75–88.

Maggi, E., Biswas, P., Del Prete, G. F., Parronchi, P., Macchia, D., Simonelli, C., Emmi, L., De Carli, M., Tiri, A., Ricci, M., and Romagnani, S. (1991). Accumulation of Th-2-like helper T cells in the conjunctiva of patients with vernal conjunctivitis. *J. Immunol.* **146**, 1169–1174.

Mande, R. (1996). Manifestations tuberculeuses chez les vaccinés. *In* "Manuel Practique de Vaccination" (R. Mande, ed.), pp. 237–240. Médicales, Flammarion, France.

Morita, C. T., Beckman, E. M., Bukowski, J. F., Tanaka, Y., Band, H., Bloom, B. R., Golan, D. E., and Brenner, M. B. (1995). Direct presentation of nonpeptide prenyl pyrophosphate antigens to human gammadelta T cells. *Immunity,* **3**, 495–507.

Mosmann, T. R., Cherwinski, H., Bond, M. W., Giedlin, M. A., and Coffman, R. L. (1986). Two types of murine helper T cell clone: I. Definition according to profiles of lymphokine activities and secreted proteins. *J. Immunol.* **136**, 2348–2357.

Mosmann, T. R., Schumacher, J. H., Street, N. F., Budd, R., O'Garra, A., Fong, T. A. T., Bond, M. W., Moore, K. W. M., Sher, A., and Fiorentino, D. F. (1991). Diversity of cytokine synthesis and function of mouse $CD4^+$ T cells. *Immunol. Rev.* **123**, 209–229.

Orme, I. M., (1988a). Induction of nonspecific acquired resistance and delayed-type hypersensitivity, but not specific acquired resistance, in mice inoculated with killed mycobacterial vaccines. *Infect. Immun.* **56**, 3310–3312.

Orme, I. M. (1988b). Characteristics and specificity of acquired immunologic memory to *Mycobacterium tuberculosis* infection. *J. Immunol.* **140**, 3589–3593.

Orme, I. M., and Collins, F. M. (1983). Protection against *Mycobacterium tuberculosis* infection by adoptive immunotherapy. *J. Exp. Med.* **158**, 74–84.

Pearlman, E., Kazura, J. W., Hazlett, Jr., F. E., and Boom, W. H . (1993). Modulation of murine cytokine responses to mycobacterial antigens by helminth-induced T helper 2 cell responses. *J. Immunol.* **151**, 4857–4864.

Pfeffer, K., Schoel, B., Plesnila, N., Lipford, G. B., Kromer, S., Deusch, K., and Wagner, H. (1992). A lectin-binding, protease-resistant mycobacterial ligand specifically activates Vgamma9+ human gammadelta T cells. *J. Immunol.* **148**, 575–583.

Porcelli, S., Morita, C. T., and Brenner, M. B. (1992). CD1b restricts the response of human $CD4^-8^-$ T lymphocytes to a microbial antigen. *Nature (London)* **360**, 593–597.

Ramsay, A. J., Husband, A. J., Ramshaw, I. A., Bao, S., Matthaei, K. I., Koehler, G., and Kopf, M. (1994). The role of interleukin-6 in mucosal IgA antibody responses *in vivo. Science* **264**, 561–563.

Rook, G. A. W., Champion, B. R., Steele, J., Varey, A. M., and Stanford, J. L. (1985). I-A restricted activation by T cell lines of anti-tuberculous activity in murine macrophages. *Clin. Exp. Immunol.* **159**, 414–420.

Rosenthal, S. R. (1980). Routes and methods of administration. *In* "BCG Vaccine: Tuberculosis–Cancer," pp. 146–175. PSG Publ., Littleton, Massachusetts.

Salgame, P., Abrams, J. S., Clayberger, C., Goldstein, H., Convit, J., Modlin, R. L., and Bloom, B. R. (1991). Differing lymphokine profiles of functional subsets of human CD4 and CD8 T cell clones. *Science* **254**, 279–282.

Sanchez, F. O., Rodriguez, J. I., Agudelo, G., and Garcia, L. F. (1994). Immune responsiveness and lymphokine production in patients with tuberculosis and healthy controls. *Infect. Immun.* **62**, 5673–5678.

Scott, P., Pearce, E., Cheever, A. W., Coffman, R. L., and Sher, A. (1989). Role of cytokines and $CD4^+$ T-cell subsets in the regulation of parasite immunity and disease. *Immunol. Rev.* **112**, 161–182.

Société des Nations (C.H.745) Organisation d'Hygiène Genèva. (1928). Rapport de la conférence technique pour l'étude de la vaccination antituberculeuse par le BCG. *Inst. Pasteur Paris,* 1–12.

Springer, T. A. (1994). Traffic signals for lymphocyte recirculation and leukocyte emigration: The multistep paradigm. *Cell (Cambridge, Mass.)* **76**, 301–314.

Tanaka, Y., Morita, C. T., Nieves, E., Brenner, M. B., and Bloom, B. R. (1995). Natural and synthetic non-peptidic antigens recognized by human gammadelta T cells. *Nature (London)* **375**, 155–158.

Tsukaguchi, K., Balaji, K. N., and Boom, W. H. (1995). $CD4^+$ alphabeta T cell and gammadelta T cell responses to *Mycobacterium tuberculosis. J. Immunol.* **154**, 1786–1796.

Vajdy, M., Kosco-Vilbois, M. H., Kopf, M., Kohler, G., and Lycke, N. (1995). Impaired mucosal immune responses in interleukin 4-targeted mice. *J. Exp. Med.* **181**, 41–53.

Van Deinse, F. (1948). Enquête sur la fréquence des adénites suppurées consécutives à la vaccination au BCG par scarifications cutanées ou par voie buccale. *In* "Premier Congrès International du BCG 1948," pp. 89–91. Institut Pasteur, Paris.

Weigert, C. (1883). Wege des tuberkelgiftes zue den serosen hauten. *Dtsch. Med. Wochenschr.* **9**, 453–462.

Weill-Halle, B. (1924). La tuberculose du nourrisson et d'essais de vaccination par le bacille bilie de Calmette–Guerin. *Monde Med.* **34**, 461–480.

Winter, N., Lagranderie, M., Rauzier, J., Timm, J., Leclerc, C., Guy, B., Kieny, M. P., Gheorghiu, M., and Gicquel, B. (1991). Expression of heterologous genes in *Mycobacterium bovis* BCG: Induction of a cellular response against HIV-1 Nef protein. *Gene* **109**, 47–54.

Winter, N., Lagranderie, M., Gangloff, S., Leclerc, C., Gheorghiu, M., and Gicquel, B. (1995). Recombinant BCG strains expressing SIVmac25*nef* gene induce proliferative and CTL responses against nef synthetic peptides in mice. *Vaccine* **13**, 471–478.

Yamamura, M., Uyemura, K., Deans, R. J., Weinberg, K., Rea, T. H., Bloom, B. R., and Modlin, R. L. (1991). Defining protective responses to pathogens: Cytokine profiles in leprosy lesions. *Science* **254**, 277–279.

Yasutomi, Y., Koenig, S., Haun, S. S., Stover, C. K., Jackson, R. K., Conard, P., Conley, A. J., Emini, E. A., Fuerst, T. R., and Letvin, N. L. (1993). Immunization with recombinant BCG-SIV elicits SIV-specific cytotoxic T lymphocytes in rhesus monkeys. *J. Immunol.* **150**, 3101–3107.

Zeyland, J., and Piasecka-Zeyland, E. (1928). Sur la penetration des bacilles a travers la paroi du tube digestif d'apres les autopsies des enfants vaccines au BCG par voie baccale. *Ann. Inst. Pasteur* **42**, 61–66.

VI

Mucosal Vaccines for Viral Diseases

21

Polioviruses and Mucosal Vaccines

CAROLYN WEEKS-LEVY
Biostar Inc.
Saskatoon, Saskatchewan S7N 3R2, Canada

PEARAY L. OGRA
Department of Pediatrics
Children's Hospital
University of Texas Medical Branch
Galveston, Texas 77555

I. Introduction

Poliovirus has been widely studied for many decades, and many significant scientific discoveries have been made during this time. However, research on specific mucosal and cellular immune responses has not been performed until very recently in the history of polio vaccines. The cellular immunity necessary for poliovirus clearance and its role in the development of the disease poliomyelitis are still not well defined. The immunological background of individuals predisposed to contract poliomyelitis is still undefined and further investigation is required to gain a comprehensive picture of the host immune status and susceptibility to polio disease. Understanding the immunological aspects of poliovirus was not necessary for the development of the oral and inactivated vaccines in the 1950s. As more vaccines are introduced into immunization schedules and formulations of combination vaccines become more complex, the necessity to understand required immunological responses will become critical. This chapter provides background information on polio vaccines, and will compare immune responses elicited by both OPV and IPV given alone and in combination schedules (IPV/OPV) as well as in direct combination with other live-attenuated or parenterally administered vaccine formulations. Effects of local immunity on outbreaks and shedding of revertant virus will also be discussed. In addition, the importance of mucosal immunity will be highlighted throughout the text. This chapter also touches on studies aimed at understanding the role of cellular immune responses and specific immunoglobulin classes in the prevention of poliovirus infection.

A. Polio Vaccines

One of the first major breakthroughs in polio vaccine development was made by John Enders and his colleagues in 1949 when they demonstrated that poliovirus could be propagated in tissue culture cells (Enders *et al.*, 1949). This discovery made the development of the inactivated (Salk) and live-attenuated (Sabin) poliovirus vaccines possible. The introduction of these vaccines during the 1950s and 1960s led to the successful control of poliomyelitis in developed countries. The advantages and disadvantages of oral and inactivated poliovirus vaccine, OPV, and IPV, respectively, will be discussed throughout the text. Table I summarizes the characteristics, advantages and disadvantages of these vaccines.

1. IPV

The inactivated poliovirus vaccine (IPV-Salk) developed by Jonas Salk was approved for public use by the U.S. Public Health Service in 1955. Inactivated polio vaccine is composed of three serotypes of wild-type poliovirus strains inactivated with formalin (Salk, 1953; Salk *et al.*, 1953). To be protected, an individual must raise immunity to all three polio serotypes. The vaccine did a tremendous job in dramatically decreasing the number of paralytic poliomyelitis cases. After the introduction of IPV, the number of paralytic polio cases decreased from 37 cases in 100,000 to 0.8 cases in 100,000 (Strebel *et al.*, 1992). However, during the first 4 years of the vaccine's use, it became evident that thousands of children continued to be infected with polio each year. IPV-Salk was administered routinely until oral poliovirus vaccine (OPV) was approved for use.

TABLE I
Characteristics, Advantages and Disadvantages of Oral Polio Vaccine (OPV) and Inactivated Polio Vaccine (IPV)

Characteristic	OPV	IPV
Composition	Live-attenuated Sabin strains of serotypes 1,2,3	Inactivated wild-type strains or inactivated Sabin strains of serotypes 1,2,3
Formulation	*WHO:* 10^6:10^5:$10^{5.8}$ (10:1:6) *US:* $10^{6.5}$:$10^{5.6}$:$10^{6.3}$ (8:1:5)	*IPV-Salk:* 20-2-4 D antigen units for types 1,2,3 respectively *EIPV:* 40-8-32 D antigen units for types 1,2,3, respectively
Countries using	United States South America China Former Soviet Union Africa Canada—some provinces All other countries not listed under IPV	Sweden Norway Finland Iceland Holland Netherlands Canada—some provinces
Countries using combined schedule	Canada (Prince Edward Island) Ireland Denmark Israel	
Advantages	Easy to administer. Confers good humoral and intestinal immunity. Relatively inexpensive to manufacture. Intestinal immunity prevents replication and spread of epidemic virus. Herd immunity.	Can be combined with other parenteral vaccines. EIPV formulation confers good humoral and some intestinal immunity. Can be used in immunocompromised individuals. Vaccine is thermally stable.
Disadvantages	Vaccine virus reverts in gut of vaccinees, may cause vaccine-associated disease. Virus can spread to unimmunized contacts. Cannot be used in immunocompromised individuals. Cold chain is required.	Need repeated boosters. Does not provide as good intestinal immunity. More expensive to produce. Wild-type strains are used, failure in the inactivation could cause disease in vaccinees.

Since then, OPV has been the recommended vaccine for immunologically competent individuals in the United States. Recently, however, investigators have become interested in employing IPV into a routine immunization schedule. A combination schedule where IPV is given prior to OPV has been under investigation since the introduction of an enhanced-potency formulation of IPV, EIPV (McBean *et al.*, 1988). Vaccination with EIPV before OPV may have a positive impact on the rate of vaccine-associated disease (see OPV below).

The classical IPV vaccine provides excellent humoral immunity but less mucosal immunity. Humoral immunity is important in stopping viremic polio spread; the mucosal immunity stops polio infection at its site of entry into the body. EIPV has an increased antigenic content of 40-8-32 D antigen units for types 1, 2, and 3 respectively. The classical IPV, however, had a D antigen content of 20-2-4 (Faden, 1993). In addition, the enhanced potency IPV has seroconversion rates of 99% after two doses in contrast to earlier IPV preparations that required three or four doses to achieve a comparable seroconversion rate (Faden *et al.*, 1990; Grenier *et al.*, 1984; McBean *et al.*, 1988; Simoes *et al.*, 1985). With its increased antigen content, EIPV was postulated to have the potential to induce mucosal immunity. The enhanced potency IPV has been examined for its ability to induce nasopharyngeal immunity. Figure 1 shows secretory antibody responses measured with respect to capsid proteins VP1, VP2, and VP3 as well as whole-virus neutralization and whole-virus ELISA (IgA) after immunization with OPV, IPV-Salk, EIPV, or IPV/OPV. Enhanced-potency IPV was able to induce ELISA antibody, neutralizing antibody activity, and S-IgA to capsid proteins VP1 and VP2 in some nasopharyngeal samples tested (Zhaori *et al.*, 1988). This is a clear advantage of the EIPV vaccine over the classical formulation; as a result of this factor, the combination of EIPV immunization followed by OPV immunization is under consideration in the United States.

Other countries have relied on the use of IPV either solely or in combination regimes with OPV. For example, the Nordic countries Sweden, Finland, Norway, Iceland, and Holland use IPV alone, while Denmark uses a mixed schedule of IPV followed by OPV (Bottiger, 1993). The vaccination rates in these countries are extremely high, and IPV has been used successfully to prevent poliomyelitis. In these countries, the general circulation of wild virus appeared to cease simultaneously with the disease. The enhanced potency IPV formulation has been introduced into the vaccination schedule based on studies comparing immune responses of the original formulation and enhanced-po-

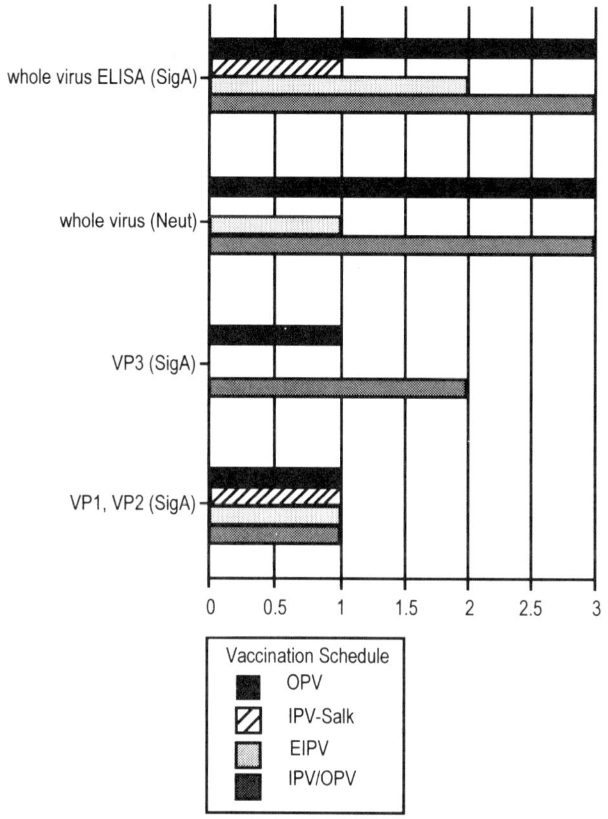

Figure 1. Comparison of secretory immune responses elicited by different vaccination schedules. Specific responses measured are indicated on the vertical axis. Positive responses are on the horizontal axis and are scored from 0 to +++ with +++ being the greatest response. This figure is adapted from Ogra and Garofalo (1990). Secretory antibody response to viral vaccines. *Prog. Med. Virol.* **37**, 156–189.

tency formulation (Mellander *et al.*, 1993). It was found that after three doses of either of the IPV formulations the enhanced-potency IPV induced higher serum neutralization titers for type 1 and type 3 poliovirus. Similar levels of secretory IgA in saliva were found in the two vaccine groups. Avidity of serum IgG antibodies was significantly higher after two doses of the enhanced formulation in comparison to avidity after thee doses of the original formulation. The enhanced potency formulation was recommended to be used in a three-dose schedule. Though the majority of the world depends on OPV (see Table I), successful reliance on an IPV immunization schedule has been achieved in well-vaccinated populations.

2. *OPV*

Research efforts continued throughout the late 1940s and 1950s in an attempt to develop another type of poliovirus vaccine based on live, weakened strains of the virus (OPV). Work was conducted in the laboratories of Drs. Hilary Koprowski, Herald Cox, and Albert Sabin in the United States. Eventually, the three polio serotypes developed by Dr. Sabin (Sabin 1, Sabin 2, Sabin 3) were approved for use by the U.S. Public Health Service in 1961 (Sabin and Boulger, 1973). The live vaccine has been the recommended vaccine for immunocompetent individuals since its introduction. One of the advantages of OPV is that it is easier to orally administer and provides both mucosal and parenteral/systemic immunity. OPV was thought to provide the recipient with lifelong immunity, but more recent studies have forced researchers to question this idea (Nishio *et al.*, 1984). An additional benefit of the OPV vaccine is that in most cases, the vaccine virus can spread from immunized individuals to those unimmunized (herd immunity). Since the introduction of OPV, the rate of poliomyelitis decreased to 0.002 cases per 100,000 in the United States (Strebel *et al.*, 1992). Now, the only cases of poliomyelitis are those termed vaccine-associated cases of paralytic polio thought to be caused by the vaccine virus (Stratton *et al.*, 1994).

In contrast to IPV, different factors come into play with respect to take rate with OPV vaccination, especially in developing countries. One major concern especially for use of OPV in the tropics is the thermostability of the vaccine. OPV requires that a cold chain is maintained during storage and transport. The virus is not stable for prolonged periods at ambient temperatures. Other factors that affect the efficacy of OPV include low-potency vaccine formulations, enteric infections, malnutrition, and breast feeding (Patriarca *et al.*, 1991). The one factor that can be controlled to some extent is the potency of the vaccine formulation. Many developing countries receive vaccine through the World Health Organization (WHO) or other organizations that formulate to WHO specifications. To address concerns of low-potency vaccine formulations, the WHO has set a higher requirement for the amount of type 3 virus in the oral poliovirus vaccine formulation. The new WHO formulation standards still set lower requirements for the amount of vaccine virus in a dose compared to that used in the United States formulation (see Table 1). The World Health Organization has also been pursuing development of a thermostable OPV formulation to help solve issues with maintaining a cold chain (Lemon and Milstein, 1994). Methods under development include freeze drying in the presence of stabilizers as well as using deuterium to stabilize the capsid proteins (Rong *et al.*, 1994). The desire is to develop an OPV formulation that can withstand temperatures of 45°C for seven days and show less than 0.5 log10 drop in titer of each poliovirus serotypes (Lemon and Milstein, 1994). This goal may not be achieved but a more thermostable formulation will likely be developed.

OPV had proven to be a safe and effective vaccine over its many years of use. However, on rare occasion the vaccine has been associated with paralytic poliomyelitis (Stratton *et al.*, 1994). Individuals at risk of

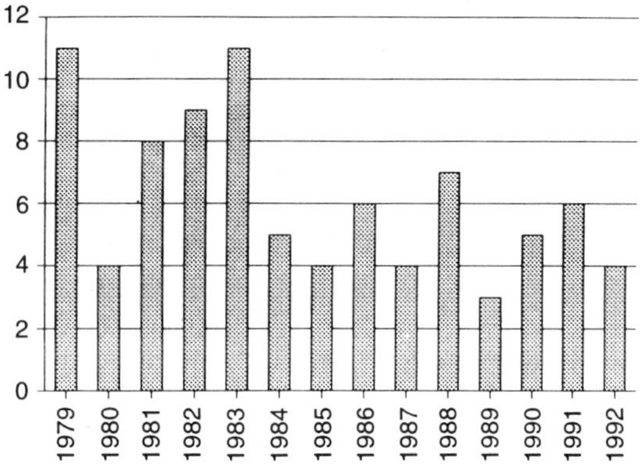

Figure 2. Confirmed cases of paralytic poliomyelitis in the United States during the time period from 1979 to 1992. Years are indicated on the horizontal axis and numbers of cases on the vertical axis. The cases include contact and vaccinee cases.

developing vaccine associated disease include: recipients of OPV (who are usually infants receiving their first dose), people in contact with OPV recipients (who are most often unvaccinated or inadequately vaccinated), and immunologically abnormal individuals. After 1964, the rate of vaccine associated polio in the United States has remained fairly stable at 3–4 cases/10 million doses distributed (Strebel *et al.*, 1992). Figure 2 illustrates the number of vaccines associated cases of all types that have occurred in the United States over the period from 1979–1992. With the decrease of circulating wild polio strains from the Americas, more emphasis has been placed on eliminating vaccine associated paralytic polio. Therefore, research has been carried out to understand the changes the virus undergoes as it replicates in the intestinal tract. It is known that with passage in the human gut that poliovirus vaccine strains have a tendency to lose their fully attenuated phenotypic characteristics (Furesz *et al.*, 1966). Early studies also revealed that poliovirus serially passaged in tissue culture became more neurovirulent with passage (Stones *et al.*, 1964). The exact genetic changes that characterized drift from fully attenuated Sabin strains to more neurovirulent strains were not known until the scientific community began to understand the molecular biology of the virus.

II. Neurovirulence and Molecular Biology of Poliovirus

A. Neurovirulence Testing of OPV

The primary safety test employed to evaluate the oral poliovirus vaccine is the monkey neurovirulence test, which is performed according to the Code of Federal Regulations (21:630.16) in the United States. Dr. Sabin chose his strains based on their inability to cause severe lesions or paralysis when introduced into the nervous tissues of monkeys. In brief, rhesus monkeys are inoculated with monovalent vaccine virus via either the intraspinal or intrathalamic route. Monkeys are observed for a 17- to 21-day test period, at the end of which they are sacrificed. The brain and spinal cord of each animal are fixed, sectioned, and stained for the evaluation of polio-specific lesions. A score is given to each batch of vaccine based on the number and severity of lesions in the monkeys tested. This score is compared to that of an attenuated reference strain and must be within a certain limit of the reference score. The intention of the test is to discover batches of vaccine that have accumulated virus with more neurovirulent potential. Investigation into the nature of the virus that causes more lesions in monkey nervous tissues continues to be defined at the molecular level.

B. Molecular Basis of Attenuation

The tools of molecular biology have been used to discover the genetic basis of attenuation of the polio vaccine strains. The discovery that the single-stranded polio genome could be transformed into an infectious cDNA (Racaniello and Baltimore, 1981) provided the means to genetically engineer the poliovirus genome. Sequences of the attenuated Sabin strains were derived in different research facilities (Nomoto *et al.*, 1982; Stanway *et al.*, 1984; Toyoda *et al.*, 1984; Weeks-Levy *et al.*, 1991) as well as sequences of wild-type strains (Racaniello and Baltimore, 1981; Stanway *et al.*, 1984). These discoveries made it possible to study genetic mutations that attenuate strains. Comparison of the sequences and construction of infectious cDNA clones containing different combinations of mutations was used to identify genetic determinants of attenuation (Racaniello, 1988). Each of the three Sabin strains was found to contain bases in their 5′ noncoding regions that were important for attenuating the strains. The important attenuating bases in the 5′ noncoding region of Sabin 1, 2, and 3 are at nucleotide positions 480, 481, and 472, respectively. These base positions are thought to play a critical role in maintaining the polio genome's secondary and tertiary structure responsible for forming the ribosomal landing pad that controls translational efficiency (Wimmer *et al.*, 1993).

Once some genetic changes that cause an increase in neurovirulence were identified, these changes were evaluated in poliovirus samples obtained after replication in the human intestinal tract. Evans *et al.* (1985) showed that a single nucleotide change in the Sabin 3 strain at position 472 was responsible for an increase in neurovirulence. Wild-type bases in the 5′ noncoding region at positions 480, 481, and 472 and at other positions are selected as the polio vaccine strains replicate in the gut of vaccinees (Kew *et al.*, 1981; Cann *et al.*, 1984;

Macadam *et al.*, 1989; Minor and Dunn, 1988; Minor *et al.*, 1986a; Tatem *et al.*, 1991). This reverted virus is presumed to have gained sufficient neurovirulence to cause paralytic polio in rare cases of recipient and contact disease.

III. Virus Shedding and Revertants

On one hand, OPV confers the benefit of herd immunity through shedding of vaccine virus by vaccinees and contact by those unimmunized. On the other hand, spread of virus by vaccinees can cause contact cases of vaccine associated poliomyelitis.

A. Shedding with a Combined IPV/OPV Schedule

The genetic reversion of bases in the 5′ noncoding region of virus isolated from individuals immunized with OPV after prior vaccination with EIPV has been evaluated and compared to that of groups receiving OPV or EIPV alone (Abraham *et al.*, 1993). Revertant poliovirus strains based on evaluation of the 5′ noncoding region were not shed by vaccinees given three or more doses of OPV. Subjects receiving three or more doses of EIPV and then challenged with OPV were found to shed revertant polio strains in 50–100% of the subjects. The incorporation of EIPV into the immunization schedule did not prevent shedding of poliovirus revertants. These results raise concerns about a combination vaccination schedule with EIPV followed by OPV. Should vaccination with EIPV increase the pools of revertant viruses in circulation, what does this mean for the unimmunized individuals in the population? If polioviruses shed by EIPV recipients are transmitted to those unimmunized and undergo further reversion, then will polio strains more closely related to wild-type strains start to emerge in the environment? These questions should be answered as combination schedules are adopted by different countries. Efforts should also be focused on increasing the percentage of the population that is immunized.

B. Analysis of Revertants from Vaccinees

Points to keep in mind when evaluating the shedding of revertant viruses include understanding the level of neurovirulence that genetic reversion confers to the strains and methods used to isolate virus for these studies. Full monkey neurovirulence testing of a Sabin 3 strain shed by a primary vaccinee has been carried out (Tatem *et al.*, 1991). The strain was reverted at base position 472 in the 5′ noncoding region and at nucleotide 2493 in capsid protein VP1, and was a mixture of bases at position 6061 in the polymerase gene. Compared to neurovirulence test results with the fully neurovirulent strain Leon, the stool isolate was highly attenuated (see Table II). The contribution to neurovirulence of reversions in the 5′ noncoding regions to Sabin vaccine strains is yet to be determined, and can only be compared to strains with varying degrees of neurovirulent properties. Another point is that isolating representative poliovirus from the stool of vaccinees can produce misleading results. Often filtrates are made from feces, and the virus is amplified on tissue culture before it is serotyped. Since certain polio strains outgrow others, this method can provide researchers with a virus population different from that found directly in feces (Buonagurio *et al.*, 1995). For this reason, methods to detect revertants directly from stool isolates must be developed to get a true picture of the revertants shed by vaccinees immunized with OPV and IPV alone and in combination schedules.

TABLE II
Neurovirulence of Stool Isolate in Comparison to Wild-Type Strain

Virus[a]	Dose[b]	Animals paralyzed	Mortality	Polio lesions[c]	Severe lesions[d]
NC 1	6.4	1/48	0/48	48/48	0/48
KW4	7.7	1/6	0/6	6/6	3/6
KW4	6.1	2/24	0/24	24/24	10/24
KW4	4.7	0/5	0/5	5/5	0/5
KW4	3.7	0/6	0/6	6/6	0/6
Leon	8.4	2/2	2/2	2/2	2/2
Leon	3.7	5/5	0/5	5/5	5/5

Note. Taken from Tatem *et al.*, 1991.
[a]NC 1 is the Sabin type 3 attenuated reference strain. KW4 is a type 3 strain isolated from stool taken 5 days postvaccination; Leon is the pathogenic parental strain of Sabin 3.
[b]Log10 TCID50 of virus injected as described in the Code of Federal Regulations 12:630.16.
[c]Number of monkeys with poliovirus-specific lesions in the brain or spinal cord/total number of test animals.
[d]Number of monkeys with ≥grade 3 (on a scale of 0–4) lesions/total number of test animals.

IV. The Immune System and Poliovirus Vaccines

The main lines of defense which mediate immunity against viral infections include circulating antibody, secretory IgA (S-IgA) mucosal antibody, and cell-mediated immunity such as natural killer cells, cytotoxic T lymphocytes (CTLs), and other lymphocyte subsets involved in effector or immunoregulatory functions. Poliovirus enters the body through the alimentary tract and replicates in tissues of the nasopharynx and intestinal tract. Development of mucosal immunity and S-IgA antibodies is important in preventing mucosally restricted enteric infections. Furthermore, circulating antibody is important for the prevention of systemic disease in those instances where there is an absence of protection against viral replication at the mucosal site of entry. The role of cell-mediated immunity in poliovirus infection is not well established.

Neutralizing antibody titers are considered the gold standard in measuring the efficacy of poliovirus vaccines (Cooper, 1979; Ogra and Karzon, 1971). Although neutralizing antibody titers have been used to determine the efficacy of oral poliovirus vaccine, other immune responses may have as much if not more relevance to the efficacy of the vaccine. Other viral-specific immune responses have been measured using different techniques. These techniques include: ELISA assays, hemagglutination inhibition, passive hemagglutination, radioimmunoassays, immunofluorescence, and T-cell proliferation assays to viral antigens or whole virus. These assays probably detect different antigenic epitopes on known antigens or completely different viral antigens of the same virus. It is not known whether antibody responses detected by these other methods, whether taken alone or in combination, are protective against disease. The ultimate test of effectiveness is still based on the success of the vaccine to prevent disease.

A. Mucosal Responses

Mucosal immunity is the first line of defense for protection against poliovirus infection. IgA was found to be the predominant immunoglobulin class in external secretions and exhibited structural differences compared to IgA found in serum. On mucosal surfaces, IgA exists mainly as a dimeric molecule that possesses a unique secretory component (s.c.). Secretory IgA also contains one J chain per four light chains (Bergmann and Waldman, 1988). The structure of S-IgA is thought to help the molecule survive in the harsh environment of low pH and proteases of the intestinal mucosa. The majority of S-IgA is synthesized locally in plasma cells found predominantly beneath the epithelium of secretory surfaces. Another component of S-IgA, the s.c., is found primarily in the mucosal epithelium. The dimer of S-IgA is produced in the plasma cells below the site where s.c. is made. As dimeric IgA passes through the epithelium, it combines with the s.c. portion. The joining of the two molecules completes the S-IgA molecule. Many studies have been performed to establish the concept of a common mucosal immune system where IgA precursor cells emigrate to different mucosal sites such as mesenteric lymph nodes, lamina propria of the small intestine and bronchi, gestational mammary glands, salivary glands, genital areas, and ocular area to provide protection at these portals of entry into the body (Bergmann and Waldman, 1988).

Salk IPV induces the production of IgM, IgG, and IgA antibodies in serum (Ogra *et al.*, 1980). IPV-Salk, however, was found not to induce a significant neutralizing secretory antibody (S-IgA) response in the alimentary tract or nasopharynx (Ogra and Karzon, 1971). IPV may not induce a good secretory immune response due to the limited amount of antigen that presents itself to the gut-associated lymphoid tissue (GALT). A booster effect has been seen in individuals previously primed with IPV-Salk upon revaccination with IPV-Salk as well as a modest secretory antibody response (Ogra, 1984). Oral poliovirus vaccine induces secretory immune and neutralizing antibody responses in the mucosal sites that are superior to those elicited by IPV. Mucosal immunization (intranasal) with IPV induces a secretory antibody response that is superior to immunization by the parenteral route (Ogra *et al.*, 1980; Ogra and Karzon, 1971). Parenteral administration of IPV-Salk induces much less mucosal immune response, although EIPV has been found to induce more of a mucosal response compared to IPV-Salk. Boosting with OPV after immunization with IPV leads to an enhanced S-IgA response. Table III summarizes the features of the immune responses induced by conventional inactivated and live vaccines administered by parenteral and mucosal

TABLE III
Nature of Immunologic Reactivity after Parenteral or Mucosal Immunization with Conventional Live or Inactivated Vaccine

	Response to immunization by indicated route and type of vaccine	
Features of response	Parenteral inactivated	Mucosal live
Immunologic response similar to natural infection	−	+
Development of systemic immune response	+	+
Persistence of systemic immune response	±	+
Detection of viral antigen in mucosal surfaces	−	+
Development of secretory immune response	±	+
Persistence of secretory immune response	−	+
Development of secretory immunity in other mucosal sites and milk	−	+
Protection against mucosal natural reinfection	−	+
Protection against systemic disease after natural reinfection	+	+
Development of herd immunity via spread of vaccine virus to contacts	−	+

Note. +, Always; ±, occasional or inconsistent; −, absent. Adapted from Ogra and Garofalo (1990).

routes, and correlates to responses to vaccination with IPV-Salk and OPV, respectively.

Immune responses have been measured in children receiving 1X enhanced potency IPV, double-strength EIPV, or quadruple-strength EIPV and compared to OPV immune responses. Responses to types 1 and 3 poliovirus in EIPV vaccinees were compared to those of infants receiving three doses of OPV at 6, 12, and 18 weeks of age. Secretory IgA responses measured in salivary samples were greater in OPV vaccinees compared to any of the IPV groups (Zaman *et al.*, 1991). Secretory IgA appears to have a role in inhibiting the replication of poliovirus at mucosal surfaces. This is examplified by a study where IgA-deficient individuals were found to shed poliovirus for prolonged periods of time after oral vaccination (Savilahti *et al.*, 1988). Even though an enhanced potency formulation of IPV induced better secretory responses compared to earlier IPV formulations, the responses still do not meet or exceed the response elicited by OPV. These data are important for illustrating the difference in immune response elicited by a live-replicating vaccine versus a parenterally administered vaccine. To gain the benefit of both vaccines, combination schedules have been investigated. Combination of IPV immunization first with OPV to follow may help prevent vaccine-associated disease while still inducing superior local immunity found with OPV vaccination.

B. T-Cell Responses

Early evidence that T-cell responses were important for polio clearance came from individuals with severe T-cell deficiency (Saulsbury *et al.*, 1975; Wood *et al.*, 1988). These individuals became chronically infected with poliovirus; one individual described in these studies came down with paralytic poliomyelitis.

Polio-specific cellular immune responses have recently been studied. The aim of these studies was to begin to understand the participation of cell-mediated immune responses in clearance of virus and in the potential destruction of nervous tissue infected with poliovirus. First steps in answering these questions have been to define T- and B-cell epitopes on the poliovirus capsid. The mouse model has been used to study T-cell responses to polio (Kutubuddin *et al.*, 1992a,b). T helper and CTL epitopes have been localized in capsid protein VP1 in areas of the protein that were identified as neutralizing antibody recognition sites. Both virus and VP1 capsid protein induced a major histocompatibility complex class I restricted T-lymphocyte response. Vaccinia recombinants expressing different portions of the polio capsid proteins VP1, VP2, VP3, and VP4 were used to define regions of the capsid proteins recognized by bulk virus-specific CTL population. The CTL population was found to recognize target cells carrying VP1 sequences but not sequences of VP2, VP3, or VP4. In contrast, peripheral blood monomolecular cells of Sabin-immunized human donors proliferated to all four capsid proteins (Simons *et al.*, 1993). This indicated the presence of T-cell epitopes located in all four capsid proteins. The contribution of CTL response to virus clearance or damage of nervous tissue remains unknown but the studies described have provided a basis to investigate these questions.

C. Immunoglobulin Isotypes/Subclasses Involved in Immunity

Investigations into immunoglobulin antibody isotypes/subclasses necessary for conferring protective immunity have been conducted in a number of research laboratories. A study in Finland examined immunoglobulin isotype composition in patients with paralytic polio, adults receiving OPV booster after primary immunization with EIPV, and children receiving their first EIPV dose (Julkunen *et al.*, 1987). All groups exhibited IgG1 and IgG3 isotypes of antibody. In the individuals with paralytic poliomyelitis, the IgG1 and IgG3 subclasses, and IgA were found in the serum and cerebrospinal fluid. IgM antibodies were detected only in the sera and not in the cerebrospinal fluid. IgG2 and IgG4 subclasses were undetectable in this group. The adults who received OPV exhibited IgG1, IgG3, IgM, IgA, IgG2, and IgG4 isotypes. The children receiving EIPV showed IgG1, IgG3, and IgM isotypes. Antibody levels in IgG2, IgG4, and IgA were observed in only a few children. The induction of IgG1 and IgG3 isotypes primarily is consistent with results found with other viral infections. It is interesting to note the lack of IgG2 and IgG4 subclasses and lack of IgM in cerebrospinal fluid in individuals with paralytic polio. The role of these specific antibodies in disease progression is not known.

Other studies have pointed to the importance of IgM in combating disease, especially in individuals deficient in the production of IgA (Savilahti *et al.*, 1988). Eight individuals, one with partial IgA deficiency and the others with IgA levels below 0.05 g/liter were given OPV. All the individuals had previously received a full course of IPV immunization prior to the study. The virus shedding patterns and antibody responses in serum and saliva were examined. Results from these individuals were compared to a control group receiving OPV. The IgA-deficient group was found to excrete poliovirus for an extended period of time compared to the controls. Another interesting finding was that a higher level of IgM was excreted into the saliva and intestine of the IgA-deficient group. This salivary IgM exhibited activity against poliovirus. This study is key in showing the importance of secretory IgA in clearing an enteric viral infection and implicating a role for IgM containing J chain and s.c. in virus clearance. Table IV shows a sum-

TABLE IV

Antibody Subclasses and/or Isotypes Induced by OPV, IPV-Salk, EIPV or IPV/OPV Vaccination Schedules or in Individuals with Paralytic Polio

Schedule	Antibody subclass and isotype induced							Reference
	IgG1	IgG2	IgG3	IgG4	IgM	IgA	S-IgA	
OPV	ND	ND	ND	ND	+	+	+	Ogra (1980) Zaman *et al.* (1991)
IPV-Salk	ND	ND	ND	ND	+	+	±	Ogra and Karzon (1971) Ogra (1980)
EIPV (first dose)	+	±	+	±	+	±	ND	Julkunen *et al.* (1987)
IPV/OPV (OPV after IPV series)	+	+	+	+	+	+	ND	Julkunen *et al.* (1987)
Patients with paralytic polio	+	−	+	−	+[a]	+	ND	Julkunen *et al.* (1987)
Patients with IgA deficiency (IPV/OPV)	+	+	+	+	+[b]	−	−	Savilahti *et al.* (1988)

Note. ND, not determined; +, always; ±, occasional or inconsistent; −, absent.
[a]IgM antibodies found in sera but not in cerebrospinal fluid.
[b]Salivary IgM found complexed to J chain and secretory component (s.c.).

mary of antibody subclasses and/or isotypes elicited by different vaccine schedules in individuals with poliomyelitis, in immunologically deficient individuals, and in immunocompetent individuals.

V. The Nature of Immune Responses to Polio Vaccines

A. Immune Responses and Outbreaks

The mucosal immunity induced by OPV leads to the inhibition of replication of poliovirus strains ingested after vaccination. In polio endemic areas this is an important feature because transmission of wild circulating poliovirus strains can be blocked (Melnick, 1992). Lack of neutralizing mucosal immunity in certain individuals immunized with IPV allows for the replication of polio in the gut should the vaccinee ingest live-attenuated or wild-type virus (Nightengale, 1977; Ogra and Karzon, 1971; Onorato *et al.*, 1991). Wild-type or attenuated polio strains can potentially circulate in fully vaccinated populations if an IPV schedule is followed. The use of an IPV schedule eliminates the possibility of vaccination via herd immunity. Refusal of vaccine, no herd immunity, and possible circulation of poliovirus in the immunized population are factors that taken together can lead to problems when an IPV schedule is used alone. This is exemplified by the outbreak of paralytic polio that occurred in the Netherlands during 1992–1993 (van Wijngaarden and van Loon, 1993). The polio cases were restricted to individuals in a religious sect who refused vaccination. These individuals had no immunity conferred by contact with polio vaccine strains in the environment. Low levels of circulating wild virus in the immunized general populace were observed. A mixed vaccination schedule using IPV and OPV has been considered as a measure to help prevent this type of outbreak in the future. An immunization schedule where IPV is used solely works well when 100% of the population is immunized. As wild-type polio is eradicated from the world, this type of outbreak will become less likely.

Antigenic sites on the poliovirion have been localized (Emini *et al.*, 1982; Evans *et al.*, 1983; Minor *et al.*, 1986b) and their susceptibility to protease cleavage *in vivo* has been studied. The major antigenic site in capsid protein VP1 of most type 3 and some type 1 polioviruses are sensitive to trypsin (Minor *et al.*, 1987). The cleaved form of VP1 is not efficient at binding site 1 specific monoclonal antibodies in these viruses (Fricks *et al.*, 1985; Icenogle *et al.*, 1986). Serum from individuals immunized solely with IPV was severely reduced in its ability to neutralize trypsin-cleaved virus (Roivainen and Hovi, 1987, 1988). These results showed that antibodies induced by IPV are targeted largely to an intact antigenic site I. The studies also indicated that host enzymes bringing about antigenic changes in poliovirus *in vivo* produce virus that can evade immunity raised to the uncleaved antigen. An example of antigenic changes in VP1 leading to disaster occurred in Finland where an outbreak of poliomyelitis happened during August 1984 to January 1986 (Hovi *et al.*, 1986). The majority of people who contracted paralytic polio from a circulating wild-type strain were immunized by IPV. The outbreak occurred for several reasons: immunization rates dropped, there was a low percentage of individuals with neutralizing antibody to the epidemic strain, and there were antigenic differences between the wild virus and the vaccine virus (Hovi *et al.*, 1986).

B. Polio Combination Vaccine Schedules

Investigations into serum-neutralizing, nasopharyngeal-neutralizing, and S-IgA antibodies of combination immunization schedules with EIPV and OPV have been carried out (Faden *et al.*, 1990). Data were compared for the following immunization schedules: OPV–OPV–OPV, IPV–IPV–IPV, IPV–OPV–OPV, and IPV–IPV–OPV. The three groups receiving EIPV in the vaccination schedule were found to have higher geometric mean titers of circulating antibody compared to the group receiving OPV. This study showed that in the OPV group (after three doses), 70–100% of the recipients developed neutralizing or IgA-specific antibodies to poliovirus in the nasopharyngeal secretions. This is in contrast to the groups receiving EIPV only. Local immune response in this group ranged from 43 to 90%. The groups receiving the combination schedules with EIPV and OPV had local responses that were in between the IPV only and OPV only groups. Another significant observation made in the Faden *et al.* (1990) and Onorato *et al.* (1991) studies was that children who received OPV after being immunized with EIPV shed virus more frequently and for a longer period of time. This result was not entirely expected because an IPV vaccine with higher potency was expected to reduce virus shedding. This observation may result from differences in humoral antibody to wild-type strains being insufficient to fully neutralize attenuated strains or modification of the attenuated vaccine strains in the gut by intestinal enzymes that significantly change the conformation of the neutralization sites. Another study conducted by Lederle Laboratories and the University of Texas at Galveston is currently ongoing to determine the shedding frequency of infants immunized with IPV produced from the attenuated Sabin strains. Immunization schedules utilizing combinations of IPV-Sabin and OPV with groups for each vaccine alone are under evaluation. It will be interesting to see if humoral immunity to Sabin IPV will also increase virus shedding with OPV administration compared to children receiving a schedule of OPV only.

VI. Polio Vaccines in Combination with Other Vaccines

With more and more vaccines becoming available, methods to combine or coadminister them are being developed. In combining live vaccines, one must consider possible interference of the replicating entities in the vaccine. Parenterally injected combination vaccines face problems stemming from the compatibility of the components. In the end, both types of combination vaccines must still provide the protective immunity of the separate components.

A. Combination with Oral Rotavirus Vaccine

A study was recently conducted to evaluate the effect of immunizing individuals with Rhesus-human reassortant tetravalent (RRV-TV) oral rotavirus vaccine at the same time as OPV or IPV (Migasena *et al.*, 1995). With the first dose of vaccine at 2 months of age, 37% of infants receiving RRV-TV with IPV and only 10% of infants vaccinated with RRV-TV and OPV had seroconverted to the rotavirus as measured by IgG ELISA. After multiple doses of RRV-TV the level of rotavirus-neutralizing IgA titers was not different between the groups receiving OPV or IPV. This exemplifies potential problems with administering vaccines which both replicate at mucosal surfaces and emphasizes the need for completion of full vaccination schedules.

B. Combination with DPT and *Haemophilus influenzae* B

Combining inactivated parenterally administered vaccines is an attractive way of assuring that infants receive as many vaccines as possible in one shot. Combining different components in one shot is a challenge from the perspective of formulation and providing fully immunogenic components. Different combinations have been made with IPV, diphtheria–tetanus–pertussis, and *Haemophilus influenzae* B vaccine components (Qureshi *et al.*, 1989; Barreto *et al.*, 1993). To date, there is no evidence that the combinations made have any deleterious effect on the immunogenicity of any of the components at the humoral level. The effect on the secretory immunity elicited by the IPV component and cellular responses in these vaccine combinations is not yet clear.

VII. Concluding Remarks

This chapter has focused on the different immune responses elicited by oral and inactivated poliovirus vaccines with an emphasis on the importance of mucosal immunity. The lessons of the past can aid in the development of new vaccines. The immune response elicited by the live-replicating polio vaccines is excellent as far as inducing mucosal immunity. Although the inactivated vaccine (EIPV) was able to induce local immunity, it was not able to induce the same quality of immunity even at 4× the dose. These types of immunological differences bear on the development of new vaccines. As vaccines become more complex in their nature and formulation, the desired immune response for a certain component may not be optimal. It is important to understand the optimal response for vaccination of single components and achieve that response in new combination vaccines or new formulations with improved components. As the understanding of the immunology of responses to vaccines progresses, the information will help researchers design better vaccines.

References

Abraham, R., Minor, P., Dunn, G., Modlin, J. F., and Ogra, P. L. (1993). Shedding of virulent poliovirus revertants during immunization with oral poliovirus vaccine after prior immunization with inactivated polio vaccine. *J. Infect. Dis.* **168**, 1105–1109.

Barreto, L., Scheifele, D., Noseworthy, G., Stratton, F., Bjornson, G., and Schaart, W. (1993). A controlled comparison of *Haemophilus influenzae* type B diphtheria toxoid conjugate vaccine given concurrently or in combination with DPT-IPV vaccine to 18-month-old children. *Immunol. Infect. Dis.* **3**, 316–320.

Bergmann, K.-C., and Waldman, R. H. (1988). Stimulation of secretory antibody following oral administration of antigen. *Rev. Infect. Dis.* **10**, 939–950.

Bottiger, M. (1993). The elimination of polio in the Scandinavian countries. *Public Health Rev. (Isr.)* **21**, 27–33.

Buonagurio, D. A., Coleman, J. W., Patibandla, S. A., Prabhakar, B. S., and Tatem, J. M. (1995). Enhanced detection of poliovirus of vaccinees by RT-PCR. Abstracts of the Interscience Conference on Antimicrobial Agents and Chemotherapy 35. San Francisco, California. p. 185.

Cann, A. J., Stanway, G., Hughes, P. J., Minor, P. D., Evans, D. M. A., Schild, G. C., and Almond, J. W. (1984). Reversion to virulence of the live-attenuated Sabin type 3 oral poliovirus vaccine. *Nucleic Acids Res.* **12**, 7787–7778.

Cooper, N. R. (1979). Humoral immunity to viruses. *In* "Comprehensive Virology" (H. Frankel-Conrat and R. R. Wagner, eds.), pp. 123–169. Plenum, New York.

Emini, E. A., Jameson, B. A., Lewis, A. J., Larsen, G. R., and Wimmer, E. (1982). Poliovirus neutralization epitopes: Analysis and localization with neutralizing monoclonal antibodies. *J. Virol.* **43**, 997–1005.

Enders, J. F., Weller, T. H., and Robbins, F. C. (1949). Cultivation of the Lansing strain of poliomyelitis virus in cultures of various human embryonic tissues. *Science* **109**, 85–87.

Evans, D. M. A., Minor, P. D., Schild, G. S., and Almond, J. W. (1983). Critical role of an eight amino acid sequence of VP1 in neutralization of poliovirus type 3. *Nature (London)* **304**, 459–462.

Evans, D. M. A., Dunn, G., Minor, P. D., Schild, G. C., Cann, A. J., Stanway, G., Almond, J. W., Currey, K., and Maizel, J. V. (1985). A single nucleotide change in the 5′ non-coding region of the genome of the Sabin type 3 poliovaccine is associated with increased neurovirulence. *Nature (London)* **314**, 548–550.

Faden, H. (1993). Poliovirus vaccination: A trilogy. *J. Infect. Dis.* **168**, 25–28.

Faden, H., Modlin, J. E., Thoms, M. L., McBean, A. M., Ferdon, M. B., and Ogra, P. L. (1990). Comparative evaluation of immunization with live attenuated and enhanced-potency inactivated trivalent poliovirus vaccines in childhood: Systemic and local immune responses. *J. Infect. Dis.* **162**, 1291–1297.

Fricks, C. E., Icenogle, J. P., and Hogle, J. M. (1985). Trypsin sensitivity of the Sabin strain of type 1 poliovirus: Cleavage sites in virions and related particles. *J. Virol.* **54**, 856–859.

Furesz, J., Armstrong, R. E., Moreau, P., Yarosh, W., and Nagler, F. P. (1966). Antigenic studies on Sabin types 1 and 3 poliovaccine virus during 1 to 7 passage in the human intestinal tract. *Am. J. Epidemiol.* **83**, 501–508.

Grenier, B., Hamza, B., Xueref, B. C., Viarme, F., and Roumaintzeff, M. (1984). Seroimmunity following vaccination in infants by an inactivated poliovirus vaccine prepared on Vero cells. *Rev. Infect. Dis.* **6**(Suppl.), S545–547.

Hovi, T., Cantell, K., Huovilainen, A., Kinnunen, E., Kuronen, T., Lapinleimu, K., Pöyry, T., Roivainen, M., Salama, N., Stenvik, M., Silander, A., Thoden, C.-J., Salminen, S., and Weckström, P. (1986). Outbreak of paralytic poliomyelitis in Finland: Widespread circulation of antigenically altered poliovirus type 3 in a vaccinated population. *Lancet* **1**, 1427–1432.

Icenogle, J. P., Minor, P. D., Ferguson, M., and Hogle, J. M. (1986). Modulation of humoral response to a 12-amino acid site on the poliovirus virion. *J. Virol.* **60**, 297–301.

Julkunen, I., Ukkonen, P., Stenvik, M., Hovi, T., Renkonen, L., and Makela, O. (1987). Proportions of immunoglobulin isotypes in paralytic poliomyelitis and after vaccination. *J. Clin. Immunol.* **7**, 319–326.

Kew, O. M., Nottay, B. K., Hatch, M. H., Nakano, J. H., and Obijecki, J. F. (1981). Multiple genetic changes can occur in the oral poliovaccines upon replication in humans. *J. Gen. Virol.* **56**, 337–347.

Kutubuddin, M., Simmons, J., and Chow, M. (1992a). Identification of thelper epitopes in the VP1 capsid protein of poliovirus. *J. Virol.* **66**, 3042–3047.

Kutubuddin, M., Simons, J., and Chow, M. (1992b). Poliovirus-specific major histocompatibility complex class I restricted cytolytic Tcell epitopes in mice localize to neutralizing antigenic regions. *J. Virol.* **66**, 5967–5974.

Lemon, S. M., and Milstein, J. B. (1994). The thermostability of vaccines. *International Journal of Technology Assessment in Health Care* **10**, 1 177–184.

Macadam, A. J., Arnold, C., Houlett, J., John, A., Mardsen, S., Taffs, F., Reeve, P., Hamada, N., Wareham, K., Almond, J., Cammack, N., and Minor, P. D. (1989). Reversion of attenuated and temperature-sensitive phenotype of the Sabin type 3 strain of poliovirus in vaccinees. *Virology* **172**, 408–414.

McBean, A. M., Thoms, M. L., Albrecht, P., Cuthie, J. C., and Bernier, R. (1988). Field staff and coordinating committee. Serologic response to oral polio vaccine and enhanced-potency inactivated polio vaccines. *Am. J. Epidemiol.* **128**, 615–628.

Mellander, L., Bottiger, M., Hanson, L. A., Taranger, J., and Carlsson, B. (1993). Avidity and titers of the antibody response to two inactivated poliovirus vaccines with different antigen content. *Acta Paediatr.* **82**, 552–556.

Melnick, J. L. (1992). Poliomyelitis: Eradication in sight. *Epidemiol. Infect.* **108**, 1–18.

Migasena, S., Simasathien, S., Samakoses, R., Pitisuttitham, P., Sangaroon, P., van Steenis, G., Beuvery, E. C., Bugg, H., Bishop, R., Davidson, B. L., and Vesikari, T. (1995). Simultaneous administration of oral rhesus–human reassortant tetravalent (RRV-TV) rotavirus vaccine and oral poliovirus vaccine (OPV) in Thai infants. *Vaccine* **13,** 168–174.

Minor, P. D., and Dunn, G. (1988). The effect of sequences in the 5′ non-coding region on the replication of polioviruses in the human gut. *J. Gen. Virol.* **69,** 1091–1096.

Minor, P. D., John, A., Ferguson, M., and Icenogle, J. F. (1986a). Antigenic and molecular evolution of the vaccine strain of type 3 poliovirus during the period of excretion by a primary vaccinee. *J. Gen. Virol.* **67,** 693–706.

Minor, P. D., Ferguson, M., Evans, D. M. A., Almond, J. W., and Icenogle, J. P. (1986b). Antigenic structure of polioviruses of serotypes 1, 2, and 3. *J. Gen. Virol.* **67,** 1283–1291.

Minor, P. D., Ferguson, M., Phillips, A., Magrath, D. I., Huovilainen, A., and Hovi, T. (1987). Conservation *in vivo* of protease cleavage sites in antigenic sites of polioviruses. *J. Gen. Virol.* **68,** 1857–1865.

Nightengale, E. O. (1977). Recommendations for a national policy on polomyelitis vaccination. *N. Engl. J. Med.* **297,** 249–253.

Nishio, O., Ishihara, Y., Sakae, K., Nonomura, Y., Kuno, A., Yasukawa, W., Inoue, H., Miyamura, K., and Kono, R. (1984). The trend of acquired immunity with live poliovirus vaccine and the effect of revaccination follow-up of vaccinees for ten years. *J. Biol. Stand.* **12,** 1–10.

Nomoto, A., Omata, T., Toyoda, H., Kuge, S., Horie, H., Kataoka, Y., Genba, Y., Nakano, Y., and Imura, N. (1982). Complete nucleotide sequence of the attenuated poliovirus Sabin 1 strains genome. *Proc. Natl. Acad. Sci. U.S.A.* **79,** 5793–5797.

Ogra, P. L. (1984). Mucosal immune response to poliovirus vaccines in childhood. *Rev. Infect. Dis.* **6,** S361–368.

Ogra, P. L., and Garofalo, R. (1990). Secretory antibody response to viral vaccines. *Prog. Med. Virol.* **37,** 156–189.

Ogra, P. L., and Karzon, D. T. (1971). Formation and function of poliovirus antibody in different tissues. *Prog. Med. Virol.* **13,** 156–193.

Ogra, P. L., Fishaut, M., and Gallaher, M. R. (1980). Viral vaccination via the mucosal route. *Rev. Infect. Dis.* **2,** 352–369.

Onorato, I. M., Modlin, J. F., McBean, A. M., Thoms, M. L., Losansky, G. A., and Bernier, R. H. (1991). Mucosal immunity induced by enhanced potency inactivated and oral polio vaccines. *J. Infect. Dis.* **163,** 1–6.

Patriarca, P. A., Wright, P. E., and John, T. J. (1991). Factors affecting the immunogenicity of oral poliovirus vaccine in developing countries: Review. *Rev. Infect. Dis.* **13,** 926–939.

Qureshi, A. W., Zulfiqar, I., Raza, A., and Siddiqi, N. (1989). Comparison of immunogenicity of combined DPT–inactivated injectable polio vaccine (DPT–IPV) and association of DPT and attenuated oral polio vaccine (DPT + OPV) in Pakistani children. *J. Pak. Med. Assoc.* **39,** 31–35.

Racanaiello, V. R. (1988). Poliovirus neurovirulence. *Adv. Virus. Res.* **34,** 217–246.

Racaniello, V. R., and Baltimore, D. (1981). Cloned poliovirus complementary DNA is infectious in mammalian cells. *Science* **214,** 916–919.

Roivainen, M., and Hovi, T. (1987). Intestinal trypsin can significantly modify antigenic properties of polioviruses: Implications for the use of inactivated poliovirus vaccine. *J. Virol.* **61,** 3749–3753.

Roivainen, M., and Hovi, T. (1988). Cleavage of VP1 and modification of antigenic site I of Type 2 polioviruses by intestinal trypsin. *J. Virol.* **62,** 3536–3539.

Rong, W., Guillot, S., Georgescu, M.-M., Balanant, J., Delpeyroux, F., and Crainic, R. (1994). Thermal stabilization of poliovaccine strain by heavy water. Abstract W3 from Europic '94. Korpilampi, Finland.

Sabin, A. B., and Boulger, L. R. (1973). History of Sabin attenuated poliovirus oral live vaccine strains. *J. Biol. Stand.* **1,** 115–118.

Salk, J. E. (1953). Recent studies in immunization against poliomyelitis. *Pediatrics* **12,** 471–482.

Salk, J. E., Bennett, B. L., Lewis, L. J., Ward, E. N., and Youngner, J. S. (1953). Studies on human subjects on active immunization against poliomyelitis. 1. A preliminary report of experiments in progress. *JAMA, J. Am. Med. Assoc.* **151,** 1081–1098.

Saulsbury, F. T., Winkelstein, J. A., Davis, L. E., Hsu, S. H., D'Souza, B. J., Gutcher, G. R., and Butler, I. J. (1975). Combined immunodeficiency and vaccine-related poliomyelitis in a child with cartilage hair hypoplasia. *J. Pediatr.* **86,** 868–872.

Savilahti, E., Klemola, T., Carlsson, B., Mellander, L., Stenvik, M., and Hovi, T. (1988). Inadequacy of mucosal IgM antibodies in selective IgA deficiency: Excretion of attenuated poliovirus is prolonged. *J. Clin. Immunol.* **8,** 89–94.

Simoes, E. A., Padmini, B., Steinhoff, M. C., Jadhav, M., and John, T. J. (1985). Antibody response of infants to two doses of inactivated poliovirus vaccine of enhanced potency. *Am. J. Dis. Child.* **139,** 977–980.

Simons, J., Kutubuddin, M., and Chow, M. (1993). Characterization of polivirus-specific T lymphocytes in the peripheral blood of Sabin-vaccinated humans. *J. Virol.* **67,** 1262–1268.

Stanway, G., Hughes, P. J., Mountford, R. C., Reeves, P., Minor, P. D., Schild, G. C., and Almond, J. W. (1984). Comparison of the complete nucleotide sequence of the genomes of the neurovirulent poliovirus P3/Leon/37 and its attenuated Sabin vaccine derivative P3/Leon/12a,b. *Proc. Natl. Acad. Sci. U.S.A.* **81,** 1539–1543.

Stones, P. B., Macdonald, C. R., McDougall, J. K., and Ramsbottom, P. F. (1964). Preparation and properties of a derivative of Sabin's type 3 poliovirus strains Leon 12a,b. 10th Symposium of the European Association against Poliomyelitis, Warsaw, pp. 390–397.

Stratton, K. R., Howe, C. J., and Johnston, R. B., Jr. (eds.) (1994). "Adverse Events Associated with Childhood Vaccines," National Academy Press, Washington, D.C., Chapt. 7, pp. 187–210.

Strebel, P. M., Sutter, R. W., Cochi, S. L., Biellik, R. J., Brink, E. W., Kew, O. M., Pallansch, M. A., Orenstein, W. A., and Hinman, A. R. (1992). Epidemiology of poliomyelitis in the United States one decade after the last reported case of indigenous wild virus-associated disease. *Clin. Infect. Dis.* **14,** 568–579.

Tatem, J. M., Weeks-Levy, C., Mento, S. J., DiMichele, S. J., Georgiu, A., Waterfield, W. F., Sheip, B., Costalas, C., Davies, T., Ritchey, M. B., and Cano, F. R. (1991). Oral poliovirus vaccine in the United States: Molecular characterization of Sabin type 3 after replication in the gut of vaccines. *J. Med. Virol.* **35,** 101–109.

Toyoda, H., Kohara, M., Kataoka, Y., Suganuma, T., Omata, T., Imura, N., and Nomoto, A. (1984). Complete nucleotide sequences of all three poliovirus serotype genomes implication for genetic relationship, gene function and antigenic determinants. *J. Mol. Biol.* **174,** 561–585.

van Wijngaarden, J. K., and van Loom, A. M. (1993). The polio epidemic in the Netherlands, 1992/1993. *Public Health Rev. (Isr.)* **21,** 107–116.

Weeks-Levy, C., Tatem, J. M., DiMichele, S. J., Waterfield, W., Georgiu, A. F., and Mento, S. J. (1991). Identification and characterization of a new base substitution in the vaccine strains of Sabin 3 poliovirus. *Virology* **185,** 934–937.

Wimmer, E., Hellen, C. U. T., and Cao, X. (1993). Genetic of poliovirus. *Annu. Rev. Genet.* **27,** 353–436.

Wood, D. J., David, T. J., Chrystie, I. L., and Totterdell, B. (1988). Chronic enteric virus infection in two T-cell immunodeficient children. *J. Med. Virol.* **24,** 435–444.

Zaman, S., Carlsson, B., Jalil, F., Mellander, L., van Wezel, A. L., Bottiger, M., and Hanson, L. A. (1991). Comparison of serum and salivary antibodies in children vaccinated with oral live or parenteral inactivated poliovirus vaccines of different antigen concentrations. *Acta Paediatr. Scand.* **80,** 1166–1173.

Zhaori, G., Sun, M., and Ogra, P. L. (1988). Characterization of the immune response to poliovirus virion polypeptides after immunization with live or inactivated polio vaccines. *J. Infect. Dis.* **158,** 160–165.

22

The Rationale for a Mucosal Approach to the Prevention of Respiratory Syncytial Virus-Associated Pulmonary Disease

PETER F. WRIGHT
Departments of Pediatrics and Microbiology and Immunology
Vanderbilt Medical Center
Nashville, Tennessee 37232

I. Introduction

Respiratory Syncytial Virus (RSV) is the leading cause of acute viral lower respiratory disease in infancy and early childhood (McIntosh and Chanock, 1990). The virus is classified as a pneumovirus and is structurally related to the parainfluenza viruses and mumps. It is a negative-sense, single-stranded RNA virus with a nonsegmented genome which codes for 10 proteins. Two surface proteins have important roles in attachment (G protein) and cell fusion (F protein). These two proteins are the major targets for neutralizing antibody. Other proteins that may be important in immune recognition include M2 and SH, small proteins on the viral surface, and the internal proteins, matrix and nucleoprotein. Presentation of individual virus proteins in the context of vaccinia expression vectors has shown that the major protection is afforded by F and G (Wertz *et al.*, 1987).

The most typical clinical manifestation of RSV is bronchiolitis, which is an inflammatory obstruction of the small airways and submucosal cellular infiltrate, epithelial necrosis, and mucous plugging (Wohl and Chernick, 1978). RSV is a highly seasonal disease with yearly epidemics during the winter months in temperate climates (Kim *et al.*, 1973a). It is spread by large particle droplets that are aerosolized or spread by direct contact to the respiratory tract.

RSV is limited in its replication to the mucosal surfaces of the respiratory tract. We know little about the actual population(s) of cells on the epithelial layer that RSV is replicating in or what limits its replication to the respiratory mucosa. There are descriptions that it may preferentially infect ciliated epithelial cells (Henderson *et al.*, 1978). The virus is released from the apical surface of cells and has no known targeting to microfold (M) cells, making it even less accessible to serum antibody and posing questions as to the pathways of antigen presentation. Furthermore, as the name syncytial implies, the virus has an effective fusion mechanism that may allow cell-to-cell spread of virus. Immune defenses may have to deal with a virus that behaves like a strict intracellular pathogen in that it can replicate and spread from cell to cell by fusion in spite of antibody in the extracellular environment.

In spite of a cohort of children from birth to 9 months going into the epidemic that has not been exposed to the virus, RSV has a unique propensity to cause more serious lower respiratory tract disease in infants between 1 and 3 months of life. An exception is that children with bronchopulmonary dysplasia and significant congenital heart disease are at particular risk of disease requiring hospitalization into the second year of life. RSV infection in the neonate is atypical with lethargy and poor feeding without wheezing or lower tract signs, yet mortality is high (Hall *et al.*, 1979).

The infection begins with upper respiratory symptoms with characteristic increases in mucous production, sneezing, and cough. Otitis media is a recognized sequelae of the upper respiratory component due to eustachian tube obstruction and perhaps direct extension of the viral infection to the middle ear space. After a varying period of time, often 3 to 5 days, there may be sudden evidence of involvement of the lower respiratory tract with prolonged expiration, tachypnea with radiographic evidence of hyperinflation, atelectasis, or pneumonia. The pneumonic process is certainly mediated by obstruction related to direct viral cellular damage and mucous secretion but may additionally have pharmacologic or immune mediated components. It is not clear if the onset of symptoms is directly related to the

MUCOSAL VACCINES

period of peak virus shedding or if it comes as the cytokine or immune response is initiated. Virus can regularly be recovered at the time of hospitalization but rapidly diminishes within days of the onset of lower respiratory tract symptoms and appearance of measurable serum antibody.

The sequelae of bronchiolitis are rare except that children hospitalized with bronchiolitis have an increased incidence of asthma later in childhood (Price, 1990). It is not clear whether bronchiolitis causes pulmonary damage that predisposes to asthma or whether bronchiolitis is the first manifestation of a propensity to reactive airway disease. As 1:100 children are hospitalized it means that a very high proportion of children, approximately 1:25, who are in the target for severe illness, 1 to 3 months of age during an epidemic, will be hospitalized.

RSV is a viral infection, occurring in a unique epidemiologic setting in early infancy, that one would like to treat or prevent. To begin to develop a rational, focused, and safe approach to such a goal it is necessary to understand what is known about the normal immune response and the correlates of immunity to RSV.

II. Is There Immunity to RSV?

There are two RSV serogroups that share fusion protein determinants but differ significantly in their glycoprotein (G protein) epitopes. Strain variation may account for some reinfection (Hall *et al.*, 1990). However, data from adults rechallenged with the same virus stock indicate that within 3 months following infection 30% can be reinfected and within 8 months two-thirds of adults could be reinfected (Hall *et al.*, 1991). Reinfection is seen frequently in children as well, although with less lower tract involvement with second and third infections (Henderson *et al.*, 1979). The very young age of acquisition means that initial infection occurs with a relatively immature immune system.

In contrast, in animal models immunity following respiratory infection is long lived (Graham *et al.*, 1991). No animal model is fully permissive for RSV infection so that immunity that would be less than complete in humans might be effective in animals. The lack of a fully permissive animal model is a major impediment to our understanding of pathogenesis, although well-standardized cotton rat and murine models exist. Live, attenuated intranasal vaccines have very different patterns of virus replication in naive and previously infected children (Wright *et al.*, 1976). In previously infected children the virus is recovered in low titer for 2–4 days while in naive children shedding is seen for 10 or more days at 100- to 1000-fold higher titer. In adults the correlates of protection are more difficult to assess as all have had multiple previous infections.

Finally, the most compelling argument for immunity in RSV infection is the very young age distribution of hospitalized patients. This strongly suggests that immunity is generated following primary infection that prevents the most serious lower respiratory tract manifestations of RSV disease. Making this assumption, one could presume to investigate what is known about the mechanisms of immunity and approach the development of a vaccine. However, the field of RSV vaccine development has been dominated by a clinical observation that a formalin-inactivated whole virus vaccine given parenterally caused enhanced illness when recipients of the vaccine were exposed to natural infection.

III. Why Was Enhanced Illness Seen following Inactivated Vaccine?

Children suffered severe illness on natural exposure to RSV subsequent to vaccination with formalin-inactivated RSV vaccine (Kim *et al.*, 1969). This is the most compelling observation for an immune-mediated component of RSV disease. The illness was a severe bronchiolitis and pneumonia with a high rate of hospitalization and death. The illness occurred in children over 6 months of age. This observation provides an important clue suggesting that the severity of illness in the very young is not simply a function of airway size and that there may be an immune component to the pathogenesis of RSV disease. However, the mechanism of vaccine-induced potentiation may be independent of events in serious primary infection. The antigenic components of the vaccine may have been altered by the inactivation process. There is evidence that the vaccine stimulated nonneutralizing and nonfusion inhibiting antibodies (Murphy and Walsh, 1988). Recent work in animal models strongly suggests that vaccines of this type and perhaps any parenteral-inactivated vaccine leads to the induction of a Th2 T-helper subset response mediated by IL-4 and IL-10 and resultant pathology on challenge. In contrast, a Th1 response is seen with live virus given intranasally. The pathway that immunity follows with the initial antigen exposure determines the response following challenge. A distinctive pathologic picture is seen on challenge with wild-type virus of alveolar neutrophilic infiltrate in the mice previously given inactivated vaccine. More severe illness is also seen on challenge. It is not established that this is the same pathophysiologic process that was present in the infants with enhanced disease, but it is suggestive that we are close to understanding the events that occurred after inactivated vaccine. The presence of eosinophilia (Chin *et al.*, 1969) and augmented lyphoproliferative response (Kim *et al.*, 1976) in children with enhanced disease is consistent with the hypothesis suggested by the murine model. Due to the debate concerning the interpretation of these observations, all vaccine approaches that are using inactivated or subunit products parenterally as RSV immunogens have been limited. Thus part of the argument for a mucosal vaccine is that by simulating natural infection it may be a safe route for induction of immunity.

IV. Role of Serum Antibody

In infants, RSV largely ignores the protective shield of passively transferred maternal serum antibody except at the highest levels (Glezen *et al.*, 1981). In experimental adult studies, no or incomplete protection by serum antibody against shedding was seen (Hall *et al.*, 1991). In animal models a high level of neutralizing antibody protects against pulmonary and to a much lesser extent nasal infection (Prince *et al.*, 1985). Depletion of B-cells in the murine model using anti-mu antisera had little effect on the duration and height of primary virus replication, although it did alter the extent of virus replication on rechallenge (Graham *et al.*, 1991a). More recent studies with an RSV hyperimmune globulin from human plasma have suggested that prophylactic use of immune globulin on a monthly basis may prevent disease in those at special risk for RSV, including those with marked prematurity and compromising cardiopulmonary disease (Groothuis *et al.*, 1993). The therapeutic use of this product and other IgA and IgG monoclonal antibody preparations are under active investigation. Consideration is being given to maternal immunization to boost humoral immunity at birth. Nevertheless, circulating antibody may be assumed to be of limited value because of the mucosal site of viral replication. Given the very young age of onset of the most severe illness, there is concern that maternal antibody may be detrimental by either antibody-mediated immunopathology or antibody suppression (Murphy *et al.*, 1986).

Immunodeficiency diseases provide some information as to the role of cellular immunity as prolonged RSV shedding is seen in HIV-infected children (King *et al.*, 1993). Significant amounts of RSV disease are now being documented in the elderly (Falsey *et al.*, 1995) and in bone marrow transplant patients (Harrington *et al.*, 1992).

V. Role of Mucosal Immunity

Although in one experimental adult study there was a statistical correlation of immunity with the presence of mucosal antibody (Mills *et al.*, 1971), it was not reported in another (Hall *et al.*, 1991). The correlation of mucosal protection against RSV with secretory IgA antibody is not nearly as strong as that seen with parainfluenza type 1 where the presence of measurable IgA specific immunity blocked experimental infection completely (Smith *et al.*, 1966). In young children given a low dose of a partially attenuated live RSV vaccine virus, shedding was significantly influenced by the presence of neutralizing nasal antibody (Wright *et al.*, 1976). In animal models the immunity induced by live vaccine administered by the mucosal route is more complete and of longer duration than that seen with parenteral whole or subunit-inactivated vaccines, in spite of comparable levels of serum antibody (Graham *et al.*, 1991b). Topical IgG antibody provides some protection against primary infection but may also lower the protection on challenge.

Theoretically, an advantage of stimulating mucosal polymeric IgA antibody to RSV is the ability of the antibody to be transcytosed across the epithelial cell with intracellular disruption of viral replication (Mazanec *et al.*, 1992). This might be of particular interest with RSV because of its syncytial spread from cell to cell. A recently described IgA monoclonal antibody significantly decreased RSV replication in experimental animal models (Weltzin *et al.*, 1994).

There is concern that protection may be compartmentalized within the respiratory tract and mechanisms of protection differ in the upper and lower tract. For example, serum antibody is more protective against pulmonary than nasal infection in animal models (Graham *et al.*, 1993). In contrast, if primary infection is limited to the upper respiratory tract the lung may remain susceptible on challenge (Graham *et al.*, 1995).

VI. Role of Cell-Mediated Immunity

Data on systemic cell mediated immune response in infants are limited, particularly in attempts to demonstrate cytotoxic lymphocyte responses (Chiba *et al.*, 1989). However, the murine model is now providing insight into the induction of immunity with RSV infection. Depletion experiments in the murine model show that both CD4 and CD8 T cell subsets play a role in termination of primary infection (Graham *et al.*, 1991c). In persistently infected mice, passively transferred cytotoxic T cells in low numbers clear infection, but in high numbers they can cause a hemorrhagic pneumonia (Cannon *et al.*, 1988). The most protective immune responses are associated with the induction of T helper cytokine profile that drives the immune response toward a Th1 response with predominant interferon gamma and IL-2 expression and diminished IL-4 response on challenge. Because the Th1 pattern should promote induction of a CD8 cytotoxic T cell (CTL) activity the argument can be made that CTLs are components of a protective response. Efforts to direct cytokine expression toward Th1-like patterns have included immunization with anti-IL-4 (Tang and Graham, 1994) or rIL-12

(Tang and Graham, 1995) used as adjuvants. Both approaches shifted cytokine expression to a Th1 pattern, but while anti-IL-4 reduced illness IL-12 did not. CD8 CTL activity was increased in the anti-IL-4 mice but was not present in mice treated with rIL-12.

Given the mucosal replication and apical expression of the virus, the question of how CTLs would mediate control of infection can be raised. There is an implication that for the lymphocytes to recognize virally infected cells, they would have to be in the extracellular environment on the surface of the epithelial compartment of the respiratory tract.

VII. Mucosal Immunization

The primary approach to induce mucosal immunity to RSV has focused on live-attenuated vaccines. Initially, there was cold-adaptation of RSV A strain by sequential passage at 26°C. This virus was attenuated in adults but caused residual illness in young seronegative children (Friedewald *et al.*, 1968; and Kim *et al.*, 1971). The rationale for the development of the next generation of live-attenuated vaccines rested on the observation that temperature-sensitive (ts) mutants could be derived (Gharpure *et al.*, 1969). They theoretically provided a further margin of safety as the ts property would limit growth in the lower respiratory tract as shown in the hamster (Wright *et al.*, 1971a). One of the ts viruses, ts-1, was evaluated sequentially in adults (Wright *et al.*, 1971b) and seropositive and seronegative infants (Wright *et al.*, 1976; Kim *et al.*, 1973b). There was a marked difference in the shedding pattern when vaccine was given to seronegative children; with the prolonged shedding that occurred in these circumstances reversion of the ts property and mild respiratory illness were seen. An alternative vaccine candidate, ts 2, with the interesting property of being nonsyncytial in its plaque morphology, proved to be overly attenuated, with doses as high as 10^6 not proving infectious (Wright *et al.*, 1982). Genetic stability was considered an essential phenotypic property of the virus and active clinical evaluation of these products stopped for 15 years. An important lesson from the early live vaccine experience was that unlike inactivated virus, enhanced illness was not seen when vaccine recipients were reexposed to natural infection in the ensuing winter.

More recently, further mutagenized RSV A strain viruses derived from both ca and ts have been assessed. These vaccine candidates have been put through an extensive evaluation in tissue culture and animal models to rank the level of attenuation and provide a series of

TABLE I
Human Experience with Respiratory Syncytial Virus Vaccines

Reference	Vaccine	Route	Age group studied			Comments
				Children		
			Adult	Prev. Inf.	Naive	
Kapikian, 1969 Kim *et al.*, 1969 Chin *et al.*, 1969 Fulginiti *et al.*, 1969	Formalin-inactivated	im		x	x	Potentiated disease on challenge in naive recipients
Belshe *et al.*, 1993 Tristram *et al.*, 1993 Paradiso *et al.*, 1994	Subunit-purified F protein	im		x		Humoral immunity No mucosal antibody Reinfection seen
Belshe *et al.*, 1982	Live virus	im		x	x	Low immunogenicity No efficacy
Friedwald *et al.*, 1968 Kim *et al.*, 1971	Cold-adapted live virus, CP-52	i.n.	x	x	x	Residual virulence in naive children
Wright *et al.*, 1971a,b Kim *et al.*, 1973b Wright *et al.*, 1976	ts live virus (ts-1)	i.n.	x	x	x	Genetic instability Residual virulence in naive children
Wright *et al.*, 1982	ts live virus (ts-2)	i.n.	x	x	x	Overly attenuated, noninfectious
McKay *et al.*, 1988 Pringle *et al.*, 1993	ts live virus	i.n.	x			Immunogenic in adults
Current trials	Further attentuated vaccines from ca and ts-1 parents	i.n.	x	x	x	Studies in progress

potential vaccines that can be evaluated in man (Crowe *et al.*, 1994). The animal modeling has included evaluation in chimpanzees, the most susceptible nonhuman primate. A similar approach is being taken to derive RSV B strain vaccines. Such candidates are currently under evaluation in man.

VIII. Summary

The goals of immunization for RSV are to prevent serious lower respiratory tract illness in infants, immunocompromised individuals, and the elderly. The history of RSV vaccines in humans is summarized in Table I. Based on current knowledge, the vaccine should produce serum and secretory antibody and should direct the immune response toward a Th1 response with the generation of CD8 CTLs. Live-attenuated vaccines offer the best current approach to the mucosal prevention of RSV. The vaccines presently being evaluated, although empirically derived, have been evaluated comprehensively in animals and build on earlier clinical trials. A major molecular advance is the recent description of progress toward the generation a cDNA copy of RSV which will allow specific mutagenesis to be directed toward attenuation (Grosfeld *et al.*, 1995). Other approaches that are being explored include live vectors suitable for mucosal delivery, subunit vaccines, and delivery systems including liposomes and microspheres.

The ultimate test of any vaccine comes with its administration to seronegative children. Such evaluation is initially carried out in children 6–24 months of age who have not experienced RSV, but the target for evaluation of safety and efficacy of vaccination is the child at 1 to 2 months of age so that immunity is induced before natural exposure. The level of immunologic maturation and the presence of maternal antibody may alter the appropriate level of attenuation for a vaccine candidate in early infancy. The imperative of the clinical impact of this disease gives little choice but to continue actively the development and assessment of the mucosal approach to the prevention of RSV. From it we will learn about the capabilities and mechanisms by which the mucosal immune system prevents respiratory viral infections that are limited to the mucosal surface.

Acknowledgments

The critical comments of Dr. David Karzon and Dr. Barney Graham are much appreciated, as are the insights provided through the years by Dr. Robert Chanock and Dr. Brian Murphy. Support for many of the studies at Vanderbilt have been provided by a series of contracts for the support of vaccine evaluation from NIAID, NIH.

References

Belshe, R. B., Van Voris, L. P., and Mufson, M. A. (1982). Parenteral administration of live respiratory syncytial virus vaccine: Results of a field trial. *J. Infect. Dis.* **145**, 311–319.

Belshe, R. B., Anderson, E. L., and Walsh, E. E. (1993). Immunogenicity of purified f glycoprotein of respiratory syncytial virus: Clinical and immune responses to subsequent natural infection in children. *J. Infect. Dis.* **168**, 1024–1029.

Cannon, M. J., Openshaw, P. J. M., and Askonas, B. A. (1988). Cytotoxic T cells clear virus but augment lung pathology in mice infected with respiratory syncytial virus. *J. Exp. Med.* **168**, 1163–1168.

Chiba, Y., Higashidate, Y., Suga, K., Honjo, K., Tsutsumi, H., and Ogra, P. L. (1989). Development of cell-mediated cytotoxic immunity to respiratory syncytial virus in human infants following naturally acquired infection. *J. Med. Virol.* **28**, 133–139.

Chin, J., Magoffin, R. L., Shearer, L. A., Schiebele, J. H., and Lennette, E. H. (1969). Field evaluation of a respiratory syncytial virus vaccine and a trivalent parainfluenza virus vaccine in a pediatric population. *Am. J. Epidemiol.* **89**, 449–463.

Crowe, J. E., Jr., Bui, P. T., London, W. T., Davis, A. R., Hung, P. P., Chanock, R. M., and Murphy, B. R. (1994). Satisfactorily attenuated and protective mutants derived from a partially attenuated cold passaged respiratory syncytial virus mutant by introduction of additional attenuating mutations during chemical mutagenesis. *Vaccine* **12**, 691–699.

Falsey, A. R., Cunningham, C. K., Barker, W. H., Kouides, R. W., Yuen, J. B., Menegus, M., Weiner, L. B., Bonville, C. A., and Betts, R. F. (1995). Respiratory syncytial virus and influenza A infections in the hospitalized elderly. *J. Infect. Dis.* **172**, 389–394.

Friedewald, W. T., Forsyth, B. R., Smith, C. B., Gharpure, M. A., and Chanock, R. M. (1968). Low-temperature grown RS virus in adult volunteers. *JAMA, J. Am. Med. Assoc.* **203**, 690–694.

Fulginiti, V. A., Eller, J. J., Sieber, O. F., Joyner, J. W., Minamitani, M., and Meiklejohn, G. (1969). Respiratory virus immunization. I. A. field trial of two inactivated respiratory virus vaccines; an aqueous trivalent parainfluenza virus vaccine and an alum-precipitated respiratory syncytial virus vaccine. *Am. J. Epidemiol.* **89**, 435–448.

Gharpure, M. A., Wright, P. F., and Chanock, R. M. (1969). Temperature-sensitive mutants of respiratory syncytial virus. *J. Virol.* **34**, 414–421.

Glezen, W. P., Paredes, A., Allison, J. E., Taber, L. H., and Frank, A. L. (1981). Risk of respiratory syncytial virus infection for infants from low-income families in relationship to age, sex, ethnic group, and maternal antibody level. *J. Pediatr.* **98**, 708–715.

Graham, B. S., Bunton, L. A., Rowland, J., Wright, P. F., and Karzon, D. T. (1991a). Respiratory syncytial virus infection in anti-mu-treated mice. *J. Virol.* **65**, 4936–4942.

Graham, B. S., Bunton, L. A., Wright, P. F., and Karzon, D. T. (1991b). Reinfection of mice with respiratory syncytial virus. *J. Med. Virol.* **34,** 7–13.

Graham, B. S., Bunton, L. A., Wright, P. F., and Karzon, D. T. (1991c). The role of T cell subsets in the pathogenesis of primary infection and reinfection with respiratory syncytial virus in mice. *J. Clin. Invest.* **88,** 1026–1033.

Graham, B. S., Davis, T. H., Tang, Y. W., Bunton, L. A., and Gruber, W. C. (1993). Immunoprophylaxis and immunotherapy of respiratory syncytial virus-infected mice with RSV-specific immune serum. *Pediatr. Res.* **21,** 270–274.

Graham, B. S., Tang, Y. W., and Gruber, W. C. (1995). Tropical prophylaxis of respiratory syncytial virus (RSV)-challenged mice with RSV-specific immune globulin. *J. Infect. Dis.* **171,** 1468–1474.

Groothuis, J. R., Simoes, E. A. F., Levin, M. J., Hall, C. B., Long, C. E., Rodrigues, W. J., Arrobio, J., Meissner, H. C., Fulton, D. R., Welliver, R. C., Tristram, D. A., Siber, G. R., Prince, G. A., Van Raden, M., and Hemming, V. G. (1993). Prophylactic administration of respiratory syncytial virus immune globulin to high-risk infants and young children. *N. Engl. J. Med.* **329,** 1524–1530.

Grosfeld, H., Hill, M. G., and Collins, P. L. (1995). RNA replication by respiratory syncytial virus (RSV) is directed by the N, P, and L proteins; transcription also occurs under these conditions but requires RSV superinfection for efficient synthesis of full-length mRNA. *J. Virol.* **69,** 5677–5686.

Hall, C. B., Kopelman, A. E., Douglas, R. G., Jr., Geiman, J. M., and Meagher, M. P. (1979). Neonatal respiratory syncytial virus infection. *N. Engl. J. Med.* **300,** 393–396.

Hall, C. B., Walsh, E. E., Schnabel, K. C., Long, C. E., McConnochie, K. M., Hildreth, S. W., and Anderson, L. J. (1990). Occurrence of groups A and B of respiratory syncytial virus over 15 years: Associated epidemiologic and clinical characteristics in hospitalized and ambulatory children. *J. Infect. Dis.* **162,** 1283–1290.

Hall, C. B., Walsh, E. E., Long, C. E., and Schnabel, K. C. (1991). Immunity to and frequency of reinfection with respiratory syncytial virus. *J. Infect. Dis.* **163,** 693–698.

Harrington, R. D., Hooton, T. M., Hackman, R. C., Storch, G. A., Osborne, B., Gleaves, C. A., Benson, A., and Meyers, J. D. (1992). An outbreak of respiratory syncytial virus in a bone marrow transplant center. *J. Infect. Dis.* **165,** 987–993.

Henderson, F. W., Hu, S. C., and Collier, A. M. (1978). Pathogenesis of respiratory syncytial virus infection in ferret and fetal human tracheas in organ culture. *Am. Rev. Respir. Dis.* **118,** 29–37.

Henderson, F. W., Collier, A. M., Clyde, W. A., Jr., and Denny, F. W. (1979). Respiratory syncytial virus infections, reinfections and immunity: A prospective, longitudinal study in young children. *N. Engl. J. Med.* **300,** 530–534.

Kapikian, A. Z., Mitchell, R. M., Chanock, R. M., Steinhoff, R. A., and Stewart, C. E. (1969). An epidemiologic study of altered clinical reactivity to respiratory syncytial (RS/virus) infection in children previously vaccinated with an inactivated RS virus vaccine. *Am. J. Epidemiol.* **89,** 405–421.

Kim, H. W., Canchola, J. G., Brandt, C. D., Pyles, G., Chanock, R. M., Jensen, K., and Parrott, R. H. (1969). Respiratory syncytial virus disease in infants despite prior administration of antigenic inactivated vaccine. *Am. J. Epidemiol.* **89,** 422–434.

Kim, H. W., Arrobio, J. O., Pyles, G. Brandt, C. D., Camargo, E., Chanock, R. M., and Parrott, R. H. (1971). Clinical and immunological response of infants and children to administration of low-temperature adapted respiratory syncytial virus. *Pediatrics* **48,** 745–755.

Kim, H. W., Arrobio, J. O., Brandt, C. D., Jefferies, B. C., Pyles, G., Reid, J. L., Chanock, R. M., and Parrott, R. H. (1973a). Epidemiology of respiratory syncytial virus infection in Washington, D.C. Importance of the virus in different respiratory tract disease syndromes and temporal distribution of infection. *Am. J. Epidemiol.* **98,** 216–225.

Kim, H. W., Arrobio, J. O., Brandt, C. D., Wright, P. F., Hodes, D., Chanock, R. M., and Parrott, R. H. (1973b). Safety and antigenicity of temperature sensitive (ts) mutant respiratory syncytial virus (RSV) in children. *Pediatrics* **52,** 56–63.

Kim, H. W., Leikin, S. L., Arrobio, J., Brandt, C. D., Chanock, R. M., and Parrott, R. H. (1976). Cell-mediated immunity to respiratory syncytial virus induced by inactivated vaccine or by infection. *Pediatr. Res.* **10,** 75–78.

King, J. C., Jr., Burke, A. R., Clemens, J. D., Nair, P., Farley, J. J., Vink, P. E., Batlas, S. R., Rao, M., and Johnson, J. P. (1993). Respiratory syncytial virus illnesses in human immunodeficiency virus- and noninfected children. *Pediatr. Infect. Dis. J.* **12,** 733–739.

McIntosh, K. M., and Chanock, R. M. (1990). Respiratory syncytial virus. *In* "Virology" (B. N. Fields, ed.), pp. 1045–1072. Raven, New York.

McKay, E., Higgins, P., Tyrrell, D., and Pringle, C. (1988). Immunogenicity and pathogenicity of temperature-sensitive modified respiratory syncytial virus in adult volunteers. *J. Med. Virol.* **25,** 411–421.

Mazanec, M. B., Kaetel, C. S., Lamm, M. E., Fletcher, D., and Nerdud, J. G. (1992). Intracellular neutralization of virus by immunoglobulin A antibodies. *Proc. Natl. Acad. Sci. U.S.A.* **89,** 6901–6905.

Mills, J. V., VanKirk, J. E., Wright, P. F., and Chanock, R. M (1971). Experimental respiratory syncytial virus infection of adults. *J. Immunol.* **107,** 123–130.

Murphy, B. R., and Walsh, E. E. (1988). Formalin-inactivated respiratory syncytial virus vaccine induces antibodies to the fusion protein that are deficient in fusion-inhibiting activity. *J. Clin. Microbiol.* **26,** 1595–1597.

Murphy, B. R., Alling, D. W., Snyder, M. H., Walsh, E. E., Prince, G. A., Chanock, R. M., Hemming, V. G., Rodriguez, W. J., Kim. H. W., Graham, B. S., and Wright, P. F. (1986). Effect of age and preexisting antibody response of infants and children to the F and G proteins during respiratory syncytial virus infection. *J. Clin. Microbiol.* **24,** 894–898.

Paradiso, P. R., Hildreth, S. W., Hogerman, D. A., Speelman, D. J., Lewin, E. B., Oren, J., and Smith, D. H. (1994). Safety and immunogenicity of a subunit respiratory syncytial virus vaccine in children 24 to 48 months old. *J. Pediatr.* **13,** 792–798.

Price, J. F. (1990). Acute and long-term effects of viral bronchiolitis in infancy (review). *Lung* **168,** 414–421.

Prince, G. A., Horswood, R. L., and Chanock, R. M. (1985). Quantitative aspects of passive immunity to respiratory syncytial virus infection in infant cotton rats. *J. Virol.* **55,** 517–520.

Pringle, C. R., Filipiuk, A. H., Robinson, B. S., Watt, P. J., Higgins, P., and Tyrell, D. A. (1993). Immunogenicity and pathogenicity of a triple temperature-sensitive modified respiratory syncytial virus in adult volunteers. *Vaccine* **11,** 473–478.

Smith, C. B., Purcell, R. H., Bellanti, J. A., and Chanock, R. M. (1966). Protective effect of antibody to parainfluenza type 1 virus. *N. Engl. J. Med.* **275,** 1145–1152.

Tang, Y. W., and Graham, B. S. (1994). Anti-IL-4 treatment at immunization modulates cytokine expression, reduces illness, and increases cytotoxic T lymphocyte activity in mice challenged with respiratory syncytial virus. *J. Clin. Invest.* **94,** 1953–1958.

Tang, Y. W., and Graham, B. S. (1995). Interleukin 12 treatment during immunization elicits a Th1-like immune response in mice challenged with respiratory syncytial virus and improves vaccine immunogenicity. *J. Infect. Dis.* **172,** 734–738.

Tristram, D. A., Welliver, R. C., Mohar, C. K., Hogerman, D. A., Hildreth, S. W., and Paradiso, P. R. (1993). Immunogenicity and safety of respiratory syncytial virus subunit vaccine in seropositive children 18–36 months old. *J. Infect. Dis.* **167,** 191–195.

Weltzin, R., Hsu, S. A., Mittler, E. S., Georgakopoulos, K., and Monath, T. P. (1994). Intranasal monoclonal immunoglobulin A against respiratory syncytial virus protects against upper and lower respiratory disease. *Antimicrobial Agents Chemother.* **38,** 2785–2791.

Wertz, G. W., Stott, E. J., Young, K., K.-Yo, King, A. M. Q., Bungham, C. R., and Ball, L. W. (1987). Respiratory syncytial virus proteins expressed from vaccinia virus vectors protect against live virus challenge in mice. *Vaccines* **87,** 360–363.

Wohl, M. E., and Chernick, V. (1978). State of the art: bronchiolitis. *Am. Rev. Respir. Dis.* **118,** 759–781.

Wright, P. F., Woodend, W. G., and Chanock, R. M. (1971a). Temperature-sensitive mutants of respiratory syncytial virus: *In vivo* studies in hamsters. *J. Infect. Dis.* **122,** 501–512.

Wright, P. F., Mills, J. V., and Chanock, R. M. (1971b). Evaluation of a temperature-sensitive mutant of respiratory syncytial virus in adults. *J. Infect. Dis.* **124,** 505–511.

Wright, P. F., Shinozaki, T., Fleet, W., Sell, S. H., Thompson, J., and Karzon, D. T. (1976). Evaluation of a live, attenuated respiratory syncytial virus vaccine in infants. *J. Pediatr.* **88,** 931–936.

Wright, P. F., Belshe, R. B., Kim, H. W., Van Voris, L. P., and Chanock, R. M. (1982). Administration of a highly attenuated, live respiratory syncytial virus vaccine to adults and children. *Infect. Immun.* **37,** 397–400.

23

Oral Immunization with Influenza Virus Vaccines

ROBERT B. COUCH
THOMAS R. CATE
WENDY A. KEITEL
Departments of Microbiology and Immunology and Medicine
Baylor College of Medicine
Houston, Texas 77030

I. Introduction

The importance of immunity at the mucosal surface of the respiratory tract for prevention of influenza was articulated decades ago. Francis provided data on influenza virus neutralizing substances in nasal secretions and subsequently proposed that these neutralizing substances were antibodies. He proposed that their primary role was to prevent infection while that for circulating antibody was to control an infection once established and thereby prevent spread, particularly to the lungs (Francis, 1940, 1943). Specific data to support this concept was later provided by Fazekas de St. Groth (1950) for influenza in a mouse challenge model. These fundamental concepts of influenza immunity have not changed; they have, however, been clarified and considerable effort has been expended on identifying the optimal manner of immunization for achieving optimal circulating and secretion antibody levels for prevention of influenza and its complications. These latter efforts have involved parenteral and respiratory vaccinations and both live-attenuated and inactivated vaccines. In this regard, the specific role and importance of cell-mediated immune responses to influenza virus at mucosal surfaces remains uncertain.

The description of a common mucosal immune system provided the rationale for proposing that immunization of the mucosal immune system at a distant site would lead to distribution of antigen-sensitized lymphocytes to all mucosal sites including the site where natural infection would occur (Couch *et al.*, 1984; Mestecky, 1987). A focus for application of this concept to immunization for influenza has been on oral immunization for inducing mucosal immunity in the respiratory tract. Not only is the oral route accepted as the most convenient route for drug administration, but the gastrointestinal (GI) tract contains the largest mucosal surface and produces about 80% of secretory IgA (S-IgA) antibodies in humans (McGhee and Kiyono, 1992). The importance of influenza as a medical problem and the availability of influenza vaccines suitable for human administration stimulated the investigation of oral immunization for prevention of influenza (Couch *et al.*, 1986).

This report will summarize the major findings derived from published animal and human studies, report findings of our recent studies evaluating the approach in humans, and comment on the status of the approach.

II. Oral Immunization with Live Virus

Oral immunization with live, partially attenuated influenza viruses was first introduced for immunization of children in Russia (Alexandrova, *et al.*, 1970). Virus grown in embryonated hens' eggs was orally administered as a liquid in an effort to reduce the reactogenicity seen in children when the same material was administered intranasally. Oral administration reduced reactogenicity without significantly altering immunogenicity and protective effects. The administration of vaccine as a liquid was evaluated after administration of vaccine in enteric-coated capsules exhibited low immunogenicity [9–25% serum hemagglutination-inhibiting (HI) antibody responses versus 53–68% for liquid] (Alexandrova, *et al.*, 1970). The basis for the difference was presumed to be infection of pharyngeal tissues among children given liquid vaccine as submandibular node enlargement was noted in many and virus was recovered from throat swab specimens from 55–68% of children, frequencies similar to those of children given vaccine intranasally. The importance of nasopharyngeal infection was suggested by other studies in mice that were allowed to drink live vaccine (estimated dose 18,000,

MUCOSAL VACCINES

1800, 180 CCA) and, in a separate experiment, inactivated vaccine (estimated dose 7200, 720, 72 CCA) (Boudreault and Pavilanis, 1972). Mean serum HI antibodies postvaccine were 143, 71, and 4, respectively, in the live vaccine group and 0 for all inactivated vaccine groups. Protection against challenge was high in the live vaccine groups (93–100%) and absent in the inactivated vaccine group (0–8%).

Antibodies in secretions were not measured in either the human or mouse studies. Nevertheless, these studies indicate that oral administration of live influenza virus vaccine can lead to induction of a high rate of protective immune responses against influenza virus infection. While infection of the upper respiratory tract occurs, the route apparently induces fewer respiratory symptoms than intranasal administration of the same vaccine.

It was reported by Bergmann, Waldman, and coworkers that administration of live influenza virus orally where the nasopharynx is bypassed can lead to protection in mice (Bergmann and Waldman, 1982, 1983; Bergmann *et al.*, 1984; Briese *et al.*, 1987; Waldman *et al.*, 1987). Live A/PR/8/34 (H1N1) virus was grown in embryonated eggs and given by intraesophageal or intragastric tube to anesthetized mice in doses that varied between 10^4 and 10^8 EID_{50} and that exhibited hemagglutination titers of 1:3–1:512. In one study the total dose was reported as 40 μg HA (Briese *et al.*, 1987). Virus was given two or three times at 8- to 14-day intervals. Despite the varied doses and schedules utilized, the results of immunization were relatively uniform. Serum HI or IgG antibody in ELISA tests and lung lavage HI or IgA antibody were induced by all regimens and doses. IgA antibody was detected in uterine fluids when sought, but no antibody was detected in bile fluids (Bergmann and Waldman, 1982; Briese *et al.*, 1987). In a study comparing results in young and old mice, serum antibody responses were much lower among old mice, while lung lavage IgA antibody was minimally reduced (Waldman *et al.*, 1987). Both age groups were significantly protected against challenge with infectious virus.

Unfortunately, no attempt was made to rule out infection of the respiratory tract in these studies; however, rectal immunization produced similar findings suggesting that respiratory infection was not necessary for induction of protection. The authors interpreted their studies as indicating that immunization had occurred via the intestinal tract and that circulating IgA antibody precursor cells had lodged in the respiratory tract and led to antibody in respiratory secretions that conveyed protection against an infectious virus challenge. The parameters of immunization that ensured success in the mouse were not explored.

A summary of the findings from these experiments with oral administration of live influenza virus vaccine is given in Table I. The experience of Russian investigators with partially attenuated live influenza virus led them to use this vaccine approach among children. The experience in mice provided encouragement to pursue the approach for humans with inactivated vaccines.

TABLE I
Oral Live Influenza Virus Immunizations

- Drinking live vaccine reduces reactogenicity in humans
- Live vaccine is highly immunogenic when given as liquid to children
- A major reduction in immunogenicity follows similar doses of vaccine given via enteric-coated capsules
- Live vaccine given intragastrically can be highly immunogenic in mice
- Intragastric live virus induces lung lavage IgA antibody
- Old mice given live virus intragastrically developed lung lavage IgA antibody responses similar to young mice but lower serum IgG responses

In order to obtain the benefits of both the humoral and cell-mediated immune responses that follow infection with an oral vaccine, Meitin *et al.* (1994) employed an orally administered recombinant vaccinia virus vaccine containing genes coding for the influenza virus HA protein. The vaccinia virus can be manufactured cheaply, is heat stable, and is easily transportable; it is, however, acid labile and must be protected during passage through the stomach. Mice given vaccinia HA vaccine into the jejunum developed IgA anti HA antibody in nasal wash fluids equal to that following intranasal immunization as well as cytotoxic lymphocyte responses by spleen cells similar to those following influenza virus infection. Following challenge, lung lavage and nasal wash virus titers were significantly and equally reduced among animals given vaccinia HA intrajejunally and intranasally. Less reduction was noted in nasal wash virus titers among animals given vaccine parenterally; they had developed high serum IgG antibody responses but little to no nasal wash IgA antibody. The authors interpreted their studies to indicate that jejunal immunization with vaccinia HA vaccine consistently leads to induction of mucosal IgA antibody, some serum IgG antibody, and specific CTL responses that can prevent or reduce the intensity of influenza virus infection. They further proposed that an enteric-coated multivalent recombinant vaccinia could be an inexpensive, safe, effective, temperature stable, and universal vaccine.

III. Oral Immunization with Inactivated Virus

A. Animal Immunizations

More variables of the immunizing procedure have been evaluated in animal immunizations with inactivated influenza virus than with live influenza virus. In a series of reports, Chen *et al.*, evaluated intragastric immunizations among mice given a histamine H_2-receptor antagonist (Tagamet) and aluminum hydroxide to inhibit gastric acid before administering antigen (Chen *et al.*, 1987; Chen and Quinnan, 1988, 1989). Under these conditions, whole virus vaccine in doses of 40–43 μg HA daily for 4 days followed by a similar regimen 3 weeks later (total 320–340 μg HA) induced a dominance of IgA antibody in lung lavage fluids, while the dominant antibody was IgG among those given vaccine parenterally (5 μg HA at 3-week intervals). Antibody in serum was predominantly IgG for both routes. *In vitro* stimulation of lung lymphocytes yielded IgA antibody only. Further studies indicated that antibody responses were similar in pattern but significantly greater after whole virus than after comparable doses of split virus vaccine and reduced with reducing doses of antigen. A dose of 160 μg HA given once was equivalent to 40 μg given on 4 successive days. IgA and IgG antibodies in pulmonary lavage fluids peaked at 1 week and persisted for 4 months. Levels in secretions were similar among mice regardless of age, whereas both serum IgA and IgG antibody levels decreased with increasing age (Chen and Quinnan, 1989). Complete protection against death from homotypic challenge was provided by both oral and parenteral immunization but was reduced for a serologically related subtype and absent for a different subtype indicating similar specificity of protection for both immunization routes.

The reduced immunogenicity for inactivated vaccine given by the oral route when compared to the parenteral route was confirmed by Farag-Mahmoud *et al.* (1988) and shown to be largely attributable to degradation of antigen in passage through the stomach. They systematically tested immunogenicity of a whole virus vaccine given in drinking water, then gelatin capsules (which should dissolve in the stomach), and then directly by injection into the lumen of the duodenum after intestinal exposure via surgical incision. When vaccine was administered in drinking water or in capsules, serum antibody was detected after a single dose of 66 μg of HA, but not 26 μg. A dose of 106 μg HA given by either of these routes induced IgA antibody in lung fluids and IgG antibody in serum, and conveyed significant protection against influenza virus infection. In contrast, when vaccine was given by the intraduodenal or intramuscular (i.m.) route, comparable serum and lavage fluid IgG responses and protection against infection were provided by vaccine doses as low as 6.6, 0.66, and 0.06 μg HA, even though no IgA antibody was detected in the latter animals using a radioimmunoassay procedure. When two doses of 6.6 μg HA were given by the i.m. or intraduodenal routes 4 weeks apart, IgA antibody was detected in intestinal secretions, but not in lung lavage fluids.

A summary of findings from oral immunization of mice with inactivated influenza virus vaccine is shown in Table II. It seems clear that inactivated influenza virus vaccine given orally can induce immune responses that convey protection to immunized animals. One study reported considerable degradation of antigenicity in passage through the stomach, not a surprising finding in view of the known lability of the influenza virus HA (Hoyle, 1960). The circulation of IgA-producing lymphocytes to the lung has been demonstrated. Moreover, the oral route offers a potential advantage for use in elderly persons who, despite a decline in serum immune responses, tend to retain mucosal immune responsiveness with advancing age (Finkelstein *et al.*, 1984). These studies further suggest that ways to obviate the large antigen dose requirement for adequate immunogenicity are needed in order for this route of immunization to achieve clinical utility.

Options for reducing the antigen dose for acceptable immunization include protecting antigen during passage through the stomach and upper intestine, enhancing uptake by M cells in the intestinal mucosa, and enhancing immune responses by inclusion of adjuvants. Some exploratory efforts of this type have been described (Table III). Influenza vaccine has been successfully incorporated into microspheres composed of polylactide-*co*-glycolide in various particle sizes. Eldridge *et al.* (1990) provided data that a heterogeneous population of microspheres could induce both systemic and mucosal immune responses to staphylococcal enterotoxin. He indicated that particles 10 μm in diameter remain at the

TABLE II
Oral-Inactivated Influenza Virus Vaccine Immunizations in Mice

- Inactivated virus vaccine is less immunogenic when given in drinking water than when the stomach is bypassed
- Intestinal immunization induces lung lavage IgA antibody
- Whole-virus vaccine could be more immunogenic than split product vaccine
- Antibody responses are more dependent on dose than frequency of doses
- Lung lavage IgA responses are similar for old and young mice but IgG responses are lower among old mice
- Specificity of protection for homotypic and heterotypic challenge is the same for oral and parenteral immunization

TABLE III
Options Evaluated in Mice for Preserving and Enhancing Immunogenicity of Oral Immunization with Influenza Virus Vaccine

- Vaccine incorporated in polylactide-*co*-glycolide microspheres
- Vaccine adsorbed to chicken enthrocyte ghosts
- Vaccine incorporated in immunostimulating complexes (ISCOMs)
- Liposomes containing vaccine and acridine, a lipoidal amine adjuvant
- Vaccine–cholera toxin B combinations

mucosal level, those of 5–10 μm pass to regional lymph nodes, and those <5 μm pass to regional nodes and into the systemic circulation. Similar preparations employing influenza virus antigen have been shown to induce similar responses in mice (Moldoveneau *et al.*, 1993). In addition, these responses induce protection of mice against influenza.

Pang *et al.* (1992) employed chicken erythrocyte ghosts as vehicles for adsorbed gamma-irradiated influenza virus. After administering sodium bicarbonate, erythrocyte antigen or control was given by feeding needle on Days 1, 3, and 5; mice were then challenged with live virus 2 weeks later. High levels of IgG antibody appeared in serum and lung extracts but only IgA was seen in nasal washings. Protection levels were high with correlations of virus yield in dose–response studies relating best to local IgG for lung virus and local IgA for nasal wash virus. Surprisingly, low doses of irradiated erythrocyte-adsorbed virus (10^{2-3} $TCID_{50}$) induced immune responses and protection. The basis for the immunogenicity of erythrocyte-adsorbed antigen was not determined.

Immunostimulating complexes (ISCOMs) given intranasally induced serum antibody responses comparable to subcutaneous administration but no antibody was detected after oral administration (Lovgren, 1988). Comparative studies of mice vaccinated intranasally or orally (intragastric administration of a sodium bicarbonate–vaccine combination) with an influenza virus vaccine–cholera toxin B combination indicated that the intranasal route was greater than 100 times more immunogenic on a dose basis for IgA antibody responses in respiratory secretions (Hirabayashi *et al.*, 1990). Finally, Bergmann reported enhanced IgA antibody responses in lung fluids when irradiated virus was mixed with liposomes containing acridine, a lipoidal amine adjuvant reported to enhance immune responses in intestinal mucosa (Bergmann and Waldman, 1988). Thus, it appears that it is possible to devise methods to reduce dosage requirements and to improve the potential utility of oral immunization with inactivated influenza vaccine, but the optimal approach remains to be determined.

B. Human Immunizations

A series of reports on experimental immunizations of humans with inactivated influenza vaccines has been provided by Waldman, Bergmann *et al.* (Bergmann *et al.*, 1986a, 1987; Lazzell *et al.*, 1984; Waldman *et al.*, 1982, 1983, 1986, 1987). A summary of immune responses reported in these studies is provided in Table IV. As can be seen, a variety of doses and regimens have been employed. Most, if not all, vaccinations employed split product vaccine. In view of the responses reported in small animal studies, the absence of any serum antibody responses is remarkable; serum responses were detected among other volunteers given low doses of vaccine i.m. at the same time. All human adults will have been primed by prior influenza virus infection and most, if not all, would have possessed serum antibody to the vaccine antigen at the time of immunizations (data not given), a circumstance known to reduce the likelihood of detecting HI antibody responses in serum. That this is not the reason for absence of serum antibody rises, however, is suggested by a similar study in unprimed monkeys where a total of 600 μg HA of inactivated virus was given by esophageal tube and no serum HI antibody responses were detected (Bergmann *et al.*, 1986b). In that

TABLE IV

Immune Responses among Persons Immunized Orally with Inactivated Influenza Virus Vaccine

Oral vaccine regimen	Total dose (HA) (μg)	No. vols.[a] Total	No. vols.[a] Oral vac.	Serum No.	Saliva No. w/increase	Saliva Mean fold increase	Nasal secretions No. w/increase	Nasal secretions Mean fold increase
7 μg HA × 10 capsules × 7 days[c]	490	24	8	0	—	—	4	2.0
14 μg HA × 7 days[c]	98	24	8	0	5	9.2	6	3.8
0.4 μg HA × 10 capsules × 6 days[c]	24	5	5	0	—	~6.0[d]	—	~8.0[d]
8 μg HA × 7 days[c]	56	24 young	8	0	6	3.7	6	5.0
8 μg HA × 7 days[c]	56	32 elderly	11	0	3	1.8	9	4.5
3.1 μg HA × 5 capsules,[e] Days 1, 4, 8, 12	62	112 children (4–16 years)	30	0	5[f]	<1.0	9[f]	<1.0

Antibody responses among oral group[b]

[a] No. in study and No. given vaccine orally.
[b] Fourfold or greater. Serum tests were HI; secretions tests were HI or ELISA.
[c] All vaccine was split product from the Parke-Davis Co.; capsules were enteric-coated.
[d] Estimated from line graphs.
[e] Vaccine was from VEB SSW Dresden, GDR, type not specified; capsules were enteric-coated.
[f] Increases restricted to "low" antibody group (22% for saliva, 53% for nasal secretions).

study, antibody responses in nasal secretions and saliva were similar to those listed in the table for humans.

As noted in the table, significant increases in antibody occurred in respiratory secretions in all studies, usually in half or more of the subjects. No regimen or dose appeared to be superior to the others and there is no suggestion of a dose response. In fact, although not studied systematically, the results suggest a threshold response that was exceeded by the lowest dose (24 μg HA) and that an increasing dose is not followed by increasing numbers of circulating, sensitized lymphocytes homing to the respiratory tract. The responses listed were at 3 or 4 weeks after immunization, or were undesignated except in two sequential studies. These studies reported peak antibody titers 7 to 10 weeks after immunization (Bergmann *et al.*, 1986a, 1987).

Thus, these exploratory studies in humans indicate that oral immunization with inactivated influenza virus vaccine can lead to IgA antibody responses in respiratory secretions. In the studies, responses were similar in secretions to those that followed i.m. vaccine but the latter also induced serum antibody. The relation of vaccine dose to responses and whether the responses will convey significant protection to humans remain uncertain.

Oral administration of inactivated influenza virus vaccine has also been tested among adults and children in Romania for induction of serum HI antibody and protection against illness (Cajal *et al.*, 1974; Coban *et al.*, 1985; Petrescu and Cajal, 1984; Petrescu *et al.*, 1976, 1977). In fact, it has apparently been distributed commercially in that country. Vaccine is given as 0.5 ml of a liquid containing about 1000 HA units in tea or on sugar. Serum HI antibody responses reportedly occur in 50 to 75% of persons and significant reductions in influenzal illness during subsequent epidemics are detected. Unless pharyngeal application of antigen is immunogenic, it is difficult to reconcile these reports with the animal and human studies described above using inactivated vaccines.

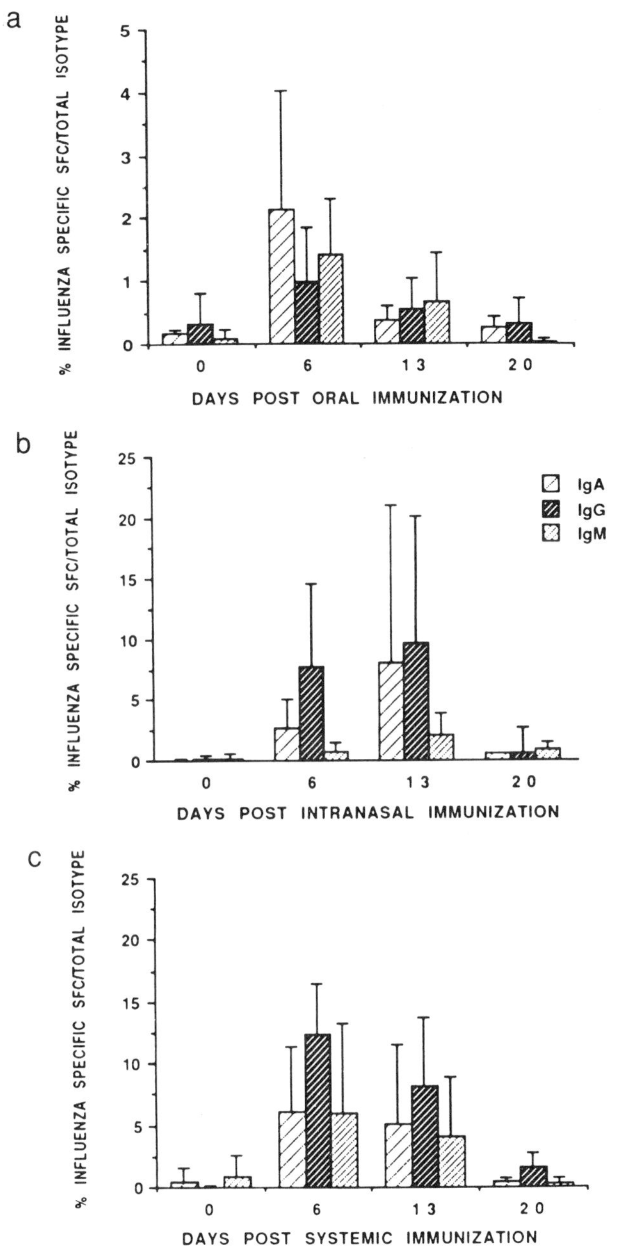

Figure 1. Kinetics and isotype distribution of influenza virus-specific spot-forming cells (SFC) in (a), orally; (b), intranasally; and (c), systemically immunized volunteers. The antibodies were assayed against HA isolated from influenza A Texas (H1H1) virus (b) or 1:100 dilution of vaccine homologous to those used in the immunization protocols (a, c). The data represent mean + S.D. of 7 (a, c), or 5 (b) individuals.

C. Recent Studies

Moldoveneau *et al.* (1995) administered inactivated influenza virus vaccine to adult volunteers via enteric-coated capsules. Volunteers were given 150-μg HA doses orally on 5 consecutive days (750 μg HA) of each component in a trivalent (H1N1, H3N2, B) vaccine; other groups were given a 15-μg HA dose of each component intramuscularly or monavalent H1N1 live attenuated vaccine intranasally. Serum, saliva, nasal secretions, and peripheral blood lymphocytes were collected 6, 13, and 20 days later. Orally vaccinated volunteers developed a significant increase in virus-specific IgA spot-forming cells (SFC) in blood on Days 6 and 13; IgM SFC were increased on Day 6 only and IgG SFC only on Day 13 (Fig. 1). Those given vaccine i.m. developed significant increases only in IgG SFC (Day 6, 13, and 20). Live virus intranasally induced both IgA and IgG SFC on Days 6 and 13. IgA antibody increased after oral vaccine in saliva and nasal wash specimens; IgG also increased in nasal specimens. Significant serum antibody increases were confined to the IgG isotype. Intranasal vaccination caused increases in IgA in saliva and both IgA and IgG in nasal secretions.

We recently undertook an evaluation of the utility

of oral immunization of humans for influenza by employing some of the more promising approaches for protection of antigen in passage through the stomach and for enhancing uptake. A dose ranging study employed an enteric-coated capsule, prepared by the Alza Corporation (Palo Alto, CA) that is designed to provide a predetermined delay in release of contents, the Chronset system. The capsules in this study contained lyophilized whole virus vaccine and were designed to release vaccine as a bolus dose within 1 to 2 hr after gastric emptying. Significant increases in antibody were detected in serum and nasal secretions but those for a standard 15-μg HA dose of vaccine given i.m. were greater than those that followed the highest oral vaccine dose (337 μg HA given twice at 7-day intervals). A dose-ranging study employing microspheres was unsuccessful because the preparation provided was defective; this promising approach awaits testing in humans. More recently, a pilot study employed subunit antigen incorporated in liposomes that was given via enteric-coated capsules at a dose of 100 μg HA. Liposome incorporated antigen had reportedly enhanced antibody responses to carbohydrate antigens in rats (Bruyere *et al.*, 1987). Antibody responses to influenza virus were detected in serum and nasal secretions but at low frequency.

TABLE V

Human Trials with Oral Administration of Inactivated Influenza Virus Vaccine in Enteric-Coated Capsules

- A high dose (compared to parenteral) is required for immunogenicity of vaccine
- IgA antibody responses are induced in nasal secretions
- Little or no IgG antibody responses appear in serum of orally immunized persons
- There is no indication of a dose-related antibody response among those immunized

IV. Comment

Published studies of oral immunization among animals clearly indicate a need to protect influenza virus antigens from degradation during passage through the stomach and also suggest that, in addition to preventing degradation, means are needed for increasing the frequency of effective responses. Also, data from these oral immunization studies in animals do not clearly identify the IgA antibody response in respiratory secretions as the mechanism of protection against virus challenge. Nevertheless, the data clearly indicate that intestinal immunization is followed by appearance of lymphocytes with a capacity for producing specific IgA antibody in respiratory secretions. Thus, the tenets of the common mucosal immune system are applicable to oral influenza vaccination.

Findings from studies in humans are summarized in Table V. Thus far results are not encouraging. It appears difficult to achieve a satisfactory immune response when either live or inactivated antigen is released into the intestinal lumen, even though IgA antibody responses do develop in respiratory secretions. Nasopharyngeal immunization with live and inactivated influenza virus vaccine has led to high frequencies of IgG antibody responses in serum and IgA antibody responses in respiratory secretions with quantities of antigen considerably lower than those used in many oral immunization trials (Kasel *et al.*, 1969). Although part of the reduced antigenicity of oral immunization may be attributed to differences in effective antigen dose, it may be that the compartmentalization of mucosal immune responses will make a respiratory vaccination route more desirable (Mestecky and McGhee, 1992; Pierce and Cray, 1981, 1982). Waldeyer's ring in the nasopharynx consists of a concentration of lymphoid tissue that is proposed as the upper respiratory equivalent of Peyer's patches in the intestine (Craig and Cebra, 1971; McGhee and Kiyono, 1992; Mestecky and McGhee, 1992). Uptake of antigen and generation of immune responses by these tissues could obviate the requirement for circulation of antigen responsive cells from distant sites for an IgA antibody response in respiratory secretions.

It should be emphasized that the primary and essential mediator for protection against influenza in humans is IgG antibody in serum (Couch *et al.*, 1984). Nevertheless, IgA antibody can contribute to prevention and control of infection at the mucosal level and is a desirable response to vaccination. Achieving maximal responses of both antibody types among vaccine recipients is preferred.

Acknowledgments

Research performed by the authors and summarized in this report was supported by Public Health Service Contract NO1-AI-15103 from the National Institute of Allergy and Infectious Diseases. The content of this publication does not necessarily reflect the views or policies of the Department of Health and Human Services, nor does mention of trade names, commercial products, or organizations imply endorsement by the U.S. Government.

References

Alexandrova, G. I., Smorodintsev, A. A., Beljaeva, N. M., Vasil'ev, B. J. A., Geft, R. A., Panteleev, V. G., Sejfer, M. A., and Selivanov, A. A. (1970). Testing the safety and effectiveness of oral administration of a live influenza vaccine. *Bull. WHO* **42,** 429–436.

Bergmann, K.-C., and Waldman, R. H. (1982). Occurrence of influenza specific antibodies in the lung after oral immunization in mice. *Poumon Coeur* **38**, 289–292.

Bergmann, K. C., and Waldman, R. H. (1983). Antibodies against influenza and stimulated macrophages in the lung lavage fluid of mice following oral immunization. *Allerg. Immunol.* **29**, 215–222.

Bergmann, K. C., Lachmann, B., and Noack, K. (1984). Lung mechanics in orally immunized mice after aerolized exposure to influenza virus. *Respiration* **46**, 218–221.

Bergmann, K. C., Waldman, R. H., Tischner, H., and Pohl, W. D. (1986a). Antibody in tears, saliva and nasal secretions following oral immunization of humans with inactivated influenza virus vaccine. *Int. Arch. Allergy Appl. Technol.* **80**, 107–109.

Bergmann, K. C., Waldman, R. H., Nordheim, W., Nguyen, H. T., Huynh, P. L., and Tischner, H. (1986b). Remote-site stimulation of influenza antibodies in monkeys following intestinal stimulation. *Immunol. Lett.* **12**, 65–67.

Bergmann, K. C., Waldman, R. H., Reinhofer, M., Pohl, W. D., Tischner, H., and Werchan, D. (1987). Oral immunization against influenza in children with asthma and chronic bronchitis. *Adv. Exp. Med. Biol.* **216B**, 1685–1690.

Bergmann, K. C., and Waldman, R. H. (1988). Enhanced murine respiratory tract IgA antibody response to oral influenza vaccine when combined with a lipoidal amine (avridine). *Int. Arch. Allergy Appl. Immunol.* **87**, 334–335.

Boudreault, A., and Pavilanis, V. (1972). Oral immunization against influenza virus. *Arch. Gesamte Virusforsch.* **38**, 177–182.

Briese, V., Polh, W.-D., Noack, K., Tischner, H., and Waldman, R. H. (1987). Influenza specific antibodies in the femal genital tract of mice after oral administration of live influenza vaccine. *Arch. Gynecol.* **240**, 153–157.

Bruyere, T., Waschmann, D., Klein, J. P., Scholler, M., and Frank, R. M. (1987). Local response in rat to liposome-associated *Streptococcus mutans* polysaccharide–protein conjugate. *Vaccine* **5**, 39–42.

Cajal, N., Sarateanu, D., Petrescu, A., Mihail, A., Popescu, A., and Teodosiu, O. (1974). Preliminary data on the efficiency of an inactivated influenza vaccine administered by oral route. *Rev. Roum. Virol.* **25**, 23–27.

Chen, K.-S., Burlington, D. B., and Quinnan, G. V., Jr. (1987). Active synthesis of hemagglutinin-specific immunoglobulin A by lung cells of mice that were immunized intragastrically with inactivated influenza virus vaccine. *J. Virol.* **61**, 2150–2154.

Chen, K.-S., and Quinnan, G. V., Jr. (1988). Induction, persistence and strain specificity of haemagglutinin-specific secretory antibodies in lungs of mice after intragastric administration of inactivated influenza virus vaccines. *J. Gen. Virol.* **69**, 2779–2784.

Chen, K.-S., and Quinnan, G. V., Jr. (1989). Secretory immunoglobulin A antibody response is conserved in aged mice following oral immunization with influenza virus vaccine. *J. Gen. Virol.* **70**, 3291–3296.

Coban, V., Mihail, A., Petrescu, A., Teodosiu, O., and Sternberg, I. (1985). Efficiency of the NIVGRIP inactivated influenza vaccine applied by oral route: Evaluation in a community of preschool children in the period 1981–84. *Rev. Roum. Med. Virol.* **36**, 79–83.

Couch, R. B., Kasel, J. A., Six, H. R., Cate, T. R., and Zahradnik, J. M. (1984). Immunological reactions and resistance to infection with influenza virus. *In* "Molecular Virology and Epidemiology of Influenza" (C. Stuart-Harris and C. Potter, eds.), pp. 119–153. Academic Press, London.

Couch, R. B., Kasel, J. A., Glezen, W. P., Six, H. R., Taber, L. H., Frank, A. L., Greenberg, S. B., Zahradnik, J. M., and Keitel, WA. (1986). Influenza: Its control in persons and populations. *J. Infect. Dis.* **153**, 431–440.

Craig, S. W., and Cebra, J. J. (1971). Peyer's patches: An enriched source of precursors for IgA-producing immunocytes in the rabbit. *J. Exp. Med.* **134**, 188–200.

Eldridge, J. H., Hammond, C. J., Meulbroek, J. A., Staas, J. K., Gilley, R. M., and Tice, T. R. (1990). Controlled vaccine release in the gut-associated lymphoid tissues. I. Orally administered biodegradable microspheres target the Peyer's Patches. *J. Controlled Release* **11**, 205–214.

Farag-Mahmoud, F. I., Wyde, P. R., Rosborough, J. P., and Six, H. R. (1988). Immunogenicity and efficacy of orally administered inactivated influenza virus vaccine in mice. *Vaccine* **6**, 262–268.

Fazekas de St. Groth, S. (1950). Influenza: A study in mice. *Lancet* **1**, 1101–1105.

Finkelstein, M. S., Tanner, M., and Freedman, L. (1984). Salivary and serum IgA levels in a geriatric outpatient population. *J. Immunol.* **4**, 85–91.

Francis, T., Jr. (1940). The inactivation of epidemic influenza virus by nasal secretions of human individuals. *Science* **91**, 198–199.

Francis, T., Jr. (1943). A rationale for studies in the control of epidemic influenza. *Science* **97**, 229–235.

Hirabayashi, T., Kurata, H., Funato, H., Nagamine, T., Aizawa, C., Tamura, S., Shimada, K., and Kurata, T. (1990). Comparison of intranasal inoculation of influenza HA vaccine combined with cholera toxin B subunit with oral or parenteral vaccination. *Vaccine* **8**, 243–248.

Hoyle, L., Reviewed in (1960). The influenza viruses. *In* "Virology Monographs," pp. 68–75. Springer-Verlag, New York.

Kasel, J. A., Rossen, R. D., Fulk, R. V., Fedson, D. S., Couch, R. B., and Brown, P. (1969). Human influenza: Aspects of the immune response to vaccination. *Ann. Int. Med.* **71**, 369–398.

Lazzell, V., Waldman, R. H., Rose, C., Khakoo, R., Jacknowitz, A., and Howard, S. (1984). Immunization against influenza in humans using an oral enteric-coated killed virus vaccine. *J. Biol. Stand.* **12**, 315–321.

Lovgren, K. (1988). The serum antibody response distributed in subclasses and isotypes after intranasal and subcutaneous immunization with influenza virus immunostimulating complexes. *Scand. J. Immunol.* **27**, 241–245.

McGhee, J. R., and Kiyono, H. (1992). Mucosal immunity to vaccines: Current concepts for vaccine development and immune response analysis. *In* "Genetically Engineered Vaccines" (J. E. Ciardi, J. R. McGhee, and J. M. Keith, eds.), pp. 3–12. Plenum, New York.

Meitin, C. A., Bender, B. S., and Small, P. A., Jr. (1994). Enteric immunization of mice against influenza with recombinant vaccinia. *Proc. Natl. Acad. Sci. U.S.A.* **91,** 11187–11191.

Mestecky, J. (1987). The common mucosal immune system and current strategies for induction of immune responses in external secretions. *J. Clin. Immun.* 7, 265–276.

Mestecky, J., and McGhee, J. (1992). Prospects for human mucosal vaccines. *In* "Genetically Engineered Vaccines" (J. E. Ciardi, J. R. McGhee, and J. M. Keith, eds.), pp. 13–23. Plenum, New York.

Moldoveneau, Z., Novak, M., Huang, W.-Q., Gilley, R. M., Staas, J. K., Schafer, D. P., Compans, R. W., and Mestecky, J. (1993). Oral immunization with influenza virus in microspheres. *J. Infect. Dis.* **167,** 84–90.

Moldoveneau, Z., Clements, M. L., Prince, S. J., Murphy, B. R., and Mestecky. J. (1995). Human immune responses to influenza virus vaccines administered by systemic or mucosal routes. *Vaccine* **13,** 1006–1012.

Pang, G. T., Clancy, R. L., O'Reilly, S. E., and Cripps, A. W. (1992). A novel particulate influenza vaccine induces long-term and broad-based immunity in mice after oral immunization. *J. Virol.* **66,** 1162–1170.

Petrescu, A., and Cajal, N. (1984). Results obtained with the NIVGRIP inactivated influenza vaccine applicable by nasal and/or oral route. *Rev. Roum. Med. Virol.* **4,** 307–314.

Petrescu, A. L., Milhail, A., Popescu, A., and Cojita, J. 76). Bivalent influenza vaccination with inactivated vaccines administered by nasal or oral route. *Rev. Roum. Med. Virol.* **27,** 41.

Petrescu, A. L., Cajal, N., Bronitki, A. L., Mihail, A., Teodosiu, O., Popescu, G., Isaia, G., and Popescu, A. (1977). The experience of the "Stefan S. Nicolau" Institute of Virology in the preparation and administration of inactivated influenza vaccines applicable by nasal or oral route. *Rev. Roum. Med. Virol.* **28,** 213–217.

Pierce, N. F., and Cray, W. C., Jr. (1981). Cellular dissemination of priming for a mucosal immune response to cholera toxin in rats. *J. Immunol.* **127,** 2461–2464.

Pierce, N. F., and Cray, W. C., Jr. (1982). Determinants of the localization, magnitude, and duration of a specific mucosal IgA plasma cell response in enterically immunized rats. *J. Immunol.* **128,** 1311–1315.

Waldman, R. H., Lazell, V. A., Bergmann, K.-C., Khakoo, R., Jacknowitz, A. I., Howard, S. A., and Rose, C. (1982). Oral immunization against influenza. *Poumon Cour* **38,** 293–296.

Waldman, R. H., Stone, J., Lazzell, V., Bergmann, K. C., Khakoo, R., Jacknowitz, A., Howard, S., and Rose, C. (1983). Oral route as method for immunizing against mucosal pathogens. *Ann. N.Y. Med. Sci.* **409,** 510–516.

Waldman, R. H., Stone, J., Bergmann, K.-C., Khakoo, R., Lazzell, V., Jacknowitz, A., Waldman, E. R., and Howard, S. (1986). Secretory antibody following oral influenza immunization. *Am. J. Med. Sci.* **292,** 367–371.

Waldman, R. H., Bergmann, K.-C., Stone, J., Howard, S., Chiodo, V., Jacknowitz, A., Waldman, E. R., and Khakoo, R. (1987). Age-dependent antibody response in mice and humans following oral influenza immunization. *J. Clin. Immunol.* 7, 327–332.

24

Parainfluenza Virus Vaccines

ROBERT B. BELSHE
FRANCES K. NEWMAN
RANJIT RAY
Division of Infectious Diseases and Immunology
Saint Louis University Health Sciences Center
St. Louis, Missouri 63110

I. Introduction

The human parainfluenza viruses (HPIV), types 1, 2, and 3, are important pathogens in infants and young children (Chanock and McIntosh, 1990; Wright, 1991). HPIV routinely cause otitis media, pharyngitis, and the common cold. These upper respiratory tract infections (URI) occur commonly and may be associated with lower respiratory infections (LRI) including croup, pneumonia, and bronchiolitis. Primary infection in young children is associated with lower respiratory disease and often leads to hospitalization. As a group, the parainfluenza viruses are the second most common cause of hospital admission for respiratory infection and are second only to respiratory syncytial virus as a significant pathogen in young children. Parainfluenza type 3 is unique among the parainfluenza viruses in its ability to commonly infect young infants less than 6 months of age. Bronchiolitis and pneumonia are common in infants infected with this type; in this regard, HPIV-3 is similar to respiratory syncytial virus.

A number of reviews on HPIV have recently been published (Ray and Compans, 1990; Kingsbury, 1991; Henrickson *et al.*, 1994) concerning the various aspects of these virus infections. This chapter is an overview on these important viral pathogens and describes recent developments with parainfluenza virus type 3 vaccine.

II. Virology

All of the HPIV are very similar in structural, physicochemical, and biological characteristics. HPIV is composed of a single RNA strand of negative polarity surrounded by a lipid envelope of host cell origin. These are pleiomorphic viruses which have an average diameter of 150–250 nm. The typical HPIV genome contains approximately 15,000 nucleotides of genetic information (Storey *et al.*, 1984; Wechsler *et al.*, 1985) and encodes at least six structural proteins [3′-NP-P(+C)-M-F-HN-L-5′] (Storey *et al.*, 1984; Galinski *et al.*, 1986; Spriggs and Collins, 1986a,b). In addition, HPIV-1, 2, and 3 encode for a nonstructural protein "C" and HPIV-2 for a protein "v." These proteins are produced from overlapping reading frames within the P gene and may require editing of the mRNA (Ohgimoto *et al.*, 1990; Southern *et al.*, 1990; Matsuoka *et al.*, 1991).

The most abundant nucleocapsid protein (NP) encapsidates the genomic RNA to maintain the structural integrity and the template function of the RNA genome (Galinski *et al.*, 1991). The other two proteins, large protein (L) and the phosphoprotein (P), associate with the NP-RNA template and constitute the RNA polymerase complex. L is likely to be the RNA polymerase, whereas P is an auxiliary protein essential for the function of L (Sanchez and Banerjee, 1985). During the transcriptive phase, the L–P complex interacts with the NP-RNA template to transcribe the genome RNA into mRNAs (De *et al.*, 1990). On the other hand, during the replication step *in vivo,* NP forms a soluble complex with P, and the resulting NP–P complex interacts with the transcribing RNP to switch transcription reaction to replication (Horikami *et al.*, 1992). NP and P of HPIV-3 have been shown recently to interact very strongly *in vivo* through specific domains (Zhao and Banerjee, 1995). Additionally, a domain with P has been characterized that seems to act as a negative regulator in its interaction with NP.

The M protein is involved with the insertion as well as aggregation of the viral glycoproteins HN and F on the surface of the host cell and with the attraction of completed nucleocapsids to these areas that will soon bud to become virions (Choppin *et al.*, 1981; Ray *et al.*,

MUCOSAL VACCINES

1991). The HN protein (hemagglutinin-neuraminidase) functions in virus–host cell attachment via sialic acid receptors and has neuraminidase activity. The F (fusion) protein is involved in virus–host cell membrane fusion (syncytium formation) which is required for host cell infection by entry of the nucleocapsid. The ability of the F protein to induce both fusion and hemolysis may vary among the different parainfluenza viruses (Moscona and Peluso, 1991; Ebata *et al.*, 1991). HN protein has been suggested to play a role in cell fusion by specific interaction with the F protein (Ebata *et al.*, 1991; Moscona and Peluso, 1991; Hu *et al.*, 1992).

III. Epidemiology

HPIV are pervasive pathogens that have been found throughout the world. In the United States, HPIV-1, 2, and 3 cause approximately one-third of the estimated five million lower respiratory infections (LRI) that occur each year in children under the age of 5 (Glezen *et al.*, 1971; Denny and Clyde, 1986). They also cause upper respiratory infections in infants, children, and adults, and to a lesser extent, cause LRI in the immunocompromised and elderly. In pediatric hospitals, 3–18% of admissions are often the result of acute LRI. Depending on the time of year, HPIV infection can be detected in 9–67% of these admissions (Downham *et al.*, 1974; Murphy *et al.*, 1980; Henrickson *et al.*, 1996).

HPIV-1 occurs in biennial epidemics during the fall in both hemispheres (Denny *et al.*, 1983; Denny and Clyde, 1986). At least 50% of laryngotracheobronchitis (croup) can be linked to HPIV-1. Epidemiologic studies over multiple seasons have been used to estimate that on average more than 580,000 cases of croup occur each year in the United States in children under 5 years of age. The majority of croup cases occur every other year in parallel with the HPIV-1 epidemic (Rocchi *et al.*, 1970; Roman *et al.*, 1978). This virus also causes bronchiolitis, tracheobronchitis, pneumonia, and febrile and afebrile wheezing, predominantly in children 7–36 months of age with a peak incidence in the second and third year of life. HPIV-1 can cause LRI in young infants but is rarely seen in infants less than 4 weeks old. A higher incidence in white children has been reported for both HPIV-1 and croup (Downham *et al.*, 1974). Similarly, a higher incidence in boys has been reported for infection with this virus and the clinical syndrome of croup. It has been estimated that in the United States 97,000 children under 5 years of age are seen in emergency rooms and 35,000 children are admitted to hospitals per biennial epidemic of HPIV-1 (Downham *et al.*, 1974).

The epidemiology of HPIV-2 has not been investigated to the extent of HPIV-1. Infection with this virus has been reported to occur biennially with HPIV-1 or to alternate years with HPIV-1. However, infection with HPIV-2 occurs in yearly outbreaks in the United States (Downham *et al.*, 1974; Murphy *et al.*, 1980; Wright *et al.*, 1984). This pathogen has a peak incidence in the fall to early winter with a slightly longer "season" than HPIV-1. Croup is the most frequent LRI caused by this virus, but it can also cause any of the other respiratory illnesses associated with HPIV-1. The peak incidence of HPIV-2 infections occurs in the second year of life with approximately 60% of infections taking place in children less than 5 years of age. Of interest is the observation in one study that more girls than boys were symptomatic with LRI caused by HPIV-2, than LRI caused by HPIV-1 or 3 (Downham *et al.*, 1974). LRI caused by HPIV-2 has been reported less frequently than with HPIV-1 and HPIV-3. Recent reports have indicated that either geographic differences or differences in isolation and detection techniques may play a role in under-reporting this virus (Downham *et al.*, 1974; Henrickson *et al.*, 1994, 1996). It has been estimated that during the 1991 epidemic, there could have been as many as 157,000 children under the age of 5 seen in emergency rooms, and 35,000 children admitted to hospitals in the United States with HPIV-2 infection. This resulted in almost $200 million of direct patient care costs for HPIV-1 and -2 combined.

HPIV-3 is unique among the parainfluenza viruses in its ability to infect young infants less than 6 months of age. This virus causes the majority (approximately 40%) of its infections in the first 12 months of life with bronchiolitis and pneumonia being the most common clinical syndromes. It is second only to RSV as a cause of LRI in neonates and young infants. Approximately 20,000 infants and children are hospitalized each year in the United States because of LRI caused by HPIV-3. Boys develop LRI more frequently than girls (Glezen *et al.*, 1984). Although endemic throughout the world, this virus also occurs in spring epidemics in North America; epidemics may be related to climate conditions (Glezen *et al.*, 1984; de Silva and Cloonan, 1991).

HPIV-4 has been isolated from a very small number of children and adults and few epidemiologic reports have been conducted (Killgore and Dowdle, 1970; Gardner, 1969). Approximately one-third of the cases have been in infants less than 1 year of age, one-third in preschool children, and one-third in school age children and adults. Seroprevalence studies have demonstrated that 60–84% of infants have significant antibody levels after birth, presumably maternal in origin. These levels drop to 7–9% by 7–12 months of age and remain low for several years before increasing to about 50% by 3–5 years of age. Antibody levels to HPIV-4 continue to rise throughout childhood until approximately 95% of adults have antibody to HPIV-4 A and 75% have antibody to HPIV-4 B (McIntosh *et al.*, 1984). The majority of HPIV-4 clinical isolates appear to be subtype B. All of the different respiratory tract syndromes can also be caused by HPIV-4. Based on the seroprevalence data, infection with HPIV-4 is almost universal but disease is either rare or difficult to detect.

IV. Reinfection

Reinfections are common with these agents but generally milder than primary infection; 43% of children less than 5 years of age will develop a second infection with HPIV-3, and 12% will have more than two infections during this time period (Wong *et al.*, 1988). Reinfection by HPIV-1 and HPIV-2 occurs regularly but at a lower rate than HPIV-3 in young children (Welliver *et al.*, 1982). All four types of HPIV cause URI in older children and adults, and can cause reinfections throughout life. Approximately 10% of acute respiratory disease in adults (>25 years of age) can be caused by HPIV (Tumova *et al.*, 1988).

V. Pathogenesis

Mucous membranes of the nose and throat are the initial site of parainfluenza virus infection. Patients with mild disease may have limited involvement of the bronchi as well. Larynx and upper trachea are involved in more extensive infections with HPIV-1 and HPIV-2, and result in the croup syndrome. Infections may also extend to the lower trachea and bronchi, with accumulation of inspissated mucus and resultant atelectasis and pneumonia (71). When PHPIV-3 produces severe disease, infection of the small air passages is likely with the development of bronchopneumonia, bronchiolitis, or bronchitis (Parrott *et al.*, 1959, 1962; Welliver *et al.*, 1986). Otitis media occurs more frequently with HPIV-3. A study with incompletely attenuated HPIV inoculated into seronegative children demonstrated that virus shedding occurs up to Day 11 (Wright *et al.*, 1977). Longer virus shedding is observed in immunocompromised hosts, suggesting the importance of immunological factors in controlling virus replication in the respiratory tract. Severe acute croup, which is the most dramatic and serious manifestation of initial parainfluenza virus infection, is noted in 2–3% of primary type 1 or type 2 infections (Chanock *et al.*, 1963; Glezen *et al.*, 1982). Croup is also the predominant form of illness in HPIV epidemics. A majority of the children undergoing primary infection with HPIV-3 develop a febrile illness. In some cases involvement of the lower respiratory tract results in either pneumonia or bronchitis (Chanock *et al.*, 1963).

The possible contribution of the immune response to pathogenesis of illness is suggested by the observation that infants and children who develop parainfluenza virus croup produce local, virus-specific IgE antibodies earlier and in larger amounts than patients of comparable age who develop infections restricted to the upper respiratory tract (Welliver *et al.*, 1982). Cell-mediated immune responses to parainfluenza viral antigens, as well as parainfluenza virus-specific IgE antibody responses, have been reported to be greater among infants with parainfluenza virus bronchiolitis than among infected infants who develop only upper respiratory illnesses. A prolonged carrier state of HPIV-3 is observed in patients with chronic bronchitis and emphysema (Gross *et al.*, 1973). It has been suggested that healthy adults may shed infectious viruses intermittently and infect susceptible individuals; furthermore, investigators have also suggested that persistent infection might occur (Parkinson *et al.*, 1980).

The hamster provides an animal model for HPIV infection. Infected animals develop recognizable pathologic changes in the lung which are not altered by passive administration of antibodies (Glezen and Femald, 1976; Buthala and Soret, 1964; Metzgar *et al.*, 1974). Infected hamsters do not show visible signs of respiratory illness or a significant weight loss during infection. Ferrets have also been shown to be readily infected with HPIV3 (Metzgar *et al.*, 1974). Replication of HPIV 3 in cotton rats has been studied and two different species of cotton rats are suggested to offer separate models for the two major pulmonary manifestations of HPIV-3 infection (Porter *et al.*, 1991).

VI. Antigenic Composition

There are five major serotypes within the paramyxovirus genus. These serotypes can be grouped antigenically into two divisions: (1) HPIV-1 and HPIV-3, and (2) HPIV-2, HPIV-4, and mumps (Ray and Compans, 1986; Tsurudome *et al.*, 1989; Henrickson, 1991). HPIV all share common antigens and variable levels of heterotypic antibody are often detected during infection. Thus, it is difficult to determine whether the heterotypic responses are anamnestic in nature or simply cross reactions to similar antigens during serologic testing. However, specific hyperimmune animal serum in the past and more recently monoclonal antibodies have been employed to differentiate these viruses in standard assays (Sarkkinen *et al.*, 1981).

HPIV-1 and HPIV-3 have had subgroups (A and B) reported in which progressive antigenic changes have taken place (Henrickson, 1991; Prinoski *et al.*, 1992). Furthermore, HPIV-1 strains isolated over the last 10 years demonstrate persistent antigenic and genetic differences compared to the 1957 type strain (Henrickson, 1991; Henrickson and Savatski, 1992; Komada *et al.*, 1992). Antigenic differences exist among mouse, bovine, and human strains of parainfluenza viruses (Ray and Compans, 1986; Rydbeck *et al.*, 1987). Antigenic stability and conservation of neutralizing epitopes of the HN glycoprotein of numerous HPIV-3 strains have been suggested (Coelingh *et al.*, 1988; Al-Ahdal *et al.*, 1985). However, two of the four neutralizing domains of the F glycoprotein vary among clinical isolates (Coelingh *et al.*, 1988). Antigenic variation in hemagglutinin and neuraminidase epitopes has been observed with HPIV-2 (Ray *et al.*, 1992). However, these variations may not significantly influence the protective immune response against related strains of HPIV-2.

VII. Immune Responses

Both hemagglutinin neuraminidase (HN) and the fusion (F) proteins have been shown to induce neutralizing antibody (Kasel *et al.*, 1984; Ray *et al.*, 1988a,b; Coelingh *et al.*, 1988; Spriggs *et al.*, 1988) and cytotoxic T cells (Randall and Young, 1988; Al-Ahdal *et al.*, 1985). The nucleocapsid (NP) and the matrix (M) protein have also been shown to induce cytotoxic T cells (Randall and Young, 1988). HPIV-3-mediated immunoregulation of human T lymphocytes has been suggested to play an important role in the failure of the virus to induce lifelong immunity (Sieg *et al.*, 1994). Serological studies with children naturally infected with HPIV-3 have demonstrated that the antibody response to the HN glycoprotein is seen with initial infection and progressively rises with the number of infections (Kasel *et al.*, 1984). In contrast, an antibody response to the F glycoprotein is detected only after repeated infections, which may reflect the lower immunogenicity of this protein. Development of serum antibodies to both glycoproteins of HPIV-3 appears to correlate with protection from infection. Nasal IgA antibodies to HPIV-3 probably play an important role in resistance to infection (Ray *et al.*, 1988a). Investigation concerning the induction of type-specific and cross-protective immune responses against HPIV following intranasal immunization with isolated envelope glycoproteins or primary infection with live virus suggested that a type-specific protective immune response is generated in experimental animals (Ray *et al.*, 1990). This result indicates that a multivalent parainfluenza virus vaccine is required for protection against natural HPIV infection.

VIII. Progress in Vaccine Development

Early attempts to immunize infants with formalin-inactivated HPIV-3 showed increases in serum antibodies without significant protection against disease (Fulginiti *et al.*, 1967; Norrby and Gollmar, 1975). This may result from the loss of important antigenic sites on the vaccine during formalin inactivation, as has been suggested for Sendai, mumps, and measles viruses (Parrott *et al.*, 1967; Örvell and Norrby, 1977; Norrby and Penttinen, 1978). However, significant progress has been made in recent years toward the development of candidate vaccines against human parainfluenza virus infection.

Hamsters subcutaneously immunized with the isolated HN and F glycoprotein preparation (Ray *et al.*, 1985) showed complete protection from infection after challenge with live virus. The efficacy of immunization with the purified viral glycoproteins (Ray and Compans, 1987) either alone or in combination was tested as a subunit vaccine in hamsters (Ray *et al.*, 1988b). Results of virus recovery following challenge infection suggested that although immunization with HN or F alone induced an antibody response to the respective glycoproteins, it did not provide a significant level of protection. However, immunization with a mixture of both the glycoproteins induced higher virus-neutralizing activity and afforded complete protection from infection. Intranasal administration of HPIV-3 glycoproteins in hamsters induced a significantly higher local IgA response and correlated with protection from challenge infection with live virus (Ray *et al.*, 1988a,b). Both of the envelope glycoproteins of HPIV-3 have been suggested to be essential components of a subunit vaccine. Efforts are underway to increase the antigenicity of the HPIV proteins by microencapsulation (Ray *et al.*, 1993) or by the addition of a suitable adjuvant for optimal systemic and local protective immune responses.

Recombinant HPIV-3 glycoproteins expressed in insect cells using a baculovirus expression vector were also tested as vaccine candidates in experimental animals. Cotton rats immunized intraperitoneally with recombinant HN showed reduction of virus replication in the upper respiratory tract (Coelingh *et al.*, 1987). On the other hand, using a similar approach with the recombinant baculovirus expressing the F glycoprotein, hamsters and cotton rats were observed to be moderately protected against HPIV-3 challenge (Ray *et al.*, 1989; Hall *et al.*, 1991). Recombinant vaccinia virus expressing HPIV-3 surface glycoproteins, when inoculated intradermally into Patas Monkeys or cotton rats, were shown to offer significant resistance to challenge infection (Spriggs *et al.*, 1987, 1988).

Bovine HPIV-3 as a candidate live virus vaccine is under investigation (Coelingh *et al.*, 1988; Clemens *et al.*, 1991). Replication of bovine and human HPIV-3 and cross-protective effects of the bovine virus were evaluated in nonhuman primates. Replication of bovine HPIV-3 was restricted in old-world monkeys, and infection with the bovine strain provided significant protection to HPIV-3 challenge.

Live-attenuated HPIV-3 vaccine candidates have been developed by serial passage of wild-type HPIV-3 at suboptimal temperature (Belshe and Hissom, 1982).

These cold-passaged vaccine candidates possess three phenotypic markers including the cold-adapted (ca) property, the temperature-sensitive (ts) property, and tiny plaque (tp) morphology. These properties are not associated with the wild-type parent virus. These intranasally administered vaccine candidates may prevent serious respiratory illness from subsequent natural HPIV-3 infection by stimulating an immune response similar to a wild-type infection without causing illness.

IX. Development of Live-Attenuated HPIV-3 Vaccine

The JS strain of the human parainfluenza virus type 3 (HPIV-3), the wild-type (wt) parent virus of several live attenuated vaccine candidates, was originally recovered from a 1-year-old child with a febrile respiratory illness. After 14 passages at the permissive temperature of 37°C the wt parent strain was biologically cloned by plaque purification prior to being cold-adapted. The resulting plaque-purified wt parent clone, designated C127, was passaged at 33.5°C for 3 additional passages prior to serial passages at suboptimal temperatures to produce cold-adapted strains (Fig. 1) (Belshe and Hissom, 1982). Virus plaques selected from cold passage (cp) levels 7, 12, 18, and 45 were evaluated for phenotypic markers including the ts, tp, and ca properties. The ts phenotype was determined by comparing the titer of the wt parent, C127, with each of the cold passaged clones at 32 and 39°C in L-132 cells, a human embryonic lung continuous cell line. If the plaque assay titer of the virus at 39°C was ≥100-fold less than the titer at 32°C, the virus was considered to be ts. A virus with a plaque size of less than one half the size of the wt virus plaque at 32°C was considered to be a tiny plaque mutant. The cold-adapted phenotype was determined by comparing the growth of the wt parent virus with each of the mutants at 20 and 32°C. Viruses were inoculated into cell

TABLE I

Prevalence of Temperature-Sensitive (ts), Tiny-Plaque (tp), and Cold-Adapted (ca) Clones among the Populations of Parainfluenza 3 Virus in Relationship to Tissue Culture Passage History at Suboptimal Temperature

Cold passage level	Number of ts clones/ number tested	Number of tp clones/ number tested[a]	Number of ca clones/ number tested[a]
0 (wild-type)	0/21	0/21	0/7
7	1/9[b]	1/9[b]	5/6[b]
12	3/12[b]	3/12[b]	7/12[b]
18	8/10[b]	8/10[b]	10/10[b]
45	13/13	13/13	13/13

[a]The same clones were tested for the ts property.
[b]The same clones manifested the ts, tp, and ca properties. Some clones were ca but not ts or tp.

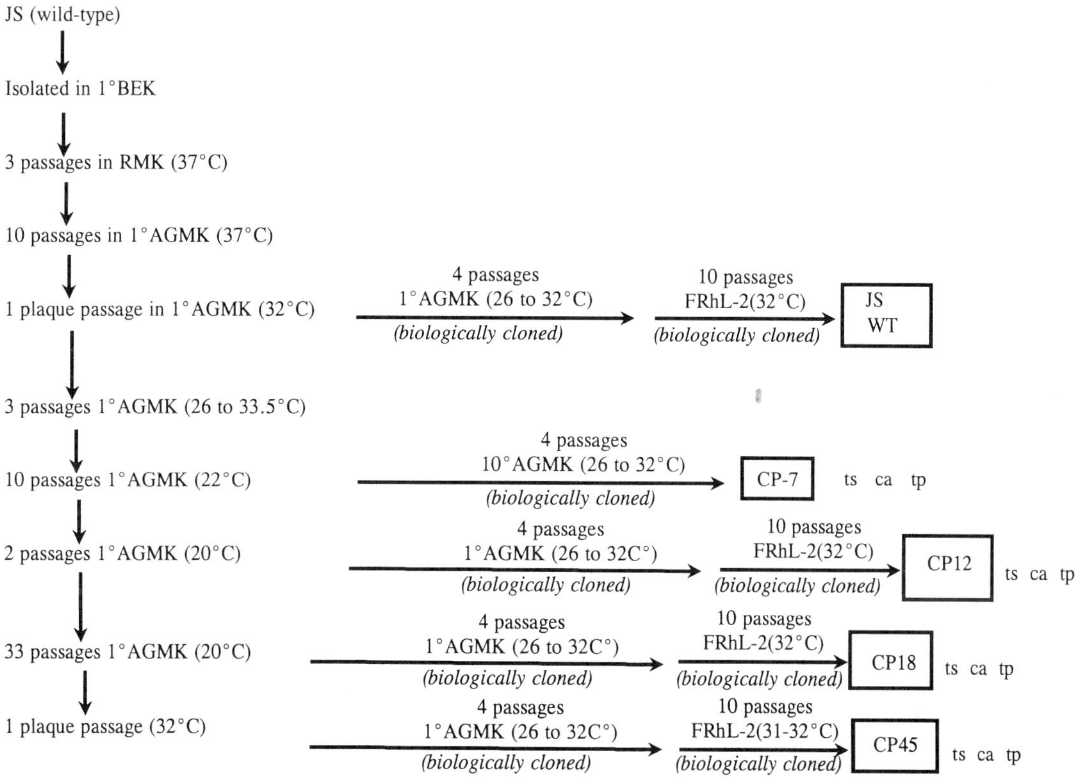

Figure 1. Passage history of the JS parent and cold passaged mutant vaccine viruses CP7, CP12, CP18, and CP45.

culture tubes of primary AGMK cells and incubated at 20 and 32°C. When the titer of replication at 20 was within > 1% of the titer of growth at 32°C, the virus was assigned the cold-adapted phenotype.

The proportion of ts and ca clones selected from the various cold passage levels was directly related to the number of cold passage levels; the percentage of ts and ca clones increased as the number of levels increased (Table I). Each of the ts clones was cold-adapted and exhibited the tiny plaque morphology; however, not all of the ca clones were ts, suggesting that the ts and ca mutations were not linked.

X. Evaluation of Cold-Passaged Vaccine Strains in Animals

Based on *in vitro* characterization, five clones were selected for evaluation in weanling hamsters: one from cp7, cp12, and cp45, and two from cp18 (Crookshanks and Belshe, 1984). Weanling hamsters were intranasally inoculated with either the wt parent virus (C127) or one of the five mutants. Attenuation of the clones in hamsters was directly related to the cold passage level of the mutant; cold passage 7 virus was the least attenuated and cp45 was the most attenuated. All of the viruses recovered from the animals inoculated with the HPIV-3 ca mutants from cp12 and cp18 were genetically stable, i.e., they retained their ts phenotype and did not form plaques at 39°C. The results of the hamster experiments suggested that the multiple mutations accumulated by cold adaptation were associated with genetic stability and attenuation in hamsters. Efficacy of the vaccine candidates in hamsters was determined by a challenge experiment (Crookshanks-Newman and Belshe, 1986).

Cold passage 12, cp18, and cp45 viruses were evaluated in seronegative rhesus monkeys for attenuation, replication in the nasopharynx and trachea, and genetic stability after replication *in vivo* (Hall *et al.*, 1992). Following intratracheal inoculation of rhesus monkeys with cp12 or cp18 virus, the titer of virus recovered from the upper and lower respiratory tract of the animals was greatly restricted when compared with the wt HPIV-3. Cold passage 45 virus was not recovered from the monkeys that received the intratracheal inoculation. However, in a separate study a group of rhesus monkeys were intratracheally and intranasally inoculated with the cp45 virus. Virus was recovered from the upper respiratory tract of these animals in similar quantities as the cp12 and cp18 viruses but there was a substantial restriction of the replication in the lower respiratory tract. cp45 virus exhibited both ts and non-ts phenotypes which contributed to the attenuation of the virus as determined by replication in the rhesus monkeys.

Based on results of a chimpanzee study with cp12 and the rhesus monkey experiment with cp12, cp18, and cp45, the HPIV-3 vaccine from cp45 was tested in seronegative chimpanzees to assess attenuation, level of replication in the nasopharynx and trachea, genetic stability following *in vivo* replication, and efficacy against wt HPIV-3 challenge (Hall *et al.*, 1993). Animals intranasally and intratracheally inoculated with 10^4 $TCID_{50}$ of either wild-type HPIV-3 or cp45 vaccine were observed for signs of rhinorrhea and had nasopharyngeal swabs and tracheal lavage samples collected several times throughout the 14-day observation period following inoculation. Results from the animals inoculated with cp45 virus included a reduction in both the duration and the severity of rhinorrhea and a 500-fold decrease in replication in the nasopharynx and trachea in comparison with the wt HPIV-3. Phenotypic characterization of the viruses recovered from these animals indicated that *in vivo* replication did not cause reversion to the wt phenotype. However, based on an increase in the cut-off temperature of the isolates (>39°C) compared with the cp45 parent virus (cut-off temperature 38°C), partial loss of the ts property was observed (data not shown).

Further characterization of the genetic stability of cp45 viruses following *in vivo* replication was evaluated by inoculating two chimpanzees with an isolate recovered from one of the chimpanzees vaccinated with cp45. The quantity of virus recovered from the nasopharynx and trachea of these animals was restricted in comparison with the wt HPIV-3; however, the cut-off temperature of the isolates increased from 39°C (cut-off temperature of the inoculum) to ≥40°C. Although partial loss of the ts phenotype was observed, i.e., the increase in the cut-off temperature, the cp45 vaccine retained its attenuation phenotype.

XI. Human Studies

Vaccine pools were produced for the wt HPIV-3 (C127) as well as cold-adapted strains from cp12, cp18, and cp45 which had been evaluated in hamsters. The wt HPIV-3 vaccine and vaccine from cp12 and cp18 were evaluated in adults with low levels of IgA to HPIV-3 in order to determine safety and immunogenicity (Clemens *et al.*, 1991). Each of the strains, including the wt, was poorly infectious for adults.

The cold passage 18 vaccine which was intermediately attenuated in the hamster model and highly attenuated in adults was chosen for evaluation in children (Belshe *et al.*, 1992). Healthy seropositive children (hemagglutination inhibition antibody titer to HPIV-3 of greater than 8) from two age groups, 3 to 10 years of age and 6 to 36 months of age, were enrolled in a placebo-controlled study of cp18. The vaccine virus was not recovered and there were no increased antibody levels in any of the 3- to 10-year-old children following vaccination with the cp18 virus. Although the seropositive infants, 6 to 36 months of age, were more susceptible to infection with the cp18 virus, the vaccine was attenuated and immunogenic. Four seronegative infants 6 to 36 months of age were vaccinated with the cp18 vaccine. Each infant shed the vaccine virus and had an antibody rise. None of them developed a fever but two of them exhibited mild upper respiratory symptoms and mild wheezing (detectable only with a stethoscope). The cp18 vaccine was considered to be insufficiently attenuated for seronegative infants due to mild wheezing.

A number of studies have been initiated with the most attenuated of the cold-adapted parainfluenza virus strains, cp45 vaccine, in children 6 months to 10 years of age (Karron *et al.*, 1995). Initially, forty-one healthy children who were seropositive for HPIV-3 were vaccinated with 10^5 or 10^6 $TCID_{50}$ of the cp45 vaccine and 15 children received placebo. The cp45 vaccine was safe but very few of the seropositive children were infected with the vaccine. This finding was expected to be seen in children with preexisting antibody.

Forty-four seronegative children were vaccinated with the cp45 vaccine in doses ranging from 10^2 to 10^6 $TCID_{50}$; an additional 14 volunteers received placebo (Table II). Ninety percent of the seronegative volunteers who received either 10^4 or 10^5 $TCID_{50}$ of vaccine were infected with cp45 (Table II). Infected vaccinees shed a mean peak titer of $10^{2.4}$ pfu/ml (plaque forming units/ml) of cp45, which was 100-fold less than the amount of virus recovered from placebo recipients who shed wt HPIV-3. The vaccine was safe (Table III) although the cp45 vaccine replication was somewhat restricted; 81% of the children who received the 10^5 $TCID_{50}$ dose of the vaccine had a serum HAI antibody response to HPIV-3 with a geometric mean titer of 1:32 which has been shown to be protective in nonhuman primates (Clemens *et al.*, 1991).

Earlier studies with the cp18 HPIV-3 vaccine candidate showed a loss of the ts property in some of the isolates from vaccinated children. In contrast, the cp45 HPIV-3 vaccine retained its ts and ca phenotype following replication in seronegative children as demonstrated by the characterization of 86 isolates of the vaccine collected from 25 children. The importance of retaining the ts property is significant; both ts and non-ts mutations play a role in the attenuation phenotype of cp45 in rhesus monkeys. Live attenuated HPIV-3 cp45 vaccine is safe, immunogenic, and genetically stable in seronegative children. Additional studies are planned to assess the duration of antibody and to determine if a second dose of vaccine is needed. Since the target age for vaccination with a HPIV-3 vaccine is under 6 months, cp45 will be evaluated in children as young as 1 month of age in order to assess the safety and the effect of maternal antibody on vaccine replication.

TABLE III

Evaluation of CP45 in Seronegative Young Children, Clinical Events

Dose	*N*	% with			
		Fever	URI	LRI	Otitis Media
10^2	8	0	38	0	25
10^3	7	14	28	0	14
10^4	13	38	46	8	8
10^5	16	18	31	0	13
Placebo	14	21	50	0	14

TABLE II

Evaluation of CP45 in Seronegative Young Children, Infectivity and Vaccine Virus Shedding, and Antibody Response

Dose	*N*	% Infected	Virus isolation			% with HAI antibody response
			% Shedding	Mean duration (days)	Mean peak titer (log^{10})	
10^2	8	75	62	11	1.0	50
10^3	7	43	43	14	2.3	43
10^4	13	85	85	11	2.1	54
10^5	16	94	87	10	2.4	81
Placebo	14	7[a]	0	0	—	0

[a]One placebo recipient had a nasal wash EIA antibody response but not a serum antibody response.

XII. Molecular Characterization of the Candidate Vaccine Strain

The molecular basis of attenuation for a number of viruses is not clearly known. Attenuation associated with many point mutations introduced by multiple passage of the morbilli virus into tissue culture or nonnatural host has been suggested (Barrett *et al.*, 1991). An analysis of several Edmonston-derived vaccine strains showed that the Edmonston–Zagreb vaccine was heavily contaminated with defective-interfering (DI) particles. It is not clear whether the presence of DI particles contributes to the attenuated phenotype; however, the potentially harmful effects resulting from the DI particles role in establishing a persistent infection raises questions regarding vaccine safety (Calain and Roux, 1988). Characterization of the temperature-sensitive and live-attenuated HPIV-3 strain (cp45) grown at a permissive temperature (32°C) suggested that the virus efficiently multiplies in cell lines and retains antigenic and functional properties of the envelope glycoproteins (Ray *et al.*, 1995). When grown at a nonpermissive temperature (39.5°C), the cp45 virus exhibited poor replication; however, shifting to permissive temperature allowed virus growth. Although at a nonpermissive temperature the virus polypeptide synthesis was significantly reduced, the HN and F glycoproteins were transported to cell surfaces. Antigenic sites of the envelope glycoproteins, previously defined by panels of monoclonal antibodies (Coelingh and Tierney, 1989; Coelingh *et al.*, 1985; Ray and Compans, 1986, 1987), reacted similarly to the parent wild-type virus and biological activity of the virus envelope glycoproteins appeared to remain unaffected as a result of cold adaptation. However, the biological activity of the individual functional domains of the virus proteins has not been investigated. Studies of mRNA synthesis from the P gene suggested a poor transcriptional activity of the cp45 virus at a nonpermissive temperature. Virus mRNA synthesis is markedly reduced at a nonpermissive temperature and as a result the polypeptide synthesis and virus growth are significantly affected. Although the transcriptional activity of cp45 is reduced, virus glycoproteins are transported to infected cell surfaces and have limited viral morphogenesis at the nonpermissive temperature. Results from this study indicate that the temperature sensitivity of cp45 virus is related to altered transcriptional activity and a marked reduction in virus polypeptide synthesis.

Characterization of ts Sendai virus mutants has suggested a defect in the hemagglutinin protein affecting infectivity of progeny virus particles when grown at nonpermissive temperature (Portner *et al.*, 1975; Thompson and Portner, 1987). The ts mutants of Newcastle disease virus (NDV) have been shown to be sensitive for fusion and hemadsorption properties (Tsipis and Bratt, 1976; Peeples and Bratt, 1982; Peeples *et al.*, 1982). At permissive temperature, biological properties of ts RNA+ mutants showed lower HA, NA, and hemolysis activities as compared to the wild-type virus. However, these mutants showed infectivities similar to that of wild-type virus. A recent study (Shibata *et al.*, 1993) of a ts mutant of influenza B virus suggested that viral proteins were produced at nonpermissive temperature. However, the ts mutant did not display enzymatic or hemagglutinating activity, but produced noninfectious virus particles which become infectious after treatment with trypsin. Characterization of a cold-adapted influenza A virus vaccine strain suggested conformational changes in the RNA structure facilitating advantageous growth at 25°C (Herlocher *et al.*, 1993). Results from studies with cp45 did not reveal detectable changes in the biological properties of the virus glycoproteins when grown at permissive or nonpermissive temperatures. Comparison of the nucleotide and predicted amino acid sequences of cp45 and the parent wild-type virus suggested seven amino acid substitutions in genes encoding four different polypeptides, M, F, HN, and L (Stokes *et al.*, 1993). Apart from the other changes, three unique substitutions in the L protein of cp45 have been noted. Furthermore, the 3′ leader region, important in gene regulation and in virus propagation, exhibited nucleotide changes. Mutations in the noncoding regulatory regions, resulting from the attenuation process, have been suggested to affect transcription and/or replication of polio viruses (Westrop *et al.*, 1989; Bouchard *et al.*, 1995). Recently, mutations within the 3′ noncoding terminal sequences of Sendai virus have been shown to be sensitive to mutagenesis (Harty and Palese, 1995). Additional studies will be required to determine if the nucleotide changes in the 3′ leader region of cp45 has any effect on the ts or attenuation properties. Temperature-sensitivity of cp45 virus was further investigated by complementation of a specific gene function (Ray *et al.*, 1996). CV1 cells were transfected with cloned genes from wild-type HPIV-3 encoding the large protein (L), phosphoprotein (P), and nucleocapsid protein (NP), alone or together, for expression of biologically active proteins. L gene-transfected cells when infected with cp45 virus and incubated at nonpermissive temperature (39.5°C) supported the growth of cp45. The virus titers obtained by complementation of the L protein were in the order of 190 to 2300 pfu/ml of culture medium as compared to the undetectable growth of the cp45 temperature-sensitive mutant at the nonpermissive temperature. Virus produced following complementation of the L protein still maintained the temperature-sensitive genotype. Results from this study suggest that the temperature sensitivity of cp45 candidate vaccine strain is primarily related to the L protein and can be complemented with that of wild-type virus for replication. Additionally, further studies with this mutant virus indicated the important role of the L protein for RNA polymerase activity in virus replication. The molecular mechanism of attenuation of the cp45 virus will facilitate further characterization of this promising live virus vaccine strain.

XIII. Potential Use of Reverse Genetics in Vaccine Development

Cold-adapted live influenza virus vaccines have been investigated extensively and hold promise for use in the general population. The major concern associated with the cold-adapted live virus vaccines is that the limited number of attenuating mutations could permit the generation of a revertant virus, despite the fact that in clinical trials the viruses have maintained the attenuating phenotype. One way to avoid this drawback would be to introduce multiple attenuating mutations into the viral genes or make recombinants of proven vaccines expressing envelope glycoproteins of target viruses. For a single-stranded negative-sense RNA virus, it is difficult to engineer mutations directly into the viral genome as is possible for many DNA viruses and positive strand RNA viruses. However, a reverse-genetics approach developed with influenza A virus has allowed direct genetic manipulation of specific viral genes (Enami *et al.*, 1990). This general approach has been adapted and used successfully to establish similar transfection systems employing parainfluenza viruses (Park *et al.*, 1991; Park and Krystal, 1992; De and Banerjee, 1993; Dimmock and Collins, 1993; Calain *et al.*, 1992; Calain and Roux, 1993) and respiratory syncytial virus (Collins *et al.*, 1991, 1993). In addition to the transfection systems using reporter genes, transfection systems employing defective interfering RNAs to examine RNA replication have been established (Pattnaik *et al.*, 1992; Calain *et al.*, 1992; Calain and Roux, 1993). Recent success with the generation of infectious rabies virus and vesicular stomatitis virus (Schnell *et al.*, 1994; Lawson *et al.*, 1995; Whelan *et al.*, 1995) by reverse-genetics holds promise for a similar accomplishment with HPIV-3. This will allow us to answer a number of important fundamental questions regarding further characterization of specific mutations in the viral genome of cp45 and to make recombinants of cp45 expressing antigens of other paramyxovirus types.

XIV. Concluding Remarks

For some time, the scientific community has desired to develop HPIV vaccines for pediatric population. Children are most vulnerable to this viral agent, and immunoprophylaxis at an early stage of life needs to be considered. As discussed in this chapter, several approaches were taken in the last three decades to understand the basis of protective immune responses and for the development of vaccines for immunization against HPIV infection. However, concerns for safety and cost-effective issues for community use are valid elements associated with the majority of these approaches. Live-attenuated viral vaccines are generally believed to induce long-term protection among the great majority of individuals. The vaccine strain would not be useful if the virus does not undergo limited replication in vaccinated humans for stimulation of appropriate immune responses. The live-attenuated HPIV3 vaccine strain (cp45), developed as a result of serial passage and adaptation at cold temperature, is attenuated in primates and humans. All of the available results from clinical trials indicate that the vaccine strain is safe and induces protective immune responses. However, some areas, especially detailed analyses of mucosal and systemic antibody as well as cellular immune responses in the vaccinated children, remain to be investigated. Furthermore, additional studies should address the optimal age for vaccinating infants and determine if multiple doses are necessary. Our recent studies indicated multiple changes in the genome and temperature sensitivity of the polymerase gene in this vaccine strain. Additional work is necessary for further characterization of the attenuating property.

Although antigenic composition of HPIV is relatively stable, the mechanisms for reinfection with HPIV are not clearly understood. The increasing awareness of the postnatal development of infant's immune system should help to understand the nature of interaction of the virus with host immune system. HPIV infections are limited to epithelial surfaces and do not spread systemically. Effort to provide protection at the mucosal surface, a natural site of HPIV entry and spread of infection, would be most appropriate. Although induction of long-term protection at the mucosal surface is relatively difficult against this viral agent, partial protection would both eliminate the severity of the disease manifested by HPIV and alleviate suffering.

References

Al-Ahdal, M. N., Nakamura, L., and Flanagan, T. D. (1985). Cytotoxic T-lymphocyte reactivity with individual Sendai virus glycoproteins. *J. Virol.* **54**, 53–57.

Barrett, T., Subbarao, S. M., Belsham, G. J., and Mahy, B. W. J. (1991). The molecular biology of the morbilliviruses. *In* "The Paramyxoviruses" (D. W. Kingsbury, ed.), pp. 83–102. Plenum, New York.

Belshe, R. B., and Hissom, F. K. (1982). Cold adaptation of parainfluenza virus type 3: Induction of three phenotypic markers. *J. Med. Virol.* **10**, 235–242.

Belshe, R. B., Karron, R. A., Newman, F. K., Anderson, E. L., Nugent, S. L., Steinhoff, M., Clemens, M. L., Wilson, M. H., Hall, S. L., Tierney, E. L., and Murphy, B. R. (1992). Evaluation of a live attenuated, cold-adapted parainfluenza virus type 3 vaccine in children. *J. Clin. Microbiol.* **30**, 2064–2070.

Bouchard, M. J., Lam, D.-H., and Racaniello, V. (1995). Determinants of attenuation and temperature sensitivity in the type 1 poliovirus Sabin vaccine. *J. Virol.* **69**, 4972–4978.

Buthala, D. A., and Soret, M. G. (1964). Parainfluenza type 3 virus infection in hamsters. Virologic, serologic and pathologic studies. *J. Infect. Dis.* **114**, 226–231.

Calain, P., and Roux, L. (1988). Generation of measles virus defective interfering particles and their presence in a preparation of attenuated live-virus vaccine. *J. Virol.* **62**, 2859–2866.

Calain, P., and Roux, L. (1993). The rule of six, a basic feature for efficient replication Sendai virus defective interfering RNA. *J. Virol.* **67**, 4822–4830.

Calain, P., Curran, J., Kolakofsky, D., and Roux, L. (1992). Molecular cloning of natural paramyxovirus copy-back defective interfering RNAs and their expression from DNA. *Virology* **191**, 62–71.

Chanock, R. M., and McIntosh, K. (1990). Parainfluenza viruses. *In* "Virology" (B. N. Fields, ed.), pp. 963–988. Raven, New York.

Chanock, R. M., Parrott, R. H., Johnson, K. M., Kapikian, A. Z., and Bell, J. A. (1963). Myxoviruses: Parainfluenza. *Am. Rev. Respir. Dis.* **88**, 152–166.

Choppin, P. W., Richardson, C. D., Merz, C. D., Hall, W. W., and Scheid, A. (1981). The functions and inhibition of the membrane glycoproteins of paramyxoviruses and myxoviruses and the role of the measles virus M protein in subacute schlerosing panencephalitis. *J. Infect. Dis.* **143**, 352–362.

Clemens, M. L., Belshe, R. B., King, J., Newman, F., Westblom, T. U., Tierney, E. L., London, W. T., and Murphy, B. R (1991). Evaluation of bovine, cold-adapted human, and wild-type human parainfluenza type 3 viruses in adult volunteers and in chimpanzees. *J. Clin. Microbiol.* **29**, 1175–1182.

Coelingh, K. V., and Tierney, E. I. (1989). Antigenic and functional organization of human parainfluenza virus type 3 fusion glycoprotein. *J. Virol.* **63**, 375–382.

Coelingh, K. V., Winter, C. C., and Murphy, B. R. (1985). Antigenic variation in the hemagglutinin–neuraminidase protein of human parainfluenza type 3 virus. *Virology* **143**, 569–582.

Coelingh, K. V., Murphy, B. R., Collins, P. L., LeBacq-Verheyden, A. M., and Battey, J. F. (1987). Expression of biologically active and antigenically authentic parainfluenza type 3 virus hemagglutinin–neuraminidase glycoprotein by a recombinant baculovirus. *Virology* **160**, 465–472.

Coelingh, K. V., Winter, C. C., Tiemey, E. L., London, W. T., and Murphy, B. R. (1988). Attenuation of bovine parainfluenza virus type 3 in nonhuman primates and its ability to confer immunity to human parainfluenza virus type 3 challenge. *J. Infect. Dis.* **157**, 655–662.

Collins, P. L., Mink, M. S., and Stec, D. S. (1991). Rescue of synthetic analogs of respiratory syncytial virus genomic RNA and effect of truncations and mutations on the expression of a foreign reporter gene. *Proc. Natl. Acad. Sci. U.S.A.* **88**, 9663–9667.

Collins, P. L., Mink, M. A., Hill, M. G., Camargo, E., Grosfeld, H., and Stec, D. S. (1993). Rescue of a 7502-nucleotide (49.3% of full-length) synthetic analog of respiratory syncytial virus genomic RNA. *Virology* **195**, 252–256.

Crookshanks, F. K., and Belshe, R. B. (1984). Evaluation of cold-adapted and temperature-sensitive mutants of parainfluenza virus type 3 in weanling hamsters. *J. Med. Virol.* **13**, 243–249.

Crookshanks-Newman, F. K., and Belshe, R. B. (1986). Protection of weanling hamsters from experimental infection with wild-type parainfluenza virus type 3 (para 3) by cold-adapted mutants of para 3. *J. Med. Virol.* **18**, 131–137.

de Silva, L. M., and Cloonan, M. J. (1991). Brief report: Parainfluenza virus type 3 infections: Findings in Sydney and some observations on variations in seasonality worldwide. *J. Med. Virol.* **35**, 19–21.

De, B. P., and Banerjee, A. K. (1993). Rescue of synthetic analogs of genome RNA of parainfluenza virus type 3. *Virology* **196**, 344–348.

De, B. P., Galinski, M. S., and Banerjee, A. K. (1990). Characterization of an *in vitro* system for the synthesis of mRNA from human parainfluenza virus type 3. *J. Virol.* **64**, 1135–1142.

Denny, F. W., and Clyde, W. A., Jr. (1986). Acute lower respiratory infections in nonhospitalized children. *J. Pediatr.* **108**, 635–46.

Denny, F. W., Murphy, T. F., Clyde, W. A., Jr., Collier, A. M., and Henderson, F. W. (1983). Croup: An 11-year study in a pediatric practice. *Pediatrics* **71**, 871–876.

Dimmock, K., and Collins, P. L. (1993). Rescue of synthetic analogs of genomic RNA and replicative-intermediate RNA of human parainfluenza virus type 3. *J. Virol.* **67**, 2772–2778.

Downham, M. A., McQuillin, J., and Gardner, P. S. (1974). Diagnosis and clinical significance of parainfluenza virus infections in children. *Arch. Dis. Child.* **49**, 8–15.

Ebata, S. N., Cote, M. J., Kang, C. Y., and Dimock, K. (1991). The fusion and hemagglutinin–neuraminidase glycoproteins of human parainfluenza virus 3 are both required for fusion. *Virology* **183**, 437–441.

Enami, M., Luytjes, W., Krystal, M. M., and Palese, P. (1990). Introduction of site-specific mutations into the genome of influenza virus. *Proc. Natl. Acad. Sci., U.S.A.* **87**, 3802–3805.

Fulginiti, V. A., Amer, J., Eller, J. J., Joyner, J. W., Sr., and Askin, P. (1967). Parainfluenza virus immunication. IV. Simultaneous immunization with parazinfluenza types 1, 2, and 3 aqueous vaccines. *Am. J. Dis. Child.* **114**, 26–28.

Galinski, M. S., Mink, M. A., Lambert, S. L., Wechsler, S. L., and Pons, M. W. (1986). Molecular cloning and sequence analysis of the human parainfluenza 3 virus mRNA encoding the P and C proteins. *Virology* **154**, 46–60.

Galinski, M. S., and Wechsler, S. L. (1991). The molecular biology of the paramyxoviruos genus. *In* "The Paramyxovirus" (D. W. Kingsbury, ed.), pp. 41–82. Plenum, New York.

Gardner, S. D. (1969). The isolation of parainfluenza 4 subtypes A and B in England and serological studies of their prevalence. *J. Hyg.* **67,** 545–550.

Glezen, W. P., and Femald, G. W. (1976). Effect of passive antibody on parainfluenza virus type 3 pneumonia in hamsters. *Infect. Immun.* **14,** 212–216.

Glezen, W. P., Loda, F. A., Clyde, W. A., Jr., Senior, R. J., Sheaffer, C. I., Conley, W. G., and Denny, F. W. (1971). Epidemiologic patterns of acute lower respiratory disease of children in a pediatric group practice. *J. Pediatr.* **78,** 397–406.

Glezen, W. P., Loda, F. A., and Denny, F. W. (1982). Parainfluenza viruses. *In* "Viral Infections of Humans. Epidemiology and Control" (A. S. Evans, ed.), pp. 441–454. Plenum, New York.

Glezen, W. P., Frank, A. L., Taber, L. H., and Kasel, J. A. (1984). Parainfluenza virus type 3: Seasonality and risk of infection and reinfection in young children. *J. Infect. Dis.* **150,** 851–857.

Gross, P. A., Green, R. H., and McCrearren, M. G. (1973). Persistent infection with parainfluenza type 3 virus in man. *Am. Rev. Respir. Dis.* **108,** 894–898.

Hall, S. L., Murphy, B. R., and van Wyke Coelingh, K. L. (1991). Protection of cotton rats by immunization with the human parainfluenza virus type 3 fusion (F) glycoprotein expressed on the surface of insect cells infected with a recombinant baculovirus. *Vaccine* **9,** 659–667.

Hall, S. L., Stokes, A., Tierney, E. L., London, W. T., Belshe, R. B., Newman, F. K., and Murphy, B. R. (1992). Cold passaged human parainfluenza 3 viruses contain ts and non-ts mutations leading to attenuation in rhesus monkeys. *Virus. Res.* **22,** 173–184.

Hall, S. L., Sarris, C. M., Tiemey, E. L., London, W. T., and Murphy, B. R. (1993). A cold-adapted mutant of parainfluenza virus type 3 is attenuated and protective in chimpanzees. *J. Infect. Dis.* **167,** 958–962.

Henrickson, K. J. (1991). Monoclonal antibodies to human parainfluenza virus type 1 detect major antigenic changes in clinical isolates. *J. Infect. Dis.* **164,** 1128–1134.

Henrickson, K. J. (1996). Isolation and detection methods useful for efficient recovery of human parainfluenza virus types one and two. *J. Virol. Methods* in press.

Henrickson, K. J., and Savatski, L. (1992). Genetic variation and evolution of human parainfluenza virus type 1 hemagglutinin neuraminidase: Analysis of 12 clinical isolates. *J. Infect. Dis.* **166,** 995–1005.

Henrickson, K. J., Ray, R., and Belshe, R. B. (1994). Parainfluenza Virus. *In* "Principals and Practice of Infectious Diseases" (G. L. Mandell, R. G. Douglas, and J. E. Bennett, eds.), 4th Ed., pp. 177–184. Churchill and Livingstone, New York.

Henrickson, K. J., Kuhn, S. M., and Savatski, L. L. (1994). Epidemiology and cost of infection with human parainfluenza virus types 1 and 2 in young children. *Clin. Infect. Dis.* **18,** 770–779.

Herlocher, M. L., Massab, H. N., and Webster, R. G. (1993). Molecular and biological changes in the cold-adapted "master strain" A/AA/6/60(H2N2) influenza virus. *Proc. Natl. Acad. Sci. U.S.A.* **90,** 6032–6036.

Horikami, S. M., Curran, J., Kolakofsky, D., and Moyer, S. A. (1992). Complexes of Sendai virus NP-P and P-L proteins are required for defective interfering particle genome replication *in vitro*. *J. Virol.* **66,** 4901–4908.

Hu, X., Ray, R., and Compans, R. W. (1992). Functional interactions between the fusion protein and hemagglutinin-neuraminidase of human parainfluenza viruses. *J. Virol.* **66,** 1528–1534.

Karron, R. A., Wright, P. F., Newman, F. K., Makhene, M., Thompson, J., Samorodin, R., Wilson, M. H., Clemens, M. L., Murphy, B. R., and Belshe, R. B. (1995). A live attenuated human parainfluenza type 3 virus vaccine is safe, infectious, immunogenic and phenotypically stable in healthy infants and children. *J. Infect. Dis.* **172,** 1445–1450.

Kasel, J. A., Frank, A. L., Keitel, W. A., Taber, L. H., and Glezen, W. P. (1984). Acquisition of serum antibodies to specific viral glycoproteins of parainfluenza virus 3 in children. *J. Virol.* **52,** 828–832.

Killgore, G. E., and Dowdle, W. R. (1970). Antigenic characterization of parainfluenza 4A and 4B by the hemagglutination-inhibition test and distribution of HI antibody in human sera. *Am. J. Epidemiol.* **91,** 308–316.

Kingsbury, D. W. (1991). The paramyxoviruses. Plenum, New York.

Komada, H., Kusagawa, S., Orvell, C., Tsurudome, M., Nishio, M., Bando, H., Kawano, M., Matsumara, H., Norrby, E., and Yasuhiko, I. (1992). Antigenic diversity of human parainfluenza virus type 1 isolates and their immunological relationship with Sendai virus revealed by monoclonal antibodies. *J. Gen. Virol.* **73,** 875–884.

Lawson, N. D., Stillman, E. A., Whitt, M. A., and Rose, J. K. (1995). Recombinant vesicular stomatitis viruses from DNA. *Proc. Natl. Acad. Sci., U.S.A.* **92,** 4477–4481.

McIntosh, K., Kurachek, S. C., Cairns, L. M., Burns, J. C., and Goodspeed, B. (1984). Treatment of respiratory viral infection in an immunodeficient infant with ribavirin aerosol. *Am. J. Dis. Child.* **138,** 305–308.

Matsuoka, Y., Curran, J., Pelet, T., Kolakofsky, D., Ray, R., and Compans, R. W. (1991). The P gene of human parainfluenza virus type 1 encodes P and C proteins but not a cysteine-rich V protein. *J. Virol.* **65,** 3406–3410.

Metzgar, D. P., Gower, T. A., Larson, E. F., Fuscaldo, A. A., and Mascoli, C. C. (1974). The effect of parainfluenza virus type 3 on newborn ferrets. *J. Biol. Stand.* **2,** 273–282.

Moscona, A., and Peluso, R. W. (1991). Fusion properties of cells persistently infected with human parainfluenza virus type 3: Participation of hemagglutinin–neuraminidase in membrane fusion. *J. Virol.* **65,** 2773–2777.

Murphy, B., Phelan, P. D., Jack, I., and Uren, E. (1980). Seasonal pattern in childhood viral lower respiratory tract infections in Melbourne. *Med. J. Aust.* **1,** 22–24.

Norrby, E., and Gollmar, Y. (1975). Identification of measles virus-specific hemolysis-inhibiting antibodies separate from hemagglutination-inhibiting antibodies. *Infect. Immun.* **11,** 231–239.

Norrby, E., and Penttinen, K. (1978). Differences in antibodies to the surface components of mumps virus after immunization with formalin-inactivated and live virus vaccines. *J. Infect. Dis.* **138,** 672–676.

Ohgimoto, S., Bando, H., Kawano, M., Okoamoto, K., Kondo, K., Tsurudome, M., Nishino, M., and Ito, Y. (1990). Sequence analysis of P gene of human parainfluenza type 2 virus: P and cysteine-rich proteins are translated by two mRNAs that differ by two nontemplated G residues. *Virology* **177**, 116–123.

Örvell, C., and Norrby, E. (1977). Immunologic properties of purified Sendai virus glycoproteins. *J. Immunol.* **119**, 1882–1887.

Park, K. H., and Krystal, M. (1992). *In vivo* model for pseudotemplated transcription in Sendai virus. *J. Virol.* **66**, 7033–7039.

Park, K. H., Huang, R., Correia, F. F., and Krystal, M. (1991). Rescue of a foreign gene by Senda virus. *Proc. Natl. Acad. Sci. U.S.A.* **88**, 5537–5541.

Parkinson, A. J., Muchmore, H. G., McConnell, T. A., Scott, L. V., and Miles, J. A. R. (1980). Serological evidence for parainfluenza virus infection during isolation at South Pole Station, Antarctica. *Am. J. Epidemiol.* **112**, 334–340.

Parrott, R. H., Vargosko, A. J., Luckey, A., Kim, H. W., Cumming, C., and Chanock, R. (1959). Clinical features of infection with hemadsorption viruses. *N. Engl. J. Med.* **260**, 731–738.

Parrott, R. H., Vargosko, A. J., Kim, H. W., Bell, J. A., and Chanock, R. M. (1962). Myxoviruses. 111. Parainfluenza. *Am. J. Public Health* **52**, 907–917.

Parrott, R. H., Kim, H. W., Arrobio, J. O., Canchola, J. G., Brandt, C. D., DeMeio, J. L., Jensen, K. E., and Chanock, R. M. (1967). "First International Conference on Vaccines against Viral and Rickettsial Diseases of Man," pp. 35–41. Plenum, New York.

Pattnaik, A. K., Ball, L. A., LeGrone, A. W., and Wertz, G. W. (1992). Infectious defective interfering particles of VSV from transcripts of a cDNA clone. *Cell (Cambridge, Mass.)* **69**, 1011–1020.

Peeples, M. E., and Bratt, M. A. (1982). Virion functions of RNA^+ temperature-sensitive mutants of Newcastle disease virus. *J. Virol.* **42**, 440–446.

Peeples, M. E., Rasenas, L. L., and Bratt, M. A. (1982). RNA synthesis by Newcastle disease virus temperature-sensitive mutants in two RNA-negative complementation groups. *J. Virol.* **42**, 996–1006.

Porter, D. D., Prince, G. A., Hemming, V. G., and Porter, H. G. (1991). Pathogenesis of human parainfluenza virus 3 infection in two species of cotton rats: Sigmodon hispidus develops bronchiolitis, while Sigmodon fulviventer develops interstitial pneumonia. *J. Virol.* **65**, 103–111.

Portner, A., Scroggs, R. A., Marx, P. A., and Kingsbury, D. W. (1975). A temperature-sensitive mutant of Sendai virus with an altered hemagglutinin–neuraminidase polypeptide: Consequences for virus assembly and cytopathology. *Virology* **67**, 179–187.

Prinoski, K., Cote, M. J., Kang, C. Y., and Dimock, K. (1992). Evolution of the fusion protein gene of human parainfluenza virus 3. *Virus Res.* **22**, 55–69.

Randall, R. E., and Young, D. F. (1988). Humoral and cytotoxic T cell immune responses to internal and external structural proteins of simian virus 5 induced by immunization with solid matrixantibody–antigen complexes. *J. Gen. Virol.* **69**, 2505–2516.

Ray R., and Compans, R. W. (1986). Monoclonal antibodies reveal extensive antigenic differences between the hemagglutinin–neuraminidase glycoproteins of human and bovine parainfluenza 3 viruses. *Virology* **148**, 232–236.

Ray, R., and Compans, R. W. (1987). Glycoproteins of human parainfluenza virus type 3: Affinity purification, antigenic characterization and reconstitution into lipid vesicles. *J. Gen. Virol.* **68**, 409–418.

Ray, R., Brown, V. E., and Compans, R. W. (1985). Glycoproteins of human parainfluenza virus type 3: Characterization and evaluation as a subunit vaccine. *J. Infect. Dis.* **152**, 1219–1230.

Ray, R., and Compans, R. W. (1990). Immunochemistry of paramyxoviruses. *In* "Immunochemistry of Viruses II" (M. V. H. Van Regenmortel and A. R. Neurath, eds.), pp. 215–234. Elsevier, Amsterdam.

Ray, R., Glaze, B. J., Moldoveanu, Z., and Compans, R. W. (1988a). Intranasal immunization of hamsters with envelope glycoproteins of human parainfluenza virus type 3. *J. Infect. Dis.* **157**, 648–654.

Ray, R., Glaze, B. J., and Compans, R. W. (1988b). Role of individual glycoproteins of human parainfluenza virus type 3 in the induction of a protective immune response. *J. Virol.* **62**, 783–787.

Ray, R., Galinski, M., and Compans, R. W. (1989). Expression of the fusion glycoprotein of human parainfluenza type 3 virus in insect cells by a recombinant baculovirus and analysis of its immunogenic property. *Virus Res.* **12**, 169–180.

Ray, R., Matsuoka, Y., Burnett, T. L., Glaze, B. J., and Compans, R. W. (1990). Human parainfluenza virus induces a type-specific protective immune response. *J. Infect. Dis.* **162**, 746–749.

Ray, R., Roux, L., and Compans, R. W. (1991). Intracellular targeting and assembly of paramyxovirus proteins. *In* "Paramyxovirus" (D. W. Kingsbury, ed.), pp. 457–479. Plenum, New York.

Ray, R., Duncan, J., Quinn, R., and Matsuoka, Y. (1992). Distinct hemagglutinin and neuraminidase epitopes involved in antigenic variation of recent human parainfluenza virus type 2 isolates. *Virus Res.* **24**, 107–113.

Ray, R., Novak, M., Duncan, J. D., Matsuoka, Y., and Compans, R. W. (1993). Microencapsulated human parainfluenza virus induces a protective immune response. *J. Infect. Dis.* **167**, 752–755.

Ray, R., Meyer, K., Newman, F., and Belshe, R. B. (1995). Characterization of a live, attenuated human parainfluenza type 3 virus candidate vaccine strain. *J. Virol.* **69**, 1959–1963.

Ray, R., Galinski, M. S., Hemingway, B. R., Meyer, K., Newman, F. K., and Belshe, R. B. (1996). Temperature-sensitive phenotype of the human parainfluenza virus type 3 candidate vaccine strain (cp45) correlates with a defect in the L gene. *J. Virol.* **70**, 580–584.

Rocchi, G., Arangio-Ruiz, G., Giannini, V., Jemolo, A. M., Andreoni, G., and Archetti, I. (1970). Detection of viraemia in acute respiratory disease of man. *Acta. Virol.* **14**, 405–407.

Roman, G., Phillips, C. A., and Poser, C. M. (1978). Parainfluenza virus type 3: Isolation from CSF of a patient with Gullain–Barre syndrome. *JAMA, J. Am. Med. Assoc.* **240,** 1613–1615.

Rydbeck, R., Love, A., Ovell, C., and Norrby, E. (1987). Antigenic analysis of human and bovine parainfluenza virus type 3 strains with monoclonal antibodies. *J. Gen. Virol.* **68,** 2153–2160.

Sanchez, A., and Banerjee, A. K. (1985). Studies on human parainfluenza virus 3: Characterization of the structural proteins and *in vitro* synthesized proteins coded by mRNAs isolated from infected cells. *Virology* **143,** 45–54.

Sarkkinen, H. K., Halonen, P. E., and Salmi, A. A. (1981). Type-specific detection of parainfluenza viruses by enzyme-immunoassay and radioimmunoassay in nasopharyngeal specimens of patients with acute respiratory disease. *J. Gen. Virol.* **56,** 49–57.

Schnell, M. J., Mebatsion, T., and Conzelmann, K. K. (1994). Infectious rabies viruses from cloned cDNA. *EMBO J* **13,** 4195–4203.

Shibata, S., Yamamoto-Goshima, F., Maeno, K., Hanaichi, T., Fujita, Y., Nakajima, K., Imai, M., Komatsu, T., and Sugiura, S. (1993). Characterization of a temperature-sensitive influenza B virus mutant defective in neuraminidase. *J. Virol.* **67,** 3264–3273.

Sieg, S., Muro-Cacho, C., Robertson, S., Huang, Y., and Kaplan, D. (1994). Infection and immunoregulation of T lymphocytes by parainfluenza virus type 3. *Proc. Natl. Acad. Sci., U.S.A.* **91,** 6293–6297.

Southern, J. A., Precious, B., and Randall, R. E. (1990). Two nonplated nucleotide additions are required to generate the P mRNA of parainfluenza virus type 2 since the RNA genome encodes protein V. *Virology* **177,** 388–390.

Spriggs, M. K., and Collins, P. L. (1986a). Human parainfluenza virus type 3: Messenger RNAs, polypeptide coding assignments, intergenic sequences, and genetic map. *J. Virol.* **59,** 646–654.

Spriggs, M. K., and Collins, P. L. (1986b). Sequence analysis of the P and C protein genes of human parainfluenza virus type 3: Patterns of amino acid sequence homology among paramyxovirus proteins. *J. Gen. Virol.* **67,** 2705–2719.

Spriggs, M. K., Murphy, B. R., Prince, G. A., Olmstead, R. A., and Collins, P. L. (1987). Expression of the F and HN glycoproteins of human parainfluenza virus type 3 by recombinant vaccinia viruses: Contributions of the individual proteins to host immunity. *J. Virol.* **61,** 3416–3423.

Spriggs, M. K., Collins, P. L., Tiemey, E., London, W. T., and Murphy, B. R (1988). Immunization with vaccinia virus recombinants that express the surface glycoproteins of human parainfluenza virus type 3 (PIV3) protects patas monkeys against PIV3 infection. *J. Virol.* **62,** 1293–1296.

Stokes, A., Tierney, E. L., Carris, C. M., Murphy, B. R., and Hall, S. L. (1993). The complete nucleotide sequence of two-cold-adapted, temperature-sensitive attenuated mutant vaccine viruses (cp12 and cp45) derived from the JS strain of human parainfluenza virus type 3 (PIV3). *Virus Res.* **30,** 43–52.

Storey, D. G., Dimock, K., and Kang, C. Y. (1984). Structural characterization of virion proteins and genomic RNA of human parainfluenza virus 3. *J. Virol.* **52,** 761–766.

Thompson, S. D., and Portner, A. (1987). Localization of functional sites on the hemagglutinin–neuraminidase glycoprotein of Sendai virus by sequence analysis of antigenic and temperature-sensitive mutants. *Virology* **160,** 1–8.

Tsipis, J. E., and Bratt, M. A. (1976). Isolation and primary characterization of temperature-sensitive mutants of Newcastle disease virus. *J. Virol.* **18,** 848–855.

Tsurudome, M., Nishio, M., Komada, H., Bando, H., and Ito, Y. (1989). Extensive antigenic diversity among human parainfluenza type 2 virus isolates and immunological relationships among paramyxoviruses revealed by monoclonal antibodies. *Virology* **171,** 38–48.

Tumova, B., Heinz, F., Syrucek, L., Bruchova, M., Fedova, D., Kunzova, L., and Strizova, V. (1988). Occurrence and aetiology of acute respiratory diseases: Results of a long-term surveillance programme. *Acta Virol.* **33,** 50–62.

Wechsler, S. L., Lambert, D. M., Galinski, M. S., Heineke, B. E., and Pons, M. W. (1985). Human parainfluenza virus 3: Purification and characterization of subviral components, viral proteins and viral RNA. *Virus Res.* **3,** 339–351.

Welliver, R. C., Wong, D. T., Middleton, E. J., Sun, M., McCarthy, N., and Ogra, P. L. (1982). Role of parainfluenza virus-specific IgE in pathogenesis of croup and wheezing subsequent to infection. *J. Pediatr.* **101,** 889–896.

Welliver, R. C., Wong, D. T., Sun, M., and McCarthy, N. (1986). Parainfluenza virus bronchiolitis: Epidemiology and pathology. *Am. J. Dis. Child.* **140,** 34–40.

Westrop, G. D., Wareham, K. A., Evans, D. M. A., Dunn, G., Minor, P. D., McGrath, D. I., Taffs, F., Marsden, S., Skinner, M. A., Schild, G. C., and Almond, J. W. (1989). Genetic basis of attenuation of the Sabin type 3 oral polio virus vaccine. *J. Virol.* **63,** 1338–1344.

Whelan, S. P. J., Ball, L. A., Barr, J. N., and Wertz, G. T. W. (1995). Efficient recovery of infectious vesicular stomatitis virus entirely from cDNA clones. *Proc. Natl. Acad. Sci. U.S.A.* **92,** 8388–8392.

Wong, V. K., Steinberg, E., and Warford, A. (1988). Parainfluenza virus type 3 meningitis in an 11-month-old infant. *Pediatr. Infect. Dis. J.* **7,** 300–301.

Wright, F. P. (1991). Parainfluenza viruses. *In* "Textbook of Human Virology" (R. B. Belshe, ed.), 2nd Ed., pp. 342–350. Mosby Year Book, St. Louis, Missouri.

Wright, F. P., Meguro, H., Thompson, J., Torrence, A. E., and Karzon, D. T. (1977). Live parainfluenza type 3 vaccine in children. *Pediatr. Res.* **11,** 509.

Wright *et al.* (1984).

Zhao, H., and Banerjee, A. K. (1995). Interaction between the nucleocapsid protein and the phosphoprotein of human parainfluenza virus 3. *J. Biol. Chem.* **270,** 12485–12490.

25

Development of a Mucosal Rotavirus Vaccine

MARGARET E. CONNER
Division of Molecular Virology
Baylor College of Medicine
Houston VA Medical Center
Houston, Texas 77030

MARY K. ESTES
Division of Molecular Virology
Baylor College of Medicine
Houston, Texas 77030

PAUL A. OFFIT
Section of Infectious Diseases
The Children's Hospital of Philadelphia
Philadelphia, Pennsylvania 19104

H. FRED CLARK
Department of Pediatrics
University of Pennsylvania School of Medicine
Philadelphia, Pennsylvania 19104

MANUEL FRANCO
NINGGUO FENG
HARRY B. GREENBERG
Division of Gastroenterology
Stanford School of Medicine
Stanford, California 94305; and
Palo Alto VA Medical Center
Palo Alto, California 94304

I. Introduction

Diarrhea is the most prevalent infectious disease in developing countries and ranks second only to respiratory disease in developed countries. The majority of diarrheal illness and deaths occurs in children less than 5 years of age (Institute of Medicine, 1986). During the first 5 years of life, the average child contracts diarrheal illness multiple times and rotaviruses are the single most important cause of severe dehydrating diarrheal disease in young children worldwide (Glass *et al.*, 1994; Bern and Glass, 1994). Mortality due to rotavirus infection occurs primarily in developing nations and is thought to approach one million deaths per year (Institute of Medicine, 1986). Rotavirus infection of human infants also causes extensive morbidity worldwide. In the United States alone, the cost of hospitalizations due to rotavirus infections has been estimated to be $352 million annually (Matson and Estes, 1990). Recent cost-effectiveness analysis of a rotavirus immunization program in the United States, presuming a vaccine efficacy rate of 50%, indicates a rotavirus vaccine would annually prevent more than one million cases of rotavirus diarrhea, 58,000 hospitalizations, and 82 deaths and yield a net

MUCOSAL VACCINES

savings of $79 million to health care and $466 million to society (Smith *et al.*, 1995). The medical importance of rotavirus infection provides a compelling rationale for development of effective vaccination programs.

Rotavirus also is an important cause of diarrhea in animals including most species of domestic and laboratory animals (Saif *et al.*, 1994). In animals, protection from severe disease is required in the first few weeks of life before active vaccination is effective. Therefore, rotavirus vaccines in animals are based on maternal vaccination and passive transfer of antibody through the colostrum and milk to newborn animals (Conner *et al.*, 1994b). This review focuses on immunity to rotavirus infection and the development of a rotavirus vaccine for humans.

Rotaviruses are members of the Reoviridae family. Rotaviruses contain 11 segments of dsRNA, each of which codes for one protein. Six structural proteins exist in the virus particle and five nonstructural proteins are only expressed in infected cells. Rotaviruses are structurally complex with three concentric capsid layers. The capsid layers from inside to outside are composed of (i) VP2, (ii) VP6, and (iii) VP7 from which spikes of VP4 emanate. Two outer capsid proteins, VP4 (the spike protein) and VP7 (a glycoprotein), induce neutralizing antibodies; consequently rotaviruses have a binary serotype designation which describes P (VP4) and G (VP7) types.

Rotaviruses were first recognized as a causative agent of gastroenteritis in children by Bishop *et al.* (1973). Rotavirus infections are primarily limited to the nondividing mature epithelial cells on the villi of the small intestine, although this tropism is not absolute (Conner and Ramig, 1996). Infection can result in clinical signs including watery diarrhea, anorexia, depression, dehydration, and vomiting primarily in young children. Subclinical infections also are common in all age groups. Symptomatic infections can occur in adults but tend to be mild; severe disease has been reported in the elderly. Loss of fluids from diarrhea and vomiting can result in fatal dehydration. Malnutrition, concomitant infections, and depressed immunity may exacerbate disease. Diarrhea is thought to be due to viral replication leading to enterocyte destruction which results in malabsorption (Conner and Ramig, 1996). A new mechanism of rotavirus-induced disease has been postulated, where the nonstructural protein NSP4 functions as a viral enterotoxin that induces disease (Ball *et al.*, 1996b).

The incubation period for rotavirus infection is short, generally 1–2 days; virus is shed in stools in high quantities (up to 10^{10}–10^{11} particles per 1 g of stool) for variable duration but typically for 3–7 days. The tremendous amount of virus shed in feces, the duration of shedding, and the stability of rotavirus in the environment can result in extensive contamination of the environment. Infection is transmitted by the fecal–oral route or by contact with contaminated fomites. In temperate climates, rotavirus infections occur primarily in the winter months, while in tropical climates they predominate in the dry season.

Development of a rotavirus vaccine is complicated by a number of factors relating to the epidemiology of rotavirus infections. Currently 14 G and 10 P serotypes are known, and an additional 10 P types have been classified based on amino acid sequence homology (Estes, 1996). In humans, 9 G and 8 P types have been identified, but the majority of infections are due to rotaviruses of G 1–4 and P1A[8] or P1B[4] serotypes [genotypes]. Unlike influenza, multiple serotypes or strains of rotavirus often circulate in a given community at the same time or within the same year; different serotypes can circulate in different locations and the serotype of virus circulating cannot be predicted. Multivalent vaccines are being developed, since some studies have shown limited cross-protection between viruses of different G serotypes. Rotavirus infection occurs in all age groups, but disease primarily occurs in young children (6 months to 2 years) requiring vaccines to be safe and immunogenic when administered to the young. Since rotavirus infections are ubiquitous, virtually 100% of the adult population has antibody to rotavirus. The presence of maternally derived antibodies in young children may interfere with the immune response to a vaccine.

Developing a clear understanding of the factors which regulate the resolution of primary rotavirus infection and the induction of immunity to reinfection is a critical step in identifying the best vaccine strategy. Studies in both children and animal models which have yielded important information about immunity to rotavirus infection are reviewed below.

II. Immunologic Determinants of Protection against Rotavirus-Induced Gastroenteritis in Humans

Because rotaviruses represent mucosal pathogens, protection against rotavirus disease will most likely be mediated by an immune response which is active at the intestinal mucosal surface. A consequence of mucosal pathogens replicating only at the initial portal of entry is that incubation periods are relatively short, often only 1–2 days. Therefore, the time required for activation and differentiation of memory T and B cells to effector cells is longer than the period of incubation. Protection against mucosal infections may, therefore, be mediated primarily by virus-specific effector functions [i.e., virus-specific secretory IgA (S-IgA) or cytotoxic T lymphocytes] present at the mucosal surface at the time of infection. This may in part explain why protection after natural infection with mucosal pathogens is often short-lived and incomplete (i.e., protection is effective against moderate-to-severe but not mild infections). Obviously, where natural infection does not induce complete and long-lasting protection, development of a successful vaccine is difficult.

A. Immune Response to Natural Infection

Recognition that natural infection leads to reduced disease on rechallenge has stimulated efforts to understand what constitutes protective immunity. Knowledge of the location, isotypes, and longevity of virus-specific antibodies induced after rotavirus infection of infants and young children is beginning to provide useful information about what are the likely determinants of protection against challenge (Coulson *et al.*, 1990; Davidson *et al.*, 1983; Grimwood *et al.*, 1988). Virus-specific S-IgA at the duodenal mucosal surface and in the feces is detected within 1 month of infection and persists for approximately 4 months; levels of virus-specific IgA in the circulation parallel those found for S-IgA at the intestinal mucosal surface. Virus-specific IgG is not routinely detected either at the duodenal mucosal surface or in the feces. However, high titers of virus-specific IgG are detected in the circulation acutely after infection. Therefore, the presence and duration of virus-specific S-IgA at the mucosal surface parallels the epidemiological observation that although children are rarely infected within the same rotavirus season (lasting approximately 4–5 months in temperate climates), it is not uncommon for children to be reinfected during the following rotavirus season. Because high titers of virus-specific IgG in serum are detected 1 year after infection, circulating virus-specific IgG appears to serve as a marker for past infection, but not as a correlate of protection against disease.

B. Immunologic Determinants of Protection against Disease Induced by Natural Infection

Studies of neonates asymptomatically infected with rotavirus provided the first evidence that infection may afford protection against symptoms associated with subsequent infection (Bishop *et al.*, 1983). Although a rotavirus infection in the neonatal period did not decrease the risk of subsequent infection, there was a marked decrease in the percentage of infants with symptomatic reinfection (38 vs 85%). In addition, neonatal rotavirus infection significantly decreased the rate of hospitalization associated with subsequent infection (8 vs 0%). These studies have been extended to include infants and young children with the additional observation that protection is afforded after either symptomatic or asymptomatic infection (Bernstein *et al.*, 1991; Ward and Bernstein, 1994).

These epidemiological observations predict that the critical determinant of protection against rotavirus challenge is the level of virus-specific S-IgA in feces at the time of infection. This prediction has been confirmed in subsequent epidemiological studies of natural rotavirus infections; children with higher levels of fecal antibody are protected against relatively severe disease (Coulson *et al.*, 1992; Matson *et al.*, 1993, 1996; O'Ryan *et al.*, 1994).

C. Importance of Virus Serotype in Protection against Reinfection Following Natural Infection

The degree to which virus-neutralizing antibodies in serum or feces are predictive of protection against reinfection has not been clearly established. Some studies have found that protection from diarrhea is greatest following reinfection with a homotypic virus, virus with the same G type, and that virus-neutralizing antibodies in serum and feces following natural infection correlate with protection against relatively severe disease (Chiba *et al.*, 1986, 1993; O'Ryan *et al.*, 1994). The relative capacities of VP4 and VP7 to evoke protection against natural reinfection remain unknown since studies of natural infection have not included determination of the VP4 type of the infecting rotavirus strains.

III. Current Live Rotavirus Vaccines for Children

Efforts toward development of effective rotavirus vaccines began shortly after rotaviruses were first recognized as a cause of severe dehydrating diarrhea in animals in the late 1960s and early 1970s (see Chapter 26). The first attempt at development of an attenuated vaccine was for bovine rotavirus infections in cows. Although the bovine vaccine had limited efficacy in cows, this was thought to reflect the need to prevent severe disease in calves in the first few weeks of life and the inability to induce effective active immunity before infection occurred (Conner *et al.*, 1994b). Ultimately, one of the strains originally developed for a bovine vaccine was the first candidate vaccine tested for humans. Thus, development of rotavirus vaccines for children initially focused on administration of live oral rotaviruses from heterologous (nonhuman) species, a "Jennerian" vaccine approach. Efforts to develop a vaccine for human rotavirus disease continued without prior testing of candidate vaccines in animal model systems. Therefore, trial and error has played a major part in development of current candidate rotavirus vaccines for children. As data were generated from the clinical and field trials of the various vaccine formulations, vaccine formulations were modified and retested. Currently several vaccine formulations are being tested in field trials, and they are expected to be proposed for licensure soon.

A. First Generation (Animal Origin) Vaccines

1. *Bovine Rotaviruses*

The first tests of a rotavirus vaccine for humans evaluated oral inoculation of live vaccines (simian P5[3] G3 RRV and bovine P6[1] G6 NCDV and WC3). These viruses were assumed to be attenuated because of their origin from heterologous (nonhuman) species. At that time, a clear understanding of rotavirus immunity was lacking and assumptions that animal rotavirus isolates might be protective were based upon seeing extensive serologic cross-reactivity among most group A animal and human rotaviruses by virus antigen:antibody binding tests (ELISA, RIA). In addition, antibody which reacted with multiple strains of rotavirus was detected following rotavirus infection. Later, cross-neutralization antibody reactions defined distinct rotavirus serotypes and studies in animals indicated that primary immune responses are generally homotypic (Snodgrass *et al.*, 1991; Conner *et al.*, 1991). However, protection studies in animals have failed to unequivocally establish the importance of serotype-specific immune responses in protection against disease (reviewed in Clark and Offit, 1994).

The bovine rotavirus vaccine NCDV, renamed as strain RIT4237, was totally nonreactogenic when orally administered to infants in doses as high as $10^{8.0}$ $TCID_{50}$ (Vesikari *et al.*, 1983). In early clinical trials in Finland, RIT4237 efficiently induced serum antibodies, especially in seronegative infants. However, the strain specificity of the serum antibody response was exclusively homotypic (bovine serotype G6) except in infants previously seropositive to human serotype G1, who had a serotype G1 booster response (Vesikari *et al.*, 1985).

Two initial efficacy trials of RIT4237 in Finland, in which either one or two vaccine doses were administered, yielded protection rates, respectively, of 50 and 58% against all rotavirus disease, and 88 and 82% against clinically significant rotavirus disease. Selective vaccine-induced protection against more severe disease was to prove a frequent characteristic of many candidate vaccines (Vesikari, 1994). Subsequent RIT4237 vaccine trials in Rwanda and the Gambia revealed little efficacy while an intermediate level of protection was seen in a trial in Peru (De Mol *et al.*, 1986; Hanlon *et al.*, 1987; Lanata *et al.*, 1989). This vaccine ultimately was abandoned as a candidate for further application to human infants.

The WC3 strain of bovine rotavirus (also serotype G6) was developed as a vaccine candidate from a rotavirus isolated from a calf in Pennsylvania and passaged 12 times in cell culture. WC3 vaccine, like RIT4237 was totally nonreactogenic and efficiently induced only a homotypic serum neutralizing antibody response (70 to 100% of vaccinees ≤12 months old), when administered at a dose of $10^{7.0}$ to $10^{7.5}$ pfu (Clark *et al.*, 1986).

An initial efficacy trial of WC3 vaccine in Philadelphia gave 76% efficacy against all rotavirus disease and 100% protection against moderate-to-severe gastroenteritis (Clark *et al.*, 1988). Subsequent efficacy trials in Cincinnati and in the Central African Republic were characterized by no measurable protection against all rotavirus disease and minimal protection against clinically significant disease (Bernstein *et al.*, 1990; Georges-Courbot *et al.*, 1991). WC3 vaccine induced 50% protection against all rotavirus disease in a trial in Shanghai (M. S. Ho, unpublished data, 1995). This vaccine candidate is no longer being developed, although it is being used as a donor strain for the production of reassortants (see Section III.B.2. below).

2. *Simian Rotaviruses*

Rhesus rotavirus (RRV) vaccine strain MMU 18006 was isolated from a young rhesus monkey with diarrhea and evaluated as vaccine at the 16th cell culture passage level (Stuker *et al.*, 1980). This is a serotype G3 rotavirus, but the VP7 amino acid sequence and reactivity with VP7-specific monoclonal antibodies are not identical to all human G3 strains of rotavirus (Nishikawa *et al.*, 1989).

Unlike the bovine rotaviruses, RRV can undergo limited replication in the intestines of most infants. RRV is shed in the feces of more than 50% of recipients (Perez-Schael *et al.*, 1987), compared with 30% or less shedding rates with bovine rotaviruses (Vesikari *et al.*, 1986; Clark *et al.*, 1986). Although given at a lower dose of either 10^4 or 10^5 pfu than bovine rotavirus, RRV is reactogenic inducing fevers in 20% or more of vaccinees (Anderson *et al.*, 1986). The incidence of fever is much reduced in very young infants (<2 months old) and in children in developing nations. Serum antibody response rates are 70% or more and are primarily homotypic in specificity (Losonsky *et al.*, 1986, 1988).

The protective efficacy of the RRV vaccine in placebo-controlled clinical trials has varied widely. In two Scandinavian trials, protection was 48 and 38%, respectively, against all rotavirus disease and 80 and 67%, respectively, against severe disease (Vesikari *et al.*, 1990; Gothefors *et al.*, 1989). Subsequent trials in Arizona and in Rochester in the United States revealed no protection (Santosham *et al.*, 1991; Christy *et al.*, 1988), although a second trial performed 2 years later in Rochester was associated with 66% protection against all rotavirus disease (Madore *et al.*, 1992). Relatively efficient protection was observed in a Venezuelan trial in which the natural challenge strain was a homotypic serotype G3 virus. However, in this trial, similar levels of protection were also noted against rotaviruses of other serotypes

(Perez Schael *et al.*, 1990). In virtually all other trials of any rotavirus vaccine reported to date, the natural challenge virus has been predominantly serotype G1.

RRV vaccine is no longer being developed actively as a single candidate vaccine, but it is one component of a candidate tetravalent vaccine.

B. Second Generation (Animal × Human Reassortant Virus) Vaccines

Monovalent vaccines composed only of a single animal-origin rotavirus failed to consistently protect infants in repeated clinical trials. Therefore, vaccine development turned to investigation of animal rotavirus reassortants which express human rotavirus surface antigens. Cross-virus neutralization tests using sera of parenterally hyperimmunized animals suggested that the VP7 (G type) surface protein is the predominant neutralization antigen (Hoshino *et al.*, 1984). Therefore, animal rotavirus reassortants containing the gene that codes for human G serotype-specific proteins have been most intensely investigated. These reassortants apparently retain the attenuation characteristics of the parental animal virus strain which contributes to the majority of the genome segments in the virus.

1. Simian × Human Reassortant Rotaviruses

The simian virus RRV reassorted to contain human virus VP7s has been evaluated as a monotypic vaccine or in a quadrivalent mixture containing individual VP7 reassortants of G1, G2, and G4 specificity combined with native RRV as a G3 component. Alone or in combination, the RRV reassortants, like RRV, often induce transient fevers in 20–40% of recipients (Flores *et al.*, 1993). A predominant serum neutralizing antibody response to RRV is observed, accompanied by G1, G2, G3, or G4-specific responses in up to 50% (or slightly more) of vaccinees (Flores *et al.*, 1990, 1993; Lanata *et al.*, 1990).

In an initial clinical efficacy trial, the G1 reassortant of RRV provided 77% protection against all rotavirus disease compared with 65% protection induced by native RRV vaccine administered in parallel, not a significant difference (Madore *et al.*, 1992). In a subsequent efficacy trial performed in Finland, monovalent preparations of serotype 2 and of serotype 1 reassortants of RRV gave virtually identical protection, 66 and 67%, respectively, against rotavirus disease during a season when only G1 wild-type virus was identified (Vesikari *et al.*, 1992).

Two large multicenter clinical efficacy studies of the quadrivalent RRV reassortant vaccine have been conducted in the United States. Each involved a three-dose regimen of immunization. First, over 900 infants were given three doses of 10^4 pfu each of the quadrivalent vaccine, monovalent serotype G1 reassortant, or placebo. Protection rates after the first rotavirus season were 65 and 63%, respectively, for the monovalent and quadrivalent vaccine against all rotavirus disease (Sack, 1992). During a second season of observation, when nonserotype G1 rotaviruses were more prevalent, the quadrivalent vaccine was more protective (48% against all rotavirus disease) than was the monovalent vaccine (10% against all rotavirus disease).

A larger multicenter efficacy trial followed, using a protocol similar to the first except that doses of 10^5 pfu of each vaccine were administered. After the first season of observation, protection against all rotavirus disease for the monovalent vaccine was 54% and for the quadrivalent was 49% (Dennehy, 1994). Protection against moderately severe rotavirus disease was 69% for the monovalent and 80% for the quadrivalent vaccine.

Other efficacy and safety trials of the quadrivalent RRV reassortant vaccine are in progress or have been completed and are undergoing data analysis. The quadrivalent RRV vaccine is being actively developed for licensure.

2. Bovine × Human Reassortant Rotaviruses

The bovine WC3 virus, reassorted to express human rotavirus surface proteins, also is being evaluated as a candidate vaccine. WI79–9, a WC3 reassortant containing the gene for the VP7 surface protein of human P1A[8] G1 rotavirus strain, is the most extensively tested strain. No vaccine related reactogenicity has been detected in over 300 infants given a full dose of $10^{7.0}$ to $10^{7.3}$ pfu. Serum virus-neutralizing antibody responses to serotype G1 were enhanced compared to WC3 but seroconversion rates were consistently higher to WC3 (70–100%) than to the serotype G1 WI79 virus parent (22–60%) (Clark *et al.*, 1990a,b, 1992).

In an initial efficacy trial involving 77 infants in the Philadelphia area, two doses of WI79–9 induced complete protection against rotavirus diarrhea (Clark *et al.*, 1992). In a subsequent larger trial involving 329 infants in Philadelphia and Rochester, three doses of WI79–9 gave 67% protection against all rotavirus disease and 87% protection against clinically significant rotavirus disease (Treanor *et al.*, 1995).

In parallel studies, WI79–4 a WC3 reassortant bearing the human gene for the strain WI79 P1A[8] VP4 surface protein was evaluated. This reassortant was nonreactogenic in infant clinical trials, but like WI79–9, induced serum neutralizing antibody to the WC3 parent rotavirus with much greater frequency than to the WI79 (P1A[8], G1) parent virus. Nevertheless, a mixture of WI79–9 and WI79–4 monovalent reassortants efficiently induced serum virus neutralizing antibody to both WC3 virus (100%) and WI79 virus (78%) (Clark *et al.*, 1992).

The observation that a vaccine containing a mixture of WI79–4 and WI79–9 reassortants was more immunogenic than either reassortant alone led to the formulation of equal concentrations ($10^{7.0}$ pfu) of a quadrivalent vaccine containing these two reassortants, and two additional WC3 reassortants containing genes for surface VP7 components of G2 and G3 specificity (Clark *et al.*, 1995). This quadrivalent vaccine was evaluated in a placebo-controlled efficacy trial including 435 infants in 10 cities in the United States. In these trials, vaccinees exhibited an 8% excess of mild diarrheas when compared to placebo infants only after the first of three doses. Protective efficacy against all rotavirus disease was 67%. Eight placebo recipients but no vaccine recipients experienced severe rotavirus disease with a clinical score ≥17.

Development of multivalent WC3-reassortant rotavirus vaccine is continuing.

C. Additional Approaches to Live Virus Vaccine Development

Numerous other approaches to vaccine development have been proposed, some of which have reached Phase 1 clinical trials. These include the use of "newborn nursery strains" which are presumed to be naturally attenuated human rotavirus strains (Midthun *et al.*, 1991; Vesikari *et al.*, 1991) and cold adapted isolates of human rotavirus (Matsuno *et al.*, 1987). One newborn strain M37 failed to show efficacy in clinical trials and has been removed from further consideration, but others may be pursued (Vesikari, 1996).

D. Correlates of Protection from Vaccine Trials

1. *Immunologic Determinants of Protection against Challenge Induced by Immunization*

RRV, RRV × human, and WC3 × human reassortant rotaviruses have been shown to induce both virus-specific IgA in the circulation and virus-specific S-IgA in the feces (Bernstein *et al.*, 1990; Flores *et al.*, 1993; Losonsky *et al.*, 1988; Midthun *et al.*, 1989; Perez-Schael *et al.*, 1990). The presence of virus-specific IgA in serum or feces has not always predicted protection against disease in vaccine trials (Madore *et al.*, 1992; J. Treanor, unpublished data, 1994), but study designs have not always been optimal to detect correlations between virus-specific IgA and protection. These data are at variance with those found after natural infection where correlations between antibody titers and protection from clinical disease are observed (see Section II.B). One possible explanation for these differences is that the vaccines being tested are heterologous viruses which do not replicate sufficiently to induce a vigorous effective local antibody response. This idea is supported by studies in animal models where vigorous local antibody responses are seen only following infection of mice or rabbits with homologous viruses (murine and lapine viruses, respectively) or infection of mice with very high doses of heterologous viruses (M. E. Conner, unpublished, 1991; Feng *et al.*, 1994).

2. *Importance of Rotavirus Serotype in Protection against Reinfection Following Immunization*

VP4 and VP7 have each been found to be dominant in their capacity to evoke virus-specific neutralizing antibodies after immunization with animal × human rotavirus reassortants (Bernstein *et al.*, 1995; Ward *et al.*, 1990a). The importance of serotype in the development of a vaccine remains unclear, but the consensus opinion is that induction of serotype-specific immunity plays some role in protection. This opinion is supported by the observation that RRV or WC3 given alone do not consistently induce protection against disease. However, the addition of human genes (which code for outer capsid protein VP7) to either RRV or WC3 has resulted in more consistent protective efficacy, suggesting that serotype may be important in protection against human disease.

IV. Animal Models to Study Active Immunity

Understanding rotavirus infection and immunity in humans is important, but studies in humans are difficult because they are confounded by the inability of the investigator to rigorously control numerous experimental variables such as prior viral exposure. As an alternative, animal model systems have been developed to study rotavirus immunity. Most animal species are naturally infected with homologous rotaviral strains and such infections frequently cause diarrheal disease in these species. Two small-animal models and several large-animal models have been developed, and studies using these models have provided key insights into rotavirus pathogenesis and immunity (Conner and Ramig, 1996). The majority of studies examining active immunity have utilized the rabbit, mouse, and piglet models, and the following discussion will be limited to these models. Key features of the rabbit, mouse, and piglet model are compared in Table I. Although the search for an effective rotavirus vaccine began over 15 years ago, at that time a clear understanding of immunity and protection against rotavirus was not available. With this void, animal models have been useful to define basic parameters of the immune response to rotavirus infection as well as to evalu-

TABLE I
Comparison of the Rabbit, Mouse, and Pig Animal Models of Rotavirus

Parameter	Rabbit	Mouse	Pig
Cost	Moderate	Low	High
Availability (antibody-negative)	Low	High	Derived[a]
Utility for studies of mucosal immunity	High	High	High
Permissivity for human rotaviruses	Low	Low	High
Utility to study physiology	High	Moderate	High
Genetically altered strains of animals for immunological studies	Low	High	None
Feasibility of long-term immunity and protection studies	High	High	Low
Diarrhea induced following rotavirus challenge	No	No	Yes
Histopathologic lesions in small intestine following rotavirus infection	Yes	No	Yes
Vaccine studies			
(a) Homologous immunity	Yes	Yes	Yes
(b) Jennerian and modified Jennerian studies (heterologous immunity)	Yes	Yes	Yes
(c) Killed virion given parenterally	Yes	Yes	ND[b]
(d) Vaccinia, adenovirus, or baculovirus proteins	No	Yes	ND
(e) VLPs	Yes	Yes	Pending
(f) DNA	ND	Yes	ND
(g) Live-attenuated	Yes	Yes	Yes

[a]Antibody-negative piglets achieved by colstrum deprivation or derived as gnotiobiotic animals.
[b]Not done.

ate existing and new vaccine strategies. Although at least two live virus reassortant vaccines may be submitted for licensure soon, these vaccines show only ~70% efficacy against the most severe disease in developed countries (Kapikian *et al.*, 1996; Clark *et al.*, 1996). It can be anticipated that development and testing of more efficacious vaccines for use in humans will continue to depend on the use of animal models. Future efficacy studies in humans will be difficult due to the cost and large number of children required to compare the efficacy of new candidates with already licensed vaccines.

A. Studies of Rotavirus Immunity in the Rabbit Model

The rabbit was the first small animal model to be developed to examine active immunity and protection (Conner *et al.*, 1988, 1991; Thouless *et al.*, 1988). Rabbits are productively infected with homologous rabbit strains up to at least 1 year of age, which allows long-term immunity and challenge studies (Table I) (Conner *et al.*, 1988 and M. E. Conner, unpublished). At least four distinct strains of rabbit rotavirus have been described, and to date, all strains characterized are G3 serotype and P[14] genotype (Thouless *et al.*, 1986; Tanaka *et al.*, 1988; Ciarlet *et al.*, 1996). Rabbits are susceptible to infection with the heterologous SA11 virus, but this virus does not spread efficiently from rabbit to rabbit (Conner *et al.*, 1988). Although natural infections of rabbits with rotavirus result in diarrhea, experimental infections of rabbits with tissue culture adapted rotavirus strains do not result in clinical diarrhea (Conner *et al.*, 1988). Liquid intestinal contents, histopathologic lesions including shortening of villi, mild mononuclear infiltration, and vacuolation are observed following infection of rabbits from birth to over 1 year of age, but diarrhea is not observed (Estes *et al.*, 1989; Gilger *et al.*, 1988; Conner and Ramig, 1996; M. E. Conner, unpublished data). Therefore the rabbit is an infection model; protection from challenge is assessed by a decrease in virus shedding observed following virus challenge and not by protection from clinical disease. Protection from infection is thought to be a more stringent measure of protection than protection from clinical disease.

1. *Primary Immune Response in Rabbits*

The kinetics of a primary serum and mucosal immune response to rotavirus infection observed following oral inoculation of rabbits with a high dose of the rabbit (ALA) rotavirus (7.5×10^5–1×10^7 pfu) show that intestinal immune responses are detected very early; IgM, neutralizing antibody, and IgA are detected by 3, 5, and 6 days postinoculation (dpi), respectively (Conner *et al.*, 1991). The peak of virus shedding (4–6 dpi) occurs as the intestinal immune response is first detected, declining thereafter as the immune response increases. Serologic immune responses are detected as early as 7 dpi. The immune response following a single rotavirus infection of seronegative animals with a replication-efficient virus is sufficient to totally protect rabbits from infection following homologous virus challenge. In these protected animals, an anamnestic immune response is observed only by monitoring mucosal neutralizing antibodies, indicating that exposure to rotavirus is often underestimated if serum antibody titers alone are used as a measure of exposure. The immune response following a single rotavirus infection or infection and challenge of seronegative animals with a replication-efficient homologous virus is sufficient to induce durable long-lasting serologic and mucosal immune responses, up to 1.5 to 2 years (Conner *et al.*, 1991, 1996b; Conner and Estes, 1994). These studies indicate that a live homologous virus vaccine that replicates efficiently in children might be capable of stimulating higher titered and longer-lasting immune responses than heterologous, replication-restricted viruses.

Studies in rabbits also have revealed several basic concepts about the immune response to rotavirus infections that have been important for the interpretation of results from vaccine trials in children. These concepts are clear because they came from studies with animals whose exposure to specific strains of rotavirus was known and well-controlled. (i) Detection of neutralizing antibody (NAb) responses is dependent on the virus strain used in the neutralization assay. All inoculated rabbits develop detectable serum and intestinal NAb responses against the homologous infecting virus strain, but responses are detected less frequently and in lower titers against heterologous strains. (ii) NAb activity in both serum and mucosal samples is generally, but not exclusively, homotypic after an oral primary and challenge inoculation with a single virus strain. This indicates that heterotypic NAb can be induced by two infections with a single virus, probably due to common epitopes on VP4 or in the C region of VP7. An interesting question from these studies is whether even broader heterotypic responses might be induced by two oral inoculations of more than one virus strain. (iii) Heterotypic NAb responses are not always seen in both mucosal and serum samples. Therefore, measurement of heterotypic serum antibodies may not be predictive of heterotypic mucosal protection, and vaccine trials should attempt to measure mucosal antibody status. These technical points have been helpful for studies performed on characterization of the immune response of children naturally infected with rotavirus.

2. *Independence of Immune Response from Infecting Dose of Virus*

Defining the 50% infectious dose (ID_{50}) of a tissue culture adapted rabbit rotavirus (the ALA strain) in rabbits led to the discovery that the immune response to homologous rotavirus infection is not dependent on the dose of the infecting virus (Conner and Estes, 1994; Conner *et al.*, 1996b). A challenge dose of 3.5×10^5 pfu of ALA virus infects 100% of rabbits and is nearly 1000-fold higher than the ID_{50} dose (1.7×10^2 pfu). However, infection with any dose of virus sufficient to initiate infection ($\sim 10^2$ pfu) stimulates an immune response and protection from challenge analogous to infection with a high challenge dose (3.5×10^5 pfu) of virus. Similar results also have been reported in mice (Feng *et al.*, 1994).

3. *Vaccine Studies in the Rabbit Model*

The rabbit model also is being used to evaluate several vaccine strategies including inactivated parenteral and subunit vaccines. The status of these studies is discussed in Sections V.A and V.B.

B. Studies of Rotavirus Immunity in the Piglet Model

The piglet is being used as a model to study human and porcine rotavirus-induced disease. Colostrum-deprived or gnotobiotic piglets must be utilized for rotavirus studies, because rotavirus is ubiquitous in animal populations resulting in the presence of antibody to rotavirus in colostrum and milk. Compared with the other animal models, the intestinal physiology of the piglet is most analogous to humans (Saif *et al.*, 1996). Piglets become infected and develop diarrhea following infection with virulent homologous and heterologous rotaviruses up to at least 6 weeks of age, and histopathologic damage to the small intestine can be extensive (Table I). However, infection and immunity in gnotobiotic piglets may not be totally analogous to infections in children because the intestine and the immune response in gnotobiotes are underdeveloped. Although challenge studies can be performed in gnotobiotic piglets, long term immunity and protection studies are difficult because these animals must be removed from germ-free isolators at approximately 8 weeks of age. The limitations of the piglet model including cost and availability of the model hinder its extensive use, but this model is unique because it is a disease model and infection and disease are induced by infection with human rotaviruses.

1. *Infection of Piglets with Human Rotaviruses*

Piglets and calves are susceptible to infection and diarrhea following infection with human rotaviruses (Bridger *et al.*, 1975; Davidson *et al.*, 1977; Saif *et al.*, 1996; Torres-Medina *et al.*, 1976; Wyatt *et al.*, 1980; Mebus *et al.*, 1976). One of the human strains (Wa) that infects piglets has been well characterized and belongs to serotype G1, the most prevalent G rotavirus serotype and P1A[8], one of the most prevalent P types in children worldwide. This human rotavirus was inoculated directly into piglets from the original human fecal sample and has been maintained by serial passage in piglets (Wyatt *et al.*, 1980; Saif *et al.*, 1996).

Recent studies have compared the parameters of infection of piglets with heterologous piglet to piglet passaged Wa-virulent virus and tissue-culture-adapted Wa virus (Saif *et al.*, 1996). The virulent piglet-passaged Wa virus induced diarrhea, villous atrophy, and seroconversion in all inoculated piglets, and all animals were protected from homologous virus challenge. Inoculation of piglets with tissue-culture-adapted Wa virus resulted in subclinical infections with no or mild pathologic lesions, limited virus shedding in only 6% of inoculated piglets, but seroconversion of 96% of piglets. Piglets inoculated with the avirulent tissue culture adapted Wa virus were partially protected from diarrhea and virus shedding following virulent Wa virus challenge (Saif *et al.*, 1996). These results are reminiscent of results with heterologous tissue-culture-adapted rotavirus vaccine candidates, which also have limited replication and immunogenicity in children.

The piglet has been used to examine rotavirus pathogenesis by comparison of infections of piglets with virulent porcine SB1A strain, avirulent human DS-1 virus, and SB1A × DS1 single gene reassortants (Hoshino *et al.*, 1988, 1995). Early studies in piglets showed that both outer capsid proteins VP4 and VP7 induce neutralizing antibodies that can afford protection from homotypic but not against a G and P type heterotypic rotavirus challenge (Hoshino *et al.*, 1988). Recent studies have implicated VP3, VP4, VP7, or NSP4 in rotavirus virulence (diarrhea induction) and host range restriction (replication efficiency) (Hoshino *et al.*, 1995). Replacement of a single porcine SB1A gene which encodes one of these four proteins with the corresponding gene from human DS1 results in loss of virulence and failure of virus shedding in piglets. Conferment of replication efficiency and virulence to the avirulent DS1 strain required replacement of the four human virus genes encoding VP3, VP4, VP7, and NSP4 with the corresponding genes from the virulent SB1A. Several studies in mice using reassortant viruses have implicated various individual or constellations of genes in virulence and host range restriction including those coding for VP2, VP4, VP7, NSP1, NSP2, and NSP4 (Offit *et al.*, 1986a; Broome *et al.*, 1993; McNeal *et al.*, 1994). The genetic basis of virulence and host range restriction is not clearly understood and different results have been obtained from several studies. These differences are probably dependent on the strains of virus used, the genetic background of the parental virus which can influence the folding of viral proteins, the virulence and replication efficiency of the parental strains, the parameter measured as a surrogate for virulence and host range restriction, and the model system in which the studies were performed. Currently these studies are limited to the use of reassortant viruses, as a genetic rescue system for rotavirus has not yet been developed.

2. *Primary Immune Responses in Piglets*

The immune response following a primary virulent or attenuated Wa inoculation and virulent Wa virus challenge also has been assessed in piglets (Saif *et al.*, 1996). The immune response to virus infection, measured by determining the number of antibody-secreting cells (ASC) and lymphoproliferative responses (LPA), is greatest in intestinal tissues compared to systemic sites. The number of IgA ASC and the LPA induced in the small intestine by the virulent virus is significantly greater than the immune response induced following inoculation with attenuated virus. The ratios of the numbers of rotavirus specific IgG to IgA ASC detected on the day of challenge vary depending on the inoculating virus. The virulent virus induces approximately equal numbers of IgG and IgA ASC, while the attenuated Wa virus induces approximately seven times more IgG than IgA ASC. Piglets inoculated with virulent virus are fully protected from homologous virus challenge and only low transient or no increases are observed in intestinal ASC or LPA responses. Piglets originally inoculated with avirulent virus only are partially protected from virulent Wa challenge and these pigs exhibit increased ASC (six- to seven-fold) and LPA responses (two- to four-fold) following challenge. Protection from rotavirus challenge appears to correlate with the level of the local immune response generated following the primary infection.

Supplemental feeding of bovine colostrum with high levels of rotavirus-neutralizing antibody to gnotobiotic piglets effectively prevents rotavirus diarrhea when piglets are challenged with virulent porcine or human viruses (Schaller *et al.*, 1992; Bridger and Brown, 1981). Although rotavirus diarrhea and virus shedding are greatly reduced or prevented following virus challenge, development of active immunity is observed, indicating that priming of active immune responses can occur in the presence of passively acquired antibodies. Whether the level of active immunity induced is sufficient to protect against a subsequent challenge has not been evaluated.

C. Studies of Rotavirus Immunity in the Mouse Model

Two separate mouse models, in neonatal and adult animals, have been utilized to study rotavirus immunity. Mice become maturationaly resistant to rotavirus diarrheal disease at approximately 15 days of age (Eydelloth *et al.*, 1984; Wolf *et al.*, 1981). Therefore, studies of the factors that regulate immunity to disease must use passively treated suckling mice. Passive immunity can be achieved either via immunization of the dam or passive transfer of cells, serum, or milk into pups (Mackow *et al.*, 1990; Offit and Clark, 1985; Offit and Dudzik, 1990; Dunn *et al.*, 1995; Fiore *et al.*, 1996; Matsui *et al.*, 1989; Offit *et al.*, 1986b,c; Andrew *et al.*, 1992). While the passive immunity model has provided useful information, it may not provide information of direct relevance to humans, where active viral immunity is required.

An active model of rotavirus immunity to infection using adult mice was first described in 1990 (Ward *et al.*, 1990b). Although adult mice do not develop diarrhea following rotavirus infection, they are susceptible to infection with several strains of murine rotavirus, shed virus, and mount an immune response. Virus shedding is of a slightly shorter duration but in comparable quantities and the immune responses seen in adult mice are qualitatively and quantitatively similar to those seen in suckling mice (Burns *et al.*, 1995; Ishida *et al.*, 1996). Of note, adult mice do not develop intestinal pathologic lesions, but they do have increased fluid accumulation in their small bowel during primary infection, and they develop complete and long-lasting immunity to rechallenge after primary infection with a murine virus (Table I) (Burns *et al.*, 1995). At least six distinct strains of murine rotavirus have been described which infect mice. To date, all these strains are G3 serotype with two distinct P [16,20] genotypes (P genotype designation based on classification in Estes, 1996) (Greenberg *et al.*, 1986; Dunn *et al.*, 1994; Sereno and Gorziglia, 1994; Ushijima *et al.*, 1995). Mice are susceptible to infection with some heterologous rotaviruses, but these infections are always semipermissive (see below) and do not efficiently spread from mouse to mouse (Ramig, 1988).

1. *Primary Immune Responses in Mice*

a. Cellular Immune Response. The mouse model has been used extensively to study the cytotoxic and T helper immune response to primary rotavirus infection, generally with heterologous, as opposed to homologous, infection (Bruce *et al.*, 1994; Franco *et al.*, 1993; Offit and Dudzik, 1989, 1990; Offit *et al.*, 1991a,b). Although not rigorously examined, it appears that cytotoxic responses are more readily detected in mice following heterologous rather than homologous infection. Whether this paradoxical observation is an artifact of the cytotoxicity assay systems employed or a fundamental difference in immune response remains to be elucidated.

Cytotoxic T lymphocytes (CTLs) generated after heterologous infection in mice are cross-reactive, MHC-restricted, and detectable among intraepithelial as well as systemic lymphocytes (Offit and Dudzik, 1989; Offit *et al.*, 1991a). The major target of CTLs appears to be located on VP7, but other proteins (VP6, VP3) may also serve as targets (Franco *et al.*, 1993, 1994; Offit *et al.*, 1991a). Early studies indicated that passively transferred immune CD8$^+$ T cells from mice immunized with baculovirus recombinant VP1, VP4, VP6, and VP7 or infected with rotavirus were capable of clearing chronic infection in SCID mice and preventing primary illness in suckling mice (Dharakul *et al.*, 1990, 1991; Offit and Dudzik, 1990). The role of actively induced CD8$^+$ T cells in preventing infection after primary exposure is less clear (see Section C.2).

b. Humoral Immune Response. The humoral immune response to rotavirus infection in mice has not been studied extensively. Serum and intestinal antibodies to rotavirus are present 5 to 7 days following primary infection of mice with murine virus (Eydelloth *et al.*, 1984; Feng *et al.*, 1994). The relative titers of both local and systemic immune responses induced after oral infection may differ significantly in homologous and heterolgous virus infections (Feng *et al.*, 1994). After primary infection with murine viruses a mucosal IgA response develops by 6 days postinfection, and this response, not the serum IgG response, correlates with decreased antigen excretion (Burns *et al.*, 1995; Ishida *et al.*, 1996). The local primary immune response to heterologous neonatal virus infection is long-lived ($\geq$ 1 year), with the greatest number of rotavirus-specific ASC in the lamina propria (Shaw *et al.*, 1993). These results are consistent with the enduring ($>$ 1–2 years) immunity to reinfection in the mouse following a single exposure to murine virus (Burns *et al.*, 1995; McNeal and Ward, 1995). Mice, as discussed above for rabbits, develop more complete and long-lasting immunity to reinfection than humans.

2. *Immune Effector Mechanisms Involved in Resolution of Primary Infection and Prevention of Reinfection*

The resolution of primary homologous rotavirus infection is dependent on immune mechanisms, since both SCID and RAG-2 knockout mice which both lack T and B cells become chronically infected after exposure to murine rotavirus. Early studies of nude mice indicated these animals resolve rotavirus infection normally (Eiden *et al.*, 1986). Recent reexamination of this model indicates that nude mice shed virus for 2 to 3 days longer than their heterozygous littermates, but primary infection is completely resolved (Franco, unpublished results). The mechanism governing this T-cell independent resolution of primary infection is currently under study.

To better evaluate the role of CD8$^+$ T cells in rotavirus immunity, rotavirus infection in β_2 microglobulin-deficient mice treated with anti-CD8 antibody to remove residual CD8$^+$ T-cell cytotoxic activity and congeneic C57BL/6 control mice was compared (Franco and Greenberg, 1995). CD8$^+$ T-cell deficient mice, like nude mice, have a slightly delayed resolution of primary rotavirus infection, but clearance is complete. Hence, CD8$^+$ T cells appear to play a role in clearance of primary infection but are not required for this function. CD8$^+$ T-cell-depleted mice, which had cleared primary infection, were completely immune to reinfection at 6–8 weeks after primary infection (Franco and Greenberg, 1995). This immunity correlated with high levels of IgA antirotavirus antibody in the feces of immune animals. These data indicate that $CD8^+$ T cells do not appear to play a significant role in the development of active protective immunity after homologous infection in the mouse.

To directly evaluate the role of antibody in rotavirus immunity, neonatal and adult J_HD or μMT knockout mice which are incapable of producing antibody (Chen *et al.*, 1993; Kitamura *et al.*, 1991) were infected with murine rotavirus (Franco and Greenberg, 1995; McNeal *et al.*, 1995). In general, J_HD mice resolved primary rotavirus infection in a manner identical to antibody-producing mice (Franco and Greenberg, 1995; McNeal *et al.*, 1995), although 2 animals out of 29 shed virus chronically (Franco and Greenberg, 1995). μMT mice failed to fully resolve virus shedding and chronically shed low levels of virus sporadically for up to 93 days following primary infection (McNeal *et al.*, 1995). When the J_HD or μMT mice were depleted of $CD8^+$ T cells, rotavirus was shed chronically (J_HD) or rotavirus shedding was significantly elevated (μMT), indicating the $CD8^+$ T cells were involved in resolution of primary infection of these antibody deficient animals. Since μMT and some J_HD mice shed rotavirus for a prolonged period, it appears as if an antibody response is also involved in the resolution of primary infection as well as protection from reinfection. Depletion of $CD8^+$ T cells in μMT mice prior to primary virus infection had little effect on virus shedding compared to nondepleted controls, indicating that a possible third immunological effector mechanism may play a role in resolution of virus shedding (McNeal *et al.*, 1995).

J_HD knockout mice, which had resolved primary infection were rechallenged 6–12 weeks later with homologous virus (Franco and Greenberg, 1995; McNeal *et al.*, 1995). All mice became reinfected, albeit at a somewhat lower level of shedding than nonimmune controls or compared to virus shedding following primary virus infection. Therefore complete resistance to reinfection is absolutely dependent on antibody (presumably IgA) and not on $CD8^+$ T cells.

3. *Studies of Active Vaccination in the Mouse Model*

Infection with murine rotavirus fully protects against subsequent homologous virus reinfection (Burns *et al.*, 1995). Since all the murine rotaviruses examined to date appear to have related VP7s, it is impossible to directly examine the role of G-serotype specific immunity in the mouse model of homologous infection. However, it is clear that infection of mice with a murine virus expressing one P genotype is associated with immunity against a second P genotype challenge in the context of shared G types (Burns *et al.*, 1995).

The nature of protective immunity following heterologous infection in mice has been studied (Feng *et al.*, 1994). Heterologous viruses vary considerably in their abilities to induce local immune responses in mice, with RRV (G3 P5[3], simian origin) and SA11 (G3 P[2], simian origin) appearing to be the most efficient. However, in all cases, heterologous infection is much less effective than homologous infection at stimulating a local humoral response (Feng *et al.*, 1994). The ability to stimulate a local response is not directly related to virulence since attenuated murine viruses are more immunogenic than virulent heterologous strains (Feng *et al.*, 1994). Protection after heterologous infection is directly correlated with fecal or serum IgA levels but not with serum IgG responses (Feng *et al.*, 1994; McNeal *et al.*, 1994). These preliminary studies indicate that it is either the ability of a virus to replicate efficiently in the intestine or the ability to induce greater local immunogenicity, rather than viral serotype, which is the primary determinant of protection following heterologous infection (Feng *et al.*, 1996; McNeal *et al.*, 1994).

Intraperitoneal immunization of mice with live or inactivated heterologous or homologous viruses induces protection from reinfection with murine virus (McNeal *et al.*, 1992). Recent studies indicate that both IgA and IgG rotavirus specific antibody-secreting cells are induced in the lamina propria following intramuscular immunization (Coffin *et al.*, 1995). Therefore, protection from challenge following parenteral immunization is likely mediated by induction of local antibodies in the intestine; the mechanism of local antibody induction following parenteral vaccination is currently unknown.

D. Conclusions from Studies of Rotavirus Immunity in the Animal Models

Animal models have provided many insights into rotavirus immunity and pathogenesis and will continue to be important in the future to provide further knowledge in these areas as well as to compare newly developed vaccines. We have learned that antibody (presumably local Ig) appears to be the primary determinant of protection, while both $CD8^+$ T cells and antibody are involved in mediating clearance of primary infection. Following rotavirus infection, induction of humoral immunity occurs very quickly. IgA, IgM, and neutralizing antibody are detected in feces within 3–6 days which generally coincides with the peak of virus shedding which then rapidly declines. In animal models, development of intestinal immune responses appears to correlate most closely with protection.

Additionally, it has been shown in animals that heterologous infection is a far less efficient stimulator of the local immune response and protective immunity than homologous infection. Although heterologous infection can induce complete protection against challenge, protection is dependent on large viral doses (10^7 pfu in the mouse) and small decreases in immunization dose lead to a considerable loss of immunogenicity. These observations appear relevant to current human vaccine trials and also emphasize the need to carefully monitor local as well as systemic immune responses in vaccinees.

The development of heterotypic protective immunity after oral heterologous immunization has been clearly demonstrated. In fact, local immunogenicity, rather than serotype specificity, of the immunizing heterologous virus appears to be a key determinant of protection in animal models. Previous conflicting evidence on heterotypic protection obtained in animal models is likely attributable to testing different virus strains, as inoculum or challenge viruses have distinct infectious doses and replication efficiencies. The relevance of these observations to current "Jennerian" vaccine trials needs to be determined. Whether the differences in immune responses to homologous and heterologous viruses are due simply to limited replication efficiency and antigen presentation, or to host factors that regulate the difference in immune response to homologous and heterologous infection, remains to be elucidated. If the differences are due to limited replication efficiency or host restriction of the heterologous vaccine virus strains, a better vaccine strategy for live orally administered vaccines will be to use attenuated human virus strains that are capable of efficient replication but have limited virulence. Production and characterization of such strains are in progress, but it remains unclear if an effective balance between attenuation, replication efficiency, and immunogenicity will be easily obtained for a human virus. If the differences in immune response to homologous and heterologous viruses are immune regulated, the degree of Th1 and Th2 activation to these different immunogens, as well as the anatomic location at which helper T-cell activation occurs, might vary. The genetic basis for differences in local immunogenicity between homologous and heterologous viruses is currently under study.

In the rabbit and mouse model, humoral immunity following one homologous rotavirus infection is long-lasting. In children, immunity is generally not long-lived unless children have been infected multiple times. These differences in responses in rotavirus naive animal models and children may be due to the presence of potentially interfering but not protective levels of antibodies in children at the time of rotavirus infection. These antibodies, of maternal origin in very young children or actively induced in older children, may interfere with development of a vigorous long-lived active immune response. Studies of the immune responses in antibody positive animals may help to understand the immune response in children.

Key questions which remain to be answered are whether protective efficacy in small animal models (protection from infection) will correlate with protection from diarrhea in the piglet model, and whether protection in any of the animal models will accurately predict vaccine efficacy in children. The results from all the animal models have already helped define a number of parameters of immunity and pathogenesis that were difficult to address in children. These studies also have provided important technical information that has been applied to studies in children. Research on new vaccine strategies is being tested first in animal models and results from the animal models will be used to determine which strategies will be pursued in the future. Utilization of the rabbit, piglet, and mouse models to study VLPs produced in baculovirus, DNA immunization, and recombinant rotaviral proteins is currently underway. Preliminary failures to induce protective immunity in mice using live recombinant expression vectors appear to be due to the difficulty of targeting immunity to the GI tract of the mouse with these vectors. The success of future strategies may be dependent, at least in part, on the ability of the immunization to induce antirotavirus antibody in the gastrointestinal tract. The availability of genetically altered mice with specific immune defects may help elucidate why different vaccine strategies succeed or fail.

Comparison of various vaccine strategies in small animal models and the piglet model will address the question of how protective efficacy in the infection models relates to protective efficacy in a disease model. Current and future predictions of efficacious formulations or strategies from results in animal models await testing in children.

V. New Approaches to Vaccines for Children

Rotavirus does not normally cause viremia or systemic disease; infection is limited to the apical villus epithelium of the intestinal mucosa. Destruction of this epithelium or the effects of a viral toxin or both, are associated with an especially severe dehydrating diarrhea. Therefore, induction of an immune response that is effective in protecting the intestine is necessary for prevention of disease. A number of possible rotavirus vaccine candidates have been or are currently being actively pursued (Table II). The first candidate vaccines for humans have been live attenuated vaccines (see Section III.A), and this approach has continued to be pursued, albeit with extensive modification. The use of inactivated or subunit vaccines administered parenterally or orally with microencapsulation show promise based on initial testing in the rabbit and mouse models.

TABLE II
Rotavirus Vaccine Candidates

Live-attenuated vaccines
Animal or human viruses
Animal/human virus reassortants
Inactivated vaccines
Subunit vaccines
Proteins from purified virus
Proteins synthesized from cloned genes
Proteins from high-yielding expression vectors
Proteins produced in the GI tract with live vectors
Virus-like particles from expressed proteins
Synthetic peptides
Nucleic acid vaccines

A. Inactivated Vaccines

1. Parenterally Administered Vaccine

Inactivated parenteral vaccines have been pursued due to (i) safety concerns with live attenuated vaccines, (ii) low efficacy of live-attenuated vaccines in the face of maternal antibody, (iii) the need to induce heterotypic immunity to rotavirus, but interference of replication observed with early multivalent live-attenuated formulations, (iv) early data from other pathogens indicating that parenteral vaccines can be efficacious, (v) the possibility that combined parenteral/oral vaccine would elicit higher immune responses and protection than an oral vaccine alone, and (vi) the majority of current childhood vaccines are administered parenterally.

Efficacy of inactivated vaccines was first seen when rabbits or mice were administered inactivated or live rotavirus intramuscularly or intraperitoneally, respectively (Conner *et al.*, 1993; McNeal *et al.*, 1992). Protection from live homologous virus challenge is observed in both species. Examination of intestinal isotype specific antibody responses in rabbits found no IgA in the intestine of any rabbit prior to challenge (Conner *et al.*, 1993). However, IgG antibodies were induced and appeared to have mediated protection. The levels of intestinal IgG antibody and protective efficacy induced by parenteral vaccination with inactivated virus appear to be dose dependent (M. E. Conner *et al.*, unpublished, 1994). Based on recent evidence in mice showing that both IgA and IgG ASC are present in the intestine following parenteral vaccination, it is possible that some or all the IgG detected in rabbits was locally produced (Coffin *et al.*, 1995). These results indicate that parenteral rotavirus vaccines either alone or with oral live or subunit vaccines may provide protection from rotavirus infection or disease.

B. Subunit Vaccines

To date, there has been little reported success inducing active immunity with individual proteins obtained from purified virus, high-yielding expression vectors, or with synthetic peptides (reviewed in Conner *et al.*, 1994b; Conner and Ramig, 1996). These immunogens have proven to be of limited immunogenicity or failed to induce active protective immunity. These disappointments presumably are because discontinuous epitopes are important in induction of protective immunity, and native folding of the proteins or peptides is not achieved with individual soluble rotavirus proteins or the recombinant vectors are not able to efficiently target to or stimulate the enteric immune system.

Promising results have been obtained with recombinant virus-like particles (VLPs) produced by coexpression of rotavirus proteins in eukaryotic cells. Most data are available for studies using VLPs made by coexpressing rotavirus proteins in insect cells infected with baculovirus recombinants (Estes *et al.*, 1987; Labbé *et al.*, 1991; Crawford *et al.*, 1994; Sabara *et al.*, 1991). Several potential advantages of this approach include (i) display of properly folded discontinuous epitopes, (ii) presentation of particulate antigens with enhanced targeting to and uptake by the mucosal immune system, (iii) adjuvants and delivery systems might not be needed with VLPs, and (iv) rotavirus VLPs might provide a delivery vehicle for other antigens to the intestinal tract. VLPs also provide a powerful tool both for molecular biology studies (Crawford *et al.*, 1994) and to decipher the role of individual proteins in induction of protection.

Evaluation of the potential of VLPs as a vaccine is in the early stages, and both parenteral and oral routes with different formulations of rotavirus proteins and adjuvants, is being pursued (Conner *et al.*, 1996a,c). G3 VP2/6/7 and VP2/4/6/7 VLPs administered parenterally to mice and rabbits induce both neutralizing and isotype-specific antibody responses in serum and the intestine, and rabbits are totally or partially protected from ALA rotavirus challenge (Conner *et al.*, 1994a,b,c). Studies to examine the use of rotavirus VLPs as a mucosal immunogen are ongoing and preliminary results indicate that oral inoculation of mice with rotavirus VP2/6/7 VLPs with cholera toxin induce both serologic and intestinal antibody responses (Conner *et al.*, 1996b,c). Future studies will optimize mucosal delivery of rotavirus VLPs. Studies with live-attenuated vaccines in children indicate a possible need for a multivalent vaccine. Several approaches to produce a multivalent VLP vaccine show promise, such as production of chimeric VLPs that display VP7s from two or more serotypes on the same VLP and expression of rotavirus VP7s that induce neutralizing antibody to homotypic and heterotypic rotavirus strains (Crawford *et al.*, 1994; Conner *et al.*, 1995). VLPs also have proven to be a highly effective immunogen for induction of maternal lactogenic antibody in cows (Fernandez *et al.*, 1996; Conner *et al.*, 1996a).

C. Targeted Delivery of Vaccines

Administration of oral live or inactivated virus or subunit vaccines is problematic if the vaccine formulation is not stable during passage through stomach acids and exposure to pepsins, intestinal bile salts, and proteases, or if there is limited targeting or uptake of the vaccine antigens by the GALT. Many strategies have been proposed to overcome these problems. These include encapsulation of vaccine immunogens which can (i) provide protection from harsh environments, (ii) deliver a particulate formulation of specified size to better target antigen to Peyer's patches, (iii) provide a sustained release of immunogen, (iv) possibly provide an adjuvant effect, and (v) decrease the effective vaccine dose. An aqueous-based system of charged film microcapsules has recently been shown to capture infectious or inactivated rotavirus particles, penetrate to and persist in the GALT after oral inoculation, deliver greater levels of rotavirus antigen to the GALT than when free virus is orally inoculated, and enhance the virus-specific immune response after oral or parenteral immunization (Offit *et al.*, 1994; Brown *et al.*, 1995; Khoury *et al.*, 1995). Oral administration of microencapsulated live or inactivated rotavirus has induced higher levels of serologic antibodies and intestinal IgA antibodies or lamina propria IgA ASC than comparable doses of free virus. Virus-specific immune responses were detected with as little as 0.35 μg of microencapsulated virus (Khoury *et al.*, 1995). Protective efficacy remains to be assessed following immunization with microencapsulated virus. Encapsulation may provide a means to induce higher levels of antibody to live-attenuated, inactivated, or subunit vaccines with smaller doses of immunogen.

D. Nucleic Acid Vaccines

Studies are underway to evaluate the efficacy of DNA immunization in the adult mouse rotavirus model (Herrmann *et al.*, 1996). Mice vaccinated with plasmids encoding murine VP6, VP4, or VP7 developed intestinal and serologic antibody and were protected from homologous virus challenge. These results are of interest because vaccination with the same proteins in vaccinia or adenovirus vectors did not induce active protective immunity.

E. Future Vaccine Approaches

Recent identification of a rotavirus nonstructural protein, NSP4, that acts as a viral enterotoxin may provide a novel approach to induce protection from clinical rotavirus disease (Ball *et al.*, 1996b). Induction of antibodies to NSP4 may be sufficient to induce protection from clinical disease without the need to induce antibodies to the structural proteins, or induction of antibodies to both NSP4 and the structural proteins may provide enhanced levels of protection than is seen with rotavirus alone.

An additional novel approach is the possible production of an edible rotavirus vaccine. One idea is to express antigens of the major pathogens afflicting the developing world in bananas. After the initial development stage, many countries could produce their own vaccines as bananas can be grown in most developing countries. Such vaccines would cost pennies per dose, as costly and technically advanced production facilities for standard vaccine manufacturing would not be needed. Proof of concept of this approach has been shown by testing recombinant Norwalk capsid antigen expressed in tobacco and potatoes. Mice fed such preparations showed both serum and intestinal antibody responses (Ball *et al.*, 1994, 1996a; Mason *et al.*, 1996).

VII. Summary and Conclusions

Since the first attempts at development of a rotavirus vaccine, our knowledge about rotavirus infection and immunity has rapidly expanded from the interplay of basic research in molecular biology, studies of pathogenesis and immunology in animal models, epidemiology and clinical-based research in human volunteers, and natural infections in children and vaccine trials. Following several modifications of the first approach of making a live-attenuated vaccine, two live-attenuated vaccines have shown efficacy (~70%) against severe dehydrating diarrhea in children and should be submitted for licensure soon. These vaccines may significantly reduce the number of severe cases of diarrhea in developed countries, but they will only reduce the deaths due to rotavirus if they are effective in developing countries and if they are available in such settings. Even if this happens, with a vaccine that is 70% effective there may still be as many as 300,000 deaths per year due to rotavirus. Therefore, development efforts toward better rotavirus vaccines should continue. Our understanding of rotavirus infection and immunity has increased greatly in the last several decades, but development of new and even more effective rotavirus vaccines will be dependent on our gaining a better understanding of rotavirus immunity and pathogenesis coupled with developments in mucosal immunology and vaccinology.

Acknowledgments

M.E.C. and M.K.E. were supported by Grants AI24998 and DK30144 from the NIH , MIMV2718130 from the WHO, and 004949-029 from the Advanced Technology Program of the Texas Higher Education Coordinating Board. P.A.O. was supported by Grant AI 26251 from the NIH. M.F., N.F., and H.B.G. were supported by Grants R37AI21632 and DK38707 from the NIH, by a grant from WHO, and by a V. A. Merit Review Grant. H.B.G. is a medical investigator at the Palo Alto Veterans Administration Medical Center. M.A.F. is funded by a Walter V. and Idun Berry fellowship.

References

Anderson, E. L., Belshe, R. B., Bartram, J., Crookshanks-Newman, F., Chanock, R. M., and Kapikian, A. Z. (1986). Evaluation of rhesus rotavirus vaccine (MMU 18006) in infants and young children. *J. Infect. Dis.* **153,** 823–831.

Andrew, M. E., Boyle, D. B., Coupar, B. E. H., Reddy, D., Bellamy, A. R., and Both, G. W. (1992). Vaccinia-rotavirus VP7 recombinants protect mice against rotavirus-induced diarrhoea. *Vaccine* **10,** 185–191.

Ball, J. M., Hardy, M. E., Barone, C., Conner, M. E., and Estes, M. K. (1994). Oral immunization of recombinant Norwalk virus particles. *Am. Soc. Virol. 13th Annu. Meeting* **W46–11,** 269 (abstract).

Ball, J. M., Estes, M. K., Hardy, M. E., Conner, M. E., Opekun, A. R., and Graham, D. Y. (1996a). Recombinant Norwalk virus-like particles as an oral vaccine. *Arch. Virol.* in press.

Ball, J. M., Tian, P., Zeng, C. Q., Morris, A., and Estes, M. K. (1996b). Age-dependent diarrhea is induced by a viral nonstructural glycoprotein. *Science* **272,** 101–104.

Bern, C., and Glass, R. I. (1994). Impact of diarrheal diseases worldwide. *In* "Viral Infections of the Gastrointestinal Tract" (A. Z. Kapikian, ed.), pp. 1–26. Dekker, New York.

Bernstein, D. I., Smith, V. E., Sander, D. S., Pax, K. A., Schiff, G. M., and Ward, R. L. (1990). Evaluation of WC3 rotavirus vaccine and correlates of protection in healthy infants. *J. Infect. Dis.* **162,** 1055–1062.

Bernstein, D. I., Sander, D. S., Smith, V. E., Schiff, G. M., and Ward, R. L. (1991). Protection from rotavirus reinfection: 2-Year prospective study. *J. Infect. Dis.* **164,** 277–283.

Bernstein, D. I., Glass, R. I., Rodgers, G., Davidson, B. L., and Sack, D. A. (1995). Evaluation of rhesus rotavirus monovalent and tetravalent reassortant vaccines in U.S. children. U.S. Rotavirus Vaccine Efficacy Group. *JAMA, J. Am. Med. Assoc.* **273,** 1191–1196.

Bishop, R. F., Davidson, G. P., Holmes, I. H., and Ruck, B. J. (1973). Virus particles in epithelial cells of duodenal mucosa from children with acute gastroenteritis. *Lancet* **2,** 1281–1283.

Bishop, R. F., Barnes, G. L., Cipriani, E., and Lund, J. S. (1983). Clinical immunity after neonatal rotavirus infection. A prospective longitudinal study in young children. *N. Engl. J. Med.* **309,** 72–76.

Bridger, J. C., and Brown, J. F. (1981). Development of immunity to porcine rotavirus in piglets protected from disease by bovine colostrum. *Infect. Immun.* **31,** 906–910.

Bridger, J. C., Woode, G. N., Jones, J. M., Flewett, T. H., Bryden, A. S., and Davies, H. (1975). Transmission of human rotaviruses to gnotobiotic piglets. *J. Med. Microbiol.* **8,** 565–569.

Broome, R. L., Vo, P. T., Ward, R. L., Clark, H. F., and Greenberg, H. B. (1993). Murine rotavirus genes encoding outer capsid proteins VP4 and VP7 are not major determinants of host range restriction and virulence. *J. Virol.* **67,** 2448–2455.

Brown, K. A., Moser, C. A., Speaker, T. J., Khoury, C. A., Kim, J. E., and Offit, P. A. (1995). Enhancement by microencapsulation of rotavirus-specific intestinal immune responses in mice assessed by enzyme-linked immunospot assay and intestinal fragment culture. *J. Infect. Dis.* **171,** 1334–1338.

Bruce, M. G., Campbell, I., Xiong, Y., Redmond, M., and Snodgrass, D. R. (1994). Recognition of rotavirus agents by mouse L3T4-positive T helper cells. *J. Gen. Virol.* **75,** 1859–1866.

Burns, J. W., Krishnaney, A. A., Vo, P. T., Rouse, R. V., Anderson, L. J., and Greenberg, H. B. (1995). Analyses of homologous rotavirus infection in the mouse model. *Virology* **207,** 143–153.

Chen, J., Trountine, M., Alt, F. W., Young, F., Kurahara, C., Loring, J. F., and Huszar, D. (1993). Immunoglobulin gene rearrangement in B cell deficient mice generated by targeted deletion of the J_H locus. *Int. Immunol.* **5,** 647–656.

Chiba, S., Yokoyama, T., Nakata, S., Morita, Y., Urasawa, T., Taniguchi, K., Urasawa, S., and Nakao, T. (1986). Protective effect of naturally acquired homotypic and heterotypic rotavirus antibodies. *Lancet* **2,** 417–421.

Chiba, S., Nakata, S., Ukae, S., and Adachi, N. (1993). Virological and serological aspects of immune resistance to rotavirus gastroenteritis. *Clin. Infect. Dis.* **16** (Suppl. 2), S117–S121.

Christy, C., Madore, H. P., Pichichero, M. E., Gala, C., Pincus, P., Vosefski, D., Hoshino, Y., Kapikian, A., and Dolin, R. (1988). Field trial of rhesus rotavirus vaccine in infants. *Pediatr. Infect. Dis. J.* **7,** 645–650.

Ciarlet, M., Estes, M. K., and Conner, M. E. (1996). Comparative amino acid sequence analysis of the outer capsid protein VP4 from four lapine strains reveals identity with genotype P[14] human rotaviruses. Submitted for publication.

Clark, H. F., and Offit, P. A. (1994). Rotavirus vaccines. *In* "Vaccines" (S. A. Plotkin and E. A. Mortiner, eds.), pp. 809–822. Saunders, Philadelphia, Pennsylvania.

Clark, H. F., Furukawa, T., Bell, L. M., Offit, P. A., Perrella, P. A., and Plotkin, S. A. (1986). Immune response of infants and children to low-passage bovine rotavirus (strain WC3). *Am. J. Dis. Child.* **140,** 350–356.

Clark, H. F., Borian, F. E., Bell, L. M., Modesto, K., Gouvea, V., and Plotkin, S. A. (1988). Protective effect of WC3 vaccine against rotavirus diarrhea in infants during a predominantly serotype 1 rotavirus season. *J. Infect. Dis.* **158,** 570–587.

Clark, H. F., Borian, F. E., Modesto, K., and Plotkin, S. A. (1990a). Serotype 1 reassortant of bovine rotavirus WC3, strain WI79- 9, induces a polytypic antibody response in infants. *Vaccine* **8,** 327–332.

Clark, H. F., Borian, F. E., and Plotkin, S. A. (1990b). Immune protection of infants against rotavirus gastroenteritis by a serotype 1 reassortant of bovine rotavirus WC3. *J. Infect. Dis.* **161**, 1099–1104.

Clark, H. F., Welsko, D., and Offit, P. A. (1992). Infant responses to bovine rotavirus WC3 reassortants containing human rotavirus VP7, VP4, or VP7 & VP4. *ICAAC* **1394**, 343 (abstract).

Clark, H. F., White, C. J., Offit, P. A., Stinson, D., Eiden, J., Weaver, S., Cho, I., Shaw, A., Drah, D., Ellis, R., and QHBRV Study Group. (1995). Preliminary evaluation of safety and efficacy of quadrivalent human–bovine reassortant rotavirus vaccine. *Pediatr. Res.* **37**, 122A

Clark, H. F., Offit, P. A., Ellis, R. W., Krah, D., Shaw, A. R., Eiden, J. J., Pichichero, M., and Treanor, J. J. (1996). WC3 reassortant vaccines in children—a brief review. *Arch. Virol.* in press.

Coffin, S. E., Klinek, M., and Offit, P. A. (1995). Induction of virus-specific antibody production by lamina propria lymphocytes following intramuscular inoculation with rotavirus. *J. Infect. Dis.* **172**, 874–878.

Conner, M. E., and Estes, M. K. (1994). Determination of the duration of a primary immune response and the ID_{50} of Ala rabbit rotavirus in rabbits. *Am. Soc. Virol. 13th Annu. Meeting* **W4–1**, 111 (abstract).

Conner, M. E., and Ramig, R. F. (1996). Enteric diseases. *In* "Viral Pathogenesis" (N. Nathanson, ed.), Raven, New York.

Conner, M. E., Estes, M. K., and Graham, D. Y. (1988). Rabbit model of rotavirus infection. *J. Virol.* **62**, 1625–1633.

Conner, M. E., Gilger, M. A., Estes, M. K., and Graham, D. Y. (1991). Serologic and mucosal immune response to rotavirus infection in the rabbit model. *J. Virol.* **65**, 2562–2571.

Conner, M. E., Crawford, S. E., Barone, C., and Estes, M. K. (1993). Rotavirus vaccine administered parenterally induces protective immunity. *J. Virol.* **67**, 6633–6641.

Conner, M.E., Crawford, S.E., Barone, C., and Estes, M.K. (1994a). Rotavirus or virus-like particles administered parenterally induce active immunity. *In* "Vaccines 94" (E. Norrby, F. Brown, and R. M. Chanock, eds.), p. 351. Cold Spring Harbor Laboratory, Cold Spring Harbor, New York.

Conner, M. E., Matson, D. O., and Estes, M. K. (1994b). Rotavirus vaccines and vaccination potential. *In* "Rotaviruses" (R. Ramig, ed.), pp. 286–337. Springer-Verlag, Berlin.

Conner, M. E., Crawford, S. E., Barone, C., Zhou, Y.-J., and Estes, M. K. (1995). Induction of heterotypic neutralizing antibodies by serotype G1 VLPs. (Abstract W2/04) Proceedings of the Fifth International Symposium on Double-Stranded RNA Viruses, March 19–23, 1995, Jerba, Tunisia.

Conner, M. E., Crawford, S. E., Barone, C., O'Neal, C., Zhou, Y.-J., Fernandez, F., Parwani, A., Saif, L. J., Cohen, J., and Estes, M. K. (1996a). Rotavirus subunit vaccines. *Arch. Virol.* in press.

Conner, M. E., Graham, D. Y., and Estes, M. K. (1996b). Determination of the duration of a primary immune response and the ID_{50} of ALA rabbit rotavirus in rabbits. Submitted for publication.

Conner, M. E., Zarley, D., Hu, B., Parsons, S., Drabinski, D., Greiner, S., Smith, R., Jiang, B., Corsaro, B., Barniak, V., Madore, H. P., Crawford, S. E., and Estes, M. K. (1996c). Virus-like particles (VLPs) as a rotavirus subunit vaccine. *J. Inf. Dis.*, in press.

Coulson, B. S., Grimwood, K., Masendycz, P. J., Lund, J. S., Mermelstein, N., Bishop, R. F., and Barnes, G. L. (1990). Comparison of rotavirus immunoglobulin A coproconversion with other indices of rotavirus infection in a longitudinal study in childhood. *J. Clin. Microbiol.* **28**, 1367–1374.

Coulson, B. S., Grimwood, K., Hudson, I. L., Barnes, G. L., and Bishop, R. F. (1992). Role of coproantibody in clinical protection of children during reinfection with rotavirus. *J. Clin. Microbiol.* **30**, 1678–1684.

Crawford, S. E., Labbe, M., Cohen, J., Burroughs, M. H., Zhou, Y.-J., and Estes, M. K. (1994). Characterization of virus-like particles produced by the expression of rotavirus capsid proteins in insect cells. *J. Virol.* **68**, 5945–5952.

Davidson, G. P., Gall, D. G., Petric, M., Butler, D. G., and Hamilton, J. R. (1977). Human rotavirus enteritis induced in conventional piglets. Intestinal structure and transport. *J. Clin. Invest.* **60**, 1402–1409.

Davidson, G. P., Hogg, R. J., and Kirubakaran, C. P. (1983). Serum and intestinal immune response to rotavirus enteritis in children. *Infect. Immun.* **40**, 447–452.

De Mol, P., Zissis, G., Butzler, J. P., Mutwewingabo, A., and Andre, F. E. (1986). Failure of live, attenuated oral rotavirus vaccine (letter). *Lancet* **2**, 108.

Dennehy, P. H. For the U.S. Rotavirus Vaccine Efficacy Group. (1994). Safety and efficacy of an oral tetravalent rhesus rotavirus vaccine (RRV-TV) in healthy infants. *Pediatr. Res.* **35**, 1052.

Dharakul, T., Rott, L., and Greenberg, H. B. (1990). Recovery from chronic rotavirus infection in mice with severe combined immunodeficiency: Virus clearance mediated by adoptive transfer of immune $CD8^+$ T lymphocytes. *J. Virol.* **64**, 4375–4382.

Dharakul, T., Labbe, M., Cohen, J., Bellamy, A. R., Street, J. E., Mackow, E. R., Fiore, L., Rott, L., and Greenberg, H. B. (1991). Immunization with baculovirus-expressed recombinant rotavirus proteins VP1, VP4, VP6, and VP7 induces $CD8^+$ T lymphocytes that mediate clearance of chronic rotavirus infection in SCID mice. *J. Virol.* **65**, 5928–5932.

Dunn, S. J., Burns, J. W., Cross, T. I., Vo, P. T., Ward, R. L., Bremont, M., and Greenberg, H. (1994). Comparisons of VP4 and VP7 of five murine rotavirus strains. *Virology* **203**, 250–259.

Dunn, S. J., Fiore, L., Werner, R. L., Cross, T. L., Broome, R. L., Ruggeri, F. M., and Greenberg, H. B. (1995). Immunogenicity, antigenicity and protective efficacy of baculovirus expressed VP4 trypsin cleavage products, VP5(1)* and VP8* from rhesus rotavirus. *Arch. Virol.* **140**(11), 1969–1978.

Eiden, J., Lederman, H. M., Vonderfecht, S., and Yolken, R. (1986). T-cell-deficient mice display normal recovery from experimental rotavirus infection. *J. Virol.* **57**, 706–708.

Estes, M. K. (1996). Rotaviruses and their replication. *In*

"Fields Virology" (B. N. Fields, D. M. Knipe, P. M. Howley, and *et al.*, eds.), 3rd Ed., pp. 1625–1655. Lippincott–Raven, Philadelphia, Pennsylvania.

Estes, M. K., Crawford, S. E., Penaranda, M. E., Petrie, B. L., Burns, J. W., Chan, W. K., Ericson, B., Smith, G. E., and Summers, M. D. (1987). Synthesis and immunogenicity of the rotavirus major capsid antigen using a baculovirus expression system. *J. Virol.* **61,** 1488–1494.

Estes, M. K., Conner, M. E., Gilger, M. A., and Graham, D. Y. (1989). Molecular biology and immunology of rotavirus infections. *Immunol. Invest.* **18,** 571–581.

Eydelloth, R. S., Vonderfecht, S. L., Sheridan, J. F., Enders, L. D., and Yolken, R. H. (1984). Kinetics of viral replication and local and systemic immune responses in experimental rotavirus infection. *J. Virol.* **50,** 947–950.

Feng, N., Burns, J. W., Bracy, L., and Greenberg, H. (1994). Comparison of mucosal and systemic humoral immune responses and subsequent protection in mice orally inoculated with a homologous or a heterologous rotavirus. *J. Virol.* **68,** 7766–7773.

Feng, N., Vo, P. T., Chung, D., Vo, T.-V. P., Hoshino, Y., and Greenberg, H. B. (1996). Heterotypic protection following oral immunization with live heterologous rotavirus in a mouse model. Submitted for publication.

Fernandez, F. M., Conner, M. E., Parwani, A. V., Todhunter, D., Smith, K. L., Crawford, S. E., Estes, M. K., and Saif, L. J. (1996). Isotype-specific antibody responses to rotavirus and virus proteins in cows inoculated with subunit vaccines comprised of recombinant SA11 rotavirus core-like particles (CLP) or virus-like particles (VLP). *Vaccine,* in press.

Fiore, L., Dunn, S. J., Ridolfi, B., Ruggeri, M., Mackow, E. R., and Greenberg, H. B. (1995). Antigenicity, immunogenicity, and passive protection induced by immunization with the baculovirus-expressed VP7 protein from rhesus rotavirus. *J. Gen. Virol.* **76**(8), 1981–1988.

Flores, J., Perez-Schael, I., Blanco, M., White, L., Garcia, D., Vilar, M., Cunto, W., Gonzalez, R., Urbina, C., Boher, J., Mendez, M., and Kapikian, A. Z. (1990). Comparison of reactogenicity and antigenicity of M37 rotavirus vaccine and rhesus-rotavirus-based quadrivalent vaccine. *Lancet* **336,** 330–334.

Flores, J., Perez-Schael, I., Blanco, M., Rojas, A. M., Alfonzo, E., Crespo, I., Cunto, W., Pittman, A. L., and Kapikian, A. Z. (1993). Reactogenicity and immunogenicity of a high-titer rhesus rotavirus-based quadrivalent rotavirus vaccine. *J. Clin. Microbiol.* **31,** 2439–2445.

Franco, M. A., and Greenberg, H. B. (1995). Role of B cells and cytotoxic T lymphocytes in clearance of and immunity to rotavirus infection in mice. *J. Virol.* **69,** 7800–7806.

Franco, M. A., Prieto, I., Labbe, M., Poncet, D., Borras-Cuesta, F., and Cohen, J. (1993). An immunodominant cytotoxic T cell epitope on the VP7 rotavirus protein overlaps the H2 signal peptide. *J. Gen. Virol.* **74,** 2579–2586.

Franco, M. A., Lefevre, P., Willems, P., Tosser, G., Lintermanns, P., and Cohen, J. (1994). Identification of cytotoxic T cell epitopes on the VP3 and VP6 rotavirus proteins. *J. Gen. Virol.* **75,** 1–8.

Georges-Courbot, M. C., Monges, J., Siopathis, M. R., Roungou, J. P., Gresenguet, A., Bellec, L., Bouquety, I. C., Lanckviet, C., Cadoz, M., Hesel, L., Gouvea, G., Clark, H. F., and Georges, A. I. (1991). Evaluation of the efficacy of a low passage bovine rotavirus (strain WC3) vaccine in children in Central Africa. *Res. Virol.* **142,** 405–411.

Gilger, M. A., Conner, M. E., Estes, M. K., and Graham, D. Y. (1988). Effect of rotavirus infection on rabbit small intestinal structure. *Gastroenterology* **94,** A-146.

Glass, R. I., Gentsch, J., and Smith, J. C. (1994). Rotavirus vaccines: Success by reassortment? *Science* **265,** 1389–1391.

Gothefors, L., Wadell, G., Juto, P., Taniguchi, K., Kapikian, A. Z., and Glass, R. I. (1989). Prolonged efficacy of rhesus rotavirus vaccine in Swedish children. *J. Infect. Dis.* **159,** 753–757.

Greenberg, H. B., Vo, P. T., and Jones, R. (1986). Cultivation and characterization of three strains of murine rotavirus. *J. Virol.* **57,** 585–590.

Grimwood, K., Lund, J. C., Coulson, B. S., Hudson, I. L., Bishop, R. F., and Barnes, G. L. (1988). Comparison of serum and mucosal antibody responses following severe acute rotavirus gastroenteritis in young children. *J. Clin. Microbiol.* **26,** 732–738.

Hanlon, P., Hanlon, L., Marsh, V., Byass, P., Shenton, F., Hassan-King, M., Jobe, O., Sillah, H., Hayes, R., M'Boge, B. H., Whittle, H. C., and Greenwood, B. M. (1987). Trial of an attenuated bovine rotavirus vaccine (RIT 4237) in Gambian infants. *Lancet* **1,** 1342–1345.

Herrmann, J. E., Chen, S. C., Fynan, E. F., Santoro, J. C., Greenberg, H. B., and Robinson, H. L. (1996). DNA vaccines against rotavirus infections. *Arch. Virol.* in press.

Hoshino, Y., Wyatt, R. G., Greenberg, H. B., Flores, J., and Kapikian, A. Z. (1984). Serotypic similarity and diversity of rotaviruses of mammalian and avian origin as studied by plaque-reduction neutralization. *J. Infect. Dis.* **149,** 694–702.

Hoshino, Y., Saif, L. J., Sereno, M. M., Chanock, R. M., and Kapikian, A. Z. (1988). Infection immunity of piglets to either VP3 or VP7 outer capsid protein confers resistance to challenge with a virulent rotavirus bearing the corresponding antigen. *J. Virol.* **62,** 744–748.

Hoshino, Y., Saif, L. J., Kang, S.-Y., Sereno, M. M., Chen, W.-K., and Kapikian, A. Z. (1995). Identification of group A rotavirus genes associated with virulence of a porcine rotavirus and host range restriction of a human rotavirus in the gnotobiotic piglet model. *Virology* **209,** 274–280.

Institute of Medicine (1986). Prospects for immunizing against rotavirus. *In* "New Vaccine Development. Establishing Priorities. Diseases of Importance in Developing Countries," Vol. 2, pp. 308–318. National Academy Press, Washington, D.C.

Ishida, S.-I., Feng, N., Tang, B., Gilbert, J. M., and Greenberg, H. B. (1996). Quantification of the systemic and local immune responses to individual rotavirus proteins during rotavirus infection in mice. *J. Clin. Microbiol.* **34,** 1694–1700.

Kapikian, A. Z., Hoshino, Y., Chanock, R. M., and Perez-Schael, I. (1996). Jennerian and modified Jennerian approach to vaccination against rotavirus diarrhea using a quadrivalent rhesus rotavirus (RRV) and human-RRV reassortant vaccine. *Arch. Virol.* in press

Khoury, C. A., Moser, C. A., Speaker, T. J., and Offit, P. A. (1995). Oral inoculation of mice with low doses of microencapsulated, noninfectious rotavirus induces virus-specific antibodies in gut-associated lymphoid tissue. *J. Infect. Dis.* **172,** 870–874.

Kitamura, D., Roes, J., Kuhn, R., and Rajewsky, K. (1991). A B cell-deficient mouse by targeted disruption of the membrane exon of the immunoglobulin μ chain gene. *Nature (London)* **350,** 423–426.

Labbé, M., Charpilienne, A., Crawford, S. E., Estes, M. K., and Cohen, J. (1991). Expression of rotavirus VP2 produces empty corelike particles. *J. Virol.* **65,** 2946–2952.

Lanata, C. F., Black, R. E., Aguila, R., Erel, A., Verastegui, H., Gerna, G., Dlores, J., Kapikian, A. Z., and Andre, F. E. (1989). Protection of Peruvian children against rotavirus diarrhea of specific serotypes by one, two, or three dosages of the RIT 4237 attenuated bovine rotavirus vaccine. *J. Infect. Dis.* **159,** 452–459.

Lanata, C. F., Black, R. E., Burton, B., Midthun, K., and Davidson, B. (1990). Safety, immunogenicity, and efficacy of one or three doses of the rhesus tetravalent rotavirus vaccine in Lima, Peru. *Vaccine* **10,** 273.

Losonsky, G. A., Rennels, M. B., Kapikian, A. Z., Midthun, K., Ferra, P. J., Fortier, D. N., Hoffman, K. M., Baig, A., and Levine, M. M. (1986). Safety, infectivity, transmissibility and immunogenicity of rhesus rotavirus vaccine (MMU 18006) in infants. *Pediatr. Infect. Dis.* **5,** 25–29.

Losonsky, G. A., Rennels, M. B., Lim, Y., Krall, G., Kapikian, A. Z., and Levine, M. M. (1988). Systemic and mucosal immune responses to rhesus rotavirus vaccine MMU 18006. *Pediatr. Infect. Dis. J.* **7,** 388–393.

Mackow, E. R., Vo, P. T., Broome, R., Bass, D., and Greenberg, H. B. (1990). Immunization with baculovirus-expressed VP4 protein passively protects against simian and murine rotavirus challenge. *J. Virol.* **64,** 1698–1703.

McNeal, M. M., and Ward, R. L. (1995). Long-term production of rotavirus antibody and protection against reinfection following a single infection of neonatal mice with murine rotavirus. *Virology* **211,** 474–480.

McNeal, M. M., Sheridan, J. F., and Ward, R. L. (1992). Active protection against rotavirus infection of mice following intraperitoneal immunization. *Virology* **191,** 150–157.

McNeal, M. M., Broome, R. L., and Ward, R. L. (1994). Active immunity against rotavirus infection in mice is correlated with viral replication and titers of serum rotavirus IgA following vaccination. *Virology* **204,** 642–650.

McNeal, M. M., Barone, K. S., Rae, M. N., and Ward, R. L. (1995). Effector functions of antibody and $CD8^+$ cells in resolution of rotavirus infection and protection against reinfection in mice. *Virology* **214,** 387–397.

Madore, H. P., Christy, C., Pichichero, M., Long, C., Pincus, P., Vosefsky, D., Kapikian, A. Z., Dolin, R., and Elmwood, P. (1992). Field trial of rhesus rotavirus or human–rhesus rotavirus reassortant vaccine of VP7 serotype 3 or 1 specificity in infants. *J. Infect. Dis.* **166,** 235–243.

Mason H. S., Ball, J. M., Shi, J.-J., Jiang, X., Estes, M. K., and Arntzen, C. A. (1996). Expression of Norwalk virus capsid protein in transgenic tobacco and potato and its oral immunogenicity in mice. *Proc. Natl. Acad. Sci. U.S.A.* **93,** 5335–5340.

Matson, D. O., and Estes, M. K. (1990). Impact of rotavirus infection at a large pediatric hospital. *J. Infect. Dis.* **162,** 598–604.

Matson, D. O., O'Ryan, M., Herrera, I., Pickering, L., and Estes, M. K. (1993). Fecal antibody responses to symptomatic and asymptomatic rotavirus infections. *J. Infect. Dis.* **167,** 577–583.

Matson, D. O., Velazquez, F. R., Calva, J. J., Morrow, A. L., Lourdes Guerrero, L., Shults, J. N., Estes, M. K., Carter-Campbell, S., Glass, R. I., Pickering, L. K., and Ruiz-Palacios, G. M. (1996). Protective immunity against group A rotavirus infection and illness in infants. *Arch. Virol.* in press.

Matsui, S. M., Offit, P. A., Vo, P. T., Mackow, E. R., Benfield, D. A., Shaw, R. D., Padilla-Noriega, L., and Greenberg, H. B. (1989). Passive protection against rotavirus-induced diarrhea by monoclonal antibodies to the heterotypic neutralization domain of VP7 and the VP8 fragment of VP4. *J. Clin. Microbiol.* **27,** 780–782.

Matsuno, S., Murakami, S., Takagi, M., Hayashi, M., Inouye, S., Hasegawa, A., and Fukai, K. (1987). Cold-adaptation of human rotavirus. *Virus Res.* **7,** 273–280.

Mebus, C. A., Wyatt, R. G., Sharpee, R. L., Sereno, M. M., Kalica, A. R., Kapikian, A. Z., and Twiehaus, M. J. (1976). Diarrhea in gnotobiotic calves caused by the reovirus-like agent of human infantile gastroenteritis. *Infect. Immun.* **14,** 471–474.

Midthun, K., Pang, L. Z., Flores, J., and Kapikian, A. Z. (1989). Comparison of immunoglobulin A (IgA), IgG, and IgM enzyme-linked immunosorbent assays, plaque reduction neutralization assay, and complement fixation in detecting seroresponses to rotavirus vaccine candidates. *J. Clin. Microbiol.* **27,** 2799–2804.

Midthun, K., Halsey, N. A., Jett-Goheen, M., Clements, M. L., Steinhoff, M., King, J. C., Karron, R., Wilson, M., Burns, B., Perkis, V., Samorodin, R., and Kapikian, A. Z. (1991). Safety and immunogenicity of human rotavirus vaccine strain M37 in adults, children, and infants. *J. Infect. Dis.* **164,** 792–796.

Nishikawa, K., Hoshino, Y., Taniguchi, K., Green, K. Y., Greenberg, H. B., Kapikian, A. Z., Chanock, R. M., and Gorziglia, M. (1989). Rotavirus VP7 neutralization epitopes of serotype 3 strains. *Virology* **171,** 503–515.

O'Ryan, M., Matson, D., Estes, M., and Pickering, L. (1994). Anti-rotavirus G type-specific and isotype-specific antibodies in children with natural rotavirus infection. *J. Infect. Dis.* **169,** 504–511.

Offit, P. A., and Clark, H. F. (1985). Protection against rotavirus-induced gastroenteritis in a murine model by passively acquired gastrointestinal but not circulating antibodies. *J. Virol.* **54,** 58–64.

Offit, P. A., and Dudzik, K. I. (1989). Rotavirus-specific cytotoxic T lymphocytes appear at the intestinal mucosal surface after rotavirus infection. *J. Virol.* **63,** 3507–3512.

Offit, P. A., and Dudzik, K. I. (1990). Rotavirus-specific cytotoxic T lymphocytes passively protect against gastroenteritis in suckling mice. *J. Virol.* **64,** 6325–6328.

Offit, P. A., Blavat, G., Greenberg, H. B., and Clark, H. F. (1986a). Molecular basis of rotavirus virulence: Role of gene segment 4. *J. Virol.* **57,** 46–49.

Offit, P. A., Clark, H. F., Blavat, G., and Greenberg, H. B. (1986b). Reassortant rotaviruses containing structural proteins VP3 and VP7 from different parents induce antibodies protective against each parental serotype. *J. Virol.* **60,** 491–496.

Offit, P. A., Shaw, R. D., and Greenberg, H. B. (1986c). Passive protection against rotavirus-induced diarrhea by monoclonal antibodies to surface proteins VP3 and VP7. *J. Virol.* **58,** 700–703.

Offit, P. A., Boyle, D. B., Both, G. W., Hill, N. L., Svoboda, Y. M., Cunningham, S. L., Jenkins, R. J., and McCrae, M. A. (1991a). Outer capsid glycoprotein VP7 is recognized by cross-reactive, rotavirus-specific, cytotoxic T lymphocytes. *Virology* **184,** 563–568.

Offit, P. A., Cunningham, S. L., and Dudzik, K. I. (1991b). Memory and distribution of virus-specific cytotoxic T lymphocytes (CTLs) and CTL precursors after rotavirus infection. *J. Virol.* **65,** 1318–1324.

Offit, P. A., Khoury, C. A., Moser, C. A., Clark, H. F., Kim, J. E., and Speaker, T. J. (1994). Enhancement of rotavirus immunogenicity by microencapsulation. *Virology* **203,** 134–143.

Perez-Schael, I., Gonzalez, M., Daoud, N., Perez, M., Soto, I., Garcia, D., Daoud, G., Kapikian, A. Z., and Flores, J. (1987). Reactogenicity and antigenicity of the rhesus rotavirus vaccine in Venezuelan children. *J. Infect. Dis.* **155,** 334–338.

Perez-Schael, I., Blanco, M., Vilar, M., Garcia, D., White, L., Gonzalez, R., Kapikian, A. Z., and Flores, J. (1990). Clinical studies of a quadrivalent rotavirus vaccine in Venezuelan infants. *J. Clin. Microbiol.* **28,** 553–558.

Ramig, R. F. (1988). The effects of host age, virus dose, and virus strain on heterologous rotavirus infection of suckling mice. *Microbial Pathogen.* **4,** 189–202.

Sabara, M., Parker, M., Aha, P., Cosco, C., Gibbons, E., Parsons, S., and Babiuk, L. A. (1991). Assembly of double-shelled rotaviruslike particles by simultaneous expression of recombinant VP6 and VP7 proteins. *J. Virol.* **65,** 6994–6997.

Sack, P. (1992). Efficacy of rhesus rotavirus monovalent or tetravalent oral vaccines in U.S. children. *ICAAC* p. 344 (abstract).

Saif, L. J., Rosen, B. I., and Parwani, A. V. (1994). Animal rotaviruses. *In* "Viral Infections of the Gastrointestinal Tract" (A. Z. Kapikian, ed.), 2nd Ed., pp. 279–367. Dekker, New York.

Saif, L. J., Ward, L. A., Yuan, L., Rosen, B. I., and To, T. L. (1996). The gnotobiotic piglet as a model for studies of disease pathogenesis and immunity to human rotaviruses. *Arch. Virol.* in press.

Santosham, M., Letson, G. W., Wolff, M., Reid, R., Gahagan, S., Adams, R., Callahan, C., Sack, R. B., and Kapikian, A. Z. (1991). A field study of the safety and efficacy of two candidate rotavirus vaccines in a native American population. *J. Infect. Dis.* **163,** 483–487.

Schaller, J. P., Saif, L. J., Cordle, C. T., Candler, E., Winship, T. R., and Smith, K. L. (1992). Prevention of human rotavirus-induced diarrhea in gnotobiotic piglets using bovine antibody. *J. Infect. Dis.* **165,** 623–630.

Sereno, M. M., and Gorziglia, M. I. (1994). The outer capsid protein VP4 of murine rotavirus strain Eb represents a tentative new P type. *Virology* **199,** 500–504.

Shaw, R. D., Merchant, A. A., Groene, W. S., and Cheng, E. H. (1993). Persistence of intestinal antibody response to heterologous rotavirus infection in a murine model beyond 1 year. *J. Clin. Microbiol.* **31,** 188–191.

Smith, J. C., Haddix, A. C., Teutsch, S. M., and Glass, R. I. (1995). Cost-effectiveness analysis of a rotavirus immunization program for the United States. *Pediatrics* **96,** 609–615.

Snodgrass, D. R., Fitzgerald, T. A., Campbell, I., Browning, G. F., Scott, F. M. M., Hoshino, Y., and Davies, R. C. (1991). Homotypic and heterotypic serological responses to rotavirus neutralization epitopes in immunologically naive and experienced animals. *J. Clin. Microbiol.* **29,** 2668–2672.

Stuker, G., Oshiro, L. S., and Schmidt, N. J. (1980). Antigenic comparisons of two new rotaviruses from rhesus monkeys. *J. Clin. Microbiol.* **11,** 202–203.

Tanaka, T. N., Conner, M. E., Graham, D. Y., and Estes, M. K. (1988). Molecular characterization of three rabbit rotavirus strains. *Arch. Virol.* **98,** 253–265.

Thouless, M. E., DiGiacomo, R. F., and Neuman, D. S. (1986). Isolation of two lapine rotaviruses: Characterization of their subgroup, serotype and RNA electropherotypes. *Arch. Virol.* **89,** 161–170.

Thouless, M. E., DiGiacomo, R. F., Deeb, B. J., and Howard, H. (1988). Pathogenicity of rotavirus in rabbits. *J. Clin. Microbiol.* **26,** 943–947.

Torres-Medina, A., Wyatt, R. G., Mebus, C. A., Underdahl, N. R., and Kapikian, A. Z. (1976). Diarrhea caused in gnotobiotic piglets by the reovirus-like agent of human infantile gastroenteritis. *J. Infect. Dis.* **133,** 22–27.

Treanor, J. J., Clark, H. F., Pichichero, M., Christy, C., Gouvea, V., Shrager, D., Palazzo, S., and Offit, P. (1995). Evaluation of the protective efficacy of a serotype 1 bovine-human rotavirus reassortant vaccine in infants. *Pediatr. Infect. Dis. J.* **14,** 301–307.

Ushijima, H., Morikawa, S., Hasegawa, A., Mukoyama, A., Suzuki, E., Yamamoto, T., and Nishio, O. (1995). Characterization of VP4 and VP7 of murine rotavirus (YR-1) isolated in Japan. Proceedings of the Fifth International Symposium on Double-Stranded RNA Viruses, March 19–23, 1995, Jerba, Tunisia.

Vesikari, T. (1994). Bovine rotavirus-based rotavirus vaccines in humans. *In* "Viral Infections of the Gastrointestinal Tract" (A. Z. Kapikian, ed.), pp. 419–442. Dekker, New York.

Vesikari T. (1996). Trials of oral bovine and rhesus rotavirus vaccines in Finland: an historical account and present status. *Arch. Virol.* in press.

Vesikari, T., Isolauri, E., Delem, A., D'Hondt, E., Andre, F. E., and Zissis, G. (1983). Immunogenicity and safety of live oral attenuated bovine rotavirus vaccine strain RIT 4237 in adults and young children. *Lancet* **2**, 807–811.

Vesikari, T., Ruuska, T., Bogaerts, H., Delem, A., and Andre, F. (1985). Dose-response study of RIT 4237 oral rotavirus vaccine in breast-fed and formula-fed infants. *Pediatr. Infect. Dis.* **4**, 622–625.

Vesikari, T., Kapikian, A. Z., Delem, A., and Zissis, G. (1986). A comparative trial of rhesus monkey (RRV-1) and bovine (RIT 4237) oral rotavirus vaccines in young children. *J. Infect. Dis.* **153**, 832–839.

Vesikari, T., Rautanen, T., Varis, T., Beards, G. M., and Kapikian, A. Z. (1990). Clinical trial in children vaccinated between 2 and 5 months of age. *Am. J. Dis. Child.* **144**, 285–289.

Vesikari, T., Ruuska, T., Koivu, H.-P., Green, K. Y., Flores, J., and Kapikian, A. Z. (1991). Evaluation of the M37 human rotavirus vaccine in 2- to 6- month-old infants. *Pediatr. Infect. Dis. J.* **10**, 912–917.

Vesikari, T., Ruuska, T., Green, K. Y., Flores, J., and Kapikian, A. Z. (1992). Protective efficacy against serotype 1 rotavirus diarrhea by live oral rhesus–human reassortant rotavirus vaccines with human rotavirus VP7 serotype 1 or 2 specificity. *Pediatr. Infect. Dis. J.* **11**, 535–542.

Ward, R., and Bernstein, D. (1994). Protection against rotavirus disease after natural rotavirus infection. *J. Infect. Dis.* **169**, 900–904.

Ward, R. L., Knowlton, D. R., Greenberg, H. B., Schiff, G. M., and Bernstein, D. I. (1990a). Serum-neutralizing antibody to VP4 and VP7 proteins in infants following vaccination with WC3 bovine rotavirus. *J. Virol.* **64**, 2687–2691.

Ward, R. L., McNeal, M. M., and Sheridan, J. F. (1990b). Development of an adult mouse model for studies on protection against rotavirus. *J. Virol.* **64**, 5070–5075.

Wolf, J. L., Cukor, G., Blacklow, N. R., Dambrauskas, R., and Trier, J. S. (1981). Susceptibility of mice to rotavirus infection: Effects of age and administration of corticosteroids. *Infect. Immun.* **33**, 565–574.

Wyatt, R. G., James, W. D., Bohl, E. H., Theil, K. W., Saif, L. J., Kalica, A. R., Greenberg, H. B., Kapikian, A. Z., and Chanock, R. M. (1980). Human rotavirus type 2: Cultivation *in vitro*. *Science* **207**, 189–191.

26

Rotavirus Vaccine: The Clinical Experience with the Rhesus Rotavirus-Based Vaccines

Albert Z. Kapikian
Epidemiology Section, Laboratory of Infectious Diseases
National Institute of Allergy and Infectious Diseases
National Institutes of Health
Bethesda, Maryland 20892

I. Introduction: Importance of Rotavirus as a Cause of Diarrhea

Although diarrheal illnesses have been described since the dawn of recorded history, their etiology remained largely unknown until relatively recently (Kumate and Isibasi, 1986). Although bacterial agents were implicated as the cause of diarrheal illness in selected situations, the vast majority of these illnesses could not be ascribed to any etiologic agent until the early 1970s when two new groups of viruses were discovered: (i) the 27-nm Norwalk agent in 1972 (Kapikian *et al.*, 1972), which, along with related viruses, has emerged as a major cause of epidemic gastroenteritis of adults and older children (Kapikian *et al.*, 1996); and (ii) the 70-nm rotavirus in 1973 (Bishop *et al.*, 1973), which is now recognized as the single most important cause of severe diarrheal illnesses in infants and young children both in developed and developing countries, accounting for 35–50% of them (Kapikian and Chanock, 1996). The relative importance of these and other agents as a cause of severe diarrhea in infants and young children in developed and developing countries is shown in Fig. 1.

In contrast to many other enteric agents, rotaviruses can be considered to be rather egalitarian in an epidemiologic sense, as evidenced by incidence and prevalence data available from various settings: (i) about 90% of infants and young children develop rotavirus infections regardless of economic status or hygienic standards (Kapikian and Chanock, 1996); (ii) 3.5 million episodes of rotavirus gastroenteritis are estimated to occur annually in infants and young children in the United States, a risk of 1:1.2 per child per year, while in developing countries the annual number of such episodes is estimated to be 130 million, a risk of 1:1.1 per child (Glass *et al.*, 1994); (iii) in the United States, about 500,000 doctor visits are made annually because of rotavirus gastroenteritis, a risk of 1:8 per child per year, while in the developing countries approximately 18 million episodes of moderate to severe gastroenteritis occur, for a similar risk of 1:8 per child per year (Glass *et al.*, 1994). Although the rates of rotavirus infection are comparable in these disparate environmental settings, the consequences of such infections are radically different with regard to mortality: in developing countries, more than 870,000 infants and young children less than 5 years of age die because of rotavirus-associated illness annually (Institute of Medicine, 1986b), a risk of 1:160 per child, whereas in the United States 75–150 children in this same age group die because of such illness annually (Institute of Medicine, 1986a; Ho *et al.*, 1988; Glass *et al.*, 1994), a risk of 1:40,000 per child (Glass *et al.*, 1994). A major factor responsible for this striking difference in the mortality rate is attributed to the lack of adequate health care in poor areas of the world.

II. Rotavirus Vaccine Development

Because rotaviruses are an important cause of morbidity in developed countries and a major cause of mortality in developing countries, the need for a rotavirus vaccine has received international attention and support (World Health Organization, 1980). Although it became clear soon after their discovery that rotaviruses were indeed the long sought-after major etiologic agents of severe diarrhea of infants and young children, efforts to develop a vaccine were not feasible because of the inability to propagate them efficiently in cell culture. Indeed, the first bona fide cultivation of human rotavirus was accomplished by the passage of a rotavirus particle positive

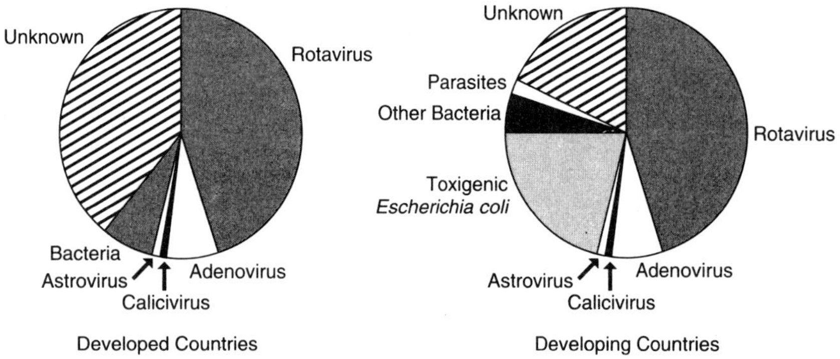

Figure 1. An estimate of the role of etiological agents in severe diarrheal illnesses requiring hospitalization of infants and young children in developed countries (left) and in developing countries (right). From Kapikian (1993).

human stool suspension (strain Wa) 11 times sequentially in gnotobiotic piglets, followed by passage and recovery of a mutant that grew efficiently in monkey kidney cell cultures (Wyatt *et al.*, 1980). With later modifications, rotaviruses could be grown in tissue culture directly from clinical specimens with relative ease (Sato *et al.*, 1980; Urasawa *et al.*, 1981), further spurring the quest for a vaccine. Later, the Wa strain was considered as a vaccine candidate and was administered to adult volunteers in Phase I safety and antigenicity studies (Kapikian *et al.*, 1983; Wyatt *et al.*, 1985). Its further development was deferred, however, in favor of the "Jennerian" approach described later in this chapter.

The oral route of administration was adopted as early animal studies demonstrated that local intestinal immunity played a major role in resistance to rotavirus disease. Especially convincing were investigations in newborn lambs, in which humoral and local antibodies could be segregated, demonstrating that local intestinal, but not humoral, antibodies were the prime determinants of resistance to rotavirus challenge (Snodgrass and Wells, 1976).

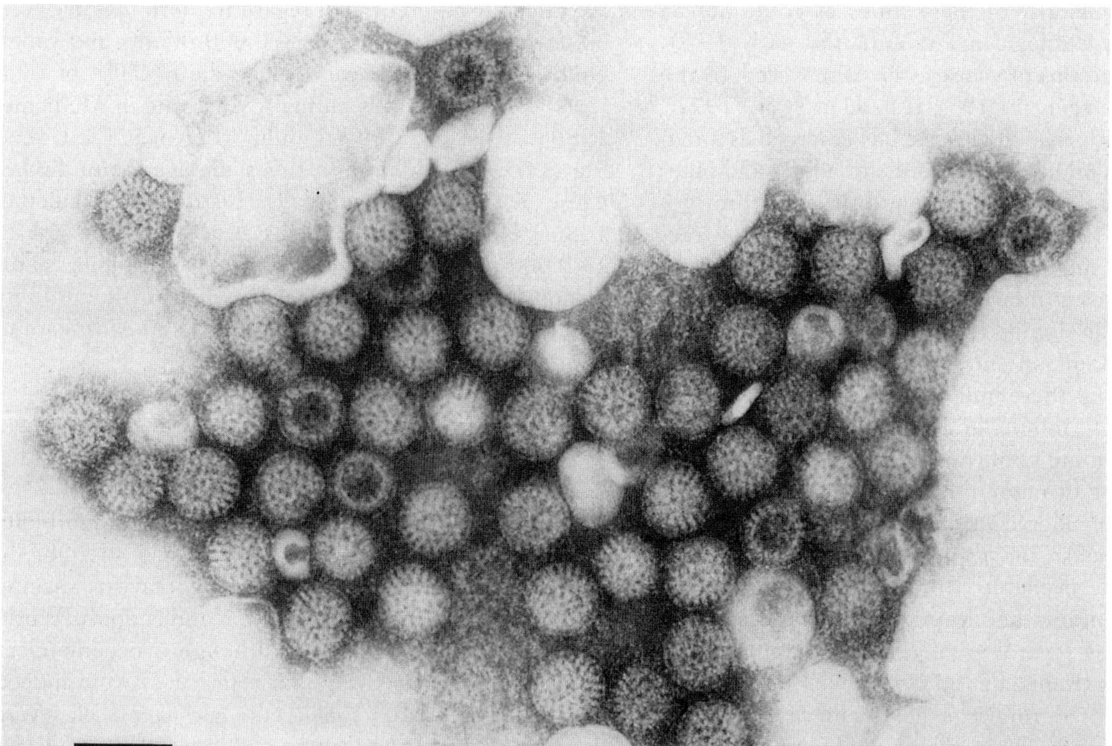

Figure 2. Rotavirus particles observed by immune electron microscopy in a stool filtrate prepared from the stool of a child with acute gastroenteritis. The bar represents 100 nm. From Kapikian *et al.* (1976).

III. Properties of Rotavirus Relevant to Vaccine Development

Rotaviruses are 70 nm in diameter, are nonenveloped, and possess a distinctive double-shelled outer capsid when viewed by negative-stain electron microscopy (Kapikian and Chanock, 1996; Mattion *et al.*, 1994; Prasad *et al.*, 1990) (Fig. 2). Within the double capsid is a third layer, the core, which contains the virus genome comprising 11 segments of double-stranded RNA, as shown schematically in Fig. 3. The segmented genome readily undergoes genetic reassortment during coinfection. Rotaviruses possess three major antigenic properties: group, subgroup, and serotype, which are mediated by various proteins (Hoshino and Kapikian, 1994a,b). Group specificity is defined predominantly by VP6, the major structural protein encoded by gene six. Subgroups are also defined by VP6 (Mattion *et al.*, 1994). Seven distinct groups (A to G) have been described with almost all human rotaviruses of epidemiologic importance belonging to group A; because of this, rotavirus vaccine development is focused on the latter group. Serotype specificity is defined by VP7 and VP4, the two major neutralization antigens located on the outer capsid; VP7, which is encoded by gene segment 7, 8, or 9 depending on the strain, is the most abundant protein located on the outer capsid. This protein forms the smooth outermost surface of the virus particle and, until recently, was considered to be the only determinant of serotype specificity. Fourteen VP7 or "G" (VP7 is a glycoprotein) human and animal rotavirus serotypes have been described; of the 14, 10 have been detected in humans, 13 in animals, and 9 in both humans and animals (Hoshino and Kapikian, 1994a,b; Mattion *et al.*, 1994). However,

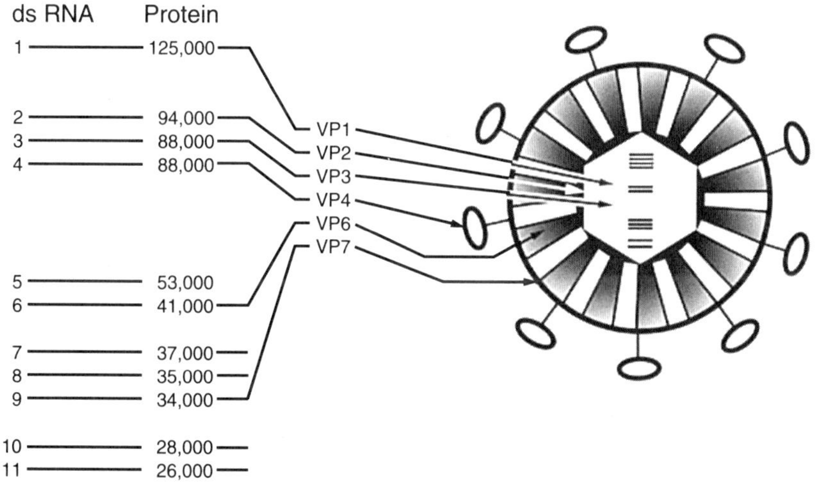

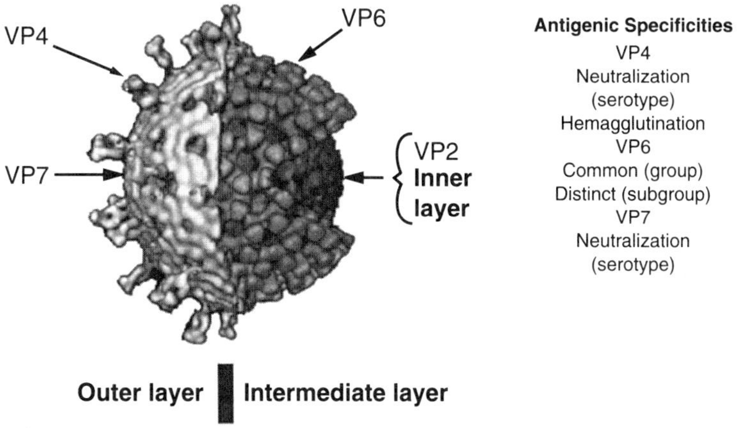

Figure 3. Top: Schematic representation of the rotavirus particle. Bottom: Surface representations of the three-dimensional structures of the outer layer of the complete particle (left) and a particle (right) in which the outer layer and a small triangular portion of the intermediate layer have been removed exposing the inner layer. Modified from Kapikian and Chanock (1996). The three-dimensional figure at the bottom is courtesy of B. V. V. Prasad.

only serotypes 1, 2, 3, and 4 are of epidemiologic importance. Overall, VP7 serotype 1 occurs most frequently, but other serotypes may predominate in certain years or seasons. The other outer capsid protein VP4 (encoded by gene 4), protrudes from the outer surface in the form of 60 discrete spikes 10–12 nm in length (Prasad *et al.*, 1990). Recently, a VP4 serotyping numbering system based on neutralization was described and coexists with the previously described VP4 genotyping numbering scheme (Estes and Cohen, 1989; Sereno and Gorziglia, 1994; Hoshino and Kapikian, 1994a,b).

Antibodies to VP4 and VP7 are each independently associated with protection against rotavirus challenge in various animal models (Hoshino and Kapikian, 1994a,b). However, the immune mechanisms for protection are not clearly established, as a result of conflicting views concerning the role of humoral antibodies. Local intestinal antibodies have been shown to be of importance in a limited number of studies (Matson *et al.*, 1993; Kapikian and Chanock, 1996). The role of cellular immunity has also aroused considerable debate (Offit, 1996).

A. The Jennerian Approach to Vaccination

Almost 200 years ago Edward Jenner described the use of cowpox material in humans as a means of preventing human smallpox. The most extensively evaluated approach to rotavirus vaccination has been the Jennerian strategy in which a related, live, attenuated virus from an animal host is used as the immunogen (Kapikian, 1994a,b). Three important observations were instrumental in its use for rotavirus immunoprophylaxis: (i) human and animal rotaviruses share a common group antigen, as antisera to various animal rotaviruses reacted with both the human and animal strains in various serologic assays (Kapikian *et al.*, 1974, 1976a; Woode *et al.*, 1976); (ii) children undergoing rotavirus infection developed a seroresponse not only to human rotavirus but also to animal rotaviruses of bovine, simian, and murine origin (Kapikian *et al.*, 1974, 1976a); and (iii) studies in gnotobiotic calves provided the major impetus when prenatal administration of a bovine rotavirus strain (NCDV) to a fetal calf *in utero* induced resistance to postnatal challenge with a human rotavirus at birth (Wyatt *et al.*, 1979).

The Jennerian approach was evaluated for efficacy using three animal rotavirus vaccine candidates: a bovine rotavirus, NCDV or WC3 (by others) (Vesikari, 1994; Clark *et al.*, 1988) or a rhesus rotavirus (RRV) strain MMU18006, isolated from a rhesus monkey with diarrhea (Stucker *et al.*, 1980) and developed as a vaccine at NIH and evaluated at numerous centers (Kapikian *et al.*, 1989; Kapikian, 1994a,b). We did not pursue studies with the bovine NCDV strain that was used in the gnotobiotic calf model due to the lack of clarity regarding the cell culture pedigree of this strain (Kapikian *et al.*, 1986). The RRV strain grew efficiently in simian tissue culture, shared VP7 serotype 3 specificity with human rotavirus serotype 3, and, in addition, was adapted to grow in DBS-FRhL$_2$ cells, a semicontinuous simian diploid cell strain developed by the Division of Biologic Standards, the predecessor of the Food and Drug Administration (Kapikian, 1994a,b; Wallace *et al.*, 1973).

This live virus vaccine was examined in Phase 1 clinical trials for safety and antigenicity beginning in adults and progressing sequentially to older and younger children, concluding in the target population of infants less than 6 months of age (Kapikian *et al.*, 1986, 1989). Prior to oral administration of vaccine, a buffer was given because rotaviruses are acid labile and are inactivated at pH < 3 (Vesikari *et al.*, 1984; Weiss and Clark, 1985). The vaccine induced an unacceptable rate of reactions in the over 6-month age group, but was found to be safe and antigenic in the target population of less than 6-month-old infants, in whom it induced a self-limited transient febrile response on the third or fourth day after vaccination in up to one-third of vaccinees. It appeared that passively acquired maternal antibodies in the <6-month age were the critical factor in modulating the reactions (Kapikian *et al.*, 1986; Rennels *et al.*, 1987).

As shown in Table I, the Jennerian approach has been evaluated in Phase 2 studies in over 1600 infants and young children at the 10^4 pfu or 10^5 pfu dose in nine placebo-controlled trials (Kapikian, 1994b). The efficacy of the vaccine has been variable, ranging from 0 to 85% against severe diarrhea. Because the overall efficacy of the vaccine was greatest in the study in Venezuela, in which the predominant infecting strain was the same VP7 serotype as the vaccine (i.e., serotype 3), the variability of protection was attributed to the failure of the vaccine to protect against heterotypic (i.e., non-serotype 3) strains (Flores *et al.*, 1987; Perez-Schael *et al.*, 1990). This was especially pronounced in the <6-month age group of vaccinees who were not primed by previous infection, and thus likely failed to develop a broadened antibody response after vaccination (Losonsky *et al.*, 1988; Green *et al.*, 1990).

B. Modified Jennerian Approach to Vaccination

A modified Jennerian strategy was adopted in an attempt to achieve broader antigenic coverage (Kapikian *et al.*, 1986; Kapikian, 1994b). Three single-gene substitution reassortant strains that possessed 10 genes from the RRV and a single gene that encodes the antigenic specificity of VP7 serotype 1, 2, or 4 were generated by coinfection of monkey kidney cells with the RRV MMU188006 and human rotavirus strains with VP7 serotype 1, 2, or 4, specificity under selective pressure

TABLE I
Protective Efficacy of a Single Oral Dose of Rhesus Rotavirus Vaccine in Phase II Field Trials

Study No.	Study site (investigators)	Age at "vaccination" (months)	No. in each group		Efficacy (%) against rotavirus diarrhea		Predominant VP7 serotype
			Vaccine[a]	Placebo	Any	Moderate to severe	
1	Baltimore–Annapolis, MD (Rennels *et al.*, 1986)	5–20	14	10	100[b]	NA[c]	NA
2	Umea, Sweden (Gothefors *et al.*, 1989)	4–12	53	51	48	80	1
3	Caracas, Venezuela (Flores *et al.*, 1987; Perez-Schael *et al.*, 1990)	1–10	151	151	64	85	3
4	Rochester, NY (Christy *et al.*, 1988)	2–4	85	88	0	0	1
5	Navajo Res., AZ (Santosham *et al.*, 1991)	2–5	108[d]	107	0	0	1
6	Central Maryland (Rennels *et al.*, 1990)	2–11	63	49	29	~29	1
7	Tampere, Finland (Vesikari *et al.*, 1990)	2–5	100	100	38	67	1, 4
8	Rochester, NY (Madore *et al.*, 1992)	2–4	76[e]	73	66	NA	1
9	Lima, Peru (Lanata *et al.*, 1996)	2	~195[f]	~196	29	34	1, 3
	Total		845	825			

Note. Adapted from Kapikian (1994b).
[a] 10^5 pfu in trials 1 and 2, 10^4 pfu in remainder
[b] Based on only three cases in placebo and none in vaccine group
[c] Not available
[d] A third group of 106 infants received RIT4237 vaccine (10^8 $TCID_{50}$ dose), also without efficacy
[e] A third group received DxRRV vaccine
[f] Other groups received DxRRV or DS-1xRRV vaccine

against the RRV (as shown schematically in Fig. 4) (Midthun *et al.*, 1985, 1986). The goal was to incorporate these three reassortants (which represented three of the four epidemiologically important human rotavirus VP7 serotypes) with RRV (representing the VP7 serotype 3 strain itself) into a single quadrivalent vaccine to achieve the broadest antigenic coverage.

Before combining the strains into a single preparation, phase 1 studies were carried out with individual reassortant strains, which demonstrated that each was safe and immunogenic, with reactions similar to those observed with the RRV strain in the target population (Flores *et al.*, 1993). Phase 2 efficacy trials with individual reassortants in Finland and Rochester were promising as a protective efficacy of 66 and 77%, respectively, was achieved against any rotavirus diarrhea (Vesikari *et al.*, 1992; Madore *et al.*, 1992). It was paradoxical that heterotypic protection was demonstrated with the DS-1 × RRV reassortant in Finland and the RRV strain in Rochester. This was difficult to explain, although "priming" by previous natural infection was a possibility in Rochester, but not likely in Finland. The failure of individual reassortants and RRV to protect against any rotavirus diarrhea and only moderately against severe diarrhea in Peru may reflect the presence of coinfecting etiologic agents or the single 10^4 PFU dose of vaccine (Lanata *et al.*, 1996).

C. The Quadrivalent Vaccine

The reassortant strains were combined into a quadrivalent formulation and evaluated in Phase 1 studies for reactogenicity and antigenicity. The combination vaccine was safe, causing self-limited febrile reactions that were similar to those observed with the RRV vaccine or individual reassortants noted earlier in the target population (Flores *et al.*, 1993). However, the vaccine failed to induce adequate neutralizing antibody responses against individual serotypes, necessitating adjustments in dosage, until finally a two-dose regimen of 10^5 pfu of each component in the vaccine was adopted as this schedule induced a "take rate" approaching or achieving an arbitrary level of 50% against each of the serotypes (Flores *et al.*, 1993; Kapikian *et al.*, 1992).

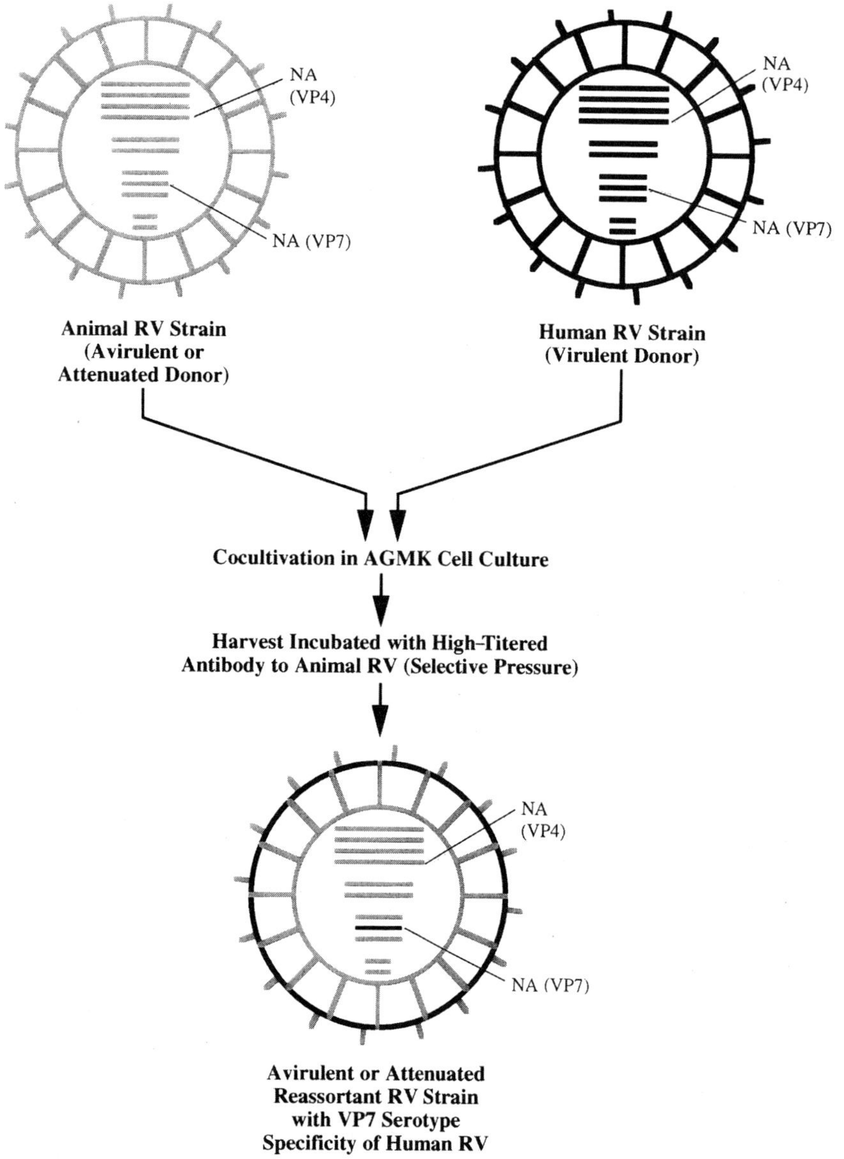

Figure 4. Production of reassortant rotavirus (RV) vaccine. NA, neutralizing antigen-encoding gene. Modified from Kapikian *et al.* (1986).

IV. Field Trials with Quadrivalent Vaccine

Eleven Phase 2 or 3 field trials in over 10,000 infants and young children, with individual reassortants or the quadrivalent vaccine, are completed, completed and being analyzed, or in progress (Table II). Two field trials with the quadrivalent vaccine have been completed and reported, with promising results, as described below.

A multicenter trial was conducted in the United States in almost 900 infants and young children who received three doses of 4×10^4 pfu of the quadrivalent vaccine or a monovalent VP7 serotype 1 reassortant vaccine (D × RRV) or a placebo at approximately 2, 4, and 6 months of age (Bernstein *et al.*, 1995). The quadrivalent vaccine was safe but mildly reactogenic, inducing a significantly greater number of febrile episodes (>38°C, rectal) than the placebo on the 4th and 5th days, and, overall, over the first 5 days after the first dose (overall, 14% in quadrivalent vaccine and 7% in placebo groups). The efficacy of the tetravalent and monovalent vaccines over two rotavirus seasons against any rotavirus diarrhea was 49 and 54%, respectively (Table III shows results with quadrivalent vaccine only). The efficacy against very severe diarrheal illness reached 73 and 82% for the monovalent and quadrivalent vaccine preparations, respectively. With regard to other parameters of

TABLE II
Phase 2 or 3 Efficacy Field Trials of Individual Human–Rhesus Rotavirus (RV) Reassortment Vaccines and Quadrivalent RV Vaccines

Study site (investigators)	Number of infants [recruitment age (Months)][a]	Number in each group: Vaccine (dose in PFU)	Placebo	Status
1. Tampere, Finland (Vesikari *et al.*, 1992)	359 (2–4)	120 DxRRV (10^4) 119 DS-1xRRV (10^5)	120	Completed
2. Rochester, NY (Madore *et al.*, 1992)	223 (2–4)	74 DxRRV (10^4) 76 RRV (10^4)	73	Completed
3. Lima, Peru (Lanata *et al.*, 1996)	782 (2)	~195 DxRRV (10^4) ~196 DS-1xRRV (10^4) ~195 RRV (10^4)	~196	Completed
4. Lima, Peru (Lanata *et al.*, 1995)	600 (2–4)	200 Quadx1 (10^4)[b] 200 Quadx3 (10^4)[b]	200	Completed (under analysis)
5. U.S. Multicenter Study (Bernstein *et al.*, 1995)	898 (2–6)	297 DxRRVx3 (4×10^4)[b] 305 Quadx3 (10^4)[b]	296	Completed
6. Yangon, Myanmar (K. Moe *et al.*, unpublished)	430 (neonates)	215 Quadx3 (10^5)[b]	215	Completed (under analysis)
7. Belem, Brazil (Linhares *et al.*, 1995)	540 (1–5)	~270 Quadx3 (10^4)	~270	Completed (under analysis)
8. Navajo Res., Arizona (Santosham *et al.*, 1995)	1051 (2–6)	356 DxRRVx3 (4×10^5)[b] 347 Quadx3 (10^5)[b]	348	Completed (under analysis)
9. U.S. Multicenter Study (Rennels *et al.*, 1996)	1187 (2–6)	404 DxRRVx3 (4×10^5)[b] 398 Quadx3 (10^5)[b]	385	Completed
10. Caracas, Venezuela (Perez-Schael *et al.*, 1995)	2223 (2–4)	~1112 Quadx3 (10^5)[b]	~1111	In progress
11. Tampere, Finland (Joensuu and Vesikari, 1995)	2285 (2–7)	~1142 Quadx3 (10^5)[b]	~1143	In progress
Total	10,578	6221	4357	

Note. Adapted from Kapikian (1994b); vaccinees given only RRV (study 2 and 3) are also included in Table 1.
[a]Age (approx.) at time of single or initial dose of vaccine; upper range indicates approx. maximum age for final dose of vaccine.
[b]Dose of each component.

severity, the quadrivalent vaccine significantly reduced the number of illnesses of greater than 3 days duration and the number of medical visits (Table III).

These studies were extended in a second multicenter study in which a 10-fold greater dose (4×10^5 pfu) of quadrivalent vaccine or 4×10^5 pfu of a monovalent VP7 serotype 1 reassortant vaccine or a placebo was administered in a three-dose regimen to over 1200 infants beginning at approximately 2 months of age (Rennels *et al.*, 1996). This higher dose of quadrivalent vaccine was safe, although a significantly greater number of fevers (>38°C axillary) was observed on the fourth day following the first dose (2.2 vs. 0.2% in vaccine and placebo recipients, respectively). This lower rate of fevers probably reflected the taking of temperatures by the axillary rather than rectal route. The protective efficacy of the quadrivalent vaccine over a single rotavirus season was 49% against any rotavirus diarrhea and 80% against severe rotavirus diarrhea (Table IV). Both the monovalent and quadrivalent vaccines induced a marked reduction in the number of dehydrating diarrheal episodes, with 13 episodes occurring in the placebo group, two in the monovalent vaccine recipients, and none in the quadrivalent vaccinees. Although serotype 1 was the most frequently detected serotype (77%) and both the monovalent and quadrivalent vaccines achieved comparable protection against this serotype (44 and 55%, respectively), protection against serotype 3 rotavirus diarrhea [the second most commonly detected serotype (19%)], was 77 and 45% for the quadrivalent and monovalent groups, respectively. This trend ($P = 0.14$) was not significant between vaccine groups, but the numbers observed were significant only for the quadrivalent vaccine when compared to the placebo group.

TABLE III

Protective Efficacy of Quadrivalent Rotavirus (RV) Vaccine (4×10^4 pfu) on the Occurrence of RV Diarrhea of Varying Severity over Two RV Seasons in the United States

Parameter	Number with indicated parameter who received: Quadrivalent vaccine (N=305)	Placebo (N=296)	Protective efficacy
RV diarrhea	29 (10%)	65 (22%)	57%[a]
Severity score of RV diarrhea[a]			
1–8	14 (5%)	24 (9%)	49%[b]
9–14	11 (4%)	25 (9%)	59%[c]
15–20	2 (1%)	11 (4%)	82%[d]
RV diarrhea >3 days duration	2 (1%)	25 (9%)	92%[e]
Medical visits	6 (2%)	27 (9%)	78%[f]

Note. Adapted from Bernstein *et al.* (1995).

*Severity score not available from two vaccinees and five controls. Individuals with score >8 excluded from 1 to 8 efficacy analysis and those with score >14 from 9 to 14 efficacy analysis.

[a]$P<0.0001$ (F.E.T.), 95% CI 35, 71%.

[b]$P<0.05$, CI 4, 73%.

[c]$P<0.001$, CI 20, 79%.

[d]$P<0.02$, CI 31, 96%.

[e]$P<0.001$, CI 71, 98%.

[f]$P<0.001$, CI 50, 91%.

Two preliminary efficacy trials of the quadrivalent vaccine in infants and young children are of particular interest: one in Belem, Brazil (Linhares *et al.,* 1995) and the other in an American Indian population in Arizona (Santosham *et al.,* 1995). Preliminary reports indicate that during the first year of surveillance, the quadrivalent vaccine achieved a protective efficacy against any rotavirus diarrhea of 57% in Brazil and 52% in Arizona. Although efficacy appeared to fade during the second year (not shown), the demonstration of efficacy in this developing area in Brazil and in the American Indian infants in whom the RRV vaccine had failed previously (Santosham *et al.*, 1991) was particularly encouraging. A trial in Peru with the monovalent or quadrivalent vaccine under analysis yielded less promising results, as shown in Table V (Lanata *et al.*, 1995). The results from the various efficacy trials, completed and under analysis, are summarized in Table V.

TABLE IV

Protective Efficacy of Quadrivalent Rotavirus (RV) Vaccine (4×10^5 pfu) on the Occurrence of RV Diarrhea of Varying Severity over One RV Season in the United States

Parameter	Number with indicated parameter who received: Quadrivalent vaccine (N=398)	Placebo (N=385)	Protective efficacy
RV diarrhea	51 (13%)	97 (25%)	49%[a]
Severity score of RV diarrhea			
>8	24 (6%)	72 (19%)	68%[b]
>14	7 (2%)	34 (9%)	80%[c]
Medical intervention	16 (4%)	58 (15%)	73%[d]
Dehydration	0 (0%)	13 (3%)	100%[e]

Note. Adapted from Rennels *et al.* (1996).

[a]$P<0.0001$ (F.E.T.), 95% CI 31, 63%.

[b]$P<0.0001$, CI 50, 79%.

[c]$P<0.0001$, CI 56, 91%.

[d]$P<0.0001$, CI 54, 84%.

[e]$P<0.001$, CI 73, 100%.

V. Other Modified Jennerian Approaches

Further modifications of the modified Jennerian approach are being pursued in case the RRV-based quadrivalent vaccine fails to yield the optimal level of protection; an underlying theme in these strategies is the incorporation of the human rotavirus VP4 into various formulations in order to enhance antigenicity (Hoshino and Kapikian, 1994b). Such approaches include single- or double-gene substitution reassortant rotaviruses. The single-gene substitution reassortment rotaviruses have a VP7 gene from human rotavirus 1, 2, 3, or 4 and the other 10 genes from the bovine rotavirus UK strain, is a formulation similar in principle to that of the RRV-based quadrivalent vaccine described above (Midthun *et al.*, 1985, 1986). These strains will be incorporated into a quadrivalent vaccine with the potential to formulate a pentavalent or hexavalent vaccine in which a reassortant with the VP4 of human Wa rotavirus (VP7:1; VP4:1A) and 10 genes from UK (for pentavalent vaccine), and a reassortant with the VP4 of human rotavirus strain DS-1(VP7:2; VP4:1B) and 10 genes from UK (for hexavalent vaccine) are added to take advantage of the antigenicity of the VP4 component of human rotaviruses (Hoshino and Kapikian, 1994b). A similar, but not identical, approach is under consideration for the RRV-based quadrivalent vaccine described earlier, if a pentavalent or hexavalent vaccine should be required (Y. Hoshino *et al.*, unpublished studies). Double-gene substitution reassortants with the VP4 gene of Wa and the VP7 gene of human rotavirus serotype 1, 2, 3, or 4 and the remaining nine genes from the UK strain have also been developed (Hoshino *et al.*, 1996). These strains would have the advantage of possessing both the VP4 and VP7 genes from a human rotavirus and the attenuation potential of the remaining genes from an animal host. Impetus for the latter approach was prompted by studies in gnotobiotic piglets that demonstrated that substitution of the 3rd (VP3), 4th (VP4), VP7, or 10th (NS28) gene of a virulent porcine rotavirus strain with that of an attenu-

TABLE V
Protective Efficacy of Rhesus Rotavirus (RRV)-Based Monovalent or Quadrivalent Vaccine in Phase 2–3 Field Trials

Vaccine, serotype, strain (Titer in pfu)	Study site (investigators)	Age (months) at vaccination [No. doses]	No. in each group		% Efficacy vs RV diarrhea		Predominant VP7 serotype
			Vaccine	Placebo	Any	Very severe	
1. Monovalent, G1, DxRRV (10^4)	Tampere, Finland	2–4 [1]	120	120	67[a]	NA[b]	1
Monovalent, G2, DS-1xRRV (10^5)	(Vesikari *et al.*, 1992)		119		66[a]	NA	
2. Monovalent, G1, DxRRV (10^4)	Rochester, NY (Madore *et al.*, 1992)	2–4 [1]	74	73	77[a]	NA	1
3. Monovalent, G1, DxRRV (10^4)	Lima, Peru	2 [1]	~195	~195	0	32	1
Monovalent, G2, DS-1xRRV (10^4)	(Lanata *et al.*, 1996)		~195		0	40	
4. Monovalent, G1, DxRRV ($4x10^4$)	U.S. Multicenter	2–6 [3]	297	296	40	73	1, 3
Quadrivalent, G1, 2, 3, 4[c] ($4x10^4$)	(Bernstein *et al.*, 1995)		305		57	82	
5. Monovalent, G1, DxRRV ($4x10^5$)	U.S. Multicenter	2–6 [3]	404	385	54	69	1, 3
Quadrivalent, G1, 2, 3, 4[c] ($4x10^5$)	(Rennels *et al.*, 1996)		398		49	80	
6. Monovalent, G1, DxRRV ($4x10^5$)	Navajo Res., AZ	2–6 [3]	356	348	29[a]	NA	NA
Quadrivalent, G1, 2, 3, 4[c] ($4x10^5$)	(Santosham *et al.*, 1995)		347		52[a]	NA	NA
7. Quadrivalent, G1, 2, 3, 4[c] ($4x10^4$)	Belem, Brazil (Linhares *et al.*, 1995)	1–5 [3]	~270	~270	57[a]	NA	NA
8. Monovalent, G1, DxRRV ($4x10^4$)	Lima, Peru	2 [1]	~200	~200	0	35–66	NA
Quadrivalent, G1, 2, 3, 4[c] ($4x10^4$)	(Lanata *et al.*, 1995)	2–4 [1]	~200				

[a]Includes only first RV "season" of longer study or first year of longer study
[b]NA, not available.
[c]Composed of DxRRV, DS-1xRRV, RRV, ST-3xRRV.

ated virus resulted in loss of virulence (Hoshino *et al.*, 1995).

VI. Non-Jennerian Approach

A cold-adapted human rotavirus serotype 1 strain was initially described in Japan (Matsuno *et al.*, 1987). Further cold-adapted human rotavirus strains of VP7 1, 2, 3, or 4 serotype and of human rotavirus-human rotavirus reassortants (Wa × DS-1 or Wa × P) with the VP4 and 9 other genes from Wa and the VP7 of DS-1 or P are available (Hoshino *et al.*, 1994c). These strains may possess the desired level of antigenicity because of the presence of all 11 human rotavirus genes and, may also be attenuated because of cold adaptation.

VII. Cost Effectiveness of Rotavirus Vaccine

As a result of advances in rotavirus vaccine development, estimates were recently made on the effects of a moderately effective rotavirus vaccine on morbidity, mortality, and cost-effectiveness on a birth cohort of 4.1 million children followed from birth to 5 years of age in the United States (Smith *et al.*, 1995). It is estimated that if a vaccine is 50% effective against rotavirus diarrhea, a vaccination program in the United States would prevent over one million cases of rotavirus diarrhea, over 400,000 physician visits, 58,000 hospitalizations, and 82 deaths per year. If the vaccine costs $30 a dose, it would yield a net savings of $79 million with regard to the health care system and $466 million from the perspective of society. Thus, not only would this development aid in the primary purpose of preventing morbidity and mortality, but from an economic viewpoint, immunization with a rotavirus vaccine would be cost-effective and cost-saving as well.

VIII. Summary

The first dose of RRV vaccine was administered to two adult volunteers in January of 1994, which began the sequential progression of studies with RRV-based vaccines in younger individuals until the target population of <6-month-old infants was reached (Kapikian *et al.*, 1989). In addition, the first dose of the DxRRV (VP7:1) reassortant vaccine was given to two adult volunteers in April 1986 (Kapikian *et al.*, 1989), which began the sequential progression to the target population and paved the way for studies with the other human-RRV reassortant strains and finally to the quadrivalent formulation (Flores *et al.*, 1990, 1993).

It should be noted that the realistic goal of a rotavirus vaccine is not to prevent rotavirus infection, or mild rotavirus diarrhea, but to prevent severe rotavirus diarrhea. This becomes apparent when studying the characteristics of naturally occuring rotavirus infection wherein prior rotavirus infection induces (i) poor protection against reinfection, (ii) a moderate degree of protection against mild illness, but (iii) a high protection against severe rotavirus illness in infants and young children (Bishop *et al.*, 1983; Kapikian, 1994b).

There is promise that within the not-too-distant future a rotavirus vaccine that has been under development for over a decade will be available for prevention of severe diarrhea in infants and young children in both developed and developing countries.

Acknowledgments

I thank Todd J. Heishman and Lisa C. White for outstanding editorial assistance.

References

Bernstein, D. I., Glass, R. I., Rogers, G., Davidson, B. L., and Sack, D. A. for the U.S. Rotavirus Vaccine Efficacy Group (1995). Evaluation of rhesus rotavirus monovalent and tetravalent reassortant vaccines in U.S. children. *JAMA, J. Am. Med. Assoc.* **273**, 1191–1196.

Bishop, R. F., Davidson, G. P., Holmes, I. H., and Ruck, B. J. (1973). Virus particles in epithelial cells of duodenal mucosa from children with viral gastroenteritis. *Lancet* **2**, 1281–1283.

Bishop, R. F., Barnes, G. L., Cipriani, E., and Lund, J. S. (1983). Clinical immunity after neonatal rotavirus infection. A prospective longitudinal study in young children. *N. Engl. J. Med.* **309**, 72–76.

Christy, C., Madore, H. P., Pichichero, M. E., Gala, C., Pincus, P., Vosefski, D., Hoshino, Y., Kapikian, A. Z., and Dolin, R. (1988). The Elmwood and Panorama Pediatric Groups: Field trial of rhesus rotavirus vaccine in infants. *Pediatr. Infect. Dis. J.* **7**, 645–650.

Clark, H. F., Borian, F. E., Bell, L. M., Modesto, K., Gouvea, V., and Plotkin, S. A. (1988). Protective effect of WC3 vaccine against rotavirus diarrhea in infants during a predominantly serotype 1 rotavirus season. *J. Infect. Dis.* **158**, 570–587.

Estes, M. K., and Cohen, J. (1989). Rotavirus gene structure and function. *Microbiol. Rev.* **53**, 410–449.

Flores, J., Perez-Schael, I., Gonzalez, M., Garcia, D., Perez, M., Daoud, N., Cunto, W., Chanock, R. M., and Kapikian, A. Z. (1987). Protection against severe rotavirus diarrhea by rhesus rotavirus vaccine in Venezuelan infants. *Lancet* **1**, 882–884.

Flores, J., Perez-Schael, I., Blanco, M., White, L., Garcia, D., Vilar, M., Cunto, W., Gonzalez, R., Urbina, C., Boher, J., Mendez, M., and Kapikian, A. Z. (1990). Comparison of reactogenicity and antigenicity of M37 rotavirus vaccine and rhesus-rotavirus-based quadrivalent vaccine. *Lancet* **336**, 330–334.

Flores, J., Perez-Schael, I., Blanco, M., Rojas, A. M., Alfonzo, E., Crespo, I., Cunto, W., Pittman, A., and Kapikian, A. Z. (1993). Reactogenicity and immunogenicity of a high-titered rhesus rotavirus-based quadrivalent rotavirus vaccine. *J. Clin. Microbiol.* **31**, 2439–2445.

Glass, R. I., Gentsch, J., and Smith, J. C. (1994). Rotavirus vaccines: Success by reassortment? *Science* **265**, 1389–1391.

Gothefors, L., Wadell, G., Juto, P., Taniguchi, K., Kapikian, A. Z., and Glass, R. I. (1989). Prolonged efficacy of rhesus rotavirus vaccine in Swedish children. *J. Infect. Dis.* **159**, 753–757.

Green, K. Y., Taniguchi, K., Mackow, E. R., and Kapikian, A. Z. (1990). Homotypic and heterotypic epitope-specific antibody responses in adult and infant rotavirus vaccinees: Implications for vaccine development. *J. Infect. Dis.* **161**, 667–669.

Ho, M.-S., Glass, R. I., Pinsky, P. F., Young-Okoh, N., Sappenfield, W. M., Buehler, J. W., Gunter, N., and Anderson, L. J. (1988). Diarrheal deaths in American children Are they preventable? *JAMA, J. Am. Med. Assoc.* **260**, 3281–3285.

Hoshino, Y., Jones, R. W., Chanock, R. M., and Kapikian, A. Z. (1996). Construction of four double gene substitution human × bovine rotavirus reassortant vaccine candidates: Each bears two outer capsid human rotavirus genes, one encoding P serotype 1A, the other encoding G sereotype 1, 2, 3, and 4 specificity. Submitted.

Hoshino, Y., and Kapikian, A. Z. (1994a). Rotavirus antigens. *Curr Top. Microbiol. Immunol.* **185**, 179–227.

Hoshino, Y., and Kapikian, A. Z. (1994b). Rotavirus vaccine development for the prevention of severe diarrhea in infants and young children. *Trends Microbiol.* **2**, 242–249.

Hoshino, Y., Kapikian, A. Z., and Chanock, R. M. (1994c). Selection of cold-adapted mutants of human rotaviruses that exhibit various degrees of growth restriction *in vitro*. *J. Virol.* **68**, 7598–7602.

Hoshino, Y., Saif, L., Kang, S.-Y., Sereno, M. M., Chen W.-K., and Kapikian, A. Z. (1995). Identification of group A rotavirus genes associated with virulence of a porcine rotavirus and host range restriction of a human rotavirus in the gnotobiotic piglet model. *Virology* **209**, 274–280.

Institute of Medicine. (1986a). Prospects for immunizing against rotavirus. *In* "New Vaccine Development. Establishing Priorities. Diseases of Importance in the United States," Vol. 1, pp. 410–423. National Academy Press, Washington, D.C.

Institute of Medicine. (1986b). The prospects for immunizing against rotavirus. *In* "New Vaccine Development. Establishing Priorities. Diseases of Importance in Developing Countries," Vol. 2, pp. 308–316. National Academy Press, Washington, D.C.

Joensuu, J., and Vesikari, T. (1995). Field trial of rhesus–human reassortant rotavirus vaccine in Finland: First results Fifth rotavirus vaccine workshop. Current issues and future development, Atlanta, Georgia, p. SIV-32. Atlanta Centers for Disease Control.

Kapikian, A. Z. (1993). Viral gastroenteritis. *JAMA, J. Am. Med. Assoc.* **269**, 627–630

Kapikian, A. Z. (1994a). Jennerian and modified Jennerian approach to vaccination against rotavirus diarrhea in infants and young children: An introduction. *In* "Viral Infections of the Gastrointestinal Tract" (A. Z. Kapikian, ed.), pp. 409–417. Dekker, New York.

Kapikian, A. Z. (1994b). Rhesus rotavirus-based human rotavirus vaccines and observations on selected non-Jennerian approaches to rotavirus vaccination. *In* "Viral Infections of the Gastrointestinal Tract" (A. Z. Kapikian, ed.), pp. 443–470. Dekker, New York.

Kapikian, A. Z., and Chanock, R. M. (1996). Rotaviruses. *In* "Virology" (B. N. Fields, Knipe, D. M., Howley, P. M., Chanock, R. M., Melnick, J. L., Monath, T. P., Roizman, B., and Straus, S., eds.), pp. 1657–1708. Lippincott/Raven, Philadelphia/New York.

Kapikian, A. Z., Wyatt, R. G., Dolin, R., Thornhill, T. S., Kalica, A. R., and Chanock, R. M. (1972). Visualization by immune electron microscopy of a 27nm particle associated with acute infectious non-bacterial gastroenteritis. *J. Virol.* **10,** 1075–1081.

Kapikian, A. Z., Kim, H. W., Wyatt, R. G., Rodriquez, W. J., Ross, S., Cline, W. L., Parrott, R. H., and Chanock, R. M. (1974). Reovirus-like agent in stools: Association with infantile diarrhea and development of serologic tests. *Science* **185,** 1049–1053.

Kapikian, A. Z., Cline, W. L., Kim, H. W., Kalica, A. R., Wyatt, R. G., Van Kirk, D. H., Chanock, R. M., James, H. D., Jr., and Vaughn, A. L. (1976a). Antigenic relationships among five reovirus-like (RVL) agents by complement-fixation (CF) and development of new substitute CF antigens for the human RVL agent of infantile gastroenteritis. *Proc. Soc. Exp. Biol. Med.* **152,** 535–539.

Kapikian, A. Z., Kim, H. W., Wyatt, R. G., Cline, W. L., Arrobio, J. O., Brandt, C. D., Rodriquez, W. J., Sack, D. A., Chanock, R. M., and Parrott, R. H. (1976b). Human reovirus-like agent as the major pathogen associated with "winter" gastroenteritis in hospitalized infants and young children. *N. Engl. J. Med.* **294,** 965–972.

Kapikian, A. Z., Wyatt, R. G., Levine, M. M., Black, R. E., Greenberg, H. B., Flores, J., Kalica, A. R., Hoshino, Y., and Chanock, R. M. (1983). Studies in volunteers with human rotaviruses. *Dev. Biol. Stand.* **53,** 209–218.

Kapikian, A. Z., Hoshino, Y., Flores, J., Midthun, K., Glass, R. I., Nakagomi, O., Nakagomi, T., Chanock, R. M., Potash, L., Levine, M. M., Dolin, R., Wright, P. F., Belshe, R. E., Anderson, E. L., Vesikari, T., Gothefors, L., Wadell, G., and Perez-Schael, I. (1986). *In* "Development of Vaccines and Drugs against Diarrhea" (J. Holmgren, A. Lindberg, and R. Mollby, eds.), 11th Nobel Conference, Stockholm 1985, pp. 192–214. Studentlitteratur, Lund, Sweden.

Kapikian, A. Z., Flores, J., Hoshino, Y., Midthun, K., Green, K. Y., Gorziglia, M., Chanock, R. M., Potash, L., Perez-Schael, I., Gonzalez, M., Vesikari, T., Gothefors, L., Wadell, G., Glass, R. I., Levine, M. M., Rennels, M. B., Losonsky, G. A., Christy, C., Dolin, R., Anderson, E. L., Belshe, R. B., Wright, P. F., Santosham, M., Halsey, N. A., Clements, M. L., Sears, S. D., Steinhoff, M. C., and Black, R. E. (1989). Rationale for the development of a rotavirus vaccine for infants and young children. *In* "Progress in Vaccinology" (G. P. Talwar, ed.), Vol. 2, pp. 151–180. Springer-Verlag, New York.

Kapikian, A. Z., Vesikari, T., Ruuska, T., Madore, H. P., Christy, C., Dolin, R., Flores, J., Green, K. Y., Davidson, B. L., Gorziglia, M., Hoshino, Y., Chanock, R. M., Midthun, K., and Perez-Schael, I. (1992). An update on the "Jennerian" and modified "Jennerian" approach to vaccination of infants and young children against rotavirus diarrhea. *Adv. Exp. Med. Biol.* **327,** 59–69.

Kapikian, A. Z., Estes, M. K., and Chanock, R. M. (1996). Norwalk group of viruses. *In* "Virology" (B. N. Fields, ed.), in press. Raven, New York.

Kumate, J., and Isibasi, A. (1986). Pediatric diarrheal diseases: A global perspective. *Pediatr. Infect. Dis.* **5,** 521–528.

Lanata, C. F., Midthun, K., Black, R. E., Butron, B., Penny, M. E., Jett-Goheen, M., and Davidson, B. L. (1995). Safety, immunogenicity and protective efficacy of one or three doses of the rhesus tetravalent rotavirus vaccine in infants from Lima, Peru. Abstracts of Fifth Rotavirus Vaccine Workshop. Current Issues and Future Development. Atlanta, Georgia, p. SIII-31.

Lanata, C., Black, R. E., Flores, J., Lazo, F., Butron, B., Linares, A., Huapaya, A., Ventura, G., Gil, A., and Kapikian, A. Z. (1996). Immunogeniciy, safety and protective efficacy of one dose of the rhesus rotavirus vaccine and serotype 1 and 2 human–rhesus rotavirus reassortants in children from Lima, Peru. *Vaccine,* in press.

Linhares, A. C., Gabbay, Y. B., de Freitas, R. B., Mascarenhas, J. D. P., Oliveira, C. S., Bellesi, N., Lainson, Z. L., Ramos, F. L. P., and Valente, S. A. (1995). Immunogenicity, safety and efficacy of rhesus–human, reassortant rotavirus (RRV-tetravalent) vaccine in Belem, Brazil. Abstract in Fifth Rotavirus Vaccine Workshop. Current Issues and Future Development, Atlanta, Georgia, p. SIII-29. Atlanta Centers for Disease Control.

Losonsky, G. A., Rennels, M. B., Lim, Y., Krall, G., Kapikian, A. Z., and Levine, M. M. (1988). Systemic and mucosal immune responses to rhesus rotavirus vaccine MMU18006. *Pediatr. Infect. Dis. J.* **7,** 388–393.

Madore, H. P., Christy, C., Pichichero, M., Long, C., Pincus, P., Vosefsky, P., Kapikian, A. Z., Dolin, R., Elmwood, Panorama, and Westfall Pediatric Groups (1992). Field trial of rhesus rotavirus or human–rhesus reassortant vaccine of VP7 serotype 3 or 1 specificity in infants. *J. Infect. Dis.* **166,** 235–243.

Matson, D. O., O'Ryan, M. L., Herrara, I., Pickering, L. K., and Estes, M. K. (1993). Fecal antibody response to symptomatic and asymptomatic rotavirus infections. *J. Infect. Dis.* **167,** 577–583.

Matsuno, S., Murakami, S., Takagi, M., Hayashi, M., Inouye, S., Hasegawa, A., and Fukai, K. (1987). Cold adaptation of human rotavirus. *Virus Res.* **7,** 273–280.

Mattion, N. M., Cohen, J., and Estes, M. K. (1994). The rotavirus proteins. *In* "Viral Infections of the Gastrointestinal Tract" (A. Z. Kapikian, ed.), pp. 169–249. Dekker, New York.

Midthun, K., Greenberg, H. B., Hoshino, Y., Kapikian, A. Z., Wyatt, R. G., and Chanock, R. M. (1985). Reassortant rotaviruses as potential live rotavirus vaccine candidates. *J. Virol.* **53,** 949–954.

Midthun, K., Hoshino, Y., Kapikian, A. Z., and Chanock, R. M. (1986). Single gene substitution rotavirus reassortants containing the major neutralization protein (VP7) of human rotavirus serotype 4. *J. Clin. Microbiol.* **24,** 822–826.

Offit, P. (1996). Immunologic determinants of protection against rotavirus disease. Proceedings of Fifth Rotavirus Vaccine Workshop. Current issues and future development, Atlanta, Georgia, p. SIII-p18. Atlanta Centers for Disease Control.

Perez-Schael, I., Garcia, D., Gonzalez, M., Gonzalez, R., Daoud, N., Perez, M., Cunto, W., Kapikian, A. Z., and Flores, J. (1990). Prospective study of diarrheal diseases in Venezuelan children to evaluate the efficacy of rhesus rotavirus vaccine. *J. Med. Virol.* **30**, 219–229.

Perez-Schael, I., Guntinas, M. J., Rojas, A. M., Fernandez, R., Perez, M., Boher, Y., Gonzalez, R., and Kapikian, A. (March, 1992–September, 1995). Current status of the quadrivalent rotavirus vaccine trial in Venezuela. Abstract in Fifth Rotavirus Vaccine Workshop. Current Issues and Future Development, Atlanta, Georgia, 1995, p. SIII-31. Atlanta Centers for Disease Control.

Prasad, B. V., Burns, J. W., Marietta, E., Estes, M. K., and Chiu, W. (1990). Localization of VP4 neutralization sites in rotavirus by three-dimensional cryo-electron microscopy. *Nature (London)* **343**, 476–479.

Rennels, M. B., Losonsky, G. A., Levine, M. M., Kapikian, A. Z., and the Clinical Study Group (Fortier, D. N., Sutton J. M., Ferra, P. J., and Hoffman, K. M.) (1986). Preliminary evaluation of the efficacy of rhesus rotavirus vaccine strain MMU18006 in young children. *Pediatr. Infect. Dis.* **5**, 587–588.

Rennels, M. B., Losonsky, G. A., Shindledecker, L., Hughes, T., Kapikian, A. Z., Levine, M. M., and the Clinical Study Group (Ferra, P. J., Fortier, D. N., Sutton J. M.). (1987). Immunogenicity and reactogenicity of lowered doses of rhesus rotavirus vaccine strain MMU18006 in young children. *Pediat. Infect. Dis. J.* **6**, 260–264.

Rennels, M. B., Losonsky, G. A., Young, A. E., Shindledecker, C. L., Kapikian, A. Z., Levine, M. M., and the Clinical Study Group. (1990). An efficacy trial of rhesus rotavirus vaccine in Maryland. *Am. J. Dis. Child.* **144**, 601–604.

Rennels, M. B., Glass, R. I., Dennehy, P. H., Bernstein, D. I., Pichichero, M. E., Zito, E. T., Mack, M. E., Davidson, B. L., and Kapikian, A. Z., for the United States Rotavirus Efficacy Group (1996). Safety and efficacy of high-dose rhesus–human reassortant rotavirus vaccines—report of the national multicenter trial. *Pediatrics* **97**, 7–13.

Santosham, M., Letson, G. W., Wolff, M., Reid, R., Gahagan, S., Adams, R., Callahan, C., Sack, R. B., and Kapikian, A. Z. (1991). A field study of the safety and efficacy of two candidate rotavirus vaccines in a Native American population *J. Infect. Dis.* **163**, 483–487.

Santosham, M., Reid, R., Croll, J., Brenneman, G., Weatherholtz, R., Moulton, L., Ward, R., and Davidson, B. (1985). A comparative study of the efficacy, safety and immunogencity of three doses of oral tetravalent rhesus rotavirus vaccine (4×10^5 pfu/dose) and serotype reassortant rhesus rotavirus vaccine (4×10^5 pfu/dose) in Native American Infants. Abstract in Fifth Rotavirus Vaccine Workshop. Current Issues and Future Development, Atlanta, Georgia, 1995, p. SIII-28. Atlanta Centers for Disease Control.

Sato, K., Inaba, Y., Shinozaki, T., Fujii, R., Matumota, M. (1981). Isolation of human rotavirus in cell cultures. *Arch. Virol.* **69**, 155–160.

Sereno, M. M., and Gorziglia, M. (1994). The outer capsid protein VP4 of murine rotavirus strain Eb represents a tentative new P type. *Virology* **199**, 500–504.

Smith, J. C., Haddix, A. C., Teutsch, S. M., and Glass, R. I. (1995). Cost effectiveness analysis of a rotavirus immunization program for the United States. *Pediatrics* **96**, 609–615.

Snodgrass, D. R., and Wells, P. W. (1976). Rotavirus infection in lambs. Studies on passive protection. *Arch. Virol.* **52**, 201–205.

Stuker, G., Oshiro, L., and Schmidt, N. J. (1980). Antigenic composition of two new rotavirus from rhesus monkeys. *J. Clin. Microbiol.* **11**, 202–203.

Urasawa, T., Urasawa, S., and Taniguchi, K. (1981). Sequential passages of human rotavirus in MA-104 cells. *Microbiol. Immunol.* **25**, 1025–1035.

Vesikari, T. (1994). Bovine rotavirus-based vaccines in humans. *In* "Viral Infections of the Gastrointestinal Tract" (A. Z. Kapikian, ed.), pp. 419–442. Dekker, New York.

Vesikari, T., Isolauri, E., D'Hondt, E., Delem, A., and Andre, F. E. (1984). Increased "take" rate of oral rotavirus vaccine in infants after milk feeding. *Lancet* **2**, 700.

Vesikari, T., Rautanen, T., Varis, T., Beards, G. M., and Kapikian, A. Z. (1990). Rhesus rotavirus candidate vaccine. Clinical trial in children vaccinated between 2 and 5 months of age. *Am. J. Dis. Child.* **144**, 285–289.

Vesikari, T., Ruuska, T., Kouvu, H. P., Green, K. Y., Flores, J., and Kapikian, A. Z. (1991). Evaluation of the M37 human rotavirus vaccine in 2- to 6-month-old infants. *Pediatr. Inf. Dis. J.* **10**, 912–917.

Vesikari, T., Ruuska, T., Green, K. Y., Flores, J., and Kapikian, A. Z. (1992). Protective efficacy against serotype 1 rotavirus diarrhea by live oral rhesus–human reassortant rotavirus vaccines with human rotavirus VP7 serotype 1 or 2 specificity. *Pediatr. Inf. Dis. J.* **11**, 535–542.

Wallace, R. E., Vasington, P. J., Petricciani, J. C., Hopps, H. E., Lorenz, D. E., and Kodanka, Z. (1973). Development of a diploid cell line from fetal rhesus monkey lung for virus vaccine production. *In Vitro* **8**, 323–332.

Weiss, C., and Clark, H. F. (1985). Rapid inactivation of rotaviruses by exposure to acidic buffer or acid gastric juice. *J. Gen. Virol.* **66**, 2725–2730.

Woode, G. N., Bridger, J. C., Jones, J. M., Flewett, T. H., Bryden, A. S., Davies, H. A., and White, G. B. B. (1976). Morphological and antigenic relationships between viruses (rotaviruses) from acute gastroentertis of children, calves, piglets, mice and foals. *Infect. Immun.* **14**, 804–810.

World Health Organization Scientific Working Group. (1980). Rotavirus and other viral diarrhoeas. *Bull. WHO* **58**, 183–198.

Wyatt, R. G., James, W. D., Bohl, E. H., Theil, K. W., Saif, L. J., Kalica, A. R., Greenberg, H. B., Kapikian, A. Z., and Chanock, R. M. (1980), Human rotavirus type 2: Cultivation *in vitro*. *Science* **207**, 189–191.

Wyatt, R. G., Kapikian, A. Z., Hoshino, Y., Flores, J., Midthun, K., Greenberg, H. B., Glass, R. I., Askaa, J., Levine, M. M., Black, R. E., Clements, M. L., Potash, L., and London, W. T. (1985). *In* "Control and Eradication of Infectious Diseases: An International Symposium" PAHO copublication series No. 1, pp. 17–28. Pan American Health Organization, Washington, D.C.

Wyatt, R. G., Mebus, C. A., Yolken, R. H., Kalica, A. R., James, H. D., Jr., Kapikian, A. Z., and Chanock, R. M. (1979). Rotaviral immunity in gnotobiotic calves: Heterologous resistance to human virus induced by bovine virus. *Science* **203**, 548–550.

27

Rectal and Genital Immunization with SIV/HIV

THOMAS LEHNER
Department of Immunology
United Medical and Dental Schools at Guy's and St. Thomase's Hospital
London SE1 9RT, England

CHRISTOPHER J. MILLER
Virology and Immunology Unit
California Regional Primate Research Center
University of California
Davis, California 95616

I. Introduction

The World Health Organization estimates that 6 to 8 million people are currently infected with HIV worldwide. The most conservative estimates predict that 15 to 20 million people will be infected with HIV by the year 2000 and most of these people will be infected through heterosexual contact. This is particularly true in the urban centers of sub-Saharan Africa and Asia (Johnson, 1988; Piot *et al.*, 1988). Most of the HIV-infected patients will develop the acquired immune deficiency syndrome (AIDS). In developed countries HIV is transmitted most commonly by homosexual contact (Winkelstein *et al.*, 1986), or through contaminated needles. Overall, more than 70% of patients are infected by HIV through the genital or rectal mucosa (European Study Group, 1992; Curran *et al.*, 1985). Despite the large number of people infected, epidemiological studies indicate that HIV is not transmitted efficiently from one individual to another by heterosexual contact (reviewed in *Miller et al.*, 1993). Because the mean period from seroconversion to AIDS is about 8–10 years (Baccheti and Moss, 1989), these individuals have the potential, through sexual contact, to disseminate HIV widely before they become aware that they are infectious. Indeed, AIDS may spread further and cause a more serious global epidemic than is currently appreciated. Vaccination against microbial agents is the most cost effective approach in reducing morbidity and mortality in a population, and because there is no cure for AIDS, it is critical to develop an effective HIV vaccine. In developing countries, with a limited medical infrastructure, vaccines may offer the only practical strategy to reduce the impact of HIV.

II. Genito-Urinary and Rectal Epithelia

Mucosal transmission of HIV may take place through the cervico-vaginal, rectal, urethral, or foreskin epithelium, during vaginal or anal sex. The possibility has also been considered, but certainly not established, that oral sex might lead to infection by HIV (Dossey, 1988; Detels and Visschers, 1988; Ho *et al.*, 1985). A comparative histological examination of the most relevant human epithelia has shown (Hussain and Lehner, 1995) that the mean thickness (±SD) of oral (263 ± 1.6 mm) or vaginal epithelium (215.5 ± 89.2 mm) is about 9 to 12 times greater than that of rectal epithelium (24.6 ± 9.7 mm). These results are consistent with the view that rectal mucosa is more likely to be breached during rectal intercourse than vaginal or oral epithelium during vaginal or oral sex. This is compounded by the trauma inflicted to the rectal mucosa during intercourse, and the rich vascular bed of the rectal mucosa which may facilitate virus entry. Quite apart from the purely morphological features, there is evidence that recurrent infections of the rectum or the cervix and the high incidence of cervical erosions, especially in high-risk groups, facilitate rectal or cervico-vaginal transmission of HIV (European Study Group, 1992; Felman, 1990), probably by providing a breach in mucosal integrity.

The male foreskin and urethra might also become infected when exposed to HIV-infected cervical secretions during heterosexual intercourse or on direct contact with infected rectal tissues during homosexual intercourse (Winkelstein *et al.*, 1986; Curran *et al.*, 1985; Mayer *et al.*, 1986; Simonsen *et al.*, 1988; Cameron *et al.*, 1989). The target cells for HIV infection of the male genitourinary tract are unclear; however the presence of foreskin in homosexual men is clearly associated with increased risk of HIV infection (Kreiss and Hopkins, 1992). In contrast, there is a lack of evidence supporting transmission of HIV by oral sex (Dossey, 1988; Detels and Visschers, 1988) or by intimate kissing between sero-positive subjects (harboring HIV in saliva) and sero-negative subjects (Ho *et al.*, 1985). It is also possible that a salivary inhibitor may inactivate HIV and prevent infection (Fox *et al.*, 1989).

III. Epithelial Cells and Receptors Involved in HIV Transmission

For HIV transmission to occur through an intact mucosal surface, the virus must initially bind to an epithelial receptor. There are five potential cells or receptors which may be involved in HIV infection.

A. CD4 Glycoprotein and Langerhans Cells

The CD4 glycoprotein is the main receptor for HIV and targets for HIV appear to be cells expressing the 55-kDa CD4 glycoprotein, such as T cells, macrophages, and dendritic and Langerhans cells (Dalgleish *et al.*, 1984; Klatzmann *et al.*, 1984). The V1 domain of the CD4 glycoprotein binds the HIV gp120 envelope glycoprotein (Maddon *et al.*, 1987; Arthos *et al.*, 1989; Peterson and Seed, 1988). The other three domains of CD4 may be involved in cell to cell fusion or syncytium formation (Camerini and Seed, 1990; Healey *et al.*, 1990). CD4 is not expressed by vaginal, rectal, urethral, oral, or foreskin epithelial cells, although $CD4^+$ mononuclear cells are present in the lamina propria of each epithelium. However, CD4 is expressed by Langerhans cells (Fig. 1) which are present in the cervico-vaginal, foreskin, and oral epithelia but not those of the rectum or urethra (Miller *et al.*, 1992c, 1994; Hussain and Lehner, 1995). There are significantly more Langerhans cells in the upper third of vaginal or foreskin epithelium than found in oral epithelium. This may be one indicator of the high risk factor in uncircumsized males contracting HIV infection (Kreiss and Hopkins, 1992), as compared with the very low risk of transmission of HIV through the normal oral mucosa during oral sex (Dossey, 1988; Detels and Visschers, 1988). Although HIV has been detected in Langerhans cells of patients with AIDS (Jarry *et al.*, 1990; Tschachler *et al.*, 1987) others have been unable to confirm this (Kanitakis *et al.*, 1989; Kalter *et al.*, 1990).

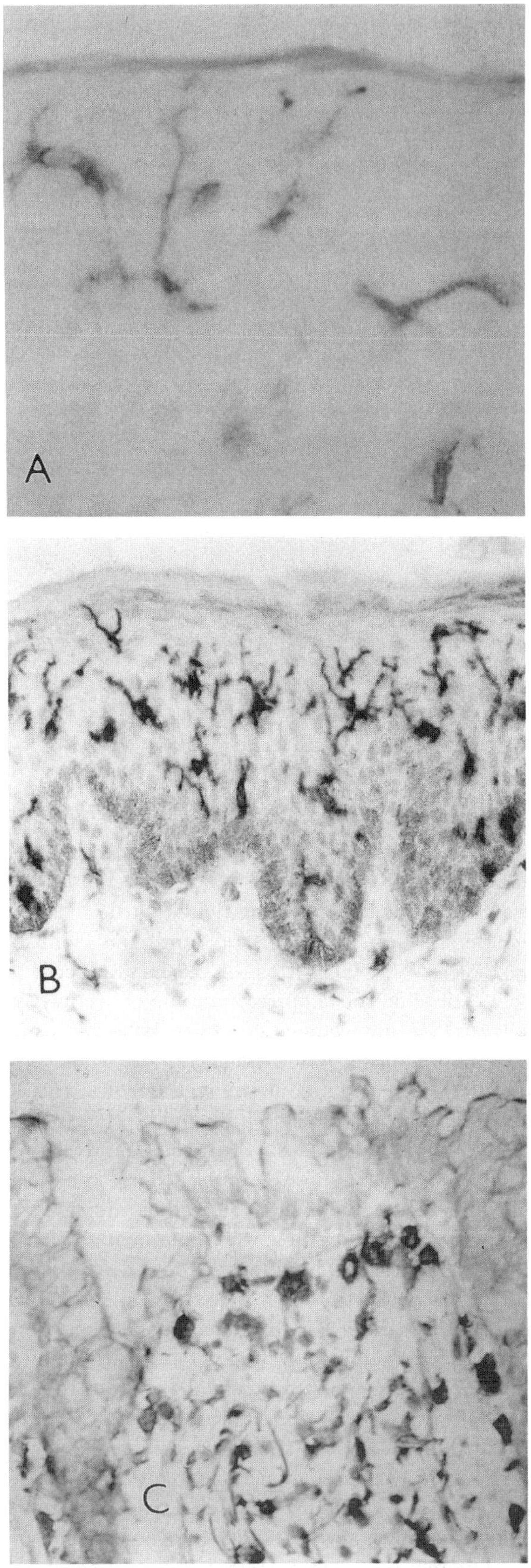

Figure 1. Langerhans cells in (A) cervico-vaginal and (B) foreskin epithelia, stained with CD1 monoclonal antibodies, compared with (C) rectal epithelium, which shows no Langerhans cells but $CD4^+$ cells in the lamina propria.

B. Microfold Cells

Microfold or M cells are found among the epithelial cells covering Peyer's patches in the intestine (Owen and Nemanic, 1978). Numerous lymphoid follicles with M cells have been reported in the rectal mucosa (O'Leary and Sweeny, 1986). Rodent M cells are capable of transmitting HIV to lymphoid cells (Amerongen *et al.*, 1991). However, HIV has yet to be identified in human M cells, though HIV nucleic acid has been detected in rectal epithelium (Nelson *et al.*, 1988; Mathijs *et al.*, 1988).

C. Galactosyl Cerebroside or Sulfatide

The galactosyl cerebroside or sulfatide has been postulated to serve as an alternative receptor for HIV-1 in human colonic epithelial cells which do not express CD4 (Yahi *et al.*, 1992). The envelope gp120 of HIV-1 binds to galactosyl cerebroside and two regions within gp120 might be involved: the V3 loop (van der Berg *et al.*, 1992) and the C2 region (AA 206–275) (Bhat *et al.*, 1993). The presence of galactosyl cerebroside or sulfatide on human colonic cells has been extended to human vaginal epithelial cells which may bind HIV-1 gp120 by means of sulfated lactosyl ceramide (Furuta *et al.*, 1994). Binding of HIV-1 to galactosyl or lactosyl ceramide might result in direct infection by HIV-1 or adhesion of infected cells expressing gp120 on their surface.

D. Fc Receptors for IgG (FcγR)

The Fc receptor for IgG (FcγR) offers an alternative mechanism for cell-free HIV infection, by enabling HIV–antibody complexes to bind via Fcγ receptors to epithelial cells (Takeda *et al.*, 1988; Homsy *et al.*, 1989). Indeed, infected seminal fluid contains HIV and IgG antibodies (Wolff *et al.*, 1992), so immune complexes can be formed. FcγII and FcγIII receptors were detected in rectal, endocervical, and urethral epithelia (Hussain *et al.*, 1991, 1992) and FcγIII and FcγI receptors were detected in the foreskin epithelium (Hussain and Lehner, 1995), which may enable HIV–antibody complexes to bind to these epithelial cells. However, FcγI and FcγII receptors were not found in oral epithelium and FcγIII receptors were confined to gingival epithelium (Hussain and Lehner, 1995). This would diminish the chances of oral HIV infection by means of HIV–antibody complexes.

E. HLA Class II Expression on Epithelial Cells

The expression of class II MHC on the epithelial cell may enable HIV-bound $CD4^+$ cells to gain access to the cells. The expression of HLA-DR was investigated in cervico-vaginal, rectal, urethral, and oral epithelia and foreskin, as HIV in seminal and cervico-vaginal fluid might be CD4 cell-associated, and CD4 glycoprotein binds HLA class II antigen (Doyle and Strominger, 1987). It is noteworthy that the epithelial cells lining the endocervical [but not vaginal or rectal tract (Hussain *et al.*, 1992)] and male genito-urinary tract can express HLA class II (DR) antigen (Ritchie *et al.*, 1984). This may be associated with T-cell activation, especially during infection. Whether HLA class II might enable CD4 cell-associated HIV to bind and facilitate infection of these epithelial cells needs to be explored.

F. Nonspecific Entry into Epithelial Cells

$CD4^-$ cervical and intestinal cells can be infected directly by HIV-infected monocytes *in vitro* (Bourinbaiar and Phillips, 1991). The mode of entry of HIV appears to be primarily by the phagocytic pathway, through membrane invagination enclosing virions, or through receptor-mediated endocytosis. Direct fusion between viral envelope and epithelial membrane has also been observed by electron microscopy (Bourinbaiar and Phillips, 1991).

G. Trauma and Infection of the Rectal Mucosa and Cervix

It has been generally assumed that trauma and/or infection may facilitate transmission of HIV due to the thin columnar epithelium of the rectum, compared with the thick stratified squamous epithelium of vaginal or oral mucosa. Indeed, as discussed above vaginal epithelium is about 9 to 12 times thicker than that of rectal epithelium, so that rectal mucosa is more vulnerable to be breached during rectal intercourse than vaginal or oral epithelia during vaginal or oral sex.

IV. Functional Biology of the Draining Lymph Nodes

The significance of lymph nodes in HIV infection has greatly increased with the realization that they appear to serve as viral reservoirs (Pantaleo *et al.*, 1993; Embretson *et al.*, 1993). Recent investigations of HIV dynamics indicate a rapid replication of HIV with a half-life of about 2 days (Ho *et al.*, 1995; Wei *et al.*, 1995). Although the location of the replicating CD4 population is not known, it does not appear to reside in the PBMC pool, and is more likely to be located in the lymphoid tissue (Pantaleo *et al.*, 1993; Embretson *et al.*, 1993).

It has been suggested that HIV is transmitted through the intact epithelium by Langerhans cells, or epithelial cells may pass the virus to macrophages or dendritic cells in the lamina propria. These cells will enter the lymphatics to drain to the local lymph nodes. The male and female genito-urinary system drains primarily into the external and internal iliac lymph nodes, and the rectum to the internal and common iliac as well as inferior mesenteric lymph nodes. We have conducted autopsy examinations of rhesus and cynomolgus macaques after mucosal genital, rectal, or targeted lymph node immunization; this revealed enlarged internal and external iliac lymph nodes containing T and B cells sensitized to the immunizing SIV p27 antigen (Lehner *et al.*, 1992a, 1993, 1994a). The internal iliac lymph nodes were also identified after vaginal submucosal administration of colloidal carbon in rhesus macaques (Miller *et al.*, 1992a) and are consistent with the lymph nodes identified by subserous immunization of the female mouse pelvis (Thapar *et al.*, 1990).

T-cell proliferative responses to p27 were elicited by the iliac and inferior mesenteric lymph nodes and the spleen, but not the superior mesenteric, bronchial, or axillary lymph nodes after mucosal or TLN immunization (Lehner *et al.*, 1994a). This pattern of responses differed from that induced by intramuscular immunization, in which only the spleen (and none of the examined lymph nodes) yielded a proliferative response to the p27 antigen.

Reconstitution experiments with enriched CD4$^+$ T cells, B cells, and macrophages separated from the spleen and iliac lymph nodes after TLN immunization elicited SIV p27-specific IgA and IgG antibodies (Lehner *et al.*, 1994b). However, although splenic cells elicited higher IgG than IgA antibodies, the iliac lymph node cells yielded comparable IgG and IgA antibodies. A comparison of TLN with the two mucosal and the intramuscular routes of immunization showed similar results with reconstituted splenic cells, in that p27-specific IgG antibodies were higher than the IgA antibodies. Reconstituted iliac lymph node cells yielded higher IgA than IgG antibodies after the two mucosal routes of immunization, similar IgA and IgG antibodies after TLN, and no antibodies after intramuscular immunization. The results suggest that all routes of immunization elicit splenic CD4$^+$ T-cell-proliferative and helper function in B-cell antibody synthesis. However, only mucosal immunization induced both T- and B-cell functions in the regional draining lymph nodes. Recently, antibody-secreting IgG and IgA cells to SIV p27 and gp120 have been identified in the iliac lymph nodes and spleen (Lehner *et al.*, 1995).

V. HIV/SIV Target Cells in the Genital and Rectal Tracts

A. Genital Tract

The identity and location of the cellular targets of HIV/SIV during genital transmission are yet to be determined. Topical application of SIV onto the intact genital mucosa of mature and immature rhesus macaques results in virus transmission, and the disease induced by this route of inoculation is indistinguishable from that seen in intravenously inoculated animals (Miller *et al.*, 1989, 1990). SIV is efficiently transmitted to hysterectomized female macaques by inoculation of cell-free virus into blind vaginal pouches (Miller *et al.*, 1992a). Since there are no CD4$^+$ T cells in the vaginal epithelium, and only a few CD4$^+$ T cells are present in the submucosa of the vagina (Miller *et al.*, 1992c; Hussain and Lehner, 1995), the most likely target cells in the vaginal mucosa are Langerhans cells or macrophages (Miller *et al.*, 1992b,c; Hussain and Lehner, 1995). In chronically infected female rhesus macaques, SIV-infected cells are present in the uterus, cervix, and vagina (Miller *et al.*, 1992b). The majority of the SIV-infected cells are located in the submucosa of the ectocervix and vagina and have a morphology consistent with T lymphocytes and monocytes/macrophages. Occasionally, SIV-infected cells are also found within the stratified squamous epithelium of the vagina (Fig. 2). Some of the

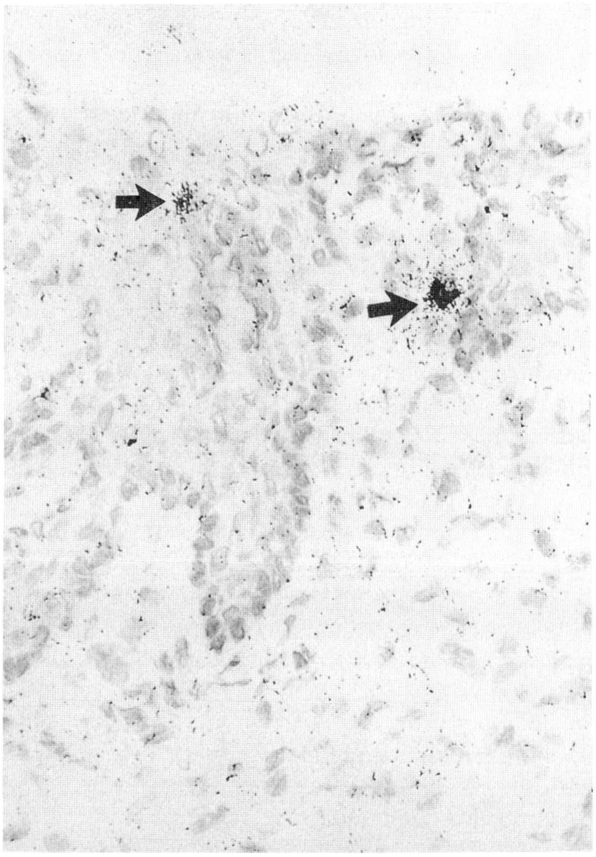

Figure 2. Vaginal mucosa from a chronically SIV-infected rhesus macaque. *In situ* hybridization for detection of SIV nucleic acid demonstrates the presence of two SIV-infected cells (arrowheads) in the stratified squamous epithelium of the mucosa. Cells with a dendritic morphology can be detected by immunohistochemical staining for SIV p27 and these might be CD4$^+$ Langerhans cells.

infected cells in this location have a dendritic cell morphology consistent with Langerhans cells (Miller *et al.*, 1992c). Langerhans cells of the skin have been reported to be infected with HIV in AIDS patients (Tschachler *et al.*, 1987; Zambruno *et al.*, 1991). In a cervical biopsy material obtained from HIV-infected women, T cells and macrophages were infected with HIV (Pomerantz *et al.*, 1988; Nuovo *et al.*, 1993). These findings are consistent with the results in SIV-infected monkeys. Although *in vitro* studies have demonstrated that HIV is capable of infecting epithelial cells, there is currently no evidence that epithelial cells are infected in the reproductive tract of either SIV-infected monkeys or HIV-in-fected humans. Many laboratories using sophisticated techniques were unable to find SIV- or HIV-infected epithelial cells in the genital tract, but a rapid transit from epithelial to lymphoid cells has not been excluded.

HIV/SIV transmission to males may involve similar types of target cells, but studies to detect the location of HIV-infected cells in the penis of infected men are lacking. However, $CD4^+$ Langerhans cells are located in the foreskin (Hussain and Lehner, 1995) and the epidemiological evidence that an intact foreskin is associated with an increased risk of HIV infection (Simonsen *et al.*, 1988; Cameron *et al.*, 1989; Kreiss and Hopkins, 1992) suggests that Langerhans cells in the foreskin may be target cells during genital transmission. There is experimental evidence in adult male rhesus macaques that they can be infected with SIV by placing cell-free virus onto their foreskins (Miller *et al.*, 1994). Furthermore, SIV nucleic acid was found in the Langerhans cells of the foreskins of SIV-infected macaques (Miller *et al.*, 1994).

These findings suggest that Langerhans cells may have a role as target cells in sexual transmission of HIV and SIV. These antigen-presenting cells are potentially efficient disseminators of virus from the genital mucosa to the draining lymph nodes. These cells transport antigen from the stratified squamous epithelium to the draining lymph nodes (Hoefsmit *et al.*, 1982; Krael *et al.*, 1986; Kripke *et al.*, 1990; Kupiec-Weglinski *et al.*, 1988; Silberberg-Sinakin *et al.*, 1976; Steinman, 1991). Blood dendritic cells (of which Langerhans cell precursors are a subset) can be infected with HIV (Patterson and Knight, 1987; Macatonia *et al.*, 1990; Steinman, 1991; Patterson *et al.*, 1991). Furthermore, when infected *in vitro,* these cells produce much higher levels of virus than T cells but do not exhibit the usual cytopathic effects associated with HIV infection (Langhoff *et al.*, 1991). Thus, Langerhans cells in the male and female genital tract (Bjerke *et al.*, 1983; Edwards and Morris, 1985; Morris *et al.*, 1983; Hussain *et al.*, 1992; Hussain and Lehner, 1995) may be especially well suited as target cells for sexual transmission of HIV and SIV (Miller *et al.*, 1992a,b).

B. Lower Intestinal and Rectal Tract

Transmission of HIV by homosexual contact involves deposition of infectious semen into the rectum. If the simple columnar epithelium of the rectum is disrupted during anal intercourse this may provide HIV direct access to the monocytes, lymphocytes, and dendritic cells in the lamina propria. Studies in SIV-infected monkeys have demonstrated that viral mRNA is commonly found in the numerous $CD4^+$ monocytes and T cells in the lamina propria of the intestinal tract (Heise *et al.*, 1993, 1994). In addition, SIV-infected intraepithelial lymphocytes were also seen in these studies, but there was no evidence of epithelial cell infection in the animals examined (Heise, 1993). Numerous studies have demonstrated that HIV is capable of infection in a variety of epithelial cells *in vitro* and some studies have identified a few HIV-infected cells in the epithelial layer of the intestine (Levy, 1993). Some investigators have interpreted this finding to indicate that the enterocytes can be targets for HIV infection; however, a convincing demonstration that the cell type involved was epithelial has not been provided in any of the reports utilizing tissues obtained from AIDS patients. It is possible, however, that there is rapid transit from $CD4^-$ enterocytes or M cells to adjacent $CD4^+$ cells, thereby decreasing the chances of HIV being found in nonlymphoid cells.

VI. Importance of Viral Variants in Sexual Transmission of HIV

Studies of HIV-1 variation have identified two phenotypes: the macrophage-tropic (M tropic) and T-cell-line tropic (T-tropic) viruses. Many or most primary patient isolates are able to replicate in both peripheral blood lymphocytes and macrophages. These viruses generally exhibit slow or low replication kinetics in peripheral blood mononuclear cells, they do not replicate in or induce the formation of syncytia in most established T-cell lines, and they exhibit a lower sensitivity to soluble CD4 than that which is observed for the T-tropic viruses. In contrast, the T-tropic viruses do not replicate efficiently in monocytes or macrophages, but do replicate efficiently in PBMC and established T-cell lines, form syncytia in T-cell lines, and are sensitive to soluble CD4. There is evidence to suggest that the virus population is homogeneous early in infection with respect to cell-tropism and nucleic acid sequence (Pang *et al.*, 1992; Zhu *et al.*, 1993; Zhang *et al.*, 1993). In a few cases where the transmitting and newly infected partners have been identified, the virus transmitted may represent a variant present at low frequency in the donor viral population that is noncytopathic and macrophage tropic (Zhu *et al.*, 1993). However, viral variability can develop rapidly after infection (Pang *et al.*, 1992; Zhu *et al.*, 1993).

Three hypotheses have been proposed to explain the discrepancy between the heterogeneous virus population in the transmitting partner and the homogeneous virus recovered from a recently infected partner. The homogeneous virus observed in a newly infected person could reflect (a) exposure to a low titer of virus from the transmitter, (b) selective amplification of one variant after entering the new host, or (c) selective transmission of viral variants across the genital mucosa (Zhu *et al.*, 1993). The observation that the transmitted virus represents a minor, noncytopathic, macrophage-tropic variant in the blood of the transmitter supports the latter explanation (Zhu *et al.*, 1993). In contrast to the above reports, results of recent studies indicate that the biological phenotype or genotype of HIV isolated from the transmitting and newly infected partner is indistinguishable (Fiore *et al.*, 1994; Albert *et al.*, 1994). Indeed, individuals with rapid/high syncytium-inducing phenotype HIV-1 variants in peripheral blood often transmit this virus phenotype (Fiore *et al.*, 1994). Furthermore, individuals who are infected with rapid/high, syncytium-inducing HIV-1 variants also tend to retain this virus phenotype and show rapid disease progression. However, there is evidence for sexual transmission of multiple HIV variants with unique sequences in the *gag* and *pol* genes (Albert *et al.*, 1994). The discrepancy between the observations from different studies may be explained by differences in the stage of disease of the transmitting individuals, the regions of the HIV genome sequenced, and the methods used for sequence analyses [direct sequencing from viral nucleic acids (Albert *et al.*, 1994) or sequencing from cloned DNA (Levy, 1993)]. These conflicting reports emphasize the need to undertake further studies in this important area.

VII. Genital and Intestinal Antibody Responses to SIV/HIV Infection

A. Antibody Responses in the Genital Tract

Anti-viral antibodies are present in the vaginal secretions of HIV-infected women (Belec *et al.*, 1989; Archibald *et al.*, 1987; Lu *et al.*, 1993) and SIV-infected rhesus macaques (Miller *et al.*, 1992d). In the vaginal secretions from the SIV-infected monkeys, the immune response consisted principally of anti-SIV IgG and the levels of total IgG were elevated in both serum and vaginal secretions. The route of transmission (vaginal or intravenous) did not affect the nature of the genital antibody responses (Miller *et al.*, 1992d). Although both IgA and IgG HIV-specific antibodies are found in the vaginal secretions of women, the majority of anti-HIV antibody secretions seems to be of the IgG isotype (Belec *et al.*, 1989; Lu *et al.*, 1993). In one study (Lu *et al.*, 1993), the total IgG, IgA, and IgM levels in the vaginal fluid of HIV-infected women were several-fold higher than the levels in controls. In these women, IgG or IgA antibodies to gp160 were present but anti-gp 160 IgG predominated. No IgM antibodies to gp160 were detected. In many of these women the levels of total IgG in the secretions correlated with the level of total serum IgG. Thus, the results both in SIV-infected rhesus macaques and in HIV-infected women suggest that transudation of serum IgG antibodies is a significant source of anti-viral antibodies in vaginal secretions.

A recent, unpublished study analyzing samples from 51 HIV-1 infected women provides some insight into the origin of HIV-specific immunoglobulin in cervico-vaginal secretions (Xusheng Lu, personal communication, 1995). The seropositive, HIV-infected women studied have significantly increased levels of immunoglobulins and serum albumin in cervico-vaginal secretions, compared with secretions from HIV-negative controls. This result confirms the conclusion that a significant amount of the anti-HIV antibody in vaginal secretions is derived from serum. However, relatively high levels of secretory IgA (S-IgA) were also found in the genital secretions of these HIV-infected women, demonstrating that S-IgA can be locally produced during natural vaginal infection. In another recent unpublished communication, S-IgA antibodies to HIV were found in vaginal secretions of a number of sero-negative women who engaged in high-risk activity (D. Anderson, personal communication). This raises the important question whether vaginal S-IgA antibodies to HIV might be protective against vaginal transmission of HIV. Furthermore, there is a report that antibodies to HIV antigens can be detected in vaginal secretions from some women that are sero-negative and HIV-negative (Belec *et al.*, 1994). This raises the possibility that these women developed a local immune response to a subinfectious dose of HIV. However, we were unable to detect anti-SIV antibodies in the serum or vaginal secretions of rhesus macaques that became transiently viremic following intravaginal inoculation of SIVmac (C. Miller and Xusheng Lu, unpublished data, 1995). The results in the monkey model support the hypothesis that vaginal HIV antibodies may have been transferred passively to the women in semen during intercourse with HIV-infected partners.

HIV antibodies have also been detected in the semen of HIV-infected men (Wolff *et al.*, 1992; Belec *et al.*, 1989). In one study both IgA and IgG directed against HIV antigens were detected (Belec *et al.*, 1989), while in the other only anti-HIV IgG was detected in semen (Wolff *et al.*, 1992). In both reports, the gp160 IgG antibody response was striking. Although the relative contribution of serum-derived as compared with locally produced antibody was not directly addressed in either study, the finding that the seminal HIV antibody titers were consistently lower than those in paired serum samples led the investigators to speculate that the antibody was serum derived (Wolff *et al.*, 1992).

B. Antibody Responses in the Intestinal Tract

HIV-specific IgA and IgG have been found in the intestinal (Mathewson *et al.*, 1994; Janoff *et al.*, 1994) and rectal (Mohamed *et al.*, 1994) secretions of HIV-infected individuals and the presence of anti-HIV S-IgA in intestinal secretions was associated with diarrhea (Mathewson *et al.*, 1994). The elevated levels of IgG and monomeric IgA1 in the intestinal secretions of HIV-infected patients suggest that there is significant transudation of serum immunoglobulins into the intestine in these patients (Janoff *et al.*, 1994). Anti-HIV immunoglobulin bound to secretory component (presumably S-IgA) was found in rectal secretions of healthy HIV-infected patients (Mohamed *et al.*, 1994), suggesting that some anti-HIV was locally produced.

The overall impression reached upon reviewing the work characterizing HIV or SIV antibody responses in the intestinal and genital tracts is that a significant component of the HIV antibody in the secretions of chronically infected subjects or macaques is serum-derived and consists largely of IgG antibodies. Although HIV-specific S-IgA responses are found in the lower intestinal and genital tracts, their role in protection from viral infection has not been determined.

VIII. Genital and Rectal Cellular Responses to HIV/SIV Infection

CD4 and CD8 T-cell responses play a central role in both antibody and cell-mediated immunity. Most proteins are dependent on CD4 helper function in eliciting both IgG and S-IgA antibodies. Furthermore, the CD4 Th2 subset of cells generates cytokines which are essential in the production of IgA antibodies. Preferential IgA antibody synthesis to SIV p27 has been recorded *in vitro* with reconstituted iliac lymph node $CD4^+$ T cells, B cells, and macrophages, as compared with corresponding splenic cells, after augmented vaginal, rectal, male genital, or TLN immunization (Lehner *et al.*, 1992b, 1993, 1994a,b). Indeed, specific SIV gp120 and p27 antibody-secreting B cells have recently been eluted from rectal tissue and the draining iliac lymph nodes in macaques immunized by the TLN route with SIV gp120 and p27 (Lehner *et al.*, 1995).

$CD8^+$ class I-restricted cytotoxic T-cell responses to gp120, p27, nef and pol proteins have been associated with HIV-1 protection (Walker *et al.*, 1987; Nixon *et al.*, 1988) and this may be particularly significant in the acute phase of HIV-1 infection (Pantaleo *et al.*, 1994). The early development of a cytotoxic response to SIV has also been seen in rhesus monkeys acutely infected with SIV; this response may control initial viral replication (Yasutomi *et al.*, 1993; Reimann *et al.*, 1994). However, a high precursor frequency of $CD8^+$ cytotoxic cells has also been recorded later in HIV sero-positive subjects (Carmichael *et al.*, 1993). There is now evidence that $CD8^+$ cytotoxic cells can be identified in simian vaginal mucosa (Lohman *et al.*, 1995), rectal mucosal, and the draining iliac lymph nodes (Klavinskis *et al.*, 1996). Hence, both CD4 helper and cytokine generating cells, as well as CD8 cytotoxic cells, may exert their protective activities at the mucosal portal of entry of HIV infection.

Recent evidence suggests that the route of immunization may generate a diversity of T-cell epitopes and may determine their hierarchy in the draining lymph node, and splenic and circulating T cells (Lehner *et al.*, 1993; Brookes *et al.*, 1995). These studies have only been conducted with SIV p27 peptides. Intramuscular immunization induced a significantly higher frequency of circulating or splenic T-cell proliferation with peptides 121–140, 41–60, or 61–80 than the corresponding cells from macaques immunized by the female or male genital route ($P < 0.05$–< 0.01). However, iliac lymph node cells showed significantly higher T-cell proliferation with peptide 121–140 or 61–80 after male or female genital or TLN immunization than after intramuscular immunization ($P < 0.05$).

The T-cell subset which responded to p27 and the synthetic peptides was then determined by stimulating enriched $CD4^+$ and $CD8^+$ T lymphocytes from peripheral blood with p27. This showed high stimulation indices and counts to p27 by the $CD4^+$ cells (SI 44.3 $\pm$ 20.3, 3340 $\pm$ 1636 cpm), with low SI and counts by the $CD8^+$ cells (SI 6.9 $\pm$ 3.5, 529 $\pm$ 210 cpm). The possibility that the differences in T-cell epitope hierarchy might be due to differences in MHC expressed by the macaques was then examined. Macaques with the same MHC DR2, 3 haplotype were immunized with p27:Ty-VLP by the five routes. The T-cell epitope hierarchies differed with the immunization route, in spite of all five macaques sharing DR2,3 antigens, suggesting that it is not the MHC DR but the route of immunization which is responsible for generating the diversity of T-cell epitopes. Differences in the ability of antigen-presenting cells to process and present certain peptides may account for the diversity of epitope hierarchies (Brookes *et al.*, 1995). Indeed, dendritic cells were more effective than macrophages in processing and presenting the native p27 antigen or the peptides when tested by the proliferative assay. The diversity of T-cell epitopes may affect the control of HIV at different anatomical sites, the route of administration of the vaccine, and selection of polypeptides or recombinant antigens for immunization.

Th1 and Th2 cytokines, as well as CAF (CD8 cell anti-viral factor), are generated by CD4 and/or CD8 subsets of T cells and have been implicated in the pathogenesis of AIDS. The view that Th1 cells are essential for protection against the development of the manifestations of AIDS and Th2 cells may not be protective or may even be harmful (Clerici and Shearer, 1993) needs to be considered in the context of progress during the latent period of HIV-infected patients. There is no evidence that HIV infection (in contrast to the disease AIDS) can be prevented by generating a Th1-type response, for this would argue against any involvement of IgA antibodies in preventing HIV infection. Mucosal immunization favors Th2 cytokines and therefore antibody responses, but as discussed above CD4/CD8 proliferative and cytotoxic responses are also elicited. It appears that protection from the initial HIV infection might require Th2 cytokines for antibodies and Th1 cytokines for the cellular functions (especially CD8 cytotoxic cells), whereas progression to clinical AIDS may be associated with a switch from Th1 to Th2 cytokines (Clerici and Shearer, 1993). IL-12 may be particularly pertinent, since it stimulates maturation of Th1 cells (Hsieh *et al.*, 1993; Afonso *et al.*, 1994). CAF is a cytokine-like factor released from a CD8-cell subset; it inhibits HIV replication in CD4 cells (Mackewicz and Levy, 1992).

There is little direct evidence of cytokine functions in the genital or rectal mucosa. Preliminary evidence of genital, rectal, or TLN immunization, however, suggests that both Th1 (IL-2 and IFNγ) and Th2 (IL-4 and IL-5) types of cytokines are generated, but that the Th2 cytokines predominate, especially when cholera toxin is used as a mucosal adjuvant (Kiyono *et al.*, 1996).

IX. Routes of Immunization That Elicit Genito-Urinary and Rectal Immunity

Immunization via the mucosal associated lymphoid tissue might be expected to elicit S-IgA antibodies in the genito-urinary and rectal tracts (McDermott and Bienenstock, 1979; Mestecky, 1987). Indeed, oral immunization in rodents induced antibodies in the genital tract, and adoptively transferred murine mesenteric lymph node cells home to the genital tissues (McDermott and Bienenstock, 1979). Direct administration of SRBC into Peyer's patches of Sprague–Dawley rats induced vaginal IgA and IgG antibodies (Wira and Sandoe, 1987, 1989). These experiments suggest that sensitized B cells may home from GALT to the genital tract. However, oral immunization in nonhuman primates with the recombinant SIV *gag* p27 fused to the yeast retrotransposon virus-like particles (p27:Ty VLP) failed to induce significant S-IgA antibodies in the genital or rectal tracts (Lehner *et al.*, 1992b). Similarly, microencapsulated formalin-treated SIV administered orally to rhesus macaques failed to elicit vaginal antibodies or protection when challenged with live SIV by the vaginal route (Marx *et al.*, 1993). However, augmenting oral immunization (or intratracheal) with prior i.m. immunization with SIV induced vaginal IgG and IgA antibodies to SIV, and five out of six macaques were protected when challenged by the vaginal route (Marx *et al.*, 1993).

A comprehensive series of experiments in macaques with SIV p27:Ty-VLP covalently linked to cholera toxin B subunit (CT-B) for its adjuvant activity suggests that for effective genito-urinary or rectal immunity, local mucosal immunization needs to be augmented by oral and then intramuscular immunization (Lehner *et al.*, 1994b). Indeed, augmenting genital by oral immunization in female (Lehner *et al.*, 1992a) or male macaques (Lehner *et al.*, 1994a) or augmenting rectal by oral immunization (Lehner *et al.*, 1993) induced S-IgA and IgG antibodies to p27 at the corresponding mucosal surface. Serum antibodies and $CD4^+$ T-cell-proliferative responses to p27 were also elicited by the three routes of immunization. Autopsy examination of these macaques showed T- and B-cell responses in the internal iliac lymph node cells, in contrast to systemic immunization.

As an alternative strategy, a subcutaneous immunization technique was developed in order to administer the vaccine in the proximity of the internal and external iliac lymph nodes (Lehner *et al.*, 1994b). The same antigen was administered as that in the augmented mucosal immunization (p27:Ty-VLP), except aluminium hydroxide was used as an adjuvant. Significant concentrations of S-IgA (and IgG) antibodies to p27 were found after the second immunization in the rectal washings and urine of both sexes, in vaginal washings of female macaques, and in urethral washings and ejaculates of male macaques (Table I). Serum IgA antibody titers to p27 were higher than the corresponding IgG titers.

TLN immunization elicited a pattern of responses to p27 in the lymph nodes similar to those elicited by the three mucosal routes (internal and external iliac, inferior mesenteric, and iliac-paraortic), in addition to the splenic and circulating T lymphocytes. The proliferative T cells belonged to the $CD4^+$ subset, irrespective of the route of immunization (Lehner *et al.*, 1992a, 1993, 1994a,b). Reconstitution experiments with enriched $CD4^+$ T cells, B cells, and macrophages separated from the spleen and iliac lymph nodes after TLN immunization elicited SIV p27-specific IgA and IgG antibodies (Lehner *et al.*, 1994b). Although splenic cells elicited

TABLE I
Comparative Quantitative Analysis of SIV Anti-p27 IgA Antibodies, Following Five Routes of Immunization in 29 Macaques with SIV p27:Ty-VLP

	Route of immunization		IgA antibodies to p27[a]					
		No.	Rectal	Vaginal	Urethral	Seminal fluid	Urine	Serum
1a	TLN (male)	5	1.70 (0.41)	—	0.61 (0.12)	3.3 (0.15)	0.78 (0.18)	3.33 (0.54)
1b	TLN (female)	4	1.63 (0.27)	3.79 (0.38)	—	—	0.77 (0.12)	3.97 (0.48)
2	Recto–oral–IM[b]	6	1.16 (0.26)	—	0	—	0	2.81 (0.12)
3	Vagino–oral–IM	5	1.7 (0.36)	2.27 (0.28)	0	0	—	3.03 (0.14)
4	Genito–oral–IM[b]	4	1.60 (0.05)	—	0.89 (0.23)	1.4	0.84 (0.11)	1.96 (0.05)
5	Intramuscular	5	0	0	0	—	0	2.34 (0.29)

[a]p27-specific IgA antibodies are expressed as a % of total IgA concentration and are given as mean % (±SEM).
[b]Male.

higher IgG than IgA antibodies, the iliac lymph node cells yielded comparable IgG and IgA antibodies.

Localization of specific T- and B cells to the draining lymph nodes of the genito-urinary and rectal tracts might be essential in preventing transmission of HIV by infected Langerhans cells, dendritic cells, or macrophages from the mucosal tissues to the lymph nodes. These T- and B-cell functions might prevent formation of a viral reservoir in the draining lymph nodes, if the mucosal immune barrier were breached. The significance of this observation has been strengthened by recent reports that HIV is found early in infection in the lymph nodes (Pantaleo *et al.*, 1993; Embretson *et al.*, 1993) and that the virus particles are bound to follicular dendritic cells as immune complexes (Armstrong and Horne, 1984; Tenner-Racz *et al.*, 1986; Biberfeld *et al.*, 1986). A central immune barrier is also induced, which is comparable to that found after i.m. immunization, in that splenic and circulating proliferative and helper T cells are found, as well as sensitized B cells and IgG and IgA antibodies.

X. Mucosal Immunity in Protection against Mucosal Challenge by Live SIV

Most of the SIV vaccine studies to date have been limited to parenteral immunization schedules and systemic routes of virus challenge. In nonhuman primates HIV-1 has been used in chimpanzees and both HIV-2 and SIV in macaques to test the efficacy of vaccines against intravenous challenge. Effective protection has resulted using inactivated whole virus, modified live virus, and envelope-based vaccines (reviewed by Gardner and Hu, 1991). Most of the SIV studies have been carried out with inactivated SIV grown in human T cells. It was later established that the immunity was due to human cellular components (HLA class I and class II) and that protection could be elicited by immunization with SIV-free human T cells (Stott, 1991; Arthur *et al.*, 1992; Chan *et al.*, 1992; Langlois *et al.*, 1992; Bergmeier *et al.*, 1994).

Systemic immunization with inactivated SIV grown in human cells has failed to protect macaques from vaginal challenge with the live SIV (Marthas *et al.*, 1992). However, an augmented mucosal systemic strategy, outlined above, has been used more successfully, in which inactivated SIV grown in human cells was prepared in microcapsules administered first i.m. and then by either the oral or intratracheal route (Marx *et al.*, 1993). Indeed, five out of six macaques were protected when challenged by the vaginal route; this protection was associated with vaginal IgA and IgG antibodies (Marx *et al.*, 1993). Nevertheless, rectal transmission with SIV was prevented by intramuscular immunization alone with inactivated SIV grown in human T cells (Cranage *et al.*, 1992). These two successful experiments suggest that at least xenogeneic anti-cell antibodies can protect vaginal or rectal transmission of SIV by augmented mucosal–systemic or systemic immunization, respectively (Marx *et al.*, 1993; Cranage *et al.*, 1992). Recently, recombinant SIV envelope gp120 and core p27 were administered by the novel targeted lymph node immunization strategy (Lehner *et al.*, 1996). This elicited S-IgA and IgG antibodies to gp120 and p27 in rectal fluid, rectal, and lymph node antibody-secreting B cells to these antigens and T-cell proliferative and cytotoxic cells. Rectal challenge with an SIV molecular clone showed either total prevention of SIV infection or decreased viral load by more than 90%. If these results are readily reproducible, a subunit vaccine strategy might be pursued.

A fundamental problem in vaccination against SIV/HIV is that the mechanism preventing infection has not been identified. Both B- and T-cell immunity have been reported, with neutralizing IgG antibodies to gp120 (Javaherian *et al.*, 1992; Moore *et al.*, 1994) and $CD8^{+}$ MHC class I-restricted cytotoxic cells to gp120 and p27 antigens (Walker *et al.*, 1987; Nixon *et al.*, 1988; Koenig *et al.*, 1988). A working hypothesis has been postulated that sexual transmission of HIV/SIV might be controlled by five successive immune barriers, with each barrier in turn either preventing infection or progressively decreasing the viral load (Lehner *et al.*, 1995). In Barrier 1, viral adhesion to mucosal surface may be prevented by S-IgA (and IgG) antibodies to gp120. If this proves ineffective, Barrier 2, consisting of intraepithelial polymeric IgA to p27 (or gp120), may prevent viral assembly. However, any virus that crosses the epithelium will encounter the subepithelial immune Barrier 3, consisting of SIV-specific B cells secreting antibodies, CD4 cells producing cytokines, and CD8 cytotoxic cells. If the rectal epithelium is not intact or is breached through trauma, the third immune barrier in the submucosa, the fourth barrier in the draining lymph nodes, and the fifth barrier in the circulation and spleen remains.

The three different immune mechanisms involved at the first three barriers seem to offer the best chance of preventing viral transmission at the site of entry. The regional lymph nodes to which any virus that has successfully breached the mucosal and submucosal barriers is carried by macrophages, Langerhans cells, or dendritic cells may not permit viral latency and formation of a viral reservoir on account of the potent CD8, CD4, and B-cell responses. Indeed, IgG-p27-C3d immune complexes may localize on the surface of follicular dendritic cells in lymphoid follicles (Armstrong and Horne, 1984; Tenner-Racz *et al.*, 1986; Biberfeld *et al.*, 1986) activate T and B cells and prevent or decrease viral load in these lymph nodes. Dissemination of any residual live virus might be arrested by the circulating serum antibodies and T-cell functions. The five successive immune barriers may utilize a fail-safe defense strategy, with site-directed differences in isotype (IgA or IgG), subunit antigen (envelope or core protein), and recognition of defined T- and B-cell epitopes. This concept is consistent with recent findings concerning the crucial role of lymph nodes as reservoirs of infection (Ho *et al.*, 1995; Wei *et al.*, 1995), the homing of specific antibody-forming B cells (Lehner *et al.*, 1995) and cytotoxic CD8 cells to the vaginal (Lohman *et al.*, 1995) or rectal mucosa (Klavinskis *et al.*, 1996), the intraepithelial mechanism of virus-neutralizing IgA antibodies (Mazanec *et al.*, 1992), and the differential T-cell epitope expression with the route of immunization (Brookes *et al.*, 1995).

References

Afonso, L. C. C., Scharton, T. M., Viera, L. Q., Wysocka, M., Trincheieri, G., and Scott, P. (1994). The adjuvant effect of interleukin-12 in a vaccine against Leichmania major. *Science* **263**, 235–237.

Albert, J., Walhberg, J., Leitner, T., Escanilla, D., and Uhlen, M. (1994). Analysis of a rape case by direct sequencing of the human immunodeficiency virus type 1 *pol* and *gag* genes. *J. Virol.* **68**, 5918–5924.

Amerongen, H. M., Weltzin, R., Farnet, C. M., Michetti, P., Haseltine, W. A., and Neutra, M. R. (1991). Transepithelial transport of HIV-1 by intestinal M cells: A mechanism for transmission of AIDS. *J. Acquired Immune Defic. Syndr.* **4**, 760–765.

Archibald, D. W., Witt, D. J., Craven, D. E., Vogt, M. W., Hirsch, M. S., and Essex, M. (1987). Antibodies to human immunodeficiency virus in cervical secretions from women at risk from AIDS. *J. Infect. Dis.* **156**, 240–241.

Armstrong, J. A., and Horne, R. (1984). Follicular dendritic cells and virus-like particles in AIDS-related lymphadenopathy. *Lancet* **1**, 370–372.

Arthos, J., Deen, K., Chaikin, M., Fornwald, J., Sathe, G., Sattentau, Q., Clapham, P., Weiss, R., McDougal, J., Pietropaolo, C., Axel, R., Truneh, A., Maddon, P., and Sweet, R. (1989). Identification of the residues in human CD4 critical for the binding of HIV. *Cell. (Cambridge)* **57**, 469–481.

Arthur, L. O., Bess, J. W., Jr., Sowder II, R. C. *et al.* (1992). Cellular proteins bound to immunodeficiency viruses: Implications for pathogenesis and vaccines. *Science* **258**, 1935–1938.

Baccheti, P., and Moss, A. R. (1989). Incubation period of AIDS in San Francisco. *Nature (London)* **338**, 251–253.

Belec, L., Georges, A., Steenman, G., and Martin, P. (1989). Antibodies to human immunodeficiency virus in vaginal secretions of heterosexual women. *J. Infect. Dis.* **160**, 385–391.

Belec, L., Tevi-Benissan, C., Gresenguet, G., Meillet, D., and Pillot, J. (1994). HIV-1 antibody serum negativity with vaginal secretions positively. *Lancet* **343**, 1047–1048.

Bergmeier, L. A., Walker, J., Tao, L., Cranage, M., and Lehner, T. (1994). Antibodies to human and non-human primate cellular and culture medium components in macaques vaccinated with the simian immunodeficiency virus. *Immunology* **83**, 213–220.

Bhat, S., Mettus, R. V., Reddy, E. P., Ugen, K. E., Srikanthan, V., Williams, W. V., and Weiner, D. B. (1993). The galactosyl ceramide/sulfatide receptor binding region of HIV-1 gp120 maps to amino acids 206–275. *AIDS Res. Hum. Retroviruses* **9**, 175–181.

Biberfeld, P., Chayt, K. J., Marselle, L. M., Biberfeld, G., Gallo, R. C., and Haper, M. E. (1986). HTLVIII expression in infected lymph nodes and relevance to pathogenesis of lymphadenopathy. *Am. J. Pathol.* **125,** 436–442.

Bjercke, S., Scott, H., Braathen, L. R., and Thorsby, E. (1983). HLA-DR expressing Langerhans like cells in vaginal and cervical epithelium. *Acta Obstet. Gynecol. Scand.* **62,** 585–589.

Bourinbaiar, A. S., and Phillips, D. M. (1991). Transmission of human immunodeficiency virus from monocytes to epithelia. *J. Acquired Immune Defic. Syndr.* **4,** 56–63.

Brookes, R., Bergmeier, L. A., Mitchell, E., Walker, J., Tao, L., Klavinskis, L., Meyers, N. J., Layton, G., Adams, S. E., and Lehner, T. (1995). Generation and diversity in the hierarchy of T-cell epitope responses following different routes of immunization with simian immunodeficiency virus protein. *AIDS* **9,** 1017–1024.

Camerini, D., and Seed, B. (1990). A CD4 domain important for HIV-mediated syncytium formation lies outside the virus binding site. *Cell. (Cambridge, Mass.)* **60,** 747.

Cameron, D. W., Simonsen, J. N., D'Costa, L. J., Ronald, A. R., Maitha, G. M., Gakinya, M. N., Cheang, M., Ndinya, A. J., Piot, P., and Brunham, R. C. (1989). Female to male transmission of human immunodeficiency virus type 1: Risk factors for seroversion in men. *Lancet* **2,** 403–407.

Carmichael, A., Jin, X., Sissons, P., and Borysiewicz, L. (1993). Quantitation analysis of the human immunodeficiency virus type 1 (HIV-1)-specific cytotoxic T lymphocyte (CTL) response at different stages of HIV-1 infection: Differential CTL responses to HIV-1 and Epstein Bar virus in late disease. *J. Exp. Med.* **177,** 249–256.

Chan, W. L., Rodgers, A., Hancock, R. D., Taffs, F., Kitchin, P., Farrar, G., and Liew, F. Y. (1992). Protection of simian immunodeficiency virus-vaccinated monkeys correlates with anti-HLA class I antibody response. *J. Exp. Med.* **176,** 1203–1207.

Clerici, M., and Shearer, G. M. (1993). A Th1 → Th2 switch is a critical step in the etiology of HIV infection. *Immunol. Today* **14,** 107–111.

Cranage, M. P., Baskerville, A., Ashworth, L. A. E., Dennis, M., Cook, N., Sharpe, S., Farrar, G., Rose, J., Kitchin, P. A., and Greenaway, P. J. (1992). Intrarectal challenge of macaques vaccinated with formalin-inactivated simian immunodeficiency virus. *Lancet* **339,** 273–274.

Curran, J. W., Morgan, W. M., Hardy, A. M., Jaffe, H. W., Darrow, W. W., and Dowdle, W. R. (1985). The epidemiology of AIDS: Current status and future prospects. *Science* **229,** 1352–1357.

Dalgleish, A. G., Beverley, P. C., Clapham, P. R., Crawford, D. H., Greaves, M. F., and Weiss, R. A. (1984). The CD4 (T4) antigen is an essential component of the receptor for the AIDS retrovirus. *Nature (London)* **312,** 763–767.

Detels, R., and Visschers, B. (1988). HIV and orogenital transmission. *Lancet* **2,** 1023.

Dossey, D. E. (1988). HIV and orogenital transmission. *Lancet* **2,** 1023.

Doyle, C., and Strominger, J. L. (1987). Interaction between CD4 and class II MHC molecules mediating cell adhesion. *Nature (London)* **330,** 256–259.

Edwards, J. N. T., and Morris, H. B. (1985). Langerhans cells and lymphocyte subsets in the female genital tract. *Br. J. Obstet. Gynecol.* **92,** 974–982.

Embretson, J. E., Zupancic, M., Ribas, J. L., Burke, A., Racz, P., Tenner-Racz, K., and Haase, A. T. (1993). Massive covert infection of helper T lymphocytes and macrophages by HIV during the incubation period of AIDS. *Nature (London)* **362,** 359–361.

European Study Group on Heterosexual Transmission of HIV. (1992). Comparison of female to male and male to female transmission of HIV in 563 stable couples. *Br. Med. J.* **304,** 809.

Felman, Y. M. (1990). Recent developments in sexually transmitted diseases: Is heterosexual transmission of HIV a major epidemiologic factor in the spread of AIDS? New York City's experience. *Sexually Transmitted Diseases* **46,** 29–31.

Fiore, J. R., Bjorndal, A., Peipke, K. A., Di Stefano, M., Angarano, G., Giuseppe, P., Gaines, H., Fenyo, E. M., and Albert, J. (1994). The biologic phenotype of HIV-1 is usually retained during and after sexual transmission. *Virology* **204,** 297–303.

Fox, P. C., Wolff, A., Yen, B-K., Atkinson, J. C., and Baum, B. J. (1989). Salivary inhibition of HIV-1 infectivity: Functional properties and distribution in men, women and children. *JADA.* **118,** 709–711.

Furuta, Y., Eriksson, K., Svennerholm, B., Fredman, P., Horal, P., Jeansson, S., Vahlne, A., Holmgren, J., and Czerkinsky, C. (1994). Infection of vaginal and colonic epithelial cells by the human immunodeficiency virus type 1 is neutralized by antibodies raised against conserved epitopes in the envelope glycoprotein gp120. *Proc. Natl. Acad. Sci. U.S.A.* **91,** 12559–12563.

Gardner, M. B., and Hu, S. L. (1991). SIV vaccines, 1991—a year in review. *AIDS* 5(Suppl. 2), S115–S127.

Healey, D., Dianda, L., Moore, J. P., McDougal, J. S., Moore, M. J., Estess, P., Buck, D., Kwong, P. D., Beverley, P. C. L., and Sattentau, Q. J. (1990). Novel anti-CD4 monoclonal antibodies separate human immunodeficiency virus infection and fusion of $CD4^+$ cells from virus binding. *J. Exp. Med.* **172,** 1233–1242.

Heise, C., Vogel, P., Miller, C. J., Halsted, C. H., and Dandekar, S. (1993). Simian immunodeficiency virus infection of the gastrointestinal tract of rhesus macaques: Functional, pathological and morphological changes. *Am. J. Pathol.* **142,** 1759–1771.

Heise, C., Miller, C. J., Lackner, A., and Dandekar, S. (1994). Primary acute simian immunodeficiency virus infection of intestinal lymphoid tissue is associated with gastrointestinal dysfunction. *J. Infect. Dis.* **169,** 1116–1120.

Ho, D. D., Byington, R. E., Schooley, R. T., Flynn, T., Rota, T. R., and Hirsch, M. (1985). Infrequency of isolation of HTLV-III virus from saliva in AIDS. *N. Engl. J. Med.* **313,** 1606.

Ho, D. D., Neumann, A. U., Perelson, A. S., Chen, W., Leonard, J. M., and Markowitz, M. (1995). Rapid turnover of plasma virions and CD4 lymphocytes in HIV-1 infection. *Nature (London)* **373,** 123–126.

Hoefsmit, E. C. M., Duijvestijn, A. M., and Kamperdijk, E. W. A. (1982). Relation between Langerhans cells, veilded cells and interdigitating cells. *Immunobiology* **161,** 255–265.

Homsy, J., Meyer, M., Tateno, M., Clarkson, S., and Levy, J. A. (1989). The Fc and not CD4 receptor mediates antibody enhancement of HIV infection in human cells. *Science* **244,** 1357–1360.

Hsieh, C. S., Macatonia, S. E., Tripp, C. S., Wolf, S. F., O'Garra, A., and Murphy, K. M. (1993). Development of Th1 CD4+ T cells through IL-12 produced by Listeria-induced macrophages. *Science* **260,** 496–497.

Hussain, L. A., and Lehner, T. (1995). Comparative investigation of Langerhans cells and potential receptors for HIV in oral, genitourinary and rectal epithelia. *Immunology* **85,** 475–484.

Hussain, L. A., Kelly, C. G., Hecht, E.-M., Fellowes, R., Jourdan, M., and Lehner, T. (1991). The expression of Fc receptors for immunoglobulin G in human rectal epithelium. *AIDS* **5,** 1089–1094.

Hussain, L. A., Kelly, C. G., Fellowes, R., Hecht E.-M., Wilson, J., Chapman, M., and Lehner, T. (1992). Expression and gene transcript of Fc receptors for IgG, HLA class II antigens and Langerhans cells in human cervicovaginal epithelium. *Clin. Exp. Immunol.* **90,** 530–538.

Janoff, E. N., Jackson, S., Wahl, S. M., Thomas, K., Peterman, J. H., and Smith, P. D. (1994). Intestinal mucosal immunoglobulins during human immunodeficiency virus infection. *J. Infect. Dis.* **170,** 200–307.

Janossy, G. (1986). HTLVIII/LAV viral antigens in lymph nodes of homosexual men with persistent generalized lymphadenopathy and AIDS. *Am. J. Pathol.* **123,** 9–15.

Jarry, A., Cortez, A., Rene, E., Muzeau, F., and Brousse, N. (1990). Infected cells and immune cells in the gastrointestinal tract of AIDS patients. An immunohistochemical study of 127 cases. *Histopathology* **16,** 133–140.

Javaherian, K., Langlois, A. J., Schmidt, S., Kaufman, M., Cates, N., Langeduk, J. P. M., Meleon, R. H., Desrosiers, R. C., Burns, D. P., Bolognesi, D. P., LaRose, G. J., and Putney, S. D. (1992). The principal neutralization determinant of simian immunodeficiency virus from that of human immunodeficiency virus type 1. *Proc. Natl. Acad. Sci. U.S.A.* **89,** 1418–1422.

Johnson, A. M. (1988). Heterosexual transmission of human immunodeficiency virus. *Br. Med. J.* **296,** 1017–120.

Kalter, D. C., Gendelman, H. E., and Meltzer, M. S. (1990). Infection of human epidermal Langerhans' cells by HIV. *AIDS* **4,** 266–268.

Kanitakis, J., Marchand, C., Su, H., Thivolet, J., Zambruno, G., Schmitt, D., and Gazzolo, L. (1989). Immunohistochemical study of normal skin of HIV-1 infected patients shows no evidence of infection of epidermal Langerhans cells by HIV. *AIDS Res. Hum. Retroviruses* **5,** 293–302.

Kiyono (1996). In preparation.

Klatzmann, D., Champagne, E., Chamaret, S., Gruest, J., Guetard, D., Hercend, T., Glukman, J. C., and Montagnier, L. (1984). T-lymphocyte T4 molecule behaves as the receptor for human retrovirus LAV. *Nature (London)* **312,** 767–768.

Klavinskis, L. S., Bergmeier, L. A., Brookes, R., Hayward, L., Layton, G., Meyers, N. S., Ward, R., and Lehner, T. (1996). Cytotoxic T lymphocytes after rectal, vaginal, oral or targetted lymph node immunization in macaques. *J. Immunol.* in press.

Koenig, S., Earl, P., Powell, D., Pantaleo, G., Merli, S., Moss, B., and Fauci, A. S. (1988). Group-specific, major histocompatibility complex class-I restricted cytotoxic responses to human immunodeficiency virus 1 (HIV-1) envelope proteins by cloned peripheral blood T cells from an HIV-1 infected individual. *Proc. Natl. Acad. Sci. U.S.A.* **85,** 8638–8642.

Kraal, G., Breel, M., Janse, M., and Bruin, G. (1986). Langerhans cells, veiled cells and intergitating cells in the mouse recognized by a monoclonal antibody. *J. Exp. Med.* **163,** 981–997.

Kreiss, J. K., and Hopkins, S. G. (1992). The association between circumcision status and human immunodeficiency virus infection among homosexual men. *J. Infect. Dis.* **168,** 1404–1408.

Kripke, M. L., Munn, C. G., Jeevan, A., Tang J.-M., and Bucana, C. (1990). Evidence that cutaneous antigen-processing cells migrate to regional lymph nodes during contact sensitization. *J. Immunol.* **145,** 2833–2837.

Kupiec-Weglinski, J., Austyn, J., and Morris, P. (1988). Migration patterns of dendritic cells in the mouse. Traffic from blood, and T-cell-dependent and independent entry into lymphoid tissue. *J. Exp. Med.* **167,** 632–645.

Langhoff, E. F., Terwilliger, E. F., Bos, H. J., Kalland, K. H., Pozansky, M. C., Bacon, O. M. L., and Haseltine, W. A. (1991). Replication of human immunodeficiency virus type 1 in primary dendritic cell cultures. *Proc. Natl. Acad. Sci. U.S.A.* **88,** 7998–8002.

Langlois, A. J., Weinhold, K. J., Matthews, T. J., Greenberg, M. L., and Bolognesi, D. P. (1992). The ability of certain SIV vaccines to provoke reactions against normal cells. *Science* **255,** 292–293.

Lehner, T., Bergmeier, L. A., Panagiotidi, C., Tao, L., Brookes, R., Klavinskis, L. S., Walker, P., Walker, J., Ward, R. G., Hussain, L., Gearing, A. J. H., and Adams, S. E. (1992a). Induction of mucosal and systemic immunity to a recombinant simian immunodeficiency viral protein. *Science* **258,** 1365–1369.

Lehner, T., Panagiotidi, C., Bergmeier, L. A., Tao, L., Brookes, R., and Adams, S. (1992b). A comparison of the immune responses following oral, vaginal or rectal route of immunization with SIV antigens in non-human primates. *Vaccine Res.* **1,** 319.

Lehner, T., Brookes, R., Panagiotidi, C., Tao, L., Bergmeier, L. A., Klavinskis, L. S., Walker, P., Walker, J., Ward, R., Hussain, L., Gearing, A. J. H., and Adams, S. E. (1993). T- and B-cell functions and epitope expression in non-human primates immunized with SIV by the rectal route. *Proc. Natl. Acad. Sci. U.S.A.* **90,** 8638–8642.

Lehner, T., Tao, L., Panagiotidi, C., Klavinskis, L. S., Brookes, R., Hussain, L., Meyers, N., Adams, S. E., Gearing, A. J. H., and Bergmeier, L. A. (1994a). Mucosal model of genital immunization in male rhesus macaques with a recombinant simian immunodeficiency virus p27 antigen. *J. Virol.* **68,** 1624–1632.

Lehner, T., Bergmeier, L. A., Tao, L., *et al.* (1994b). Targeted lymph node immunization with simian immunodeficiency virus p27 antigen to elicit genital, rectal and urinary immune responses in nonhuman primates. *J. Immunol.* **153,** 1858–1868.

Lehner, T., Wang, Y., Cranage, M., Bergmeier, L. A., Mitchell, E., Tao, L., Hall, G., Dennis, N., Cook, Brookes, R., Klavinskis, L., Jones, I., Doyle, L., and Ward, R. (1995).

Mucosal immunity elicited by targeted iliac lymph node immunization with a subunit SIV envelope and core vaccine in macaques. *Nature Med.* **2,** 767–772.

Levy, J. A. (1993). Pathogenesis of human immunodeficiency virus infection. *Microbiol. Rev.* **57,** 183–289.

Lohman, B. L., Miller, C. J., and McChesney, M. B. (1995). Antiviral cytotoxic T lymphocytes in vaginal mucosa of simian immunodeficiency virus-infected rhesus macaques. *J. Immunol.* **155,** 5855–5860.

Lu, X. S., Belec, L., and Pillot, J. (1993). Anti-gp160 IgG and IgA antibodies associated with a large increase in total IgG in cervicovaginal secretions from human immunodeficiency virus type 1 infected women. *J. Infect. Dis.* **167,** 1189–1192.

Macatonia, S., Lau, R., Patterson, S., Pinching, A., and Knight, S. (1990). Dendritic cell infection, depletion and dysfunction in HIV-infected individuals. *Immunology* **71,** 38–45.

McDermott, M. R., and Bienenstock, J. (1979). Evidence for a common mucosal system. I. Migration of B immunoblasts into intestinal, respiratory and genital tissues. *J. Immunol.* **122,** 1892–1898.

Mackewicz, C., and Levy, J. A. (1992). $CD8^+$ cell anti-HIV activity: Nonlytic suppression of virus replication. *AIDS Res. Hum. Retroviruses* **8,** 629–640.

Maddon, P., Molineaux, S. M., Maddon, D. E., Zimmerman, K. A., Godfrey, M., Alt, F. W., Chess, L., and Axel, R. (1987). Structure and expression of the human and mouse T4 genes. *Proc. Natl. Acad. Sci. U.S.A.* **84,** 9155–9159.

Marthas, M., Sutjipto, S., Miller, C., Higgins, J., Torten, J., Unger, R., Kiyono, H., McGhee, J., Marx, P., and Pedersen, N. (1992). Efficacy of live-attenuated and whole-inactivated simian immunodeficiency virus vaccines against intravenous and intravaginal challenge. *In* "Vaccines 1992" (F. Brown, R. M. Chanock, H. S. Ginsberg, and R. A. Lerner, eds.), pp. 117–122. Cold Spring Harbor Laboratory, Cold Spring Harbor, New York.

Marx, P. A., Compans, R. W., Getie, A., Staas, J. K., Gilley, R. M., Muligan, M. J., Yamshchikov, G. V., Chen, D., and Eldridge, J. H. (1993). Protection against vaginal SIV transmission with microencapsulated vaccine. *Science* **260,** 1323–1327.

Mathewson, J. J., Jiang, Z. D., DuPont, H. L., Chintu, C., Luo, N., and Zumla, A. (1994). Intestinal secretory IgA immune response against human immunodeficiency virus among infected patients with acute and chronic diarrhea. *J. Infect. Dis.* **169,** 614–617.

Mathijs, J. M., Hing, M., Grierson, J., Dwyer, D. E., Goldschmidt, C., Cooper, D. A., and Cunningham, A. L. (1988). HIV infection of the rectal mucosa. *Lancet* **1,** 1111.

Mayer, K. H., Ayotte, D., Groopman, J. E., Stoddard, A. M., Sarrgadharan, M., and Gallo, R. (1986). Association of human T lymphotropic virus type III antibodies with sexual and other behaviour in a cohort of homosexual men from Boston with and without generalized lymphadenopathy. *Am. J. Med.* **80,** 357.

Mazanec, M. B., Kaetzel, C. S., Lamm, M. E., Fletcher, D., and Nedrud, J. G. (1992). *Proc. Natl. Acad. Sci. U.S.A.* **89,** 6901–6905.

Mestecky, J. (1987). The common mucosal immune system and current strategies for induction of immune responses in external secretions. *J. Clin. Immunol.* **7,** 265–263.

Miller, C. J., Alexander, N. J., Sutjipto, S., Lackner, A. A., Hendrickx, A. G., Gettie, A., Lowenstine, L. J., Jennings, M., and Marx, P. A. (1989). Genital mucosal transmission of simian immunodeficiency virus: Animal model for heterosexual transmission of human immunodeficiency virus. *J. Virol.* **63,** 4277–4284.

Miller, C. J., Alexander, N. J., Sutjipto, S., Hendrickx, A. G., Jennings, M., and Marx, P. A. (1990). Effect of virus dose and nonoxynol-9 on the genital transmission of SIV in rhesus macaques. *J. Med. Primatol.* **19,** 401–409.

Miller, C. J., Alexander, N. J., Vogel, P., Anderson, J., and Marx, P. A. (1992a). Mechanism of genital transmission of SIV: A hypothesis based on transmission studies and the location of SIV in the genital tract of chronically infected female rhesus macaques. *J. Med. Primatol.* **21,** 64–68.

Miller, C. J., Vogel, P., Alexander, N. J., Sutjipto, S., Hendrickx, A. G., and Marx, P. A. (1992b). Localization of SIV in the genital tract of chronically infected female rhesus macaques. *Am. J. Pathol.* **141,** 655–660.

Miller, C. J., McChesney, M., and Moore, P. F. (1992c). Langerhans cells, macrophages and lymphocyte subsets in the cervix and vagina of rhesus macaques. *Lab. Invest.* **67,** 628–634.

Miller, C., Kang, D., Marthas, M., Moldoveanu, Z., Kiyono, H., Marx, P., Eldridge, J., Mestecky, J., and McGhee, J. (1992d). Genital secretory immune response to chronic SIV infection: A comparison between intravenously and genitally inoculated rhesus macaques. *Clin. Exp. Immunol.* **88,** 520–526.

Miller, C. J., McGhee, J. R., and Gardner, M. B. (1993). Mucosal immunity, HIV transmission and AIDS. *Lab. Invest.* **68,** 129–145.

Miller, C. J., Vogel, P., Alexander, N. J., Dandekar, S., Hendrickx, A. G., and Marx, P. A. (1994). Pathology and localisation of SIV in the reproductive tract of chronically infected male rhesus macaques. *Lab. Invest.* **70,** 255–262.

Mohamed, O. A., Ashley, R., Goldstein, A., McElrath, J., Dalessio, J., and Corey, L. (1994). Detection of rectal antibodies to HIV-1 by a sensitive chemiluminescent western blot immunodetection method. *J. Acquir. Immune Defic. Syndr.* **7,** 375–380.

Moore, J. P., Cao, Y., Ho, D. D., and Koup, R. J. (1994). Development of anti-gp120 antibody response during seroconversion to human immunodeficiency virus type 1 *J. Virol.* **68,** 5142–5155.

Morris, H. H. B., Gatter, K. C., Stein, H., and Mason, D. Y. (1983). Langerhans cells in human cervical epithelium: An immunohistologic study. *Br. J. Obstet. Gynecol.* **90,** 400–411.

Nelson, J. A., Wiley, C. A., Reynolds-Kohler, C., Reese, C. E., Margaretten, W., and Levy, J. (1988). Human immunodeficiency virus detected in bowel epithelium from patients with gastrointestinal symptoms. *Lancet* **1,** 259–262.

Nixon, D. F., Townsend, A. R. M., Elvin, J. G., Rizza, C. R.,

Gallwey, J., and McMichael, A. J. (1988). HIV-1 *gag* specific cytotoxic T lymphocytes defined with recombinant vaccinia virus and synthetic peptides. *Nature (London)* **336**, 484–487.

Nuovo, G. J., Forde, A., MacConnell, P., and Farenwald, R. (1993). In situ detection of PCR-amplified HIV-1 nucleic acids and tumor necrosis factor cDNA in cervical tissues. *Am. J. Pathol.* **143**, 40–48.

O'Leary, A. D., and Sweeny, E. C. (1986). Lymphoglandular complexes of the colon: Structure and distribution. *Histopathology* **10**, 267–283.

Owen, R. L., and Nemanic, P. (1978). Antigen processing structures of the mammalian intestinal tract: An SEM study of lymphoepithelial organs. *Scanning Electron Microsc.* **2**, 367–378.

Pang, S., Shlesinger, Y., Daar, E. S., Mondgil, T., Ho, D. D., and Chen, I. S. (1992). Rapid generation of sequence variation during primary HIV-1 infection. *AIDS* **6**, 453–460 [erratum: AIDS **6**, 606ff.].

Pantaleo, G., Graziosi, C., Demarest, J. F., Butini, L., Montroni, M., Fox, C. H., Orenstein, J. M., Kotler, D. P., and Fauci, A. S. (1993). HIV infection is active and progressive in lymphoid tissue during the clinically latent stage of disease. *Nature (London)* **362**, 355–357.

Pantaleo, G., Demarest, J. F., Soudeyns, H., Graziosi, C., Denis, F., Adelsberger, J. W., Borrow, P., Saag, M. S., Shaw, G. M., Sekaly, R. P., and Fauci, A. S. (1994). Major expansion of CD8 T cells with a predominant Vβ usage during the primary immune response to HIV. *Nature (London)* **370**, 463–466.

Patterson, S., and Knight, S. C. (1987). Susceptibility of human peripheral blood dendritic cells to infection by human immunodeficiency virus. *J. Gen. Virol.* **68**, 1177–1181.

Patterson, S., Gross, J., Bedford, P., and Knight, S. C. (1991). Morphology and phenotype of dendritic cells from peripheral blood and their productive and non-productive infection with human immunodeficiency virus type-1. *Immunology* **72**, 361–367.

Peterson, A., and Seed, B. (1988). Genetic analysis of monoclonal antibody and HIV binding sites on the human lymphocyte antigen CD4. *Cell (Cambridge, Mass.)* **54**, 65–72.

Piot, P., Plummer, F. A., Mhalu, F. S., Lamboray, J.-L., Chin, J., and Mann, J. M. (1988). AIDS: An international perspective. *Science.* **239**, 537–586.

Pomerantz, R. J., de la Monte, S. M., Donegan, C. E., Rota, T. R., Vogt, M. W., Craven, D. E., and Hirsch, M. S. (1988). Human immunodeficiency virus (HIV) infection of the uterine cervix. *Ann. Int. Med.* **108**, 321–327.

Reimann, K. A., Tenner-Racz, K., Racz, P., Montefiori, D. C., Yasutomi, Y., Lin, W., Ransil, B. J., and Letvin, N. L. (1994). Immunopathogenic events in the acute infection of rhesus monkeys with simian immunodeficiency virus of macaques. *J. Virol.* **68**, 2362–2370.

Ritchie, A. W. S., Hargreave, B., James, K., and Chisholm, G. D. (1984). Intraepithelial lymphocytes in the normal epididymis. A mechanism for tolerance to sperm autoantigens. *Br. J. Urol.* **56**, 79–83.

Silberberg-Sinakin, I., Thorbecke, G. J., Baer, R. L., Rosenthal, S. A., and Berezowsky, V. (1976). Antigen-bearing Langerhans cells in skin, dermal lymphatics and in lymph nodes. *Cell. Immunol.* **25**, 137–151.

Simonsen, J. N., Cameron, D. W., Gakinya, M. N., Ndiny, A., Achola, J. O. D'Costa, L. J., Karasiva, P., Cheang, M., Ronald, A. R., Piot, P., and Plummer, F. A. (1988). Human immunodeficiency virus infection among men with sexually transmitted diseases: Experience from a center in Africa. *N. Engl. J. Med.* **319**, 274–278.

Steinman, R. M. (1991). The dendritic cell system and its role in immunogenicity. *Annu. Rev. Immunol.* **9**, 271–296.

Stott, E. J. (1991). Anti-cell antibody in macaques. *Nature (London)* **353**, 393.

Takeda, A., Tuazon, C. U., and Ennis, F. A. (1988). Antibody-enhanced infection by HIV-1 via Fc receptor-mediated entry. *Science* **242**, 580–583.

Tenner-Racz, K., Racz, P., Bofil, M., Schultz-Meyer, A., Dietrich, M., Kern, P., Weber, J., Pinching, A. J., DiMarzo-Veronese, F., Popovic, M., Klatzmann, D., Gluckman, J. C. (1987). HTLV-III/LAV viral antigens in lymph nodes of homosexual men with generalized lymphadenopathy and AIDS. *Am. J. Pathol.* **123**, 9–15.

Thapar, M. A., Parr, E. L., and Parr, M. B. (1990). Secretory immune responses in mouse vaginal fluid after pelvic, parenteral or vaginal immunization. *Immunology* **70**, 121–125.

Tschachler, E., Groh, V., Popvic, M., Mann, D. L., Konrad, K., Safai, B., Eron, L., diMarzo-Veronese, F., Wolff, K., and Stingl, G. (1987). Epidermal Langerhans cells: A target for HTLV-III/LAV infection. *J. Invest. Dermatol.* **88**, 233–237.

van der Berg, L. H., Sadiq, S., Lederman, S., and Latov, N. (1992). The gp120 glycoprotein of HIV-1 binds to sulfatide and to the myelin associated glycoprotein. *J. Neurosci. Res.* **33**, 513–518.

Walker, B. D., Chakrabarti, S., Moss, B., Paradis, T. J., Flynn, T., Durno, A. G., Blumberg, R., Kaplan, J. C., Hirsch, M. S., and Scholley, R. T. (1987). HIV-specific cytotoxic T lymphocytes in seropositive individuals. *Nature (London)* **328**, 345–348.

Wei, X., Ghosh, S. K., Tayleor, M. E., Johnson, V. A., Emini, E. A., Deutsch, P., Lifson, J. D., Bonheoffer, S., Nowak, M. A., Hahn, B. H., Saag, M. S., and Shaw, G. M. (1995). Viral dynamics in human immunodeficiency virus type 1 infection. *Nature (London)* **373**, 117–122.

Winkelstein, W., Wiley, J. A., Padian, N., and Levy, J. (1986). Potential for transmission of AIDS-associated retrovirus from bisexual men in San Francisco to their female sexual contacts. *J. Am. Med. Assoc.* **255**, 901.

Wira, C. R., and Sandoe, C. P. (1987). Specific IgA and IgG antibodies in the secretions of the female reproductive tract effects of immunization and estradiol on expression of this response *in vivo*. *J. Immunol.* **138**, 4159–4164.

Wira, C. R., and Sandoe, C. P. (1989). Effect of uterine immunization and oestradiol on specific IgA and IgG antibodies in uterine vaginal and salivary secretions. *Immunology* **68**, 24–30.

Wolff, H., Mayer, K., Seage, G., Politch, J., Horsburgh, C. R., and Anderson, D. J. (1992). A comparison of HIV-1 antibody classes, titers and specificities in paired semen and blood samples from HIV-1 seropositive men. *J. AIDS* **5**, 65–69.

Yahi, N., Baghdiguian, S., Moreau, H., and Fantini, J. (1992). Galactosyl ceramide (or a closely related molecule) is the receptor for human immunodeficiency virus type 1 on human colon epithelial HT29 cells. *J. Virol.* **66**, 4848–4854.

Yasutomi, Y., Reimann, K. A., Lord, C. I., Miller, M. D., and Letvin, N. L. (1993). Simian immunodeficiency virus-specific $CD8^+$ lymphocyte response in acutely infected rhesus monkeys. *J. Virol.* **67**, 1707–1711.

Zambruno, G., Mori, L., Marconi, A., Mongiardo, N., De Rienzo, B., Bertazzoni, U., and Giannetti, A. (1991). Detection of HIV-1 in epidermal Langerhans cells of HIV-infected patients using polymerase chain reaction. *J. Invest. Dermatol.* **96**, 979–982.

Zhang, L. Q., MacKenzie, P., Cleland, A., Holmes, E. C., Leigh Brown, A. J., and Simmonds, P. (1993). Selection for specific sequences in the external envelope protein of human immunodeficiency virus type 1 upon primary infection. *J. Virol.* **67**, 3345–3356.

Zhu, T., Mo, H., Wang, N., Nam, D. S., Cao, Y., Koup, R. A., and Ho, D. D. (1993). Genotypic and phenotypic characterization of HIV-1 patients with primary infection. *Science* **261**, 1179–1181.

VII

Site-Directed Mucosal Vaccines

28

Mucosal Immunity in the Female Reproductive Tract: Effect of Sex Hormones on Immune Recognition and Responses

CHARLES R. WIRA
CHARU KAUSHIC
Department of Physiology
Dartmouth Medical School
Lebanon, New Hampshire 03756

I. Introduction

The mucosal immune system in the reproductive tract is fundamentally similar to but distinct from that present at other mucosal surfaces throughout the body. As the first line of defense against pathogenic organisms, protection at these sites involves the successful interaction of both humoral and cellular immune systems (Vaerman and Férin, 1974; Ogra *et al.*, 1981). The uniqueness of mucosal immunity in the female reproductive tract resides in the apparent paradox that while protecting against potential bacterial and viral pathogens, this system is selectively neutral to allogenic spermatozoa and supportive of a fetal placental unit that is immunologically distinct and essential for perpetuation of our species (Harbour and Blalock, 1989; Wegmann *et al.*, 1993). To accomplish this, mucosal immunity in the reproductive tract has evolved to be responsive to the constraints of procreation while at the same time protecting the mother.

Within the reproductive tract, sexually transmitted diseases represent a major unresolved challenge (Cates, 1986; Piot *et al.*, 1988; Cooper, 1995). In particular, organisms including acquired immune deficiency syndrome virus, herpes simplex virus, group B streptococcus, human papilloma virus, hepatitis B virus, *Neisseria gonorrhoeae,* and *Chlamydia vaginalis* are a threat to the health of both adults and newborns. Transmission of these agents into men, women, and children can lead to pain and reproductive tract cancer, as well as bladder and urinary tract infections. Some of these infections in the genital tract, if untreated, can cause infertility, brain damage, paralysis, heart disease, blindness in the newborn, and death. In all cases, these organisms are highly contagious and spread through sexual contact at mucosal surfaces within an infected individual. Major efforts are being made to fully define the mucosal immune system in the female reproductive tract in recognition of the fact that sexually transmitted diseases are being observed with increasing frequency in teenagers and that, on a worldwide level, greater than 75% of new AIDS cases are the result of heterosexual transmission of HIV from men to women (Forrest, 1992). Mechanisms for heterosexual transmission of HIV-1 remain to be identified. It is unknown, for example, whether transmission of HIV-1 through the genital tract is affected by mucosal epithelial and local immune cells, or whether physical disruption of the genital epithelium is required.

Although extensive studies of mucosal surfaces have been underway for many years, very little is known about the mucosal immune systems in men and women. Whereas much progress has been made in understanding the mechanisms through which invading organisms interact with cells in the reproductive tract, very little is known about the events in the reproductive tract necessary for eliciting immune protection. Aside from the complexities of host pathogen interactions, defining mucosal immunity in the reproductive tract is further complicated by the recognition that the reproductive tract represents a critical interface between the endocrine and immune systems. It is through these interactions that immune protection and adaption to the events of fertilization, implantation, pregnancy, and parturition occurs.

This chapter builds on a previous review which defined the regulatory control by estradiol and progesterone of immunoglobulins in reproductive tract secretions (Wira *et al.*, 1994). Our intent in this chapter is to define the interplay which exists between the endocrine and immune systems in the female reproductive tract as it relates to the induction of immune responses. Our focus will be to identify those sites which contribute to humoral immunity in the reproductive tract by examining both the afferent and efferent arms of the immune system.

II. Mucosal Immunity in the Female Reproductive Tract

A. Immune Cells in Reproductive Tract Tissues

Studies during the past several decades have provided evidence to support the hypothesis that the female reproductive tract possesses both affector and effector components of the immune system. Depending on the tissue analyzed and the species involved, both components of the immune system have been demonstrated in the reproductive tract. In the mouse and rat uterus, for example, lymphatic vessels are present both in the deeper layers of the endometrium and in the myometrium, which contain a rich supply of vessels that drain to the regional lymph nodes (Fabian, 1976; Head *et al.*, 1986). Also present in the uterine endometrium is a significant population of Ia antigen bearing antigen-presenting cells (Head and Gaede, 1986). Others have demonstrated that Langerhans cells, which are present in the epithelial lining of the mouse vagina, express Ia and common leukocyte antigen (Young, 1985; Young and Hosking, 1986). T lymphocytes of both helper ($CD4^+$) and cytotoxic/suppressor ($CD8^+$) types are also found in the epithelium, sometimes in close association with Langerhans cells (Parr and Parr, 1991). Depending on the species studied, the Fallopian tube, uterus, vagina, and cervix may contain either numerous or very limited numbers of macrophages, T lymphocytes, B lymphocytes, and NK cells. For example, the presence of immunocompetent cells has been reported in the human uterus (Sen and Fox, 1967; Kamat and Isaacson, 1987). These cells exhibit cyclic distribution, representing 10–15% of stroma during follicular phase and 20–25% in the late secretory phase. The major leukocyte population is T lymphocytes and macrophages. The $CD8^+$ suppressor/cytotoxic population is predominant in the stroma as well as in the epithelial layer. In contrast, NK cells are distributed throughout the stromal layer of the endometrium. In other studies, MHC class II antigens have been described in Fallopian tubes and endometrium in the human (Natali *et al.*, 1981; Laguens *et al.*, 1990; Bjercke and Brandtzaeg, 1993). These cells reportedly make up 13–25% in the proliferative phase and 16–43% in the secretory phase of the cells in the uterine endometrium. Since the majority of these cells were not of macrophage lineage, these findings suggested that they are either a special population of connective tissue stromal cells able to express HLA-DR or reticular dendritic cells (Laguens *et al.*, 1990).

B. Humoral Immunity in the Female Reproductive Tract

A number of investigators have reported the presence of immunoglobulins and plasma cells in the female reproductive tract of various species (for reviews see Wira *et al.*, 1994; Parr and Parr, 1994). Previous studies from our laboratory have shown in the rat that the levels of IgA, IgG, and secretory component (s.c.) in both uterus and vagina are regulated by female sex hormones (Wira and Sandoe, 1977; Wira *et al.*, 1980; Sullivan *et al.*, 1983; Wira and Sullivan, 1985). The presence of immunoglobulins and hormonal regulation of the plasma cells have been described in mouse uterus as well as in the rat (Bernard *et al.*, 1981; Canning and Billington, 1983; Parr and Parr, 1985; Mitchell, 1986). In the human, the amounts of IgA and IgG present in the uterus of the female genital tract vary with the phase of the menstrual cycle, as well as with anatomical location (Tauber *et al.*, 1985). IgG levels in secretions from the uterine mucosa were highest during the peri-ovulatory phase, whereas levels in the Fallopian tube were lowest at that time. IgA and IgG levels in cervical secretions vary with the stage of the menstrual cycle with lowest levels measured at midcycle (Schumacher, 1980). Further suppression of IgA and IgG throughout the menstrual cycle was observed when women were treated with oral contraceptives. Studies carried out in our laboratory have demonstrated that the levels of s.c. in uterine secretions vary during the menstrual cycle of women (Sullivan *et al.*, 1984). Levels were low during the proliferative phase, highest during the secretory phase, and lowest during menstruation. Others have shown that lymphocytes and/or plasma cells are distributed throughout the reproductive tract with low numbers present in the uterus and vagina (Lippes *et al.*, 1970; Rebello *et al.*, 1975; Kelly and Fox, 1979). In contrast, significant numbers of IgA-, IgG-, and IgM-producing lymphocytes are found in the cervix. Depending on the tissue analyzed and the species involved, IgA and IgG may be either synthesized locally and/or of serum origin (Tourville *et al.*, 1970; Rebello *et al.*, 1975). In the uterus, endometrial gland cells stained strongly for IgA and secretory component (s.c.), the receptor responsible for transporting IgA from tissue to lumen (Tourville *et al.*, 1970; Vaerman and Férin, 1974). In other studies, s.c.-positive cells, and IgA- and IgG-producing cells have been localized in the human Fallopian tube (Hurlimann *et al.*, 1978; Kutteh *et al.*, 1988). Cooper *et al.* (1987) showed that the human Fallopian tube possesses immunoglobulin-bearing B cells, T cells, and a large number of natural killer (NK) cells. They demonstrated that infection of the Fallopian tube with

Neisseria increases the number of s.c.- and IgA-positive cells when compared to noninfected controls. In other studies, Kutteh *et al.* (1990) reported a 6- to 10-fold increase in plasma cells of all classes in infected segments of human Fallopian tube, suggesting that local immunity is important in first-line defense of the genital tract against invading organisms.

C. Experimental Induction of Immune Response in the Female Reproductive Tract

In 1974, Beer and Billingham demonstrated that histocompatible allogenic skin grafted into the uterine wall of rats survived with remarkable frequency compared to grafts which were rejected if they had been transplanted to more conventional sites. The rejection phenomenon was shown to be cell mediated, since skin allografts in the uterus of immunologically tolerant rats were promptly rejected when specifically sensitized immune cells were passively transferred into the recipient host (Beer and Billingham, 1974). Several studies have demonstrated that specific antibodies can be induced in uterine and/or vaginal secretions following local (female reproductive tract) and distal (gastrointestinal tract) immunization. Kerr (1955) and Corbeil *et al.* (1974) demonstrated that antibody titers in uterine secretions were higher than those measured in serum following *Brucella abortus* or *Vibrio fetus* infection in cattle. In studies related to contraceptive vaccine development, Shelton and Goldberg demonstrated that following intrauterine immunization with sperm-specific isozyme lactate dehydrogenase C4 (LDH-C4), female mice secreted IgA-specific antibodies specific for LDH-C4 in their uterine fluids and showed lower rates of pregnancy (Shelton and Goldberg, 1986). In earlier studies, Allardyce (1984) reported that intragastric administration of live epididymal rat sperm to adult female virgin rats resulted in short- to long-term infertility related to appearance of antisperm IgA antibodies in genital tract secretions prior to mating. Ogra and Ogra (1973) made the important observation in women that immunization with inactivated polio virus placed within the uterine lumen results in IgG antibodies in uterine secretions. As a part of these studies they demonstrated that intravaginal and oral immunization lead to systemic as well as local antibody responses in the female reproductive tract. In other studies, however, no antibody responses were detected in women following intrauterine immunization with horseradish peroxidase (Vaerman and Férin, 1974). Local antibody production following vaginal and/or cervical deposition of antigen indicates that the lower genital tract is immunologically responsive (Kerr, 1955; Yang and Schumacher, 1979; Parr and Parr, 1990). Several studies have shown that gastrointestinal and pelvic immunization resulted in accumulation of antibodies in genital tract secretions (Allardyce, 1984; Thapar *et al.*, 1990). Studies done in our laboratory demonstrated that following gastrointestinal, intrauterine, and intraperitoneal immunization, there is an accumulation of specific IgA and IgG antibodies throughout the genital tract (Wira and Sandoe, 1987b, 1989; Wira and Prabhala, 1993). Overall, these studies demonstrate the presence of specific antibodies in uterine and cervico-vaginal secretions following both distal and local (reproductive tract) exposure to antigen. Further, it suggests that antigen-specific genital tract immune responses can be induced against such pathogens as HIV-1. It therefore becomes crucial to establish the mechanism(s) by which the secretory immune system in the female genital tract is hormonally regulated in order to optimize immune responses to specific antigens.

III. Sex Hormone Regulation of Mucosal Immunity in the Female Reproductive Tract

Previous work from our laboratory has defined the central role played by the sex hormones in the female reproductive tract in regulating the efferent arm of the immune system. These studies led to the conclusion that estradiol and progesterone are the principle hormones responsible for regulating IgA, IgG, and polymeric Ig receptor (pIgR), the protein responsible for transport of polymeric immunoglobulins from tissues into secretions, in both the uterus and vagina (for review see Wira and Stern, 1992). Other studies from our group have led us to conclude that endocrine balance during the reproductive cycle, at implantation, and throughout pregnancy results in separate and distinct changes in the mucosal system that are unique to uterus, cervix, and vagina (Wira and Stern, 1992; Wira *et al.*, 1994). In this chapter, we present studies from our laboratory that examine the role of steroid hormones on the afferent and efferent arms of the immune system in the female reproductive tract. We include our most recent findings, which show that both the uterus and vagina are inductive sites for antigenic challenge and that sex hormones play a crucial role in regulating antigen presentation by uterine and vaginal cells. Also included are our findings which indicate that systemically administered sex hormones as well as locally (uterine) deposited cytokine and antigen, influence T- and B-lymphocyte proliferation in lymphoid organs distant from the reproductive tract. We have also included recent experiments which extend our previous findings to show that sex hormones regulate the mucosal immune response in the female reproductive tract at the molecular level and that epithelial cells play a key regulatory role in the control of IgA transcytosis from tissues into secretions.

A. Hormonal Control of Antibodies in Uterine and Vaginal Secretions

The important observations by Ogra and Ogra (1973) that oral, uterine and vaginal immunization of women with inactivated poliovirus led to the presence of specific antibodies in uterine and vaginal secretions led us to utilize these approaches to more fully define the role of the reproductive cycle and sex hormones in the induction of immune responses of the female genital tract. Using sheep red blood cells (SRBC), a known T-cell dependent antigen, we immunized intact rats whose uteri were ligated to ensure recovery of uterine secretions. When animals were immunized and boosted 6 days later, specific anti-SRBC IgA antibodies were found in uterine and cervico-vaginal secretions following Peyer's patches (PP) or intraperitoneal (i.p.) immunization (Wira and Sandoe, 1987a, 1987b). Anti-SRBC IgG antibodies were also found in the uterine but not in vaginal secretions following PP and i.p. immunization. Subcutaneous (s.c.) immunization resulted in weak responses for IgG in the uterus and IgA in the vagina. These studies indicated that uterine and vaginal antibody responses could be obtained following PP and i.p. immunization in intact animals under normal endocrine conditions, and suggested that oral and i.p. immunization might be effective routes for inducing uterine and cervico-vaginal immune responses.

To define the regulatory role of estradiol in reproductive tract immune responses, ovariectomized rats were immunized by PP and i.p. injection of SRBC and sacrificed 3 to 12 days postimmunization. Animals received either estradiol or saline for the last 3 days prior to sacrifice (Wira and Sandoe, 1987b; Wira and Prabhala, 1993). Table I shows that in the absence of estradiol (saline, Day 12), very few IgA and IgG antibodies are found in uterine secretions following PP immunization. In response to estradiol, IgA antibodies rose and peaked (Day 9), and then returned to baseline levels by Day 12 postimmunization. IgG antibodies in uterine secretions increased from Day 3 to Day 12 postimmunization. In contrast, when animals were i.p. immunized, only IgG antibodies accumulated in uterine secretions in response to estradiol treatment. When vaginal antibody levels were analyzed (not shown), we found that estradiol lowered IgA and IgG antibody levels in cervico-vaginal secretions in both i.p. and PP immunized rats. These results indicate that the accumulation of anti-SRBC antibodies in the uterus following PP and i.p. immunization is dependent on estradiol stimulation and, as discussed previously, is mediated through estradiol regulation of IgA transport from uterine tissue to the uterine lumen (Richardson *et al.*, 1995). In contrast, IgG most likely enters the uterus as a part of the stimulatory effect of estradiol on fluid imbibition (Sullivan and Wira, 1983, 1984). These data indicated that the appearance of specific antibodies in uterine secretions after primary immunization is estradiol-dependent.

TABLE I

Time Course of the Effect of Estradiol on Specific IgA and IgG Antibodies in Uterine Secretions following Peyer's Patch and Intraperitoneal Immunization with SRBC

		Time (hr)				
		Estradiol				Saline
Isotype	Treatment	3	6	9	12	12
IgA	i.p.	±	±	±	±	±
IgG		±	±	++	+++	±
IgA	PP	±	++	+++	++	±
IgG		±	++	+++	++++	±

Note. Ovariectomized rats were immunized by injecting packed SRBC (200 μl) directly into Peyer's patches or the peritoneal cavity. Animals were treated with either estradiol (1 μg/day) or 0.9% saline (controls: designated as Day 12) for 3 days prior to sacrifice 24 hr after the last injection at the times indicated (Days 3 through 12). Each bar represents the mean ± SE of three or four animals/group. From Wira and Sandoe (1987b) and Wira and Prabhala (1993). −, None; ±, detectable; +, low; ++, medium; +++, high; ++++, very high.

The effect of uterine immunization with SRBC on IgA and IgG antibodies in uterine secretions is shown in Table II. When animals received both primary and secondary immunizations with SRBC in the uterine lumen (ut/ut), the uterine IgA-antibody response obtained was

TABLE II

Influence of Estradiol and Route of Immunization on the Presence of Anti-SRBC-Specific IgA and IgG Antibodies in Uterine Secretions

Isotype	Treatment	Nonimmune	PP/PP	PP/ut	ut/ut
IgA	Saline	−	−	−	+++
	Estradiol	−	+**	+*	++++
IgG	Saline	−	±	±	+
	Estradiol	−	+**	+*	+

Note. Ovariectomized rats were immunized with SRBC injected into Peyer's patches (PP) or instilled into one uterine horn (ut). Animals were immunized (primary, Day 0) via the Peyer's patches and boosted (secondary, Day 13) either via the Peyer's patches (PP/PP), or the uterus (PP/ut) or were immunized and boosted by placing SRBC directly into the uterine lumen (ut/ut). Nonimmunized animals were sham-operated at the time of primary and secondary immunzation. Animals were injected with 0.1 ml saline (S) or estradiol (E_2; 1.0 μg/day) for 3 days prior to killing 24 hr after the last injection on Day 26 post-primary immunization. Bars represent the mean ± SE values of samples taken from five or six animals/group. From Wira and Sandoe (1989). −, None; ±, detectable; +, low; ++, medium; +++, high; ++++, very high.

*Significantly ($P<0.05$) greater than saline-treated immunized controls.

**Significantly ($P<0.01$) greater than saline-treated immunized controls.

10- to 30-fold greater than that seen following PP immunization and boosting (PP/PP) or when the primary immunization was PP followed by uterine boosting (PP/ut) (Wira and Sandoe, 1989). Similarly, the IgG antibody response following ut/ut immunization was 2- to 5-fold greater than that measured following PP/PP or PP/ut immunization. In these studies, we found that estradiol administered for the last 3 days prior to sacrifice of ut/ut immunized animals had no effect on IgA or IgG antibody levels. One explanation for the lack of an estradiol effect is that immune cells were no longer producing antibodies at the time of uterine sampling (26 days after primary immunization), and, therefore, were unable to respond to estradiol stimulation. These studies demonstrated that the uterus is an inductive site for immune response and indicates that, relative to other sites examined, IgA responses are most pronounced in the uterus with intrauterine immunization. More recently, local deposition of antigens in the vaginae of primates has been shown to induce IgA and IgG vaginal responses that are more pronounced than that seen following oral immunization (Wassen *et al.*, 1995; Eriksson *et al.*, 1995).

In other studies, we found that the uterine immunization results in the appearance of antibodies throughout the reproductive tract and at other mucosal surfaces of the body (Wira and Sandoe, 1989). Following SRBC immunization of one uterine horn and ligation at the utero-cervical junction to prevent secretion leakage, IgA and IgG antibodies were found in contralateral nonimmunized horns of estradiol-treated animals. Specific antibodies were also found in the vaginal secretions from saline-treated immunized animals, at levels higher than those found in estradiol-treated animals as well as in serum and saliva. These findings indicate that the genital tract, in addition to receiving immunological information from distal sites, also contributes immunological information which is distributed systemically.

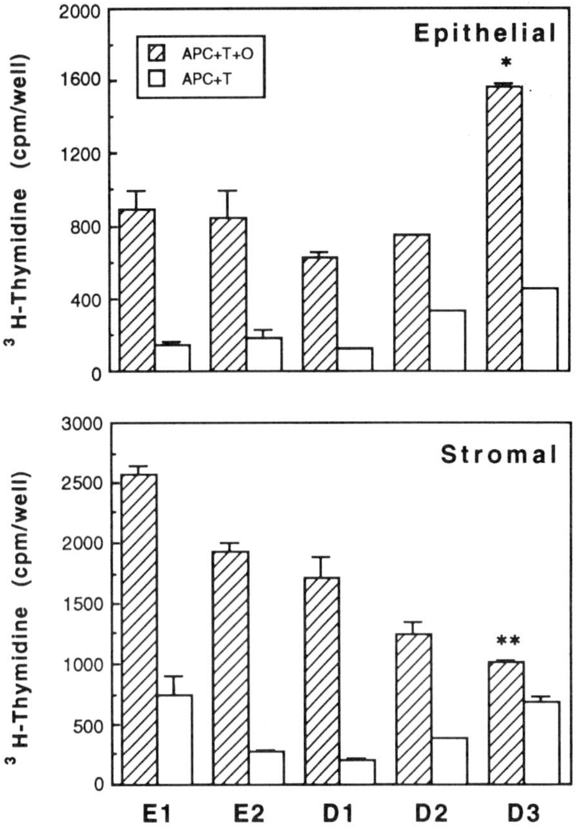

Figure 1. Influence of the estrous cycle on uterine epithelial and stromal antigen presentation. Rats were selected based on daily vaginal smears. Stages of the cycle are indicated as follows: estrus (E) days 1 and 2 and diestrus (D) days 1, 2, and 3. Uteri (4–7/group) were pooled and epithelial and stromal cells (1×10^5 cells/100 μl) were prepared. Epithelial or stromal antigen-presenting cells (APC) were incubated with OVA-sensitized T cells (1×10^5 cells/100 μl) and OVA (300 μg/ml) for 3 days. ^{3}H-Thymidine was added for the last 24 hr of incubation. Values shown are ^{3}H-thymidine incorporation for antigen presenting cells (APC) + T and APC + T + OVA (O) values. *Epithelial cell antigen presentation (D3) was significantly ($P < 0.01$) greater than D1 and D2 values. **Antigen presentation by stromal cells (D3) was significantly ($P < 0.01$) lower than E1, E2, D1, and D2 values. From Wira and Rossoll (1995a).

B. Antigen Presentation by Uterine Epithelial and Stromal Cells

Central to the tenet that a mucosal surface is an inductive site is the presence of cells that recognize antigen and are able to present it to T cells. To explore the possibility that uterine cells are able to present antigen, epithelial and stromal cells were prepared from intact rats at various stages of the reproductive cycle. As seen in Fig. 1, epithelial cells from the uteri of diestrous (D3) animals were significantly more efficient in presenting antigen to sensitized T-lymphocytes than were cells from rats at D1 and D2 stages of the estrous cycle. Our finding that antigen presentation at D3 was similar to that seen at E1 and E2 suggests that increases in antigen presentation are due to the effect of estradiol which is elevated in blood at these stages of the cycle (Shaikh, 1971). In contrast, antigen presentation at D1 and D2, when progesterone levels in blood are elevated, was significantly lower than that seen at D3. We also observed that antigen presentation by uterine stromal cells varies with the stage of the estrous cycle. In contrast to epithelial cells, antigen presentation was lowest at diestrus (D3) relative to all other stages of the cycle (Fig. 1). In other studies, we found that antigen presentation by epithelial and stromal cells is class II specific and mediated through costimulatory molecules ICAM-1 and LFA (Wira and Rossoll, 1995a). To the best of our knowledge, this is the first demonstration that uterine cells present antigen and that antigen presentation is precisely regulated throughout the reproductive cycle.

To more fully define the influence of hormones on antigen presentation, uterine cells were prepared from rats previously ovariectomized and treated with either saline or estradiol (1 μg/day) for 3 days prior to sacrifice 24 hr after the last injection. As seen in Fig. 2, antigen presentation by epithelial cells from estradiol-treated rats was significantly greater (twofold) than that seen with epithelial cells from control animals. In contrast, estradiol significantly decreased antigen presentation by stromal cells. Since antigen presentation was measured in the same groups of animals, these studies indicate that estradiol has a differential effect on epithelial and stromal cell antigen presentation, which parallels our findings in the uteri of intact animals at D3 of the estrous cycle.

C. Antigen Presentation by Vaginal Cells

In other studies, we prepared isolated cells from the vaginae of adult rats to determine whether the vaginal cells are capable of presenting antigen. Others have previously demonstrated that Langerhans cells and macrophages are present in the vagina (Parr and Parr, 1991). Cells from pooled rat vaginae were prepared by enzymatic and mechanical separation and incubated with ovalbumin (OVA)-sensitized T cells in the presence of OVA. As shown in Fig. 3, vaginal cells are able to present antigen and antigen presentation varies with the stage of the estrous cycle. Cells from the vaginae of Diestrous Day 3 animals were significantly less efficient in presenting antigen to sensitized T-lymphocytes than were cells from rats at all other stages of the estrous cycle (D3 < E1 < E2 < D2 < D1). Antigen presentation at Diestrous Day 3 was approximately sevenfold less than that seen at Diestrus Day 1. In other studies, we found that antigen presentation was MHC class II restricted and that the addition of anti-macrophage/dendritic cell antibodies inhibited antigen presentation (Wira and Rossoll, 1995b). These findings suggested that macrophages and/or dendritic cells are most likely the cells responsible for antigen presentation in the vagina. In other studies, we found that granulocytes, macrophages, and dendritic cells, with very few B and T cells, are present in vaginal tissues and that the number of class II positive cells in vaginal tissues varies with the stage of the reproductive cycle. Class II positive cells were present in greater numbers at diestrus (D1 and D2) than at estrus (E1 and E2) (C. Kaushic, E. Frauendorf, and C. R. Wira, unpublished observation) suggesting that differences in antigen presentation may be due either to

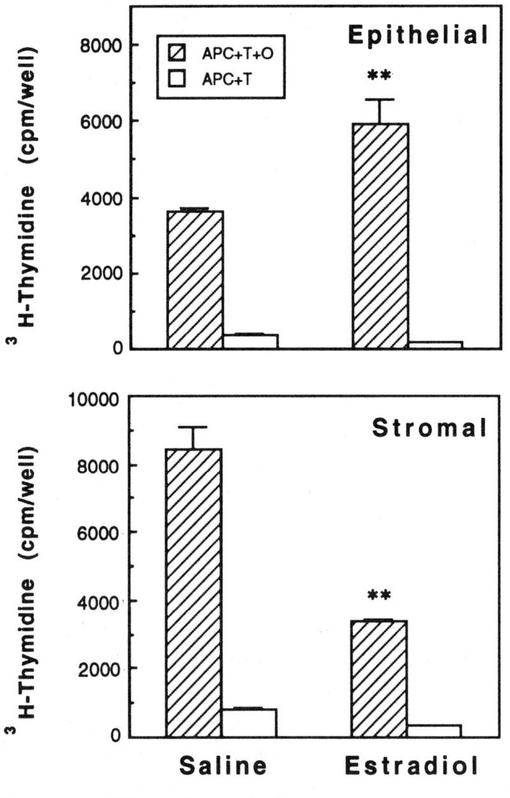

Figure 2. Effect of estradiol on antigen presentation by uterine epithelial and stromal cells. OVA-sensitized T cells were incubated with either epithelial or stromal cells from the uteri of ovariectomized rats treated with saline (0.1 ml) or estradiol (1 μg/0.1 ml/day) for 3 days prior to sacrifice 24 hr after the third injection. Antigen-presenting cells and T cells were incubated with OVA (300 μg/ml) for 3 days; ^{3}H-thymidine was added for last 24 hr of incubation. Values shown indicate ^{3}H-thymidine incorporation as described in the legend to Fig. 1. Values shown as mean ± SE of cells from six to eight animals/per group. **Significantly ($P < 0.05$) different from saline controls. From Wira and Rossoll (1995a).

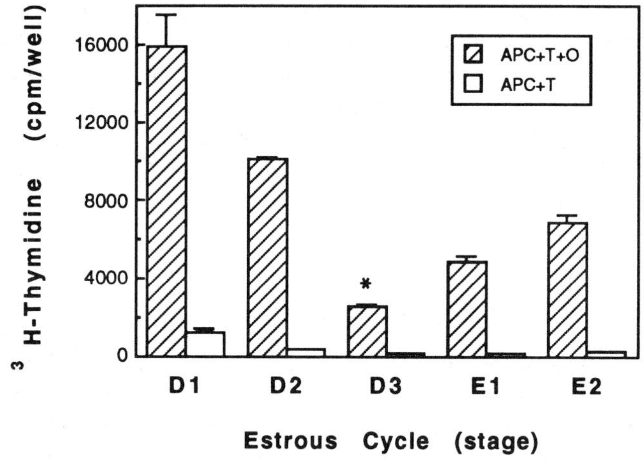

Figure 3. Effect of the reproductive cycle on antigen presentation by vaginal cells. Rats were selected based on daily vaginal smears after animals had gone through at least two normal (5-day) reproductive cycles. Stages of the cycle are indicated as follows: diestrus (D) days 1, 2, and 3; estrus (E) days 1 and 2. Vaginal tissues (three or four rats/group) were pooled, epithelial cells were prepared and incubated with T cells and OVA (300 μg/ml) for 2 days prior to ^{3}H-thymidine pulse and analysis of cell proliferation. Nonspecific control values (APC + T cell) were subtracted from wells containing OVA. *Each value (D3 < E1 < E2 < D2 < D1) is significantly ($P < 0.01$) different from other values. From Wira and Rossoll (1995b).

hormone/cytokine regulation of class II expression or to the migration of macrophages and/or dendritic cells into the vagina.

The effect of estradiol and progesterone on antigen presentation by vaginal cells is shown in Fig. 4. When administered to ovariectomized rats, estradiol, but not progesterone, inhibited antigen presentation. In contrast, when animals received progesterone prior to estradiol, the inhibitory effect of estradiol was blocked. This experiment indicates that estradiol and progesterone regulate antigen presentation in the female lower reproductive tract in a way that is different from that seen in the uterus. Overall, these findings indicate that both the uterus and the vagina are inductive sites for immune responses and that antigen presentation is hormonally regulated.

D. Effect of the Estrous Cycle and Interferon-γ on Spleen Cell Mitogenesis

To identify the role of sex hormones in modulating mucosal immune responses and to more fully define the sites of interaction between local immunity and systemic elements of the systemic immune system, studies were undertaken to measure mitogenic responses of splenic T and B lymphocytes to sex hormone and local (uterine) cytokine and antigen exposure. Animals were selected by daily vaginal smears after they had gone through at least one normal (4-day) estrous cycle. To examine the effect of the estrous cycle on the response of spleen cells to mitogens, spleen cells were prepared and incubated with Con A (1 μg/ml), PHA (5 μg/ml), or LPS (10 μg/ml) in 96-well microtiter plates for 3 days. Cell proliferation was evaluated by measuring the incorporation of ^{3}H-thymidine added to incubation wells for the last 24 hr. As seen in Fig. 5, spleen cell mitogenesis varied significantly with the stage of the estrous cycle, in that mitogenesis of T and B lymphocytes from proestrous rats in response to Con A, PHA, and LPS was significantly greater (two- to threefold) than that seen with spleen cells from animals at estrous and/or diestrous stages of the cycle. In other studies (Table III), we examined whether estradiol was responsible for changes in spleen cell mitogenesis observed during the estrous cycle (Prabhala and Wira, 1995). When ovariectomized animals were treated with estradiol for 3 days prior to sacrifice 24 hr after the third injection, estradiol treatment had a stimulatory effect on spleen cell responses to both T- and B-cell mitogens relative to saline controls. These results indicate that changes in splenic T- and B-lymphocyte mitogenesis during the estrous cycle are most likely due to estradiol which is known to be elevated at this time (Shaikh, 1971).

In other studies, we have examined the effects of cytokines and antigens placed in the uterine lumen on splenic mitogenesis and have determined that intrauterine instillation of IFNγ increases mitogen-stimulated B- and T-lymphocyte proliferation in the spleen (Prabhala and Wira, 1991). For example, when IFNγ was placed in the uterine lumen, a three- to fivefold increase in spleen cell proliferation to Con A, PHA, and LPS mitogens was observed relative to spleen cells from

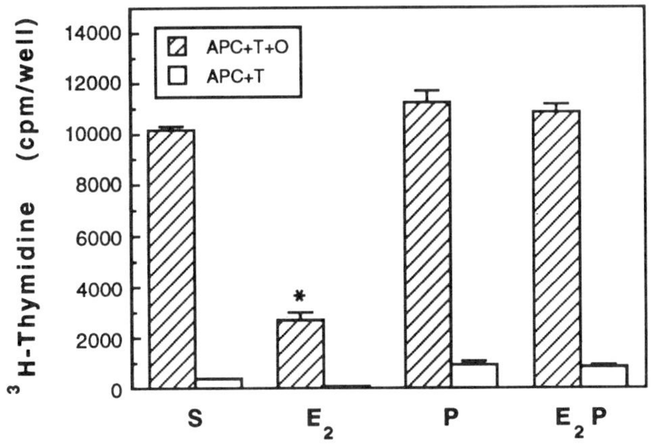

Figure 4. Effect of estradiol and progesterone on antigen presentation by vaginal cells. Ovariectomized rats were injected daily for 3 days with saline (0.1 ml) containing estradiol (E_2, 1 μg), progesterone (P, 1000 μg), or estradiol and progesterone (E_2P) and sacrificed 24 hr after the last injection. For those animals receiving both hormones, progesterone was given 30 min prior to the administration of estradiol. Control group received only saline (S). Nonspecific control values (APC + T cell) were subtracted from wells containing OVA (300 μg/ml). *Value of the estradiol group was significantly ($P < 0.001$) lower than the values of all other groups. From Wira and Rossoll (1995b).

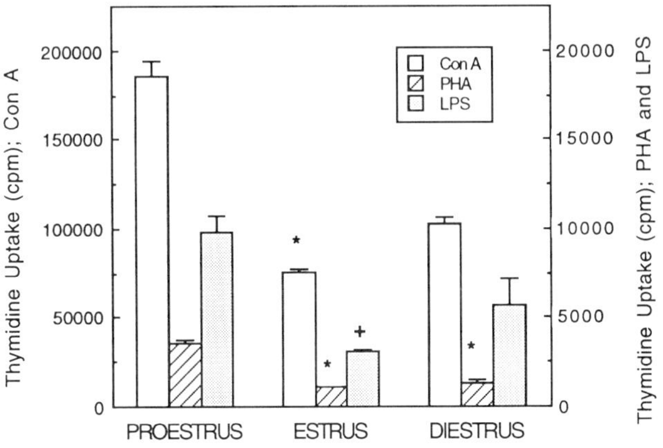

Figure 5. Mitogenic response of isolated spleen cells from intact female rats at various stages of the reproductive cycle. Animals were selected by routine vaginal smears and spleens were recovered during proestrus, estrus, and diestrus (Day 2). Splenocytes were prepared and incubated with Con A (1 μg/ml), PHA (5 μg/ml), and LPS (10 μg/ml) for 3 days. ^{3}H-thymidine was added to culture wells for the last 24 hr of each incubation. Each bar represents the mean ± SE minus background (counts per minute/well in the absence of mitogen) of splenocytes pooled from four to six animals/group. +, Significantly ($P < 0.05$) lower than proestrous values; *, Significantly ($P < 0.01$) lower than proestrous values. From Prabhala and Wira (1995).

TABLE III
Effect of Estradiol on the Mitogenic Response of Spleen Cells

Groups	Thymidine incorporation (cpm)[a] Con A	PHA	LPS
Control	++	+	+
Estradiol	++++	+++	++

[a]Results represent mean and SEM of a pool of six animals. Amount of ^{3}H-thymidine incorporation: ±very low; +low; ++medium, +++high, ++++very high. Adapted from Prabhala and Wira (1995).

TABLE IV
Time Course of the Effect of One, Two, or Three Estradiol Treatments on s.c. and IgA Content in Uterine Secretions of Ovariectomized Rats

Time (hr)	0	12	24	36	48	60	72
Treatment	E_2	—	E_2	—	E_2	—	—
IgA	–	–	–	–	+	++++	+++
s.c.	–	–	–	–	+	++++	+++

Note. Animals were injected with either estradiol (E_2, 2 μg/day) or saline (controls, indicated as 0 time point). Each value equals the mean ± SE of 4 (E_2) or 12 (saline) determinations. The levels of IgA are reported as immunocytoma (IS) units, as previously described. –, None; ±, detectable; +, low; ++, medium; +++, high; ++++, very high. Adapted from Sullivan *et al.* (1983).

control animals which received intrauterine PBS. When the same dose was given subcutaneously, no effect was observed. More recently, we found that ovalbumin placed in the uterine lumen, but not given subcutaneously, also increases mitogen-stimulated B- and T-lymphocyte proliferation in the spleen (C. R. Wira and R. Rossoll, unpublished observation). Overall, these responses to cytokines and antigen deposited in the uterine lumen demonstrate the close connection that exists between the mucosal immune system in the uterus and vagina and lymphoid tissues distant to the reproductive tract. Whether these interactions are mediated through dendritic cells, which upon hormone, cytokine, or antigen stimulation migrate to the spleen, similar to that observed in the heart and respiratory tract (Gong *et al.*, 1994), remains to be determined. What is apparent from these studies is that a previously unrecognized connection exists between the spleen and the reproductive tract.

E. Effect of Estradiol on Uterine IgA and s.c. in the Female Reproductive Tract

Since IgA is transported into secretions at mucosal surfaces by secretory component, the external domain of the polymeric IgA receptor, studies were undertaken to determine whether s.c. is also under hormonal control. As seen in Table IV, when estradiol was given to ovariectomized rats for 3 days, s.c. levels increased sharply, in parallel with IgA in uterine secretions. Subsequent studies showed that whereas IgA of blood origin enters uterine tissues within 2–4 hr after each injection of estradiol, IgA movement from tissue to lumen takes place only after uterine epithelial cells produce s.c. in response to estradiol or interferon-γ (Prabhala and Wira, 1991).

To establish whether uterine epithelial cells are able to transport IgA, epithelial cells prepared from the uteri of rats at proestrus, diestrus, and estrus were pooled and grown to confluence on Millicell chambers (Richardson *et al.*, 1993). As shown in Fig. 6, significantly more ^{125}I-IgA was recovered in apical media than in basolateral media following 20 hr of incubation when equal concentrations of ^{125}I-IgA were placed in either the basolateral or apical media and TCA precipitable counts were measured in the opposite chamber. To eliminate the possibility that either leakage or fluid phase movement was responsible for dIgA movement across the cell monolayers, equal amounts of the fluid phase marker ^{3}H-inulin were included with ^{125}I-dIgA. Our finding that ^{3}H-inulin movement in both directions occurred at the same rate indicated that dIgA is preferentially transported through uterine cells from the basolateral to the apical side.

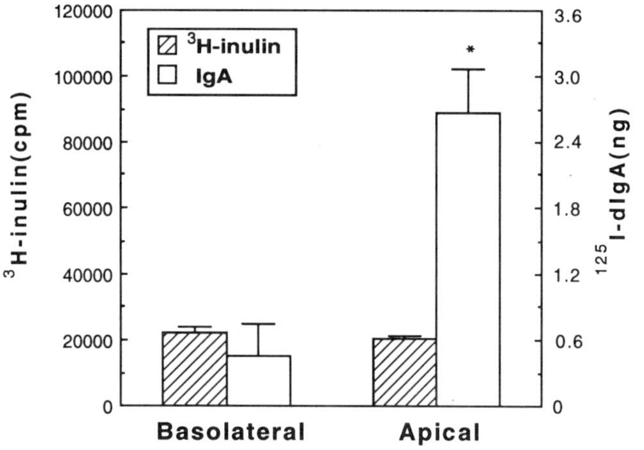

Figure 6. Transcytosis of dIgA by UEC in culture. ^{125}I-labeled dIgA and the fluid phase/leakage marker ^{3}H-inulin were added to either the basolateral or apical media of confluent UEC cultures grown on HA filters and incubated for 20 hr at 37°C. Medium from the opposite chamber of protein addition was TCA-precipitated and the pellet was counted to determine the amount of ^{125}I-dIgA that had been transcytosed (right *y* axis). ^{3}H-Inulin movement was measured by counting a sample of the media from opposite chamber (left *y* axis). Total counts/300 μl (apical) or 500 μl (basolateral) volume are shown on graph. Values represent the mean ± standard error of three wells/group. From Richardson *et al.* (1995).

To assess whether the movement of dIgA across uterine cell monolayers was receptor mediated, epithelial cells were grown to confluence on Millicell chambers prior to adding ^{125}I-IgA to the basolateral chamber either alone or in the presence of excess unlabeled dIgA (Richardson *et al.*, 1995). These studies indicated that ^{125}I-IgA movement in wells containing unlabeled dIgA was reduced by 50% relative to that seen with ^{125}I-IgA alone. To examine the specificity of dIgA transcytosis, excess unlabeled IgG was added to the basolateral media of cell cultures along with ^{125}I-dIgA. The presence of IgG had no affect on the movement of ^{125}I-IgA from basolateral to apical compartment. These findings demonstrated that dIgA transcytosis through uterine epithelial cells is receptor-mediated, saturable, and specific for polymeric IgA. To determine whether uterine s.c. is directly involved in the transport of dIgA, transcytosed ^{125}I-IgA in apical media was analyzed to determine whether s.c. was associated with ^{125}I-IgA. When rabbit anti-rat s.c. antibody was used to immunoprecipitate transcytosed ^{125}I-dIgA, significantly more radioactivity was recovered than that seen when first antibody was substituted with normal rat serum (control) (Richardson *et al.*, 1995). Overall, these studies demonstrated that dIgA is transported through uterine epithelial cells and that s.c. remains associated with dIgA after it is released into the apical medium. These studies suggest that the movement of dIgA through uterine epithelial cells is mediated by the pIg receptor which binds IgA at the basolateral surface and following transcytosis, is released into apical media as secretory IgA.

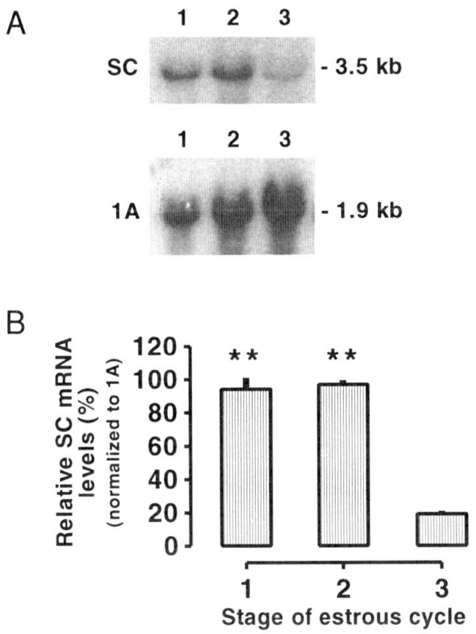

Figure 7. pIgR mRNA levels in uteri of rats at different stages of estrous cycle. (A) Northern blot analysis showing pIgR mRNA in uteri of animals at (1) proestrus, (2) estrus, and (3) diestrus. Each lane (1–3) contains 30 μg total RNA. The same blot was rehybridized with 1A probe to normalize the amount of total RNA in each lane. The size of pIgR and 1A mRNA in kilobases is indicated. (B) Relative amounts of pIgR mRNA present in uteri of animals at different stages of estrous cycle after normalization with 1A. Northern blots were quantified by densitometric analysis and relative amounts of mRNA presented as the percentage of maximum expression (see Methods for details). Results were pooled from four different experiments as mean ± SE. **Significantly ($P < 0.01$) greater than diestrus. From Kaushic *et al.* (1995).

F. Endocrine Regulation of pIgR mRNA Levels in the Female Reproductive Tract

Based on our earlier studies which suggested that estradiol effects on IgA transport were mediated through the synthesis of pIgR mRNA (Wira *et al.*, 1984), we set out to determine if pIgR mRNA could be detected in uterine tissues and whether this mRNA was hormonally controlled. Using the pIgR probe from a rat liver library which has been shown previously to detect rat pIgR mRNA in liver and kidney (Banting *et al.*, 1989), we found by Northern blot analysis that a single message species of approximately 3.5 kb is present in rat uterine tissues. To determine whether pIgR levels vary with the stage of the reproductive cycle, total RNA was extracted from uteri pooled from four to six animals at proestrus, estrus, and diestrus. As seen in Fig. 7A, Northern analysis of RNA indicated that pIgR mRNA levels in uteri were high at proestrus and estrus and low at diestrus. To normalize the amount of pIgR mRNA detected, each blot was stripped and hybridized with a probe for 1A mRNA, which is known to be constitutively produced in the uterus and is independent of estradiol regulation (Hsu *et al.*, 1988). Polymeric IgR mRNA message levels at proestrus and estrus were approximately five times higher than those present at diestrus (Fig. 7B). In immunohistochemical studies to identify the cells in uteri which express pIgR, uterine luminal and glandular epithelial cells from rats at proestrus and estrus expressed significantly more pIgR than epithelial cells in the uteri of diestrous animals (Kaushic *et al.*, 1995). These findings demonstrate that endocrine changes, which prepare the reproductive tract for ovulation, have a stimulatory effect on pIgR expression on epithelial cells. Further, it indicates that levels of pIgR mRNA correlate well with expression of pIgR on epithelial cells that line the lumen and glands of the uterus.

To determine whether estradiol-induced increases in s.c. coincide with elevated pIgR mRNA levels, ovariectomized rats received subcutaneous injections of estradiol (1 μg/day) or saline (0.1 μl/day) for 3 consecutive days and were sacrificed 4 and 12 hr after the last injection. The times selected were based on the interval of estradiol treatment we had previously observed to be necessary for s.c. to appear in uterine secretions (Table IV). As seen in Fig. 8, pIgR mRNA was detected by Northern analysis in uteri of both estradiol and saline-

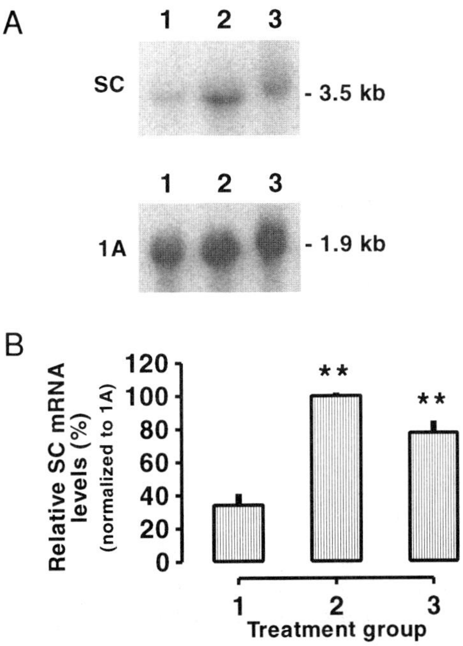

Figure 8. Influence of estradiol on pIgR mRNA levels in rat uteri. (A) Northern blot analysis showing pIgR mRNA in uteri of ovariectomized rats treated daily for 3 days with (1) saline (0.1 ml); (2) estradiol (1 μg/0.1 ml) and sacrificed 4 hr following third injection; (3) estradiol and sacrificed 12 hr after the third injection. Each lane contains 30 μg total RNA extracted from the treatment group. The same blot was rehybridized with 1A probe to normalize the amount of total RNA loaded in each lane. (B) Relative amounts of pIgR mRNA present in uteri of estradiol-treated rats. Northern blots were quantified by densitometric analysis and pIgR mRNA levels were normalized with the 1A mRNA levels for each sample. Relative mRNA levels are presented as the percentage of maximum expression. Results were obtained from two separate experiments and expressed as mean ± SE. **Significantly ($P < 0.01$) greater than the saline control. From Kaushic *et al.* (1995).

treated animals. Figure 8B shows the ratio of pIgR mRNA in the estradiol-treated rats after normalization with 1A mRNA. pIgR mRNA levels increased significantly following estradiol treatment, with high levels detected at both 4 and 12 hr after the third injection. Estradiol increased pIgR mRNA levels approximately 2.5-fold beyond that measured in saline controls. In other studies (not shown), progesterone given to ovariectomized rats lowered pIgR mRNA levels below that seen in saline controls (Kaushic *et al.*, 1995). Further, when administered along with estradiol, progesterone partially reversed the stimulatory effect of estradiol. As a part of this study, pIgR levels in uterine fluid of estradiol-treated rats were analyzed by RIA. Unexpectedly, we found that whereas pIgR levels in uterine secretions increased 200-fold (saline vs estradiol), pIgR mRNA levels increased 2- to 3-fold. Whether these differences are due to increased stability of pIgR and/or pIgR mRNA remains to be established.

A question that arose from our studies of s.c. levels in vaginal secretions was whether s.c. was produced locally in the lower reproductive tract (Wira and Sullivan, 1985). To determine whether pIgR is expressed in vaginal tissues and if expression varies with the stage of the estrous cycle, animals were selected by vaginal smears to obtain tissues representative of each stage of the cycle. Total RNA was extracted from vaginae pooled from four to six animals at proestrus, estrus, and diestrus and analyzed for pIgR mRNA. The Northern analysis of RNA in Table V indicates that pIgR mRNA levels in vaginae were highest at diestrus and lowest at proestrus and estrus (C. Kaushic and C. R. Wira, unpublished observation). When normalized to 1A, pIgR message levels at diestrus were significantly higher than that seen at proestrus and estrus. To identify the cells in vaginal tissues which express pIgR, immunohistochemical localization was undertaken with rabbit anti-rat-pIgR antibody. Of those cells present in vaginal tissues, only squamous epithelial cells expressed s.c. Vaginal epithelial cells from rats at diestrus expressed significantly more pIgR than did epithelial cells in the vaginae from animals at proestrus and estrus. Overall, these studies indicate that pIgR and pIgR mRNA are expressed in both the uterus and the vagina and that both are under hormonal control. Moreover, it indicates that endocrine control within the uterus and vagina is unique in that estradiol stimulates pIgR and pIgR mRNA in the uterus at a time when both are inhibited in the vagina.

IV. Discussion

The results presented demonstrate that both afferent and efferent arms of the mucosal immune system are

TABLE V
Polymeric IgR mRNA and s.c. Levels in Vaginal Tissue of Rats at Different Stages of the Estrous Cycle

	Stage of estrous cycle		
	Proestrus	Estrus	Diestrus
pIgR mRNA	±	+	+++
s.c. protein	+	+	+++

Note. RNA was extracted from vaginae of rats (six to nine animals/group) at different stages of the estrous cycle. Northern blotting and immunohistochemistry were done according to procedures described previously (Kaushic *et al.*, 1995). The bands obtained in Northern blots were quantitated by scanning densitometry. Amount of pIgR mRNA (as detected by Northern blotting) or s.c. protein (as detected by immunohistochemistry): ±, very low; +, low; ++, medium, +++, high.

present in the female reproductive tract, that both are regulated by sex hormones and selected cytokines, and that the nature of this regulation varies from site to site throughout the reproductive tract. For example, IgA, IgG, and s.c. levels in uterine secretions increase in response to estradiol and are antagonized by the action of progesterone. In contrast, immunoglobulins and s.c. levels are lowered in cervico-vaginal secretions in response to estradiol and progesterone. In both cases, control by sex hormones is mediated in part through s.c. mRNA levels which are differentially regulated in the uterus and vagina. Our understanding of the multiple levels at which these hormones interact with the secretory immune system indicates that in response to estradiol, antigen presentation is stimulated in the uterus and inhibited in the vagina. In other studies, we have found that in response to estradiol, lymphoid cells migrate into the reproductive tract, IgA and IgG move from blood into uterine tissue, and immunoglobulins move from tissue to lumen, in part, due to hormonal control of the IgA receptor.

Our present understanding of mucosal immune system in the female reproductive tract is depicted in Fig. 9. Based on a number of studies, it is clear that antigens, including sperm, bacteria, and viruses, make initial contact with the vaginal mucosa (VM) and then, depending on physical as well as immunological factors, ascend through the ecto-cervix (ECX), cervix (CX), uterus (ut), and Fallopian tubes (FT). Depending on the

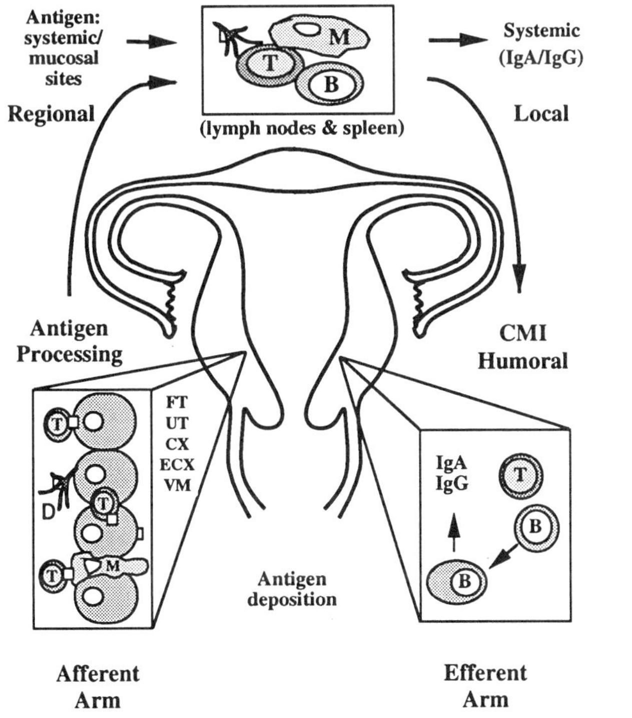

Figure 9. Schematic representation of the afferent and efferent arms of the immune system in the female reproductive tract.

stage of the reproductive cycle and the organ involved, if protection is inadequate, organisms evade immune surveillance and enter the pelvic cavity to potentially cause pelvic inflammatory disease. As seen in our model, sufficient evidence now exists to indicate that the afferent arm of the immune system is present throughout the tract and that both epithelial- and nonepithelial-antigen presenting cells capable of presenting antigen are present. Our findings demonstrate that the upper and lower regions are inductive sites for immune responses. It also indicates that immunological events in the reproductive tract involve sites distant from the reproductive site. Based on our experiments and those of others (Beer and Billingham, 1974; Head *et al.*, 1986), both lymph nodes and spleen are involved in the events that occur after antigen or cytokines are deposited in the uterine lumen. Whether this represents an evolutionary step that compensates for the absence of highly organized immune structures in the reproductive tract similar to the Peyer's patches found in the intestine is open to speculation. What is clear in our animal model is that local influences in the reproductive tract influence T- and B-lymphocyte responses in the spleen. These cells, in turn, as well as immune cells from other mucosal surfaces including the gastrointestinal tract, migrate into reproductive tract tissues to mount both humoral and CMI responses. Overall, the reproductive tract has both afferent and efferent arms of the immune system and shares with other mucosal surfaces the fundamental components necessary for recognizing and responding to antigenic challenge.

One implication of our studies is that in any strategy for vaccine development against sexually transmitted diseases, both the lower and upper reproductive tract need to be recognized as potential sites for inducing immune responses. That the reproductive tract was not considered an inductive site has dictated strategies and protocols to induce immune protection which excluded direct instillation of antigen at the site to be protected. Only recently, with the use of gels to extend the time of antigen exposure, have new findings supportive of inducing local immune responses been reexamined (Wassen *et al.*, 1995; Eriksson *et al.*, 1995). It is also important to recognize that diversity of immune function exists within the reproductive tract. For example, within a given species, the mucosal immune system in the vagina is functionally unique from that seen in the cervix, uterus, and Fallopian tube. Further, regulation of immune recognition and responsiveness by sex hormones varies from site to site. Only by considering site of antigen stimulation as well as stage of the menstrual cycle, both when immunization occurs and when responses to immunization are to be measured, can one begin to obtain a clear understanding of the effectiveness of a given vaccine.

That epitheial and stromal cells in the uterus and

vagina are able to present antigen demonstrates that the reproductive tract is an inductive site for immune responses. What remains to be determined is to whom antigen is presented. As a fixed population, antigen presentation by luminal epithelial cells is theoretically restricted to intraepithelial lymphocytes or cells which interface with epithelial cells at the basement membrane. Whether these cells lead to immune responses or tolerance similar to that seen in the intestine remains to be determined. In recent studies, we have demonstrated that glandular as well as luminal epithelial cells present antigen (Wira and Rossoll, unpublished observation). Since glandular epithelial cells responses to sex hormones are different from that seen with luminal cells, their roles in the induction of immune responses may be different. For example, whereas luminal expression of class II antigen is barely detectable, glandular cells express class II in abundance at late diestrus and estrus (Head and Gaede, 1986). Further, it is at this time that class II positive cells are found in greatest numbers in close association with glandular epithelium (Head *et al.*, 1986). As discussed previously (Wira and Rossoll, 1995a, 1995b), antigen presentation by epithelial cells may involve either local immune cells or nontraditional pathways in which dendritic or other antigen-presenting cells, following interaction with epithelial cells, transfer antigen to sites distant to the reproductive tract.

In studies attempting to more fully define the efferent arm of the immune system in the female reproductive tract, we examined the mechanism of estradiol action at the molecular level. The data summarized in this review, when considered in light of the effects of estradiol on IgA and s.c. levels in uterine and vaginal secretions, indicate that the regulatory effects of estradiol are in part mediated through the expression of pIg mRNA in epithelial cells which line the uterus and vagina. The *in vitro* studies described provide new information into the mechanism by which IgA is transported from uterine tissue into secretions. These studies, which utilized normal uterine epithelial cells grown to confluence on Millicell chambers, provide the foundation of information necessary to study the direct effects of sex hormones and cytokines and the interactions between epithelial and stromal cells that regulate epithelial cell transport of IgA.

V. Conclusions

Our studies of mucosal immunity in the female reproductive tract raise important issues about the complexity of immune protection which involves both the endocrine and immune systems. Previously, we demonstrated that endocrine balance markedly influences the efferent arm of the mucosal immune system in rodents and humans (Wira *et al.*, 1994). Both IgA, IgG, and s.c. levels in uterine and cervico-vaginal secretions and immune cell migration into the reproductive tract are hormonally controlled. Our recent findings extend these observations by demonstrating that the afferent (recognition) arm of the immune system in the reproductive tract is also hormonally regulated. Taken together, these studies demonstrate that estradiol, progesterone, and cytokines interact in a coordinated manner to regulate both the afferent and efferent arms of the immune system in the female reproductive tract. It is important to note that these studies utilize the rat as an animal model. As discussed in the Introduction, hormones clearly influence many aspects of the immune system in the human reproductive tract. Whether all of our findings can be translated directly to the human is highly unlikely, given the diversity of reproductive behavior and biology that exists within mammals. What is important is that the unique characteristics and potential within the reproductive tract be recognized as efforts are made to utilize this system in the control of population, the identification of problems of infertility, and the prevention and treatment of sexually transmitted diseases including HIV, the causative agent of AIDS.

Acknowledgments

This work was supported by Research Grants AI-13541 and AI-34478 from NIH.

References

Allardyce, R. A. (1984). Effect of ingested sperm on fecundity in the rat. *J. Exp. Med.* 159, 1548–1553.

Banting, G., Brake, B., Braghetta, P., Luzio, J. P., and Stanley, K. K. (1989). Intracellular targeting signals of polymeric immunoglobulin receptors are highly conserved between species. *FEBS Lett.* **254**, 177–183.

Beer, A., and Billingham, R. E. (1974). Host responses to intrauterine tissue, cellular and fetal allografts. *J. Reprod. Fertil.* **21**(Suppl), 59.

Bernard, O., Rachman, F., and Bennett, D. (1981). Immunoglobulins in the mouse uterus before implantation. *J. Reprod. Fertil.* **63**, 237–240.

Bjercke, S., and Brandtzaeg, P. (1993). Glandular distribution of immunoglobulins, J chain, secretory component, and HLA-DR in the human endometrium throughout the menstrual cycle. *Hum. Reprod.* **8**, 1420–1425.

Canning, M. B., and Billington, W. D. (1983). Hormonal regulation of immunoglobulins and plasma cells in the mouse uterus. *J. Endocrinol.* **97**, 419–424.

Cates, W. J. (1986). Priorities for sexually transmitted diseases in the late 1980s and beyond. *Sexually Transmitted Diseases* **13**, 114–117.

Cooper, M. D. (1995). The mucosal immune response to sexually transmitted diseases in the human female reproductive tract. *Mucosal Immunol. Update* **3**, 9–14.

Cooper, M. D., Dever, C., Tempel, K., Moticka, E. J., Hindman, T., and Stephens, D. S. (1987). Characterization of lymphoid cells from the human fallopian tube mucosa. *In* "Recent Adances in Mucosal Immunology" (J. Mestecky, J. R. McGhee, J. Bienenstock, and P. L. Ogra, eds.), pp. 387–394. Plenum, New York.

Corbeil, L. B., Duncan, J. R., Schurig, G. D., Hall, C. E., and Winter, A. J. (1974). Bovine venereal disease: Variations in the immunoglobulin class of the antibodies in genital secretions and serum. *Infect. Immun.* **10**, 1084–1090.

Eriksson, K., Quiding-Jarbrink, M., Osek, J., Moller, A., Bjork, S., Kieny, M., Holmgren, J., and Czerkinsky, C. (1995). Immunization strategies for the induction of vaginal and rectal immune responses in non-human primates. *Clin. Immunol. Immunopathol.* **76**, S-43.

Fabian, G. (1976). The lymphatic vessels of the uterus during the sexual cycles of mice. *Lymphology* **9**, 78–82.

Forrest, B. D. (1992). The need for consideration of mucosal immunity in vaccine approaches to AIDS. *Vaccine Res.* **1**, 137–142.

Gong, J. L., McCarthy, K. M., Rogers, R. A., and Schneeberger, E. E. (1994). Interstitial lung macrophages interact with dendritic cells to present antigenic peptides derived from particulate antigens to T cells. *Immunology* **81**, 343–351.

Harbour, D. V., and Blalock, J. E. (1989). Lymphocytes and lymphocytic hormones in pregnancy. *Prog. Neuroendocrinol. Immunol.* **2**, 55–63.

Head, J. R., and Gaede, S. D. (1986). Ia antigen expression in the rat uterus. *J. Reprod. Immunol.* **9**, 137–153.

Head, J. R., Miller, S. T., and Kresge, C. K. (1986). Uterine lymphatic vessels and IA+ cells: Possible role in antigen processing. *In* "Reproductive Immunology" (D. A. Clark and B. A. Croy, eds.), pp. 205–210. Elsevier, Cambridge, U.K.

Hsu, C. Y. J., Komm, B. S., Lyttle, C. R., and Frankel, F. (1988). Cloning of estrogen-regulated messenger ribonucleic acids from rat uterus. *Endocrinology* **122**, 631–639.

Hurlimann, J., Dayal, R., and Gloor, E. (1978). Immunoglobulins and secretory component in endometrium and cervix: Influence of inflammation and carcinoma. *Virch. Arch. Pathol. Anat. Histol.* **377**, 211–223.

Kamat, B. R., and Isaacson, P. G. (1987). The immunocytochemical distribution of leukocytic subpopulations in human endometrium. *Am. J. Pathol.* **127**, 66–73.

Kaushic, C., Richardson, J. M., and Wira, C. R. (1995). Regulation of polymeric immunoglobulin A receptor messenger ribonucleic acid expression in rodent uteri: Effect of sex hormones. *Endocrinology* **136**, 2836–2844.

Kelly, J. K., and Fox, H. (1979). The local immunological defense system of the human endometrium. *J. Reprod. Immunol.* **1**, 39–45.

Kerr, W. R. (1955). Vaginal and uterine antibodies in cattle with particular reference to *Brucella abortus*. *Brit. Vet. J.* **111**, 169–178.

Kutteh, W. H., Hatch, K. D., Blackwell, R. E., and Mestecky, J. (1988). Secretory immune system of the female reproductive tract: I. Immunoglobulin and secretory component-containing cells. *Obstet. Gynecol.* **71**, 56–60.

Kutteh, W. H., Blackwell, R. E., Gore, H., Kutteh, C. C., Carr, B. R., and Mestecky, J. (1990). Secretory immune system of the female reproductive tract. II. Local immune system in normal and infected Fallopian tube. *Fertil. Steril.* **54**, 51–55.

Laguens, G., Goni, J. J., Laguens, M., Goni, J. M., and Laguens, R. (1990). Demonstration and characterization of HLA-DR positive cells in the stroma of human endometrium. *J. Reprod. Immunol.* **18**, 179–186.

Lippes, J., Ogra, S., Tomasi, T. B., and Tourville, D. R. (1970). Immunohistochemical localization of γG, γA, γM, secretory piece and lactoferrin in the human female genital tract. *Contraception* **1**, 163.

Mitchell, B. S. (1986). The localization of immunoglobulins in the non-pregnant rat uterus. *J. Anat.* **146**, 237.

Natali, P. G., de Martino, C., Quaranta, V., Nicotra, M., Frezza, F., Pellegrino, M. A., and Ferrone, S. (1981). Expression of Ia-like antigens in normal human nonlymphoid tissues. *Transplantation* **31**, 75–78.

Ogra, P. L., and Ogra, S. S. (1973). Local antibody response to poliovaccine in the human female genital tract. *J. Immunol.* **110**, 1307–1311.

Ogra, P., Yamanaka, T., and Losonsky, G. A. (1981). Local immunologic defenses in the genital tract. *In* "Reproductive Immunology" (N. Fleicher, ed.), pp. 381–394. Alan R. Liss, New York.

Parr, M. B., and Parr, E. L. (1985). Immunochemical localization of immunoglobulins A, G, and M in the mouse female genital tract. *J. Reprod. Fertil.* **74**, 361–370.

Parr, E. L., and Parr, M. B. (1990). A comparison of antibody titers in mouse uterine fluid after immunization by several routes, and the effect of the uterus on antibody titres in vaginal fluid. *J. Reprod. Fertil.* **89**, 619–625.

Parr, M. B., and Parr, E. L. (1991). Langerhans cells and T lymphocyte subsets in the murine vagina and cervix. *Biol. Reprod.* **44**, 491–498.

Parr, M. B., and Parr, E. L. (1994). Mucosal immunity in the female and male reproductive tracts. *In* "Handbook of Mucosal Immunology" (P. L. Ogra, J. Mestecky, M. E. Lamm, W. Strober, J. R. McGhee, and J. Bienenstock, eds.), pp. 677–689. Academic Press, New York.

Piot, P., Plummer, F. A., Mhalu, F. S., Lamboray, J. L., Chin, J., and Mann, J. M. (1988). AIDS: An international perspective. *Science* **239**, 573–579.

Prabhala, R. H., and Wira, C. R. (1991). Cytokine regulation of the mucosal immune system: *In vivo* stimulation by interferon-gamma of secretory component and immunoglobulin A in uterine secretions and proliferation of lymphocytes from spleen. *Endocrinology* **129**, 2915–2923.

Prabhala, R. H., and Wira, C. R. (1995). Influence of estrous cycle and estradiol on mitogenic responses of splenic T- and B-lymphocytes. *Adv. Exp. Med. Biol.* **371A**, 379–381.

Rebello, R., Green, F., and Fox, H. (1975). A study of the secretory immune system of the female genital tract. *J. Obstet. Gynecol.* **82**, 812–816.

Richardson, J., Kaushic, C., and Wira, C. R. (1993). Estradiol regulation of secretory component: Expression by rat uterine epithelial cells. *J. Steroid Biochem.* **47**, 143–149.

Richardson, J. M., Kaushic, C., and Wira, C. R. (1995). Polymeric immunogloblin (Ig) receptor production and IgA transcytosis in polarized primary cultures of mature rat uterine epithelial cells. *Biol. Reprod.* **53**, 488–498.

Schumacher, G. F. B. (1980). Humoral immune factors in the female reproductive tract and their changes during the cycle. *In* "Immunological Aspects of Infertility and Fertility Control" (D. Dinsda and G. Schumacher, eds.), pp. 93–141. Elsevier, North Holland, New York.

Sen, D. K., and Fox, H. (1967). The lymphoid tissue of the endometrium. *Gynaecologia* **163**, 371–378.

Shaikh, A. A. (1971). Estrone and estradiol levels in the ovarian venous blood from rats during the estrous cycle and pregnancy. *Biol. Reprod.* **5**, 297–307.

Shelton, J. A., and Goldberg, E. (1986). Local reproductive tract immunity to sperm specific lactate dehydrogenase-C4. *Biol. Reprod.* **35**, 873–876.

Sullivan, D. A., and Wira, C. R. (1983). Hormonal regulation of immunoglobulins in the rat uterus: Uterine response to a single estradiol treatment. *Endocrinology* **112**, 260–268.

Sullivan, D. A., and Wira, C. R. (1984). Hormonal regulation of immunoglobulins in the rat uterus: Uterine response to multiple estradiol treatments. *Endocrinology* **114**, 650–658.

Sullivan, D. A., Underdown, B. J., and Wira, C. R. (1983). Steroid hormone regulation of free secretory component in the rat uterus. *Immunology* **49**, 379–386.

Sullivan, D. A., Richardson, G. S., MacLaughlin, D. T., and Wira, C. R. (1984). Variations in the levels of secretory component in human uterine fluid during the menstrual cycle. *J. Steroid Biochem.* **20**, 509–513.

Tauber, P. F., Wettich, W., Nohlen, M., and Zaneveld, L. J. D. (1985). Diffusable proteins of the mucosa of the human cervix, uterus, and fallopian tubes: Distribution and variations during the menstrual cycle. *Am. J. Obstet. Gynecol.* **15**, 1115–1125.

Thapar, M. A., Parr, E. L., and Parr, M. B. (1990). Secretory immune responses in mouse vaginal fluid after pelvic, parenteral or vaginal immunization. *Immunology* **70**, 121–125.

Tourville, D. R., Ogra, S. S., Lippes, J., and Tomasi, T. B. J. (1970). The human female reproductive tract: Immunohistological localization of A, G, M, secretory piece and lactoferrin. *Am. J. Obstet. Gynecol.* **108**, 1102–1108.

Vaerman, J.-P., and Férin, J. (1974). Local immunological response in the vagina, cervix and endometrium. *Acta Endocrinol.* **194**, 281–305.

Wassen, E., Schon, K., Holmgren, J., Jertborn, M., and Lycke, N. (1995). Local vaccination of the female genital tract is efficient. *Clin. Immunol. Immunopathol.* **76**, S-44.

Wegmann, T. G., Lin, H., Guilbert, L., and Mosmann, T. R. (1993). Bidirectional cytokine interactions in the maternal–fetal relationship: Is successful pregnancy a Th2 phenomenon? *Immunol. Today* **14**, 353–356.

Wira, C. R., and Prabhala, R. H. (1993). The female reproductive tract is an inductive site for immune responses: Effect of estradiol and antigen on antibody and secretory component levels in uterine and cervico-vaginal secretions following various routes of immunization. *In* "Scientific Basis of Fertility Regulation. Local Immunity in Reproductive Tract Tissues" (P. D. Griffin and P. M. Johnson, eds.), pp. 271–293. Oxford Univ. Press, New York.

Wira, C. R., and Rossoll, R. M. (1995a). Antigen presenting cells in the female reproductive tract: Influence of the estrous cycle on antigen presentation by uterine epithelial and stromal cells. *Endocrinology* **136**, 4526–4534.

Wira, C. R., and Rossoll, R. M. (1995b). Antigen presenting cells in the female reproductive tract: Influence of sex hormones on antigen presentation in the vagina. *Immunology* **84**, 505–508.

Wira, C. R., and Sandoe, C. P. (1977). Sex steroid hormone regulation of IgA and IgG in rat uterine secretions. *Nature (London)* **268**, 534–536.

Wira, C. R., and Sandoe, C. P. (1987a). Origin of IgA and IgG antibodies in the female reproductive tract: Regulation of the genital response by estradiol. *Adv. Exp. Med. Biol.* **216A**, 403–412.

Wira, C. R., and Sandoe, C. P. (1987b). Specific IgA and IgG antibodies in the secretions of the female reproductive tract: Effects of immunization and estradiol on expression of this response *in vivo*. *J. Immunol.* **138**, 4159–4164.

Wira, C. R., and Sandoe, C. P. (1989). Effect of uterine immunization and oestradiol on specific IgA and IgG antibodies in uterine, vaginal and salivary secretions. *Immunology* **68**, 24–30.

Wira, C. R., and Stern, J. E. (1992). Endocrine regulation of the mucosal immune system in the female reproductive tract: Control of IgA, IgG, and secretory component during the reproductive cycle, at implantation and throughout pregnancy. *In* "Hormones and Fetal Pathophysiology" (J. R. Pasqualini and R. Scholler, eds.), pp. 343–368. Dekker, New York.

Wira, C. R., and Sullivan, D. A. (1985). Estradiol and progesterone regulation of IgA, IgG and secretory component in cervico-vaginal secretions of the rat. *Biol. Reprod.* **32**, 90–95.

Wira, C. R., Hyde, E., Sandoe, C. P., Sullivan, D. A., and Spencer, S. (1980). Cellular aspects of the rat uterine IgA response to estradiol and progesterone. *J. Steroid Biochem.* **12**, 451–459.

Wira, C. R., Stern, J. E., and Colby, E. (1984). Estradiol regulation of secretory component in the uterus of the rat: Evidence for involvement of RNA synthesis. *J. Immunol.* **133**, 2624–2628.

Wira, C. R., Richardson, J., and Prabhala, R. (1994). Endocrine regulation of mucosal immunity: Effect of sex hormones and cytokines on the afferent and efferent arms of the immune system in the female reproductive tract. *In* "Handbook of Mucosal Immunology" (P. L. Ogra, J. Mestecky, M. E. Lamm, W. Strober, J. R. McGhee, and J. Bienenstock, eds.), pp. 705–718. Academic Press, New York.

Yang, S. L., and Schumacher, G. F. B. (1979). Immune response after vaginal application of antigens in the rhesus monkey. *Fertil. Steril.* **32**, 588–598.

Young, W. G. (1985). Epithelial kinetics affect Langerhan's cells of the mouse vaginal epithelium. *Anat. Rec.* **123**, 131–136.

Young, W. G., and Hosking, A. R. (1986). Langerhans cells in murine vaginal epithelium affected by oestrogen and topical vitamin A. *Anat. Rec.* **125**, 59–64.

29

Mucosal Immunity in the Urinary System

William W. Agace
Catharina Svanborg
Division of Clinical Immunology
Department of Medical Microbiology
Lund University
S-223 62 Lund, Sweden

I. The Urinary Tract as a Model System for Studies of Mucosal Immunity

The urinary tract has been discussed as an integral part of the common mucosal immune system (Hanson *et al.*, 1977). The structure of the mucosa and its cellular components differ, however, from other mucosal sites. The naive urinary tract mucosa does not contain M cells, organized lymphoid tissue, or goblet cells. Formation of Peyer's patch-like lymphoid aggregates has been reported to occur as a result of long-standing infection, but the properties of these lymphoid aggregates are poorly understood. The lower urinary tract, the urethra and trigominol area of the bladder, is lined by squamous epithelial cells. The transitional epithelium, which is unique to the urinary tract, lines the bladder, ureters, and renal pelvis. This epithelial layer is organized to permit the large volume changes of the bladder and to withstand the extreme pH and osmolarity of urine without disruption of its barrier function. Epithelial cell elements are also found in the kidney. The renal tubuli are, for example, lined by a single layer of columnar epithelial cells.

The urinary tract mucosa forms an efficient barrier to microbes and molecules in the urine. It is constantly exposed to different organic and inorganic compounds that are excreted with urine as a result of filtration through the kidney. It is not known to what extent these molecules evoke an immune response or stimulate mucosal lymphoid elements in the urinary tract. Our knowledge of mucosal immunity in the urinary tract has mainly been derived from studies of infection. This chapter will consequently be limited to mucosal immunity as it relates to urinary tract infection.

Urinary tract infections (UTI) provide an excellent model for studies of antibacterial mucosal responses. Bacteria reach this normally sterile organ system through the urethra, and establish a population of $\geq 10^5$ bacteria/ml of urine. Since most UTIs are caused by a single bacterial strain, it is possible to study the host response as a function of the virulence properties of the infecting strain. The mucosal compartment is easily accessible for study since host response molecules and cells are excreted with urine and may be collected and characterized. Studies of host–parasite interactions in the urinary tract have provided a number of insights that have proven to be relevant for infections at other mucosal sites.

II. Urinary Tract Infection—Background

UTI are one of the most common nonepidemic bacterial infections in humans. The frequency of infection varies with age, gender and predisposing factors. Acute pyelonephritis occurs in about 3% of girls and 1% of boys prior to 11 years of age (Winberg *et al.*, 1974). The frequency of acute cystitis in children is difficult to determine, however, most women have at least one episode of acute cystitis within their lifetime. Asymptomatic bacteriuria (ABU) is found in 1% of girls, 2–11% of pregnant women, and 15–20% of elderly individuals (Kunin, 1987).

Escherichia coli is the dominating etiological agent in UTI; however, infections with other species including *Proteus, Klebsiella, Enterobacter,* and *Staphylococcus saprophyticus* occur with varying frequency. Most uropathogens colonize the large intestine, spread to the vaginal and periurethral areas and ascend into the urinary tract to establish bacteriuria (Bettelheim and Taylor, 1969; Grüneberg, 1969; Lidin-Janson *et al.*, 1977; Plos *et al.*, 1995). To colonize the urinary tract, bacteria must resist elimination by the urine flow and bacterici-

MUCOSAL VACCINES

dal components in urine and in the mucosa. Bacterial colonization is aided by specific binding of bacterial adherence factors (P, type 1, Dr, and S fimbriae) to mucosal host receptors. Once established in the urinary tract the bacteria may persist asymptomatically or induce a host response leading to symptomatic infection. In about 30% of patients with acute pyelonephritis bacteria invade through the mucosa into the blood stream and cause bacteremia.

The severity of infection depends on the virulence of the infecting strain. *E. coli* clones that cause the most severe form of UTI (acute pyelonephritis) possess a number of virulence factors that are infrequent among the strains that cause ABU. These include adherence determinants (predominantly P fimbriae), endo- and exotoxins (specific LPS types, hemolysin), iron binding proteins (aerobactin), and specific capsular polysaccharides (Svanborg-Edén and de Man, 1987; Svanborg-Edén *et al.*, 1988; Johnson, 1991). The strongest association with acute pyelonephritis is seen with P fimbriae. P fimbriation is thought to enhance *E. coli* virulence for the urinary tract in several ways (Svanborg *et al.*, 1994). P fimbriated *E. coli* adhere to human colonic epithelial cells *in vitro* and persist longer in the large intestine of UTI prone children than other *E. coli* strains (Wold *et al.*, 1988b, 1992). P-fimbriated *E. coli* also adhere to uroepithelial cells and activate a cytokine response in those cells (Hedges *et al.*, 1990, 1992b; Agace *et al.*, 1993a).

While the factors which determine bacterial virulence for the urinary tract have received extensive attention, the important host defense mechanisms that contribute to the clearance of infection remain largely unknown. Furthermore, it remains to be shown whether absence of bacteriuria is due to lack of exposure to uropathogenic bacteria or to efficient defense mechanisms in the urinary tract of resistant individuals. In this chapter we will discuss mucosal immune response to infection in the urinary tract, and the host factors thought to be of importance in the antibacterial defense of the urinary tract mucosa.

III. Mechanisms of Resistance to Bacterial Colonization

Adherence is important for the colonization of the intestinal reservoir, the vaginal and periurethral areas, and for induction of symptoms within the urinary tract. The differential expression of adherence factors by the bacteria facilitates their interaction with the mucosa during the different stages of colonization and infection. A number of host factors act to modify or prevent bacterial attachment to the urinary tract mucosa: (A) Mechanic defenses and bactericidal activities exert a nonspecific barrier to bacterial establishment. (B) Host receptor expression influences the ability of bacteria to attach. (C) Anti-adhesive molecules are secreted into the urine.

A. Mechanic Defenses and Bactericidal Effects of Urine and the Mucosa

The urine flow and bladder voiding are important mechanisms of removing bacteria from the urinary tract. Patients with inborn or induced changes in urine flow have an increased frequency of UTI and are often infected with other species and bacteria of lower virulence. Early experiments by Norden and co-workers (1968) showed that 99.9% of a 10^9 bacterial inoculum, given intravesically into guinea pigs, was removed by voiding. In an artificial bladder model, O'Grady and Pennington (1966) studied the effects of bacterial multiplication rates, urine flow rates, bladder volume, and frequency of bladder voiding. They proposed a model with critical values which must be achieved if a bacterial population is to successfully colonize the urinary tract (O'Grady and Pennington, 1966). It was concluded that liquid with a bacterial content of 10^5/ml that wet the bladder surface after voiding was sufficient to reinoculate the next portion of urine and thus result in the persistence of bacteriuria. In contrast to these results, Cox and Hinman (1961) showed that an inoculum of 10^7 *E. coli* was cleared from the bladders of healthy adult males within 72 hr. These conflicting *in vitro* and *in vivo* observations indicate the importance of mechanisms in addition to the urine flow in maintaining the sterility of the urinary tract.

Urine can support bacterial growth (Pasteur, 1863); however, not all *E. coli* strains are capable of growth in this medium (Kaye, 1968). While *E. coli* urinary isolates from patients with UTI were found to multiply in urine and to reach high cell densities, fecal isolates were killed. These observations demonstrated that urine contains antibacterial molecules, and suggested that strains causing UTI are selected, in part, due to resistance to these factors (Gordon and Riley, 1992).

The antibacterial activity of urine is influenced by a number of factors including urea and ammonium concentration, pH, and osmolarity (Asscher *et al.*, 1966) (Kaye, 1968). *E. coli* growth in urine is inhibited by extremes of pH, and high osmolarity (Asscher *et al.*, 1966). One principal antibacterial osmolyte is urea. Its activity can be modulated by pH and the concentration of electrolytes (Kaye, 1968).

Early studies by Norden and co-workers (1968) indicated that the bladder mucosa exhibits bactericidal activity. They showed that a fraction of an *E. coli* inoculum was killed by bladder mucosa in guinea pigs. The antibacterial activity of the bladder mucosa was not paralleled by an antibacterial activity of urine, or by phagocytosis by leukocytes. Schulte-Wisserman (1985) confirmed that urinary tract epithelial cells produce bactericidal molecules *in vitro* and suggested that these bactericidal molecules were present in lower levels in UTI prone individuals. Recently, Connell and co-workers (1996) isolated a bactericidal hydrophilic, weakly cationic low-molecular-weight amine containing compound (between 500 and 1000 MW) from human urine. At physiologic concentrations, this compound was bactericidal for fecal but not urinary tract isolates.

Molecules with bactericidal activity have been detected at different mucosal sites. After the discovery of the cecropins in insects, the defensins were described in granulocytes (for review see Boman, 1991). Peptides belonging to this family have subsequently been isolated from the intestinal mucosa and the oral cavity (Pattersson-Delafield *et al.*, 1980; Zasloff, 1987; Lee *et al.*, 1989; Eisenhauer *et al.*, 1992). The defensins and molecules with similar activity can be predicted to emerge as essential constituents of innate mucosal immunity. The molecular nature of the urinary tract defensins, and their contribution to the antibacterial defense within the urinary tract, requires further study.

B. Host Susceptibility to Bacterial Colonization Is Influenced by the Expression of Mucosal Receptors for Attaching Bacteria

The susceptibility to infection with attaching bacteria may be influenced by the availability of mucosal receptors for the bacterial adhesins. Early studies suggested an association between vaginal colonization and the susceptibility to UTI (Stamey *et al.*, 1971; Stamey and Sexton, 1975; Fowler *et al.*, 1977). Bacteria showed increased attachment to vaginal epithelial cells from women with recurrent UTI compared to controls *in vitro.* Subsequent studies confirmed that vaginal and uroepithelial cells from women and children with recurrent UTI have higher receptor activity for attaching bacteria than cells from healthy controls (Fowler and Stamey, 1977; Källenius and Winberg, 1978; Svanborg-Edén and Jodal, 1979; Schaeffer *et al.*, 1981). These observations have prompted studies at the molecular level to try to define the mechanisms of increased adherence (Schaeffer *et al.*, 1981).

E. coli P fimbriae recognize as receptors Galα1-4Galβ and GalNAcβ1-3Galα1-4Galβ containing oligosaccharide sequences in the globoseries of glycolipids (Leffler and Svanborg-Edén, 1980). These glycolipids are present in epithelial and nonepithelial cells of the urinary bladder and ureters (Leffler and Svanborg-Edén, 1981; Breimer *et al.*, 1985) and on erythrocytes (Källenius *et al.*, 1980). The structural prerequisites for P fimbrial–receptor interactions are therefore present along the urinary tract. However, individual variations in receptor expression exist. The globoseries of glycolipids are antigens in the P blood group system. The expression of these antigens on uroepithelial cells varies depending on the P blood group, ABH blood group, and secretor state of the individual (Marcus *et al.*, 1981). Based on comparative studies of blood group and glycolipid expression, the P blood group can be used to predict the receptor repertoire for P-fimbriated bacteria on epithelial cells in the urinary tract. In addition, the P blood group of an individual can be used in epidemiological studies to analyze the role of receptor expression for the susceptibility to infection.

1. *Absence of Receptors for P Fimbriae*

Individuals of the p blood group fail to synthesize functional Galα1-4Galβ containing glycolipids (Marcus *et al.*, 1981), and therefore lack receptors for P fimbriated *E. coli* on their uroepithelial cells (Leffler and Svanborg-Edén, 1981) and erythrocytes (Källenius *et al.*, 1980; Leffler and Svanborg-Edén, 1981). As a result p individuals should be resistant to infection with P-fimbriated *E. coli.* The low frequency of p individuals in the population has, however, precluded an evaluation of the relative morbidity in infections due to P-fimbriated *E. coli* in individuals of the p and P_1/P_2 blood group phenotypes.

2. *P_1 Blood Group and Acute Pyelonephritis*

Individuals of blood group P_1 run an 11-fold higher risk of attracting recurrent episodes of acute pyelonephritis with P-fimbriated *E. coli* than P_2 individuals (Lomberg *et al.*, 1981, 1983). This difference does not reflect an increase in the number of receptors for P-fimbriated *E. coli* on uroepithelial cells (Lomberg *et al.*, 1986b). Instead, P_1 individuals have an increased tendency to carry P-fimbriated *E. coli* strains in the fecal flora compared to individuals of the P_2 blood group (Plos *et al.*, 1995). The mechanism of this increased carriage is not clear. We have proposed that P_1 individuals express more or better receptors for P-fimbriated *E. coli* in the large intestine, and consequently run an increased risk of UTI due to these bacteria.

3. *P and ABH Blood Group Dependent Expression of Receptors for prsG$_{J96}$ Positive Strains*

P fimbriae are encoded by the *pap* chromosomal gene cluster (Hull *et al.*, 1981). The *pap*G adhesin sequences determine the receptor specificity (Lindberg *et al.*, 1984; Lund *et al.*, 1988). Several G adhesin variants exist (Marklund, 1991), which share the specificity for the globoseries of glycolipid receptors but differ in isoreceptor specificity, in binding to epithelial cells, and in disease association (Lund *et al.*, 1988; Senior *et al.*,

1988; Lindstedt *et al.*, 1989; Strömberg *et al.*, 1990; Johanson *et al.*, 1992). Most G adhesins recognize Galα1-4Galβ containing glycolipids, and attach to uroepithelial cells from P_1 an P_2 positive individuals, regardless of their ABH blood group or secretor state (Johanson *et al.*, 1992). The $prsG_{J96}$ adhesin prefers a receptor epitope composed of a GalNAcα linked to a globoseries core (Leffler and Svanborg-Edén, 1981; Lund *et al.*, 1988; Senior *et al.*, 1988; Lindstedt *et al.*, 1989, 1991; Strömberg *et al.*, 1990; Johanson *et al.*, 1992). Strains expressing this adhesin recognize the globo-A glycolipid expressed on uroepithelial cells from A_1 secretor individuals (Lindstedt *et al.*, 1989, 1991), and attach to uroepithelial cells from these individuals *in vitro*. This receptor specificity has been shown to influence the host range of uropathogenic *E. coli in vivo*. Individuals infected with strains exclusively binding globo-A were 100% A_1 positive compared to 43% in the population at large (Lindstedt *et al.*, 1991).

4. *Secretor State*

The secretor state influences the derivatization of epithelial glycoconjugates with the A, B, H, blood group determinants. Nonsecretors lack the glycosyl-transferase(s) required to elongate the globoseries core structure with ABH determinants. Nonsecretor individuals run an increased risk of contracting mucosal infections, including *Hemophilus influenzae, Streptococcus pneumoniae,* and superficial candida infections (Blackwell *et al.*, 1986a–c). In addition, nonsecretor individuals are overrepresented among women with a history of recurrent UTI and among children with UTI who develop renal scarring (Kinane *et al.*, 1982). The mechanism of this association is not known. Attachment to squamous uroepithelial cells has been investigated because the secretor state influences epithelial cell glycosylation and receptor expression. The binding of P-fimbriated *E. coli* to squamous uroepithelial cells of nonsecretors is increased compared to secretors (Lomberg *et al.*, 1989). In a recent study, vaginal epithelial cells from nonsecretors were found to express two extended globo-series glycosphingolipids with receptor activity for P-fimbriated *E. coli* (Stapleton *et al.*, 1992). These glycosphingolipids were not present on cells from secretors and were assumed to be a sialylated form of the globopenta glycolipid, which in secretors is fucosylated and processed to ABH antigens. The two receptors may provide additional binding sites for P fimbriae during UTI; however, they are not likely to explain the increased scarring in nonsecretors, since strains causing renal scarring do not often express P fimbriae.

C. Secreted Inhibitors of Bacterial Adherence

Mucosal secretions contain a variety of molecules that can interfere with bacterial attachment. Urine contains a number of oligosaccharides and glycoproteins with receptor activity for bacterial adhesins.

1. *Tamm Horsfall Protein*

The Tamm Horsfall glycoprotein (THP; Uromodulin) is produced by the luminal cells of the thick ascending loop of Henlé and the early distal tubules as a 76-kDa glycoprotein containing approximately 25–30% carbohydrate (Fletcher *et al.*, 1970a,b; Sikri *et al.*, 1979). It forms the uromucoid or urinary slime that is thought to replace the goblet cell mucins present at other mucosal sites. THP is found at the epithelial surface as high-molecular-weight aggregates (7×10^7 kDa) and is the most abundant protein of normal human urine (Fletcher *et al.*, 1970a,b; Sikri *et al.*, 1979). In addition, THP contains terminal mannose residues, that are recognized by fimH, which is the fimbriae associated adhesin of type 1 fimbriae and can inhibit the binding of type 1 fimbriated *E. coli* to urinary tract epithelial cells *in vitro* (Svanborg-Edén *et al.*, 1981). Early studies by Ørskov and coworkers (1980) showed that type 1 fimbriated *E. coli* adhere to urinary slime containing THP. However, type 1 fimbriae bind better to immobilized THP than soluble THP (Parkkinen *et al.*, 1988). This may be of consequence in the binding of type 1 fimbriated strains to renal tissue.

Soluble THP blocks S fimbriae-mediated agglutination of human erythrocytes, presumably as it contains NeuAc(α2-3)Gal(β1-4)GlcNAc, a receptor active epitope for S fimbriae (Parkkinen *et al.*, 1988). THP does not, however, interfere with P fimbriae-mediated adherence to epithelial cells. This may explain the lower virulence of S-fimbriated strains, despite the ability of S fimbriae to bind the same uroepithelial tissues as P fimbriae *in vitro* (Korhonen *et al.*, 1986). Soluble inhibitors of P fimbrial attachment have not been isolated from urine.

Interestingly, THP also binds to neutrophils. Binding is calcium-dependent and RGD-mediated and requires metabolically active cells. THP increases phagocytosis, complement expression, and arachidonic acid metabolism, and may play an important role in mediating neutrophil/bacterial interactions in the urinary tract (Toma *et al.*, 1994).

2. *Low-Molecular-Weight Compounds*

Urine contains numerous low-molecular-weight (200–2000 MW) oligosaccharides that strongly inhibit *E. coli* type 1-mediated hemagglutination of guinea pig erythrocytes (Parkkinen *et al.*, 1988). The α mannosidase treatment of the oligosaccharides decreased their inhibitory activity, suggesting a mannose-dependent interaction with the adhesin of type 1 fimbriae.

3. *Oligosaccharide of Secretory IgA*

Secretory IgA (S-IgA) antibodies with specificity for bacterial surface structures are potent inhibitors of bacterial attachment (see below). In addition, S-IgA and IgA myeloma proteins, particularly those of the IgA2 subclass, carry oligosaccharide sequences with terminal mannose residues, that can interact with the mannose specific adhesin of type 1-fimbriated *E. coli.* Myeloma proteins were found to agglutinate type 1-fimbriated *E. coli* and to inhibit its attachment to urinary tract epithelial cells *in vitro* (Wold *et al.*, 1988a, 1990).

Despite the reported *in vitro* activities of many of these receptor analogs and inhibitors of attachment, additional studies assessing their role in the protection against UTI *in vivo* are required.

IV. Mucosal Inflammation

A. Mucosal Cytokine Responses in the Urinary Tract

The existence of a mucosal cytokine response to UTI was first recognized in the urinary tract of mice. IL-6 was found to be secreted into the urine within minutes of intravesical instillation of *E. coli* (de Man *et al.*, 1989). Similar observations were made during bacterial colonization of the human urinary tract, where intravesical instillation of bacteria induced rapid secretion of IL-6 and IL-8 into the urine (Hedges *et al.*, 1991; Agace *et al.*, 1993b); however, IL-1α, IL-1β, and TNFα were not detected (unpublished observations). Serum IL-6 or IL-8 levels were not elevated suggesting that these cytokines were of mucosal origin and were not being excreted through the kidneys.

The mucosal cytokine response to UTI has subsequently been studied in different patient groups with UTI. Most adults with acute pyelonephritis and asymptomatic bacteriuria (86%) had elevated urinary IL-6 levels at the time of diagnosis. In contrast, serum IL-6 was only detected in the patients with acute pyelonephritis (50%) (Hedges *et al.*, 1992a). Ko and co-workers (1993) showed that urinary IL-8 levels were raised in 112 of 113 adult patients with different forms of UTI, caused both by gram-positive and gram-negative bacteria. IL-1β has been detected in the urine of patients with bacterial cystitis but not in the urine of healthy controls or individuals suffering from interstitial cystitis. Serum IL-1β levels were not measured (Martins *et al.*, 1994). Children with UTI show a more differentiated urinary cytokine response. Those with acute pyelonephritis have high urine cytokine levels, while those with ABU have low or absent urine cytokine responses (Benson *et al.*, 1994).

1. *Role of Urinary Tract Epithelial Cells in Mucosal Cytokine Production*

Epithelial cells are the first to encounter the infecting bacterial strain. The epithelial cell response is therefore likely to precede that of other cell types at the mucosa. We have shown that uropathogenic *E. coli* stimulate cytokine production in human bladder and kidney cell lines and in freshly isolated uroepithelial cells (Hedges *et al.*, 1990, 1992b; Agace *et al.*, 1993a,b). The bacteria activated *de novo* synthesis of cytokine-specific mRNA (IL-1α, IL-1β, IL-6, IL-8, but not TNFα) (Hedges *et al.*, 1994). The cytokines detected in the supernatants of *E. coli*-stimulated epithelial cells in culture (IL-6 and IL-8) are the same as those found in the urine of individuals after deliberate colonization with *E. coli.* These observations suggest that epithelial cells are an important source of mucosal cytokines at the onset of UTI [for review see (Hedges *et al.*, 1995)].

2. *Mechanism of E. coli-induced Epithelial Cytokine Production*

The mechanisms by which *E. coli* induce urinary epithelial cytokine secretion are not fully understood. Lipopolysaccharide (LPS), a potent inducer of cytokine production in monocytes, is a poor stimulant of epithelial cytokine production. LPS concentrations 1000-fold higher than those used to stimulate monocytes were found to induce only low-level cytokine production (Hedges *et al.*, 1992b). Recent evidence has suggested that soluble CD14 greatly enhances epithelial cell responsiveness to LPS (Pugin *et al.*, 1993). The lack of CD14 receptors on urinary tract epithelial cells may explain, in part, their resistance to LPS stimulation.

Bacterial attachment enhances the epithelial cytokine response. IL-6 and IL-8 secretion were significantly higher in cells stimulated with attaching *E. coli* strains (type 1 fimbriated, P-fimbriated) than after exposure to isogenic nonfimbriated strains (Hedges *et al.*, 1992b; Agace *et al.*, 1993b; Svensson *et al.*, 1994). Various mechanisms may be proposed to explain the increased cytokine secretion to attaching strains: (1) binding of bacteria may increase the concentration at the epithelial surface of bacterial substance(s) able to activate a cytokine response, (2) the binding of fimbriae to glycoconjugate receptors may induce additional transmembrane signaling events leading to cytokine production. Recent studies have shown that P fimbriated *E. coli* induce the release of ceramide and activate its phosphorylation to ceramide-1-phosphate through serine–threonine protein kinases (Hedlund *et al.*, 1996).

3. *Mucosal Cytokine Networks Regulate the Epithelial Cytokine Response to Bacteria*

Nonepithelial cells resident at or recruited to the urinary tract mucosa during the inflammatory process are likely to contribute to the mucosal cytokine response to infection. For example, neutrophils produce IL-8 after stimulation with *E. coli* and are a likely second source of this cytokine during UTI [W. W. Agace and C. Svanborg, (1996) unpublished observation]. In addition, neutrophils have been reported to secrete IL-1, TNF, and IL-6 after stimulation with LPS, IL-1, or TNF (for review see Lloyd and Oppenheim, 1992). T cells resident within the urinary tract mucosa are likely additional participants in the mucosal cytokine response during the course of infection. Exogenous cytokines have recently been shown to modify the epithelial cytokine response to bacteria. IL-1 acted in synergy with *E. coli* as an inducer of epithelial IL-6 and IL-8 responses (Hedges *et al.*, 1994). IL-4, IL-5, IL-12, IL-13, TGFβ1 and IFNγ enhanced the *E. coli* induced IL-6 response, while IL-5, IL-12, and TGFβ1 marginally enhanced IL-8 responses (Hedges *et al.*, 1995). The strongest effects were observed in conjunction with IL-4 and IFNγ. IL-4 induced IL-6 production in synergy with *E. coli,* while IFNγ both enhanced and inhibited IL-6 and IL-8 responses, depending on the order in which the stimulants were added.

B. Neutrophil Recruitment in Response to UTI

Bacteriuria causes a rapid neutrophil influx into the urine. Neutrophil recruitment during UTI involves the generation of a chemotactic gradient from the urinary tract mucosa, adherence of neutrophils to the endothelial vessel wall, and their extravasation into the lamina propria. Finally, neutrophils cross the urinary tract epithelium into the urine. The molecular mechanisms underlying the increase in urinary neutrophil numbers are gradually becoming understood.

1. Neutrophil Chemoattractants

The role of complement and bacterial chemotactic formyl peptides in inducing neutrophil migration have been examined in a rat UTI model. Intravenous injection of cobra venom factor (complement depletion) or addition of phenylbutazone (a competitive antagonist of bacterial chemotactic formyl peptides) significantly reduced neutrophil recruitment into rat kidney tissue 32 hr after infection with *E. coli* (Meylan and Glauser, 1989).

Recent identification of a neutrophil chemotactic cytokine family has led to the examination of their role in neutrophil migration during UTI. IL-8 is the best characterized member of the α chemokine family (CXC) of cytokines with chemotactic activity for neutrophils (for review see Baggiolini *et al.*, 1994). In patients with UTI and patients deliberately colonized with *E. coli* in the urinary tract, levels of urinary IL-8 correlate strongly with urinary neutrophil numbers (Agace *et al.*, 1993b; Ko *et al.*, 1993). The neutrophil chemotactic activity of infected urine was reduced by 50% *in vitro* by monoclonal antibodies to IL-8 (Ko *et al.*, 1993). The role of CXC chemokines during UTI *in vivo* remains to be assessed.

Taken together, these observations suggest that neutrophil migration during UTI is a complex event mediated by an array of chemoattractants originating from the host and bacterial pathogen.

2. Role of Epithelial Cells in Neutrophil Migration

While neutrophil migration across endothelial vessels has been extensively studied, few studies examining neutrophil migration across urinary tract epithelium into urine have been conducted. We have recently shown that urinary tract epithelial cells participate in the induction of neutrophil migration in two ways: (a) by the secretion of neutrophil chemoattractants and (b) by the expression of cell adhesion molecules. *E. coli* and IL-1 were recently shown to induce neutrophil migration across kidney and bladder epithelial layers upon epithelial cell activation (Agace *et al.*, 1995). *E. coli* and IL-1-induced epithelial IL-8 secretion and anti-IL-8 antibody completely blocked the IL-1- and *E. coli*-induced transepithelial migration (Agace *et al.*, 1996). Specific neutrophil/epithelial interactions, mediated by cell adhesion molecules, were also required. Epithelial cell lines and normal urinary tract epithelial cells were found to express intercellular adhesion molecule-1 (ICAM-1), but not ICAM-2, P-selectin, or E-selectin. *E. coli* and IL-1 upregulated the expression of ICAM-1 on the epithelial cell surface and antibodies to ICAM-1 blocked from 60 to 80% of *E. coli*-induced transepithelial neutrophil migration. The neutrophil receptor for ICAM-1 was tentatively identified as the β_2 integrin CD11b/CD18 (Mac-1) since antibodies to CD11b and CD18 but not to CD11a blocked the *E. coli* induced transepithelial neutrophil migration (Agace *et al.*, 1995).

C. Role of Mucosal Inflammation and Neutrophil Influx in the Clearance of UTI

Mucosal inflammation is thought to play an essential role in the resistance of the urinary tract to infection. This was first indicated by studies in a murine UTI model. C3H/HeJ mice, which have a defective response to LPS, were found to be highly susceptible to intravesical infection with *E. coli* compared to C3H/HeN normal mice (Hagberg *et al.*, 1984a). Analysis of their mucosal inflammatory responses revealed that the urinary neutrophil and IL-6 levels were significantly lower in C3H/HeJ mice (Shahin *et al.*, 1987; de Man *et al.*, 1989). C57BL/10ScCr (LPS hyporesponder) mice are also more susceptible to experimental UTI, and have a reduced inflammatory response compared to normal C57BL/6J mice (Agace *et al.*, 1992). The presence of neutrophils in the urine in both mouse backgrounds corresponded with clearance of infection. Further studies showed that pharmacological inhibitors of inflammation (Dexamethasone, diclofenac, and indomethacin) severely inhibited the ability of C3H/HeN mice to clear acute UTI (Linder *et al.*, 1990). A role for neutrophils in the clearance of UTI was confirmed by Miller and co-workers (1987) who showed that treatment of rats with anti-neutrophil serum led to a 1000-fold increase in bacterial numbers in infected kidneys.

Macrophages make up only a small proportion of the total cellular infiltrate during UTI. Evidence from rat UTI models have shown that depletion of macrophages with silica and carrageenan had little effect on the clearance of acute or chronic pyelonephritis (Miller *et al.*, 1987). This conclusion was also supported by studies in A/J mice which, despite a deficient macrophage function, were as able to clear acute kidney infection as their normal counterparts (Svanborg-Edén *et al.*, 1984).

V. Specific Immunity in Urinary Tract Infection

A. Cell-Mediated Immunity

The normal urinary tract mucosa contains few T cells. $CD8^+$ T cells are sparsely scattered within the uroepithelium while $CD8^+$ and to a lesser extent $CD4^+$ T cells are present in the submucosa/lamina propria (Gardiner *et al.*, 1986; Christmas, 1994). γδ T cells have not been found in bladder, renal, ureter, and urethra biopsies from healthy individuals (Vroom *et al.*, 1991; Christmas, 1994).

Early studies by Smith and co-workers (1975) demonstrated the presence of T cells in the cellular infiltrate in experimental pyelonephritis in rabbits. T cells, primarily of the T-helper phenotype, are also found in pyelonephritic lesions. In patients with bacterial cystitis, the uroepithelium and submucosa are infiltrated predominantly with $CD4^+$ T cells while γδ T cells were detected only occasionally in sections (Christmas, 1994). In a rat model of ascending acute pyelonephritis, Kurnick and co-workers (1988) observed a predominant mononuclear cell influx in the kidney interstitium 4, 8, 15, 21, and 25 days after bacterial inoculation. Most of these cells were $CD4^+$ T cells with a small proportion of $CD8^+$ cells. The cell infiltrate contained T cells specific for the infecting strain. T-cell expansion in response to *E. coli* was MHC restricted and was greater to non-P-fimbriated than P-fimbriated *E. coli*.

Studies examining the role of cell-mediated immunity in UTI have compared the ability of athymic animals with their normal counterparts to clear experimental infection. In an acute UTI model in mice, Swiss (nu/nu) and BALB/c (nu/nu) mice showed similar resistance to intravesical infection as their normal counterparts (Svanborg-Edén *et al.*, 1984). Similarly, in chronic UTI models using T-cell-depleted and athymic rats, absence of thymus-dependent T cells did not influence the course of infection or the development of pyelonephritic lesions (Coles *et al.*, 1974; Miller *et al.*, 1986). The lack of T-cell involvement in these models was recently brought into question when Bandeira and co-workers (1991) found the majority of murine intraepithelial lymphocytes (IEL) to be T cells of extrathymic origin. Congenitally athymic nude mice, however, have far fewer extrathymically derived IELs than normal mice (Lin *et al.*, 1993). The role of T cells of extrathymic origin for the clearance of infection in normal animals needs further study.

B. Humoral Immunity

1. *Serum Antibody Response to UTI*

Specific antibodies to *E. coli* antigens are found in the circulation of most individuals; however, levels increase during episodes of acute UTI (Winberg *et al.*, 1963; Vosti *et al.*, 1965; Andersen, 1966; Holmgren and Smith, 1975). The serum antibody response to UTI is dominated by IgM and IgG antibodies (Winberg *et al.*, 1963). *E. coli*-induced pyelonephritis stimulates a specific serum antibody response to the O and in a few cases the K antigen of the infecting strain (Kaijser *et al.*, 1977b, 1983). Anti-lipid A antibodies of the IgG class are elevated in girls with acute pyelonephritis, acute cystitis, and asymptomatic bacteriuria (Mattsby-Baltzer *et al.*, 1981). Antibodies directed against *E. coli* fimbriae are also detected in the serum of patients with UTI (Svanborg-Edén *et al.*, 1982a). Antibodies to type 1 fimbriae are found in the serum of patients with cystitis and acute pyelonephritis (Rene *et al.*, 1982; Rene and Silverblatt, 1982). More recently specific serum antibodies to P fimbriae were shown to be produced in patients suffering from pyelonephritis with P-fimbriated *E. coli* (De Ree and van den Bosch, 1987). Anti-P fimbrial antibodies were not detected in the serum of healthy controls. These antibodies appeared to be directed against the major P fimbrial subunit and not the minor adhesin component since they were unable to inhibit mannose resistant hemagglutination. It is unclear to what extent the G adhesin is immunogenic and can give rise to antibodies that block bacterial interactions with the cell surface receptors.

2. *Urine Antibody Response to UTI*

Immunoglobulins and their fragments constitute a portion of the protein excreted daily into the urine of most individuals (Hanson and Tan, 1965; Bienenstock and Tomasi, 1968). These molecules have little specific activity against the bacterial pathogens that cause UTI, and are therefore unlikely to contribute to the early defense against invading pathogens. Once established, however, infections of the urinary tract elicit a specific urinary antibody response. A primary antibody response occurs within 7–10 days of diagnosis in children with their first episode of acute pyelonephritis (Jodal *et al.*, 1974; Sohl-Åkelund *et al.*, 1979). The antibodies are primarily of the S-IgA type suggesting a mucosal origin of these antibodies but levels of monomeric IgA and IgG also increase in urine during UTI (Hanson *et al.*, 1977; Svanborg-Edén *et al.*, 1985).

The sites of antibody production within the urinary tract have been examined. The kidney is considered a major site of IgA production, since higher antibody responses occur in patients with acute pyelonephritis than in cystitis (Hanson *et al.*, 1977). Morphologic studies comparing IgA B lymphocyte populations in different parts of the urinary tract are, however, not available. The bladder mucosa and lower urinary tract can clearly produce S-IgA (Burdon, 1970, 1971). The "bladder sweat" collected from anephric patients was shown to contain such immunoglobulins (Bienenstock and Tomasi, 1968; Feldman *et al.*, 1971). Furthermore, antigenic challenge in the lower urinary tract was shown to induce a significant local immune response (Burdon, 1970). Recently, Christmas (1994) observed significantly higher levels of IgA producing plasma cells in the urothelium and submucosa of patients with bacterial cystitis compared to healthy controls, confirming the presence of these cells at the mucosa during infection.

The urinary antibodies are directed against a variety of bacterial surface antigens. The most extensive studies have been performed using different LPS preparations. Antibodies to the O polysaccharide are commonly detected (Winberg *et al.*, 1963; Holmgren *et al.*, 1968; Neter, 1975; Sohl-Åkelund *et al.*, 1979). These antibodies are specific for each O antigen type, and have been suggested to exert a selective force against reinfection with strains of the same serotype in patients with recurrent UTI (Bergström *et al.*, 1967; Andersen, 1968; Neter, 1975). Antibodies to "common antigen" epitopes in the LPS core structure, with broad cross-reactivity against most *E. coli* strains have also been detected (Kunin, 1987). Antibodies to lipid A [I. Mattsby-Baltzer, (1980) unpublished observation] and the capsular antigens (Kaijser *et al.*, 1977) occur, but do not appear to be a common finding in the urine of patients with UTI. Urinary antibodies directed against type 1 and P fimbriae have been described in children (Svanborg-Edén *et al.*, 1982a).

3. *Role of Antibodies in Protection Against Infection*

Despite numerous studies reporting specific antibody responses to UTI, their contribution to the resistance of infection is not well understood. IgA antibodies isolated from the urine of patients with acute pyelonephritis have been shown to block the adherence of *E. coli* to urinary tract epithelial cells *in vitro* (Svanborg-Edén and Svennerholm, 1978). Whether IgA antibodies have a similar role during UTI remains to be shown. Circumstantial evidence for a role of humoral immunity has come from vaccination studies in experimental animal models. Vaccine preparations of whole bacterial and isolated bacterial components such as LPS, capsular polysaccharide, and fimbriae induce protection to subsequent challenge with strains carrying the vaccine antigen (Kaijser *et al.*, 1978; Kaijser and Olling, 1973; Brooks *et al.*, 1974; Mattsby-Baltzer *et al.*, 1982; O'Hanley *et al.*, 1985; Pecha *et al.*, 1989). Although these studies infer a role of specific immunity in protection from subsequent infection, it remains unclear to what extent specific antibodies are involved.

Passive immunization studies suggest that specific antibodies at sufficiently high serum titers can influence the course of infection. Intraperitoneal injection of pooled ascites fluid containing monoclonal antibodies directed to *E. coli* K13 gave slight protection from intravesical challenge with *E. coli* O6:K13:H1 in rats (Kaijser *et al.*, 1983). Anti-P fimbrial antibodies protected mice from experimental infection (Silverblatt and Cohen, 1979; Svanborg-Edén *et al.*, 1983). In contrast, immunization with antisera to lipid A antibody had no effect on the outcome of infection in rats (Mattsby-Baltzer *et al.*, 1982). In all of these studies, high-serum antibody titers were required for maximum protection.

The role of humoral immunity in protection of UTI remains controversial for a number of reasons. First, levels of specific circulating and local antibodies in individual mice after exposure to antigen show no correlation with outcome of infection (Hagberg *et al.*, 1984b). Second, in human infections bacteria often persist despite the presence of high titers of type-specific antibody (Vosti *et al.*, 1965). Third, CBA/N (*xid;* B-lymphocyte subsest deficient) mice are equally adept at clearing experimental UTI as their normal counterparts (Svanborg-Edén *et al.*, 1984). Fourth, the frequency of UTI is not increased in patients with antibody deficiencies such as hypogammaglobulinemia.

VI. Prevention of Urinary Tract Infection

A. Receptor Analogs

The fimbriae-mediated attachment to epithelial cells can be blocked by the addition of soluble receptors. The binding of type 1 fimbriae is inhibited by mannose and different structural variants of mannosylated oligosaccharides (Firon *et al.*, 1982, 1983). Aronson and coworkers (1979) successfully used mannose to inhibit experimental UTI due to type 1-fimbriated *E. coli.*

The attachment of P fimbriated *E. coli* to epithelial cells is inhibited by Galα1-4Galβ-containing oligosaccharides (Leffler and Svanborg-Edén, 1980). Synthetic derivatives of Galα1-4Galβ containing oligosaccharides with even higher inhibitory activity have been made (Kihlberg *et al.*, 1988). Addition of globotetraose to a P-fimbriated bacterial inoculum reduced the recovery of P fimbriated *E. coli* in an acute UTI mouse model (Svanborg-Edén *et al.*, 1982b). It remains to be seen whether globotetraose given to animals intravesically or orally effects the outcome of an ongoing infection with P-fimbriated *E. coli*.

Cranberry juice has long been recommended in the treatment and prevention of UTI; however, data supporting its efficacy have been conflicting. A recent report confirmed the benefits of this treatment in elderly women suffering from recurrent infections (Avon *et al.*, 1994). Its mechanism of action is not known; however, cranberry juice and the urine of mice fed cranberry juice prevented *E. coli* adhesion to uroepithelial cells (Sobota, 1984; Schmidt and Sobota, 1988). Zafriri and colleagues (1989) suggested that activity was due to the presence of fructose and a nondialyzable polymeric compound that inhibited type 1- and P-fimbriated adherence, respectively.

B. Vaccination in Acute UTI

The early observation that vaccination with heat or formalin-killed *E. coli* induced high levels of antibody in rats and prevented retrograde pyelonephritis (Brooks *et al.*, 1974) has led to hopes of vaccine development for UTI. Immunization of experimental animals with whole bacteria gave O type-specific protection (Kaijser *et al.*, 1978). The large variation in O antigens coupled with the risk for adverse reactions upon immunization with antigens containing endotoxin led to trials with other *E. coli* antigens. The capsular or K antigens are fewer in number and elicit greater protection in experimental models than O antigens (Kaijser and Ahlstedt, 1977a). Unfortunately, K antigens are poor immunogens in man (Hanson *et al.*, 1977). Immunization with purified P fimbriae was shown to protect mice and monkeys against experimental pyelonephritis with homologous and heterologous P-fimbriated *E. coli* (Roberts *et al.*, 1984; O'Hanley *et al.*, 1985; Pecha *et al.*, 1989).

The design of a UTI vaccine is complicated by the antigenic variability of uropathogenic *E. coli*. Surveys of patient populations with UTI show that considerable differences exist between the antigenic properties of strains causing first time and recurrent episodes of acute pyelonephritis and between strains from patients with and without underlying defects of their host defenses against UTI (Bergström *et al.*, 1967; Lomberg *et al.*, 1983, 1984). Sporadic episodes of uncomplicated acute pyelonephritis are caused by a selected group of virulent *E. coli*, 90% of which are P fimbriated. Treatment with receptor analogs or vaccination with the P fimbriae of *E. coli* would therefore be predicted to work in children and adults with sporadic episodes of acute pyelonephritis.

C. Vaccination in Recurrent UTI

Recurrent episodes of acute pyelonephritis are caused by a more diverse array of bacteria than the acute infections. Strains causing recurrent acute cystitis or acute pyelonephritis with renal scarring (where arguably vaccination is most needed) express a diverse range of O and K antigens. In addition, only 40% and 29% are P-fimbriated, respectively (Lomberg *et al.*, 1983, 1984, 1986a, 1989). The antigenic diversity of the strains that cause UTI makes it difficult to define a protective antigen or a set of antigens that will give protection in these patient groups. During the 1960s there was extensive activity to try to identify the "common antigen," shared by acute and recurrent bacteriuria strains, that could be used to generate a broadly cross-reactive immune response to protect the urinary tract. This line of work has not yet had practical applications. Prevention of recurrent infection is therefore likely to require approaches other than vaccination. Two such approaches are briefly discussed below.

1. Deliberate Colonization of the Urinary Tract with Nonvirulent Bacteria

Asymtomatic bacteriuria (ABU) in childhood is commonly left untreated (Lindberg *et al.*, 1978). It has been noted that the frequency of symtomatic "break through" recurrences of UTI is lower in those with ABU than in a treated group (Hansson *et al.*, 1989). Furthermore the asymtomatic carrier state did not jeopardize the health of the child or renal development. This led to the assumption that ABU was protecting the urinary tract, by competitive exclusion of more virulent bacterial strains. The use of avirulent bacteria to establish a state of artificial ABU has therefore been discussed as an approach to the prevention of infection in patients suffering recurrent urinary tract infection where other treatments are not successful. Initially, patients were colonized with a strain from their own intestinal flora, devoid of virulence factors (Hagberg *et al.*, 1986). Subsequently, a strain for more general use was selected. This strain lacked the known virulence factors associated with pyelonephritic strains and did not attach to the urinary tract epithelium. Still this *E. coli* strain was able to persist in the bladders of patients for long periods of time without causing adverse effects. So far, patients carrying this strain have not contracted symptomatic UTI with other uropathogens (Anderson *et al.*, 1991) [H. Connell, (1996) personal communication].

2. *Mucosal Inflammation*

Studies examining host defense in the urinary tract have highlighted the importance of mucosal inflammation as opposed to specific immunity. While further investigation concerning the processes involved in the mucosal inflammatory response is required, identifying the inflammatory parameters involved in clearance may help us to design new ways of boosting immunity in susceptible individuals.

Acknowledgments

These studies were supported by: The Medical Faculty, Lund University; the Swedish Medical Research Council (Grants 7934, 9823); the Österlund and Crafoord foundations; and the Royal Physiographic Society. W.A. is supported by a Swedish Medical Research Council Scholarship.

References

Agace, W., Hedges, S., and Svanborg, C. (1992). Lps genotype in the C57 black mouse background and its influence on the interleukin-6 response *to E. coli* urinary tract infection. *Scand. J. Immunol.* **35**, 531–538.

Agace, W., Hedges, S., Andersson, U., Andersson, J., Ceska, M., and Svanborg, C. (1993a). Selective cytokine production by epithelial cells following exposure to *Escherichia coli. Infect. Immun.* **61**, 602–609.

Agace, W., Hedges, S., Ceska, M., and Svanborg, C. (1993b). IL-8 and the neutrophil response to mucosal Gram negative infection. *J. Clin. Invest.* **92**, 780–785.

Agace, W., Patarroyo, M., Svensson, M., Carlemalm, E., and Svanborg, C. (1995a). *Escherichia coli* induce transuroepithelial neutrophil migration by an ICAM-1 dependant mechanism. *Infect. Immun.* **63**, 4054–4062.

Agace, W., Godaly, G., Ceska, S., and Svanborg, C. (1996). *Escherichia coli* induced trans-uroepithelial migration is IL-8 dependent. In preparation.

Andersen, H. (1966). Studies of urinary tract infections in infancy and childhood. VII. The relation of *E. coli* antibody in pyelonephritis as measured by homologous and common (Kunin) antigens. *J. Pediatr.* **68**, 542–550.

Andersen, H. (1968). Clinical studies in the antibody response to *E. coli* O antigens in infants and children with urinary tract infection, using a passive haemagglutination technique. *Acta Paediatr. Scand. Suppl.*, **180**, 8–28.

Anderson, P., Engberg, I., Lidin-Janson, G., Lincoln, K., Hull, R., Hull, S., and Svanborg-Edén, C. (1991). Persistence of *Escherichia coli* bacteriuria not determined by bacterial adherence. *Infect. Immun.* **59**, 2915–2921.

Aronson, M., Medalia, O., Schori, L., Mirelman, D., Sharon, N., and Ofek, I. (1979). Prevention of colonization of the urinary tract of mice with *Escherichia coli* by blocking of bacterial adherence with methyl alpha-D-mannopyranoside. *J. Infect. Dis.* **139**, 329–332.

Asscher, A. W., Sussman, M., Waters, W., Harvard Davis, R., and Chick, S. (1966). Urine as a medium for bacterial growth. *Lancet* **2**, 1037–1041.

Avon, J., Monane, M., Gurwitz, J., Glynn, R., Choodnovkiy, I., and Lipsitz, L. (1994). Reduction of Bacteriuria and Pyuria after ingestion of cranberry juice. *JAMA, J. Am. Med. Assoc.* **271**, 751–754.

Baggiolini, M., Dewald, B., and Moser, B. (1994). Interleukin-8 and related chemotactic cytokines-CXC and CC chemokines. *Adv. Immunol.* **55**, 97–179.

Bandiera, A., Itohara, S., Bonneville, M., Burlen-Derranoux, O., Mota-Santos, T., Coutinho, A., and Tonegawa, S. (1991). Extrathymic origin of intestinal intraepithelial lymphocytes bearing T-cell antigen receptor $\gamma\delta$. *Proc. Natl. Acad. Sci. U.S.A.* **88**, 43–47.

Benson, M., Andreasson, A., Jodal, U., Karlsson, Å., Rydberg, J., and Svanborg, C. (1994). Interleukin 6 in childhood urinary tract infection. *Pediatr. Infect. Dis. J.* **13**, 612–616.

Bergström, T., Lincoln, K., Ørskov, F., Ørskov, I., and Winberg, J. (1967). Studies of urinary tract infections in infancy and childhood. VIII. Reinfection vs. relapse in recurrent urinary tract infection. Evaluation by means of identification of infecting organisms. *J. Pediatr.* **71**, 13–20.

Bettelheim, K. A., and Taylor, J. (1969). A study of *Escherichia coli* isolated from chronic urinary tract infection. *J. Med. Microbiol.* **2**, 225–236.

Bienenstock, J., and Tomasi, T. (1968). S-IgA in normal urine. *J. Clin. Invest.* **47**, 1162–1167.

Blackwell, C., Jonsdottir, K., Hanson, M., Todd, W., Chaudhuri, A., Mathew, B., Bettle, R., and Weir, D. (1986a). Non-secretion of ABO blood group antigens predisposing to infection by *Neisseria meningitidis* and *Streptococcus pneumoniae. Lancet* **2**, 284–285.

Blackwell, C., Jonsdottir, K., Hanson, M., and Weir, D. (1986b). Non-secretion of ABO blood group antigens predisposing to infection by *Haemophilus influenzae. Lancet* **2**, 687.

Blackwell, C., Thom, S., Lawrie, O., Weir, D., Wray, D., and Kinane, D. (1986c). Non-secretion of blood group antigens and susceptibility to oral infections by *Candida albicans. J. Dent. Res.* **64**, 502.

Boman, H. (1991). Antibacterial peptides: Key components needed in immunity. *Cell (Cambridge, Mass.)* **65**, 205–207.

Breimer, M. E., Hansson, G. C., and Leffler, H. (1985). The specific glycosphingolipid composition of human urethral epithelial cells. *J. Biochem. (Tokyo)* **98**, 1169–1180.

Brooks, S., Lyons, J., and Braude, A. (1974). Immunization against retrograde pyelonephritis. *Am. J. Pathol.* **74**, 345–354.

Burdon, D. (1970). Quantitative studies of urinary immunoglobulins in hospital patients including patients with urinary tract infection. *Clin. Exp. Immunol.* **6**, 189–196.

Burdon, D. (1971). Immunoglobulins of normal human urine and urethral secretions. *Immunology* **21**, 363–368.

Christmas, T. (1994). Lymphocyte populations in the bladder wall in normal bladder, bacterial cystitis and interstitial cystitis. *Br. J. Urol.* **73**, 508–515.

Coles, G., Chick, S., Hopkins, M., Ling, R., and Radford, N. (1974). The role of the T-cell in experimental pyelonephritis. *Clin. Exp Immunol.* **16,** 629–636.

Connell, H., Wilson, I., Sabharwal, H., Persson, L., Kockum, I., Zasloff, M., and Svanborg, C. (1996). Determinants of *Escherichia coli* growth in human urine. *Chemotherapy* in press.

Cox, C., and Hinman, F. (1961). Experiments with induced bacteriuria, vesical emptying and bacterial growth on the mechanism of bladder defense to infection. *J. Urol.* **86,** 739–748.

de Man, P., van Kooten, C., Aarden, L., Engberg, I., Linder, H., and Svanborg Eden, C. (1989). Interleukin-6 induced at mucosal surfaces by gram-negative bacterial infection. *Infect. Immun.* **57,** 3383–3388.

De Ree, J., and van den Bosch, J. (1987). Serological response to the P fimbriae of uropathogenic *Escherichia coli* in pyelonephritis. *Infect. Immun.* **55,** 2204–2207.

Eisenhauer, P., Harwig, S., and Lehrer, R. (1992). Cryptdins: Antibacterial defensins of the murine small intestine. *Infect. Immun.* **60,** 3556–3565.

Feldman, B., Hedman, R., and Hong, R. (1971). Local immunomechanisms of the urinary tract. *Invest. Urol.* **8,** 575–582.

Firon, N., Ofek, I., and Sharon, N. (1982). Interaction of mannose-containing oligosaccharides with the fimbrial lectin of *Escherichia coli. Biochem. Biophys. Res. Commun.* **105,** 1426–1432.

Firon, N., Ofek, I., and Sharon, N. (1983). Carbohydrate specificity of the surface lectins of *Escherichia coli, Klebsiella pneumoniae,* and *Salmonella typhimurium. Biochem. Biophys. Res. Commun.* **105,** 1426–1432.

Fletcher, A., Neuberger, A., and Ratcliffe, A. (1970a). Tamm–Horsfall urinary glycoprotein: The chemical composition. *Biochem. J.* **120,** 417–424.

Fletcher, A., Neuberger, A., and Ratcliffe, W. (1970b). Tamm–Horsfall urinary glycoprotein: The subunit structure. *Biochem. J.* **120,** 425–432.

Fowler, J., and Stamey, E. (1977). Studies of introital colonization in women with recurrent urinary tract infection. VII. The role of bacterial adherence. *J. Urol.* **117,** 472.

Gardiner, R., Seymour, G., Lavin, M., Strutton, M. G., Gemmell, E., and Hazan, G. (1986). Immunohistochemical analysis of the human bladder. *Br. J. Urol.* **58,** 19–25.

Gordon, D., and Riley, M. (1992). A theoretical and experimental analysis of bacterial growth in the bladder. *Mol. Microbiol.* **6,** 555–562.

Grüneberg, R. (1969). Relationship of infecting urinary organisms to the faecal flora in patients with symptomatic urinary infections. *Lancet* **2,** 766–768.

Hagberg, L., Hull, R., Hull, S., McGhee, J. R., Michalek, S. M., and Svanborg-Edén, C. (1984a). Difference in susceptibility to gram-negative urinary tract infection between C3H/HeJ. and C3H/HeN mice. *Infect. Immun.* **46,** 839–844.

Hagberg, L., Leffler, H., and Svanborg-Edén, C. (1984b). Non-antibiotic prevention of urinary tract infection. *Infection* **12,** 132–137.

Hagberg, L., Bruce, A., Reid, G., Svanorg-Edén, C., Lincoln, K., and Lidin-Janson, G. (1986). Colonization of the urinary tract with bacteria from the normal fecal and urethral flora in patients with recurrent urinary tract infections. *In* "Host–Parasite Interactions in Urinary Tract Infections" (E. Cass and C. Svanborg-Edén, eds.), pp. 194–297. Univ. Chicago Press, Chicago.

Hanson, L., and Tan, E. (1965). Characterization of antibodies in human urine. *J. Clin. Invest.* **44,** 703–715.

Hanson, L., Ahlstedt, S., Fasth, A., Jodal, U., Kaijser, B., Larsson, P., Lindberg, U., Olling, S., Sohl-Åkerlund, A., and Svanborg-Edén, C. (1977). Antigens of *Escherichia coli,* human immune response and the pathogenesis of urinary tract infections. *J. Infect. Dis.* **135,** 144–149.

Hansson, S., Caugant, D., Jodal, U., and Svanborg-Edén, C. (1989). Untreated asymptomatic bacteriuria in girls: I-stability of urinary isolates. *Br. Med. J.* **298,** 853–855.

Hedges, S., de Man, P., Linder, H., van Kooten, C., and Svanborg-Edén, C. (1990). Interleukin-6 is secreted by epithelial cells in response to Gram-negative bacterial challenge. *In* "Advances in Mucosal Immunology. International Conference of Mucosal Immunity" (T. Macdonald, ed.), pp. 144–148. Kluwer, London.

Hedges, S., Anderson, P., Lidin-Janson, G., de Man, P., and Svanborg, C. (1991). Interleukin-6 response to deliberate colonization of the human urinary tract with gram-negative bacteria. *Infect. Immun.* **59,** 421–427.

Hedges, S., Stenquist, K., Lidin-Janson, G., Martinell, J., Sandberg, T., and Svanborg, C. (1992a). Comparison of urine and serum concentrations of interleukin-6 in women with acute pyelonephritis or asymptomatic bacteriuria. *J. Infect. Dis.* **166,** 653–656.

Hedges, S., Svensson, M., and Svanborg, C. (1992b). Interleukin-6 response of epithelial cell lines to bacterial stimulation *in vitro. Infect. Immun.* **60,** 1295–1301.

Hedges, S., Agace, W, Svensson, M., Sjögren, A.-C., Ceska, M., and Svanborg, C. (1994). Uropithelial cells are a part of a mucosal cytokine network. *Infect. Immun.* **62,** 2315–2321.

Hedges, S., Agace, W., and Svanborg, C. (1995). Epithelial cytokine responses and mucosal cytokine networks. *Trends Microbiol.* **3,** 266–270.

Hedges, S., Bjarnadottir, M., Agace, W., and Svanborg, C. (1996). Interleukin-4 and gamma interferon modify the epithelial cell cytokine response to Gram-negative bacteria. *Cytokine.* In press.

Hedlund, M., Svensson, M., Nilsson, Å., Duan, R., and Svanborg, C. (1996). Role of the ceramide signalling pathway in cytokine responses to P fimbriated *Escherichia coli. J. Exp. Med.* **183,** 1–8.

Holmgren, J., Eggertsen, G., Hanson, L., Jodal, U., Lincoln, K., and Winberg, J. (1968). The antibody response of children with pyelonephritis to different antigens of *E. coli. Acta Pathol. Microbiol. Scand.* **72,** 457.

Holmgren, J., and Smith, J. (1975). Immunological aspects of urinary tract infection. *Prog. Allergy* **18,** 289–352.

Hull, R. A., Gill, R. E., Hsu, P., Minshew, B. H., and Falkow, S. (1981). Construction and expression of recombinant plasmids encoding type 1 or D-mannose resistant pili from the urinary tract infection *Escherichia coli* isolate. *Infect. Immun.* **33,** 933–938.

Jodal, U., Ahlstedt, S., Carlsson, B., Hanson, L. A., Lindberg, U., and Sohl, A. (1974). Local antibodies in childhood urinary tract infection: A preliminary study. *Int. Arch. Allergy Appl. Immunol.* **47,** 537–46.

Johanson, I., Lindstedt, R., and Svanborg, C. (1992). The role of the *pap* and *prs* encoded adhesins in *Escherichia coli* adherence to human epithelial cells. *Infect. Immun.* **60,** 3416–3422.

Johnson, J. (1991). Virulence factors in *Escherichia coli* urinary tract infection. *Clin. Microbial Rev.* **4,** 80–128.

Kaijser, B., and Olling, S. (1973). Experimental hemotagous pyelonephritis due to *Escherichia coli* in rabbits. The antibody response and its protective capacity. *J. Infect. Dis.* **128,** 41–49.

Kaijser, B., and Ahlstedt, S. (1977). Protective capacity of antibodies against *Escherichia coli* O and K antigens. *Infect. Immun.* **17,** 286–289.

Kaijser, B., Hanson, L. A., Jodal, U., Lidin, J. G., and Robbins, J. B. (1977). Frequency of *Escherichia coli* K antigens in urinary-tract infections in children. *Lancet* **1,** 663–666.

Kaijser, B., Larsson, P., and Olling, S. (1978). Protection against ascending *Escherichia coli* pyelonephritis in rats and significance of local immunity. *Infect. Immun.* **20,** 78–81.

Kaijser, B., Larsson, P., Nimmick, W., and Söderström, T. (1983). Antibodies to *Escherichia coli* K and O antigens in protection against acute pyelonephritis. *Prog. Allergy* **33,** 275–288.

Källenius, G., and Winberg, J. (1978). Bacterial adherence to periurethral epithelial cells in girls prone to urinary tract infection. *Lancet* **2,** 540–542.

Källenius, G., Möllby, R., Svensson, S. B., Winberg, J., Lundblad, S., Svensson, S., and Cedergren, B. (1980). The Pk antigen as a receptor for the hemaglutination of pyelonephritogenic *E. coli. FEMS Microbiol. Lett.* **7,** 297–302.

Kaye, D. (1968). Antibacterial activity of human urine. *J. Clin. Invest.* **47,** 2374–2390.

Kihlberg, J., Freijd, T., Janson, K., Sundin, A., and Magnusson, L. (1988). Synthetic receptor analogues: Preparation and calculated conformations of the 2-deoxy-6-Me, 6-deoxy, and 6-deoxy-6 flow dericatives of methyl-4-O-α-D-galactopyranosyl-β-D-galactopyranoside (methyl-β-D-galabioside). *Carbohydr. Res.* **176,** 271–286.

Kinane, E., Blackwell, C., Brettle, R., Weir, D., Winstanley, F., and Elton, R. (1982). ABO blood group, secretor state and susceptibility to recurrent urinary tract infection in women. *Br. Med. J.* **285,** 7–9.

Ko, Y. C., Mukaida, N., Ishiyama, S., Tokue, A., Kawai, T., Matsushima, K., and Kasahara, T. (1993). Elevated interleukin-8 levels in the urine of patients with urinary tract infections. *Infect. Immun.* **61,** 1307–1314.

Korhonen, T., Väisänen, V., Saxen, H., Hultberg, H., and Svenson, S. (1986). Binding of *Escherichia coli* S fimbriae to human kidney epithelium. *Infect. Immun.* **37,** 286–291.

Kunin, C. (1987). "Detection, Prevention and Management of Urinary Tract Infections." Lea & Febiger, Philadelphia, Pennsylvania.

Kurnick, J., McCluskey, R., Bhan, A., Wright, K., Wilkinson, R., and Rubin, H. (1988). *Escherichia coli*-specific T lymphocytes in experimental pyelonephritis. *J. Immunol.* **141,** 3220–3226.

Lee, J.-Y., Boman, A., Chuanxin, S., Andersson, M., Jörnvall, H., Mutt, V., and Boman, H. (1989). Antibacterial peptides from pig intestine: Isolation of a mammalian cecropin. *Proc. Natl. Acad. Sci. U.S.A.* **86,** 9159–9162.

Leffler, H., and Svanborg-Edén, C. (1980). Chemical identification of a glycosphingolipid receptor for *Escherichia coli* attaching to human urinary tract epithelial cells and agglutinating human erythrocytes. *FEMS Microbiol. Lett.* **8,** 127–134.

Leffler, H., and Svanborg-Edén, C. (1981). Glycolipid receptors for uropathogenic *Escherichia coli* on human erythrocytes and uroepithelial cells. *Infect. Immun.* **34,** 920–929.

Lidin-Janson, G., Hanson, L., and Kaijser, B. (1977). Comparison of *Escherichia coli* from bacteriuric patients with those from feces of healthy school children. *J. Infect. Dis.* **136,** 346–353.

Lin, T., Matsuzaki, G., Nakamura, T., and Nomoto, K. (1993). Thymus influences the development of extrathymically derived intestinal intraepithelial lymphocytes. *Eur. J. Immunol.* **23,** 1968–1974.

Lindberg, F., Lund, B., and Normark, S. (1984). Genes of pyelonephrithogenic *Escherichia coli* required for digalactoside specific agglutination of human cells. *EMBO J.* **3,** 1167–1173.

Lindberg, U., Claesson, I., Hanson, L. A., and Jodal, U. (1978). Asymptomatic bacteriuria in schoolgirls. VIII. Clinical course during a 3-year follow-up. *J. Pediatr.* **92,** 194–199.

Linder, H., Engberg, I., van, K. C., de, M. P., and Svanborg, E. C. (1990). Effects of anti-inflammatory agents on mucosal inflammation induced by infection with gram-negative bacteria. *Infect. Immun.* **58,** 2056–2060.

Lindstedt, R., Falk, P., Hull, R., Hull, S., Leffler, H., Svanborg, Edén, C., and Larson, G. (1989). Binding specificities of wild-type and cloned *Escherichia coli* strains that recognize globo-A. *Infect. Immun.* **57,** 3389–3394.

Lindstedt, R., Larson, G., Falk, P., Jodal, U., Leffler, H., and Svanborg, Edén. C. (1991). The receptor repetoire defines the host range for attaching *E. coli* recognizing globo-A. *Infect. Immun.* **59,** 1086–1092.

Lloyd, A., and Oppenheim, J. (1992). Poly's lament: The neglected role of the polymorphonuclear neutrophil in the afferent limb of the immune response. *Immunol. Today* **13,** 169–172.

Lomberg, H., Jodal, U., Svanborg-Edén, C., Leffler, H., and Samuelsson, B. (1981). P1 blood group and urinary tract infection. *Lancet* **1,** 551–552.

Lomberg, H., Hanson, L., Jacobsson, B., Jodal, U., Leffler, H., and Svanborg-Edén, C. (1983). Correlation of P blood group phenotype, vesicoureteral reflux and bacterial attachment in patients with recurrent pyelonephritis. *N. Engl. J. Med.* **308,** 1189–1192.

Lomberg, H., Hellström, M., Jodal, U., Leffler, H., Lincoln, K., and Svanborg-Edén, C. (1984). Virulence-associated traits in *Escherichia coli* causing first and recurrent episodes of urinary tract infection in children with or without vesicoureteral reflux. *J. Infect. Dis.* **150,** 561–569.

Lomberg, H., Hellström, M., Jodal, U., and Svanborg-Edén, C. (1986a). Renal scarring and non-attaching bacteria. *Lancet* **2,** 1341.

Lomberg, H., Cedergren, B., Leffler, H., Nilsson, B., Carlström, A.-S., and Svanborg-Edén, C. (1986b). Influence of blood group on the availability of receptors for attachment of uropathogenic *Escherichia coli*. *Infect. Immun.* **51**, 919–926.

Lomberg, H., Hellström, M., Jodal, U., Ørskov, I., and Svanborg, E. C. (1989). Properties of *Escherichia coli* in patients with renal scarring. *J. Infect. Dis.* **159**, 579–582.

Lund, B., Marklund, B. I., Str:omberg, N., Lindberg, F., Karlsson, K. A., and Normark, S. (1988). Uropathogenic *Escherichia coli* can express serologically identical pili of different receptor binding specificities. *Mol. Microbiol.* **2**, 255–263.

Marcus, D., Kundu, S., and Suguki, A. (1981). The P blood group system: Recent progress in immunochemistry and genetics. *Semin. Hematol.* **18**, 63–71.

Marklund, B. (1991). Structural and functional variation among Galα1-4Gal adhesins of uropathogenic *Escherichia coli*. PhD Thesis, University of Umeå, Umeå, Sweden.

Martins, S., Darlin, D., Lad, P., and Zimmern, P. (1994). Interleukin-1β: A clinically relevant urinary marker. *J. Urol.* **151**, 1198–1201.

Mattsby-Baltzer, I., Claësson, I., Hanson, L., Jodal, U., Kaijser, B., Lindberg, U., and Peterson, H. (1981). Antibodies to lipid A during urinary tract infection. *J. Infect. Dis.* **144**, 319–328.

Mattsby-Baltzer, I., Hanson, L., Kaijser, B., and Olling, S. (1982). Experimental *Escherichia coli* ascending pyelonephritis in rats: Active peroral immunization with live *E. coli* O6K13H1 and passively transferred anti-lipid A antibodies. *Infect. Immun.* **35**, 647–653.

Meylan, P., and Glauser, M. (1989). Role of complement derived and bacterial formylpeptide chemotactic factors in the *in vivo* migration of neutrophils in experimental *Escherichia coli* pyelonephritis in rats. *J. Infect. Dis.* **5**, 959–965.

Miller, T., Findon, G., and Cawley, S. (1986). Cellular basis of host defence in pyelonephritis. I. Chronic infection. *Br. J. Exp. Pathol.* **67**, 12–23.

Miller, T., Findon, G., and Cawley, S. (1987). Cellular basis of host defence in pyelonephritis. III. Deletion of individual components. *Br. J. Exp. Pathol.* **68**, 377–388.

Neter, E. (1975). Estimation of *E. coli* antibodies in urinary tract infection. *Kidney Int.* **4**, 523–527.

Norden, C., Green, G., and Kass, E. (1968). Antibacterial mechanisms of the urinary bladder. *J. Clin. Invest.* **47**, 2689–2700.

O'Grady, F., and Pennington, J. (1966). Bacterial growth in an *in vitro* system simulating conditions in the urinary bladder. *Br. J. Exp. Pathol.* **47**, 283–290.

O'Hanley, P., Lark, P., Falkow, S., and Schoolnik, G. (1985). Molecular basis of *Escherichia coli* colonization of the upper urinary tract in BALB/c mice. *J. Clin. Invest.* **75**, 347–360.

Ørskov, F., Ørskov, I., Jann, B., and Jann, K. (1980). Tamm–Horsfall protein or uromucoid is the normal urinary slime that traps type 1 fimbriated *Escherichia coli*. *Lancet* **1**, 887.

Parkkinen, J., Virkola, R., and Korhonen, T. (1988). Identification of factors in urine that inhibit the binding of *Escherichia coli* adhesins. *Infect. Immun.* **56**, 2623–2629.

Pasteur, L. (1863). Exam du rôle attribué au gaz oxygène atmosphérique dans la destruction des matières animales et végétales après la mort. *C. R. Acad. Sci.* **56**, 734–740.

Pattersson-Delafield, J., Martinez, R., and Lehrer, R. (1980). Microbicidal cationic proteins in rabbit alveolar macrophages: A potential host defense mechanism. *Infect. Immun.* **30**, 180–192.

Pecha, B., Low, D., and O'Hanley, P. (1989). Gal-Gal pili vaccines prevent pyelonephritis by piliated *Escherichia coli* in a murine model. Single-component Gal-Gal pili vaccines prevent pyelonephritis by homologous and heterologous piliated *E. coli* strains. *J. Clin. Invest.* **83**, 2102–2108.

Plos, K., Connell, H., Jodal, U., Marklund, B.-I., Mårild, S., Wettergren, B., and Svanborg, C. (1995). Intestinal carriage of P fimbriated *Escherichia coli* and the susceptibility to urinary tract infection in young children. *J. Infect. Dis.* **171**, 625–631.

Pugin, J., Schürer, M. C., Leturcq, D., Moriarty, A., Ulevitch, R. J., and Tobias, P. S. (1993). Lipopolysaccharide activation of human endothelial and epithelial cells is mediated by lipopolysaccharide-binding protein and soluble CD14. *Proc. Natl. Acad. Sci. U.S.A.* **90**, 2744–2748.

Rene, P., and Silverblatt, F. (1982). Serological response to *Escherichia coli* pili in pyelonephritis. *Infect. Immun.* **37**, 749–754.

Rene, P., Dinolfo, M., and Silverblatt, F. (1982). Seum and urogenital antibody responses to *Escherichia coli* pili in cystitis. *Infect. Immun.* **38**, 542–547.

Roberts, J., Hardaway, B., Kaack, E., Fussell, E., and Baskin, G. (1984). Prevention of pyelonephritis by immunization with P-fimbriae. *J. Urol.* **131**, 602–607.

Schaeffer, A., Jones, J., and Dunn, J. (1981). Association of *in vitro Escherichia coli* adherence to vaginal and buccal epithelial cells with susceptibility of women to recurrent urinary tract infection. *N. Engl. J. Med.* **304**, 1062–1066.

Schmidt, D., and Sobota, A. (1988). An examination of the antiadherence activity of cranberry juice on urinary and non urinary bacterial isolates. *Microbios* **55**, 173–181.

Schulte-Wissermann, H., Mannhardt, W., Schwarz, J., Zepp, F., and Bitter-Sauermann, D. (1985). Comparison of the antibacterial effect of uroepithelial cells from healthy donors and children of asymptomatic bacteriuria. *Eur. J. Pediatr.* **144**, 230–233.

Senior, D., Baker, N., Cedergren, B., Falk, P., Larson, G., Lindstedt, R., and Svanborg-Edén, C. (1988). Globo-A—a new receptor specificity for attaching *Escherichia coli*. *FEBS Lett.* **237**, 123–127.

Shahin, R. D., Engberg, I., Hagberg, L., and Svanborg-Edén, C. (1987). Neutrophil recruitment and bacterial clearance correlated with LPS responsiveness in local gram-negative infection. *J. Immunol.* **138**, 3475–3480.

Sikri, K., Foster, C., Bloomfield, F., and Marshall, R. (1979). Locolization by immunofluorescence and by light- and electronmicroscopic immunoperoxidase techniques of Tamm–Horsfall glycoprotein in adult hamster kidney. *Biochem. J.* **181**, 525–532.

Silverblatt, F., and Cohen, L. (1979). Antipili antibody affords protection against experimental ascending pyelonephritis. *J. Clin. Invest.* **64**, 333–336.

Smith, J., Adkins, M., and McGreary, D. (1975). Local immune response in experimental pyelonephritis in the rabbit. *Immunology* **29**, 1067–1076.

Sobota, A. (1984). Inhibition of bacterial adherence by cranberry juice: Potential use for the treatment of urinary tract infections. *J. Urol.* **131**, 1013–1016.

Sohl-Åkelund, A., Ahlstedt, S., Hanson, L., and Jodal, U. (1979). Antibody responses in urine and serum against *Escherichia coli* O antigen in childhood urinary tract infection. *Acta Pathol. Microbiol. Scand. Sect. C* **87**, 29–36.

Stamey, T., Timothy, M., Miller, M., and Mihara, G. (1971). Recurrent urinary tract infections in adult women. The role of introital enterobacteria. *Calif. Med.* **115**, 1–19.

Stamey, T., and Sexton, C. (1975). The role of vaginal colonization with enterobacteriacea in recurrent urinary tract infections. *J. Urol.* **113**, 214–217.

Stapleton, A., Nudelman, E., Clausen, H., Hakomori, S., and Stamm, W. E. (1992). Binding of uropathogenic *Escherichia coli* R45 to glycolipids extracted from vaginal epithelial cells is dependent on histo-blood group secretor status. *J. Clin. Invest.* **90**, 965–972.

Strömberg, N., Marklund, B., Lund, B., Ilver, D., Hamers, A., Gaastra, W., Karlsson, K., and Normark, S. (1990). Host-specificity of uropathogenic *Escherichia coli* depends on differences in binding specificity to Galα-4Galβ-containing isoreceptors. *EMBO J.* **9**, 2001–2010.

Svanborg-Edén, C., and de Man, P. (1987). Bacterial virulence in urinary tract infection. *Infect. Dis. Clin. North Am.* **1**, 731–750.

Svanborg-Edén, C., and Svennerholm, A.-M. (1978). Secretory immunoglobulin A and G antibodies prevent adhesion of *Escherichia coli* to human urinary tract epithelial cells. *Infect. Immun.* **22**, 790–797.

Svanborg-Edén, C., and Jodal, U. (1979). Attachment of *Escherichia coli* to urinary sediment cells from urinary tract infection prone and healthy children. *Infect. Immun.* **26**, 837–840.

Svanborg-Edén, C., Fasth, A., Hagberg, L., Hanson, L., Korhonen, T., and Leffler, H. (1981). Host interaction with *Escherichia coli* in the urinary tract. *In* "Bacterial Vaccines" (J. Robbins, J. Hill, and J. Sadoff, eds.), Vol. 4, pp. 113–133. Theime-Stratton, New York.

Svanborg-Edén, C., Hanson, L., Jodal, U., Leffler, H., Mårild, S., Korhonen, T., Brinton, C., Jann, B., Jann, K., and Silverblatt, F. (1982a). Receptor analogues and antipili antibodies as inhibitors of attachment of uropathogenic *Escherichia coli*. *In* "Recent Advances in Mucosal Immunity" (W. Strober, L. Hanson and K. Sell, eds.), pp. 355–369. Raven, New York.

Svanborg-Edén, C., Freter, R., Hagberg, L., Hull, R., Hull, S., Leffler, H., and Schoolnik, G. (1982b). Inhibition of experimental ascending urinary tract infection by a receptor analogue. *Nature (London)* **298**, 560–562.

Svanborg-Edén, Andersson, B., Hagberg, L., Hanson, L. A., Leffler, H., Magnusson, G., Noori, G., Dahmen, J., and Söderström, T. (1983). Receptor analogues and anti-pili antibodies as inhibitors of bacterial attachment *in vivo* and *in vitro*. *Ann. N.Y. Acad. Sci.* **409**, 580–592.

Svanborg-Edén, C., Briles, D., Hagberg, L., McGhee, J., and Michalek, S. (1984). Genetic factors in host resistance to urinary tract infection. *Infection* **12**, 118–123.

Svanborg-Edén, Kulhavy, R., Mårild, S., Prince, S. J., and Mestecky, J. (1985). Urinary immunoglobulins in healthy individuals and children with acute pyelonephritis. *Scand. J. Immunol.* **21**, 305–313.

Svanborg-Edén, C., Hansson, S., Jodal, U., Lidin-Janson, G., Lincoln, K., Linder, H., Lomberg, H., de Man, P., Mårild, S., Martinell, J., Plos, K., Sandberg, T., and Stenquist, K. (1988). Host-parasite interaction in the urinary tract. *J. Infect. Dis.* **157**, 421–426.

Svanborg, C., Ørskov, F., and Ørskov, I. (1994). Fimbriae and disease. *In* "Bacterial Fimbriae" (P. Klemm, ed.), pp. 253–266. CRC Press, Boca Raton, Florida.

Svensson, M., Lindstedt, R., Radin, N., and Svanborg, C. (1994). Epithelial glucosphingolipid expression as a determinant of bacterial adherence and cytokine production. *Infect. Immun.* **62**, 4404–4410.

Toma, G., Bates, J., and Kumar, S. (1994). Uromodulin (Tamm–Horsfall protein) is a leucocyte adhesion molecule. *Biochem. Biophys. Res. Commun.* **200**, 275–282.

Vosti, K., Monto, A., and Rantz, L. (1965). Host–parasite interaction in patients with infections due to *Escherichia coli*. II. Serologic response of the host. *J. Lab. Clin. Med.* **66**, 612–626.

Vroom, T. M., Scholte, G., Ossendorp, F., and Borst, J. (1991). Tissue distribution of human γδ T cells: No evidence for general epithelial tropism. *J. Clin. Pathol.* **44**, 1012–1017.

Winberg, J., Anderson, H., Hanson, L., and Lincoln, K. (1963). Studies of urinary tract infection in infancy and childhood. I. Antibody response in different types of urinary tract infections caused by coliform bacteria. *Br. Med. J.* **2**, 524.

Winberg, J., Andersen, H., Bergström, T., Jacobsson, B., Larsson, H., and Lincoln, K. (1974). Epidemiology of symptomatic urinary tract infection in childhood. *Acta Pediatr. Scand. Suppl.* **252**, 1–20.

Wold, A. E., Mestecky, J., and Svanborg, E. C. (1988a). Agglutination of *Escherichia coli* by secretory IgA-a result of interaction between bacterial mannose-specific adhesins and immunoglobulin carbohydrate? *Monogr. Allergy* **24**, 307–309.

Wold, A. E., Thorssén, M., Hull, S., and Svanborg, C. (1988b). Attachment of *Escherichia coli* via mannose of Galα1-4Galβ containing receptors to human colonic epithelial cells. *Infect. Immun.* **56**, 2531–2537.

Wold, A., Mestecky, J., Tomana, M., Kobata, A., Ohbayashi, H., Endo, T., and Svanborg-Edén, C. (1990). Secretory immunoglobulin A carries oligosaccharide receptors for *Escherichia coli* Type 1 fimbrial lectin. *Infect. Immun.* **58**, 3073–3077.

Zafriri, D., Ofek, I., Adar, R., Pocino, M., and Sharon, N. (1989). Inhibitory activity of cranberry juice on adherence of type 1 and P fimbriated *Escherichia coli* to eukaryotic cells. *Antimicrob. Agents Chemother.* **33**, 92–98.

Zasloff, M. (1987). Maganins, a class of antimicrobial peptides from *Xenopus* skin: Isolation, characterization of two active forms, and partial cDNA sequence of a precursor. *Proc. Natl. Acad. Sci. U.S.A.* **84**, 5449–5453.

30

Mucosal Immunity in the Ocular System

PAUL C. MONTGOMERY
Department of Immunology and Microbiology
School of Medicine
Wayne State University
Detroit, Michigan 48201

JUDITH WHITTUM-HUDSON
The Wilmer Institute
School of Medicine
Johns Hopkins University
Baltimore, Maryland 21287

I. Introduction

Acquired immunity at the ocular surface is mediated primarily by the mucosal immune system. The linkage of ocular subcompartments to the mucosal immune network is now well established (Mestecky *et al.*, 1978; Montgomery *et al.*, 1983, 1985; Gregory and Allansmith, 1986). Since no vaccines currently use the mucosal immune system to specifically target ocular diseases, this chapter will review ocular mucosal immunobiology, examine approaches for inducing ocular mucosal immune responses, and identify target organisms for use in potential vaccination against selected ocular infections. Additional information on ocular mucosal immunity, including the impact of ocular infection on the structure and function of this system, is contained in an excellent review (Sullivan, 1994). It is important to note that other aspects of ocular immunobiology do not involve the mucosal immune system. Descriptions of anterior chamber-associated immune deviation and retinal immunology are provided in a number of other reviews (Gery *et al.*, 1986; Streilein, 1987, 1990, 1993; Rocha *et al.*, 1992; Niederkorn and Ferguson, 1996).

II. Ocular Mucosal Immunobiology

A. Tissues and Cells

The conjunctiva and lacrimal gland are the primary ocular tissues that are considered part of the mucosal immune system. The conjunctiva is a mucous membrane consisting of an outer squamous epithelial cell layer (two to five cells thick) interspersed with goblet cells, a basement membrane, and the underlying connective tissue of the substantia propria (stroma). Figure 1 diagrams the major features of the human conjunctiva. Bulbar conjunctiva overlies the sclera between the corneal limbus and the conjunctival fornix. Multiple sebaceous glands within the deeper stroma contribute to the corneal tear film and the lubrication of the conjunctiva (Fine and Yanoff, 1979). Mast cells have been identified in the conjunctiva of humans, other primates, and several rodents (Allansmith *et al.*, 1977; Fine and Yanoff, 1979). These are particularly prominent in trauma-induced and allergic conjunctivitis. There are no microfold (M) cells in the conjunctiva and the normal conjunctiva is relatively free of lymphocytes. However, similar to gastrointestinal-associated lymphoid tissue (GALT), intraepithelial lymphocytes (IEL) have been identified in human and mouse conjunctiva (Dua *et al.*, 1994; J. A. Whittum-Hudson, unpublished observations). Human conjunctival IEL are T cells and express the mucosal lymphocyte antigen HML-1 and CD8 (Dua *et al.*, 1994). Another study found that the majority of conjunctival T cells expressed αβ TCR (Soukiasian *et al.*, 1992). The murine equivalent IEL is $CD3^+$, $CD8^+$ and TCR $\gamma\delta^+$ (J. A. Whittum-Hudson, unpublished observations). Few T cells and essentially no B cells are found in the substantia propria of normal human, monkey, or mouse conjunctiva (Reacher *et al.*, 1991; Soukiasian *et al.*, 1992; Dua *et al.*, 1994; Whittum-Hudson *et al.*, 1995a). The majority of the substantia propria T lymphocytes are $CD8^+$ cells in man and monkey and lie subepithelially. In the lower fornix of human conjunctiva, clusters of unorganized (nonfollicular) lym-

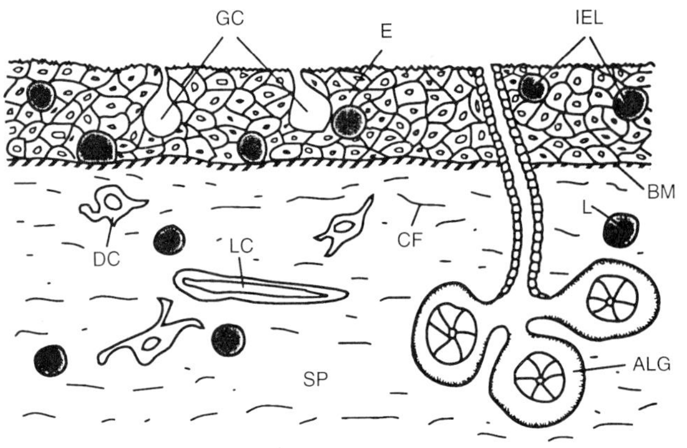

Figure 1. Diagrammatic representation of human conjunctiva showing the conjunctival stratified columnar epithelium (E), intraepithelial lymphocytes (IEL), mucous-producing goblet cells (GC), basement membrane (BM), an accessory lacrimal gland of Krause (ALG), as well as lymphatic channels (LC), collagen fibrils (CF), lymphocytes (L), and dendritic cells (DC) within the substantia propria (SP). (This figure has been adapted from Sacks *et al.*, 1986.)

phocytes may be found (Fine and Yanoff, 1979). Some species such as rabbit and guinea pigs may exhibit true follicles in the lower fornices (Shimada and Silverstein, 1975; Chandler and Gillette, 1983; Sullivan, 1994). These may develop due to persistent exposure to exogenous antigens, or reflect a nonspecific response to the environment.

Lacrimal glands also play a major role in ocular mucosal defense. In humans, lacrimal glands are found in the anterior, superolateral area of the orbit. Smaller accessory lacrimal glands (see Fig. 1) also may be found in the upper and lower conjunctiva. Ducts from the major lacrimal gland drain into the superotemporal conjunctival cul-de-sac, while ducts from accessory glands drain directly through the epithelium of the conjunctiva adjacent to their location. Lacrimal glands of other species are found in different areas both within and outside the orbit. Histological examination shows that the glands are made up of acinar units which are interconnected by ductules and that these interconnected acinar units form the lobes of the gland. Each acinar unit consists of secretory acinar epithelial cells, which are surrounded by a basement membrane, and the glandular ducts are lined with pseudostratified epithelium. Lymphatic channels also are present in the gland, and these drain into the cervical and preauricular lymph nodes. In addition to epithelial cells, a variety of other cell types such as plasma cells, B and T lymphocytes, macrophages, and dendritic cells have been identified in the interstitial connective tissue between the acinar units and ducts. In human, rabbit, rat, and mouse lacrimal glands, IgA plasma cells predominate, although IgG and IgM plasma cells are present and, in human, IgD and IgE plasma cells have been found (Franklin *et al.*, 1973; 1979; Shimada and Silverstein, 1975; Allansmith *et al.*, 1976; Brandtzaeg *et al.*, 1979; 1987; Gillette *et al.*, 1980; Crago *et al.*, 1984; Damato *et al.*, 1984; McGee and Franklin, 1984; Gudmundsson *et al.*, 1984; Brandtzaeg, 1985; Kett *et al.*, 1986; Wieczorek *et al.*, 1988; Ebersole *et al.*, 1988; Pappo *et al.*, 1988b; Hann *et al.*, 1988; Montgomery *et al.*, 1989). B cells bearing various surface immunoglobulin isotypes also have been found in smaller numbers in humans and rodents (McGee and Franklin, 1984; Pappo *et al.*, 1988b; Wieczorek *et al.*, 1988; Montgomery *et al.*, 1989, 1990; Pepose *et al.*, 1990). Both $CD4^+$ and $CD8^+$ T cells also have been identified in human and rat (Ebersole *et al.*, 1988; Gudmundsson *et al.*, 1988; Wieczorek *et al.*, 1988; Pappo *et al.*, 1988b; Pepose *et al.*, 1990; Montgomery *et al.*, 1989, 1990). Of the $CD3^+$ T cells isolated from rat lacrimal gland, 89% bear the $\alpha\beta$ and 7% express $\gamma\delta$ TCR (C. A. Skandera and P. C. Montgomery, unpublished observations). Macrophages have been demonstrated in both human and rat (Wieczorek *et al.*, 1988; Pappo *et al.*, 1988a; Montgomery *et al.*, 1989; Pepose *et al.*, 1990) and Langerhans-type dendritic cells identified in human lacrimal gland (Wieczorek *et al.*, 1988; Pepose *et al.*, 1990). These various cell types contribute a number of biologically active molecules which are important for defense at the ocular surface. The acinar epithelial cells produce lysozyme and lactoferrin which are naturally occurring tear components with bactericidal properties (Franklin *et al.*, 1973; Gillette and Allansmith, 1980; Gillette *et al.*, 1981; McGill *et al.*, 1984). In addition, the plasma cells are the main source of tear S-IgA antibodies (Sullivan and Allansmith, 1984; Peppard and Montgomery, 1987; Franklin, 1989; Sullivan, 1994) which are produced in response to antigenic challenge and are major effector molecules in mucosal defense (Mestecky and McGhee, 1987; Childers *et al.*, 1989; McGhee and Mestecky, 1990).

B. Relationship to the Mucosal Network

Although it has been postulated that the conjunctiva functions both as a mucosal inductive and effector site (Chandler and Gillette, 1983; Franklin and Remus, 1984; Franklin, 1989), the precise relationship of the conjunctiva to the mucosal immune network requires further clarification (Sullivan, 1994). With respect to inductive capabilities, the presence of lymphoid follicles containing T and B cells in rabbit (Shimada and Silverstein, 1975; Franklin *et al.*, 1979; Franklin and Remus, 1984) and, in humans, the presence of Langerhans cells, dendritic cells, and macrophages (Sacks *et al.*, 1986), as well as lymphatic channels (Srinivasan *et al.*, 1990), support the potential to process and perhaps respond to antigen. Normal conjunctival epithelial cells do not express MHC class II; however, the presence of class II^+ Langerhans cells in the epithelium and dendritic cells in the stroma suggests that antigen presentation may occur in conjunctiva. Further support for the inductive function comes from studies showing that topical application of antigen to the conjunctiva is an effective means of eliciting tear IgA antibody responses (Montgomery *et al.*, 1984a,b; Peppard *et al.*, 1988). Recent investigations have suggested that nasal-associated lymphoid tissue (NALT) may also function as an inductive site following ocular topical antigen application (Carr *et al.*, submitted; see Section III.A). With the exception of rabbit conjunctiva, which contains substantial numbers of IgA plasma cells and epithelial cells that synthesize secretory component (Franklin *et al.*, 1973, 1979; Liu *et al.*, 1981), the conjunctiva of most species does not display the typical features of a mucosal effector site. However, it should be noted that studies in at least two species, rat and monkey, have documented lymphocyte traffic from gastrointestinal-associated lymphoid tissue (GALT) to conjunctiva (Zhang *et al.*, 1983; Taylor *et al.*, 1985). These data indicate that the functional role of the conjunctiva in the mucosal network may vary significantly between species.

An abundance of evidence now indicates that the lacrimal gland is a functional part of the mucosal immune network. As has been demonstrated for other mucosal effector tissues and described above (see Section II.A), the lacrimal glands of many species contain a predominance of IgA$^+$ plasma cells. In addition, lacrimal acinar epithelial cells produce secretory component (Franklin *et al.*, 1973; Sullivan *et al.*, 1984b, 1990; Gudmundsson *et al.*, 1985; Hann *et al.*, 1991), which functions as part of the polymeric immunoglobulin receptor to mediate transport of IgA into external secretions (Solari and Kraehenbuhl, 1985). Figure 2 diagrams the biosynthetic events within lacrimal gland that lead to the production and transport of IgA into tears. Linkage of the lacrimal gland to the mucosal network occurs via trafficking lymphocyte populations. While both B and T lymphocytes traffic to mucosal tissues including lacrimal gland, B cells have been studied more extensively than T cells. IgA bearing lymphocytes from GALT (e.g., mesenteric lymph nodes) and glandular mucosal tissues have been shown to seed lacrimal glands (Montgomery *et al.*, 1983, 1985) in a manner similar to other effector sites in the mucosal immune system (Roux *et al.*, 1977; McDermott and Bienenstock, 1979; Weisz-Carrington *et al.*, 1979). Tear IgA antibodies with specificity for oral microbes (Burns *et al.*, 1982; Gregory and Allansmith,

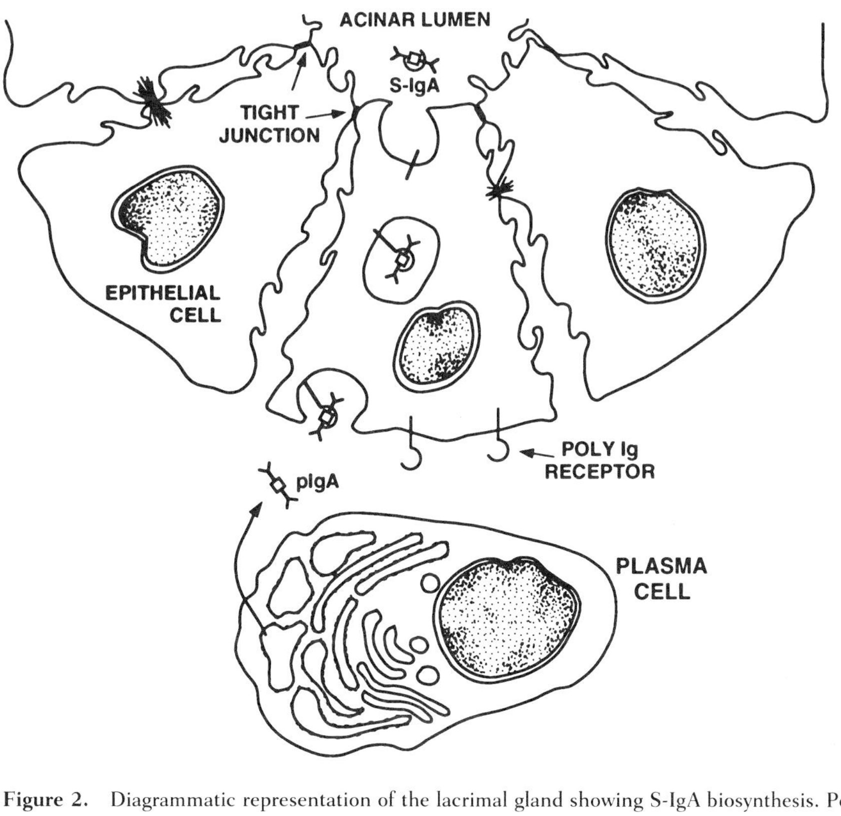

Figure 2. Diagrammatic representation of the lacrimal gland showing S-IgA biosynthesis. Polymeric IgA (pIgA) is synthesized in plasma cells located adjacent to the acinar epithelial cells. pIgA interacts with the polymeric immunoglobulin (poly-Ig) receptor on the basolateral surface of the acinar epithelial cells, is internalized and transported to the apical surface, and is released into the glandular lumen. Prior to release of the S-IgA molecule, the poly-Ig receptor is cleaved, leaving behind the cytoplasmic domain. The remainder of the poly-Ig receptor remains associated with the S-IgA molecule and is designated secretory component (s.c.). (This figure has been reproduced from Franklin and Montgomery (1996) and published courtesy of Mosby.)

1986, 1987) as well as demonstrations that gastrointestinal immunization induced tear IgA antibodies (Mestecky *et al.*, 1978; Montgomery *et al.*, 1983; Gregory and Filler, 1987; Waldman and Bergmann, 1987) have provided further support for this linkage. Figure 3 shows the interrelationship of various compartments of the mucosal network and summarizes events leading to mucosal IgA induction following GALT immunization.

The mechanism accounting for the preferential localization or retention of specific lymphoid populations in ocular mucosal tissues is an issue of central importance in understanding the regulation of ocular mucosal immunity. Lymphocyte–high endothelial venule (HEV) interactions control lymphocyte trafficking into organized lymphoid tissue and lymph nodes (Butcher, 1986; Woodruff *et al.*, 1987, Stoolman, 1989; Chin *et al.*, 1991b; Picker and Butcher, 1992; Shimizu *et al.*, 1992; Bevilacqua, 1993) as well as into organized mucosal lymphoid tissues (Jalkanen *et al.*, 1989; Chin *et al.*, 1991a). In general, these interactions involve lymphocyte homing receptors which interact with vascular addressins on HEVs and other specialized endothelial cells. Although little is known regarding the mechanisms involved in cell trafficking to conjunctival tissue, the parameters regulating lymphocyte localization within the lacrimal gland are beginning to be defined. With respect to glandular structures, the control of lymphocyte traffic could occur on two levels: (1) at exit from the vasculature, or (2) within the stroma of the glandular tissue. There are no HEVs in lacrimal gland and no selective interactions with glandular endothelium have yet been demonstrated. Therefore, it appears that lymphocyte entry into lacrimal gland is random (McGee and Franklin, 1984). Current evidence suggests that lymphocyte populations are selectively retained based on interactions that occur within the lacrimal tissue microenvironment. Early studies indicated that B-cell retention, particularly those committed to IgA production, resulted from a direct interaction with T cells located in lacrimal tissue (Franklin and Shepard, 1990). Recently, an *in vitro* binding assay has been used to show that circulating lymphocyte populations preferentially adhere to lacrimal gland acinar epithelium (O'Sullivan and Montgomery, 1990). Both B and T lymphocytes participate in this interaction with B cells binding in greater numbers (O'Sullivan *et al.*, 1994a). Studies with biochemical inhibitors and antibodies directed against various adhesion molecules initially suggested the involvement of L-selectin (O'Sullivan *et al.*, 1994a,b). Other data indicated that pretreatment of lymphocytes with certain cytokines (IL-4 and TGFβ) reduced the capacity of those cells to interact with lacrimal gland but not lymph node or Peyer's patches (Elfaki *et al.*, 1994). These latter data provided the initial support for the involvement of a receptor distinct from those mediating interactions with lymph node and Peyer's patch HEVs. The characterization of the lymphocyte receptor is still ongoing, but an 85-kDa factor has been identified which specifically inhibits lymphocyte interactions with lacrimal and salivary gland tissues (Montgomery and Liberati, 1995). Current studies are focused on defining the relationship of this molecule to other lymphocyte surface determinants and adhesion molecules, as well as on the identification of the acinar epithelial cell ligand or counter receptor. With respect to the ligand, recent studies using cultured rat lacrimal gland acinar cells suggest that this molecule is shed into the culture medium (O'Sullivan *et al.*, 1995) and has led to the speculation that trafficking lymphocytes may also interact with secreted ligand accessing the interstitial glandular spaces. Although the ligand or counter receptor has not yet been isolated, it appears to be a 20- or 21-kDa glycoprotein (R. Raja and P. C. Montgomery, unpublished observations).

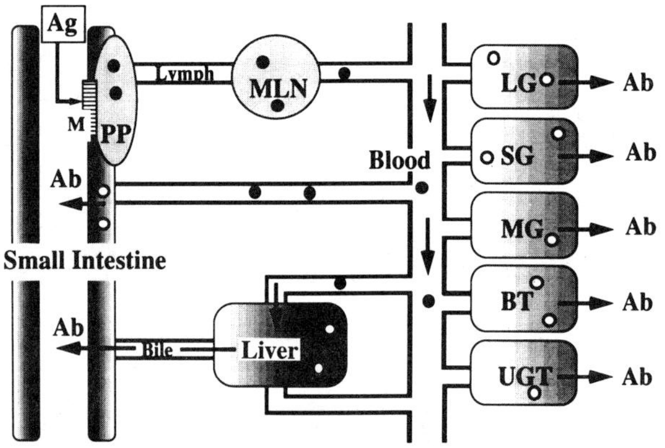

Figure 3. Schematic representation of the major features of the mucosal immune network as they relate to gastrointestinal-associated lymphoid tissue (GALT). Intestinal antigens (Ag) are taken up by microfold (M) cells overlying Peyer's patches (PP) and are delivered to lymphoid cells in the PP. T cells and IgA committed B cells (●) migrate to the mesenteric lymph nodes (MLN), enter the circulation, and traffic to the lacrimal (LG), salivary (SG), mammary (MG) glands as well as to the lamina propria of the small intestine, the bronchial (BT) and urogenital (UGT) tracts, and liver. B lymphocytes lodging in mucosal tissues differentiate into IgA secreting plasma cells (○), producing pIgA which is transported into external secretions as S-IgA antibody (Ab). In some species the liver directly transports significant quantities of pIgA from the circulation into bile. (This figure has been reproduced from Montgomery *et al.* (1994) and published courtesy of Plenum.)

III. Induction of Ocular Mucosal Immune Responses

Regulatory events leading to the induction and expression of ocular mucosal immune responses are not completely defined. However, it is clear that many factors governing immune responses at other mucosal sites (Kiyono *et al.*, 1992; Walker, 1994) have general applicability to mucosal immune responses at the ocular surface. The immunization route is of primary importance with local (e.g., topical application to the eye) and remote site (e.g., oral or gastrointestinal) routes generating tear IgA antibody responses. Combinations of routes and their sequence of administration can also affect antibody induction in tears. Not surprisingly for replicating microbes, tissue tropism and invasive properties influence the outcome of mucosal responses. When dealing with nonreplicating immunogens, particulate antigens are more effective at inducing ocular mucosal immune responses than soluble antigens. Thus far, traditional mucosal adjuvants such as cholera toxin, delivered topically to the eye with antigen, do not appear to enhance ocular antibody responses (Peppard and Montgomery, 1990). Helper T (Th) cells and T-cell products such as cytokines appear to play key roles in regulating ocular mucosal IgA responses, but the direct role of cytotoxic T (Tc) cells in ocular mucosal immunity is currently not clear.

As noted above (see Section II.B), lymphocyte traffic from mucosal inductive to effector sites is a central feature of the ocular mucosal system. Antigen-presenting cells (e.g., macrophages and dendritic cells) are also required, but their participation in ocular mucosal responses has yet to be delineated. The neuroendocrine system also plays a role in regulating ocular mucosal responses affecting both secretory component synthesis *in vivo* (Sullivan *et al.*, 1984a) and cultured lacrimal gland acinar cells (Kelleher *et al.*, 1991) as well as tear IgA production (Sullivan and Allansmith, 1985; Sullivan, 1988). Neuroendocrine regulation is reviewed in detail elsewhere (Stanisz *et al.*, 1989; Sullivan, 1990, 1994). Although these as well as other factors yet to be identified impact ocular mucosal immune responses, our focus will be on selected parameters relevant to the development of ocular vaccination strategies. Therefore, the effects of immunization route, immune potentiators and delivery vehicles on the induction of ocular mucosal responses, in particular IgA antibody production, will be examined in detail.

A. Immunization Routes

In humans, most investigations have focused on use of the oral or gastrointestinal (GI) immunization route. Ingestion of heat-killed *Streptococcus mutans* elicited IgA antibodies in tears and saliva, but not serum antibodies (Mestecky *et al.*, 1978). In addition, a second oral immunization markedly increased tear and salivary IgA responses. Other studies using inactivated S. *mutans* have generally confirmed these initial observations (Gregory *et al.*, 1984; Gregory and Filler, 1987; Czerkinsky *et al.*, 1987). Human tear IgA antibody responses have also been noted following oral immunization with influenza vaccine (Bergmann *et al.*, 1986, 1987; Waldman and Bergmann, 1987) as well as following intranasal immunization with live rhinovirus (Douglas *et al.*, 1967; Knopf *et al.*, 1970).

The rat model has been employed to directly compare the effectiveness of antigen application to the conjunctiva (ocular topical, ot) and administration by the oral or gastrointestinal (GI) route using the nonreplicating particulate antigen, dinitrophenylated type III pneumococcus (DNP-Pn). These studies have shown: (1) both the immunization route and the sequence of stimulation play a role in tear antibody expression (Montgomery *et al.*, 1984b); (2) long-term repeated ot stimulation leads to an eventual downregulation of tear IgA antibody levels (Montgomery *et al.*, 1984a,b); (3) the ot route generally yields higher tear IgA antibody levels than GI immunization (Peppard *et al.*, 1988); and (4) coadministration of antigen and cytokines by the ot route enhances tear IgA antibody levels (Pockley and Montgomery, 1991; see Section III.B). The rat model also has been used to study the effect of immunization route on the kinetics of serum and tear antibody responses to live *Chlamydia trachomatis* (Davidson *et al.*, 1993). This study compared the effectiveness of ot, GI, subconjunctival, and intraperitoneal immunization and showed that ot application was the most effective route for eliciting IgA antibody response in tears. Interestingly, subconjunctival injection of chlamydia yielded a vigorous serum IgG response and minimal tear IgA antibodies, which is consistent with responses to other antigens delivered by this route (Cousins *et al.*, 1991). The explanation for this latter finding is not clear, but subconjunctival delivery may bypass an essential ocular mucosal processing step during antigen uptake or allow live organisms to gain access to the circulation.

Although the precise mechanism by which ot immunization elicits tear IgA antibody responses is not known, it appears that the inductive process could involve at least two pathways: (1) antigen uptake, processing, and triggering of B cells in the conjunctival substantia propria or (2) antigen drainage *via* the nasolacrimal canal, uptake by NALT M cells, processing and triggering of resident B cells in NALT (Carr *et al.*, submitted). The schematic details of these two pathways are shown in Fig. 4. Not shown in this figure is the option for antigen drainage *via* the nasolacrimal canal to access GALT or other alternatives which may be applicable to primates. In humans and monkeys, antigen may reach the accessory lacrimal glands directly or gain access to potential ductal associated lymphoid tissue as has been shown for minor salivary glands (Nair and Schroeder, 1986). However, since it is not clear how antigen would be processed within the acinar units of the accessory lacrimal glands and ductal-associated lymphoid tissue has not been identified for these glandular structures, these latter alternatives appear unlikely.

Several animal models have also been used to eval-

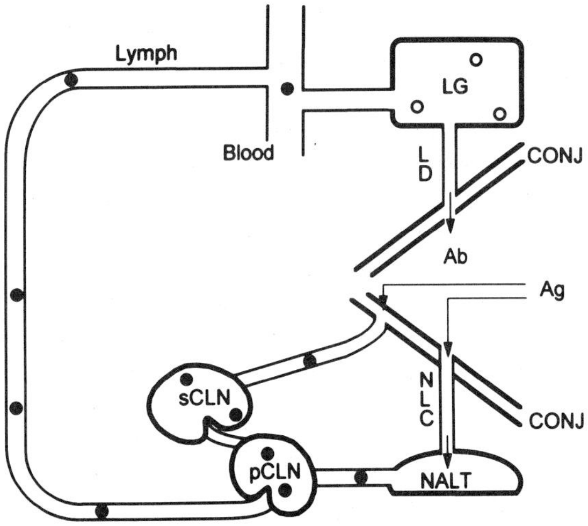

Figure 4. Schematic representation of the major components of the ocular mucosal immune system showing possible pathways for antigenic stimulation at the ocular surface. 1. Antigen may gain access to the conjunctival (CONJ) substantia propria where dendritic cells would present it to resident lymphocytes (see Fig. 1). Once triggered, B cells (●) would traffic to the superior cervical lymph node (sCLN) and gain access to lymph. 2. Ag may drain *via* the nasolacrimal canal (NLC), be taken up by M cells, and gain access to the nasal-associated lymphoid tissue (NALT) where presentation and B-cell triggering would occur. B cells (●) would traffic to the posterior cervical lymph node (pCLN) and gain access to lymph. B cells reaching lymph from either pathway would enter the circulation, traffic to the major lacrimal gland (LG), and differentiate into IgA antibody-secreting plasma cells (○). The IgA would be processed as shown in Fig. 2 and reach the ocular surface *via* the lacrimal duct (LD).

uate tear antibody responses after immunization or infection at ocular surfaces with chlamydia and other pathogens. In guinea pigs, only ocular immunization with live *Chlamydia psittaci* (GPIC) induced tear IgA (and in some cases IgG) antibodies (Murray *et al.*, 1973; Watson *et al.*, 1977; Rank and Whittum-Hudson, 1994). Killed organisms administered *via* ocular topical (Murray *et al.*, 1973) or intraperitoneal routes (Malaty *et al.*, 1981) failed to induce tear antibodies. However, similar studies with human biovars of *C. trachomatis* in owl monkeys suggested that inactivated chlamydia could indeed induce tear antibodies (MacDonald *et al.*, 1984). In the cynomolgus monkey model, ocular infection with the chlamydial organism induced vigorous IgA, IgG, and IgM responses in both serum and tears (reviewed by Taylor, 1990). Only oral immunization with live L_2 biovar of chlamydia, but not ocular serotypes, successfully induced mucosal and systemic immunity, which partially protected the host from subsequent infectious challenge (Taylor *et al.*, 1987b).

Cynomolgus monkeys develop conjunctival disease similar to that observed in humans (Whittum-Hudson and Taylor, 1984). An intense mononuclear infiltrate appears in infected conjunctiva (Whittum-Hudson *et al.*, 1986a,b; Whittum-Hudson and Taylor, 1989) and is composed of high frequencies of chlamydia-specific T and B lymphocytes (Pal *et al.*, 1992). Supporting the importance of regional draining cervical lymph nodes in conjunctival responses to pathogens, essentially identical frequencies of antigen-specific cells were detected in these lymph nodes and the conjunctivae after infection, and in "ocular-immune" animals which were topically challenged with the chlamydial hsp60 antigen (Pal *et al.*, 1990b, 1992). Serologic responses to chlamydial hsp60 and hsp70 are vigorous during chronic chlamydial infections in man and animals (Newhall *et al.*, 1982; Pal *et al.*, 1990a), although neither of these proteins delivered by the ot route immunized naive monkeys (Taylor *et al.*, 1987b, 1990). In contrast, ot boosting after systemic or oral immunization with purified or recombinant chlamydial antigens induced vigorous tear IgA and IgG and serum antibodies (Campos *et al.*, 1995; O'Brien *et al.*, 1994). It remains unclear whether the initial dosage of some antigens is too small to induce typical primary secretory immune responses when presented to the mucosal immune system by ot delivery, or if an antigen must replicate and/or be invasive to adequately prime experimental animals. Nevertheless, ocular boosting with purified antigens or infectious ocular challenge of systemically primed animals has demonstrated that anamnestic tear antibody responses occur rapidly for chlamydia (Campos *et al.*, 1995). Combined oral and subcutaneous priming with a chlamydial fusion protein of a major outer membrane protein (MOMP) variable domain incorporated into liposomes also primed for mucosal immune responses (O'Brien *et al.*, 1994).

The rabbit model has also been used to test ocular immune responses to other organisms. Live herpes simplex virus type 1 administered by the ocular route elicited tear IgA, but no IgG or IgM antibodies (Willey *et al.*, 1985). In contrast, application to scarified cornea induced tear IgA, IgG, and IgM responses (Centifanto *et al.*, 1989). Whether these differing results relate to virus strain invasiveness or access to underlying dendritic cells is unclear. Live *Staphylococcus aureus* administered ot elicited tear IgA and IgG antibodies as did a *S. aureus* subunit (peptidoglycan-ribitol teichoic acid) vaccine administered by the intradermal or subconjunctival routes with complete Freund's adjuvant (Mondino *et al.*, 1987a,b, 1991). However, given the severe inflammatory properties of Freund's adjuvant and the restrictions on its use, this latter approach is impractical as a vaccination strategy.

B. Immune Potentiators

Immune potentiators, or adjuvants, have been used to enhance antibody responses in both humans and animal models. Although the mechanisms responsible for response enhancement vary and are often not well defined, adjuvants appear to function by one or a combination of mechanisms: (1) increasing the influx of inflammatory cells; (2) promotion of antigen presentation; and/or (3) enhancing antigen uptake. Consideration of immune potentiators to enhance ocular mucosal responses requires selection of compounds which will not promote ocular inflammation and pathology.

The most widely studied mucosal adjuvant has been cholera toxin (Lycke and Holmgren, 1968) although its effects on ocular immunity are less defined. Enhancement of mucosal responses depends on the binding of the cholera toxin B subunit to the G_{M1} ganglioside displayed on the luminal surface of enterocytes such as M cells as well as potential modulatory effects of the toxin on the B, T, and antigen-presenting cells (Dertzbaugh and Elson, 1990; Elson and Dertzbaugh, 1994). Cholera toxin enhances antibody responses when coadministered with many antigens, whereas the B subunit apparently requires conjugation to antigen to function optimally. Oral immunization with cholera toxin induced the appearance of toxin-specific antibody-forming cells in rat conjunctiva (Zhang *et al.*, 1983) and toxin-specific antibodies in tears of monkeys (Campos *et al.*, 1995). However, ot administration of cholera toxin with the DNP-Pn antigen did not enhance tear IgA antibody responses in the rat model (Peppard and Montgomery, 1990), but the effects of oral or ocular administration of antigens conjugated to the B subunit on tear IgA responses have not been fully investigated. Based on recent data suggesting that nasal associated lymphoid tissue can serve as an inductive site for tear IgA antibody responses (Carr *et al.*, submitted) and the ability of the B subunit to serve as an adjuvant when coupled to antigens administered by the intranasal route (Bessen and Fischetti, 1990; Wu and Russell, 1993), this immunization protocol requires rigorous testing. Two other mucosal adjuvants, avridine and muramyl tripeptide, administered topically by the ocular route with DNP-Pn, did not enhance tear IgA antibody responses (Peppard *et al.*, 1988).

Cytokines also appear to exert important regulatory effects on mucosal IgA responses including those at ocular sites. Interleukin (IL)-6 knock-out mice have greatly reduced numbers of IgA producing cells at mucosae and exhibit grossly deficient local antibody responses to mucosal challenge (Ramsay *et al.*, 1994). In addition, transforming growth factor-β (TGFβ), IL-5, and IL-6 have been shown to enhance *in vitro* IgA responses in murine B-cell cultures. TGFβ appears to increase IgA synthesis by inducing B cells to switch to IgA production (Coffman *et al.*, 1989; Ehrhardt *et al.*, 1992), whereas IL-5 and IL-6 induce IgA^{+} B cells to terminally differentiate into IgA producing plasma cells (Coffman *et al.*, 1987; Beagley *et al.*, 1988, 1989; Harriman *et al.*, 1988). IL-5, IL-6, and TGFβ have been shown to specifically enhance IgA production *in vitro* in a rat lacrimal gland tissue fragment culture system (Pockley and Montgomery, 1990; Rafferty and Montgomery, 1993). Further, IL-5 and IL-6 in combination with antigen have been shown to enhance specific tear IgA antibody responses in rats following ot administration without affecting serum IgG antibody levels (Pockley and Montgomery, 1991). Recent studies indicate that these enhanced tear IgA antibody responses persist following restimulation with antigen in the absence of IL-5 and IL-6 (Montgomery *et al.*, 1994). Although the mechanism(s) underlying this *in vivo* cytokine-mediated enhancement is not yet known, it is clear that the regulatory roles and therapeutic potential of these and other cytokines to modulate ocular mucosal antibody responses require further investigation.

C. Delivery Vehicles

Although the oral or GI immunization route triggers IgA antibody responses at both intestinal and distal mucosal sites and represents a safe, convenient alternative for vaccine administration, it is often difficult to present intact antigen to GALT-inductive sites. Particulate antigens, including viable organisms, generally appear to be the most effective immunogens, probably due to their ability to survive the pH extremes and enzymatic degradation that occur along the alimentary tract. Since many potential vaccine candidates are microbial components or subunits and are not viable organisms or particulate immunogens, considerable effort has focused on the development of delivery systems. Such delivery systems include liposomes and biodegradable microparticles, as well as recombinant bacterial and viral vectors. Strategies for vehicle development have included not only delivery of intact immunogens and genes that code for relevant antigens, but also systems that promote uptake by relevant cells (e.g., M cells) at GALT inductive sites. Detailed information on antigen delivery systems can be found in several recent reviews (Eldridge *et al.*, 1993; Michalek *et al.*, 1994, 1995). Although many of these delivery systems may be relevant to the induction of mucosal antibody responses owing to their ability to induce vigorous responses at GALT effector sites, information is more limited on the potential to employ these vehicles to induce ocular mucosal immune responses. Based on recent observations indicating that microparticle-encapsulated antigens evoke ocular mucosal responses, discussion will be confined to this delivery vehicle.

Poly(lactide-*co*-glycolide) (PLG) microparticles are biodegradable under physiological conditions and represent an important candidate vehicle for delivery and controlled release of vaccine components (O'Hagan *et al.*, 1991; O'Hagan, 1994). PLG has been used for suture material (Wise *et al.*, 1979) and as a delivery system for drugs (Hutchinson and Furr, 1985). PLG does not evoke a tissue response (Visscher *et al.*, 1987) and has been certified by the FDA for human use. Recently, PLG microparticles have been used for ocular drug delivery without provoking histological or electrophysiological changes to the eye (Moritera *et al.*, 1992). In addition, PLG encapsulated antigens induce sustained systemic and secretory immune responses following oral administration (Challacombe *et al.*, 1992; Maloy *et al.*, 1994). Based on these data as well as observations that the cytokines IL-5 and IL-6 enhanced tear IgA antibody responses following topical application to the eye (Pockley and Montgomery, 1991; see Section III.B), PLG microparticles appear to be an appropriate vehicle to deliver antigens and immune potentiators to ocular mucosal inductive sites. Studies indicate that DNP–bovine serum albumin as well as IL-5 and IL-6 can be encapsulated in PLG microparticles without significant loss of activity. In addition, ot delivery of encapsulated antigen and cytokines evokes long-term mucosal antibody responses in tears and distal secretions as well as circulating antibodies in the rat model (Rafferty *et al.*, 1996). Further, oral delivery of a poly(lactide) encapsulated chlamydia candidate vaccine in mice induced antigen specific serologic responses and conferred partial protection against ocular challenge (Whittum-Hudson *et al.*, 1995b; see Section IV.A). While further studies are required to define the regulatory parameters and events leading to these responses, microparticles clearly are promising candidate delivery vehicles to elicit ocular mucosal immune responses.

IV. Targets for Vaccine Development

The conjunctiva is the most commonly infected tissue of the eye (Syed and Hyndiuk, 1992; Tabbara and Hyndiuk, 1995). Infection may be limited to the conjunctiva only or may be part of a lid or corneal infection. Most conjunctival infections are not vision-threatening, but most notable exceptions are *Neisseria gonorrheae* and herpes simplex virus. Conjunctivitis associated with tularemia (adults) (Knorr and Weber, 1994) and haemophilus infections (infants) (Syed and Hyndiuk, 1992) are potentially fatal because of systemic dissemination. The profile of pathogens isolated from normal and diseased human conjunctiva may vary depending upon geographic locale (Syed and Hyndiuk, 1992). Similarly, some veterinary pathogens of the conjunctiva/lacrimal gland are geographically confined (Lepper *et al.*, 1993; Rogers *et al.*, 1993). Chronic inflammation of the conjunctiva may lead to scar formation and is termed chronic progressive conjunctival cicatrisation (Bernauer *et al.*, 1993). Cicatricial diseases often progress to involve the lacrimal and meibomian glands. The combination of altered tear film, scar contraction, and corneal trauma from trichiasis may lead to blindness. Although there are noninfectious etiologies for many cicatrical disorders including pemphigoid, chlamydial infections of the conjunctiva are a classic example of the blinding sequelae of infection.

As discussed above and elsewhere (Sullivan, 1994), there are physical and biochemical barriers to help prevent ocular infection. For extracellular ocular bacterial infections, antibodies are a major component of protective immunization. Both antibody and cell-mediated immunity are believed to be important in protection against intracellular pathogens including viruses, chlamydia, and mycobacteria. Antibodies would block infection and clear free organisms, whereas $CD8^+$ cytotoxic T cells would clear infected cells and prevent full differentiation and spread from lysed host cells. There is little *in vivo* evidence from ocular sites that cytotoxic T lymphocytes are important in clearance of infectious pathogens. However, CD4 T cells serve as antigen presenting cells for B-cell responses and both CD4 and CD8 T cells produce cytokines that facilitate B- and T-cell responses. Many bacteria, viruses, and parasites are targets for vaccine development to prevent respiratory, genital tract, or other infections. If protective mucosal immunization is induced at one or more of these latter sites, it is probable that the ocular mucosal surfaces would also be protected.

A. Bacterial Infections

A variety of bacteria can infect ocular tissues. Table I lists some of the bacterial pathogens that are known to cause conjunctivitis. Bacterial conjunctivitis is most commonly caused by *S. aureus. Streptococcus* sp. are common conjunctival pathogens, except for β-hemolytic streptococci (*S. pyogenes*), while other members of this group are part of the normal conjunctival flora. These bacteria and *Haemophilus influenzae* are the most common agents causing dacryocystitis (lacrimal gland infection). *Corynebacterium diphtheriae* is a rare ocular pathogen, but can cause conjunctival scarring and associated problems. For the most part, bacterial infections of the conjunctiva are self-limiting and nonvision threatening. *Neisseria gonorrhoeae* is an exception, and this organism is the leading cause of hyperacute conjunctivitis particularly in developing countries (Syed and Hyndiuk, 1992). *N. meningitis* conjunctivitis, which cannot be distinguished clinically from *N. gonorrhoeae,* also may be associated with systemic disease. *H. influenzae* conjunctivitis occurs in children as well as adults, and one could predict a decline in the incidence of this ocular disease now that the Hib vaccine is available. Anaerobic organisms compose another part of the normal flora of the conjunctival sac. As for other infectious pathogens, the incidence of conjunctival infections with abnormal anaerobic organisms is increased in patients

TABLE I
Major Bacterial Pathogens Causing Conjunctivitis

Organism	References[a]
Staphylococcus aureus	Holzberg *et al.*, 1992
Neisseria gonorrheae	Syed and Hyndiuk, 1992
Streptococcus sp.	Murphy *et al.*, 1991
Haemophilus influenzae, *H. meningitidis*	Syed and Hyndiuk, 1992
Borellia burgdorferi	Aaberg, 1989; Zaidman, 1993
Francisella tularensis	Knorr and Weber, 1994
Chlamydia trachomatis	Wills *et al.*, 1987; Taylor *et al.*, 1992; Heggie and Lass, 1994; Brunham and Peeling, 1994;
C. psittaci	Dhingra and Mahajan, 1991
Pseudomonas aeruginosa[b]	King *et al.*, 1988; Brook and Hulburd, 1993
Shigella flexneri, *S. sonnei*[c]	Linde *et al.*, 1993
Brucella melitensis[d]	Young, 1983; Zundel *et al.*, 1992

[a]Selected primary articles and/or reviews of bacterial ocular pathogens.

[b]May cause conjunctivitis, but usually is associated with corneal infections following abrasion or tissue injury (Hazlett *et al.*, 1976; Ramphal *et al.*, 1981).

[c]Guinea pig ocular challenge model is used to test for protective immunity induced by anti-Shigella vaccine, because corneal/conjunctival epithelium is similar to intestinal epithelium in susceptibility to invasion by *Shigella*.

[d]Infects conjunctival mucosa, but is more of a problem for abortion in ewes and goats; however, vaccination *via* the conjunctiva reduced spontaneous abortions compared to systemic immunization.

with AIDS (Dugel and Rao, 1993; Campos *et al.*, 1994). Similarly, some cases of microsporidial conjunctivitis have been reported in AIDS patients (Lacey *et al.*, 1992; Lowder, 1993; Weber *et al.*, 1993).

Chlamydia trachomatis, an obligate intracellular bacterium, has received a great deal of attention with respect to vaccine development. While chlamydia has gained notoriety in recent years as a major sexually transmitted pathogen, it is, in fact, the leading cause of preventable blindness. Trachoma, resulting from chronic chlamydial infection of the conjunctiva, has been known since ancient times. Studies of patients in several endemic areas worldwide yielded valuable information regarding the epidemiologic, microbiologic, and serologic characteristics of trachoma (Nichols *et al.*, 1973; Grayston *et al.*, 1985; Dawson *et al.*, 1989; Mabey *et al.*, 1992; Taylor *et al.*, 1992). Two major animals models have been used for immunologic studies of chlamydial ocular infections: a guinea pig model which can be infected with *C. psittaci* causing guinea pig inclusion conjunctivitis (GPIC), and subhuman primates, including owl monkeys and cynomolgus monkeys, which can be infected with several biovars of *C. trachomatis,* the usual human ocular pathogen (Patton, 1990; Rank and Whittum-Hudson, 1994). More recently, a mouse model of ocular infection was developed using a human ocular biovar (Whittum-Hudson *et al.*, 1995a); this model should aid in immunologic studies which have not been possible with the other outbred species.

Vaccine development for this bacterium has been hampered by several key factors: (1) no protective antigen or epitope(s) has been conclusively identified from the plethora of immunogenic proteins; (2) no chlamydial target antigens have been shown convincingly to be expressed on the surface of infected host cells, and (3) chlamydia-induced disease sequelae are immune-mediated, though only the 57-kDa chlamydial heat-shock protein has been associated with immunopathogenic responses (Watkins *et al.*, 1986; Taylor *et al.*, 1987a; Morrison *et al.*, 1989a,b).

Various permutations of the chlamydial major outer membrane protein (MOMP) have been tested for immunogenicity and their ability to induce protective immunity in experimental animals. Biochemically extracted native MOMP, recombinant MOMP, or its variable domains have been presented by systemic and mucosal routes. In some cases, protection was tested by infectious challenge at the ocular mucosal surface or other sites (genital tract, lung, etc.). Table II lists some of the chlamydial vaccine candidates tested experimentally over the past two decades. In most cases, whole MOMP or subunits were highly immunogenic as measured primarily by serologic responses, but no significant *in vivo* protection against ocular infection was observed after direct immunization. Studies by several groups (Ward et al., 1986; Stephens, 1990; Mabey *et al.*, 1991; Stagg *et al.*, 1993; Murdin *et al.*, 1993, 1995; Tuffrey, 1994) have identified important MOMP peptide epitopes to which immune responses have been induced. None of these have been tested in ocular infection models as yet, but several have been at least partially protective in chlamydial genital infection models (reviewed by Tuffrey, 1994).

Other chlamydial antigens such as the chlamydial lipopolysaccharide (LPS) have been shown to be immunogenic but not protective in an ocular infection model (Taylor and Prendergast, 1987). An additional chlamydial antigen, the exoglycolipid antigen (GLXA) (Stuart and MacDonald, 1989), is also expressed by chlamydia and secreted from infected cell *in vitro* (Stuart *et al.*, 1991, 1994; Wyrick *et al.*, 1994). Monoclonal anti-idiotypic (Id) antibodies to GLXA have been shown to immunize and protect mice against subsequent infectious ocular challenge with a human biovar of chlamydia (Whittum-Hudson *et al.*, 1994). Oral immunization of BALB/c mice with poly(lactide) encapsulated anti-Id antibodies to GLXA was shown recently to be even more protective than the soluble antibody since 25-fold less antibody presented in microspheres induced equivalent or better reduction in microbiologic disease. In both cases, mice developed serum antibodies to the

TABLE II
Potential Chlamydial Vaccine Antigens Tested in Ocular or Extraocular Models

Antigen[a]	Delivery route[b] 1°/2°	Adjuvant/carrier[c]	References
Whole organism	i.n.		Pal *et al.*, 1994
	Oral		Taylor *et al.*, 1987b
Whole organism extracts	i.m. or s.c.	Oil emulsion	Grayston *et al.*, 1962; Nichols *et al.*, 1966, 1969; Soldati *et al.*, 1971; Schachter, 1985
MOMP (TX100)	s.c.	CFA	Taylor *et al.*, 1987a
	Oral		Taylor *et al.*, 1988
MOMP (OGP)	s.c.	CFA	Batteiger *et al.*, 1993; Campos *et al.*, 1995
	Oral/ot	CT	Campos *et al.*, 1995
rMOMP subunit	ot		Wong *et al.*, 1990
	Oral/ot	CT-B conjugate	Taylor *et al.*, 1989
MOMP/rMOMP subunits	s.c./Peyer's patches	Alum	Tuffrey, 1994
rMOMP subunit fusion protein	s.c./s.c. (EB)	Titermax	Allen and Stephens, 1993
rMOMP subunit fusion protein	Oral/oral ot	CT/liposomes	O'Brien *et al.*, 1994; Whittum-Hudson *et al.*, 1995a
	s.c./s.c.		
	i.d.	Alum/*Salmonella typhimurium*	Hayes *et al.*, 1991
rMOMP hybrid	s.c./s.c.	Poliovirus hybrid	Murdin *et al.*, 1993, 1995
hsp 70	s.c. or ot		Taylor *et al.*, 1990
hsp 60	ot		Taylor *et al.*, 1990
	s.c./ot		Rank *et al.*, 1995
Anti-idiotypic antibodies to	s.c./s.c.	Alumina (Maalox)	Whittum-Hudson and Taylor, 1994; Whittum-Hudson *et al.*, 1995a,b
chlamydial exoglycolipid	Oral/oral	Encapsulated (microspheres)	

[a]MOMP, major outer membrane protein; TX100, Triton X-100; OGP, octyl glucosyl pyranoside; rMOMP, recombinant MOMP; hsp, heat shock protein.

[b]s.c., subcutaneous; i.n., intranasal; ot, ocular topical; i.d., intradermal; i.m., intramuscular.

[c]CFA, complete Freund's adjuvant; CT, cholera toxin; CT-B, cholera toxin B subunit; IFA, incomplete Freund's adjuvant; EB, chlamydial elementary bodies.

GLXA and these antibodies were neutralizing for *in vitro* infectivity (Whittum-Hudson *et al.*, 1995b; Whittum-Hudson *et al.*, submitted). This type of vaccine approach has potential value for chlamydial infections at other sites, and against other biovars since the GLXA antigen is genus-specific as opposed to being serovar-specific.

It has been hypothesized by several investigators that protective immunity against chlamydia will require induction of neutralizing antibody in tears and it is assumed that this will be S-IgA. IgA in tears from patients with trachoma passively neutralized chlamydia and reduced disease in eyes of owl monkeys (Nichols *et al.*, 1973; Barenfanger and MacDonald, 1974). This was consistent with observations in guinea pigs ocularly infected with *C. psittaci* (Orenstein *et al.*, 1973; Malaty *et al.*, 1981). The dilemma with the chlamydial pathogen is that individuals who have had a previous ocular (or other site) infection with chlamydia are not significantly protected against subsequent ocular infections. This lack of protective immunity is seen despite evidence of vigorous antibody responses to many chlamydial antigens in tears and serum and *in vitro* lymphocyte proliferative responses to whole organism or purified antigens (Newhall *et al.*, 1982; Ward *et al.*, 1986; Whittum-Hudson and Taylor, 1989; Taylor, 1990). Several clinical studies have shown a poor correlation of acquisition of genital chlamydial infection with the presence of neutralizing serum antibodies (Jones and Van der Pol, 1994).

Cytotoxic T cells have not yet been associated directly with ocular protective immunity, nor with the immunopathogenesis of chlamydia ocular infection. It has been argued that the lack of exposure of chlamydial antigens on the surface of infected host cells would prevent them from serving as immunologic targets and may explain the failure to induce T-cell-mediated immunity. However, recent electron microscopic studies of human endometrial cells have shown that chlamydial MOMP, LPS, and the GLXA (Wyrick *et al.*, 1994) all pass from the inclusion body through the cytoplasm to the cell membrane. LPS are GLXA and both known to exit infected cells (Brade *et al.*, 1986; Stuart *et al.*, 1991;

Lukacova *et al.*, 1994). In addition, recent studies demonstrated CD8 mediated cytotoxic killing by chlamydia-primed T cells *in vitro* and some *in vivo* protection after experimental genital infection (Beatty and Stephens, 1994; Starnbach *et al.*, 1994). Thus, it is possible that chlamydial antigen presentation to $CD8^+$ effector T cells may occur in the context of MHC class I.

B. Viral and Parasitic Infections

Table III lists many of the viral and parasitic pathogens known to infect ocular tissues. With respect to viruses, such infections frequently result in conjunctivitis in both children and adults and these highly contagious infections (epidemic keratoconjunctivitis) resolve spontaneously over 2–3 weeks. The most common viral pathogen of the conjunctiva is adenovirus. Several adenovirus types (3, 7, 8, 19) may be associated with conjunctivitis, though corneal involvement is often seen (Murrah, 1988).

Ocular herpesvirus infections, though most often affecting the cornea, may cause conjunctivitis during primary infection. However, conjunctivitis is rare during recurrent infections with herpes simplex virus (Holzberg *et al.*, 1992). Herpes zoster ophthalmicus may develop in patients with latent varicella-zoster virus infections, and the conjunctivia is one of several ocular sites most often affected (Liesegang, 1993). Since at present there is no vaccine for herpesviruses, antiviral drugs remain the therapeutic option. There is a large literature concerning anti-herpesvirus vaccine development strategies, and this information is detailed in several reviews (Rouse and Lopez, 1984; Dix, 1987; Mader and Stulting, 1992; Stanberry, 1994). In addition to the fact that herpesviruses are ubiquitous and that the majority of individuals have been exposed previously, vaccine development strategies for ocular and extraocular herpes virus infections must deal with a number of questions: (1) Can recurrence of latent infections be ablated by vaccination or must primary infection be prevented? (2) Will herpesvirus-induced immunosuppression be overcome by appropriate immunization? (3) Will a combination subunit vaccine be required? and (4) Is systemic rather than mucosal immunization required? Table IV lists some recent herpes simplex virus vaccine candidates. A number of viral glycoproteins have been targeted for vaccines (e.g., Burke *et al.*, 1994), although there are some examples of better protection being conferred by vaccination with live organisms (Ghiasi *et al.*, 1995). Studies which directly tested for protection against ocular herpes simplex virus infections have used various viral constructs ranging from single or multiple glycoprotein constructs and deletion mutants delivered with or without adjuvant. Avirulent constructs have been tested in a variety of experimental models and clinical trials. While most immunizations have been *via* systemic routes (subcutaneous or intraperitoneal), a recent study using the rabbit model of recurrent ocular herpes infection showed that subconjunctival immunization with recombinant gB and gD after establishment of latent infection reduced spontaneous recurrences (Nesburn *et al.*, 1994). Promising results have been

TABLE III
Major Viral and Parasitic Pathogens of Ocular Tissues

Organisms	References[a]
Coronavirus[b]	Wickham *et al.*, 1994
Herpesviruses	Syed and Hyndiuk, 1992; Tabarra and Hyndiuk, 1995
Cytomegalovirus	Huang *et al.*, 1994
Epstein-Barr virus	Pepose, 1994; Jones *et al.*, 1994
Herpes simplex	Holzberg *et al.*, 1992; Pepose, 1994
Adenoviris (Types 3,7,8,19)	Holzberg *et al.*, 1992; Syed and Hyndiuk, 1992
Papillomavirus 16	McDonnell *et al.*, 1992
Picornaviruses (Coxsackie virus A24)	Syed and Hyndiuk, 1992
Simian immunodeficiency virus	Conway *et al.*, 1991
Feline immunodeficiency virus	Callanan *et al.*, 1992
Onchocerca vulva	Taylor, 1994
Rhinosporidium seeberi	Gori and Scasso, 1994

[a]Selected primary articles and/or reviews of nonbacterial ocular pathogens.

[b]Infects and replicates in cultured rat lacrimal gland acinar cells; but its capacity to infect *in vivo* is not known.

TABLE IV
Recent Herpes Simplex Virus Vaccine Candidates

Vaccine	References[a]
Purified or synthetic glycoproteins	
gB, gC	Chan, 1983
gB, gC	Roberts *et al.*, 1985
gD-1, gD-2	Long *et al.*, 1984
gB-1, gD-1,-2	Dix and Mills, 1985
gD	Ishizaka and Mishkin, 1991; Burke *et al.*, 1994
Baculovirus-expressed glycoproteins	
gB, gI, gC, gE, gG, and/or gH	Ghiasi *et al.*, 1995
gB-2, gD-2	Nesburn *et al.*, 1994
Adenovirus-expressed glycoproteins	
gB	Gallichan *et al.*, 1993
Vaccina virus-expressed glycoproteins	Aurelian *et al.*, 1991; Rooney *et al.*, 1991; Banks *et al.*, 1994; Fleck *et al.*, 1994
Deletion mutants (gH)	Farrell *et al.*, 1994
Anti-sense nucleic acids	Cantin *et al.*, 1992

[a]Selected references; see also Rouse and Lopez, 1984; Dix, 1987; Mader and Stulting, 1992; Stanberry, 1994.

shown in extraocular infection models by several groups. These have included strategies of mucosal vaccination with recombinant adenovirus expressing herpes simplex virus gB (Gallichan *et al.*, 1993), subcutaneous immunization with virus constructs missing an essential glycoprotein (e.g., gH; Farrell *et al.*, 1994), and systemic delivery of synthetic peptides. Other approaches have included use of anti-sense nucleic acids (Cantin *et al.*, 1992) and use of other expression systems (e.g., baculovirus and vaccinia). Recent studies of cytokine responses associated with *in vivo* or *in vitro* anti-viral protection have implicated IL-6, IL-10, and TNFα in either recovery from or reduced herpes infection (Chen *et al.*, 1994; Tumpey *et al.*, 1994; Babu *et al.*, 1995). Further investigations are required to distinguish between T-cell-mediated immunopathologic effects (Newell *et al.*, 1989; Hendricks and Tumpey, 1990; Hendricks *et al.*, 1992) and the potential requirement for individual T-cell subsets in vaccine-induced immunity.

Several common parasitic infections may cause conjunctivitis. These include *Mulluscum contagiosum, Onchocerca vulva, Verruca vulgaris,* and *Trypanosoma cruzi.* In some cases, the conjunctival mucosa may be the portal of entry (e.g., *T. cruzi*). The pathologic results of trypanosomiasis include the oculoglandular or ophthalmoganglionar complex composed of lid edema, granulomatous conjunctivitis, follicles, and inflammation of the lacrimal gland. Parinaud's oculoglandular syndrome is rare, and may also be caused by additional viral or bacterial agents (e.g., *F. tularensis, M. tuberculosis*) (Syed and Hynduik, 1992).

Experimental models of conjunctival and lacrimal gland infections have been used for many years both to identify pathogenic and protective immune responses and, more recently, to evaluate vaccine candidates. Recent advances include new rat and rabbit models of adenovirus ocular infections, which should help in evaluation of immune-mediated responses to these pathogens (Tsai *et al.*, 1992; Gordon *et al.*, 1994).

V. Summary

It is clear that events taking place both in conjunctival tissue and lacrimal gland are relevant to ocular mucosal vaccination strategies. While the lacrimal gland functions as a primary effector site for mucosal IgA antibody responses, the precise relationship of the conjunctiva to the mucosal network requires further study. It appears that the conjunctiva plays a role in the induction of mucosal antibody responses as well as serving as an effector site for cell-mediated responses. A variety of factors are involved in the regulation of ocular mucosal antibody responses and many options such as immunization routes, delivery vehicles, and immune potentiators have been investigated. Although the development of appropriate immunization strategies will depend on the properties of each potential vaccine candidate as well as the target ocular pathogen, the appropriate technology is now available to elicit mucosal antibody responses at the ocular surface. The current challenge is to identify and select the vaccine component(s) that can be used to elicit long-term protective responses to ocular pathogens.

Acknowledgments

Studies from our laboratories which are summarized in this chapter were supported in part by NIH Grants EY05133, EY04068, and EY03324, and by Edna McConnell Clark Foundation Grants 10993, 11092, and 13594. The authors thank Linda Hazlett, Nancy O'Sullivan, Robert Prendergast, and Robert Swanborg for their critical assessment of this chapter and Nancy Hynous for secretarial support.

References

Aaberg, T. M. (1989). The expanding ophthalmologic spectrum of Lyme disease. *Am. J. Ophthalmol.* **107,** 77–80.

Allansmith, M. R., Kajiyama, G., Abelson, M. B., and Simon, M. A. (1976). Plasma cell content of main and accessory lacrimal glands and conjunctiva. *Am. J. Ophthalmol.* **82,** 819–826.

Allansmith, M. R., Korb, D. R., Greiner, J. V., Henriquez, A. S., Simon, M. A., and Finnemore, V. M. (1977). Giant papillary conjunctivitis in contact lens wearers. *Am. J. Ophthalmol.* **83,** 697–708.

Allen, J. E., and Stephens, R. S. (1993). An intermolecular mechanism of T cell help for the production of antibodies to the bacterial pathogen, *Chlamydia trachomatis. Eur. J. Immunol.* **23,** 1169–1172.

Aurelian, L., Smith, C. C., Wachsman, M., and Paoletti, E. (1991). Immune responses to herpes simplex virus in guinea pigs (footpad model) and mice immunized with vaccinia virus recombinants containing herpes simplex virus glycoprotein D. *Rev. Infect. Dis.* **13,** 924–934.

Babu, J. S., Kanangat, S., and Rouse, B. T. (1995). Cell cytokine mRNA expression during the course of the immunopathologic ocular disease herpetic stromal keratitis. *J. Immunol.* **154,** 4822–4829.

Banks, T. A., Jenkins, F. J., Kanagat, S., Nair, S., Dasgupta, S., Foster, C. M., and Rouse, B. T. (1994). Vaccination with the immediate-early protein ICP47 of herpes simplex virus-type 1 (HSV-1) induces virus-specific lymphoproliferation, but fails to protect against lethal challenge. *Virology* **200,** 236–245.

Barenfanger, J., and MacDonald, A. B. (1974). The role of immunoglobulin in the neutralization of trachoma infectivity. *J. Immunol.* **113,** 1607–1671.

Batteiger, B. E., Rank, R. G., Bavoil, P. M., and Soderberg,

L. S. F. (1993). Partial protection against genital reinfection by immunization of guinea pigs with isolated outer membrane proteins of the chlamydial agent guinea pig inclusion conjunctivitis. *J. Gen. Microbiol.* **139,** 2965–2972.

Beagley, K. W., Eldridge, J. H., Kiyono, H., Everson, M. P., Koopman, W. J., Honjo, T., and McGhee, J. R. (1988). Recombinant murine IL-5 induces high rate IgA synthesis in cycling IgA-positive Peyer's patch B cells. *J. Immunol.* **141,** 2035–2042.

Beagley, K. W., Eldridge, J. H., Lee, F., Kiyono, H., Everson, M. P., Koopman, W. J., Hirano, T., Kishimoto, T., and McGhee, J. R. (1989). Interleukins and IgA synthesis. Human and murine interleukin 6 induce high rate IgA secretion in IgA-committed B cells. *J. Exp. Med.* **169,** 2133–2148.

Beatty, P. R., and Stephens, R. S. (1994). $CD8^+$ T lymphocyte-mediated lysis of chlamydia-infected L cells using an endogenous antigen pathway. *J. Immunol.* **153,** 4588–4595.

Bergmann, K. C., Waldman, R. H., Tischner, H., and Pohl, W. D. (1986). Antibody in tears, saliva and nasal secretions following oral immunization of humans with inactivated influenza vaccine. *Int. Arch. Allergy Appl. Immunol.* **80,** 107–109.

Bergmann, K. C., Waldman, R. H., Reinhöfer, W. D., Pohl, W. D., Tischner, H., and Werchan, D. (1987). Oral immunization against influenza in children with asthma and chronic bronchitis. *Adv. Exp. Med. Biol.* **216,** 1685–1690.

Bernauer, W., Broadway, D. C., and Wright, P. (1993). Chronic progressive conjunctival cicatrisation. *Eye* **7,** 371–378.

Bessen, D., and Fischetti, V. A. (1988). Influence of intranasal immunization with synthetic peptides corresponding to conserved epitopes of M protein on mucosal colonization by group A streptococci. *Infect. Immun.* **56,** 2666–2672.

Bevilacqua, M. P. (1993). Endothelial–leukocyte adhesion molecules. *Annu. Rev. Immunol.* **11,** 767–804.

Brade, L., Schramek, S., Schade, U., and Brade, H. (1986). Chemical, biological and immunochemical properties of the *Chlamydial psittaci* lipopolysaccharide. *Infect. Immun.* **54,** 568–574.

Brandtzaeg, P. (1985). Role of J chain and secretory component in receptor-mediated glandular and hepatic transport of immunoglobulins in man. *Scand. J. Immunol.* **22,** 111–145.

Brandtzaeg, P., Gjeruldsen, S. T., Korsrud, F., Baklian, K., Berdal, P., and Ek, J. (1979). The human secretory immune system shows striking heterogeneity with regard to involvement of J chain-positive IgD immunocytes. *J. Immunol.* **122,** 503–510.

Brandtzaeg, P., Kett, K., and Rognum, T. O. (1987). Subclass distribution of IgG- and IgA-producing cells in secretory tissues and alterations related to gut diseases. *Adv. Exp. Med. Biol.* **216,** 321–333.

Brook, I., and Hulburd, C. S. (1993). *Pseudomonas aeruginosa* iatrogenic blepharoconjunctivitis. *Arch. Ophthalmol.* **111,** 26–27.

Brunham, R. C., and Peeling, R. W. (1994). *Chlamydia trachomatis* antigens: Role in immunity and pathogenesis. *Inf. Agents Dis.* **3,** 218–233.

Burke, R. L., Goldbeck, C., Ng, P., Stanberry, L., Ott, G., and Van Nest, G. (1994). The influence of adjuvant on the therapeutic efficacy of a recombinant genital herpes vaccine. *J. Infect. Dis.* **170,** 1110–1119.

Burns, C. A., Ebersole, J. L., and Allansmith, M. R. (1982). Immunoglobulin A antibody levels in human tears, saliva, and serum. *Infect. Immun.* **36,** 1019–1022.

Butcher, E. C. (1986). The regulation of lymphocyte traffic. *Curr. Top. Microbiol. Immunol.* **128,** 85–122.

Callanan, J. J., Thompson, H., Toth, S. R., O'Neil, B., Lawrence, C. E., Willett, B., and Jarrett, O. (1992). Clinical and pathological findings in feline immunodeficiency virus experimental infection. *Vet. Immunol. Immunopathol.* **35,** 3–13.

Campos, M. S., Campos e Silva, L deQ., Rehder, J. R., Lee, M. B., O'Brien, T., and McDonnell, P. J. (1994). Anaerobic flora of the conjunctival sac in patients with AIDS and with anophthalmia compared with normal eyes. *Acta Ophthalmol.* **72,** 241–245.

Campos, M., Pal S., O'Brien, T. P., Taylor, H. R., Prendergast, R. A., and Whittum-Hudson, J. A. (1995). A *chlamydial* major outer membrane protein extract as a trachoma vaccine candidate. *Invest. Ophthalmol. Visual Sci.* **36,** 1477–1491.

Cantin, E. M., Podsakoff, G., Willey, D. E., and Openshaw, H. (1992). Antiviral effects of herpes simplex virus specific anti-sense nucleic acids. *Adv. Exp. Med. Biol.* **312,** 139–149.

Carr, R. M., Lolachi, C. M., Albaran, R. G., Ridley, D. M., Montgomery, P. C., and O'Sullivan, N. L. (1996). Nasal-associated lymphoid tissue is an inductive site for rat tear IgA antibody responses. Submitted for publication.

Centifanto, Y., Norrild, B., Andersen, S. M., Karcioglu, Z. A., Porretta, E., and Caldwell, D. R. (1989). Herpes simplex virus-specific antibodies present in tears during herpes keratitis. *Proc. Soc. Exp. Biol. Med.* **192,** 87–94.

Challacombe, S. J., Rahman, D., Jeffrey, H., Davis, S. S., and O'Hagan, D. T. (1992). Enhanced secretory IgA and systemic IgG antibody response after oral immunization with biodegradable microparticles containing antigen. *Immunology* **76,** 164–168.

Chan, W. L. (1983). Protective immunization of mice with specific HSV-1 glycoprotein. *Immunology* **49,** 343–352.

Chandler, J. W., and Gillette, T. E. (1983). Immunologic defense mechanisms of the ocular surface. *Ophthalmology* **90,** 585–591.

Chen, S. H., Oakes, J. E., and Lausch, R. N. (1994). Synergistic anti-herpes effect of TNF-α and IFN-γ in human corneal epithelial cells compared with that in corneal fibroblasts. *Antiviral Res.* **25,** 201–213.

Childers, N. K., Bruce, M. G., and McGhee, J. R. (1989). Molecular mechanisms of immunoglobulin A defense. *Annu. Rev. Microbiol.* **43,** 503–536.

Chin, Y. H., Cai, J. P., and Hieselar, T. (1991a). Lymphocyte migration into mucosal lymphoid tissues: Mechanism and modulation. *Immunol. Rev.* **10,** 271–278.

Chin, Y. H., Sackstein, R., and Cai, J. P. (1991b). Lymphocyte homing receptors and preferential migration pathways. *Proc. Soc. Exp. Biol. Med.* **196,** 374–380.

Coffman, R. L., Shrader, B., Carty, J., Mosmann, T. R., and Bond, M. W. (1987). A mouse T cell product that preferentially enhances IgA production. I. Biologic characterization. *J. Immunol.* **139**, 3685–3690.

Coffman, R. L., Lebman, D. A., and Shrader, B. (1989). Transforming growth factor β specifically enhances IgA production by lipopolysaccharide-stimulated murine B lymphocytes. *J. Exp. Med.* **170**, 1039–1044.

Conway, M. D., Davison-Fairburn, B., Martin, L. N., Insler, M. S., and Murphey-Corb, M. (1991). Infection of rhesus monkeys with topical instillation of simian immunodeficiency virus (SIV) B670 into the conjunctival sac. *J. Med. Primatol.* **20**, 152–155.

Cousins, S. W., Trattler, W. B., and Streilein, J. W. (1991). Immune privilege and suppression of immunogenic inflammation in the anterior chamber of the eye. *Curr. Eye Res.* **10**, 287–297.

Crago, S. S., Kutteh, W. H., Moro, I., Allansmith, M. R., Radl, J., Haaijman, J. J., and Mestecky, J. (1984). Distribution of IgA1-, IgA2-, and J chain-containing cells in human tissues. *J. Immunol.* **132**, 16–18.

Czerkinsky, C., Prince, S. J., Michalek, S. M., Jackson, S., Moldoveanu, Z., Russell, M. W., McGhee, J. R., and Mestecky, J. (1987). Oral immunization with bacterial antigen induces IgA-secreting cells in peripheral blood in humans. *Adv. Exp. Med. Biol.* **216**, 1709–1719.

Damato, B. E., Allan, D., Murray, S. B., and Lee, W. R. (1984). Senile atrophy of the human lacrimal gland: The contribution of chronic inflammatory disease. *Br. J. Ophthalmol.* **68**, 674–680.

Davidson, H. J., Byrnes, S. A., and Montgomery, P. C. (1993). The effect of immunization on rat serum and tear antibody responses to *Chlamydia trachomatis. Reg. Immunol.* **5**, 114–119.

Dawson, C. R., Juster, R., Marx, R., Daghfous, M. T., and Ben Djerad, A. (1989). Limbal disease in trachoma and other ocular chlamydial infections: Risk factors for corneal vascularisation. *Eye* **3**, 204–209.

Dertzbaugh, M. T., and Elson, C. O. (1990). Cholera toxin as a mucosal adjuvant. *In* "Topics in Vaccine Adjuvant Research" (D. R. Spriggs and W. C. Koff, eds.), pp. 119–131. CRC Press, Boca Raton, Florida.

Dhingra, P. N., and Mahajan, V. M. (1991). Ocular chlamydial zoonosis: An experimental study in monkeys. *Comp. Immunol. Microbiol. Infect. Dis.* **14**, 235–241.

Dix, R. D. (1987). Prospects for a vaccine against herpes simplex virus type 1 and 2. *Prog. Med. Virol.* **34**, 89–128.

Dix, R. D., and Mills, J. (1985). Acute and latent herpes simplex virus neurological disease in mice immunized with purified virus-specific glycoproteins gB and gD. *J. Med. Virol.* **17**, 9–18.

Douglas, R. G., Rossen, R. D., Butler, W. T., and Couch, R. B. (1967). Rhinovirus neutralizing antibody in tears, parotid saliva, nasal secretions and serum. *J. Immunol.* **99**, 297–303.

Dua, H. S., Gomes, J. A., Jindall, V. K., Appa, S. N., Schwarting, R., Eagle, R. C. Jr., Donoso, L. A., and Laibson, P. R. (1994). Mucosa specific lymphocytes in human conjunctiva, corneoscleral limbus, and lacrimal gland. *Curr. Eye Res.* **13**, 87–93.

Dugel, P. U., and Rao, N. A. (1993). Ocular infections in the acquired immunodeficiency syndrome. *In* "New and Evolving Ocular Infections" (G. Smolin and M. H. Friedlander, eds.), pp. 103–127. Little, Brown, Boston.

Ebersole, J. L., Steffen, M. J., and Pappo, J. (1988). Secretory immune responses in aging rats. II. Phenotype distribution of lymphocytes in secretory and lymphoid tissues. *Immunology* **64**, 289–294.

Ehrhardt, R. O., Strober, W., and Harriman, G. R. (1992). Effect of transforming growth factor (TGF)-β1 on IgA isotype production. *J. Immunol.* **148**, 3830–3836.

Eldridge, J. H., Stass, J. K., Chen, D., Marx, P. A., Tice, T. R., and Gilley, R. M. (1993). New advances in vaccine delivery systems. *Semin. Hematol.* **30**, 16–24.

Elfaki, M. G., O'Sullivan, N. L., Skandera, C. A., and Montgomery, P. C. (1994). Inhibition of lymphocyte adherence to rat lacrimal gland acinar epithelium by interleukin-4 and transforming growth factor-β. *Cell. Immunol.* **153**, 154–162.

Elson, C. O., and Dertzbaugh, M. T. (1994). Mucosal adjuvants. *In* "Handbook of Mucosal Immunology" (P. L. Ogra, M. E. Lamm, J. R. McGhee, J. Mestecky, W. Strober, and J. Bienenstock, eds.), pp. 391–402. Academic Press, New York.

Farrell, H. E., McLean, C. S., Harley, C., Efstathiou, S., Inglis, S., and Minson, A. C. (1994). Vaccine potential of a herpes simplex virus type 1 mutant with an essential glycoprotein deleted. *J. Virol.* **68**, 927–932.

Fine, B. S., and Yanoff, M. (1979). "Ocular Histology." Harper and Row, Hagerstown, Maryland.

Fleck, M., Podlech, J., Weise, K., and Falke, D. (1994). A vaccinia virus–herpes simplex virus (HSV) glycoprotein B1 recombinant or an HSV vaccine overcome the HSV type 2 induced humoral immunosuppression and protect against vaginal challenge in BALB/c mice. *Med. Microbiol. Immunol.* **183**, 87–94.

Franklin, R. M. (1989). The ocular secretory immune system: A review. *Curr. Eye Res.* **8**, 599–606.

Franklin, R. M., and Montgomery, P. C. (1996). Lacrimal Gland Immunology. *In* "Ocular Infection and Immunity" (J. Pepose, G. Holland, and K. Wilhelmus, eds.), pp. 133–140. Mosby Year Book, Philadelphia.

Franklin, R. M., and Remus, L. E. (1984). Conjunctival-associated lymphoid tissue: Evidence for a role in the secretory immune system. *Invest. Ophthalmol. Visual Sci.* **25**, 181–187.

Franklin, R. M., and Shepard, K. F. (1990). T-cell adherence to lacrimal gland: The event responsible for IgA plasma cell predominance in lacrimal gland. *Regional Immunology* **3**, 213–216.

Franklin, R. M., Kenyon, K. R., and Tomasi, T. B. (1973). Immunohistologic studies of human lacrimal gland: Localization of immunoglobulins, secretory component and lactoferrin. *J. Immunol.* **110**, 984–992.

Franklin, R. M., Prendergast, R. A., and Silverstein, A. M. (1979). Secretory immune system of rabbit ocular adnexa. *Invest. Ophthalmol. Visual Sci.* **18**, 1093–1096.

Gallichan, W. S., Johnson, D. C., Graham, F. L., and Rosenthal, K. L. (1993). Mucosal immunity and protection after intranasal immunization with recombinant adenovirus expressing herpes simplex virus glycoprotein B. *J. Infect. Dis.* **168**, 622–662.

Gery, I., Mochizuki, M., and Nussenblatt, R. B. (1986). Retinal specific antigens and immunopathogenic processes they provoke. *In* "Progress in Retinal Research" (N. Osborne and J. Chader, eds.), pp. 75–109. Pergamon, New York.

Ghiasi, H., Bahri, S., Nesburn, A. B., and Wechsler, S. L. (1995). Protection against herpes simplex virus-induced eye disease after vaccination with seven individually expressed herpes simplex virus 1 glycoproteins. *Invest. Ophthalmol. Visual Sci.* **36,** 1352–1360.

Gillette, T. E., and Allansmith, M. R. (1980). Lactoferrin in human ocular tissues. *Am. J. Ophthalmol.* **90,** 30–37.

Gillette, T. E., Allansmith, M. R., Greiner, J. V., and Janusz, M. (1980). Histologic and immunohistologic comparison of main and accessory lacrimal tissue. *Am. J. Ophthalmol.* **89,** 724–730.

Gillette, T. E., Greiner, J. V., and Allansmith, M. R. (1981). Immunohistochemical localization of human tear lysozyme. *Arch. Ophthalmol.* **99,** 298–300.

Gordon, Y. J., Romanowski, E. G., and Araulio-Cruz, T. (1994). Topical HPMPC inhibits adenovirus type 5 in the New Zealand rabbit ocular replication model. *Invest. Ophthalmol. Visual Sci.* **35,** 4135–4143.

Gori, S., and Scasso, A. (1994). Cytologic and differential diagnosis of rhinosporidiosis. *Acta Cytol.* **38,** 361–366.

Grayston, J. T., Woolridge, R. L., and Wang, S. (1962). Trachoma vaccine studies on Taiwan. *Ann. N.Y. Acad. Sci.* **98,** 352–367.

Grayston, J. T., Wang, S. P., Yeh, L. J., and Kuo, C. C. (1985). Importance of reinfection in the pathogenesis of trachoma. *Rev. Infect. Dis.* **7,** 717–725.

Gregory, R. L., and Allansmith, M. R. (1986). Naturally occurring IgA antibodies to ocular and oral microorganisms in tears, saliva, and colostrum: Evidence for a common mucosal immune system and local immune response. *Exp. Eye Res.* **43,** 739–749.

Gregory, R. L., and Allansmith, M. R. (1987). Local immune responses in the ocular secretory immune system of humans. *Adv. Exp. Med. Biol.* **216,** 1749–1757.

Gregory, R. L., and Filler, S. J. (1987). Protective secretory immunoglobulin A antibodies in humans following oral immunization with *Streptococcus mutans*. *Infect. Immun.* **55,** 2409–2415.

Gregory, R. L., Scholler, M., Filler, S. J., Crago, S. S., Prince, S. J., Allansmith, M. R., Michalek, S. M., Mestecky, J., and McGhee, J. R. (1984). IgA antibodies to oral and ocular bacteria in human external secretions. *Protides Biol. Fluids* **32,** 53–56.

Gudmundsson, O. G., Cohen, E. J., Greiner, J. V., Taubman, M. A., and Allansmith, M. R. (1984). Mononuclear and IgA-containing cells in the lacrimal gland of germ-free and conventional rats. *Exp. Eye Res.* **39,** 575–581.

Gudmundsson, O. G., Sullivan, D. A., Bloch, K. J., and Allansmith, M. R. (1985). The ocular secretory immune system of the rat. *Exp. Eye Res.* **40,** 231–238.

Gudmundsson, O. G., Bjornsson, J., Olafsdottir, K., Bloch, K. J., Allansmith, M. R., and Sullivan, D. A. (1988). T cell populations in the lacrimal gland during aging. *Acta Ophthalmol.* **66,** 490–497.

Hann, L. E., Allansmith, M. R., and Sullivan, D. A. (1988). Impact of aging and gender on the Ig-containing cell profile of the lacrimal gland. *Acta Ophthalmol.* **66,** 87–92.

Hann, L. E., Kelleher, R. S., and Sullivan, D. A. (1991). Influence of culture conditions on the androgen control of secretory component production by acinar cells from the lacrimal gland. *Invest. Ophthalmol. Visual Sci.* **32,** 2610–2621.

Harriman, G. R., Kuminoto, D. Y., Elliot, J. F., Paetkau, V., and Strober, W. (1988). The role of IL-5 in IgA B cell differentiation. *J. Immunol.* **140,** 3033–3039.

Hayes, L. J., Conlan, J. W., Everson, J. S., Ward, M. E., and Clarke, I. N. (1991). *Chlamydia trachomatis* major outer membrane protein epitopes expressed as fusion with LamB in an attenuated aro A strain of *Salmonella typhimurium;* their application as potential immunogens. *J. Gen. Microbiol.* **137,** 1557–1564.

Hazlett, L. D., Rosen, D., and Berk, R. S. (1976). Experimental eye infections caused by *Pseudomonas aeruginosa*. *Ophthalm. Res.* **6,** 311–318.

Heggie, A. D., and Lass, J. H. (1994). Chlamydial infections. *In* "Principles and Practice of Ophthalmology: Basic Sciences" (D. M. Albert and F. A. Jakobiec, eds.), pp. 840–854. Saunders, Philadelphia, Pennsylvania.

Hendricks, R. L., and Tumpey, T. M. (1990). Contribution of virus and immune factors to herpes simplex virus type 1 induced corneal pathology. *Invest. Ophthalmol. Visual Sci.* **31,** 1929–1939.

Hendricks, R. L., Janowicz, M., and Tumpey, T. M. (1992). Critical role of Langerhans cells in the CD4- but not CD8-mediated immunopathology in herpes simplex virus-1 infected mouse corneas. *J. Immunol.* **148,** 2522–2529.

Holzberg, M., Stulting, D., and Drake, L. A. (1992). Ocular and periocular infections. *In* "Dermatologic Clinics: Oculocutaneous Diseases II" (M. M. Grant-Kels, M. J. Rothe, and B. D. Kels, eds.), pp. 741–761. Saunders, Philadelphia, Pennsylvania.

Huang, Z., Lambert, R. W., Wickham, L. A., and Sullivan, D. A. (1993). Influence of the endocrine environment on herpes virus infection in rat lacrimal gland acinar cells. *In* "Lacrimal Gland, Tear Film and Dry Eye Syndromes: Basic Science and Clinical Relevance" (D. A. Sullivan, ed.), pp. 189–192. Plenum, New York.

Hutchinson, F. G., and Furr, B. J. A. (1985). Biodegradable polymers for the sustained release of peptides. *Biochem. Soc. Trans.* **13,** 520–523.

Ishizaka, S. T., and Mishkin, E. M. (1991). Native HSV glycoprotein D subunit vaccine: Analysis of *in vitro* T-cell activation and antigen presentation. *Viral Immunol.* **4,** 187–193.

Jalkanen, S., Nash, G. S., De los Toyes, J., MacDermott, R. P., and Butcher, E. C. (1989). Human lamina propria lymphocytes bear homing receptors and bind selectively to mucosal high endothelium. *Eur. J. Immunol.* **19,** 63–68.

Jones, R. B., and Van der Pol, R. (1994). Lack of correlation between acquisition of infection and ability of serum to neutralize chlamydial infection *in vivo*. *In* "Chlamydial Infections: Proceedings of the 8th International Symposium on Human Chlamydial Infections" (J. Orfila, G. I. Byrne, M. A. Chernesky, J. T. Grayston, R. B. Jones, G. L. Ridgway, P. Saikku, J. Schachter, W. E. Stamm, and R. S. Stephens, eds.), pp. 95–98. Societa Editrice Escalapio, Bologna, Italy.

Jones, D. T., Monroy, D., Ji, Z., Atherton, S. S., and Pflungfelder, S. C. (1994). Sjögren's syndrome: Cytokine and Epstein-Barr viral expression within the conjunctival epithelium. *Invest. Ophthalmol. Visual Sci.* **35**, 3493–3504.

Kelleher, R. S., Hann, L. E., Edwards, J. A., and Sullivan, D. A. (1991). Endocrine, neural and immune control of secretory component output by lacrimal gland acinar cells. *J. Immunol.* **146**, 3405–3412.

Kett, K., Brandtzaeg, P., Radl, J., and Haiijman, J. J. (1986). Different subclass distribution of IgA-producing cells in human lymphoid organs and various secretory tissues. *J. Immunol.* **136**, 3631–3635.

King, S., Devi, S. P., Mindoff, C., Patrick, M. L., Gold, R., and Ford-Jones, E. L. (1988). Noscorneal *Pseudomonas aeruginosa* conjunctivitis in a pediatric hospital. *Infect. Control Hosp. Epidemol.* **9**, 77–80.

Kiyono, H., Bienenstock, J., McGhee, J. R., and Ernst, P. B. (1992). The mucosal immune system: Features of inductive and effector sites to consider in mucosal immunization and vaccine development. *Regional Immunology* **4**, 54–62.

Knopf, H. L. S., Bertran, D. M., and Kapikian, A. Z. (1970). Demonstration and characterization of antibody in tears following intranasal vaccination with inactivated type 13 rhinovirus: A preliminary report. *Invest. Ophthalmol.* **9**, 727–734.

Knorr, H. L. J., and Weber, A. (1994). Zoonoses and ocular infections. *In* "Infectious Diseases of the Eye" (A. A. Bialasiewicz and K. P. Schaal, eds.), pp. 362–372. Aeolus Press, Buren, The Netherlands.

Lacey, C. J., Clarke, A. M., Fraser, P., Metcalfe, T., Bonsor, G., and Curry, A. (1992). Chronic microsporidial infection of the nasal mucosae, sinuses, and conjunctivae in HIV disease. *Genitourin. Med.* **68**, 179–181.

Lepper, A. W., Elleman, T. C., Hoyne, P. A., Lehrbach, P. R., Atwell, J. L., Schwartzkoff, C. L., Egerton, J. R., and Tennent, J. M. (1993). A *Moraxella bovis* pili vaccine produced by recombinant DNA technology for the prevention of infectious bovine keratoconjunctivitis. *Vet. Microbiol.* **36**, 175–183.

Liesegang, T. J. (1993). The biology of herpes simplex and varicella zoster virus infection. *In* "New and Evolving Ocular Infections" (G. Smolin and M. H. Friedlander, eds.), pp. 81–93. Little, Brown, Boston.

Linde, K., Randhagen, B., Beer, J., Dentchev, V., Marinova, S., Vassilev, T., and Bratoyeva, M. (1993). *Shigella flexneri* 2a and *sonnei* 1 vaccine with two attenuating markers: Construction, tolerability, and immunogenicity in 143 children aged 13–17 years. *Vaccine* **11**, 197–199.

Liu, S. H., Tagawa, Y., Prendergast, R. A., Franklin, R. M., and Silverstein, A. M. (1981). Secretory component of IgA: A marker for differentiation of ocular epithelium. *Invest. Ophthalmol. Visual Sci.* **20**, 100–119.

Long, D., Madara, T., Ponce de Leon, M., Cohen, G. H., Montgomery, P. C., and Eisenberg, R. J. (1984). Glycoprotein D protects mice against lethal challenge with herpes simplex virus types 1 and 2. *Invest. Immun.* **37**, 761–764.

Lowder, C. Y. (1993). Ocular microsporidiosis. *In* "New and Evolving Ocular Infections" (G. Smolin and M. H. Friedlander, eds.), pp. 145–151. Little, Brown, Boston.

Lukacova, M., Baumann, M., Brade, L., Mamat, U., and Brade, H. (1994). Lipopolysaccharide smooth–rough phase variation in bacteria of the genus *Chlamydia*. *Infect. Immun.* **62**, 2270–2276.

Lycke, N., and Holmgren, J. (1986). Strong adjuvant properties of cholera toxin on gut mucosal immune responses to orally presented antigens. *Immunology* **59**, 301–308.

MacDonald, A. B., McComb, D., and Howard, L. (1984). Immune response of owl monkeys to topical vaccination with irradiated *Chlamydia trachomatis*. *J. Infect. Dis.* **149**, 439–442.

McDermott, M. R., and Bienenstock, J. B. (1979). Evidence for a common mucosal immunologic system. I Migration of B immunoblasts into intestinal, respiratory and genital tissues. *J. Immunol.* **122**, 1892–1898.

McDonnell, J. M., McDonnell, P. J., and Sun, Y. Y. (1992). Human papillomavirus DNA in tissues and ocular surface swabs of patients with conjunctival epithelial neoplasia. *Invest. Ophthalmol. Visual Sci.* **33**, 184–189.

McGee, D. W., and Franklin, R. M. (1984). Lymphocyte migration into the lacrimal gland is random. *Cell Immunol.* **86**, 75–82.

McGhee, J. R., and Mestecky, J. (1990). In defense of mucosal surfaces. Development of novel vaccines for IgA responses protective at the portals of entry of microbial pathogens. *Infect. Dis. Clinics N. Am.* **4**, 315–341.

McGill, J. I., Liakos, G. M., Goulding, N., and Seal, D. V. (1984). Normal tear protein profiles and age-related changes. *Br. J. Ophthalmol.* **68**, 316–320.

Mabey, D. C., Holland, M. J., Viswalingam, N. D., Goh, B. T., Estreich, S., Macfarlane, A., Dockrell, H. M., and Treharne, J. D. (1991). Lymphocyte proliferative responses to chlamydial antigens in human chlamydial eye infections. *Clin. Exp. Immunol.* **86**, 37–42.

Mabey, D. C., Bailey, R. L., Ward, M. E., and Whittle, H. C. (1992). A longitudinal study of trachoma in a Gambian village: Implications concerning the pathogenesis of chlamydial infection. *Epidemiol. Infect.* **108**, 343–351.

Mader, T. H., and Stulting, R. D. (1992). Viral keratitis. *Infect. Dis. Clin. North Am.* **6**, 831–849.

Malaty, R., Dawson, C. R., Wong, I., Lyon, C., and Schechter, J. (1981). Serum and tear antibodies to chlamydia after reinfection with guinea pig inclusion conjunctivitis agent. *Invest. Ophthalmol. Visual Sci.* **21**, 833–841.

Maloy, K. J., Donachie, A. M., O'Hagan, D. T., and Mowat, A. McI. (1994). Induction of mucosal and systemic immune responses by immunization with ovalbumin entrapped in poly(lactide-co-glycolide) microparticles. *Immunology* **81**, 661–667.

Mestecky, J., and McGhee, J. R. (1987). Immunoglobulin A (IgA): Molecular and cellular interactions involved in IgA biosynthesis and immune response. *Adv. Immunol.* **40**, 153–245.

Mestecky, J., McGhee, J. R., Arnold, R. R., Michalek, S. M., Prince, S. J., and Babb, J. C. (1978). Selective induction of an immune response in human external secretions by ingestion of bacterial antigen. *J. Clin. Invest.* **61**, 731–737.

Michalek, S. M., Eldridge, J. H., Curtiss, R., and Rosenthal, K. (1994). Antigen delivery systems. New approaches to mucosal immunization. *In* "Handbook of Mucosal Immunology" (P. L. Ogra, M. E. Lamm, J. R. McGhee, J.

Mestecky, W. Strober, and J. Bienenstock, eds.), pp. 373–390. Academic Press, New York.

Michalek, S. M., Childers, N. K., and Dertzbaugh, M. T. (1995). Vaccination strategies for mucosal pathogens. *In* "Virulence Mechanisms of Bacterial pathogens" (J. A. Roth, C. Bolin, K. Brogden, C. Minion, and M. Wannemuehaler, eds.), pp. 269–301. American Society for Microbiology, Washington, D.C.

Mondino, B. J., Brawman-Mintzer, O., and Adamu, S. A. (1987a). Corneal antibody levels to ribitol teichoic acid in rabbits immunized with staphylococcal antigens using various routes. *Invest. Ophthalmol. Visual Sci.* **28,** 1553–1558.

Mondino, B. J., Laheji, A. J., and Adamu, S. A. (1987b). Ocular immunity to *Staphylococcus aureus. Invest. Ophthalmol. Visual Sci.* **28,** 560–564.

Mondino, B. J., Adamu, S. A., and Pitchekian-Halabi, H. (1991). Antibody studies in a rabbit model corneal phlyctenulosis and catarrhal infiltrates related to *Staphylococcus aureus. Invest. Ophthalmol. Visual Sci.* **32,** 1854–1863.

Montgomery, P. C., and Liberati, D. M. (1995). A lymph derived fraction inhibits lymphocyte adherence to lacrimal gland acinar epithelium. *Invest. Ophthalmol. Visual Sci. Suppl.* **36,** 651.

Montgomery, P. C., Ayyildiz, A., Lemaitre-Coelho, I. M., Vaerman, J. P., and Rockey, J. H. (1983). Induction and expression of antibodies in secretions. The ocular immune system. *Ann. N.Y. Acad. Sci.* **409,** 428–440.

Montgomery, P. C., Rockey, J. H., Majumdar, A. S., Lemaitre-Coelho, I. M., Vaerman, J. P., and Ayyildiz, A. (1984a). Parameters influencing the expression of IgA antibodies in tears. *Invest. Ophthalmol. Visual Sci.* **25,** 369–373.

Montgomery, P. C., Majumdar, A. S., Skandera, C. A., and Rockey, J. H. (1984b). The effect of immunization route and sequence of stimulation on the induction of IgA antibodies in tears. *Curr. Eye Res.* **3,** 861–865.

Montgomery, P. C., Skandera, C. A., and Majumdar, A. S. (1985). Evidence for migration of IgA bearing lymphocytes between peripheral mucosal sites. *Protides Biol. Fluids* **32,** 43–46.

Montgomery, P. C., Peppard, J. V., and Skandera, C. A. (1989). Isolation and characterization of mononuclear cell populations from lacrimal glands. *In* "Modern Trends in Immunology and Immunopathology of the Eye" (A. G. Secchi and I. A. Fregona, eds.), pp. 339–343. Masson, Milano, Italy.

Montgomery, P. C., Peppard, J. V., and Skandera, C. A. (1990). A comparison of lymphocyte subset distribution in rat lacrimal glands with cells from tissues of mucosal and non-mucosal origin. *Curr. Eye Res.* **9,** 85–93.

Montgomery, P. C., O'Sullivan, N. L., Martin, L. B., Skandera, C. A., Peppard, J. V., and Pockley, A. G. (1994). Regulation of lacrimal gland immune responses. *In* "Lacrimal Gland, Tear Film, and Dry Eye Syndromes. Basic Science and Clinical Relevance." (D. A. Sullivan, ed.), pp. 161–168. Plenum, New York.

Moritera, T., Ogura, Y., Yoshimura, N., Honda, Y., Wada, R., Hyon, S.-H., and Ikada, Y. (1992). Biodegradable microspheres containing adriamycin in the treatment of proliferative vitreoretinopathy. *Invest. Ophthalmol. Visual Sci.* **33,** 3125–3130.

Morrison, R. P., Belland, R. J., Lyng, K., and Caldwell, H. D. (1989a). Chlamydial disease pathogenesis. The 57-kD chlamydial hypersensitivity antigen is a stress response protein. *J. Exp. Med.* **170,** 1271–1283.

Morrison, R. P., Lyng, K., and Caldwell, H. D. (1989b). Chlamydial disease pathogenesis. Ocular hypersensitivity elicited by a genus-specific 57-kD protein. *J. Exp. Med.* **169,** 663–675.

Murdin, A. D., Su, H., Manning, D. S., Klein, M. H., Parnell, M. J., and Caldwell, H. D. (1993). A poliovirus hybrid expressing a neutralization epitope from the major outer membrane protein of *Chlamydia trachomatis* is highly immunogenic. *Infect. Immun.* **61,** 4406–4414.

Murdin, A. D., Su, H., Klein, M. H., and Caldwell, H. D. (1995). Poliovirus hybrids expressing neutralization epitopes from variable domains I and IV of the major outer membrane protein of *Chlamydia trachomatis* elicit broadly cross-reactive *C. trachomatis*-neutralizing antibodies. *Infect. Immun.* **63,** 1116–1121.

Murphy, J. C., Ackerman, J. I., Marini, R. P., and Fox, J. G. (1991). Cervical lymphadenitis in guinea pigs: Infection via intact ocular and nasal mucosa by *Streptococcus zooepidemicus. Lab. Anim. Sci.* **41,** 251–254.

Murrah, W. F. (1988). Epidemic keratoconjunctivitis. *Ann. Ophthalmol.* **20,** 36–38.

Murray, E. S., Charbonnet, L. T., and MacDonald, A. B. (1973). Immunity to chlamydial infections of the eye. I. The role of circulatory and secretory antibodies in resistance to reinfection with guinea pig inclusion conjunctivitis. *J. Immunol.* **110,** 1518–1525.

Nair, P. N. R., and Schroeder, H. E. (1986). Duct-associated lymphoid tissue (DALT) of minor salivary glands and mucosal immunity. *Immunology* **57,** 171–180.

Nesburn, A. B., Burke, R. L., Ghiasi, H., Slanina, S., Bahri, S., and Wechsler, S. L. (1994). Vaccine therapy for ocular herpes simplex virus (HSV) infection: Periocular vaccination reduces spontaneous ocular HSV type 1 shedding in latently infected rabbits. *J. Virol.* **68,** 5084–5092.

Newell, C. K., Martin, S., Sendeli, D., Mercadal, C. M., and Rouse, B. T. (1989). Herpes simplex virus-induced stromal keratitis: Role of T-lymphocyte subsets in immunopathology. *J. Virol.* **63,** 769–775.

Newhall, W. J., Batteiger, B., and Jones, R. B. (1982). Analysis of human serological responses to proteins of *Chlamydia trachomatis. Infect. Immun.* **38,** 1181–1189.

Nichols, R. L., Bell, S. D., Jr., Murray, E. S., Haddad, N. A., and Bobb, A. A. (1966). Studies on trachoma. V. Clinical observations in a field of bivalent trachoma vaccine at three dosage levels in Saudi Arabia. *Am. J. Trop. Med. Hyg.* **15,** 639–647.

Nichols, R. L., Bell, S. D., Jr., Haddad, N. A., and Bobb, A. A. (1969). Studies on trachoma. VI. Microbiological observations in a field trial in Saudi Arabia of bivalent trachoma vaccine at three dosage levels. *Am. J. Trop. Med. Hyg.* **18,** 723–730.

Nichols, R. L., Oertley, R. E., Fraser, C. E. O., MacDonald, A. B., and McComb, D. E. (1973). Immunity to chlamydial infections of the eye. VI. Homologous neutralization of trachoma infectivity for the owl monkey conjunctivae by eye secretions from humans with trachoma. *J. Infect. Dis.* **127,** 429–431.

Niederkorn, J. Y., and Ferguson, T. A. (1996). Anterior chamber associated immune deviation (ACAID). *In* "Ocular Infection and Immunity" (J. S. Pepose, G. N. Holland, and K. R. Wilhelmus, eds.) pp. 96–103. Mosby Year Book, Philadelphia.

O'Brien, T. P., Maclean, I., Edidin, M., Prendergast, R. A., and Whittum-Hudson, J. A. (1994). Immunogenicity and partial protection against ocular chlamydia with a MOMP VD4-fusion protein. *Invest. Ophthalmol. Visual Sci. Suppl.* **35,** 1301.

O'Hagan, D. T. (1994). Microparticles as oral vaccines. *In* "Novel Delivery Systems for Oral Vaccines" (D. T. O'Hagan, ed.), pp. 175–205. CRC Press, Boca Raton, Florida.

O'Hagan, D. T., Rahman, D., McGee, J. P., Jeffrey, H., Davies, M. C., Williams, P., Davis, S. S., and Challacombe, S. J. (1991). Biodegradable microparticles as controlled release antigen delivery systems. *Immunology* **73,** 239–242.

Orenstein, N. S., Mull, J. D., and Thompson III, S. E. (1973). Immunity to chlamydial infections of the eye. V. Passive transfer of antitrachoma antibodies to owl monkeys. *Infect. Immun.* **7,** 600–603.

O'Sullivan, N. L., and Montgomery, P. C. (1990). Selective interactions of lymphocytes with neonatal and adult lacrimal tissues. *Invest. Ophthalmol. Visual Sci.* **31,** 1615–1622.

O'Sullivan, N. L., Skandera, C. A., Chin, Y. H., and Montgomery, P. C. (1994a). *In vitro* adhesive interactions between rat lymphocytes and lacrimal gland epithelium. Phenotype of adherent lymphocytes and involvement of adhesion molecules. *J. Immunol.* **152,** 1684–1692.

O'Sullivan, N. L., Raja, R., and Montgomery, P. C. (1994b). Lymphocyte adhesive interaction with lacrimal gland acinar epithelium involves carbohydrate recognition. *In* "Lacrimal Gland, Tear Film, and Dry Eye Syndromes: Basic Science and Clinical Relevance" (D. A. Sullivan, ed.), pp. 181–184. Plenum, New York.

O'Sullivan, N. L., Raja, R., and Montgomery, P. C. (1995). Lymphocyte adhesive interactions with lacrimal gland acinar epithelial cells in primary culture. *Invest. Ophthal. Visual Sci.* **36,** 2246–2253.

Pal, S., Taylor, H. R., and Whittum-Hudson, J. A. (1990a). Identification of fine antigenic specificities of antibody responses in experimental *Chlamydia trachomatis* infection. *Invest. Ophthalmol. Visual Sci. Suppl.* **31,** 448.

Pal, S., Pu, Z., Huneke, R. B., Taylor, H. R., and Whittum-Hudson, J. A. (1990b). Chlamydia-specific lymphocytes in conjunctiva during ocular infection: Limiting dilution analysis. *Regional Immunology* **3,** 171–178.

Pal, S., Taylor, H. R., Huneke, R. B., Prendergast, R. A., and Whittum-Hudson, J. A. (1992). Frequency of antigen-specific B cells during experimental ocular *Chlamydia trachomatis* infection. *Infect. Immun.* **60,** 5294–5297.

Pal, S., Fielder, T. J., Peterson, E. M., and de la Maza, L. M. (1994). Protection against infertility in a BALB/c mouse salpingitis model by intranasal immunization with the mouse pneumonitis biovar of *Chlamydia trachomatis. Infect. Immun.* **62,** 3354–3362.

Pappo, J., Ebersole, J. L., and Taubman, M. A. (1988a). Resident salivary gland macrophages function as accessory cells in antigen-dependent T-cell proliferation. *Immunology* **63,** 95–104.

Pappo, J., Ebersole, J. L., and Taubman, M. A. (1988b). Phenotype and mononuclear leucocytes resident in rat major salivary and lacrimal glands. *Immunology* **64,** 295–300.

Patton, D. L. (1990). Experimental systems. *In* "Chlamydial Infections" (W. R. Bowie, H. D. Caldwell, R. P. Jones, P. Mardh, G. L. Ridgeway, J. Schachter, W. E. Stamm, and M. E. Ward, eds.), pp. 223–231. Cambridge Univ. Press, New York.

Pepose, J. S. (1994). Ocular features of sexually transmitted herpetic infections. *In* "Infectious Diseases of the Eye" (A. A. Bialasiewicz and K. P. Schaal eds.), pp. 535–544. Aeolus Press, Buren, The Netherlands.

Pepose, J. S., Akata, R. F., Pflugfelder, S. C., and Voigt, W. (1990). Mononuclear cell phenotypes and immunoglobulin gene rearrangements in lacrimal gland biopsies from patients with Sjögren's syndrome. *Ophthalmology* **97,** 1599–1605.

Peppard, J. V., and Montgomery, P. C. (1987). Studies on the origin and composition of IgA in rat tears. *Immunology* **62,** 194–198.

Peppard, J. V., and Montgomery, P. C. (1990). Optimising the expression of antibody in tears: Manipulation of the common mucosal immune response? *In* "Advances in Mucosal Immunology" (T. T. MacDonald, S. J. Challacombe, P. W. Bland, C. R. Stokes, R. V. Heatley, and A.McI. Mowat, eds.), pp. 513–517. Kluwer, London.

Peppard, J. V., Mann, R. V., and Montgomery, P. C. (1988). Antibody production in rats following ocular–topical or gastrointestinal immunization: Kinetics of local and systemic antibody production. *Curr. Eye Res.* **7,** 471–481.

Picker, L. J., and Butcher, E. C. (1992). Physiological and molecular mechanisms of lymphocyte homing. *Annu. Rev. Immunol.* **10,** 561–591.

Pockley, A. G., and Montgomery, P. C. (1990). The effects of interleukins 5 and 6 on immunoglobulin production in rat lacrimal glands. *Regional Immunology* **3,** 242–246.

Pockley, A. G., and Montgomery, P. C. (1991). *In vivo* adjuvant effects of interleukins 5 and 6 on rat tear IgA antibody responses. *Immunology* **73,** 19–23.

Rafferty, D. E., and Montgomery, P. C. (1993). The effects of transforming growth factor-β on immunoglobulin production in cultured rat lacrimal gland tissue fragments. *Regional Immunology* **5,** 312–316.

Rafferty, D. E., Elfaki, M. G., and Montgomery, P. C. (1996). Preparation and characterization of a biodegradable microparticle antigen/cytokine delivery system. *Vaccine* **14,** 532–538.

Ramphal, R. R., McNiecc, M. T., and Polack, F. M. (1981). Adherence of *Pseudomonas aeruginosa* to the injured cornea: A step in the pathogenesis of corneal infections. *Ann. Ophthalmol.* **13,** 421–425.

Ramsay, A. J., Husband, A. J., Ramshaw, I. A., Bas, S., Matthaei, K. I., Koehler, G., and Kopf, M. (1994). The role of interleukin-6 in the mucosal IgA antibody responses *in vivo. Science* **264,** 561–563.

Rank, R., and Whittum-Hudson, J. A. (1994). Animal models for ocular infection. *In* "Methods in Enzymology, Volume 235: Bacterial Pathogenesis" (V. L. Clark and P. M. Bavoli, eds.), pp. 69–83. Academic Press, New York.

Rank, R. G., Dascher, C., Bowlin, A. K., and Bavoil, P. M. (1995). Systemic immunization with Hsp60 alters the development of chlamydial ocular disease. *Invest. Ophthalmol. Visual Sci.* **36,** 1344–1351.

Reacher, M. H., Pe'er, J., Rapoza, P. A., Whittum-Hudson, J. A., and Taylor, H. R. (1991). T cells and trachoma. Their role in cicatricial disease. *Ophthalmology* **98,** 334–341.

Roberts, P. L., Duncan, B. E., Raybould, T. J. G., and Watson, D. H. (1985). Purification of herpes simplex virus glycoproteins B and C using monoclonal antibodies and their ability to protect mice against lethal challenge. *J. Gen. Virol.* **66,** 1073–1085.

Rocha, G., Baines, M. G., and Deschenes, J. (1992). The immunology of the eye and its systemic interactions. *Crit. Rev. Immunol.* **12,** 81–100.

Rogers, D. G., Anderson, A. A., Hogg, A., Nielsen, D. L., and Huebert, M. A. (1993). Conjunctivitis and keratoconjunctivitis associated with chlamydiae in swine. *J. Am. Vet. Med. Assoc.* **203,** 1321–1323.

Rooney, J. F., Wohlenberg, C. R., Moss, B., and Notkins, A. L. (1991). Live vaccinia virus recombinants expressing herpes simplex virus genes. *Rev. Infect. Dis.* **13,** 898–903.

Rouse, B. T., and Lopez, C. (1984). Strategies for immune intervention against herpes simplex virus. *In* "Immunobiology of Herpes Simplex Virus Infection" (B. T. Rouse and C. Lopez, eds.), pp. 145–156. CRC Press, Boca Raton, Florida.

Roux, M. E., McWilliams, M., Phillips-Quagliata, J. M., and Lamm, M. E. (1977). Origin of IgA-secreting cells in the mammary gland. *J. Exp. Med.* **146,** 1311–1322.

Sacks, E. H., Wieczorek, R., Jakobiec, F. A., and Knowles, D. M. (1986). Lymphocytic subpopulations in the normal human conjunctiva. A monoclonal antibody study. *Ophthalmology* **93,** 1276–1283.

Schachter, J. (1985). Overview of *Chlamydia trachomatis* infection and the requirements for a vaccine. *Rev. Infect. Dis.* **7,** 713–716.

Shimada, K., and Silverstein, A. M. (1975). Local antibody formation within the eye: A study of immunoglobulin class and antibody specificity. *Invest. Ophthalmol.* **14,** 573–583.

Shimizu, Y., Newman, W., Tanaka, Y., and Shaw, S. (1992). Lymphocyte interactions with endothelial cells. *Immunol. Today* **13,** 106–112.

Solari, R., and Kraehenbuhl, J. P. (1985). The biosynthesis of secretory component and its role in the transepithelial transport of IgA dimer. *Immunol. Today* **6,** 17–20.

Soldati, M., Verini, M. A., Isetta, A. M., and Ghione, M. (1971). Immunization research in the field of trachoma. Some laboratory and clinical contributions. *In* "Trachoma and Related Disorders" (R. L. Nichols, ed.), pp. 407–417. Excerpta Medica, Amsterdam.

Soukiasian, S. H., Rice, B., Foster, C. S., and Lee, S. J. (1992). The T cell receptor in normal and inflamed human conjunctiva. *Invest. Ophthalmol. Visual Sci.* **33,** 453–459.

Srinivasan, B. D., Jakobiec, F. A., and Iwamoto, T. (1990). Conjunctiva. *In* "Duanes's Biomedical Foundations of Ophthalmology" (W. Tasman and E. A. Jaeger, eds.), pp. 1–28. Lippincott, New York.

Stagg, A. J., Elsley, W. A., Pickett, M. A., Ward, M. E., and Knight, S. C. (1993). Primary human T-cell responses to the major outer membrane protein of *Chlamydia trachomatis. Immunology* **79,** 1–9.

Stanberry, L. R. (1994). The concept of immune-based therapies in chronic viral infections. *J. Acquired Immune Defic. Syndr.* **7,** 1–5.

Stanisz, A. M., Bienenstock, J., and Agro, A. (1989). Neuromodulation of mucosal immunity. *Regional Immunology* **2,** 414–419.

Starnbach, M. N., Bevan, M. J., and Lampe, M. F. (1994). Protective cytotoxic T lymphocytes are induced during murine infection with *Chlamydia trachomatis. J. Immunol.* **153,** 5183–5189.

Stephens, R. S. (1990). Molecular genetics of chlamydia. *In* "Chlamydial Infections" (W. R. Bowie, H. D. Caldwell, R. P. Jones, P. Mardh, G. L. Ridgway, J. Schachter, W. E. Stamm, and M. E. Ward, eds.), pp. 64–72. Cambridge Univ. Press, Cambridge.

Stoolman, L. M. (1989). Adhesion molecules controlling lymphocyte migration. *Cell (Cambridge, Mass.)* **56,** 907–910.

Streilein, J. W. (1987). Immune regulation and the eye: A dangerous compromise. *FASEB J.* **1,** 199–208.

Streilein, J. W. (1990). Anterior chamber associated immune deviation: the privilege of immunity in the eye. *Ophthalmology* **35,** 67–73.

Streilein, J. W. (1993). Immune privilege as the result of local tissue barriers and immunosuppressive microenvironments. *Curr. Opin. Immunol.* **5,** 428–432.

Stuart, E. S., and MacDonald, A. B. (1989). Some characteristics of a secreted chlamydial antigen recognized by IgG from *Chlamydia trachomatis* patient sera. *Immunology* **68,** 469–473.

Stuart, E. S., Wyrick, P. B., Choong, J., Stoler, S. B., and MacDonald, A. B. (1991). Examination of chlamydial glycolipid with monoclonal antibodies: Cellular distribution and epitope binding. *Immunology* **74,** 740–747.

Stuart, E. S., Troidle, K. M., and MacDonald, A. B. (1994). Chlamydial glycolipid antigen: Extracellular accumulation, biological activity, and antibody recognition. *Curr. Microbiol.* **28,** 85–90.

Sullivan, D. A. (1988). Influence of the hypothalamic-pituitary axis on the androgen regulation of the ocular secretory immune system. *J. Steroid Biochem.* **30,** 429–433.

Sullivan, D. A. (1990). Hormonal influence on the secretory immune system of the eye. *In* "The Neuroendocrine-Immune Network" (S. Freier, ed.), pp. 199–237. CRC Press, Boca Raton, Florida.

Sullivan, D. A. (1994). Ocular mucosal immunity. *In* "Handbook of Mucosal Immunology" (P. L. Ogra, M. E. Lamm, J. R. McGhee, J. Mestecky, W. Stober, and J. Bienenstock, eds.), pp. 569–597. Academic Press, New York.

Sullivan, D. A., and Allansmith, M. R. (1984). Source of IgA in tears of rats. *Immunology* **53,** 791–799.

Sullivan, D. A., and Allansmith, M. R. (1985). Hormonal influence on the secretory immune system of the eye: Androgen modulation of IgA levels in tears of rats. *J. Immunol.* **134,** 2978–2982.

Sullivan, D. A., Bloch, K. J., and Allansmith, M. R. (1984a). Hormonal influence on the secretory immune system of the eye: Androgen regulation of secretory component levels in rat tears. *J. Immunol.* **132,** 1130–1135.

Sullivan, D. A., Bloch, K. J., and Allansmith, M. R. (1984b). Hormonal influence on the secretory immune system of the eye: Androgen control of secretory component production by the rat exorbital gland. *Immunology* **52,** 239–246.

Sullivan, D. A., Kelleher, R. S., Vaerman, J. P., and Hann, L. E. (1990). Androgen regulation of secretory component synthesis by lacrimal gland acinar cells *in vitro. J. Immunol.* **145,** 4238–4244.

Syed, N. A., and Hyndiuk, R. A. (1992). Infectious conjunctivitis. *Infect. Dis. Clinics N. Am.* **6,** 789–805.

Tabbara, K. F., and Hyndiuk, R. A. (1995). "Infections of the Eye." Little, Brown, Boston.

Taylor, H. R. (1990). Development of immunity to ocular chlamydial infection. *Am. J. Trop. Med. Hyg.* **42,** 358–364.

Taylor, H. R. (1994). Onchocerciasis: Clinical features. *In* "Infectious Diseases of the Eye" (A. A. Bialasiewicz and K. P. Schaal, eds.), pp. 623–628. Aeolus Press, Buren, The Netherlands.

Taylor, H. R., and Prendergast, R. A. (1987). Attempted oral immunization with chlamydial lipopolysaccharide subunit vaccine. *Invest. Ophthalmol. Visual Sci.* **28,** 1722–1726.

Taylor, H. R., Pierce, N. F., Zhang, P., Schachter, J., Silverstein, A. M., and Prendergast, R. A. (1985). Secretory immune cellular traffic between the gut and the eye. *In* "Advances in Immunology and Immunopathology of the Eye" (G. R. O'Connor and J. W. Chandler, eds.), pp. 208–211. Masson Publishing, New York.

Taylor, H. R., Johnson, S. L., Schachter, J., Caldwell, H. D., and Prendergast, R. A. (1987a). Pathogenesis of trachoma: The stimulus for inflammation. *J. Immunol.* **138,** 3023–3027.

Taylor, H. R., Young, E., MacDonald, A. B., Schachter, J., and Prendergast, R. A. (1987b). Oral immunization against chlamydial eye infection. *Invest. Ophthalmol. Visual Sci.* **28,** 249–258.

Taylor, H. R., Whittum-Hudson, J., Schachter, J., Caldwell, H. D., and Prendergast, R. A. (1988). Oral immunization with chlamydial major outer membrane protein (MOMP). *Invest. Ophthalmol. Visual Sci.* **29,** 1847–1853.

Taylor, H. R., Stephens, R. S., Whittum-Hudson, J. A., and Prendergast, R. A. (1989). Initial evaluation of trachoma subunit vaccines. *Invest. Ophthalmol. Visual Sci. Suppl.* **30,** 381.

Taylor, H. R., Maclean, I. W., Brunham, R. C., Pal, S., and Whittum-Hudson, J. (1990). Chlamydial heat shock proteins and trachoma. *Infect. Immun.* **58,** 3061–3063.

Taylor, H. R., Siler, J. A., Mkocha, H. A., Munoz, B., and West, S. (1992). The natural history of endemic trachoma: A longitudinal study. *Am. J. Trop. Med. Hyg.* **46,** 552–559.

Tsai, J. C., Garlinghouse, G., McDonnell, P. J., and Trousdale, M. D. (1992). An experimental animal model of adenovirus-induced ocular disease. The cotton rat. *Arch. Ophthalmol.* **110,** 1167–1170.

Tuffrey, M. (1994). The use of animal models to study human chlamydial diseases. *In* "Chlamydial Infections: Proceedings of the 8th International Symposium on Human Chlamydial Infections" (J. Orfila, G. I. Byrne, M. A. Chernesky, J. T. Grayston, R. B. Jones, G. L. Ridgway, P. Saikku, W. E. Stamm, J. Schachter, and R. S. Stephens, eds.), pp. 513–524. Societa Editrice Esculapio, Bologna, Italy.

Tumpey, T. M., Elner, V. M., Chen, S. H., Oakes, J. E., and Lausch, R. N. (1994). Interleukin-10 treatment can suppress stromal keratitis induced by herpes simplex virus type 1. *J. Immunol.* **153,** 2258–2265.

Visscher, G. E., Robinson, R. L., and Argentieri, G. J. (1987). Tissue response to biodegradable injectable microcapsules. *J. Biomater. Appl.* **2,** 118–131.

Waldman, R. H., and Bergmann, K. C. (1987). Stimulation of secretory antibody following oral antigen administration. *Adv. Exp. Med. Biol.* **216,** 1677–1684.

Walker, R. I. (1994). New strategies for using mucosal vaccination to achieve more effective immunization. *Vaccine* **12,** 387–400.

Ward, M. E., Treharne, J. D., and Murray, A. (1986). Antigenic specificity of human antibody to chlamydia in trachoma and lymphogranuloma venereum. *J. Gen. Microbiol.* **132,** 1599–1610.

Watkins, N. G., Hadlow, W. J., Moos, A. B., and Caldwell, H. D. (1986). Ocular delayed hypersensitivity; a pathogenic mechanism of chlamydial conjunctivitis in guinea pigs. *Proc. Natl. Acad. Sci. U.S.A.* **83,** 7480–7484.

Watson, R. R., Horton, R. G., and Clinton, J. M. (1977). Suppression of secretory IgA antibodies in protein malnourished guinea pigs following a chlamydial eye and vaginal infection. *Fed. Proc.* **36,** 1251.

Weber, R., Kuster, H., Visvesvara, G. S., Bryan, R. T., Schwartz, D. A., and Luthy, R. (1993). Disseminated microsporidiosis due to *Encephalitozoon hellem:* Pulmonary colonization, microhematuria, and mild conjunctivitis in a patient with AIDS. *Clin. Infect. Dis.* **17,** 415–419.

Weisz-Carrington, P., Roux, M. E., McWilliams, M., Phillips-Quagliata, J. M., and Lamm, M. E. (1979). Organ and isotype distribution of plasma cells producing specific antibody after oral immunization: Evidence for a generalized secretory immune system. *J. Immunol.* **123,** 1705–1708.

Whittum-Hudson, J. A., and Taylor, H. R. (1989). Antichlamydial specificity of conjunctival lymphocytes during experimental ocular infection. *Infect. Immun.* **57,** 2977–2983.

Whittum-Hudson, J. A., and Taylor, H. R. (1994). The immunology of trachoma. *In* "Infectious Diseases of the Eye" (A. A. Bialasiewicz and K. P. Schaal, eds.), pp. 605–614. Aeolus Press, Buren, The Netherlands.

Whittum-Hudson, J. A., Prendergast, R. A., and Taylor, H. R. (1986a). Changes in conjunctival lymphocyte populations induced by oral immunization with *Chlamydia trachomatis. Curr. Eye Res.* **5,** 973–979.

Whittum-Hudson, J. A., Taylor, H. R., Farazdaghi, M., and Prendergast, R. A. (1986b). Immunohistochemical study of the local inflammatory response to chlamydial ocular infection. *Invest. Ophthalmol. Visual Sci.* **27,** 64–69.

Whittum-Hudson, J. A., MacDonald, A. B., Prendergast, R. A., O'Brien, T. P., and An, L. (1994). Protection against ocular chlamydial infection with an anti-idiotypic antibody. *Invest. Ophthalmol. Visual Sci. Suppl.* **35,** 1301.

Whittum-Hudson, J. A., O'Brien, T. P., and Prendergast, R. A. (1995a). Murine model of ocular infection by a human biovar of *Chlamydia trachomatis*. *Invest. Ophthalmol. Visual Sci.* **36,** 1976–1997.

Whittum-Hudson, J. A., Saltzman, W. M., O'Brien, T. P., Prendergast, R. A., and MacDonald, A. B. (1995b). Oral immunization with anti-idiotypic antibodies protects against ocular chlamydial infection. *Invest. Ophthalmol. Visual Sci. Suppl.* **36,** 1030.

Whittum-Hudson, J. A., An, L. L., Saltzman, W. M., Prendergast, R. A., and MacDonald, A. B. (1996). Oral immunization with an anti-idiotypic antibody to the exoglycolipid antigen protects against experimental *Chlamydia trachomatis* infection. Submitted for publication.

Wickham, L. A., Huang, Z., Lambert, R. W., and Sullivan, D. A. (1994). Sialodacryoadenitis virus infection of rat lacrimal gland acinar cells. *In* "Lacrimal Gland, Tear Film and Dry Eye Syndromes: Basic Science and Clinical Relevance" (D. A. Sullivan, ed.), pp. 193–196. Plenum, New York.

Wieczorek, R., Jakobiec, F. A., Sacks, E. H., and Knowles, D. M. (1988). The immunoarchitecture of the normal human lacrimal gland. Relevancy for understanding pathologic conditions. *Ophthalmology* **95,** 100–109.

Willey, D. E., Smith, M. D., Nesburn, A. B., and Trousdale, M. D. (1985). Sequential analysis of antibody responses in serum, aqueous humor and tear film during latent and induced recurrent HSV infections. *Curr. Eye Res.* **4,** 1235–1240.

Wills, J. M., Gruffydd-Jones, T. J., Richmond, S. J., Gaskell, R. M., and Bourne, F. J. (1987). Effect of vaccination on feline *Chlamydia psittaci* infection. *Infect. Immun.* **55,** 2653–2657.

Wise, D. L., Fellman, T. D., Sanderson, J. E., and Wentworth, R. L. (1979). Lactic/glycolic acid polymers. *In* "Drug Carriers in Biology and Medicine" (G. Gregoridis, ed.), pp. 237–270. Academic Press, London.

Wong, E., Pribnow, J. A., and Stephens, R. (1990). Topical ocular immunization with defined *Chlamydia trachomatis* major outer membrane epitopes. *Invest. Ophthalmol. Visual Sci. Suppl.* **31,** 571.

Woodruff, J. J., Clarke, L. M., and Chin, Y. H. (1987). Specific cell-adhesion mechanisms determining migration pathways of recirculating lymphocytes. *Annu. Rev. Immunol.* **5,** 201–222.

Wu, H. Y., and Russell, M. W. (1993). Induction of mucosal immunity by intranasal application of a streptococcal surface protein antigen with cholera toxin B subunit. *Infect. Immun.* **61,** 314–322.

Wyrick, P., Choong, J., Knight, S. T., Goyeau, D., Stuart, E. S., and MacDoland, A. B. (1994). *Chlamydia trachomatis* antigens on the surface of human endometrial cells. *Immunol. Infect. Dis.* **4,** 131–141.

Young, E. J. (1983). Human brucellosis. *Rev. Infect. Dis.* **5,** 821–842.

Zaidman, G. W. (1993). The ocular manifestations of Lyme disease. *In* "New and Evolving Ocular Infections" (G. Smolin and M. H. Friedlander eds.), pp. 9–22. Little, Brown, Boston.

Zhang, P., Pierce, N. F., Silverstein, A. M., and Prendergast, R. A. (1983). Conjunctival immunity: Compared effects of ocular or intestinal immunization in rats. *Invest. Ophthalmol.* **24,** 1411–1412.

Zundel, E., Verger, J. M., Grayon, M., and Michel, R. (1992). Conjunctival vaccination of pregnant ewes and goats with *Brucella melitensis* Rev. 1 vaccine: Safety and serological responses. *Ann. Rech. Vet.* **23,** 177–188.

31

Intranasal Immunization with Influenza Vaccine

Shin-ichi Tamura
Takeshi Kurata
Department of Pathology
National Institute of Health
Tokyo 162, Japan

I. Introduction

A. Current Inactivated Influenza Vaccine

Influenza is a highly contagious acute respiratory disease, caused by influenza virus infecting the host at the respiratory mucosal surfaces. Due to the short incubation period, the immunity raised within several days after infection cannot prevent the onset of the respiratory symptoms. Therefore, an effective immunity must be induced in advance by vaccination in order to prevent the disease. The influenza virus is an enveloped virus with two surface glycoproteins, hemagglutinin (HA) and neuraminidase (NA), and five internal proteins [matrix (M), nucleoprotein (NP), and three polymerases] (Murphy and Webster, 1990). The HA glycoprotein is responsible for the initiation of infection by receptor binding and membrane fusion, and the antibodies to the HA molecules neutralize the infectivity of the virus. The antibodies to NA efficiently prevent the release of the virus from the infected cells. The T-cell responses to the internal viral proteins reduce the level and duration of virus replication. Thus, antibody responses to HA are primarily responsible for preventing infection, whereas the antibody to NA or T cell response specific to influenza antigens contribute to recovery from infection (Ada and Jones, 1986).

To control influenza, inactivated vaccines, which are either viruses inactivated with formalin or chemically disrupted viral components, are currently used in many countries. The vaccines are licensed for parenteral administration. With these vaccines, high levels of serum anti-HA IgG antibodies are induced. In spite of the availability of influenza vaccines, influenza remains a serious infectious disease. Influenza A virus has been implicated in worldwide pandemics of respiratory diseases, and influenza B virus is involved in local outbreaks every year. These recurrences take place because influenza virus can alter the antigenic properties of HA and NA, thus escaping the presence of preexisting immunity. The influenza viruses are divided into three types, A and B, which are of epidemiologic significance, and C, based on the antigenic differences in M and NP. Human influenza A viruses have caused two major antigenic shifts in HA and a major shift in NA since 1933, resulting in three subtypes of HA (H1, H2, and H3) and two subtypes of NA (N1 and N2). Moreover, within a subtype of A viruses and within B viruses, variant viruses with minor differences due to antigenic drift have occurred every year (Wilson and Cox, 1990).

These facts suggest that the current inactivated vaccines will be effective in protecting both infection and disease if the vaccine strains include one strain whose HA is immunologically the same as the currently prevalent virus. However, the protective efficacy will be low if the vaccine strains are immunologically different from the epidemic strain (Hoskins *et al.*, 1974; Mayer *et al.*, 1978).

B. Attempts To Improve the Efficacy of the Current Vaccine

Natural influenza virus has been shown to be superior to inactivated vaccines in inducing cross-protection against variants within a subtype of A-type virus (Schulman and Kilbourne, 1965; Couch and Kasel, 1983). The cross-protection induced by natural infection appears to primarily result from the induction of cross-reacting IgA antibodies in the respiratory tract (Liew *et al.*, 1984). The cross-reactivity is derived from the polymeric nature of secretory IgA antibodies, which generate more increased overall avidity for influenza virus than occurs with serum IgG (Waldman *et al.*, 1970; Shvartsman and Zykov, 1976; Underdown and Schiff, 1986). These facts support the assertion that live vaccines elicit better immunity than inactivated vaccines. In this regard, cold-

MUCOSAL VACCINES

adapted living influenza vaccine has been developed (Maassab, 1967; Clements *et al.*, 1984; Murphy and Clements, 1989). On the other hand, these facts suggest that development of an immunization procedure to stimulate mucosal IgA antibody production would improve the protective efficacy of the current inactivated vaccine. Intranasal (i.n.) immunization with inactivated vaccine has been advocated as a means for inducing secretory IgA (S-IgA) and systemic IgG antibodies against influenza for over 20 years (Waldman and Ganguly, 1974); however, the i.n. immunization with inactivated vaccine alone cannot easily induce S-IgA antibodies.

In such circumstances, we attempted to inoculate mice intranasally with the current inactivated vaccine together with a potent adjuvant, cholera toxin B subunit (CT-B) containing a trace amount of cholera toxin (CT) (around 0.1%) (Tamura *et al.*, 1988b, 1994b). The results demonstrated that i.n. administration of the adjuvant-combined vaccine into mice can mimic the efficacy of live virus in inducing cross-protection against challenge with variant viruses. Moreover, our first field trial in humans demonstrated that nasal vaccination is feasible for humans with a significant increase in the S-IgA antibody level (Hashigucci *et al.*, 1996). In this chapter, our recent studies concerning the protective efficacy and usefulness of i.n. immunization with adjuvant-combined influenza vaccine are presented together with the background studies.

II. Protection against Influenza Virus Infection by Intranasal Immunization with the Adjuvant-Combined Vaccine

A. Protective Effects of Intranasal Immunization Are Superior to Those of Other Immunization Routes

1. *Cross-Protective Effects of Intranasal Immunization Are Superior to Those of Subcutaneous Immunization*

We systematically compared the effects of an adjuvant-combined vaccine on protection by i.n. immunization and those by subcutaneous (s.c.) immunization in BALB/c mice (Tamura *et al.*, 1992a). Mice were immunized intranasally (a 10-μl volume) or subcutaneously with various vaccines along with CT-B* (CT-B containing approx. 0.1% CT). Four weeks later, some of the immunized mice were killed to obtain both nasal and lung (bronchoalveolar) washes for measuring IgA and IgG antibodies to HA molecules of a mouse-adapted A/Guizhou/54/89 × A/Puerto Rico/8/34 (A/Guizhou-X) virus (H3N2) by ELISA. Other immunized mice were challenged intranasally by two separate methods based on the site of infection (Yetter *et al.*, 1980); either a small (nasal site-restricted) volume (2 μl; 1 μl into each nostril) or a large volume (20 μl) of A/Guizhou-X virus suspension, containing 2×10^4 EID_{50}/mouse ($10 \times LD_{50}$). Figure 1 shows virus-shedding kinetics from virgin mice infected with a mouse-adapted A/PR/8/34 (A/PR8) virus (H1N1). The viruses shed from the virgin mice infected with a small volume were first detected in the nasal washes on Day 1 and peaked on Day 3, while the virus titers of the lung washes were low on Day 3, peaked on Day 7, and declined thereafter. Thus, the small volume infection caused initial nasal infection and late lung infection. The small volume infection caused fewer deaths in the infected animals. On the other hand, the large-volume infection caused a lung-predominant infection. Under these conditions, more than 90% of the mice died in 6 to 10 days. The virus titer changed depending on the infection sites, corresponding to the severity of the disease, and ranged from mild upper respiratory infection and tracheobronchitis to severe viral pneumonia. In the subsequent experiments, the nasal virus titer resulting from the small-volume infection and the lung virus titer resulting from the large-volume infection, which were assayed 3 days after infection, were used as indices of protection in upper and lower respiratory tract of immunized mice, respectively.

Table I summarizes the nasal virus titers resulting from the small-volume infection with A/Guizhou-X virus (H3N2) as protection in the upper respiratory tract in intranasally or subcutaneously immunized mice. The i.n. immunization with A/Guizhou-X vaccine produced the lowest level of virus titer which meant almost complete protection (++++ in Table I). A vaccine, derived from a variant within the same subtype, A/Fukuoka/C29/85 (A/Fukuoka) or A/Sichuan/2/87 (A/Sichuan) virus, also provided almost complete cross-protection. A different subtype virus vaccine, A/PR8 (H1N1) vaccine, gave a slight cross-protection, whereas a different type of virus vaccine failed to deliver any protection. On the other hand, the s.c. immunization with A/Guizhou-X vaccine provided almost complete protection, whereas A/Fukuoka or A/Sichuan vaccine, as well as A/PR8 and B/Ibaraki/2/85 (B/Ibaraki) vaccine, failed to provide any cross-protection. In mice given the large volume infection, either i.n. or s.c. immunization with A/Guizhou-X vaccine provided almost complete protection, while both i.n. or s.c. immunization with A/Fukuoka or A/Sichuan vaccine afforded only a partial cross-protection (not shown in Table I). Neither i.n. nor s.c. immunization with A/PR8 or B/Ibaraki vaccine conferred any cross-protection.

Table I also summarizes production of A/Guizhou-X HA-reactive antibodies at the nasal site. The i.n. immunization with A/Fukuoka or A/Sichuan vaccine pro-

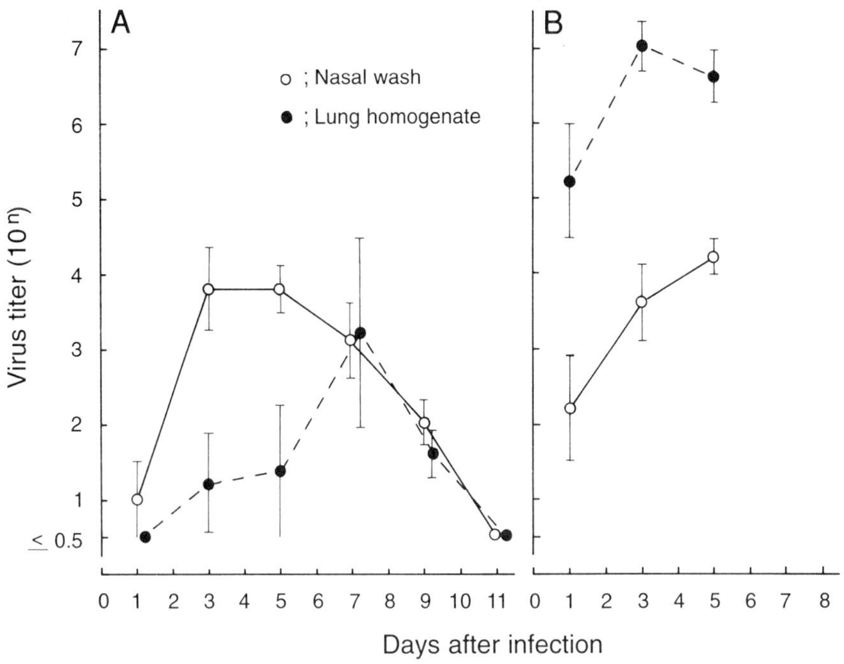

Figure 1. Kinetics of virus titers in naive mice, infected intranasally with a small (2 μl; A) or a large volume (10 μl; B) of a dilution of mouse-adapted PR8 virus containing $10^{4.1}$ EID_{50} under light anesthesia. At specific intervals six mice from each group were sacrificed, and nasal washings (○) and 10% lung homogenates (●) were titrated for virus and expressed in EID_{50}. Each point represents the mean ± SD of nasal wash or lung homogenate virus titers from all mice in each group of six.

TABLE I

Protection Against Influenza A Virus Infection and Production of Cross-Reactive Anti-HA IgA and IgG Antibodies in the Nasal Washes in Mice Immunized Intranasally or Subcutaneously with Different Adjuvant-Combined Vaccines

Immunization[a]		Challenge[b] with A/Guizhou-X	A/Ghuizhou-X HA reactive Ab[c] in nasal wash		Protection[d] in upper respiratory tract
Vaccine with CT-B*	Route		IgA	IgG	
—	i.n.	+	–	–	–
A/Guizhou-X (H3N2)	i.n.	+	++++	++++	++++
A/Fukuoka (H3N2)	i.n.	+	++	–	++++
A/Sichuan (H3N2)	i.n.	+	++	–	++++
A/PR8 (H1N1)	i.n.	+	+	–	++
B/Ibaraki	i.n.	+	–	–	–
—	s.c.	+	–	–	–
A/Guizhou-X	s.c.	+	–	++++	++++
A/Fukuoka	s.c.	+	–	–	–
A/Sichuan	s.c.	+	–	–	–
A/PR8	s.c.	+	–	–	–
B/Ibaraki	s.c.	+	–	–	–

[a]Mice had been immunized intranasally (i.n.) or subcutaneously (s.c.) with 0.15 μg of a vaccine together with 1 μg of CT-B containing around 0.1% of CT (CT-B*) 4 weeks previously.

[b]The immunized mice were infected intranasally with a small volume (1 μl×2) of a mouse-adapted A/Guizhou-X virus suspension.

[c]Antibody amounts, represented by arbitrary units, were from the nasal washes 4 weeks after immunization. Adapted from Tamura *et al.* (1992a).

[d]Protection was estimated by the nasal virus titers assayed 3 days after infection. Complete protection was represented by arbitrary units (++++). Adapted from Tamura *et al.* (1992a).

duced a relatively high level of cross-reacting IgA antibodies with almost no cross-reacting IgG antibodies in nasal washes. On the other hand, the s.c. immunization with A/Fukuoka or A/Sichuan vaccine failed to produce any cross-reacting IgA or IgG antibodies. Regarding the antibodies at the lung site, both i.n. and sc immunization produced a relatively high level of cross-reacting IgG antibodies (not shown in Table I).

In summary, the i.n. vaccination was more effective than the s.c. vaccination for providing cross-protection against infection with a variant virus within the same subtype in the upper respiratory tract, while the i.n. vaccination was equivalent to the s.c. vaccination for providing the cross-protection in the lower respiratory tract. Cross-protection was also provided against B-type virus challenge in mice immunized with variant virus vaccines within B type (Kikuta *et al.*, 1990b). Some of these findings are supported by the concept that mucosal IgA antibodies are primarily responsible for protection against upper respiratory tract infection, whereas serum IgG antibodies, which can diffuse into the lower respiratory tract, are predominantly responsible for protection of the lower respiratory tract (Ramphal *et al.*, 1979; Kris *et al.*, 1985; Nedrud *et al.*, 1987).

2. *Protective Effect of Intranasal Immunization Is Superior to Oral Immunization*

Our research team compared the antibody responses and protective efficacy of i.n. immunization with CT-B*-combined vaccine with groups orally immunized (Hirabayashi *et al.*, 1990). Mice were immunized intranasally or orally with various doses of the adjuvant-combined PR8 HA vaccine. Four weeks later, some of the immunized mice were killed to obtain nasal, bronchoalveolar and intestinal washes for measuring IgA and IgG antibodies of the vaccine. Other immunized mice were challenged with a lethal dose of A/PR8 virus. The results showed that a single-dose i.n. immunization was more than 100 times as effective as the oral immunization in inducing antiviral IgA antibodies in the respiratory tract. Moreover, the i.n. immunization was 10–100 times as effective on a dose basis as the oral immunization for inducing a similar level of antibodies in the intestinal secretion. In parallel with the induction of respiratory tract IgA, a greater protective effect against virus challenge was seen in the intranasally immunized mice than in those orally immunized (data not shown).

It is known that specific populations of mucosal lymphoid cells, induced by antigenic stimulation at one mucosal site, migrate not only to the site of origin but also to other mucosal sites via the homing pathways, collectively referred to as the common mucosal immune system (Bienenstock and Befus, 1980). Compartmentalization, however, exists within this system (McGhee and Kiyono, 1993; Haneberg *et al.*, 1994). Therefore, identification of the inductive sites that most effectively elicit IgA at the mucosal sites requiring protection seems essential for the development of effective vaccines. The results described above suggest that i.n. immunization is superior to oral immunization in inducing secretory IgA not only in the respiratory tract but also in the gastrointestinal tract. Thus, nasal-associated and/or bronchus-associated lymphoid tissue (NALT and/or BALT) seems to be the inductive sites that most effectively provide secretory IgA in the respiratory tract requiring protection against influenza virus infection. In addition, these results suggest that the i.n. route is most practical for other vaccines whose protective sites are the mucosal sites other than the respiratory tract and that are sensitive to gastrointestinal conditions such as acid and proteolytic enzymes (Walker, 1994).

B. Practical Approaches to Improving the Efficacy of Intranasal Immunization

1. *Vaccination with the Volume Confined in the Nasal Site in a Two-Dose Regimen*

To provide a practical basis for nasal vaccination by i.n. dropping or spraying in humans, we investigated the effects of i.n. immunization with a small volume of the vaccine (1 μl into each nostril) on cross-protection against virus challenge. In addition, the i.n. immunization was performed in a two-dose regimen, composed of a primary adjuvant-combined vaccine and the subsequent vaccine alone 4 weeks later (Tamura *et al.*, 1992b). In this regard, we have already shown that a two-dose rather than a single-dose regimen of nasal vaccination can be recommended to reduce the amounts of vaccine and adjuvant required for effective protection and to maintain the high protective antibody level (Tamura *et al.*, 1989b). As summarized in Table II, the primary immunization alone with a variant H3N2 vaccine, A/Fukuoka or A/Sichuan vaccine, provided no cross-protection against small-volume infection with A/Guizhou-X virus, and a slight cross-protection against large-volume infection. On the other hand, the secondary inoculation with another H3N2 strain (A/Sichuan) vaccine provided complete cross-protection against the small-volume infection. Moreover, the second vaccination provided partial or complete cross-protection against the large-volume infection. Table II also summarizes that the high efficacy to provide the cross-protection was maintained for more than 12 weeks after the second vaccination. These results indicate that a nasal site-confined volume of vaccine is sufficient in inducing effective cross-protection against infection with a variant virus and that the two-dose regimen is superior to a single-dose regimen in providing effective cross-protection against either a small- or large-volume infection

TABLE II

Cross-Protection against A/Guizhou-X Virus Challenge and Its Continuation in Mice Having Received a Primary and Secondary Intranasal Immunization of Different H3N2 Subtype Virus Vaccines

Intranasal Immunization[a]				Protection[c]	
Primary vaccine with CT-B*	Secondary vaccine	Challenge with A/Guizhou-X	Weeks between 2nd vaccine and challenge[b]	Upper respiratory tract	Lower respiratory tract
—	—	+		–	–
A/Guizhou-X	—	+		++++	++++
A/Fukuoka	—	+		–	+
A/Sichuan	—	+		–	+
A/Guizhou-X	A/Sichuan	+	2	++++	++++
A/Fukuoka	A/Sichuan	+	2	++++	++++
A/Sichuan	A/Sichuan	+	2	++++	++++
—	A/Sichuan	+	2	–	–
—	—	+		–	–
A/Guizhou-X	—	+	12	++++	++++
A/Guizhou-X	A/Sichuan	+	12	++++	++++
A/Fukuoka	A/Sichuan	+	12	++++	++++
A/Sichuan	A/Sichuan	+	12	++++	++++
—	A/Sichuan	+	12	–	–

[a]Mice received a primary immunization with a small volume (2 μl) of different H3N2 subtype vaccine (0.03 μg), prepared from A/Guizhou-X, A/Fukuoka, or A/Sichuan virus strain, with CT-B* (0.2 μg) and 4 weeks later a second immunization with a small volume (2 μl) of A/Sichuan virus vaccine (0.3 μg).

[b]Two or 12 weeks after the second immunization, mice were challenged intranasally with a small (2 μl) or large volume (20 μl) of A/Guizhou-X virus at the same doses (2×10^4 EID_{50}).

[c]Protection was estimated by the nasal and lung virus titers assayed 3 days after infection. Complete protection was represented by arbitrary units (++++). Adapted from Tamura *et al.* (1992b).

with a variant virus within the same subtype. These results also suggest that effective nasal vaccination of influenza can be attained by i.n. dropping or spraying of a small volume of a vaccine solution under a two-dose regimen in humans.

2. *Trivalent Influenza Vaccines*

The vaccines currently employed are trivalent inactivated vaccines containing influenza A viruses of different subtypes (H1N1, H3N2) and B viruses to protect the prevalence of viruses of different subtypes or types. Therefore, we examined i.n. immunization using a two-dose regimen with a small volume of CT-B*-combined trivalent vaccine for the effects on cross-protection against challenge (Tamura *et al.*, 1992b). Table III summarizes cross-protection in mice that received a primary inoculation with one trivalent vaccine together with CT-B*, and then another trivalent vaccine 4 weeks later. The primary trivalent vaccine was composed of A/Yamagata/120/86 (A/Yamagata) (H1N1), A/Sichuan (H3N2), and B/Nagasaki/1/87 (B/Nagasaki) virus vaccines, together with CT-B*, while the second trivalent vaccine was composed of A/Bangkok/10/83 (A/Bangkok) (H1N1), A/Fukuoka (H3N2), and B/Aichi/5/88 (B/Aichi) virus vaccines. The results show that the two doses of trivalent vaccine provided almost complete cross-protection against a small-volume infection with A/PR8 (H1N1), A/Guizhou-X (H3N2), or B/Ibaraki virus, and a slight, almost complete and partial cross-protection against a large-volume infection with A/PR8, A/Guizhou-X, and B/Ibaraki virus, respectively. These results suggest that i.n. immunization with the adjuvant-combined trivalent vaccine provides cross-protection against a broad range of viruses.

3. *Vaccine Strains for Providing Effective Cross-Protection*

The vaccine should be formulated as to adequately immunize humans to unique epitopes of a new epidemic virus strain. We attempted to formulate a nasal vaccine of A type virus for providing cross-protection most effectively (Tamura *et al.*, 1994a). Mice were immunized intranasally with various vaccines, prepared from some of H1N1 subtype viruses which were circulating in humans from 1934 to 1986, together with CT-B*. Four weeks later, the mice were challenged intranasally with a lethal dose of either A/PR8 (H1N1) which was circulating in 1934 or A/Yamagata (H1N1) which was circulating in 1986. Replacement of approximately 50 amino acid residues in the HA1 region (329 amino acids) of HA was estimated between PR8 and Yamagata/86 viruses used here (Winter *et al.*, 1981; Robertson, 1987).

TABLE III

Cross-Protection against Different Influenza Viruses in Mice Having Received a Primary and Secondary Intranasal Immunization of a Trivalent Virus Vaccine

Intranasal Immunization[a]			Cross-Protection	
Primary vaccine with CT-B*	Secondary vaccine	Challenge[b] virus	Upper respiratory tract	Lower respiratory tract
—	—	A/PR8	−	−
Y.+ S.+ N.	—	A/PR8	+	N.D.
—	B.+ F.+ A.	A/PR8	−	N.D.
Y.+ S.+ N.	B.+ F.+ A.	A/PR8	++	+
—	—	A/Guizhou-X	−	−
Y.+ S.+ N.	—	A/Guizhou-X	++	N.D.
—	B.+ F.+ A.	A/Guizhou-X	−	N.D.
Y.+ S.+ N.	B.+ F.+ A.	A/Guizhou-X	++++	++++
—	—	B/Ibaraki	−	−
Y.+ S.+ N.	—	B/Ibaraki	++	N.D.
—	B.+ F.+ A.	B/Ibaraki	−	N.D.
Y.+ S.+ N.	B.+ F.+ A.	B/Ibaraki	++++	++

[a]Mice received a primary immunization with a small volume of a trivalent vaccine (0.03 μg × 3) (Y.+ S.+ N.) composed of A/Yamagata (H1N1), A/Sichuan (H3N2) and B/Nagasaki irus vaccines, together with CT-B* (0.2 μg) and 4 weeks later a second immunization with a small volume (2 μl) of another trivalent virus vaccine (0.3 μg × 3) (B.+ F.+ A.) composed of A/Bangkok (H1N1), A/Fukuoka (H3N2), and B/Aichi virus vaccines.

[b]Two weeks after the second immunization, mice were challenged intranasally with a small (2 μl) or large volume (20 μl) of A/PR8 virus, A/Guizhou-X virus or B/Ibaraki virus. For further details, see the footnote to Table I. Adapted from Tamura *et al.* (1992b).

The i.n. immunization with the adjuvant-combined vaccines, prepared from variant H1N1 viruses which were recently circulating in humans, A/Kumamoto/37/79 (A/Kumamoto) and A/Bangkok/10/83, provided a higher degree of cross-protection against a challenge with A/Yamagata than with A/PR8. A booster with another variant virus vaccine given 4 weeks after the primary immunization increased the protection against A/Yamagata; the effect was higher when mice were immunized with a recently circulating strain as the second antigen than when boosted with the A/PR8 vaccine. These results suggest that vaccination with a later strain followed by another later strain under a two-dose regimen gives effective cross-protection against the virus strains involved in the current epidemic.

Field isolates of influenza A viruses have been examined to determine the evolutionary pattern (Both *et al.*, 1983; Raymond *et al.*, 1986; Yamashita *et al.*, 1988). Analyses of the sequences of various genes demonstrated that variants of A viruses arise from only one lineage because of the dominating effects of favorable variants. Thus, A-type virus strains that circulated more recently in humans retain many changes of the epitopes of the earlier viruses. These facts suggest that the latest virus strains give more effective cross-protection against new epidemic virus strains than the earliest ones. The results described above support this observation.

III. Immunological Basis of Protective Effect of Intranasal Immunization with Adjuvant-Combined Vaccine

A. Characterization of Respiratory Tract IgA Antibodies against HA Molecules

Among the antiviral antibodies which are developed during infection with influenza virus, antibodies to HA glycoprotein are the major protective factor associated with resistance to the infection and/or illness in humans (Murphy and Webster, 1990). Moreover, the above section suggests that IgA antibodies cross-reacting to HA glycoprotein are the major factor associated with cross-protection against the infection with a variant virus in the upper respiratory tract. To confirm this finding, we isolated HA glycoproteins from several viruses (Phelan *et al.*, 1980) and examined the IgA antibodies for cross-reactivity to the HA molecules in the mice immunized intranasally with CT-B*-combined purified HA molecules in a two-dose regimen (Tamura *et al.*, 1990, 1991). The results demonstrated that the HA-immunized mice possessed not only a high level of IgA antibodies, specific for HA used for immunization, but also a moderate level of IgA antibodies cross-reactive to the

HA from a variant virus within the same subtype and a low level of IgA antibodies cross-reactive to HA from a different subtype virus in the nasal washes. Moreover, the content of nasal wash IgA was higher than that of IgG and the degree of cross-reactivity of HA-specific IgA was greater than that of HA-specific IgG.

B. Protection with Anti-HA IgA Antibodies Administered into the Respiratory Tract

We examined respiratory tract anti-HA IgA antibodies for the functional role in cross-protection by passive transfer experiments (Tamura *et al.*, 1990, 1991). The respiratory tract IgA was first purified from pooled nasal and lung washes by passing through an affinity column constructed by coupling goat anti-mouse α chain-specific antibody to Sepharose. The molecular form of IgA was predominantly polymeric with a small portion in monomeric form, although the IgG was predominantly monomeric. The purified IgA was administered intranasally to naive mice; the mice were infected intranasally with a lethal dose of PR8 virus 3 hr later. Three days after infection, the virus titers of lung homogenate were determined as indices of protection. The physiological amount of IgA to A/PR8 HA was able to protect the naive host against a A/PR8 virus challenge. The IgA from A/Yamagata HA-immunized mice, containing a moderate level of antibodies cross-reacting to A/PR8 HA, was found to significantly protect naive mice from A/PR8 challenge. On the other hand, the respiratory tract IgA from the A/Fukuoka HA-immunized mice, containing only a low level of antibodies reacting to A/PR8 HA, failed to protect naive mice against A/PR8 infection. Thus, an adequate amount of cross-reacting anti-HA IgA mediated cross-protection against a variant virus infection. Other experiments showed that the duration of the ability of the transferred IgA to protect the viral infection in the respiratory tract correlated well with the amount of IgA remaining in the respiratory tract (Tamura *et al.*, 1991). These findings clearly demonstrate that IgA antibodies to influenza virus HA by themselves play a pivotal role in defense against not only homologous but also heterologous virus infection in the respiratory tract.

IV. Usefulness of CT-B Containing a Trace Amount of CT as an Adjuvant for Intranasal Immunization with Vaccine

A. Mechanism of Adjuvant Action of CT-B Supplemented with CT

CT is produced by *Vibrio cholerae* adhering to and colonizing in the small intestine. CT consists of a pentameric B subunit that binds to the specific receptor, G_{M1} ganglioside, on the cell membrane, and an A subunit that can ADP-ribosylate the G_s subunit of adenylate cyclase (Holmgren, 1981). ADP-ribosylation of adenylate cyclase results in increased intracellular cyclic AMP, which leads to various biological effects, including diarrhea. Probably by the same mechanism, CT works not only as a potent gut immunogen but also as a potent adjuvant that can augment both local and systemic antibody responses as well as cell-mediated immune responses (Holmgren and Svennerholm, 1984; Elson and Ealding, 1984; Tamura *et al.*, 1988a; Lycke *et al.*, 1992). *In vitro* and *in vivo* studies with isolated macrophages and T and B cells have shown that CT can affect all the cells engaged in immune responses, suggesting that the mechanisms responsible for the adjuvant action involve more than one step in the immune response (Dertzbaugh and Elson, 1991; Holmgren *et al.*, 1993).

Although CT enhances the immune responses to antigens given orally or intranasally, the use of holotoxin is not feasible due to its toxicity from a practical standpoint. One approach being explored to resolve this problem is to use the nontoxic component, CT-B, coupled chemically or by the gene fusion technology to foreign antigens (McKenzie and Halsey, 1984; Dertzbaugh *et al.*, 1990). Another approach is either to use a mutated toxin that is devoid of toxicity but retains the adjuvant action, or to use CT-B containing a trace amount of CT, by mixing with foreign antigens (Wilson *et al.*, 1990).

In our previous studies, we used a commercial CT-B preparation, which was estimated to contain approximately 0.1% of CT, as a potent adjuvant that augments both antibody responses and delayed-type hypersensitivity responses (Tamura *et al.*, 1988b, 1989a–c, 1990, 1991, 1992a,b, 1994a,b; Kikuta *et al.*, 1990a,b; Hirabayashi *et al.*, 1990, 1991, 1992; Gizurarson *et al.*, 1991, 1992). Recently, we examined the effectiveness of combination of purified CT-B (or recombinant *Escherichia coli* heat-labile enterotoxin B subunit; rLT-B) and a trace amount of CT (or recombinant *E. coli* heat-labile toxin; rLT) as an adjuvant for nasal influenza vaccine (Tamura *et al*, 1994b,c). LT has been shown to have a similar subunit structure and to work by a similar mechanism to CT (Clements and Finkelstein, 1979, 1980, 1988; Takeda *et al.*, 1981). The results we obtained showed that i.n. immunization with 5 μg of HA vaccine and 2 μg of purified CT-B (or rLT-B) supplemented with 0.02–2 ng of CT (or rLT) enhanced the primary and secondary anti-HA IgA and IgG antibody responses in either nasal wash or serum, although the vaccine with either 0.02–2 ng of CT (or rLT) alone or purified CT-B (or rLT-B) alone failed to induce apparent antibody production.

It is important to clarify the mechanism by which CT-B containing a trace amount of CT enhances immune responses, because the safety of CT-containing

CT-B as an adjuvant for nasal influenza vaccine should be assessed in detail before human use. The ability of CT-B containing a trace amount of CT to augment immune responses to vaccine was generated only when the adjuvant was given to mice simultaneously with the vaccine via the same route (Tamura *et al.*, 1989a). Thus, the adjuvant seems to act on the respiratory mucosa and its immune system to activate those cells which participate in the earliest events in the immune responses. In this regard, the adjuvant was able to enhance the flux of HA molecules from the nasal cavity into the mucosal tissue in the experiments with the isolated rabbit nasal mucosa (Gizurarson *et al.*, 1992). The increased transepithelial flux of antigens may explain one of the mechanisms by which the adjuvant stimulates the mucosal immune responses to the vaccine. Moreover, the adjuvant enhanced the function of antigen-presenting cells (APC); it enhanced the *in vitro* anti-KLH antibody response by acting on early events in the responses, especially by acting on APC to secrete IL-1 (Hirabayashi *et al.*, 1992). We also examined the mechanism by which CT-B and a trace amount of CT enhance synergistically the immune responses. The ability of vaccine-pulsed peritoneal macrophages to transfer the immune responses to naive mice was enhanced by the synergistic action of a trace amount of CT and a relatively large amount of CT-B, accompanying an enhancement of the intracellular cyclic AMP activity (Tamura *et al.*, 1995). Thus, the mechanism could be explained by the enhancement of the CT action on macrophages or by the efficient binding of a trace amount of CT to APC in the presence of a relatively large amount of CT-B. These results suggest that the mechanism of adjuvanticity of CT-B with a trace amount of CT involves multiple aspects of immune induction in the nasal mucosa, including an enhancement of the APC activity as the major action.

B. Effects of CT-Containing CT-B for Nasal Vaccination

Whether a trace amount of CT with CT-B can be used safely for nasal influenza vaccine should be assessed before human use. We demonstrated that around 2 ng of CT induced the maximal synergistic effect as an adjuvant in combination with CT-B when given intranasally to mice with the vaccine (Tamura *et al.*, 1994b). The dose of CT is far smaller than that which causes brain damage, so-called encephalopathy, when injected intracerebrally into the mice (more than 1 μg of CT) (Sato and Sato, 1988) and that which causes net fluid secretion in mice (more than 1.5 μg of CT) (Richardson *et al.*, 1984). Moreover, the commercial CT-B containing CT in a concentration of 0.08% of CT at a dose of 100 μg per rabbit caused little damage histologically on the nasal mucosal membrane in rabbits (Gizurarson *et al.*, 1991). In a preliminary experiment, no damage resulted when volunteers received nasal immunizations of 100 μg of CT-B containing 100 ng of CT in a 200 μl volume (unpublished data). On the other hand, Levine *et al.* (1983) reported that no diarrhea was induced in the volunteers orally given less than 2.5 μg of purified CT, whereas doses greater than 5 μg caused diarrhea. In addition, CT-B (1 mg/dose) was administered orally to individuals in Bangladesh together with killed whole *Vibrio cholerae* as a cholera vaccine without any injurious effect (Clements *et al.*, 1987). Thus, about 100 ng of CT together with a large amount of CT-B could be used as a clinically safe adjuvant for the nasal influenza vaccine.

We have demonstrated that CT could be repeatedly administered into mice as an adjuvant for nasal vaccination, without inhibition by preexisting immunity to the toxin (Tamura *et al.*, 1989c). Similar results demonstrating lack of interference with the adjuvant-enhanced intranasal immunization with a bacterial antigen by preexisting anti-CT immunity have recently been reported (Wu and Russell, 1994). Moreover, we have demonstrated that the adjuvant effect of the toxin-containing CT-B was not genetically restricted by MHC gene (Hirabayashi *et al.*, 1991). This confirmed the suggestion that the adjuvant effect of CT was not H-2-restricted (Wilson *et al.*, 1989). This fact would be favorable to application of the current vaccine together with the toxin-containing CT-B to genetically heterogeneous humans.

A potential drawback in the use of the CT-adjuvant is the possibility of unwanted immune responses to bystander antigens (Snider *et al.*, 1994). We have shown that the CT-adjuvant augments IgE antibody response to ovalbumin (OVA) and abrogates the unresponsiveness when administered orally or intranasally into mice together with OVA, regardless of the H-2 haplotype of the mice (Tamura *et al.*, 1994d). The vaccine used was an ether-split product prepared from influenza viruses grown in eggs. These facts suggest that OVA contaminating the adjuvant-combined influenza vaccine would lead to allergy against OVA. However, we failed to detect anti-OVA IgE antibody in BALB/c mice that received three successive doses of intranasal adjuvant-combined influenza vaccine at 10-day intervals and the challenge immunization with OVA in aluminum hydroxide gel. The current split-product influenza vaccine containing only a negligible amount of OVA would minimize the potential risk of allergy, even when inoculated intranasally together with CT-adjuvant.

V. Perspective

We can draw the following conclusions on the basis of the results presented in this chapter. (1) The cross-protective effect of i.n. immunization with the adjuvant-combined influenza vaccine, which is superior to s.c. vaccination, is largely due to the induction of cross-reacting anti-HA IgA antibodies which prevent infection in the upper respiratory tract, as well as the IgG antibodies which prevent infection in the lower respiratory tract (Table IV). (2) Effective nasal vaccination against influenza could be accomplished by i.n. dropping or spraying a small volume of the adjuvant-combined trivalent vaccine under a two-dose regimen in humans. (3) The degree of cross-protection seems to be dependent on the antigenic similarities between the vaccine strains and challenge virus. Therefore, if certain viruses with surface antigens (HA and NA) most like those of the epidemic strains in circulation are selected as vaccine strains, the i.n. immunization with the adjuvant-combined trivalent vaccines will provide cross-protection against all epidemic strains in humans. (4) CT-B (or LT-B) containing about 0.1% of CT (or LT) seems to be a potent and safe adjuvant for nasal vaccination against influenza. It augments the production of not only antiviral antibodies but also anti-CT-B antibodies; however, it can be used repeatedly as an adjuvant.

In these circumstances, we need field trials to confirm the effectiveness of i.n. immunization with the current adjuvant-combined influenza vaccine in humans. Our first field trial has revealed that the nasal vaccine together with LT-containing LT-B induces a significantly high level of anti-HA antibody as compared with the vaccine alone (Hashigucci *et al.*, 1995). On the other hand, the protective efficacy of the adjuvant-combined nasal vaccine would be further improved by analyzing the roles of vaccine components other than HA and NA in defense against influenza, since the analyses would lead to development of a cocktail vaccine composed of effective protective components. The viral internal proteins, such as NP and M, which are highly conserved within a type of influenza virus, are recognized by helper and cytotoxic T cells which are involved in recovery from influenza, although antibodies to either component seem to have no significant role in immunity to influenza (Ada and Jones, 1986). Both application of the adjuvant-combined vaccine to humans and analyses of the vaccine components for the roles in defense against influenza are currently under investigation.

Acknowledgments

The authors are grateful to Dr. A. Oya, the former Director-General, National Institute of Health, and Dr. C. Aizawa, the Director of the Research Center for Biologicals, the Kitasato Institute, for their invaluable advice and encouragement. The authors are also very grateful to our colleagues who have participated in the studies described in this chapter.

References

Ada, G. L., and Jones, P. D. (1986). The immune response to influenza infection. *Curr. Top. Microbiol. Immunol.* **128,** 1–54.

Bienenstock and Befus (1980). Mucosal immunology. *Immunology* **42,** 249–270.

Both, G. M., Sleigh, M. J., Coe, N. J., and Kendal, A. P. (1983). Antigenic drift in influenza virus H3 haemagglutinin from 1986 to 1980: Multiple evolutionary pathways and sequential amino acid changes at key antigenic sites. *J. Virol.* **48,** 52–60.

Clements, J. D., and Finkelstein, R. A. (1979). Isolation and characterization of homogeneous heat-labile enterotoxins with high specific activity from *Escherichia coli* cultures. *Infect. Immun.* **24,** 760–769.

Clements, J. D., Yancey, R. L., and Finkelstein, R. A. (1980). Properties of homogeneous heat-labile enterotoxin from *Escherichia coli. Infect. Immun.* **29,** 91–97.

Clements, J. D., Staton, B. F., Chakraborty, J., Sack, D. A., Khan, M. R., Huda, S., Ahmed, F., Harris, J. R., Yunusa, M., Khan, M. U., Svennerholm, A.-M., Jertborn, M., and Holmgren, J. (1987). B-subunit-whole cell and

TABLE IV

Comparison of Cross-Protective Effect of Intranasal Immunization of the Adjuvant-Combined Influenza Vaccine with That of Subcutaneous Immunization

Relation between vaccine strain and challenge virus	Infection site (respiratory tract)	Intranasal immunization		Subcutaneous immunization	
		Antibody production	Protection	Antibody production	Protection
Same strain	Upper	IgA > IgG	++++	IgG	++++
	Lower	IgA < IgG	++++	IgG	++++
Same subtype	Upper	IgA > IgG	++++	–	–
(Drift virus)	Lower	IgA < IgG	+	IgG	+
Different subtype	Upper	IgA	+	–	–
(Shift virus)	Lower	—	–	–	–
Different type	Upper	–	–	–	–
	Lower	–	–	–	–

whole cell-only oral vaccines against cholera: Studies on reactogenicity and immunogenicity. *J. Infect. Dis.* **155,** 79–85.

Clements, J. D., Hartzog, N. M., and Lyon, F. L. (1988). Adjuvant activity of *Escherichia coli* heat-labile enterotoxin and effect on the induction of oral tolerance in mice to unrelated protein antigens. *Vaccine* **6,** 269–277.

Clements, M. L., Betts, R. F., and Murphy, B. R. (1984). Advantage of live attenuated cold-adapted influenza A virus over inactivated vaccine for A/Washington/80 (H3N2) wild-type virus infection. *Lancet* **1,** 844–850.

Couch, R. B., and Kasel, J. A. (1983). Immunity to influenza in man. *Annu. Rev. Microbiol.* **37,** 529–549.

Dertzbaugh, M. T., and Elson, C. O. (1991). Cholera toxin as a mucosal adjuvant. *In* "Topics in Vaccine Adjuvant Research" (D. R. Spriggs, and W. O. Koff, eds.), pp. 119–131. CRC Press, Boca Raton, Florida.

Dertzbaugh, M. T., Peterson, D. L., and Macrina, F. L. (1990). Cholera toxin B-subunit gene fusion: Structural and functional analysis of the chimeric protein. *Infect. Immun.* **58,** 70–79.

Elson, C. D., and Ealding, W. (1984). Generalized systemic and mucosal immunity in mice after mucosal stimulation with cholera toxin. *J. Immunol.* **132,** 27–36.

Gizurarson, S., Tamura, S.-I., Kurata, T., Hashiguchi, K., and Ogawa, H. (1991). The effect of cholera toxin and cholera toxin B subunit on the nasal mucosal membrane. *Vaccine* **9,** 825–832.

Gizurarson, S., Tamura, S.-I., Aizawa, C., and Kurata, T. (1992). Stimulation of the transepithelial flux of influenza HA vaccine by cholera toxin B subunit. *Vaccine* **10,** 101–106.

Haneberg, B., Kendall, D., Amerongen, H. M., Apter, F. M., Kraehenbuhl, J.-P., and Neutra, M. R. (1994). Induction of specific immunoglobulin A in the small intestine, colon-rectum, and vagina measured by a new method for collection of secretions from local mucosal surfaces. *Infect. Immun.* **62,** 15–23.

Hashigucci, K., Ogawa, H., Ishidate, T., Yamashita, R., Kamiya, H., Watanabe, K., Hattori, N., Sato, T., Suzuki, Y., Nagamine, T., Aizawa, C., Tamura, S.-I., Kurata, T., and Oya, A. (1996). Antibody responses in volunteers induced by nasal influenza vaccine combined with *Escherichia coli* heat-labile enterotoxin B subunit containing a trace amount of the holotoxin. *Vaccine* **14,** 113–119.

Hirabayashi, Y., Kurata, H., Funato, H., Nagamine, T., Aizawa, C., Tamura S.-I., Shimada, K., and Kurata, T. (1990). Comparison of a nasal inoculation of influenza HA vaccine combined with cholera toxin B subunit with oral or parenteral vaccination. *Vaccine* **8,** 243–248.

Hirabayashi, Y., Tamura, S.-I., Suzuki, Y., Nagamine, T., Aizawa, C., Shimada, K., and Kurata, T. (1991). H-2-unrestricted adjuvant effect of cholera toxin B subunit on murine antibody responses to influenza virus haemagglutinin. *Immunology* **72,** 329–335.

Hirabayashi, Y., Tamura, S.-I., Shimada, K., and Kurata, T. (1992). Involvement of antigen-presenting cells in the enhancement of the *in vitro* antibody responses by cholera toxin B subunit. *Immunology* **75,** 493–498.

Holmgren, J. (1981). Actions of cholera toxin and the prevention and treatment of cholera. *Nature (London)* **292,** 413–417.

Holmgren, J., and Svennerholm, A.-M. (1984). Cholera and the immune response. *Prog. Allergy* **33,** 106–114.

Holmgren, J., Lycke, N., and Czerkinsky, C. (1993). Cholera toxin and cholera B subunit as oral-mucosal adjuvant and antigen vector systems. *Vaccine* **11,** 1179–1184.

Hoskins, T. W., Davies, J. R., Smith, A. J., Allchin, A., Miller, C. L., and Pollock, T. M. (1974). Influenza at Christ's Hospital. *Lancet* **1,** 105–106.

Kikuta, K., Kurata, H., Nagamine, T., Aizawa, C., Ueno, Y., Kurata, T., and Tamura, S.-I. (1990a). Enhancement of DTH response by cholera toxin B subunit inoculated intranasally together with influenza HA vaccine. *Microbiol. Immunol.* **34,** 337–346.

Kikuta, K., Hirabayashi, Y., Nagamine, T., Aizawa, C., Ueno, Y., Oya, A., Kurata, T., and Tamura, S.-I. (1990b). Cross-protection against influenza B type virus infection by intranasal inoculation of the HA vaccines combined with cholera toxin B subunit. *Vaccine* **8,** 595–599.

Kris, R. M., Asofsky, R., Evans, C. B., and Small, P. A., Jr. (1985). Protection and recovery in influenza virus-infected mice immunosuppressed with anti-IgM. *J. Immunol.* **134,** 1230–1235.

Levine, M. M., Kaper, J. D., Black, R. E., and Clements, M. L. (1983). New knowledge on pathogenesis of bacterial enteric infections as applied to vaccine development. *Microbiol. Rev.* **47,** 510–530.

Liew, F. Y., Russell, S. M., Appleyard, G., Brand, C. M., and Beale, J. (1984). Cross-protection in mice infected with influenza A virus by the respiratory route is correlated with local IgA antibody rather than serum antibody or cytotoxic T cell activity. *Eur. J. Immunol.* **14,** 350–356.

Lycke, N., Tsuji, T., and Holmgren, J. (1992). The adjuvant effect of *Vibrio cholerae* and *E. coli* heat labile enterotoxins is linked to the ability to stimulate cAMP. *Eur. J. Immunol.* **22,** 2277–2281.

Maassab, H. F. (1967). Adaptation and growth characteristics of influenza virus at 25°C. *Nature (London)* **213,** 612–614.

McGhee, J. R., and Kiyono, H. (1993). New perspectives in vaccine development: Mucosal immunity to infections. *Infect. Agents Dis.* **2,** 55–73.

McKenzie, S. J., and Halsey, J. H. (1984). Cholera toxin B subunit as a carrier protein to stimulate a mucosal immune response. *J. Immunol.* **133,** 1818–1824.

Mayer, H. M., Jr., Hopps, H. E., Parleman, P. D., and Ennis, F. A. (1978). Review of existing vaccines for influenza. *Am. J. Clin. Pathol.* **70,** 146–152.

Murphy, B. R., and Clements, M. L. (1989). The systemic and mucosal immune response of humans to influenza A virus. *Curr. Top. Microbiol. Immunol.* **146,** 107–116.

Murphy, B. R., and Webster, R. G. (1990). Orthomyxoviruses. *In* "Virology" (B. N. Fields, D. M. Knipe, R. M. Chanock, M. S. Hirsch, and J. L. Melnick, eds.), pp. 1091–1152. Raven, New York.

Nedrud, J. G., Liang, X.-P., Hague, N., and Lamm, M. E. (1987). Combined oral/nasal immunization protects mice from Sendai virus infection. *J. Immunol.* **139,** 3484–3492.

Phelan, M. A., Mayner, R. E., Bucker, D. J., and Ennis, F. A. (1980). Purification of influenza virus glycoproteins for the preparation and standardization of immunological potency testing reagents. *J. Biol. Stand.* **8,** 233–242.

Ramphal, R., Cogliano, R. C., Shands, J. W., Jr., and Small, P. A., Jr. (1979). Serum antibody prevents lethal murine influenza pneumonitis but not tracheitis. *Infect. Immun.* **25**, 992–997.

Raymond, F. L., Canton, A. J., Cox, N. J., Kendal, A. P., and Brownlee, G. G. (1986). The antigenicity and evolution of influenza H1 haemagglutinin, from 1950–1957 and 1977–1983: Two pathways from one gene. *Virology* **148**, 275–287.

Richardson, S. H., Giles, J. C., and Krucker, K. S. (1984). Sealed adult mice: New model for enterotoxin evaluation. *Infect. Immun.* **43**, 482–486.

Robertson, J. S. (1987). Sequence analysis of the haemagglutinin of A/Taiwan/1/86, a new variant of human influenza A (H1N1) virus. *J. Gen. Virol.* **68**, 1205–1208.

Sato, H., and Sato, Y. (1988). An attempt to introduce encephalopathy with pertussis toxin in mice. *Jpn. J. Med. Sci. Biol.* **41**, 235–236.

Schulman, J. L., and Kilbourne, E. D. (1965). Induction of partial specific heterotypic immunity in mice by a single infection with influenza A virus. *J. Bacteriol.* **89**, 170–174.

Shvartsman, Ya. S., and Zykov, M. P. (1976). Secretory Anti-influenza Immunity. *Adv. Immunol.* **22**, 291–330.

Snider, D. P., Marshall, J. S., Perdue, M. H., and Liang, H. (1994). Production of IgE antibody and allergic sensitization of intestinal and peripheral tissues after oral immunization with protein Ag and cholera toxin. *J. Immunol.* **153**, 647–657.

Takeda, Y., Honda, T., Taga, S., and Miwatani, T. (1981). *In vitro* formation of hybrid toxins between subunits of *Escherichia coli* heat-labile enterotoxin and those of cholera enterotoxin. *Infect. Immun.* **34**, 341–346.

Tamura, S.-I., Samegai, Y., Kurata, H., and Kurata, T. (1988a). Effects of cholera toxin on delayed-type hypersensitivity to sheep red blood cells inoculated intranasally into mice. *Microbiol. Immunol.* **32**, 1145–1161.

Tamura, S.-I., Samegai, Y., Kurata, H., Nagamine, T., Aizawa, C., and Kurata, T. (1988b). Protection against influenza virus infection by vaccine inoculated intranasally with cholera toxin B subunit. *Vaccine* **6**, 409–413.

Tamura, S.-I., Samegai, Y., Kurata, H., Kikuta, K., Nagamine, T., Aizawa, C., and Kurata, T. (1989a). Enhancement of protective antibody responses by cholera toxin B subunit inoculated intranasally with influenza vaccine. *Vaccine* **7**, 257–262.

Tamura, S.-I., Funato, H., Nagamine, T., Aizawa, C., and Kurata, T. (1989b). Protection against influenza virus infection by two-dose regimen of nasal vaccination using vaccines combined with cholera toxin B subunit. *Vaccine* **7**, 314–320.

Tamura, S.-I., Funato, H., Nagamine, T., Aizawa, C., and Kurata, T. (1989c). Effectiveness of cholera toxin B subunit as an adjuvant for nasal influenza vaccination despite preexisting immunity to CT-B. *Vaccine* **7**, 503–505.

Tamura, S.-I., Funato, H., Hirabayashi, Y., Kikuta, K., Suzuki, Y., Nagamine, T., Aizawa, C., Nakagawa, M., and Kurata, T. (1990). Functional role of respiratory tract haemagglutinin-specific IgA antibodies in protection against influenza. *Vaccine* **8**, 476–486.

Tamura, S.-I., Funato, H., Hirabayashi, Y., Suzuki, Y., Nagamine, T., Aizawa, C., and Kurata, T. (1991). Cross-protection against influenza A virus infection by passively transferred respiratory tract IgA antibodies to different haemagglutinin molecules. *Eur. J. Immunol.* **21**, 1337–1344.

Tamura, S.-I., Asanuma, H., Ito, Y., Hirabayashi, Y., Nagamine, T., Aizawa, C., Kurata, T., and Oya, A. (1992a). Superior cross-protective effect of nasal vaccination to subcutaneous inoculation with influenza HA vaccine. *Eur. J. Immunol.* **22**, 477–481.

Tamura, S.-I., Ito, Y., Asanuma, H., Hirabayashi, Y., Suzuki, Y., Nagamine, T., Aizawa, C., and Kurata, T. (1992b). Cross-protection against influenza virus infection afforded by trivalent inactivated vaccines inoculated intranasally with cholera toxin B subunit. *J. Immunol.* **149**, 981–988.

Tamura, S.-I., Asanuma, H., Ito, Y., Yoshizawa, K., Nagamine, T., Aizawa, C., and Kurata, T. (1994a). Formulation of inactivated influenza vaccines for providing effective cross-protection by intranasal vaccination in mice. *Vaccine* **12**, 310–316.

Tamura, S.-I., Yamanaka, A., Shimohara, M., Tomita, T., Komase, K., Tsuda, Y., Suzuki, Y., Nagamine, T., Kawahara, K., Danbara, H., Aizawa, C., Oya, A., and Kurata, T. (1994b). Synergistic action of cholera toxin B subunit (and *E. coli* heat-labile toxin B subunit) and a trace amount of cholera whole toxin as an adjuvant for nasal influenza vaccine. *Vaccine* **12**, 419–426.

Tamura, S.-I., Asanuma, H., Tomita, T., Komase, K., Kawahara, K., Danbara, H., Hattori, N., Watanabe, K., Suzuki, Y., Nagamine, T., Aizawa, C., Oya, A., and Kurata, T. (1994c). *Escherichia coli* heat-labile enterotoxin B subunits supplemented with a trace amount of the holotoxin as an adjuvant for nasal influenza vaccine. *Vaccine* **12**, 1083–1089.

Tamura, S.-I., Shoji, Y., Hashiguchi, K., Aizawa, C., and Kurata, T. (1994d). Effects of cholera toxin adjuvant on IgE antibody response to orally or nasally administered ovalbumin. *Vaccine* **12**, 1238–1240.

Tamura, S.-I., Ishihara, K., Miyata, K., Aizawa, C., and Kurata, T. (1995). Mechanism of enhancement of the immune responses to influenza vaccine with cholera toxin B subunit and a trace amount of holotoxin. *Vaccine* **13**, 339–341.

Underdown, B. J., and Schiff, J. M. (1986). Immunoglobulin A: Strategic defense initiative at the mucosal surface. *Annu. Rev. Immunol.* **4**, 389–417.

Waldman, R. H. and Ganguly, R. (1974). Immunity to infections on secretory surfaces. *J. Infect. Dis.* **130**, 419–440.

Waldman, R. H., Wigley, F. M., and Small, P. A., Jr. (1970). Specificity of respiratory secretion antibody against influenza virus. *J. Immunol.* **105**, 1477–1483.

Walker, R. I. (1994). New strategies for using mucosal vaccination to achieve more effective immunization. *Vaccine* **12**, 387–400.

Wilson, A. D., Stokes, C. R., and Bourne, F. J. (1989). Adjuvant effect of cholera toxin on the mucosal immune response to soluble proteins. Differences between mouse strains and protein antigens. *Scand. J. Immunol.* **29**, 739–745.

Wilson, A. D., Clarke, C. J., and Stokes, C. R. (1990). Whole cholera toxin and B subunit act synergistically as an adjuvant for the mucosal immune response of mice to keyhole limpet haemocyanin. *Scand. J. Immunol.* **31**, 443–451.

Wilson, I. R., and Cox, J. C. (1990). Structural basis of immune recognition of influenza virus hemagglutinin. *Annu. Rev. Immunol.* **8**, 737–771.

Winter, G., Fields, S., and Brownlee, G. G. (1981). Nucleotide sequence of the haemagglutinin gene of a human influenza virus H1 subtype. *Nature (London)* **292**, 72–75.

Wu, H.-Y., and Russell, M. W. (1994). Comparison of systemic and mucosal priming for mucosal immune responses to a bacterial protein antigen given with or coupled to cholera toxin (CT) B subunit, and effects of pre-existing anti-CT immunity. *Vaccine* **12**, 215–222.

Yamashita, M., Krystal, M., Fitch, W. M., and Palese, P. (1988). Influenza B virus evolution: Co-circulating lineages and comparison of evolutionary pattern with those of influenza A and C viruses. *Virology* **163**, 112–122.

Yetter, R. A., Kehrer, S., Ramphal, R., and Small, P. A., Jr. (1980). Outcome of influenza infection: Effect of site of initial infection and heterotypic immunity. *Infect. Immun.* **29**, 654–662.

32

Mucosal Immunity and Periodontitis

ROY C. PAGE
Research Center in Oral Biology
University of Washington
Seattle, Washington 98195

ROBERT GENCO
Department of Oral Biology
School of Dental Medicine
State University of New York
Buffalo, New York 14214

I. Introduction

Periodontitis is a destructive chronic inflammatory disease of the connective tissues and bone housing the teeth. The disease has an infectious etiology and is a major cause of tooth loss in adults. The prevalence of periodontal diseases in the American population is relatively high (Brown and Löe, 1993), with moderate periodontitis affecting about one-half of working adults 18–65 years or age. In contrast, progressive periodontal destruction of a magnitude sufficient to endanger the survival of the dentition occurs in a smaller but significant proportion of the population (Brown and Löe, 1993). This is true for populations in Sri Lanka and Africa where dental care traditionally has not been available (Löe *et al.*, 1986; Pilot *et al.*, 1986), for populations of treated patients maintained on recall where deterioration continues in 5 to 15% (Hirshfeld and Wasserman, 1978), and for untreated patients monitored for periods of 1 to 6 years where deterioration is infrequent and the majority of active lesions was observed in 5–10% of the study population (Lindhe *et al.*, 1983). Thus, a discrete but significant proportion of the general population, as well as patients receiving adequate periodontal therapy, is considered to be at high risk, and recent studies provide guidance in identifying those in this category for periodontal disease (Grossi *et al.*, 1994, 1995; Genco and Löe, 1993). Accordingly, the use of a vaccine for such groups would seem to be more practical, cost-effective, and workable than measures designed to be applied to entire populations.

The microbial etiology of periodontitis in humans and animals is now well established, with several species of putative periodontal pathogens having been identified (Tanner *et al.*, 1979; Slots, 1986; Loesche, 1988; Zambon *et al.*, 1988a,b). Species most strongly implicated in the etiology of the disease include *Actinobacillus actinomycetemcomitans* (especially serotype b), *Porphyromonas gingivalis, Bacteroides forsythus, Treponema denticola,* and possibly *Prevotella intermedia, Eikenella corrodens, Campylobacter rectus, Fusobacterium nucleatum, Peptostreptococcus micros,* and *Eubacterium* species (Haffajee and Socransky, 1994).

II. Humoral Immune Response in Periodontitis Patients

Numerous studies have demonstrated that many, although not all, patients with periodontitis mount a humoral immune response during the course of their spontaneous periodontal infection (Genco *et al.*, 1980; Mouton *et al.*, 1981; Tew *et al.*, 1985; Vincent *et al.*, 1987; Ebersole *et al.*, 1986; Ishikawa *et al.*, 1988; Murayama *et al.*, 1988; Zambon *et al.*, 1988a,b; Ogawa *et al.*, 1990; Chen *et al.*, 1991; Whitney et al., 1992; Ling et al., 1993). The reason some patients respond by producing serum antibodies reactive with antigens of their infecting bacteria while others do not remains unclear, as is the role such antibodies may play in the onset and progression of the disease. A growing body of evidence supports the idea that antibodies produced during the course of periodontal infection may be relatively ineffective in protecting against periodontal disease. For example, antibodies of the IgG2 subclass, followed by IgG3, IgG1, and IgG4, often predominate in the sera in both localized juvenile periodontitis (LJP) and RPP patients to antigens of *A. actinomycetemcomitans* and *P. gingivalis,* respectively (Whitney *et al.*, 1992; Ling *et al.*, 1993). IgG2 antibodies do not fix complement nor enhance opsonization and phagocytosis and killing by neutrophils as effectively as IgG1 (Roitt *et al.*, 1989). However, recent studies show that IgG2 antibodies in LJP are effective opsonins when used with phagocytes expressing the proper allotype of the low-affinity IgG (Fc) receptor (CD32) (Wilson *et al.*, 1995).

Although serum antibody titers may be rather high in some patients, measures of antibody function (such as avidity and enhancement of killing) are relatively low (Chen *et al.*, 1991; Sjöstrom *et al.*, 1992, 1994). Indeed, in a study by Sjöstrom *et al.* (1992), low-titer sera from periodontally normal individuals were more effective at enhancing phagocytosis and killing than were low-titer sera from RPP patients, suggesting that immediately following infection, normal subjects may produce antibodies that are effective in clearing the organisms prior to clinical signs of infection; however, individuals who are susceptible to periodontitis are unable to do so, and clinical disease develops. On the other hand, Baker and Wilson (1989) found opsonic IgG antibodies in high titered sera from LJP patients.

In spite of the above observations, evidence for antibody protection has been reported in some studies. Ranney *et al.* (1982) observed fewer affected teeth and less severe disease in young adults having high levels of precipitating serum antibodies to antigens of periodontopathic bacteria than in subjects with lower titers. Similarly, Gunsolley *et al.* (1987) found an inverse relationship between levels of serum antibodies reactive with antigens of *A. actinomycetemcomitans* and *P. gingivalis,* and the number of teeth having attachment loss. In addition, a negative correlation between specific serum IgG antibody and the number of pockets deeper than 4 mm has been reported (Schenck *et al.*, 1987).

Periodontal therapy appears to have a marked effect on humoral immune responses to antigens of periodontopathic bacteria (Ebersole *et al.*, 1985; Vincent *et al.*, 1987; Murayama *et al.*, 1988). Treatment by scaling and root planing or by surgery significantly enhances serum antibody titers and avidities to antigens of *P. gingivalis* and induces seronegative patients to seroconvert (Ebersole *et al.*, 1985; Chen *et al.*, 1991; Sjöstrom *et al.*, 1994). A statistically significant positive correlation was observed between titer to whole-cell sonicate of *P. gingivalis* and both mean pocket depth and mean bone loss, and a significant negative correlation exists between avidity to the whole-cell sonicate and mean bone loss and mean pocket depth (Chen *et al.*, 1991).

In another study, RPP patients treated only by scaling and root planing manifested significantly elevated serum antibody titers and avidities to antigens of *A. actinomycetemcomitans,* and at 12 months post-treatment, sera significantly enhanced chemiluminescence, phagocytosis, and killing relative to pretreatment sera (Sjöstrom *et al.*, 1994). Thus, conventional therapeutic approaches such as scaling and root planing, which are known to result in transient bacteremias, appear to elicit the production of antibodies that may be more protective than antibodies produced before treatment of the spontaneously occurring infection.

III. Prospects for a Vaccine

The observations described above, as well as data obtained from animal experiments to be described later, support the idea that development of a vaccine for control and prevention of periodontitis may be possible. However, severe challenges involved in development of a safe and effective periodontal vaccine exist. Periodontitis is a multifactorial disease in which host defense mechanisms and poorly understood genetic factors play a major role. The possibility exists that systemic immunity may contribute to the pathogenic processes leading to tissue destruction, in which case induction of mucosal immunity may be a safer approach. The presence of periodontopathic bacteria in the subgingival flora is essential but insufficient for periodontitis to occur. Of equal importance, numerous bacterial species appear to be involved, with five to seven different species strongly implicated in the etiology (Haffajee and Socransky, 1994).

The complexity may not be as great as previously thought. Not all of the implicated microbial species may be essential for the disease to occur. Most may be bystanders or species that participate only after disease has been established, while one or two species may be essential for disease initiation. Notably, in a recent epidemiologic study of 1426 patients, Grossi *et al.* (1994, 1995) observed that *P. gingivalis* and *B. forsythus* were the only subgingival species studied that were significantly linked to adult periodontitis. Second, species participating in the etiology may express shared antigenic epitopes. Most of the putative periodontal pathogens are gram-negative and therefore have lipopolysaccharide (LPS). Antigenic epitopes in LPS, especially in lipid A and to a lesser extent in core carbohydrates, are highly conserved and may be shared among gram negative bacteria (Aydintug *et al.*, 1989; DiPadova *et al.*, 1993). Evidence for epitopes that are shared between *P. gingivalis* and *B. forsythus* has been presented; immunization of *Macaca fascicularis* with a vaccine containing *P. gingivalis* induces serum antibodies reactive with LPS of both *P. gingivalis* and *B. forsythus* (Persson et al., 1994; Vasel *et al.*, 1996). These results may be explained by the polyclonal B-cell activating properties of LPS rather than the induction of specific immunity. Finally, even if several species are essential to the etiology of periodontitis, a successful vaccine may still be possible. Characterization of the antigenic epitopes of each species responsible for induction of protective immunity to that species could result in determination of the peptide sequences containing the necessary epitopes. Using known sequences and recombinant DNA technology an appropriate antigenic sequence (or series of sequences) could be constructed to induce immunity to several of the important periodontal pathogens.

In developing an experimental plan for producing a vaccine against periodontopathic bacteria, a choice had to be made early on as to the use of a traditional injectable vaccine aimed at inducing high titers of serum IgG antibodies, or an oral vaccine targeting the gut associated lymphoid tissue (GALT), production of secretory IgA (S-IgA) antibodies, and induction of mucosal immunity. The two strategies differ greatly, and each has advantages and disadvantages.

The intestine is the largest immunological organ in the body. It has 70 to 80% of all of the immunoglobulin-producing cells, about 10 to 20% of which end up outside of the gut mucosa. The cells produce 50–100 mg/kg/day of immunoglobulin, considerably more than the remaining antibody-producing cells (McGhee and Mestecky, 1990; Holmgren, 1991). S-IgA antibodies function at mucosal surfaces including the oral cavity to neutralize bacterial toxins and viruses and to inhibit attachment, adherence and colonization of the mucosal and tooth surfaces (McGhee and Mestecky, 1990; Michalek and Childers, 1990). Very small amounts of antigen are required and several excellent vehicles and adjuvants which target IgA B cells in Peyer's patches have been developed. Attenuated strains of bacteria such as *Salmonella* have been used as vectors for targeted delivery. *S. typhimurium* carrying Ag I/II or glucosyltransferase of *S. mutans* and *S. typhi* expressing lipopolysaccharide from another bacterium have been used for oral immunization in animals and humans, respectively. These induce serum as well as secretory antibodies and protection (Mestecky and Eldridge, 1991). Other bacterial antigens including M protein of streptococci and bacterial fimbriae have also been expressed in recombinant strains of *Salmonella.* Liposomes, phospholipid membrane vesicles, microspheres of poly-DL-lactide-*co*-glycolide, and antigen linked to the B subunit of cholera toxin have been successfully used as targeted vehicles (Moldoveanu *et al.*, 1993; McGhee and Mestecky, 1990; Holmgren, 1991).

An oral vaccine designed to induce S-IgA in saliva could be effective in interfering with bacterial adherence and colonization of the oral mucosa and teeth by putative periodontal pathogens without inducing significant humoral immunity which may contribute to periodontal pathology. The bacteria of concern are, however, mostly anaerobic or facultative and they are found mostly in periodontal pockets which are not accessible to salivary components. Thus, while salivary antibodies could interfere with initial mucosal colonization, they would not have access to bacteria in the subgingival flora.

In contrast to saliva, gingival crevicular fluid (GCF) is a blood-derived exudate containing serum immunoglobulins as well as immunoglobulins produced by plasma cells in the periodontal pocket wall. GCF traverses periodontal pockets where it bathes the bacteria and exudes into the mouth. Thus, GCF is an ideal vehicle for transporting specific antibodies to the subgingival bacteria as well as to the supragingival region around the necks of the teeth. It is for these reasons that investigators working to develop periodontal vaccines have considered traditional injectable as well as oral vaccines as complementary approaches to inducing protective immunity.

IV. Studies in Rodents

Rodent models of periodontal disease include germfree rats monoinfected with *Porphyromonas gingivalis* (Klausen *et al.*, 1993), mice infected with *P. gingivalis* (Baker *et al.*, 1994), ligated hamster teeth (Okuda *et al.*, 1988), subcutaneous abscess in mice (van Steenbergen *et al.*, 1982), and subcutaneous chamber models in mice and rabbits (Dahlén and Slots, 1989; Genco *et al.*, 1991). The subcutaneous abscess and chamber models are suitable for investigations concerning virulence once bacteria have entered the tissue. Factors such as colonization and destruction of periodontal bone and ligament, of course, cannot be studied in these models. However, colonization and destruction of periodontal bone and ligament can be studied in the gnotobiotic rat model monoinfected with *P. gingivalis* alone (Klausen *et al.*, 1991; Evans *et al.*, 1992a–c) or *P. gingivalis* in the presence of a controlled flora (Chang *et al.*, 1988), and in mice infected with *P. gingivalis* (Baker *et al.*, 1994).

Rats are remarkably similar to man with respect to periodontal structures as well as pathogenesis of periodontal disease (Klausen, 1991; Page and Schroeder, 1982). In addition, rats have been established as reliable models for the assessment of periodontal bone loss (Klausen *et al.*, 1989). Although it is difficult to establish *P. gingivalis* in rats for more than a few weeks (Evans *et al.*, 1992c) as is the problem with primates, several studies have shown that this infection time is sufficient to induce detectable periodontal bone loss without ligation (Klausen *et al.*, 1991; Evans *et al.*, 1992a–c).

Various antigens of *P. gingivalis* have been used in immunization studies in the rat. For example, heat-killed whole cells (Klausen *et al.*, 1991; Evans *et al.*, 1992c), and fimbrial antigens [crude preparations

(Evans *et al.*, 1992c), the 43-kDa pure preparation (Evans *et al.*, 1992c), or the 20-mer synthetic peptide (Evans *et al.*, 1992a)] have been used. Other antigens used include the 75-kDa antigen obtained from the cell surface of *P. gingivalis* (Evans *et al.*, 1992c). Whole cells, either live (Chen *et al.*, 1987, 1990) or heat-killed (Chen *et al.*, 1987; Genco *et al.*, 1992; Kesavalu *et al.*, 1992), and formalinized whole cells (Kesavalu *et al.*, 1992) have been used in the mouse abscess or chamber model. The 41-kDa fimbriae has also been used in the mouse (Ogawa *et al.*, 1989; Shimauchi *et al.*, 1991), as has a LIS extract (Chen *et al.*, 1990), LPS (Kesavalu *et al.*, 1992), and outer membrane vesicles (Chen *et al.*, 1990; Kesavalu *et al.*, 1992).

Most of these studies demonstrated a protective effect of immunization with *P. gingivalis* antigens on *P. gingivalis*-induced pathology. For example, in subcutaneous models in mice, immunization with whole *P. gingivalis* cells generally reduces the size of the primary lesion and inhibits or prevents invasion of bacteria. In fact, subsequent death of the animals upon challenge with *P. gingivalis* is also prevented (Chen *et al.*, 1987, 1990; Genco *et al.*, 1992; Kesavalu *et al.*, 1992). In rabbits, immunization led to elimination of *P. gingivalis* in the subcutaneous chamber (Dahlén and Slots, 1989). In ligated hamsters, subcutaneous administration of whole formalinized *P. gingivalis* cells resulted in reduction in the number of *P. gingivalis.* A strong effect was seen after repeated passive immunization with rabbit antisera against *P. gingivalis* cells (Okuda *et al.*, 1988).

In monoinfected rats, marked protection against *P. gingivalis*-induced periodontal bone loss was found after immunization with whole cells of *P. gingivalis* (Klausen *et al.*, 1991; Evans *et al.*, 1992c). Immunization also reduced the activity of gingival collagenase and cysteine proteinases. The controls (sham-immunized *P. gingivalis*-infected rats) had significantly higher bone loss and high gingival enzyme activities (Klausen *et al.*, 1991; Evans *et al.*, 1992c).

Several antigen extracts and purified antigens from *P. gingivalis* have been applied in immunization studies with varying results. For example, immunization with purified hemagglutinin of *P. gingivalis* appeared as effective as immunization with whole cells in reducing the recovery of *P. gingivalis* in ligated hamsters (Okuda *et al.*, 1988). Passive immunization with rabbit antiserum against hemagglutinin also resulted in marked reduction of *P. gingivalis* cultivable from ligated teeth (Okuda *et al.*, 1988). In the mouse abscess model, lipopolysaccharide, which was found to be a weak immunogen, did not interfere with the disease process. However, the lithium di-iodosalicylate (LIS) extract of membranes from *P. gingivalis* reduced the incidence of secondary lesions, but could not prevent invasion of tissues in all animals (Chen *et al.*, 1990). In another mouse abscess study, immunization with LPS slightly decreased the size of lesions and reduced the lethality to 60% of the control level (Kesavalu *et al.*, 1992). Immunization with a preparation of outer membrane vesicles of *P. gingivalis* resulted in reduction of lethality and slight reduction in the size of the mouse abscesses (Kesavalu *et al.*, 1992).

Fimbrial antigen structures, crucial for the adherence of *P. gingivalis* to oral tissues (Okuda *et al.*, 1981; Lee *et al.*, 1992), have been studied extensively in the *P. gingivalis* monoinfected rat model. *P. gingivalis* fimbriae are highly immunogenic (Ogawa *et al.*, 1989; Klausen *et al.*, 1991; Shimauchi *et al.*, 1991) and biochemically well characterized (Yoshimura *et al.*, 1985; Lee *et al.*, 1991). The fimbrillin 43-kDa subunit has been cloned and sequenced (Dickinson *et al.*, 1988). Rats immunized with purified fimbriae and with purified 43-kDa fimbrial subunit were found to be protected from *P. gingivalis* induced periodontal destruction as efficiently as rats immunized with whole *P. gingivalis* cells (Evans *et al.*, 1992c) (Fig. 1). In addition, gingival collagenase and cysteine proteinases were also reduced to control levels in the *P. gingivalis* fimbrial immunized rats (Evans *et al.*, 1992c). Animals immunized with purified fimbriae of *P. gingivalis* had both salivary and serum antibodies to this antigen (Evans *et al.*, 1992c). The salivary antibodies were elevated in the protected groups only to the *P. gingivalis* fimbrilin (Fig. 2). Similar results were obtained by immunization with a synthetic 20-amino acid peptide epitope based on the known structure of the 43-kDa fimbrial protein (Evans *et al.*, 1992a), open-

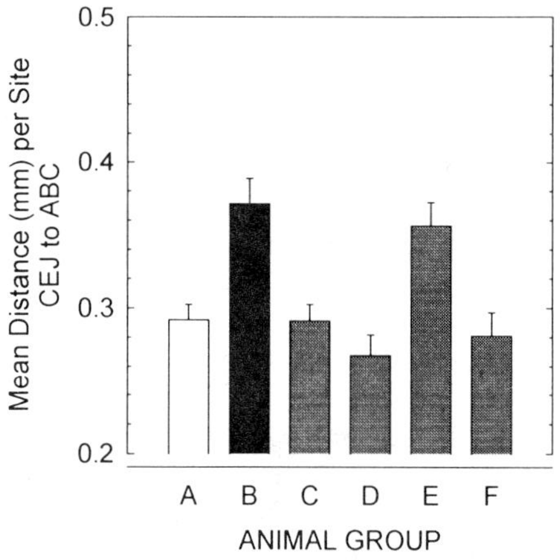

Figure 1. Alveolar bone levels measured from the cementoenamel junction to the alveolar crest presented as mean ± the standard error of the mean. Group A: Germ-free rats. B: Rats monoinfected with *P. gingivalis*. C: Rats with *P. gingivalis* and immunized with whole cells of *P. gingivalis*. D: Rats infected with *P. gingivalis* and immunized with purified 43-kDa fimbriae. E: Rats infected with *P. gingivalis* and immunized with purified 75-kDa component of *P. gingivalis*. F: Rats infected with *P. gingivalis* and immunized with a crude extract of *P. gingivalis* rich in fimbriae. Groups B and E showed statistically greater alveolar bone loss than group A ($P < 0.005$). Groups C, D, and F showed lower alveolar bone loss than group B, the infected control. From Evans *et al.* (1992c), with permission.

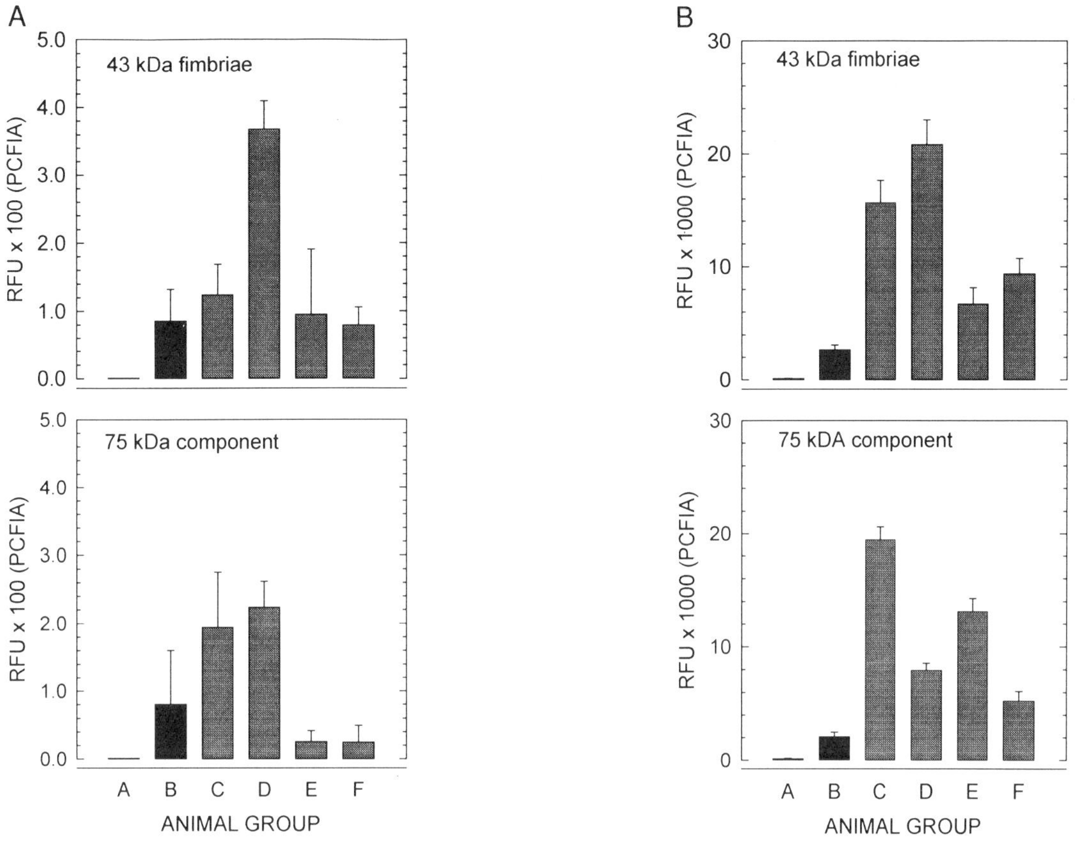

Figure 2. Salivary antibody levels to the 43-kDa fimbriae and the 75-kDa outer membrane component of *P. gingivalis*. Group A: Germfree rats. B: Rats monoinfected with *P. gingivalis*. C: Rats infected with *P. gingivalis* and immunized with whole cells of *P. gingivalis*. D: Rats infected with *P. gingivalis* and immunized with purified 43-kDa fimbriae. E: Rats infected with *P. gingivalis* and immunized with purified 75-kDa component of *P. gingivalis*. F: Rats infected with *P. gingivalis* and immunized with a crude extract of *P. gingivalis* rich in fimbriae. The saliva from each individual was diluted to 1:5 prior to testing by PCFIA. RFU, relative fluorescent unit. From Evans *et al.* (1992c), with permission.

ing the way for the development of genetically engineered or synthetic fimbrial vaccines. More recently, recombinant fimbriae have been shown to induce immunity also in the monoinfected rat model (Evans *et al.*, 1992a). Protection induced by immunization with *P. gingivalis* fimbriae appears to be specific since rats immunized with a purified 75-kDa outer membrane protein did not induce protection against *P. gingivalis*-induced periodontal bone loss in the *P. gingivalis* monoinfected animal (Evans *et al.*, 1992c) (Fig. 1).

Antigens may be strain specific and consequently not confer protection against other strains in the species. However, this does not appear to be the case with *P. gingivalis* fimbriae, since immunization of rats with whole cells from five different strains consistently induced antibodies against a component in the 43-kDa region (Genco *et al.*, 1992). Furthermore, Brant *et al.* (1995) and Lee *et al.* (1991) have shown that fimbriae share many common antigenic determinants, immunity to which may be protective.

The mechanism of immunity to *P. gingivalis* fimbriae is unknown. There are several possibilities: (1) antibodies in the secretory immune system, which are known to be induced in the *P. gingivalis*-immunized animal, may confer protection against initial colonization; (2) serum-mediated antibodies or humoral cell-mediated immunity may reduce other activities of the fimbriae such as stimulation of macrophage production of histiolytic enzymes and proinflammatory cytokines; or (3) cell-mediated immunity to *P. gingivalis* may be protective.

V. Studies in Nonhuman Primates

Several immunization studies have been performed in nonhuman primates. McArthur and co-workers (1989) immunized squirrel monkeys (*Saimiri scuireus*) using a vaccine containing 10^9 *Porphyromonas gingivalis* I-372 and incomplete Freund's adjuvant. Booster injections containing 10^9 CFU without incomplete Freund's adjuvant were given 26 and 31 weeks later. Prior to immunization the animals had no detectable black pigmenting bacteria and manifested very low serum levels of anti-*P. gingivalis* or anti-*P. intermedia* IgG, IgM, and IgA antibodies. Five teeth in the mandibular right quadrant

(quadrant 4) were ligated with silk suture material previously soaked in 10^{10} *P. gingivalis* I-372. Immediately following ligation 10^{10} viable *P. gingivalis* I-372 were applied to the gingival margin throughout the entire mouth of each animal. As shown in Table I relative to the sham-immunized group, the immunized animals manifested high serum IgG titers to antigens of the immunizing microorganism. Titers were about 100-fold greater in the immunized animals than in the sham immunized animals at 1 week postligation. Titers were, however, highly variable from animal to animal, and they were not enduring; titers decreased greatly by 7 weeks postligation. Interestingly, at 7 weeks postligation anti-*P. gingivalis* IgG serum titers had increased in the sham-immunized animals, presumably as a result of ligation and oral inoculation. Mean black pigmented *Bacteroides* (BPB) levels and mean BPB percentages of total microbiota for 10 sampling times following ligation were reported by quadrant. Although statistically significant differences at the $P < 0.05$ level could not be demonstrated, there was a strong trend toward reduction in the mean values for *P. gingivalis* in the ligated and the directly opposing quadrants. No trends could be established in the contralateral quadrants. Thus, immunization appears to affect colonization by *P. gingivalis* in this primate model.

An additional study on colonization by *P. intermedia* in the squirrel monkey was reported by Clark *et al.* (1991). Twelve squirrel monkeys were divided equally into immunized and sham-immunized groups. Most quadrants in most animals harbored *P. intermedia* prior to the beginning of the study. To reduce or eliminate the organism, the animals were treated by prophylaxis combined with administration of 20 mg/kg of tetracycline three times each day for 10 days. Following this regimen, *P. intermedia* was detected in only 1 of 48 quadrants and accounted for <1% of the sample. The animals were immunized with a vaccine containing 10^9 CFU formalinized *P. intermedia* 1447 previously isolated from a squirrel monkey in incomplete Freund's adjuvant. Over a period of 180 days, three booster injections containing 10^9 bacteria were given. As shown in Table II, very high titers of antibody were induced, although there were large variations from animal to animal. Titers appear to have persisted to a greater extent than those observed by McArthur *et al.* (1989) in animals immunized with *P. gingivalis.* Titers were roughly 22-fold greater than mean IgG reactive with *P. intermedia* 1447 levels in the sham-immunized animals. Between the second and third booster injections, animals were sampled five times and shown to be essentially free of *P. intermedia.* One hundred-eighty days following the first injection, teeth in the mandibular right quadrant were ligated with sterile silk sutures. At 14-day intervals following ligation, animals were sampled over a period of 120 days. Two weeks after ligation, *P. intermedia* could be detected in five of the six sham-immunized and three of six immunized animals. Over a period of 100 days, the percentage of immunized animals infected in the ligated quadrant remained significantly lower than for sham-immunized group. Thus immunization is associated with a reduction in the reemergence of indigenous *P. intermedia.*

Ebersole *et al.* (1991) evaluated the effect of immunization on the progression of periodontal tissue destruction using the ligature induced periodontitis model in *Macaca fascicularis.* Animals were separated into four groups of five each. Vaccines were prepared using *P. gingivalis* 3079.03 (monkey isolate), *P. intermedia* 6235.2 (monkey isolate), and the nonoral bacterium *Bacteroides fragilis* ATCC 25285, and incomplete Freund's adjuvant. One group of five animals was immunized with each vaccine and the fourth group received placebo vaccine containing adjuvant but no bacteria. Animals were immunized at 10, 12, and 14 weeks after baseline. The teeth were ligated at 16 weeks, and clinical and radiographic data were collected and microbial samples and blood harvested at intervals through 51 weeks. Three adjacent teeth in the mandibular left quadrant were ligated and the contralateral teeth served as nonligated controls.

TABLE I

Anti-*P. gingivalis* Antibody Levels in Squirrel Monkeys Sham-Immunized or Immunized with *P. gingivalis* 1-372

Week[a]	Sham immunized	Immunized
−2	12 (6–21)[b]	3,246 (1174–3278)
1	8 (4–12)	2,675 (2409–3088)
7	75 (47–114)	924 (634–1500)
9	76 (35–111)	886 (846–1202)
12[c]	89 (52–123)	781 (526–1057)

Note. Modified from McArthur *et al.* (1989).

[a]Number of weeks before (−) or after the initial ligation and infection.

[b]$n=5$ for sham-immunized and immunized groups.

[c]Two weeks after removal of ligatures.

TABLE II

Anti-*P. intermedia* 1447 IgG Antibody Levels

Bleeding time (days postligation)	U of IgG/ml of serum[a] [mean (range)]	
	Immunized	Sham immunized
0	5813.2 (3430–8867)	30.7 (10–66)
35	4043.7 (2167–6983)	104.8 (19–197)
70	3181.0 (1974–4750)	145.7 (14–362)
91	2479.5 (1598–3602)	111.3 (23–298)

Note. From Clark *et al.* (1991).

[a]IgG anti-*P. intermedia* 1447 levels were determined with an ELISA, using *P. intermedia* 1447 sonic extract as the antigen.

Specific antibody levels in serum were measured and are shown in Fig. 3. Significant increase in serum antibody of all three isotypes was observed in the immunized animals. Increases to *P. gingivalis* and *P. intermedia* occurred in both the IgG and IgA isotypes with lesser increases in levels of IgM. Titer increases were greatest in IgM in animals immunized with *B. fragilis*. As reported by others, titers were not enduring and had returned to near baseline levels by Week 51. Immunization with *P. gingivalis* not only resulted in a significant decrease in *P. gingivalis* at both ligated and nonligated sites but also caused significant reductions in *P. intermedia.* Immunization had little to no effect on several other microorganisms monitored. Immunization with *P. gingivalis* and *B. fragilis* resulted in a significant overgrowth of *A actinomycetemcomitans* at ligated sites. Overgrowth of *E. corrodens* and *C. rectus* was also observed.

No statistically significant differences were observed between immunized and nonimmunized groups with regard to plaque index, bleeding on probing, probing depth, or attachment level. While alveolar bone loss around ligated teeth in the placebo group animals as assessed by radiographic density remained stable throughout the study, significant bone loss occurred around ligated teeth in all three groups of immunized animals. The authors concluded that immunization with *P. gingivalis, P. intermedia,* and even the nonoral species *B. fragilis* enhance the progression of periodontal deterioration as assessed by bone loss in this primate model.

An additional nonhuman primate immunization study was performed by Page and co-workers (Persson *et al.*, 1994). Their study was designed to answer two questions: can immunization clear *P. gingivalis* from the subgingival flora, and can immunization alter the progression of experimental periodontitis? Ten adult monkeys (*M. fascicularis*) were enrolled in an experimental (to be immunized) group and 10 into a control (to be given adjuvant only) group. Mean age was 7.4 years. All of the animals were colonized with *P. gingivalis* and all had low titers of anti-*P. gingivalis* serum IgG antibodies. The experimental group was immunized using vaccine containing formalinized *P. gingivalis* 5083 (monkey isolate) and Syntex Adjuvant Formulation-M (SAF-M) adjuvant (Chiron, Inc., Emeryville, CA) at baseline and Weeks 3, 6, and 16. At Week 16, ligatures were placed around the second premolar and first and second molars in one mandibular and the contralateral maxillary quadrants.

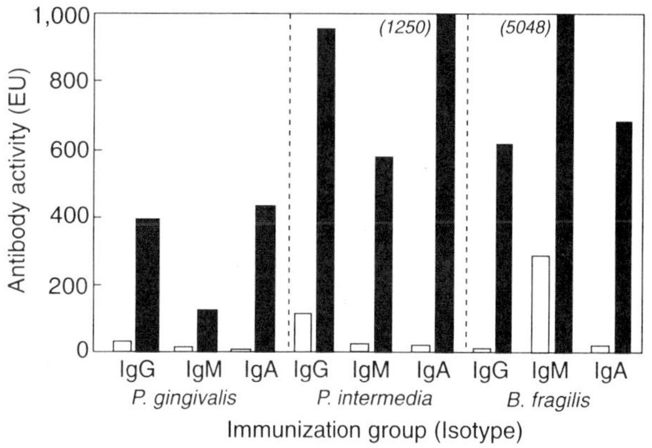

Figure 3. Serum antibody responses in nonhuman primates following active immunization. Open bars denote baseline and the black bars postimmunization. Bars denote mean levels of antibody against the homologous antigen. From Ebersole *et al.* (1991), with permission.

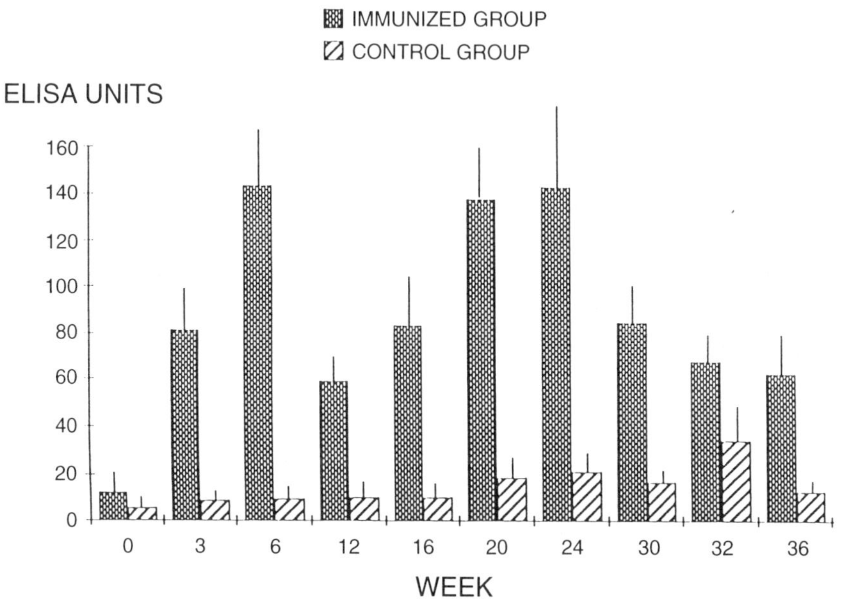

Figure 4. Mean serum antibody titers reported as ELISA units (EU) and standard error bars for control and immunized animals at baseline and for Weeks 3 through 36 following vaccination. From Persson *et al.* (1994), with permission.

Over an experimental period of 36 weeks, subgingival plaque samples and blood were harvested and clinical and radiographic data collected from ligated and nonligated teeth. Alveolar bone status as assessed by digital subtraction radiography was the primary outcome variable.

The mean serum anti-*P. gingivalis* IgG response is shown in Fig. 4. Mean titer peaked at 140 EU at Week 6, then fell to less than half that value by Week 12 and peaked again at 138 EU following the booster injection at Week 16. Mean titers were not enduring. A small, although statistically significant, increase in anti-*P. gingivalis* titer was observed in control animals following placement of ligatures. A major feature was the extreme variability in immune responsiveness among the animals.

P. gingivalis in the subgingival flora of ligated teeth, reported as micrograms *P. gingivalis* DNA measured by slot blot using DNA probes (MicroProbe Corp., Bothell, WA), is shown in Fig. 5. Prior to ligation, values were low and did not differ significantly for control and immunized animals. Following ligation at Week 16, values increased greatly and by Week 30 and thereafter they were greater for control than for immunized animals. The immunized animals segregated into two groups, 5 with *P. gingivalis* values <0.1 μg DNA (group A) and 5 >0.1 μg DNA (group B). For animals in group A serum antibody titers were significantly higher ($P < 0.001$) and the number of *P. gingivalis* cells significantly lower ($P < 0.001$) than in controls. Thus, immunization with *P. gingivalis* could reduce *P. gingivalis* in the subgingival flora but could not eliminate it.

Immunization did alter the progress of periodontal disease destruction around ligated teeth as assessed by digital subtraction radiography (Fig. 6). At both 30 and 36 weeks the control animals manifested more than twice the amount of alveolar bone loss as the immunized animals. Bone loss in vaccinated animals did not progress significantly between Week 30 and 36 in the vaccinated animals, and the amount observed may have been caused by the trauma of ligature placement. Three control and three vaccinated animals were superinfected with a slurry of viable *P. gingivalis* at Week 36 and observed at Week 44. Superinfection had no effect on bone status in the immunized animals, but induced rapid bone loss in controls. Thus, immunization in this primate model can suppress or block the progression of periodontitis as assessed by alveolar bone status.

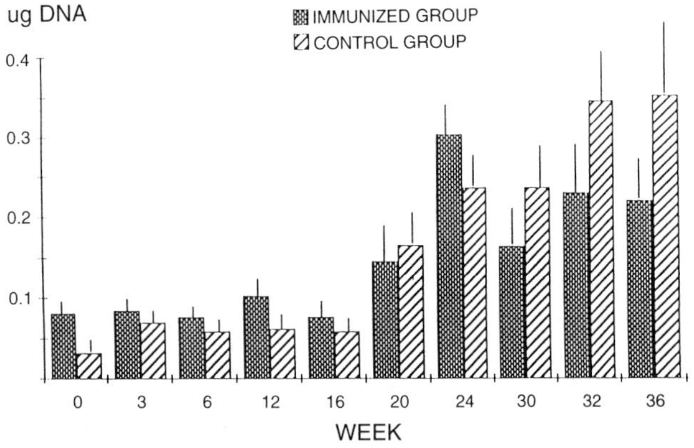

Figure 5. Mean amount of *P. gingivalis* present and standard error bars for the subgingival microflora of immunized and control animals from ligated sextants at baseline and at 3 through 36 weeks, reported as micrograms of *P. gingivalis*-specific DNA per sample measured by slot blot with a *P. gingivalis*-specific DNA probe. From Persson *et al.* (1994), with permission.

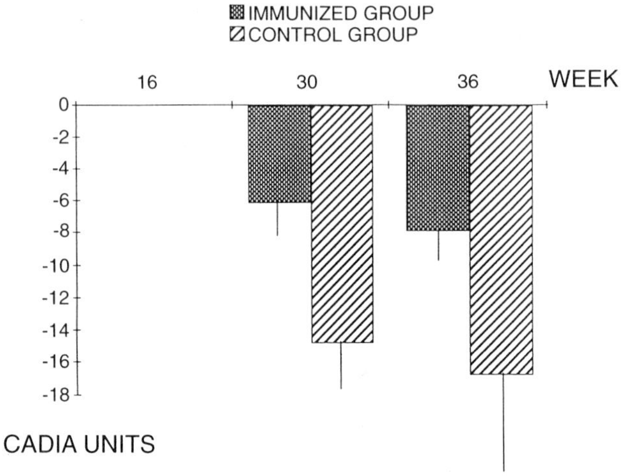

Figure 6. Mean change and standard error bars in alveolar bone housing mandibular test teeth, reported in terms of CADIA units from Week 16 when the ligatures were placed to Week 36 (values at Week 16 were considered as 0). From Persson *et al.* (1994), with permission.

VI. Discussion

A. Vaccination Studies in Rodents

Taken together, the vaccination studies in rodents clearly show that protective immunity against specific periodontal pathogens, such as *Porphyromonas gingivalis*, can be obtained by inducing an immune response to whole cells or various antigens of periodontopathic bacteria prior to inoculation of the animal with the specific pathogen. The mechanism of action of protective immunity is unclear, however, in one study in ligated hamsters (Okuda *et al.*, 1988), passively administered antibody did confer a measure of protection against *P. gingivalis*-induced pathology.

Potential mechanisms of protective immunity against periodontal pathogens include the following.

(1) Mucosal immunity mediated by secretory antibodies. In higher species, this would be mainly secretory IgA, but in rodents, IgG in saliva as well as s-IgA may

play a role. These antibodies mediate their effects by inhibiting initial colonization, hence limiting infection of the oral cavity and adjacent tissues by the periodontal pathogens.

(2) Mucosal immunity mediated by humoral antibodies. These antibodies in the serum easily find their way into the gingival tissue and could be effective at enhancing phagocytosis by neutrophils in the gingiva, the gingival crevice, or periodontal pocket. In addition, humoral antibodies could exert their protective effects by neutralizing toxic-like activities of the periodontopathic bacteria. Toxins such as the leukotoxin of *Actinobacillus* have been shown to be neutralized by antibody. In the presence of opsonic antibody, *Actinobacillus* is opsonized and phagocytosed by neutrophils. In the absence of neutralizing antibody and opsonic antibody, *Actinobacillus* leukotoxin kills the neutrophil. There are other mechanisms by which antibodies may exert protective effects such as neutralizing histiolytic enzymes (e.g., the proteases produced by *P. gingivalis*), or inhibiting factors which trigger host cells. The LPS or fimbrial stimulation of macrophages results in release of tissue-destructive factors and proinflammatory cytokines such as IL-1, which in turn would cause tissue destruction. Antibodies could block this reaction by blocking the LPS, fimbriae, or other triggering agents.

(3) Celluar immunity induced to a specific organism. This could result in enhanced phagocytosis and killing of the organisms by macrophages, or antibody-dependent cellular cytotoxicity mechanisms could be operative to protect against the periodontal pathogen.

All of these are possible mechanisms of action in the rodent experiments; definitive evidence as to which single or combination of mechanisms are operative is still needed.

One can propose that in developing a vaccine an attempt should be made to maximize the potential for mucosal immunity since this could be intrinsically the safest method of immunization. Specific induction of mucosal immunity mediated by s-IgA in the absence of or with low levels of humoral or cellular immunity could provide protection without adverse immunopathologic effects that could be exerted by humoral antibodies or by cellular immunity to the periodontal pathogens.

B. Selection of Antigen for Periodontal Vaccine

There are several approaches to the selection of antigen. One is to evaluate humans with various levels of periodontal disease in an attempt to determine whether antibodies to a particular antigen or groups of antigens are seen at a time when the disease is in remission or when patients appear to be protected. This approach has not been useful in humans so far, as most individuals who have periodontal disease suffer from episodes of tissue destruction at a time when their antibody levels to periodontal pathogens appear to be high.

A second approach is to screen various candidate antigens that are virulence factors or colonization factors in simple animal models to determine which are effective. This has been done, for example, with *P. gingivalis* fimbriae, and clear protection is obtained. A next step in this approach would be to test this antigen in higher animals such as nonhuman primates, and particularly to develop this antigen in vaccines such that it stimulates the mucosal immune system. A final step would be to test the specific antigen, possibly the genetically engineered portion or a synthetic peptide derived from this antigen, in humans to evaluate the immune response. For reasons described above, it might be prudent to engineer this vaccine such that a specific secretory immune response in the absence of significant humoral or cellular immune response is induced.

This is an orderly progression of experiments from simple gnotobiotic rodent animals using pure antigens or genetically engineered antigens, to more complex models such as the beagle dog or nonhuman primates, to humans with an emphasis on the development of mucosal immunity.

C. Vaccination Studies in Primates

Although the protocols and many details of the immunization studies that have been performed using nonhuman primates differed greatly, many of the observations were consistent. In all of the studies, reasonably high titers of serum IgG antibodies reactive with the immunizing species were observed, although titers varied enormously from animal to animal. Wide interanimal variation in immune responsiveness was reported by others conducting immunization studies in nonhuman primates. In the study by Persson *et al.* (1994), titers in the least responsive animals were not much greater than titers observed in control animals; some animals manifested a peak response after the initial two injections followed by a secondary response following booster injections. In other cases no response was observed until the third or fourth injection and then only a single peak was observed. In all of the studies, observed titers were not enduring. For example, in the study by Ebersole *et al.* (1991) titers had returned to baseline levels by Week 51 and in the study by Persson *et al.* (1994) mean titers at the end of the experiment at Week 36 were less than half peak values. The fact that the titers are not enduring may pose problems for development of a vaccine for use in humans. However, the humoral immune response in humans may be completely different from that observed in nonhuman primates, and responses induced with vaccines containing highly purified antigen may differ greatly from those induced with whole cell vaccines.

The observation by Ebersole *et al.* (1991) that immunization with *P. gingivalis* resulted not only in suppression of the immunizing organism but also of *P. intermedia* and overgrowth of *A. actinomycetemcomitans* and to a lesser extent *E. corrodens* and *C. rectus* is intriguing. The suppression of *P. intermedia* could have resulted from the presence of antigenic epitopes shared with *P. gingivalis,* from changes in the subgingival environment, or from altered interspecies interactions which are known to occur. The possibility that shared antigenic epitopes may exist is supported by the fact that epitopes, especially those in the lipid A and core carbohydrate components of LPS of gram-negative bacteria, are highly conserved (Aydintug *et al.*, 1989; Di-Padova *et al.*, 1993). It is also notable that in the study conducted by Persson *et al.* (1994), animals immunized with *P. gingivalis* manifested serum antibody titers reactive not only with the immunizing species but also with *B. forsythus,* and these antibodies were cross-reactive with antigens in LPS of the two species (Vasel *et al.*, 1996). Identification and characterization of shared epitopes could lead to development of a vaccine that targets multiple gram-negative species. The observed overgrowth of *A. actinomycetemcomitans* and other species seen by Ebersole *et al.* (1991) most likely resulted from altered interspecies interactions and other environmental factors.

All of the nonhuman primate studies demonstrate that immunization can affect composition of the subgingival microflora although immunization did not in any study clear the immunizing species from the subgingival flora. Clearance would be unlikely regardless of the effectiveness of the immunization because of the presence of the ligatures which serve as foreign bodies. However, at least in the Persson *et al.* (1994) study, immunization did not clear *P. gingivalis* from the subgingival flora of nonligated teeth. The study by Clark *et al.* (1991) supports the idea but does not prove that immunization may have the potential to suppress recolonization or reemergence of pathogenic species which have been previously eliminated or greatly suppressed.

In the studies by McArthur *et al.* (1989), Clark *et al.* (1991), and Persson *et al.* (1994), beneficial effects of immunization manifested either by a suppressive effect on the pathogenic flora or suppression or inhibition of the progression of periodontal destruction were observed. In contrast, the Ebersole *et al.* (1991) study concluded on the basis of radiographic measurements of alveolar bone status that immunization enhanced periodontal tissue destruction. This result is difficult to explain. Alveolar bone loss in *M. fascicularis* is known to occur over time following ligation of teeth (Kornman *et al.*, 1990; Offenbacher *et al.*, 1987). Notably, that did not occur in the Ebersole *et al.* (1991) study in the nonimmunized animals. This observation remains unexplained. The Ebersole *et al.* (1991) study and the study performed by Persson *et al.* (1994) used the same immunogen and the same animal model. The major differences in the two studies were that Persson *et al.* (1994) used SAF-M adjuvant and immunized 10 animals, while Ebersole *et al.* (1991) used Freund's incomplete adjuvant and immunized only five animals with *P. gingivalis.* The adjuvant may have accounted for the observed differences in the two studies. SAF-M contains muramyl dipeptide, squaline, and pluronic acid, and is known to suppress the production of IgE and minimize hypersensitivity reactions (Allison and Byars, 1986).

VII. Conclusions

Studies performed in humans and experimental animals support the hypothesis that immunization has significant potential as an effective form of intervention for the prevention and control of periodontitis. Many periodontitis patients exhibit a humoral immune response during the course of their spontaneous infection. Most of those who are seronegative convert to seropositive following routine periodontal therapy. The antibodies, however, have relatively low avidity and capacity to opsonize. Nevertheless, there is evidence for immune protection. Taken as a whole, immunization studies demonstrate that immunization can have a suppressive effect on the pathogenic subgingival flora, even in the presence of ligatures, and high specific antibody titers can alter the progression of periodontal tissue destruction. Systematic evaluation of both oral and systemic vaccines needs to be explored, and the role of systemic and mucosal immunity in preventing or altering the course of periodontitis remains unknown.

References

Allison, A. C., and Byars, N. E. (1986). An adjuvant formulation that selectively elicits the formation of antibodies of protective isotypes and cell-mediated immunity. *J. Immunol. Methods* **95,** 157–168.

Aydintug, M. K., Inzana, T. H., Letonja, T., Davis, W. E., and Corbeil, L. B. (1989). Cross-reactivity of monoclonal antibodies to *Escherichia coli* J5 with heterologous gram-negative bacteria and extracted lipopolysaccharides. *J. Infect. Dis.* **160,** 846–857.

Baker, P. J., and Wilson, M. E. (1989). Opsonic IgG antibody against *Actinobacillus actinomycetemcomitans* in localized juvenile periodontitis. *Oral Microbiol. Immunol.* **4,** 98–105.

Baker, P. J., Evans, R. T., and Roopenian, D. C. (1994). Oral infection with *Porphyromonas gingivalis* and induced alveolar bone loss in immunocompetent and severe combined immunodeficient mice. *Arch. Oral Biol.* **39,** 1035–1040.

Brant, E., Sojar, H. T., Sharma, A., Bedi, G.S., Genco, R. J., and De Nardin, E. (1995). Identification of linear antigenic sites on the *Porphyromonas gingivalis* 43 kDa fimbrillin subunit. *Oral Microbiol. Immunol.* **10**, 146–150.

Brown, L. J., and Löe, H. (1993). Prevalence, extent, severity, and progression of periodontal disease. *Periodontology 2000* **4**, Chapter 6.

Chang, K. M., Ramamurthy, N. S., McNamara, T. F., Genco, R. J., and Golub, L. M. (1988). Infection with a gram-negative organism stimulates gingival collagenase production in non-diabetic and diabetic germfree rats. *J. Periodontal Res.* **23**, 239–244.

Chen, H. A., Johnson, B. D., Sims, T. J., Darveau, R. P., Moncla, B. J., Whitney, C. W., Engel, L. D., and Page, R. C. (1991). Humoral immune response to *P. gingivalis* before and following therapy in rapidly progressive periodontitis patients. *J. Periodontol.* **62**, 781–791.

Chen, P. B., Neiders, M. E., Millar, S. J., Reynolds, H. S., and Zambon, J. J. (1987). Effect of immunization on experimental *Bacteroides gingivalis* infection in a murine model. *Infect. Immun.* **55**, 2534–2537.

Chen, P. B., Davern, L. B., Schifferle, R., and Zambon, J. J. (1990). Protective immunization against experimental *Bacteroides* (*Porphyromonas gingivalis*) infection. *Infect. Immun.* **58**, 3394–3400.

Clark, W. B., Magnusson, I., Beem, J. E., Jung, J. M., Marks, R. G., and McArthur, W. P. (1991). Immune modulation of *Prevotella intermedia* colonization in squirrel monkeys. *Infect. Immun.* **59**, 1927–1931.

Dahlén, G., and Slots, J. (1989). Experimental infections by *Bacteroides gingivalis* in nonimmunized and immunized rabbits. *Oral Microbiol. Immunol.* **4**, 6–11.

Dickinson, D. P., Kubiniec, M. A., Yoshimura, F., and Genco, R. J. (1988). Molecular cloning and sequencing of the gene encoding the fimbrial subunit protein of *Bacteroides gingivalis. J. Bacteriol.* **170**, 1658–1665.

DiPadova, F. E., Brade, H., Barclay, G. R., Poxton, I. R., Liehl, E., Schuetze, E., Kocher, H. P., Ramsay, F., Schreier, H., Brian, D., McClellan, L., and Rietschel, E. T. (1993). A broadly cross-protective monoclonal antibody binding to *Escherichia coli* and *Salmonella lipopolysaccharides. Infect. Immun.* **61**, 3863–3872.

Ebersole, J. L., Taubman, M. A., Smith, D. J., and Haffajee, A. D. (1985). Effect of subgingival scaling on systemic antibody responses to oral microorganisms. *Infect. Immun.* **48**, 534–539.

Ebersole, J. L., Taubman, M. A., Smith, D. J., and Frey, D. E. (1986). Human immune responses to oral microorganisms: Patterns of systemic antibody levels to *Bacteroides* species. *Infect. Immun.* **51**, 507–513.

Ebersole, J. L., Brunsvold, M., Steffensen, B., Wood, R., and Holt, S. C. (1991). Effects of immunization with *Porphyromonas gingivalis* and *Prevotella intermedia* on progression of ligature-induced periodontitis in the nonhuman primate *Macaca fascicularis. Infect. Immun.* **59**, 3351–3359.

Evans, R. T., Klausen, B., and Genco, R. J. (1992a). Immunization with fimbrial protein and peptide protects against *Porphyromonas gingivalis*-induced periodontal tissue destruction. *In* "Genetically Engineered Vaccines: Prospects for Oral Disease Prevention" (J. Keith and J. McGhee, eds.), pp. 255–262. Plenum, New York.

Evans, R. T., Klausen, B., Ramamurthy, N. S., Golub, L. M., Sfintescu, C., and Genco, R. J. (1992b). Periodontopathic potential of two strains of *Porphyromonas gingivalis* in gnotobiotic rats. *Arch. Oral Biol.* **37**, 813–819.

Evans, R. T., Klausen, B., Sojar, H. T., Bedi, G. S., Sfintescu, C., Ramamurthy, N. S., Bolug, L. M., and Genco, R. J. (1992c). Immunization with *Porphyromonas (Bacteroides) gingivalis* fimbriae protects against periodontal destruction. *Infect. Immun.* **60**, 2926–2935.

Genco, C. A., Cutler, C. W., Kapczynski, D. R., Maloney, K., and Arnold, R. R. (1991). A novel mouse model to study the virulence of and host response to *Porphyromonas (Bacteroides) gingivalis. Infect. Immun.* **59**, 1255–1263.

Genco, C. A., Kapczynski, D. R., Cutler, C. W., Arko, R. J., and Arnold, R. R. (1992). Influence of immunization on *Porphyromonas gingivalis* colonization and invasion in the mouse chamber model. *Infect. Immun.* **60**, 1447–1454.

Genco, R. J., and Löe, H. (1993). The role of systemic conditions and disorders in periodontal disease. *Periodontology 2000* **2**, 98–116.

Genco, R. J., Slots, J., Mouton, C., and Murray, P. (1980) Systemic immune responses to oral anaerobic organisms. *In* "Anaerobic Bacteria: Selected Topics" (D. W. Lambe, Jr., R. J. Genco, and K. J. Mayberry-Carson, eds.), pp. 277–293. Plenum, New York.

Grossi, S. G., Zambon, J. J., Ho, A. W., Koch, G., Dunford, R. G., Machtei, E. E., Norderyd, O. M., and Genco, R. J. (1994). Assessment of risk for periodontal disease. I. Risk indicators for attachment loss. *J. Periodontol.* **65**, 260–267.

Grossi, S. G., Genco, R. J., Machtei, E. E., Ho, A. W., Koch, G., Dunford, R., Zambon, J. J., and Hausmann, R. (1995). Assessment of risk for periodontal disease. II. Risk indicators for alveolar bone loss. *J. Periodontol.* **66**, 23–29.

Gunsolley, J. C., Burmeister, J. A., Tew, J. G., Best, A. M., and Ranney, R.R. (1987). Relationship of serum antibody to attachment level patterns in young adults with juvenile periodontitis or generalized severe periodontitis. *J. Periodontol.* **58**, 314–320.

Haffajee, A. D., and Socransky, S. S. (1994). Microbial etiologic agents of destructive periodontal disease. *Periodontology 2000* **5**, 78–111.

Hirshfeld, L., and Wasserman, B. (1978). A long-term survey of tooth loss in 600 treated periodontal patients. *J. Periodontal* **49**, 225–237.

Holmgren, J. (1991). Mucosal immunity and vaccination FEMS. *Microbiol. Immunol.* **89**, 1–10.

Ishikawa, I., Watanabe, H., Horibe, M., and Izumi, Y. (1988). Diversity of IgG antibody responses in patients with various types of periodontitis. *Adv. Dent. Res.* **2**, 334–338.

Kesavalu, L., Ebersole, J. L., Machen, R. L., and Holt, S. C. (1992). *Porphyromonas gingivalis* virulence in mice: Induction of immunity to bacterial components. *Infect. Immun.* **60**, 1455–1464.

Klausen, B. (1991). Microbiological and immunological aspects of experimental periodontal disease in rats. *J. Periodontol.* **62**, 59–73.

Klausen, B., Evans, R. T., and Sfintescu, C. (1989). Two complementary methods of assessing periodontal bone level in rats. *Scand. J. Dent. Res.* **97**, 494–499.

Klausen, B., Evans, R. T., Ramamurthy, N. S., Golub, L. M., Sfintescu, C., Lee, J.-Y., Bedi, G., Zambon, J. J., and Genco, R. J. (1991). Periodontal bone level and gingival proteinase activity in gnotobiotic rats immunized with *Bacteroides gingivalis. Oral Microbiol. Immunol.* **6**, 193–201.

Klausen, B., Evans, R. T., and Genco, R. J. (1993). Vaccination against *Porphyromonas gingivalis* in experimental animals. *In* "Biology of the Species *Porphyromonas gingivalis*" (H. N. Shah, D. Mayrand, and R. J. Genco, eds.), CRC Press, Boca Raton, Florida.

Kornman, K. S., Blodgett, R. F., Brunsvold, M., and Holt, S. C. (1990). Effects of topical applications of meclofenamic acid and ibuprofen on bone loss, subgingival microbiota and gingival PMN response in the primate *Macaca fascicularis. J. Periodontal Res.* **25**, 300–307.

Lee, J.-Y., Sojar, H. T., Bedi, G. S., and Genco, R. J. (1991). *Porphyromonas (Bacteroides) gingivalis* fimbrillin: Size, amino-terminal sequence, and antigenic heterogeneity. *Infect. Immun.* **59**, 383–385.

Lee, J.-Y., Sojar, H. T., Bedi, G. S., and Genco, R. J. (1992). Synthetic peptides analogous to the fimbrillin sequence inhibit adherence of *Porphyromonas gingivalis. Infect. Immun.* **60**, 1662–1670.

Lindhe, J., Haffajee, A. D., and Socransky, S. S. (1983). Progression of periodontal disease in adult subjects in the absence of periodontal therapy. *J. Clin. Periodontol.* **10**, 443–452.

Ling, T. Y., Sims, T. J., Chen, H. A., Whitney, C., Moncla, B., Engel, L. D., and Page, R. C. (1993). Titer and subclass distribution of serum IgG antibody reactive with *Actinobacillus acrinomycetemcomitans* in localized juvenile periodontitis. *J. Clin. Immunol.* **13**, 100–111.

Löe, H., Anerud, A., Boysen, H., and Morrison, E. (1986). Natural history of periodontal disease in man. *J. Clin. Periodontol.* **13**, 431–330.

Loesche, W. J. (1988). The role of spirochetes in periodontal disease. *Adv. Dent. Res.* **2**, 275–283.

McArthur, W. P., Magnusson, I., Marks, R. G., and Clark, W. B. (1989). Modification of colonization by black-pigmented *Bacteroides* species in squirrel monkeys by immunization with *Bacteroides gingivalis. Infect. Immun.* **57**, 2313–2317.

McGhee, J. R., and Mestecky, J. (1990). In defense of mucosal surfaces. Development of novel vaccines for IgA responses protective of the portals of entry of microbial pathogens. *Infect. Dis. Clin. North Am.* **4**, 315–341.

Mestecky, J., and Eldridge, J. H. (1991). Targeting and controlled release of antigens for the effective induction of secretory antibody responses. *Curr. Opin. Immunol.* **3**, 492–495.

Michalek, S. M., and Childers, N. K. (1990). Development and outlook for a caries vaccine. *Crit. Rev. Oral Biol. Med.* **1**, 37–53.

Moldoveanu, A., Novak, M., Huang, W.-Q., Gilley, R. M., Stass, J. K., Schafer, D., Compans, R. W., and Mestecky, J. (1993). Oral immunization with influenza virus in biodegradable microsphers. *J. Infect. Dis.* **167**, 84–90.

Mouton, C., Hammond, P. G., Slots, J., and Genco, R. J. (1981). Serum antibodies to oral *Bacteroides asaccharolyticus* (*Bacteroides gingivalis*): Relationship to age and periodontal disease. *Infect. Immun.* **31**, 182–192.

Murayama, Y., Nagai, A., Okamura, K., Kurihara, H., Nomura, Y., Kokeguchi, S., and Kato, K. (1988). Serum immunoglobulin G antibody to periodontal bacteria. *Adv. Dent. Res.* **2**, 339–345.

Offenbacher, S., Braswell, L. D., Loos, A. S., Johnson, H. G., Hall, C. M., McClure, H., Orkin, J. L., Strobert, E. A., Green, M. D., and Odle, B. M. (1987). Effects of flurbiprofen on the progression of periodontitis in *Macaca mulatta. J. Periodontal. Res.* **22**, 473–481.

Ogawa, T., Shimauchi, H., and Hamada, S. (1989). Mucosal and systemic immune responses in BALB/c mice to *Bacteroides gingivalis* fimbriae administered orally. *Infect. Immun.* **57**, 3466–3471.

Ogawa, T., Kusumoto, Y., Hamada, S., McGhee, J. R., and Kiyono, H. (1990). *Bacteroides gingivalis*-specific serum IgG and IgA subclass antibodies in periodontal diseases. *Clin. Exp. Immunol.* **82**, 318–325.

Okuda, K., Slots, J., and Genco, R. J. (1981). *Bacteroides gingivalis, Bacteroides asaccharolyticus,* and *Bacteroides melaninogenicus* subspecies: Cell surface morphology and adherence to erythrocytes and human buccal epithelial cells. *Curr. Microbiol.* **6**, 7–12.

Okuda, K., Kato, T., Naito, Y., Takazoe, I., Kikuchi, Y., Nakamura, T., Kiyoshige, T., and Sasaki, S. (1988). Protective efficacy of active and passive immunization against experimental infection with *Bacteroides gingivalis* in ligated hamsters. *J. Dent. Res.* **67**, 807–811.

Page, R. C., and Schroeder, H. E. (1982). "Periodontitis in Man and Other Animals." Karger, Basel.

Persson, G. R., Engel, D., Whitney, C., Darveau, R., Weinberg, A., Brunsvold, M., and Page, R. C. (1994). Immunization against *Porphyromonas gingivalis* inhibits progression of periodontitis in nonhuman primates. *Infect. Immun.* **62**, 1026–1031.

Pilot, T., Barmes, D. E., Leclercq, M. H., McCombie, B. J., and Infirri, J. S. (1986). Periodontal conditions in adults, 34–44 years of age: An overview of CPITN data in the WHO global oral data bank. *Commun. Dent. Oral Epidemiol.* **14**, 310–312.

Ranney, R. R., Yanni, N. R., Burmeister, J. A., and Tew, J. G. (1982). Relationship between attachment loss and precipitating serum antibody to *Actinobaccilus actinomycetemcomitans* in adolescents and young adults having severe periodontal destruction. *J. Periodontol.* **53**, 1–7.

Roitt, I., Brostoff, J., and Male, D. (1989). "Immunology," 2nd Ed., p. 75. Mosby, St. Louis, Missouri.

Schenck, K., Helgeland, K., and Tollefsen, T. (1987). Antibodies against lipopolysaccharide from *Bacteroides gingivalis* before and after periodontal treatment. *Scand. J. Dent. Res.* **95**, 112–118.

Shimauchi, H., Ogawa, T., and Hamada, S. (1991). Immune response gene regulation of the humoral immune response to *Porphyromonas gingivalis* fimbriae in mice. *Immunology* **74**, 362–364.

Sjöström, K., Darveau, R., Page, R. C., Whitney, C., and Engel, D. (1992). Opsonic antibody activity against *Actinobaccilus actinomycetemcomitans* in patients with rapidly progressive periodontitis. *Infect. Immun.* **60,** 4819–4852.

Sjöström, K., Ou, J., Whitney, C., Johnson, B., Darveau, R., Engel, D., and Page, R. C. (1994). Effect of treatment on titer, function, and antigen recognition of serum antibodies to *Actinobaccilus actinomycetemcomitans* in patients with rapidly progressive periodontitis. *Infect. Immun.* **62,** 145–151.

Slots, J. (1986). Bacterial specificity in adult periodontitis. A summary of recent work. *J. Clin. Periodontol.* **13,** 912–917.

Tanner, A. C. R., Haffer, C., Brathall, G. T., and Visconti, R. A. (1979). A study of the bacteria associated with advancing periodontitis in man. *J. Clin. Periodontol.* **6,** 278–307.

Tew, J. G., Marshall, D. R., Moore, W. E. C., Best, A. M., Palcanis, K. G., and Ranney, R. R. (1985). Serum antibody reactive with predominant organisms in the subgingival flora of young adults with generalized severe periodontitis. *Infect. Immun.* **48,** 303–311.

van Steenbergen, T. J. M., Kastelein, P., Touw, J. J. A., and de Graaff, J. (1982). Virulence of black-pigmented *Bacteroides* strains from periodontal pockets and other sites in experimentally induced skin lesions in mice. *J. Periodontal Res.* **17,** 41–49

Vasel, D., Sim, T. J., Bainbridge, B., Houston, L., Darveau, R., and Page, R. C. (1996). Shared antigens of *Porphyromonas gingivalis* and *Bacteroides gingivalis. Oral Microbial. Immunol.* in press.

Vincent, J. W., Falker, W. A., Cornett, W. C., and Suzuki, J. B. (1987). Effect of periodontal therapy on specific antibody responses to suspected periodontopathogens. *J. Clin. Periodontol.* **14,** 412–417.

Whitney, C., Ant, J., Moncla, B., Johnson, B., Page, R. C., and Engel, D. (1992). Serum immunoglobulin G antibody to *Porphyromonas gingivalis* in rapidly progressive periodontitis: Titer, avidity, and subclass distribution. *Infect. Immun.* **60,** 2194–2200.

Wilson, M. E., Bronson, P. M., and Hamilton, R. G. (1995). Immunoglobulin G2 antibodies promote neutrophil killing of *Actinobacillus actinomycetemcomitans. Infect. Immun.* **63,** 1070–1075.

Yoshimura, F., Takasawa, T., Yoneyama, M., Yamaguchi, T., Shiokawa, H., and Suzuki, T. (1985). Fimbriae from the oral anaerobe *Bacteroides gingivalis:* Physical, chemical, and immunological properties. *J. Bacteriol.* **163,** 730–734.

Zambon, J. J., Reynolds, H., Fisher, J. G., Shlossman, M., Dunford, R., and Genco, R. J. (1988a). Microbiological and immunological studies of adult periodontitis in patients with noninsulin-dependent diabetes mellitus. *J. Periodontol.* **59,** 23–31.

Zambon, J. J., Umemoto, T., DeNardin, E., Nakazawa, F., Christersson, L. A., and Genco, R. J. (1988b). *Actinobaccilus actinomycetemcomitans* in the pathogenesis of human periodontal disease. *Adv. Dent. Res.* **2,** 269–274.

33

Mucosal Immunity of the Middle Ear

YUICHI KURONO
GORO MOGI
Department of Otolaryngology
Oita Medical University
Oita 879-55, Japan

I. Introduction

The study of mucosal immunity in the middle ear has been the focus of many investigations. Liu *et al.* (1975) demonstrated that the levels of immunoglobulin and lysozyme in the middle ear effusions (MEEs) are not only much higher than those in sera, but also increase with age—thus reflecting the development of the local middle ear immune system.

Earlier studies in which Mogi *et al.* (1974) isolated secretory IgA (S-IgA) from pooled MEEs revealed that the antigenicity and subunit structure of S-IgA are either identical or very similar to S-IgA obtained from other external secretions like saliva, nasal secretion, colostrum, and bronchial fluid. In addition, Ogra *et al.* (1974) demonstrated that specific antibody activity in MEEs against mumps, measles, rubella, and polio virus is limited to IgA. Another important observation was that fluorescent antibody staining of tympanic mucosa showed characteristic staining for a secretory component in the surface epithelium (Mogi *et al.*, 1974; Ogra *et al.*, 1974). These findings suggest that the middle ear contains a distinct mucosal immune system which in some instances exhibits similar characteristics to immune systems present at other mucosal sites.

This chapter reviews available data on mucosal immunity in the middle ear against microbial pathogens as well as applications of mucosal vaccines for otitis media with effusion (OME).

II. Immunocompetent Cells in the Middle Ear Mucosa

Although few immunocompetent cells are found in the normal middle ear mucosa, during acute or chronic inflammation, large quantities of lymphocytes, plasma cells, macrophages, leukocytes, and other inflammatory cells become present (Lim, 1974; Mogi *et al.*, 1980; Takahashi *et al.*, 1989; Ichimiya *et al.*, 1990). In order to further investigate this response, Ichimiya *et al.* (1990) quantitatively analyzed the immunocompetent cells in the middle ear mucosa of mice bred under germ-free, specific pathogen-free, and conventional conditions to demonstrate that mast cells and Mac-1$^+$ cells exist in the middle ear of these experimental models under all three conditions. After conducting the analysis the investigators found that the level of mast cells in the middle ear was the highest followed by Mac-1$^+$ cells and lymphocytes. In addition, the investigators found that the number of lymphocyte subsets were fewer in the middle ear mucosa in comparison to the subsets present in the nasal mucosa. Furthermore, although IgA-positive (IgA$^+$), IgM$^+$, and Lyt-1$^+$ cells were found in the middle ear mucosa of conventional mice, only IgM$^+$ cells were present in the mucosa of specific pathogen-free and germ-free mice. These findings indicate that the middle ear is not exposed to antigenic stimulation as often as other areas of the upper respiratory tract.

In another study, investigators noted that when nontypeable *Haemophilus influenzae* or lipopolysaccharide (LPS) purified from *H. influenzae* was injected into the middle ear of mice, Mac-1$^+$ cells were dominant. Although the numbers of IgM$^+$ and Lyt-1$^+$ cells increased markedly, the numbers of other lymphocyte subsets did not increase until 14 days after inoculation (Ichimiya *et al.*, 1990). Takahashi *et al.* (1992) induced immune-mediated otitis media in mice using keyhole limpet hemocyanin (KLH), and observed immunocytes appearing in the middle ear and Eustachian tube. Their results showed that Mac-1$^+$ cells were dominant, followed by helper T cells, IgG$^+$, IgA$^+$, and IgM$^+$ cells, suggesting that middle ear is a potentially immunocompetent organ that can be activated with appropriate antigenic stimulation.

III. Microorganisms in MEEs and Nasopharyngeal Secretions

Streptococcus pneumoniae, nontypeable *H. influenzae,* and *Moraxella catarrhalis* are the most common causative bacteria for otitis media (Kurono *et al.*, 1988). *S. pneumoniae* is cultured from MEE in more than 50% of patients with acute otitis media. Nontypeable *H. influenzae* (NTHi) and *M. catarrhalis* are in 10 to 20%, respectively. In OME, characterized by persistent MEE without any clinical symptoms of acute inflammation such as otalgia and fever rise, nontypeable *H. influenzae* is most frequently cultured from MEE.

Since the pathogens ascend into the middle ear from the nasopharynx through the Eustachian tube, nasopharyngeal colonization with those bacteria is considered the prerequisite for otitis media. In fact, most of the pathogens cultured from MEEs are identical to those found in the nasopharynx (Kurono *et al.*, 1988). The carriage rate of *H. influenzae* in the nasopharynx is higher in patients with OME than in healthy children, and the intensity of the colonization is associated with the occurrence of this disease (Faden *et al.*, 1991). Ueyama *et al.* (1995) investigated the presence P6 gene DNA of *H. influenzae* in nasopharyngeal secretions by PCR and demonstrated that the incidence was 86% in patients with OME and 46% in controls. They also reported that P6 gene DNA was detected in more than half of MEEs and was found in all nasopharyngeal secretions of patients with OME who had P6 gene DNA in MEEs. Those findings suggest that *H. influenzae* in the nasopharynx, as well as that in the middle ear, play an important role in the pathogenesis of OME.

It is acknowledged that most cases of acute otitis media are preceded by a viral upper respiratory infection. Rhinovirus, respiratory syncytial virus (RSV), adenovirus, influenza and parainfluenza viruses are detected in MEE of 17 to 24% of children with acute otitis media, either alone or in combination with bacteria (Sung *et al.*, 1993; Chonmaitree *et al.*, 1992). Okamoto *et al.* (1993) detected genomic sequences of RSV in the samples of MEE by RT-PCR. In those patients from whose nasopharynges RSV was isolated, the viral sequences were highly detectable in the effusions. Ruuskanen *et al.* (1989) demonstrated a clear association between RSV epidemics and otitis media. RSV infection increases the colonization of nontypeable *H. influenzae* in the nasopharynx of a cotton rat model (Patel *et al.*, 1992). Suzuki and Bakaletz (1994) also demonstrated synergistic effects between adenovirus and nontypeable *H. influenzae* in experimental otitis media. Moreover, Heikkinen *et al.* (1991) reported that vaccination for influenza A reduced the incidence of acute otitis media during a 6-week epidemic of influenza A. Those results indicate that viral infection might be the sole etiology of otitis media in some children and that preceding viral infection alter the defenses to prevent bacterial invasion into the middle ear.

IV. Systemic Immune Responses against Bacterial Antigen

Serum antibody, mainly IgG, accounts for pathogenic bacteria and resolves the infection. Serum bactericidal antibody assays showed that the immune response to nontypeable *H. influenzae* in OME is strain-specific (Faden *et al.*, 1989a). All patients with OME who lacked bactericidal antibody against the organism causing the second episode possessed bactericidal antibody against the first strain at the time of the second episode. The occurrence of second episodes of OME due to different strains of NTHi in the face of preexisting heterologous bactericidal antibody suggests a lack of cross-protection. Moreover, although antibody titers in MEE declined over time, serum antibody titers remained stable and persisted for several months. Yamanaka and Faden (1993b) demonstrated that the concentration of P6-specific IgG in MEE was directly related to the concentration of anti-P6 antibody in serum and that the concentration of P6-specific IgG in MEE was inversely related to the number of bacteria in MEE. Those findings suggest that the local immunity against NTHi in the middle ear partly reflects systemic immunity. P6 is highly conserved among strains of NTHi, and serves as a target for bactericidal antibody. The failure to recognize P6 as a specific immunogen may account for recurrent OME (Yamanaka and Faden, 1993a). Children who are not otitis-prone appear to make a good response to P6. These data suggest that there may be genetic and environmental reasons for the development of P6 antibodies in both serum and MEE.

Although specific IgG antibodies are protective against the invasion of bacterial antigen into the middle ear, some evidence suggests that an immune mechanism may be involved in inducing or sustaining MEE. Experimentally, inoculation of protein antigen into the middle ear after systemic sensitization of the host with the same antigen-induced immune-mediated otitis media (Ryan *et al.*, 1986). Immune-mediated otitis media is also produced by injecting a protein antigen into the middle ear of animals that are sensitized passively with antigen-specific IgG antibodies (Ryan and Catanzaro, 1983). Mravec *et al.* (1978) produced inflammatory response in the middle ear by inoculation of the chinchilla bulla with immune complexes. Formation of immune complexes, followed by complement activation and the release of granulocyte protease from neutrophils, is the key factor in the production of immune-mediated OME (Suzuki *et al.* 1988). Inoculation of immune complexes of pneumococcal antigens into the middle ear of nonsensitized chinchilla also produced MEE. Palva *et al.* (1985) found pneumococcal immune complexes in at least 25% of MEE in patients with chronic OME. Moreover, in an animal model, acute otitis media becomes chronic OME in certain cases. Ueyama and colleagues (1993) reported that when chinchillas were inoculated with live *Streptococcus pneumoniae* after systemic immunization with killed bacteria of the same strain, 7 out of 20 animals became chronic OME. The findings suggest that the activation of the complement system may contribute to the initiation and persistence of inflammatory reactions, though the activation of the formation of the immune complex itself can be a host defense mechanism (Fig. 1). Therefore, systemic immune reactions can, at the same time, contribute to the pathogenesis of chronic OME.

V. Local Immune Response in the Middle Ear

Although pathogenic bacteria are only occasionally demonstrated in MEE, investigations of specific antibodies in the effusion against those bacteria have contributed to our understanding of the mucosal immune system in the middle ear. Liu and colleagues (1975) found that IgA levels are significantly higher in the culture-negative MEEs than in the positive MEEs, and that bacterial recovery rate is related inversely to the increase the levels of IgA and IgG in MEEs. Sloyer *et al.* (1974, 1975) found specific IgG, IgM, and IgA antibodies against causative pnemococcal serotype in 27% of effusions of patients with acute otitis media, and IgA antibodies were detected more often in MEEs without the simultaneous presence in serum. They also found the same results in acute otitis media caused by *H. influenzae*. On the other hand, Faden and co-workers (1989a,b) reported that specific antibody titers in MEEs against nontypeable *H. influenzae* was much higher for the IgG class than for the IgM and IgA classes.

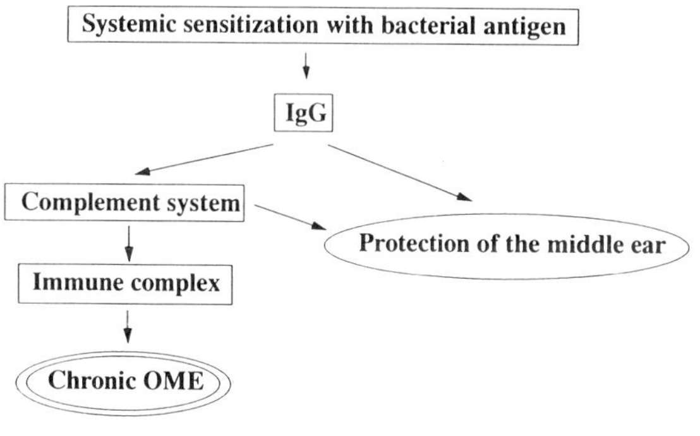

Figure 1. The role of systemic immune reactions in the pathogenesis of chronic OME.

Yamanaka and Fadden (1993b) measured antibody activities in MEEs to P6 of nontypeable *H. influenzae*, and reported that IgG specific to P6 was detected more frequently than IgM, IgA, and S-IgA antibodies. Concentration of P6-specific IgG in MEE was directly related to the concentration in the serum, and inversely related to the number of bacteria present. These findings suggest that the local immunity in the middle ear plays an important role in OME in conjunction with systemic immune system.

VI. Immunoregulation in the Middle Ear

Several studies have demonstrated the presence of cytokines in MEE which are known to regulate the immune response. Yellon *et al.* (1991) found IL-1, IL-2, and TNFα in MEEs from children with OME, and suggested that the presence of these cytokines in MEE is responsible for the persistence of OME. Juhn *et al.* (1993) also reported that the levels of IL-1β and TNFα in MEEs were higher in younger children than in older children.

Since mucosal immune responses are also regulated by the cytokine network, increases of IgA antibody seen in chronic middle ear response may arise because of a change in local immunoregulation mediated by cytokines. It is known that TGFβ stimulates class switching of IgM B cells to an IgA phenotype, and that IL-5 preferentially stimulates the production of IgA B cells already committed to that isotype. In contrast, IL-2 and IL-4 function primarily as general immune activators in immunoglobulin production, stimulating B cells already committed to IgM, IgG, or IgA to increase antibody production and differentiate into plasma cells. IL-4 is also implicated in class switching to IgG1 and IgE. Bikhazi and Ryan (1995) investigate the expression of cytokines associated with the production of different antibody isotypes in experimental acute and chronic OME, using *in situ* mRNA hybridization. The results showed that cells producing IL-2 and IL-4, but not IL-5, were present during acute OME. However, in chronic OME, IL-2 and IL-4 producing cells were less prevalent, but cells producing IL-5 were numerous. These data are consistent with the enhancement of IgG production in acute OME and increased local production of IgA during chronic OME.

Children at risk for OME have subtle immunological defects such as depressed helper–suppressor ratios, defective IL-2 production, and a decreased mitogenic response of T and B lymphocytes to stimulation with specific and nonspecific mitogens (Bernstein *et al.*, 1985). Yamanaka *et al.* (1983) reported that MEEs from patients with OME inhibit the lymphoproliferative response of peripheral blood lymphocytes or adenoidal lymphocytes. Kakiuchi and co-workers (1988) found immunosuppressive acidic protein in MEE at levels exceeding the serum concentrations. The presence of an inhibitor of the lymphoproliferative response in MEE was confirmed in an experimental animal model (Diven *et al.*, 1992). Experimental otitis media was created in the chinchilla by direct middle ear challenge with *Escherichia coli* endotoxin, *S. pneumoniae, H. influenzae,* or *Pseudomonas aeruginosa.* The effusions recovered from all four groups inhibited the lymphoproliferative response of peripheral blood lymphocytes to stimulation with phytohemagglutinin. Moreover, lymphocytes from middle ears infected with bacteria but not middle ears challenged with endotoxin were hyporesponsive or nonresponsive to the stimulation.

VII. Source of IgA Precursors in the Middle Ear

Past studies have demonstrated that the middle ear is a part of the common mucosal immune system, although considerable amounts of circulating IgG antibodies exude to the tympanic cavity in otitis media. Keithley *et al.* (1990) and Yamanaka and Fadden (1993a) suggested that IgA antibodies were produced in the middle ear by recurrent or persistent antigenic stimulation in both experimental animals and children. The manner in which lymphocytes gain access to the middle ear cavity was addressed in several studies.

Mucosal antigenic stimuli applied intraduodenally or intratracheally, induced antigen-specific IgA-forming cells in the tympanic mucosa, suggesting that the mucosa-associated lymphoid tissues are a source of lymphocytes to the tympanic cavity (Watanabe *et al.*, 1988). Tonsils and adenoids are considered to be Peyer's patch-like structures in upper respiratory tract, and J-chain-positive IgA-B cells have been suggested to arise from the tonsils and adenoids and home to sites in the upper respiratory tract such as lacrimal and parotid glands, and the nasal mucosa (Brandtzaeg, 1987). This supposition was supported by the finding that specific B cells against *Streptococcus mutans* are present in both tonsil and middle ear mucosa, since *S. mutans* is an organism that is never found in the middle ear space in otitis media (Bernstein *et al.*, 1988). Nadal *et al.* (1991) demonstrated that engraftment of human tonsil lymphocytes in the SCID mouse resulted in engraftment in the lungs but not in the gastrointestinal tract, thus indicating preferential homing of tonsil lymphocytes to the upper respiratory tract rather than to the gastrointestinal tract. They suggested that middle ear mucosa may receive lymphocytes from the tonsil during inflammation. These findings suggest that tonsils and adenoids are mucosa associated lymphoid tissue, supplying lymphocytes to the upper respiratory tract mucosa, including middle ear mucosa. Tonsils are very similar to Peyer's patches in structure. There are abundant Ig-forming cells in tonsils. However, an inductive site of the common mucosal immune system, such as Peyer's patches, has significantly fewer plasma cells than other sites of the gut mucosa which are the effector site of mucosal immune system. Although recent studies by Quiding-Järbrink and colleagues (1995) suggested that human palatine tonsils serve as powerful inductive sites for immune responses expressed in the upper aerodigestive tract, further studies should be made to clarify whether or not the tonsil is the inductive site, serving as the source of IgA precursors to the upper respiratory mucosa, as well as the tubotympanic mucosa. This information is important in the establishment of mucosal vaccine therapy for otitis media.

Previously, antigen-specific IgA-forming cells were induced in the middle ear mucosa in otitis media (Watanabe *et al.*, 1988), even though there are few lymphocytes and other immunocompetent cells in the normal middle ear mucosa. Ryan *et al.* (1990) and Kato *et al.* (1994) suggested that lymphocyte migration to the middle ear mucosa from the blood circulation was independent of the origin of lymphocytes and antigenic stimulation on the mucosal surface of the middle ear. It was also suggested that, in the early stage of inflammation, circulating lymphocytes may be recruited from the circulation to the inflamed middle ear mucosa by nonspecific inflammatory processes which may mask antigen-specific factors in lymphocyte migration (Watanabe *et al.* 1992). The extravasation of lymphocytes may be regulated by several mechanisms, such as interaction between lymphocyte receptors and endothelial adhesion molecules of high endothelium venules; and the receptor–ligand interaction between lymphocytes and lacrimal gland (O'Sullivan and Montgomery, 1990). Many lymphocytes from Peyer's patches and hilar lymphocytes adhered on the inflamed middle ear mucosa, while those cells did not bind to normal middle ear mucosa (Watanabe *et al.*, 1992). Bundo and fellow investigators (1996) isolated lymphocytes from Peyer's patches and spleen of guinea pigs immunized with DNP-ovalbumin mucosally or systemically and carried out an *in vitro* lymphocyte binding assay on the inflamed middle ear mucosa (Table I). They found that the number of binding lymphocytes obtained from Peyer's patches was significantly greater than lymphocytes from the spleen and that treatment of lymphocytes with anti-IgA antibodies reduced the number of lymphocytes binding to the mucosa. These findings suggested that many lymphocytes obtained from Peyer's patches were IgA precursors. They also observed adhesion molecules (ICAM-1) in middle ear mucosa from patients with chronic otitis media. Endothelial cells of newly grown vessels showed strong expression of ICAM-1 and weak expression of platelet endothelial cell adhesion molecule (PECAM-1)

TABLE I
Binding Ability of Lymphocytes to the Middle Ear Mucosa of Guinea Pigs after Mucosal or Systemic Immunization

	Lymphocytes	
Immunization	Peyer's patch	Spleen
Mucosal	+++	+
Systemic	+	+

and ELAM-1. Many lymphocytes bound mainly to endothelial cells in these regions and few cells were observed to bind to the basal portion of epithelial cells. The binding of lymphocytes was specific, and was not completely inhibited by anti-ICAM-1 antibody. These results suggest that the activation of Peyer's patch lymphocytes resulted in new and/or increased expression of some receptors on those cells. Those receptors may bind with organ-specific binding factors in the inflamed mucosa and play an important role in the local lodging and retention of B cells in local sites after extravasation. However, immunochemical and immunohistochemical features of those organ-specific binding factors on the inflamed middle ear mucosa and their receptors on activated lymphocytes still remain unknown.

VIII. Mucosal Immunity in the Nasopharynx

It has been reported that nasopharyngeal colonization with pathogens predisposes for the occurrence of otitis media. Stenfors and Raisanen (1992) examined the attachment of bacteria to nonciliated cells of nasopharyngeal epithelium in otitis-prone and non-otitis-prone children. In otitis-prone children, there was a significant preponderance of epithelial cells having greater than 50 attached bacteria and of epithelial cells attached with *S. pneumoniae* and *H. influenzae*. They emphasized that abundant attachment of pathogens to the epithelial cells close to the nasopharyngeal orifice of the Eustachian tube is a significant factor for the development of the otitis-prone condition. Shimamura *et al.* (1990) have performed studies that suggest that differences in the ability of bacterial pathogens to colonize the nasopharynx of different individuals may partially explain why certain individuals become infected and others do not. They demonstrated that strains of *H. influenzae* and *S. pneumoniae* adhered better to nasopharyngeal epithelial cells of children than those of adults. Furthermore, the adherence was significantly greater in children with OME than in control children.

Several studies demonstrated that IgA and S-IgA in nasopharygeal secretions influence the colonization of bacteria in the nasopharynx. Shimamura *et al.* (1990) found that the presence of pathogen-specific S-IgA in nasopharyngeal secretions decreased adherence of the pathogen to nasopharyngeal epithelial cells. Kurono *et al.* (1991) found that inhibiting activity of the adherence of both bacteria is significantly greater in nasopharyngeal secretions with S-IgA antibody activity than in those with no activity *in vitro*. Harabuchi *et al.* (1994) examined the relationship between nasopharyngeal colonization with nontypeable *H. influenzae* and recurrent otitis media in a large cohort of children followed prospectively from birth through 12 months of age. They reported that reduction or elimination of the organism was associated with a better S-IgA response to the P6 outer membrane protein than was persistence in the nasopharynx. The frequency of otitis media episodes was directly related to the frequency of colonization. The inhibitory effect of IgA antibody against nasopharyngeal colonization was confirmed by animal experiment (Kurono *et al.*, 1992). Oral immunization of BALB/c mice with whole cells or outer membrane proteins of *H. influenzae* increased pathogen-specific IgA antibody in saliva and in nasopharyngeal secretions, and enhanced the ability to clear the live bacteria inoculated into the nasopharynx (Table II). IgA antibody titers against the bacteria were inversely related to the number of bacteria in the nasopharynx (Kodama *et al.* 1995). Subcutaneous administration of vaccine affected neither salivary IgA antibody activity nor nasopharyngeal colonization by *H. influenzae* (Kurono *et al.*, 1993). These findings suggest that nasopharyngeal colonization patterns are strongly related to the occurrence of otitis media, and mucosal immune response is important in elimination of potential pathogens from the nasopharynx.

IX. Prevention of Otitis Media by Mucosal Vaccination

Prevention of OME through mucosal immunization with microbial vaccines is the most important area for the investigation of mucosal immunity of the middle ear. Watanabe and fellow investigators (1988) succeeded in

TABLE II
Antibody Activities after Oral or Systemic Immunization and Colonization by *H. influenzae* Inoculated into the Nasopharynx following the Immunization

	Saliva		Serum		Nasopharyngeal colonization
Mice	IgA	IgG	IgA	IgG	by *H. influenzae*
Oral immunization	++	−	+	+	+
Systemic immunization	−	−	+	+++	+++

inducing antigen-specific IgA-forming cells into the tubotympanal mucosa of guinea pigs by administration of antigen onto the mucosal surfaces of the duodenum. They also demonstrated that the occurrence of immune-mediated otitis media can be prevented by mucosal immunization (Watanabe *et al.*, 1989). Yoshimura *et al.* (1991) used enteric capsules for intragastric immunization of guinea pigs with *S. pneumoniae,* and investigated the efficacy against pneumococcal otitis media. With intratympanic inoculation of 10^5 and 10^6 live *S. pneumoniae,* the occurrence of otitis media was decreased in the animals that received intragastric immunization. In these guinea pigs, the values of salivary IgA antibody titers against *S. pneumoniae* were increased significantly, and histologic changes of the middle ear mucosa were slighter compared to control animals. Clinically, Clancy and colleagues (1983) administered enteric-coated polyvalent vaccines of *S. pnemoniae* and *H. influenzae* to patients for 3 months and found an increase of antigen-specific IgA titers in saliva. These findings suggest that clinical application of oral vaccination with bacterial antigen might be effective in preventing pnemococcal middle ear infection.

Recently, several studies have shown the effectiveness of intranasal immunization to enhance mucosal immunity in the upper respiratory tract. Hotomi *et al.* (1995) and Xiao *et al.* (1994) demonstrated that intranasal immunization of mice with P6 purified from *H. influenzae* or HRP mixed with cholera toxin increased antigen-specific IgA antibody in nasopharyngeal secretions. Tamura and co-workers (1992) examined the effect of intranasal immunization with influenza hemagglutinin vaccine. They demonstrated that intranasal immunization induced cross-reacting anti-hemagglutinin IgA antibody as well as IgG antibody in nasal and broncho-alveolar washes, and that the effect was superior to subcutaneous immunization. These findings suggest that intranasal immunization might also be a useful rout for mucosal vaccination to protect middle ear infection.

Acknowledgments

The studies on mucosal immunity in the nasopharynx and prevention of otitis media by mucosal vaccination were supported in part by Grant-in-Aid for General Scientific Research (B) 07457403 and (C) 06671724 from the Ministry of Education, Science and Culture of Japan.

References

Bernstein, J. M., Yamanaka, T., Cumella, J., Ogra, P. L., and Park, B. (1985). Some observations on lymphocyte and macrophage function in middle ear effusions. *In* "Immunobiology, Autoimmunity, Transplantation in Otorhinolaryngology" (L. E. Veldman, B. F. McCabe, E. H. Huizing, and N. Mygind, eds.), p. 51. Kugler, Amsterdam.

Bernstein, J. M., Scheeren, R., Schoenfeld, E., and Albini, B. (1988). The distribution of immunocompetent cells in the compartments of palatine tonsils in bacterial and viral infections of the upper respiratory tract. *Acta Oto-Laryngol.* **454**(Suppl. 1), 53–62.

Bikhazi, P., and Ryan, A. F. (1995). Expression of immunoregulatory cytokines during acute and chronic middle ear immune response. *Laryngoscope* **105**, 629–634.

Brandtzaeg, P. (1987). Immune functions and immunopathology of the palatine and nasopharyngeal tonsils. *In* "Immunology of the Ear" (J. M. Bernstein, and P. L. Ogra, eds.), pp. 63–106. Raven, New York.

Bundo, J., Watanabe, N., Yoshida, K., and Mogi, G. (1996). Study on adhesion factors in lymphocyte migration to the middle ear mucosa. *Ann. Otol. Rhinol. Laryngol.* in press.

Chonmaitree, T., Owen, M. J., Patel, J. A., Hedgpeth, D., Horlick, D., and Howie, V. M. (1992). Effect of viral respiratory tract infection on outcome of acute otitis media. *J. Pediatr.* **120**, 856–862.

Clancy, R. L., Cripps, A. W., Husband, A. J., and Buckley, D. (1983). Specific immune response in the respiratory tract after administration of oral polyvalent bacterial vaccine. *Infect. Immun.* **39**, 491–496.

Diven, W. F., Zeevi, A., and Doyle, W. J. (1992). Inhibition of lymphoprolilferation by middle ear effusion in experimental otitis media. *Arch. Otolaryngol. Head Neck Surg.* **118**, 749–752.

Faden, H. Bernstein, J., Brodsky, L., Stanievich, J., Krystofik, D., Shuff, C., Hong, J. J., Ogra, P. L. (1989a). Otitis media in children. I. The systemic immune response to nontypeable *H. influenzae. J. Infect. Dis.* **160**, 999–1004.

Faden, H., Brodsky, L., Bernstein, J., Stanievich, J., Krystofik, D., Shuff, C., Hong, J. J., Ogra, P. L. (1989b). Otitis media in Children: Local immune response to nontypeable *H. influenzae. Infect. Immun.* **57**, 3555–3559.

Faden, H., Waz, M. J., Bernstein, J. M., Brodsky, L., Stanievich, J., and Ogra, P. L. (1991). Nasopharyngeal flora in the first three years of life in normal and otitis prone children. *Ann. Otol. Rhinol. Laryngol.* **100**, 612–615.

Harabuchi, Y., Faden, H., Yamanaka, N., Duffy, L., Wolf, J., Krystofik, D., and Tonawanda/Williamsville Pediatrics (1994). Nasopharyngeal colonization with nontypeable *Haemophilus influenzae* and recurrent otitis media. *J. Infect. Dis.* **170**, 862–866.

Heikkinen, T., Ruuskanen, O., Waris, M., Ziegler, T., Arola, M., and Halonen, P. (1991). Influenza vaccination in the prevention of acute otitis media in children. *Am. J. Dis. Child.* **145**, 445–448.

Hotomi, M., Kuki, K., Yamamoto, R., and Yamanaka, N. (1995). Induction of specific mucosal immunity by intranasal application of a *Haemophilus influenzae* outer membrane protein P6 mixed with the cholera toxin B subunit. *In* "Abstracts of the Sixth International Symposium on Recent Advances in Otitis Media," abstract 160, p. 272. Ft. Lauderdale, Florida.

Ichimiya, I., Kawauchi, H., and Mogi, G. (1990). Analysis of immunocompetent cells in the middle ear mucosa. *Arch. Otolaryngol. Head Neck Surg.* **116**, 324–330.

Juhn, S. K., Lees C., Amesara, R., Kim, Y., Le, C. T., and Giebink, S. (1993). Role of cytokines in the pathogenesis of otitis media. *In* "Recent Advances in Otitis" (D. J. Lim, C. D. Bluestone, J. O. Klein, J. D. Nelson, and P. L. Ogra, eds.), pp. 431–434. Decker, Toronto, Ontario.

Kakiuchi, H., Dake, Y., and Tabata, T. (1988). Immunogenesis of otitis media with effusion: With special reference to immunosuppressive factors in the middle ear. *In* "Recent Advances in Otitis Media" (D. J. Lim, C. D. Bluestone, J. O. Klein, and J. D. Nelson, eds.), pp. 153–156. Decker, Toronto, Ontario.

Kato, H., Watanabe, N., Bundo, J., and Mogi, G. (1994). Lymphocyte migration to the middle ear mucosa. *Ann. Otol. Rhinol. Laryngol.* **103**, 118–124.

Keithley, E. M., Krekorian, T. D., Sharp, P. A., Harris, J. P., and Ryan, A. F. (1990). Comparison of immune-mediated models of acute and chronic otitis media. *Eur. Arch. Oto-Rhiono-Laryngol.* **247**, 247–251.

Kodama, S., Kurono, Y., Shigemi, H., and Mogi, G. (1995). Oral vaccination with outer membrane proteins of nontypeable *Haemophilus influenzae* in mice. *In* "Abstracts of the Sixth International Symposium on Recent Advances in Otitis Media," abstract 158, p. 270. Ft. Lauderdale, Florida.

Kurono, Y., Tomonaga, K., and Mogi, G. (1988). *Staphylococcus epidermidis* and *Staphylococcus aureus* in otitis media with effusion. *Arch. Otolaryngol. Head Neck Surg.* **114**, 1262–1265.

Kurono, Y., Shimamura, K., Shigemi, H., and Mogi, G. (1991). Inhibition of bacterial adherence by nasopharyngeal secretions. *Ann. Otol. Rhinol. Laryngol.* **100**, 455–458.

Kurono, Y., Shimamura, K., and Mogi, G. (1992). Inhibition of nasopharyngeal colonization of *Haemophilus influenzae* by oral immunization. *Ann. Otol. Rhinol. Laryngol.* **101**(Suppl. 157), 11–15.

Kurono, Y., Shimamura, K., and Mogi, G. (1993). The effect of mucosal and systemic immunization on nasopharyngeal colonization by nontypeable *Haemophilus influenzae* in BALB/c mice. *In* "Recent Advances in Otitis Media" (G. Mogi, I. Honjo, T. Ishii, and T. Takasaka, eds.), pp. 479–483. Kugler, Amsterdam and New York.

Lim, D. J. (1974). Functional morphology of the lining membranes of the middle ear and Eustachian tube. An overview. *Ann. Otol. Rhinol. Laryngol.* **83**(Suppl. 11), 5–22.

Liu, Y. S., Lim, D. J., Lang, R. W., and Birck, H. G. (1975). Chronic middle ear effusions. Immunochemical and bacteriological investigations. *Arch. Otolaryngol.* **101**, 278–286.

Mogi, G., Honjo, S., Maeda, S., Yoshida, T., and Watanabe, N. (1974). Secretory immunoglobulin A (S-IgA) in middle ear effusions. A further report. *Ann. Otol. Rhinol. Laryngol.* **83**, 92–101.

Mogi, G., Maeda, S., and Watanabe, N. (1980). The development of mucosal immunity in guinea pig middle ears. *Int. J. Pediatr. Otolaryngol.* **1**, 331–349.

Mravec, J., Lewis, D. M., and Lim, D. J. (1978). Experimental otitis media: An immune-complex-mediated response. *Trans. Am. Acad. Ophthalmol. Otolaryngol.* **86**, 258–268.

Nadal, D., Albini, B., Chen, C., Schlapfer, E., Bernstein, J. M., and Ogra, P. L. (1991). Distribution and engraftment patterns of human tonsillar mononuclear cells in mice with severe combined immunodeficiency: The role of Epstein-Barr virus. *Int. Arch. Allergy Appl. Immunol.* **95**, 341–351.

Ogra, P. L., Bernstein, J. M., Yurchak, A. M., Coppola, P. R., and Tomasi, T. B., Jr. (1974). Characteristic of secretory immune system in human middle ear: Implications in otitis media. *J. Immunol.* **112**, 488–495.

Okamoto, Y., Kudo, K., Ishikawa, K., Ito, E., Togawa, K., Saito, I., Moro, I., Patel, J. A., and Ogra, P. L. (1993). Presence of respiratory syncytial virus genomic sequences in middle ear fluid and its relationship to expression of cytokines and cell adhesion molecules. *J. Infect. Dis.* **168**, 1277–1281.

O'Sullivan, N. L., and Montgomery, P. C. (1990). Characterization of lymphocyte–glandular mucosal tissues interaction using an *in vitro* assay. *In* "Advances in Mucosal Immunology" (T. T. MacDonald, S. T. Challacombe, P. W. Bland, C. R. Stokes, R. V. Heatley, and A. M. Mowat, eds.), pp. 222–226. Kluwer, Boston.

Patel, J. A., Faden, H., Sharma, S., and Ogra, P. L. (1992). Effect of respiratory syncytial virus on adherence, colonization, and immunity of nontypeable *Haemophilus influenzae*: Implication in otitis media. *Int. J. Pediatr. Oto-Rhino-Laryngol.* **23**, 15–23.

Palva, T., Tuohimaa, P., and Lehtinen, T. (1985). Pneumococcal immune complexes and clinical course of secretory otitis media. *Int. J. Pediatr. Otorhinolaryngol.* **10**, 21–26.

Quiding-Järbrink, M., Granström, G., Nordström, I., Holmgren, J., and Czerkinsky, C. (1995). Induction of compartmentalized B-cell responses in human tonsils. *Infect. Immun.* **63**, 853–857.

Ruuskanen, O., Arola, M., Putto-Laurila, A., Mertsola, J., Meurman, O., Viljanen, M. K., and Halonen, P. (1989). Acute otitis media and respiratory virus infections. *Pediatr. Infect. Dis. J.* **8**, 94–99.

Ryan, A. F., and Catanzaro, A. (1983). Passive transfer of immune-mediated middle ear inflammation and effusion. *Acta Oto-Laryngol.* **95**, 123–130.

Ryan, A. F., Catanzaro, A., Wasserman, S. I., and Harris, J. P. (1986). Secondary immune response in the middle ear: Immunological, morphological, and physiological observations. *Ann. Otol. Rhinol. Laryngol.* **95**, 242–249.

Ryan, A. F., Sharp, P. A., and Harris, J. P. (1990). Lymphocyte circulation to the middle ear. *Acta Oto-Laryngol.* **109**, 278–287.

Shimamura, K., Shigemi, H., Kurono, Y., and Mogi, G. (1990). The role of bacterial adherence in otitis media with effusion. *Arch. Otolaryngol. Head Neck Surg.* **116**, 1143–1146.

Sloyer, J. L., Howie, V. M., Ploussard, J. H., Amman, A. J., Austrian, R., and Johnston, R. B. (1974). Immune response to acute otitis media in children. I. Serotypes isolated and serum and middle ear fluid antibody in pneumococcal otitis media. *Infect. Immun.* **9**, 1028–1032.

Sloyer, J. L., Howie, V. M., Ploussard, J. H., and Johnston,

R. B. (1975). The immune response to acute otitis media in children. II. Serum and middle ear fluid antibody in otitis media due to *Haemophilus influenzae*. *J. Infect. Dis.* **132**, 685–688.

Stenfors, L. E., and Raisanen, S. (1992). Abundant attachment of bacteria to nasopharyngeal epithelium in otitis-prone children. *J. Infect. Dis.* **165**, 1148–1150.

Sung, B. S., Chonmaitree, T., Broemeling, L. D., Owen, M. J., Patel, J. A., Hedgpeth, D. C., and Howie, V. M. (1993). Association of rhinovirus infection with poor bacteriologic outcome of bacterial–viral otitis media. *Clin. Infect. Dis.* **17**, 38–42.

Suzuki, K., and Bakaletz, L. O. (1994). Synergistic effect of adenovirus type 1 and nontypeable *Haemophilu influenzae* in a chinchilla model of experimental otitis media. *Infect. Immun.* **62**, 1710–1718.

Suzuki, M., Kawauchi, H., and Mogi, G. (1988). Immune-mediated otitis media with effusion. *Am. J. Otolaryngol.* **9**, 199–209.

Takahashi, M., Peppard, J., and Harris, J. P. (1989). Immunohistochemical study of murine middle ear and Eustachian tube. *Acta Oto-Laryngol.* **107**, 97–103.

Takahashi, M., Kanai, N., Watanabe, A., Oshima, O., and Ryan, A. F. (1992). Lymphocyte subsets in immune-mediated otitis media with effusion. *Eur. Arch. Oto-Rhino-Laryngol.* **249**, 24–27.

Tamura, S.-I., Asanuma, H., Ito, Y., Hirabayashi, Y., Suzuki, Y., Nagamine, T., Aizawa, C., Kurata, T., Oya, A. (1992). Superior cross-protective effect of nasal vaccination to subcutaneous inoculation with influenza hemagglutinin vaccine. *Eur. J. Immunol.* **22**, 477–481.

Ueyama, S., Kawauchi, H., and Mogi, G. (1993). Experimental otitis media with effusion following pneumococcal middle ear infection. *In* "Recent Advances in Otitis Media" (G. Mogi, I. Honjo, T. Ishii, and T. Takasaka, eds.), pp. 197–201. Kugler, Amsterdam and New York.

Ueyama, T., Kurono, Y. Shirabe, K., Takeshita, M., and Mogi, G. (1995). High incidence of *Haemophilus influenzae* in nasopharyngeal secretions and middle ear effusions as detected by PCR. *J. Clin. Microbiol.* **33**, 1835–1838.

Watanabe, N., Yoshimura, H., and Mogi, G. (1988). Induction of antigen-specific IgA forming cells in the middle ear mucosa. *Arch. Otolaryngol. Head Neck Surg.* **114**, 758–762.

Watanabe, N., Kato, H., and Mogi, G. (1989). Induction of antigen-specific IgA-forming cells in the upper respiratory mucosa. *Ann. Otol. Rhinol. Laryngol.* **98**, 523–529.

Watanabe, N., Yoshimura, H., Shinoda, M., Bundo, J., and Mogi, G. (1992). Lymphocyte–mucosa interaction of the middle ear mucosa. *Acta Oto-Laryngol.* **493**, 137–140.

Xiao, Y., Kawauchi, H., Ichimiya, I., Sakamoto, N., and Mogi G. (1994). Immune response of the nasal mucosa. *In* "Immunobiology in Otorhinolaryngology: Progress of a Decade" (G. Mogi, J. E. Veldman, and H. Kawauchi, eds.). Kugler, Amsterdam and New York.

Yamanaka, N., and Faden, H. (1993a). Antibody response to outer membrane protein of non-typeable *Haemophulus influenzae* in otitis-prone children. *J. Pediatr.* **122**, 212–218.

Yamanaka, N., and Faden, H. (1993b). Local antibody response to P6 of nontypeable *Haemophilus influenzae* in otitis-prone and normal children. *Acta Oto-Laryngol.* **113**, 524–529.

Yamanaka, T., Cumella, J., Parker, C., Bernstein, J. M., and Ogra, P. L. (1983). Immunologic aspects of otitis media with effusion. II: Nature of cell-mediated immunosuppressive activity in middle ear fluid. *J. Infect. Dis.* **147**, 794–799.

Yellon, R. F., Leonard, G., Marucha, P. T., Craven, R., Carpenter, R. J., Lehmann, W. B., Burleson J. A., and Kreutzer, D. L. (1991). Characterization of cytokines present in middle ear effusions. *Laryngoscope* **101**, 165–169.

Yoshimura, H., Watanabe, N., Bundo, J., Shinoda, M., and Mogi, G. (1991). Oral vaccine therapy for pneumococcal otitis media in an animal model. *Arch. Otolaryngol. Head Neck Surg.* **117**, 889–894.

Index